The Clinician's Handbook of
NATURAL
HEALING

The Clinician's Handbook of
NATURAL HEALING

Gary Null, Ph.D.

Kensington Books
http://www.kensingtonbooks.com

KENSINGTON BOOKS are published by

Kensington Publishing Corp.
850 Third Avenue
New York, NY 10022

Library of Congress Card Catalog Number: TO COME
ISBN 1-57566-284-1

First Kensington Hardcover Printing: March, 1998
10   9   8   7   6   5   4   3   2   1

Printed in the United States of America

CONTENTS

NUTRIENTS

HERBAL SUPERSTARS

ADDITIONAL HERBS

THERAPEUTIC AMINO ACIDS

ESSENTIAL AMINO ACIDS

PHYTOCHEMICALS

APPENDIXES

NUTRIENTS

■ ACETYL-L-CARNITINE

Aging

Results of this study showed that the administration of acetyl-L-carnitine to aged rats for 6 months significantly decreased the percentage of myelinated fibers characterized by age-dependent morphological alterations.

> —C. De Angelis, et al., "Acetyl-L-carnitine Prevents Age-dependent Structural Alterations in Rat Peripheral Nerves and Promotes Regeneration Following Sciatic Nerve Injury in Young and Senescent Rats," *Exp Neurol,* 128(1), July 1994, p. 103-114.

Results of this study showed that aged rats with behavioral impairments receiving acetyl-L-carnitine experienced an enhancement in spatial acquisition in a novel environment.

> —A. Caprioli, et al., "Acetyl-L-Carnitine: Chronic Treatment Improves Spatial Acquisition in a New Environment in Aged Rats," *J Gerontol A Biol Sci Med Sci,* 50(4), July 1995, p. B232-B236.

Results of this study indicated that the administration of 10 mg/kg per day of L-acetylcarnitine for 4 months had both neuroprotective and neurotrophic effects in aging rats.

> —L. Fiore & L. Rampello, "L-acetylcarnitine Attenuates the Age-dependent Decrease of NMDA-Sensitive Glutamate Receptors in Rat Hippocampus," *Acta Neurol,* 11(5), October 1989, p. 346-350.

Results of this study showed that acetyl-L-carnitine may be effective in ameliorating receptor functionality in the aging rat brain due to its ability to preserve the receptor-mediated functional Ach release response.

> —A. Imperato, et al., "In Vivo Probing of the Brain Cholinergic System in the Aged Rat. Effects of Long Term Treatment with Acetyl-L-carnitine," *Annals of the New York Academy of Science,* 621, 1991, p. 90-97.

This study examined the effects of aging and the administration of acetyl-L-carnitine on rat plasma lipid composition and erythrocytes. Aging was found to increase free and esterified levels of cholesterol while fatty acid plasma patterns showed major alterations in aged rats relative to controls. Three hours following acetyl-L-carnitine treatment, results showed such changes were back to normal.

> —F.M. Ruggiero, et al., "Effect of Aging and Acetyl-L-carnitine on the Lipid Composition of Rat Plasma and Erythrocytes," *Biochem Biophys Res Commun,* 170(2), July 31, 1990, p. 621-626.

Results of this study indicate acetyl-L-carnitine has a direct action on p75NGFR expression in the central nervous system of aged rodents.

> —G. Taglialatela, et al., "Stimulation of Nerve Growth Factor Receptors in PC12 by Acetyl-L-carnitine," *Biochem Pharmacol,* 44(3), August 4, 1992, p. 577-585.

This study examined the effects of acetyl-L-carnitine administration for 37 weeks on lipopigment in the Purkinje neurons of rats. Results showed acetyl-L-carnitine to have prophylactive effects against adverse effects of cerebral aging.

> —J.H. Dowson, et al., "The Morphology of Lipopigment in Rat Purkinje Neurons after Chronic Acetyl-L-carnitine Administration: A Reduction in Aging-related Changes," *Biol Psychiatry,* 32(2), July 15, 1992, p. 179-187.

Results of this study showed that acetyl-L-carnitine administered in 50-100 mg/kg daily doses improved neuronal bioenergetic mechanisms in rats.

> —C. Bertoni-Freddari, et al., "Dynamic Morphology of the Synaptic Junctional Areas During Aging: The Effect of Chronic Acetyl-L-carnitine Administration," *Brain Research,* 656(2), September 12, 1994, p. 359-366.

Results of this double-blind, placebo-controlled study indicated that the administration of 1500 mg per day of acetyl-L-carnitine to elderly patients with mild mental impairments proved to be beneficial against cognitive and emotional-affective mental impairment.

> —C. Cipolli & G. Chiari, [Effects of L-acetylcarnitine on Mental Deterioration in the Aged: Initial Results], *Clin Ter,* 132(6 Suppl), March 31, 1990, p. 479-510.

This study examined the effects of treatment with 75 mg/kg per day for 11 months on the optic nerve and brain morphology in rats. Results showed that treatment improved the structural organization of the cerebral areas in question and increased the volume densities of pyramidal neurons of the prefrontal cortex layers. Results also showed the treatment reduced the level of impairment of myelination of the pyramidal tract and optic nerve.

> —M.T. Ramacci, et al., "Effect of Long-term Treatment with Acetyl-L-carnitine on Structural Changes of Aging Rat Brain," *Drugs Exp Clin Res,* 14(9), 1988, p. 593-601.

This single-blind, placebo-controlled study examined the effects of 1500 mg per day of acetyl-L-carnitine for 90 days on elderly subjects with mild mental impairment. Results showed the treatment to be effective with respect to improvements on cognitive performance, and behavioral measures.

> —G. Salvioli & M. Neri, "L-acetylcarnitine Treatment of Mental Decline in the Elderly," *Drugs Exp Clin Res,* 20(4), 1994, p. 169-176.

This study examined the effects of acetyl-L-carnitine on brain adenylate cyclase activity in rats. Results showed that the treatment enhanced receptor-stimulated AC response in the frontal cortex of rats of all ages.

> —T. Florio, et al., "Effect of Acetyl-L-carnitine Treatment on Brain Adenylate Cyclase Activity in Young and Aged Rats," *European Neuropsychopharmacology,* 3(2), June 1993, p. 95-101.

Results of this study found that acetyl-L-carnitine increased nerve growth factor levels and utilization in aged rats' central nervous systems.

> —G. Taglialatela, et al., "Acetyl-L-carnitine Treatment Increases Nerve Growth Factor Levels and Choline Acetyltransferase Activity in the Central Nervous System of Aged Rats," *Exp Gerontol,* 29(1), January-February 1994, p. 55-66.

This study examined the effects of acetyl-L-carnitine on NMDA receptors in aged rats. Results showed significant reductions of NDMA in old rats relative to young were attenuated by treatment with acetyl-L-carnitine for 6 months. Single-dose treatment increased the Bmax value in old rats by 35%.

> —M. Castorina, et al., "A Cluster Analysis Study of Acetyl-L-carnitine Effect on NMDA Receptors in Aging," *Exp Gerontol,* 28(6), November-December 1993, p. 537-548.

This study examined the effects of aging and the administration of acetyl-L-carnitine on the activity of cytochrome oxidase and adenine nucleotide translocase in the heart mitochondria of rats. In aged rats, 30% reductions were found for the activity of both mitochondrial proteins systems with acetyl-L-carnitine totally reversing such effects.

> —G. Paradies, et al., "Effect of Aging and Acetyl-L-carnitine on the Activity of Cytochrome Oxidase and Adenine Nucleotide Translocase in Rat Heart Mitochondria," *FEBS Letters,* 350(2-3), August 22, 1994, p. 213-215.

Results of this study showed that the administration of acetyl-L-carnitine significantly improved the acquisition and retention of avoidance responses in aged rats.

> —C. Valerio, et al., "The Effects of Acetyl-L-carnitine on Experimental Models of Learning and Memory Deficits in the Old Rat," *Funct Neurol,* 4(4), October-December 1989, p. 387-390.

Results of this double-blind, placebo-controlled study showed that the administration of 3 g per day of acetyl-L-carnitine for 30-60 days significantly reduced the severity of symptoms associated with depression relative to controls in senile subjects between the ages of 60-80.

> —R. Bella, et al., "Effect of Acetyl-L-carnitine on Geriatric Patients Suffering from Dysthymic Disorders," *International Journal of Clinical Pharmacology Research,* 10(6), 1990, p. 355-360.

Results of this double-blind, placebo-controlled study showed that the administration of 2 g per day of acetyl-L-carnitine for three months led to significant improvements in elderly patients suffering from mental impairment.

> —M. Passeri, et al., "Acetyl-L-carnitine in the Treatment of Mildly Demented Elderly Patients," *International Journal of Clinical Pharmacology Research,* 10(1-2), 1990, p. 75-79.

Results of this study showed that 80 mg per day of acetyl-L-carnitine attenuated age-related cognitive deficits in rats when administered long term.

> —A.L. Markowska & D.S. Olton, ''Dietary Acetyl-L-carnitine Improves Spatial Behaviour of Old Rats,'' *International Journal of Clinical Pharmacology Research,* 10(1-2), 1990, p. 65-68.

This study examined the effects of L-carnitine and acetyl-L-carnitine on cell proliferation in peripheral blood lymphocytes from donors varying in age. Results found that phytohaemagglutinin-induced peripheral blood lymphocyte proliferation increased significantly in L-carnitine- or acetyl-L-carnitine-preloaded lymphocytes from subject of all ages, but with the strongest increases seen in older subjects.

> —C. Franceschi, et al., ''Immunological Parameters in Aging: Studies on Natural Immunomo-dulatory and Immunoprotective Substances,'' *International Journal of Clinical Pharmacology Research,* 10(1-2), 1990, p. 53-57.

Results of this study showed that the administration of acetyl-L-carnitine had positive effects on age-related changes in the dopaminergic system of mice.

> —H. Sershen, et al., ''Effect of Acetyl-L-carnitine on the Dopaminergic System in Aging Brain,'' *Journal of Neuroscience Research,* 30(3), November 1991, p. 555-559.

Results of this study showed that the administration of acetyl-L-carnitine for 7 months had positive effects on age-related changes in the hippocampus of rats.

> —F.R. Patacchioli, et al., ''Acetyl-L-carnitine Reduces the Age-dependent Loss of Glucocorti-coid Receptors in the Rat Hippocampus: An Autoradiographic Study,'' *Journal of Neuroscience Research,* 23(4), August 1989, p. 462-466.

Results of this study showed that the administration of acetyl-L-carnitine ameliorated age-induced cognitive deficits in rats.

> —L. Angelucci, et al., ''Nerve Growth Factor Binding in Aged Rat Central Nervous System: Effect of Acetyl-L-carnitine,'' *Journal of Neuroscience Research,* 20(4), August 1988, p. 491-496.

This review article cites studies supporting the efficacy of acetyl-L-carnitine in counteracting negative age-induced effects on physiological and pathological brain modifications in rats.

> —M. Castorina & L. Ferraris, ''Acetyl-L-carnitine Affects Aged Brain Receptorial System in Rodents,'' *Life Science,* 54(17), 1994, p. 1205-1214.

This study examined the effects of aging and the administration of 50 mg/kg per day of acetyl-L-carnitine on the bioenergetics and cholinergic metabolism in non-synaptic mitochondria and synaptosomes isolated from the cerebral cortex, hippocampus and striatum of rats. Results showed that acetyl-L-carnitine increased the high-affinity choline uptake in rat cerebral cortex as well as increased cytochrome oxidase activity in the hippocampus.

> —D. Curti, et al., ''Effect of Aging and Acetyl-L-carnitine on Energetic and Cholinergic Metabolism in Rat Brain Regions,'' *Mech Ageing Development,* 47(1), January 1989, p. 39-45.

Results of this study showed that the administration of acetyl-L-carnitine for 6 months improved memory performance in aged rats relative to controls.

—C.A. Barnes, et al., "Acetyl-L-carnitine. 2: Effects on Learning and Memory Performance of Aged Rats in Simple and Complex Mazes," *Neurobiological Aging,* 11(5), September-October 1990, p. 499-506.

Results of this study showed that the in vivo administration of L-acetylcarnitine reduced the enzyme activities associated with Krebs' cycle of synaptic rat mitochondria and increased the cytochrome oxidase activity of synaptic and non-synaptic mitochondria.

—R.F. Villa & A. Gorini, "Action of L-acetylcarnitine on Different Cerebral Mitochondrial Populations from Hippocampus and Striatum During Aging," *Neurochem Research,* 16(10), October 1991, p. 1125-1132.

Results of this study showed that treatment with acetyl-L-carnitine via drinking water led to significant reductions in the decline in the number of hippocampus NMDA receptors in the frontal cortex and striatum of rats relative to controls.

—M. Castornia, et al., "Age-dependent Loss of NMDA Receptors in Hippocampus, Striatum, and Frontal Cortex of the Rat: Prevention by Acetyl-L-carnitine," *Neurochem Research,* 19(7), July 1994, p. 795-798.

This review article notes that studies have confirmed acetyl-L-carnitine's ability to counteract the age-dependent reduction of several receptors in rodent central nervous systems.

—M. Castorina & L. Ferraris, "Acetyl-L-carnitine Affects Aged Brain Receptorial System in Rodents," *Life Science,* 54(17), 1994, p. 1205-1214.

Results of this study showed that the administration of acetyl-L-carnitine led to significant improvements in discrimination learning tasks in rats relative to controls.

—O. Ghirardi, et al., "Effect of Acetyl-l-carnitine Chronic Treatment on Discrimination Models in Aged Rats," *Physiol Behavior,* 44(6), 1988, p. 769-773.

Results of this study showed that the long-term administration of acetyl-L-carnitine antagonized the deterioration of learning ability in old rats due to aging.

—A. Caprioli, et al., "Age-dependent Deficits in Radial Maze Performance in the Rat: Effect of Chronic Treatment with Acetyl-L-Carnitine," *Prog Neuropsychopharmacol Biol Psychiatry,* 14(3), 1990, p. 359-369.

Results of this study showed that the administration of acetyl-L-carnitine for 8 months antagonized the deterioration the acquisition ability of a spatial learning task in old rats due to aging.

—O. Ghirardi, et al., "Long-term Acetyl-L-carnitine Preserves Spatial Learning in the Senescent Rat," *Prog Neuropsychopharmacol Biol Psychiatry,* 13(1-2), 1989, p. 237-245.

AIDS/HIV

Results of this study showed that 6 g per day of L-carnitine for two weeks was effective in ameliorating lipid metabolism as well as immune response in AIDS patients receiving AZT.

—C. De Simone, et al., "High Dose L-carnitine Improves Immunologic and Metabolic

Parameters in AIDS Patients," *Immunopharmacol Immunotoxicol,* 15(1), January 1993, p. 1-12.

Alcoholism

Results of this double-blind, placebo-controlled study indicated that acetyl-L-carnitine may have beneficial effects with respect to the cognitive dysfunctions associated with chronic alcoholism.

> —E. Tempesta, et al., "Role of Acetyl-L-carnitine in the Treatment of Cognitive Deficit in Chronic Alcoholism," *International Journal of Clinical Pharmacology Research,* 10(1-2), 1990, p. 101-107.

Alzheimer's Disease

This double-blind, placebo-controlled study examined the effects of 2.5 g per day of acetyl levocarnitine hypochloride for 3 months followed by 3 g for 3 months on mild to moderately demented Alzheimer's patients. Results showed those receiving the treatment experienced significantly less deterioration in timed cancellation tasks and digit span.

> —M. Sano, et al., "Double-blind Parallel Design Pilot Study of Acetyl Levocarnitine in Patients with Alzheimer's Disease," *Arch Neurol,* 49(11), November 1992, p. 1137-1141.

This double-blind, placebo-controlled study examined the effects of acetyl-L-carnitine treatment administered to patients with Alzheimer's disease for one year. Results found the treatment significantly slowed the rate of deterioration relative to controls.

> —A. Spagnoli, et al., "Long-term Acetyl-L-carnitine Treatment in Alzheimer's Disease," *Neurology,* 41(11), November 1991, p. 1726-1732.

This review article argues that acetyl-L-carnitine possesses numerous pharmacologic properties which offer protection against neurodegeneration due to aging and thus it may be effective in reducing the development of Alzheimer's disease.

> —A. Carta & M. Calvani, "Acetyl-L-carnitine: A Drug Able to Slow the Progress of Alzheimer's Disease?," *Annals of the New York Academy of Science,* 640, 1991, p. 228-232.

Results of this double-blind, placebo-controlled study found that treatment with 2 g of acetyl-L-carnitine per day for 24 weeks had beneficial short-term memory effects on patients with Alzheimer-type dementia.

> —G. Rai, et al., "Double-blind, Placebo Controlled Study of Acetyl-L-carnitine in Patients with Alzheimer's Dementia," *Curr Med Res Opin,* 11(10), 1990, p. 638-647.

Results of this study showed that the oral and intravenous administration of acetyl-L-carnitine increased CSF and plasma concentrations in Alzheimer's patients.

> —L. Parnetti, et al., "Pharmacokinetics of IV and Oral Acetyl-L-carnitine in a Multiple Dose Regimen in Patients with Senile Dementia of Alzheimer Type," *European Journal of Clinical Pharmacology,* 42(1), 1992, p. 89-93.

Results of this double-blind, placebo-controlled study found that patients treated with acetyl-L-carnitine experienced significantly less deterioration in mental status than controls.

> —J.W. Pettegrew, et al., "Clinical and Neurochemical Effects of Acetyl-L-carnitine in Alzheimer's Disease," *Neurobiol Aging,* 16(1), January-February 1995, p. 1-4.

Amenorrhea

In this study, hypothalamic amenorrhea patients received 2 g per day of acetyl-L-carnitine for 6 months. Results showed the treatment had a significant, positive impact on menstruation.

—A.D. Genazzani, et al., "Acetyl-l-carnitine as Possible Drug in the Treatment of Hypothalamic Amenorrhea," *Acta Obstet Gynecol Scand,* 70(6), 1991, p. 487-492.

Cancer

Results of this study showed that the addition of 100 microM L-acetylcarnitine to P19 teratoma cells in an N2 synthetic, serum free medium, enhanced cell survival by slowing DNA fragmentation and nuclear condensation.

—G. Galli & M. Fratelli, "Activation of Apoptosis by Serum Deprivation in a Teratocarcinoma Cell Line: Inhibition by L-acetylcarnitine," *Exp Cell Res,* 204(1), January 1993, p. 54-60.

Cardiovascular/Coronary Heart Disease

Results of this study showed that the administration of acetyl-L-carnitine (2 mg/kg iv plus 1 mg/kg/min for 30 min) to aged rats led to restoration of cardiolipin levels to levels of young rats as well as a decrease in age-induced reductions in phosphate carrier activity in rat heart mitochondria.

—G. Paradies, et al., "The Effect of Aging and Acetyl-L-carnitine on the Activity of the Phosphate Carrier and on the Phospholipid Composition in Rat Heart Mitochondria," *Biochim Biophys Acta,* 1103(2), January 31, 1992, p. 324-326.

This study administered 3 mg per day of acetyl-L-carnitine intravenously to five patients undergoing aortic reconstructive surgery prior to ischemia induction. Results indicated acetyl-L-carnitine may have positive effects on the amelioration of human skeletal muscle damage induced by ischemia-reperfusion.

—C. Adembri, et al., "Ischemia-reperfusion of Human Skeletal Muscle During Aortoiliac Surgery: Effects of Acetylcarnitine," *Histol Histopathol,* 9(4), October 1994, p. 683-690.

Dementia

Results of this study showed acetyl-L-carnitine administration for 10 weeks led to significant behavioral improvements in dementia patients relative to controls.

—E. Sinforiani, et al., "Neuropsychological Changes in Demented Patients Treated with Acetyl-L-Carnitine," *International Journal of Clinical Pharmacology Research,* 10(1-2), 1990, p. 69-74.

This double-blind, placebo-controlled study examined the effects of 1000 mg per day of L-acetylcarnitine on the senile human brain. Results showed treatment led to significant improvements relative to controls with few side effects.

—E. Bonavita, "Study of the Efficacy and Tolerability of L-acetylcarnitine Therapy in the Senile Brain," *International Journal of Clinical and Pharmacol Ther Toxicol,* 24(9), September 1986, p. 511-516.

Depression

Results of this double-blind, placebo-controlled study found that the administration of 1500 mg per day of acetyl-L-carnitine led to significant improvements in patients between the ages of 70 and 80 suffering from symptoms of depression.

> —G. Garzya, et al., "Evaluation of the Effects of L-acetylcarnitine on Senile Patients Suffering from Depression," *Drugs Exp Clin Res,* 16(2), 1990, p. 101-106.

Results of this study showed the administration of acetyl-L-carnitine to be significantly effective relative to controls in reducing depressive symptoms among elderly patients hospitalized for depression.

> —G. Garzya, et al., "Evaluation of the Effects of L-acetylcarnitine on Senile Patients Suffering from Depression," *Drugs Exp Clin Res,* 16(2), 1990, p. 101-106.

Diabetes

Results of this study found an association between metabolic and functional abnormalities related to diabetic polyneuropathy in rats and imbalances in carnitine metabolism. Treatment with acetyl-L-carnitine prevented such abnormalities.

> —Y. Ido, et al., "Neural Dysfunction and Metabolic Imbalances in Diabetic Rats. Prevention by Acetyl-L-carnitine," *Diabetes,* 43(12), December 1994, p. p. 1469-1477.

Results of this study showed that the administration of acetyl-L-carnitine to rats prevented acute Na+/-K+ ATPase defect and had corrective effects on PGE1 in diabetic nerves.

> —A.A. Sima, et al., "Primary Preventive and Secondary Interventionary Effects of Acetyl-L-Carnitine on Diabetic Neuropathy in the Bio-breeding Worcester Rat," *Journal of Clinical Investigations,* 97(8), April 15, 1996, p. 1900-1917.

This study examined the effects of acetyl-L-carnitine and proprionyl-L-carnitine on motor and sensory nerve conduction in diabetic rats. Results showed that treatment for 2 months following diabetes induction significantly attenuated the development of sciatic motor nerve conduction velocity deficits.

> —M.A. Cotter, et al., "Effects of Acetyl- and Proprionyl-L-carnitine on Peripheral Nerve Function and Vascular Supply in Experimental Diabetes," *Metabolism,* 44(9), September 1995, p. 1209-1214.

This case-control study examined the effects of 50 mg/kg per day on the diminished nerve conduction velocity (NCV) of streptozotocin-induced hyperglycemic rats. Results showed an association between acetyl-L-carnitine and a decrease in the content of diabetic sciatic nerve which indicated a reduction in lipid peroxidation.

> —S. Lowitt, et al., "Acetyl-L-carnitine Corrects the Altered Peripheral Nerve Function of Experimental Diabetes," *Metabolism,* 44(5), May 1995, p. 677-680.

Results of this study showed that treatment with acetyl-L-carnitine or sorbinil reduced structural, functional and biochemical changes in the myelin sheath of rats due to hypoglycemia.

> —J.I. Malone, et al., "The Effects of Acetyl-L-carnitine and Sorbinil on Peripheral Nerve Structure, Chemistry, and Function in Experimental Diabetes," *Metabolism,* 45(7), July 1996, p. 902-907.

Results of this study showed that the oral administration of 250 mg/kg of acetyl-L-carnitine to diabetic rats led to improvements in nerve conduction velocity after 6 weeks of treatment.

—E. Morabito, et al., "Acetyl-L-carnitine Effect on Nerve Conduction Velocity in Streptozotocin-diabetic Rats," *Arzneimittelforschung,* 43(3), March 1993, p. 343-346.

Results of this study showed that acetyl-alpha-carnitine had a more pronounced effect on hypoglycemic action than did chloropropamide in diabetic rabbits. In addition, results showed that acetyl-alpha-carnitine significantly enhanced chloropropamide's effects.

—E.K. Kim, et al., [A Comparative Evaluation of the Hypoglycemic Activity of Acetyl-alpha-carnitine and Chlorpropamide in Experimental Diabetes], *Eksp Klin Farmakol,* 57(4), July-August 1994, p. 52-53.

Results of this study indicated acetyl-L-carnitine can prevent reductions in levels of substance P and methionine-enkephalin in the intestine, making it a promising treatment for autonomic neuropathies associated with diabetes.

—A. Gorio, et al., "Peptide Alterations in Autonomic Diabetic Neuropathy Prevented by Acetyl-L-Carnitine," *International Journal of Clinical Pharmacology Research,* 12(5-6), 1992, p. 225-230.

Down's Syndrome

Results of this study showed significant improvement in visual memory and attention in Down's Syndrome patients relative to controls following treatment with acetyl-L-carnitine for 90 days.

—F.A. De Falco, et al., [Effect of the Chronic Treatment with L-acetylcarnitine in Down's Syndrome], *Clin Ter,* 144(2), February 1994, p. 123-127.

Neurological Function

Results of this double-blind, placebo-controlled study found that the oral administration of 3 g per day of acetyl-L-carnitine coupled with 50 mg of methylprednisolone for 14 days led to significant functional recovery of the nerves in patients suffering from idiopathic facial paralysis.

—C. Mezzina, et al., "Idiopathic Facial Paralysis: New Therapeutic Prospects with Acetyl-L-carnitine," *International Journal of Clinical Pharmacology Research,* 12(5-6), 1992, p. 299-304.

Results of this study showed that the administration of acetyl-L-carnitine significantly increased rat sensory neuron survival time in primary cultures for up to 40 days.

—A. Formenti, et al., "Effects of Acetyl-L-carnitine on the Survival of Adult Rat Sensory Neurons in Primary Cultures," *International Journal of Dev Neuroscience,* 10(3), June 1992, p. 207-214.

This study examined the effects of 10-50 microM of acetyl-L-carnitine administered for 10 days on primary cell cultures from hippocampal formation and cerebral cortex of 17-day-old rat embryos. Results showed the treatment had neuroprotective effects.

—G. Forloni, et al., "Neuroprotective Activity of Acetyl-L-carnitine: Studies in Vitro," *Journal of Neuroscience Research,* 37(1), January 1994, p. 92-96.

Results of this study showed that the administration of acetyl-L-carnitine for 10 months had positive neuroprotective effects on aged rats.

—S. Davis, et al., "Acetyl-L-carnitine: Behavioral, Electrophysiological, and Neurochemical Effects," *Neurobiol Aging,* 14(1), January-February 1993, p. 107-115.

Results of this study indicated that pre-ischemic administration of acetyl-L-carnitine in gerbils had neuroprotective effects.

—A. Shuaib, et al., "Acetyl-L-carnitine Attenuates Neuronal Damage in Gerbils with Transient Forebrain Ischemia Only When Given Before the Insult," *Neurochem Research,* 20(9), September 1995, p. 1021-1025.

This study assayed the in vitro effects of acetyl-L-carnitine on spontaneous and induced lipoperoxidation in rat skeletal muscle. Results showed that 10-40 mM of acetyl-L-carntine present in the medium produced significant reductions in MDA and conjugated diene formation in rat skeletal muscle.

—C. Di Giacomo, et al., "Effect of Acetyl-L-carnitine on Lipid Peroxidation and Xanthine Oxidase Activity in Rat Skeletal Muscle," *Neurochem Research,* 18(11), November 1993, p. 1157-1162.

Results of this study indicated that the administration of L-acetylcarnitine had positive effects on sciatic nerve regeneration in rats.

—E. Fernandez, et al., "Effects of L-carnitine, L-acetylcarnitine and Gangliosides on the Regeneration of the Transected Sciatic Nerve in Rats," *Neurol Research,* 11(1), March 1989, p. 57-62.

This study examined the effects of intravenous L-acetylcarnitine on Renshaw cell activity in spastic paraparesis patients. Results showed L-acetylcarnitine significantly increased recurrent inhibition levels.

—R. Mazzocchio, et al., "Enhancement of Recurrent Inhibition by Intravenous Administration of L-Acetylcarnitine in Spastic Patients," *Journal of Neurol Neurosurg Psychiatry,* 53(4), April 1990, p. 321-326.

Results of this study involving a canine model of global cerebral ischemia and reperfusion showed that the postischemic administration of acetyl-L-carnitine potentiated the normalization of brain energy metabolites and produced marked improvements in neurological outcome.

—R.E. Rosenthal, et al., "Prevention of Postischemic Canine Neurological Injury through Potentiation of Brain Energy Metabolism by Acetyl-L-carnitine," *Stroke,* 23(9), September 1992, p. 1312-1317.

Results of this study showed that the administration of acetyl-L-carnitine led to significant reductions in lipofuscin accumulation within pyramidal neurons of the prefontal cortex and hippocampus of rats.

—F. Amenta, et al., "Reduced Lipofuscin Accumulation in Senescent Rat Brain by Long-term Acetyl-L-carnitine Treatment," *Arch Gerontol Geriatr,* 9(2), September-October 1989, p. 147-153.

Parkinson's Disease

Results of this study indicated that the administration of either 1 g or 2 g per day for seven days of acetyl-L-carnitine led to improvements in H response, sleep stages and spindling activity in Parkinson's disease patients.

> —F.M. Puca, et al., "Clinical Pharmacodynamics of Acetyl-L-carnitine in Patients with Parkinson's Disease," *International Journal of Clinical Pharmacology Research,* 10(1-2), 1990, p. 139-143.

Results of this study showed monkeys pretreated with acetyl-L-carnitine did not exhibit symptoms of Parkinsonism normally associated with exposure to 1-methyl, 4-phenyl- 1,2,3,6-tetrahydropyridine (MPTP).

> —I. Bodis-Wollner, et al., "Acetyl-levo-carnitine Protects Against MPTP-induced Parkinsonism in Primates," *Journal of Neural Transm Park Dis Dement Sect,* 3(1), 1991, p. 63-72.

Reproductive Function

This study examined the effects of L-acetyl-L-carnitine on the male reproductive functions of rats made oligoasthenospermic with dibromochloropropane (DBCP). Results showed that one injection of L-acetyl-L-carnitine led to sperm count recovery and that L-acetyl-L-carnitine stimulated the production of testosterone.

> —S. Palmero, et al., "The Effect of L-acetylcarnitine on Some Reproductive Functions in the Oligoasthenospermic Rat," *Horm Metab Res* (1990 Dec) 22(12):622-6

Senility

Results of this study showed that acetyl-L-carnitine administered at high levels can have positive effects on the release of amino acids as well as neurotransmitters such as dopamine and acetylcholine in the brain of rats.

> —E. Toth, et al., "Effect of Acetyl-L-carnitine on Extracellular Amino Acid Levels in Vivo in Rat Brain Regions," *Neurochem Research,* 18(5), May 1993, p. 573-578.

Stroke

Results of this double-blind, placebo-controlled study showed that acetyl-L-carnitine had significant positive effects on memory and cognitive performance tasks in elderly patients with cerebrovascular insufficiency.

> —A. Arrigo, et al., "Effects of Acetyl-L-carnitine on Reaction Times in Patients with Cerebrovascular Insufficiency," *International Journal of Clinical Pharmacology Research,* 10(1-2), 1990, p. 133-137.

Results of this study showed that the intravenous administration of 1.5 g of acetyl-L-carnitine led to improvements in cerebral blood flow in cerebrovasular disease patients who had suffered from a stroke at least 6 months prior to treatment.

> —A. Postiglione, et al., "Cerebral Blood Flow in Patients with Chronic Cerebrovascular Disease: Effect of Acetyl-L-Carnitine," *International Journal of Clinical Pharmacology Research,* 10(1-2), 1990, p. 129-132.

Results of this study found that the intravenous administration of 1500 mg of acetyl-L-carnitine had beneficial effects on 4 out of 10 patients suffering from brain ischaemia.

> —G. Rosadini, et al., "Acute Effects of Acetyl-L-carnitine on Regional Cerebral Blood Flow in Patients with Brain Ischaemia," *International Journal of Clinical Pharmacology Research,* 10(1-2), 1990, p. 123-128.

This study examined the effects 1.5 g of intravenous L-acetyl-L-carnitine on cerebral blood flow in patients with chronic cerebrovascular disease. Results showed the treatment led to significant enhancements in cerebral blood flow.

> —A. Postiglione, et al., "Effect of Acute Administration of L-acetyl Carnitine on Cerebral Blood Flow in Patients with Chronic Cerebral Infarct," *Pharmacology Research,* 23(3), April 1991, p. 241-246.

■ ACIDOPHILUS

AIDS/HIV

Results of this study found that the survival of HIV in the female genital tract and possible transmission may be inhibited by Lactobacillus acidophilus-peroxidase-halide system activity in the vagina.

> —S.J. Klebanoff & R.W. Coombs, "Viricidal Effect of Lactobacillus Acidophilus on Human Immunodeficiency Virus Type 1: Possible Role in Heterosexual Transmission," *Journal of Exp Medicine,* 174(1), July 1, 1991, p. 289-292.

Bowel/Gastrointestinal Disorders

This article notes that preparations containing viable lactic acid bacteria of human origin may be of value in restoring normal microbial function and reducing symptoms in patients suffering from gastrointestinal infection and related conditions.

> —S. Salminen & M. Deighton, "Lactic Acid Bacteria in the Gut in Normal and Disordered States," *Digestive Disorders,* 10(4), 1992, p. 227-238.

Results of this study showed that a multibacterial combination consisting of Lactobacillus acidophilus (10(9)) and Bifidobacterium bifidum (10(9)) administered to elderly patients with bowel disorders proved effective with respect to restoration of duodenal bacterial flora and subsidence of clinical symptoms.

> —G. Pecorella, et al., [The Effect of Lactobacillus Acidophilus and Bifidobacterium Bifidum on the Intestinal Ecosystem of the Elderly Patient], *Clin Ter,* 140(1), January 1992, p. 3-10.

This study examined the effects of oral bacterial therapy on elderly patients suffering from bowel disorders involving symptoms of diarrhea, abdominal pain, and meteorism. Following a 7 day washout period, all patients were given 6 capsules per days consisting of live lyophilized Lactobacillus acidophilus (10(9) CFU/ml). Results showed significant relief of symptoms in all 60 patients receiving the treatment.

> —L. Motta, et al., [Study on the Activity of a Therapeutic Bacterial Combination in Intestinal Motility Disorders in the Aged], *Clin Ter,* 138(1), July 15, 1991, p. 27-35.

This study examined the potential of a live mix of Lactobacillus acidophilus 10(9) and Bifidobacterium bifidum 10(9) to act as an ecological therapy for gastritis and duodenitis in subjects suffering from these disorders stemming from C. pylori. Results showed the treatment was effective in improving upon the results obtained through more conventional means.

> —M.R. Gismondo, et al., [Competitive Activity of a Bacterial Preparation on Colonization and Pathogenicity of C. pylori. A Clinical Study], *Clin Ter,* 134(1), July 15, 1990, p. 41-46.

This study examined the effects of Lactobacillus acidophilus on gastrointestinal side effects of oral broad-spectrum antibiotic therapy in outpatients with ear, sinus, or throat infections. Results showed that Lactobacillus acdiophilus in combination with amoxicillin/clavulanate was correlated with a significant decrease in patient complaints of gastrointestinal side effects and yeast superinfection with 89% reporting the elimination of infection.

> —D.L. Witsell, et al., "Effect of Lactobacillus Acidophilus on Antibiotic-associated Gastrointestinal Morbidity: A Prospective Randomized Trial," *Journal of Otolaryngol,* 24(4), August 1995, p. 230-233.

This article reports on an Acidophilus milk that has been introduced as therapy in different disorders of the gastrointestinal tract and showed a clear response in patients suffering from intestinal disorders due to an application of antibiotics and in patients with constipations.

> —L. Alm, [Acidophilus Milk for Therapy in Gastrointestinal Disorders], *Nahrung,* 28(6-7), 1984, p. 683-684.

Results of this study showed that the administration of biopreparations containing lacto-or bifidobacteria produced a clinico-microbiological response rate above 90% in 37 patients with intestinal yersiniosis or pseudotuberculosis.

> —V.F. Kuznetsov, et al., [Intestinal Dysbacteriosis in Yersiniosis Patients and the Possibility of its Correction with Biopreparations], *Ter Arkh,* 66(11), 1994, p. 17-18.

Cancer

Results of this study showed that meat-eating rats fed supplements of Lactobacillus acidophilus experienced a significant reduction in fecal nitroreductase and azoreductase activity. Such findings, the authors conclude, may be relevant to the prevention of large bowel cancer.

> —B. Goldin & S.L. Gorbach, "Alterations in Fecal Microflora Enzymes Related to Diet, Age, Lactobacillus Supplements, and Dimethylhydrazine," *Cancer,* 40(5 Suppl), November 1977, p. 421-426.

In this case-control study, patients suffering from gynaecological malignancies who were scheduled for internal and external irradiation of the pelvic area received dietary counseling in addition 150 ml of a fermented milk test product containing a minimum of 2 X 10(9) live Lactobacillus acidophilus bacteria daily and 6.5% lactulose as substrate for the bacteria. Controls received counseling only. Results found that the test product prevented radiotherapy-associated diarrhea.

> —E. Salminen, et al., "Preservation of Intestinal Integrity During Radiotherapy Using Live Lactobacillus Acidophilus Cultures," *Clinical Radiology,* 39(4), July 1988, p. 435-437.

This case-control study examined the effects of Lactobacillus acidophilus supplementation on chemical-induced colon cancer in rats. Results found that, at 26 weeks into the 40 week study, supplementation of Lactobacillus acidophilus delayed chemical-induced colon tumor initiation. Results of related in vitro experiments part of the same study indicated that a large amount intestinal L acidophilus may inhibit the onset of colon cancer in humans as well.

—H. Lee, "Effect of Lactobacillus Acidophilus on Colon Carcinogenesis," *Dissertation Abstracts International,* 50(6), 1989, p. 2225.

Results of this study showed that meat eating rats administered viable cultures of Lactobacillus acidophilus and exposed to chemical carcinogens experienced a lower colon cancer rate after 20 weeks than rats not administered the Lactobacillus acidophillus.

—B.R. Goldin & S.L. Gorbach, "Effect of Lactobacillus Acidophilus Dietary Supplements on 1,2-Dimethylhydrazine Dihydrochloride-induced intestinal Cancer in Rats," *Journal of the Nationall Cancer Institute,* 64(2), February 1990, p. 263-265.

This study examined the effects of Lactobacillus acidophilus supplements and diet on human microflora enzyme activity. Results found that the supplements added to the diets of meat eaters led to a significant decrease in fecal bacterial beta-glucuronidase and nitroreductase activities.

—B.R. Goldin, et al., "Effect of Diet and Lactobacillus Acidophilus Supplements on Human Fecal Bacterial Enzymes," *Journal of the National Cancer Institute,* 64(2), February 1990, p. 255-261.

Results of this study showed that meat eating rats administered Lactobacillus acidophilus with 2-nitrofluorene or 2-naphthylamine-N-D-glucuronide, experienced significantly lower free amines and higher concentrations of conjugates in their feces relative to meat eating controls. Such findings demonstrated that intestinal flora can convert exogenously administered aromatic nitro and azo compounds and an amine-glucuronide compound to free amines with the rate of such conversions being affected by diet and by oral administration of antibiotics and lactobacilli.

—B.R. Goldin & S.L. Gorbach, "Alterations of the Intestinal Microflora by Diet, Oral Antibiotics, and Lactobacillus: Decreased Production of Free Amines from Aomatic Nitro Compounds, Azo Dyes, and Glucuronides," *Journal of the National Cancer Institute,* 73(3), September 1984, p. 689-695.

Results of this study showed that the administration bifidobacteria and Lactobacillus acidophilus had significant inhibitory effects on both aberrant crypt formation and C. perfringens in rats exposed to chemical carcinogens.

—D.D. Gallaher, et al., "Probiotics, Cecal Microflora, and Aberrant Crypts in the Rat Colon," *Journal of Nutrition,* 126(5), May 1996, p. 1362-1371.

Results of this study showed that the administration of intestinal bacteria including Bifodiobacterium longum, Lactobacillus acidophilus, and Eubacterium rectale in mice suppressed liver tumorigenesis which had been promoted with a bacterial mix of Escherichia coli, Streptococcus faecalis, and Clostridium paraputrificum.

—T. Mizutani & T. Mitsuoka, "Inhibitory Effect of Some Intestinal Bacteria on Liver Tumorigenesis in Gnotobiotic C3H/He Male Mice," *Cancer Letters,* 11(2), December 1980, p. 89-95.

This review article cites studies noting that colon cancer patients administered Lactobacillus acidophilus fermented milk experienced a significant increase in numbers of intestinal lactobacilli and dietary calcium intake, while also showing decreasing trends in levels of both soluble faecal bile acids and faecal bacterial enzymes, both being colon cancer risk factors. Results of in vitro studies have found that lactobacilli and other lactic acid bacteria can absorb cooked food mutagens. Human studies have demonstrated that Lactobacillus acidophilus consumption can significantly reduce mutagen excretion following fried meat consumption.

>   —A. Lidbeck, et al., "Lactobacilli, Anticarcinogenic Activities and Human Intestinal Microflora," *European Journal of Cancer Prevention,* 1(5), August 1992, p. 341-353.

Cardiovascular/Coronary Heart Disease

Results of this study found that specific Lactobacillus acidophilus strain RP32 acted directly on cholesterol in the GI tract of pigs, making them potentially beneficial in decreasing the overall levels of serum cholesterol

>   —S.E. Gilliland, et al., "Assimilation of Cholesterol by Lactobacillus Acidophilus," *Appl Environ Microbiol.* 49(2), February 1985, p. 377-381.

Diarrhea

Results of this study found that human Lactobacillus acidophilus strains had an inhibitory effect against the cell association of enterotoxigenic, diffusely adhering and enteropathogenic Escherichia coli, and Salmonella typhimuirum; and against cell invasion by enteropathogenic Escherichia coli, Yersinia pseuodotuberculosis, and Salmonella typhimurium. Results also showed that Lactobacillus incubations before and together with enteroviulent E coli proved more successful relative to incubation following E. coli.

>   —M.F. Bernet, et al., "Lactobacillus Acidophilus LA 1 Binds to Cultured Human Intestinal Cell Lines and Inhibits Cell Attachment and Cell Invasion by Enterovirulent Bacteria," *Gut,* 35(4), April 1994, p. 483-489.

Results of this double-blind, placebo-controlled study showed that prophylactic administration of commercial lactobacillus preparations can help prevent ampicillin-induced diarrhea in humans.

>   —V. Gotz, et al., "Prophylaxis Against Ampicillin-associated Diarrhea with a Lactobacillus Preparation," *American Journal of Hosp Pharm,* 36(6), June 1979, p. 754-757.

Results of this study showed that oral lactobacilli therapy was effective in the prevention of amoxycillin-induced diarrhea in infants.

>   —I. Contardi, [Oral Bacterial Therapy in Prevention of Antibiotic-induced Diarrhea in Childhood], *Clin Ter,* 136(6), March 31, 1991, p. 409-413.

Dyspepsia

In this study, Lactobacillus acidophilus capsules were administered to patients with dyspepsia caused by dysbacteriosis of the gastrointestinal tract. Results showed that effects were achieved the quickest in dysbioses following antibiotics, with normalization taking place within 3-4 days after going off the antibiotics. Results also showed that, in cases of malidigestion, bloating, flatulence, abdominal pain

and pressure in the epigastrium improved after 1 week of treatment and improved further after two weeks. Dairy tolerance improved in patients with lactose intolerance.
— J. Kocian, [Lactobacilli in the Treatment of Dyspepsia Due to Dysmicrobia of Various Causes], *Vnitr Lek,* 40(2), February 1994, p. 79-83.

General

This study examined the effects of Lactobacillus acidophilus supplements on fecal bacterial enzyme activity in 21 subjects. Results found significant reductions of 2- to 4-fold in the activities of the three fecal enzymes were during the lactobacilli feeding period in all subjects.
— B.R. Goldin & S.L. Gorbach, "The Effect of Milk and Lactobacillus Feeding on Human Intestinal Bacterial Enzyme Activity," *American Journal of Clinical Nutrition,* 39(5), May 1984, p. 756-761.

Results of this study found that 15 mg of erythromycin and 80 mg of heat-killed L. acidophilus administered per os daily to germ-free mice proved effective in the treatment of Campylobacter jejuni infection.
— E.N. Moyen, et al., [Modification of Intestinal Colonization and Translocation of Campylobacter Jejuni by Erythromycin and an Extract of Lactobacillus Acidophilus in Axenic Mice], *Ann Inst Pasteur Microbiol,* 137A(2), March-April 1986, p. 199-207.

This review article cites numerous studies supporting the health benefits of lactic acid bacteria found in fermented dairy products including the lowering of serum cholesterol levels, inhibition of tumor growth, inhibition of intestinal infections, and the treatment of diarrhea.
— S.L. Gorbach, et al., "Lactic Acid Bacteria and Human Health," *Ann Med,* 22(1), February 1990, p. 37-41.

This study compared the efficacy of an oral lyophilized preparation of heat-killed Lactobacillus acidophilus with sterile water on the mortality rate of newborn mice exposed to lethal doses of Eschericia coli. Results showed that the heat-killed L. acidophilus administration significantly enhanced survival time of infected suckling mice.
— J. Fourniat, et al., [Effect of the Administration of Killed Lactobacillus Acidophilus on the Survival of Suckling Mice Infected with a Strain of Enterotoxigenic Escherichia Coli], *Ann Rech Vet,* 17(4), 1986, p. 401-407.

Results of this study showed that heat-killed Lactobacillus acidophilus inhibited the adhesion of Escherichia coli B41 to HeLa 229 cells in a dose-dependent fashion.
— J. Fourniat, et al., "Heat-killed Lactobacillus Acidophilus Inhibits Adhesion of Escherichia Coli B41 to HeLa Cells," *Ann Rech Vet,* 23(4), 1992, p. 361-370.

Results of this study showed that Lactobacillus casei ssp. rhamnosus GR-1 and Lactobacillus acidophilus 76 exerted an inhibitory effect on pyelonephritogenic mutant Escherichia coli Hu 734 and E. coli ATCC 25922.
— J.A. McGroarty & G. Reid, "Detection of a Lactobacillus Substance that Inhibits Escherichia Coli," *Can Journal of Microbiology,* 34(8), August 1988, p. 974-978.

Results of this study found that Lactobacillus prevents development of the Klebsiella infection in mice and provides protection against excessive action upon the immune system.

—O.P. Kostiuk, et al., [Protective Effect of Lactobacillus Acidophilus on Development of Infection, Caused by Klebsiella Pneumoniae], *Fiziol Zh*, 39(4), July-August 1993, p. 62-68.

In this study, 444 women with trichomoniasis vaginalis were treated with Solcotrichovac, a vaccine containing at least 7 x 10(9) inactivated microorganisms of various strains of lactobacillus acidophilus in each 0.5 ml dose. Results showed that 92.5% of the patients were cured of clinical symptoms one year after the first vaccination.

—M.S. Litschgi, et al., [Effectiveness of a Lactobacillus Vaccine on Trichomonas Infections in Women. Preliminary Results], *Fortschr Med,* 98(41), November 6, 1980, p. 1624-1627.

This double-blind, placebo-controlled study administered lyophilized Bifidobacterium bifidum and Lactobacillus acidophilus capsules to 15 elderly subjects 4 times per day for a total of 28 days. Results found that both Bifidobacterium bifidum and Lactobacillus acidophilus lead to modulation of the immunological and inflammatory response in elderly subjects.

—C. De Simone, et al., "Effect of Bifidobacterium Bifidum and Lactobacillus Acidophilus on Gut Mucosa and Peripheral Blood B Lymphocytes," *Immunopharmacol Immunotoxico,* 14(1-2), 1992, p. 331-340.

In this study, Lactobacillus acidophilus was administered to ten healthy subjects as a fermented milk product following administration of enoacin and clindamycin, two antimicrobial agents. On the seventh day of enoaxacin administration, results showed enterobacteria were eliminated in nine of ten subjects while enterococci was eliminated or decreased significantly in five subjects. L. acidophilus supplementation produced a significant increase in the number of Escherichia coli in one subject, and, in all subjects, enterococci returned to the same level as before enoxacin.

—A. Lidbeck, et al., "Impact of Lactobacillus Acidophilus on the Normal Intestinal Microflora after Administration of Two Antimicrobial Agents," *Infection,* 16(6), 1988, p. 329-336.

Results of this in vitro study found that Lactobacillus strains employed in fermented milk can be used to inhibit the growth of Shigella sonnei.

—M.C. Apella, et al., "In Vitro Studies on the Growth of Shigella Sonnei by Lactobacillus Casei and Lact. Acidophilus," *Journal of Applied Bacteriology,* 73(6), December 1992, p. 480-483.

This study examined the protective effects of feeding mice milk fermented with a mixture of Lactobacillus casei and Lact. acidophilus against Shigella sonnei. Results showed a 100% survival rate in mice fed for 8 days with fermented milk and then administered Shigella sonnei orally relative to a 60% survival rate in controls after 21 days. Results also showed a significant inhibition in the colonization of the liver and with Shigella sonnei by pretreatment with fermented milk. Taken as a whole, the findings from the this study indicated that milk fermented with Lactobacilus casei and Lactobacilis acidophilus may be an effective prophylactic against gastrointestinal shigellas infections.

—M.E. Nader de Macias, et al., "Inhibition of Shigella sonnei by Lactobacillus casei and Lact. acidophilus," *Journal of Applied Bacteriol,* 73(5), November 1992, p. 407-411.

Results of this study found that L. acidophilus inhibited the growth of seven isolates of C. pylori in vitro.

> —S.J. Bhatia, et al., "Lactobacillus Acidophilus Inhibits Growth of Campylobacter Pylori in Vitro," *Journal of Clinical Microbiology,* 27(10), October 1989, p. 2328-2330.

This study examined the protective effects of feeding milk fermented with a mixture of Lactobacillus casei sp. and Lb. acidophilus sp. against Salmonella typhimurium infection in mice was compared with that obtained feeding milks fermented with these microorganisms individually. Results showed that the survival rate obtained after oral infection with Sal. typhimurium was 100% in mice pretreated by feeding during 8 days with the mixture of Lb. casei and Lb. acidophilus fermented milks in contrast to treatments with the individual milks which were ineffective.

> —G. Perdigon, et al., "Prevention of Gastrointestinal Infection Using Immunobiological Methods with Milk Fermented with Lactobacillus Casei and Lactobacillus Acidophilus," *Journal of Dairy Research,* 57(2), May 1990, p. 255-264.

This study examined the inhibitory effects of cultured milk using 76 strains of lactic acid bacteria isolated from milk products were investigated on the mutagenicity of 3-amino-1-methyl-5H-pyrido [4,3-b]indole (Trp-P2), a tryptophan pyrolysate for Salmonella typhimurium TA98. Results found that the milk cultured with Lactobacillus acidophilus LA106 exhibited the strongest inhibition with milk samples cultured with Lactococcus lactis subsp. lactis, Lll103 (10-3) and Lll102 (KM) also exhibiting high inhibition percentages.

> —M. Hosoda, et al., "Studies on Antimutagenic Effect of Milk Cultured with Lactic Acid Bacteria on the Trp-P2-induced Mutagenicity to TA98 Strain of Salmonella Typhimurium," *Journal of Dairy Research,* 59(4), November 1992, p. 543-549.

Results of this study showed that Candida albicans grew at pH 4.6 or above in nutrient broth containing 5% glucose but was retarded at pH 7.7 by filtrates of Lactobacillus acidophilus grown in casitone broth.

> —E.B. Collins & P. Hardt, "Inhibition of Candida Albicans by Lactobacillus Acidophilus," *Journal of Dairy Sciences,* 63(5), May 1980, p. 830-832.

Results of this study showed that several strains of Lactobacillis gasseri exhibited inhibitory activity against the various stains of food-borne enteric pathogenic bacteria.

> —T. Itoh, et al., "Inhibition of Food-borne Pathogenic Bacteria by Bacteriocins from Lactobacillus Gasseri," *Lett Appl Microbiol,* 21(3), September 1995, p. 137-141.

Results of this study found Lactobacillus acidophilus AC1 produced a proteinic inhibitor having a molecular weight of 5.4 kd, active against both Gram-positive and Gram-negative bacteria.

> —A.M. Mehta, et al., "Purification and Properties of the Inhibitory Protein Isolated from Lactobacillus Acidophilus AC1," *Microbios,* 38(152), 1983, p. 73-81.

Results of this study found that Lactobacillus acidophilus inhibits Candida albicans when grown on MRS agar plates.

> —M. Jack, et al., "Evidence for the Involvement of Thiocyanate in the Inhibition of Candida Albicans by Lactobacillus Acidophilus," *Microbios,* 62(250), 1990, p. 37-46.

This case-control study administered pure cultures of specially selected strains of Lactobacillus acidophilus to 60 neonates at high risk for dysbacterioses while they were still at the puerperal room. Results showed that the Lactobacillus acidophilus raised the efficacy of the preventive measures, with more than 60% of the neonates being released from the maternity home with a normally formed intestinal microflora, 60% with normal microflora in the fauces, 8% in the nose, and 70% showing normal skin microflora.

> —P.S. Moshchich, et al., [Prevention of Dysbacteriosis in the Early Neonatal Period Using a Pure Culture of Acidophilic Bacteria], *Pediatriia*, (3), 1989, p. 25-30.

In this study, chicks were hatched germfree in gnotobiotic isolators to determine Lactobacillus acidophilus' effects towards pathogeneic Escherichia coli in vivo. Results found that initial dosing with L. acidophilus prevented high levels of mortality in chick exposed to E. coli while continued dosing reduced the pH in the crop, cecum, and rectum irregardless of whether chicks were initially given L. acidophilus or E. coli.

> —B.A. Watkins, et al., "In Vivo Inhibitory Effects of Lactobacillus Acidophilus Against Pathogenic Escherichia Coli in Gnotobiotic Chicks," *Poultry Science,* 61(7), July 1982, p. 1298-1308.

This double-blind, placebo-controlled study examined the effects of lactic acid producing bacteria on intestinal microflora during amplicillin treatment in healthy subjects. Results showed that bacteroides strains were recovered in higher numbers and faster in the lactic acid producing bacteria group than controls compared to the placebo group.

> —F. Black, et al., "Effect of Lactic Acid Producing Bacteria on the Human Intestinal Microflora During Ampicillin Treatment," *Scandinavian Journal of Infectious Disease,* 23(2), 1991, p. 247-254.

This study examined the effects of Lactobacillus acidophilus supplements (fermented milk product containing 5 X 10(8)-2 X 10(9) CFU/ml in a dose of 250 ml twice a day for 7 days) on oropharyngeal and intestinal microflora in healthy subjects. Results showed slight changes in the number of aerobic and anaerobic microorganisms in the oropharynx, no change in the number of lactobacilli, a reduction in the number of Escherichia coli, and a significant increase in the number of lactobacilli. As a whole, results indicate L. acidophilus needs to be continuously administered so as to maintain high levels of intestinal lactobacilli.

> —A. Lidbeck, et al., "Impact of Lactobacillus Acidophilus Supplements on the Human Oropharyngeal and Intestinal Microflora," *Scandinavian Journal of Infectious Disease,* 19(5), 1987, p. 531-537.

In this double-blind, placebo-controlled study, 60 women with bacterial vaginosis received treatment with lyophilized Lactobacillus acidophilus. Results showed that 16 of the 28 women receiving the treatment had normal vaginal wet smear readings relative to 0 of the 29 controls. Results also found that bacteriocides were eliminated from the vagina in 12 of 16 women following treatment.

> —A. Hallen, et al., "Treatment of Bacterial Vaginosis with Lactobacilli," *Sexually Transmitted Diseases,* 19(3), May-June 1992, p. 146-148.

This article notes that Lactobacillus acidophilus strain Lat 11/83 Solco has been used for the normalization of intestinal microflora in experimental post-irradiation intestinal dysbacteriosis in mice. Results of such investigations have shown that live Solco lactobacteria, administered intragastrically, enhanced survival rate of irradiated mice and the normalization of microflora in their gastrointestinal tract.

—V. Bossart, et al., [The Effect of a Preparation Made from Solco Lactobacteria on the Survival Rate and Intestinal Microflora of Irradiated Animals], *Zh Mikrobiol Epidemiol Immunobiol*, (11), November 1990, p. 6-9.

Results of this study showed that Lactobacillus acidophilus strain Lat 11/83 is an active antagonist for the prophylaxis and intestinal dysbacteriosis in germ free mice.

—S. Popova-Barzashka, et al., [The Determination of the Antagonistic Activity of Solco Lactobacteria (Lactobacillus Acidophilus Lat 11/83) Using Gnotobiotic Technology], *Zh Mikrobiol Epidemiol Immunobiol*, (9), September 1990, p. 3-6.

Immune Enhancement

Results of this study found that Lactobacillus casei and Lactobacillus acidophilus, associated with intestinal mucosae, enhanced the activation levels of murine immune systems.

—G. Perdigon, et al., "Systemic Augmentation of the Immune Response in Mice by Feeding Fermented Milks with Lactobacillus Casei and Lactobacillus Acidophilus," *Immunology*, 63(1), January 1988, p. 17-23.

In this case-control study, subjects consumed a fermented milk containing L. acidophilus La1 and bifidobacteria over a three week period during which an attenuated Salmonella typhi Ty21a was administered to mimic an enteropathogenic infection. Results showed that lactic acid bacteria prevalent in the gastrointestinal tract acts as an adjuvant to the humoral immune response in man.

—H. Link-Amster, et al., "Modulation of a Specific Humoral Immune Response and Changes in Intestinal Flora Mediated Through Fermented Milk Intake," *FEMS Immunol Med Microbiol*, 10(1), November 1994, p. 55-63.

Results of this found that mice administered 50 micrograms per day of viable cultures of Lactobacillus acidophilus and Streptococcus thermophilus for 8 consecutive days experienced significant enhancement in their immune systems.

—G. Perdigon, et al., "Enhancement of Immune Response in Mice Fed with Streptococcus Thermophilus and Lactobacillus Acidophilus," *Journal of Dairy Science*, 70(5), May 1987, p. 919-926.

Iron Absorption

Results of this study showed that Lactobacillus acidophilus SBT 2062 increased the bioavailability or iron in rats.

—T. Oda, et al., "Effect of Lactobacillus Acidophilus on Iron Bioavailability in Rats," *Journal of Nutr Sci Vitaminol,* 40(6), December 1994, p. 613-616.

Lactose Intolerance

This study examined the relative efficacy of yogurt, sweet acidophilus milk, hydrolyzed-lactose milk, a lactase tablet, and whole milk in black subjects with lactose intolerance. Results showed that mean breath hydrogen excretion for yogurt = 12, sweet acidophulus milk = 37, hydrolyzed-lactose milk = 29, lactase tablet = 18, and whole milk = 33. A significant correlation was found between mean peak breath hydrogen excretion and reported symptoms with results also demonstrating that microbial endogenous lactase in yogurt was more effective than exogenous commercial lactase in alleviating lactose maldigestion.

—C.I. Onwulata, et al., "Relative Efficiency of Yogurt, Sweet Acidophilus Milk, Hydrolyzed-lactose Milk, and a Commercial Lactase Tablet in Alleviating Lactose Maldigestion," *American Journal of Clinical Nutruition,* 49(6), June 1989, p. 1233-1237.

This study examined the effects of Lactobacillus acidophulus on human lactose utilization by comparing the hydrogen breath excretion levels following the consumption of milk containing either 0, 2.5 X 10(6), 2.5 X 10(7), or 2.5 X 10(8) Lactobacillus acidophilus/ml daily for 6 days. Results showed that consumption of milk without cells of Lactobacillus acidophilus for 1 week did not affect lactose utilization while milk containing either 2.5 X 10(6) or 2.5 X 10(8) Lactobacillus acidophilus/ml improved lactose utilization. Lactobacillus acidophilus's effects were shown to be immediate and did not require that milk be consumed daily.

—H.S. Kim & S.E. Gilliland, "Lactobacillus Acidophilus as a Dietary Adjunct for Milk to Aid Lactose Digestion in Humans," *Journal of Dairy Science,* 66(5), May 1983, p. 959-966.

Menopause

Results of this double-blind trial involving 15 postmenopausal women found that local treatment with vaginal tablets containing 0.03 mg of estriol was equal to dosages of 0.5 mg. Gynoflor E induced significant proliferation of the vaginal epithelium and provided total restoration of the vaginal environment while simultaneous implantation of Lactobacillus acidophilus restored an acid vaginal milieu.

—B. Kanne and J. Jenny, [Local Administration of Low-dose Estriol and Vital Lactobacillus Acidophilus in Postmenopause], *Gynakol Rundsch,* 31(1), 1991, p. 7-13.

Vaginitis

In this study, 28 women with chronic nonspecific vaginitis were given Solco Trichovac, a commercial product containing at least 7 X 10(9) inactivated microorganisms of various strains of Lactobacillus acidophilus in each 0.5 ml dose. Results showed treatment produced a significant improvement 4 weeks after completion with a one year follow-up finding that close to 80% of the patients were grade I to II and the vaginal flora was clinically cured or significantly improved in 85.6% of patients.

—G. Muller & H. Salzer, [Long-term Experience in the Therapy and Prevention of Unspecific

Vaginal Discharge with a Lactobacillus Vaccine], *Wien Klin Wochenschr* 95(11), May 27, 1983, p. 371-374.

Results of this case-control study showed that consumption of 8 ounces of yogurt per day containing Lactobacillus acidophilus for six months reduced candidal colonization and infection in women with recurring candidal vaginitis.
—E. Hilton, et al., "Ingestion of Yogurt Containing Lactobacillus Acidophilus as Prophylaxis for Candidal Vaginitis," *Annals of Internal Medicine,* 116(5), March 1, 1992, p. 353-357.

■ ALPHA-LIPOIC ACID

AIDS/HIV

Results of this study indicated alpha-lipoic acid exhibited anti-HIV activity both in vitro and in vivo.
—A. Baur, et al., "Inhibition of HIV-infectivity and Replication by Alpha-lipoic Acid," *International Conference on AIDS,* 7(1), June 16-21, 1991, p. 110.

Results of this study indicated alpha-lipoic acid inhibited HIV-1 replication in vitro.
—A. Baur, et al., "Alpha-lipoic Acid is an Effective Inhibitor of Human Immuno-deficiency Virus (HIV-1) Replication," *Klin Wochenschr,* 69(15), October 2, 1991, p. 722-724.

Cancer

Results of this study showed that the ALPHA-lipoic acid derivatives 1,2-dithiocyclo pentane-4- semicarbazone (Ph 800/l), 1,2-dithio cyclopentane-3,5-dicarboxylic acid (Ph 800/8) and 1,2-dithiocyclopentane-4-thiosemicarbazone (Ph 800/18) inhibited the growth of mouse Ehrlich carcinoma cells in vitro and of Ehrlich ascites carcinoma in vivo.
—J. Kieler & B. Biczowa, "The Effects of Structural Analogues of the Effect of Structural Analogues of Alpha-Lipoic Acid on the Growth and Metabolism of L-Firboblasts and Ehrlic Cells," *Arch Immunol Ther Exp,* 15(1), 1967, p. 106-111.

Cerebral Ischemia

Results of this study showed that alpha-lipoic acid was effective in improving survival and protecting the rat brain from cerebral ischemia-induced reperfusion injury.
—M. Panigrahi, et al., "Alpha-Lipoic Acid Protects Against Reperfusion Injury Following Cerebral Ischemia in Rats," *Brain Research,* 717(1-2), April 22, 1996, p. 184-188.

Results of this study showed that intraperitoneal injections of alpha-lipoic acid provided neuroprotective effects against ischemia/reperfusion evoked cerebral injury in gerbils.
—X. Cao & J.W. Phillis, "The Free Radical Scavenger, Alpha-Lipoic Acid, Protects Against Cerebral Ischemia-Reperfusion Injury in Gerbils," *Free Radical Research,* 23(4), October 1995, p. 365-370.

Diabetes

Results of this study showed that antioxidant therapy including 600 mg of alpha-lipoic acid or 100 mcg of sodium selenite per day or 1200 IE of D-alpha-tocopherol over a period of 3 months led to improvements in symptoms of distal symmetric neuropathy in patients suffering from long-term diabetic late syndrome.

> —W. Kahler, et al., "Diabetes Mellitus — a Free Radical-Associated Disease. Results of Adjuvant Antioxidant Supplementation," *Z.Gesamte Inn Med,* 48(5), May 1993, p. 223-232.

Results of this study showed that lipoic acid improved symptoms associated with streptozotocine-induced diabetic neuropathy in rats.

> —N. Nagamatsu, et al., "Lipoic Acid Improves Nerve Blood Flow, Reduces Oxidative Stress, and Improves Distal Nerve Conduction in Experimental Diabetic Neuropathy," *Diabetes Care,* 18(8), August 1995, p. 1160-1167.

Results of this study showed that the parenteral administration of alpha-lipoic acid significantly enhanced the capacity of the insulin-stimulatable glucose transport system and of both oxidative and nonoxidative pathways of glucose metabolism in insulin-resistant rat skeletal muscle.

> —S. Jacob, et al., "The Antioxidant Alpha-lipoic Acid Enhances Insulin-stimulated Glucose Metabolism in Insulin-resistant Rat Skeletal Muscle," *Diabetes,* 45(8), August 1996, p. 1024-1029.

Results of this double-blind, placebo-controlled study indicated that the administration of 1000 mg of alpha-lipoic acid significantly increased insulin stimulated glucose disposal in NIDDM patients.

> —S. Jacob, et al., "Enhancement of Glucose Disposal in Patients with Type 2 Diabetes by Alpha-lipoic Acid," *Arzneimittelforschung,* 45(8), August 1995, p. 872-874.

Results of this double-blind, placebo-controlled study showed that the intravenous administration of 600 mg per day of alpha-lipoic acid over a period of 3 weeks reduced symptoms associated with diabetic peripheral neuropathy in NIDDM patients.

> —D. Ziegler, et al., "Treatment of Symptomatic Diabetic Peripheral Neuropathy with the Anti-oxidant Alpha-lipoic Acid. A 3-week Multicentre Randomized Controlled Trial," *Diabetologia,* 38(12), December 1995, p. 1425-1433.

Results of this study indicated that the oral administration of thiotic acid at doses of either 2 x 50 mg or 2 x 100 mg per day proved to be a successful treatment for diabetic neuropathy in human patients.

> —W. Klein, [Treatment of Diabetic Neuropathy with Oral Alpha-lipoic Acid], *MMW Munch Med Wochenschr,* 117(22), May 30, 1975, p. 957-958.

General

Results of this study showed that alpha-lipoic acid counteracted glycollate-induced free radical toxicity in rats.

> —R. Sumathi, et al., "Effect of DL Alpha-lipoic Acid on Tissue Lipid Peroxidation and Antioxidant Systems in Normal and Glycollate Treated Rats," *Pharmacol Res,* 27(4), May-June 1993, p. 309-318.

Results of this study showed that the administration of 600 mg of lipoic acid per day for one month led to increases in available brain energy levels and skeletal muscle energy levels in a woman affected by chronic progressive external opthalmoplegia and muscle mitochondria DNA deletion.

> —B. Barbirolli, et al., "Lipoic (thiotic) Acid Increases Brain Energy Availability and Skeletal Muscle Performance as Shown by in Vivo 31P-MRS in a Patient with Mitochondrial Cytopathy," *Journal of Neurology,* 242(7), July 1995, p. 472-477.

Glaucoma

Results of this study found that the administration of 0.15 g per day of lipoic acid for 1 month led to improvements of biochemical parameters, visual function, and of the coefficient of efficacy of liquid discharge in patients with stages I and II open-angle glaucoma. Positive effects were most frequent among stage II patients.

> —A.A. Filina, et al., "Lipoic Acid as a Means of Metabolic Therapy of Open-Angle Glaucoma," *Vestn Oftalmol,* 111(4), Oct-Dec 1995, p. 6-8.

Memory

Results of this study showed that alpha-lipoic acid improved memory in aged mice.

> —S. Stoll, et al., "The Potent Free Radical Scavenger Alpha-lipoic Acid Improves Memory in Aged Mice: Putative Relationship to NMDA Receptor Deficits," *Pharmacol Biochem Behav,* 46(4), December 1993, p. 799-805.

■ BETAINE

Anticonvulsive Effects

Results of this study showed that the IP administration of betaine to rats blocked pentylenetetrazol-induced seizures.

> —E.H. Ghoz & W.J. Freed, "Effects of Betaine on Seizures in the Rat," *Pharmacol Biochem Behav,* 22(4), 1985, p. 635-640.

In this study, betaine blocked the induction of convulsions induced by electroconvulsive shock and pentylenetetrazol.

> —W.J. Freed, et al., "Anticonvulsant Properties of Betaine," *Epilepsia,* 20(3), June 1979, p. 209-213.

General

Results of this series of experiments showed that when betaine was added to tissue cultures of renal medullary cells in hypertonic medium its resultant uptake by the cells replaced the decrease in sorbitol induced by aldose reductase inhibitors and restored cloning efficiency.

> —T. Moriyama, et al., "Intracellular Betaine Substitutes for Sorbitol in Protecting Renal Medullary Cells from Hypertonicity," *American Journal of Physiology,* 260(4 Pt 2), April 1991, p. F494-497.

Results of this study indicated betaine modified urea's effects on erythrocyte Ca(2+)-ATPase, via specific solute-induced conformational changes that protect the enzyme's energy-transduction capacity.

—T. Coelho-Sampaio, et al., "Betaine Counteracts Urea-induced Conformational Changes and Uncoupling of the Human Erythrocyte Ca2+ pump," *European Journal of Biochemistry*, 221(3), May 1, 1994, p. 1103-1110.

Homocystinuria

This article reports on the single case of a 24-day-old girl with homocystinuria and hypomethioninaemia due to methylenetetrahydrofolate reductase who was suffering from encephalopathy and myopathy. Treatment with betaine led to a near total recovery.

—E. Holme, et al., "Betaine for Treatment of Homocystinuria Caused by Methylenetetrahydrofolate Reductase Deficiency," *Arch Dis Child*, 64(7), July 1989, p. 1061-1064.

Results of this study found that 6 grams per day of betaine proved to be an effective alternative therapy for the treatment of homocystinuria.

—B.C. Montero, et al., [Homocystinuria: Effectiveness of the Treatment with Pyridoxine, Folic Acid, and Betaine], *An Esp Pediatr*, 39(1), July 1993, p. 37-41.

This article reports on the single case of a 3-year-old retarded girl with homocystinuria who experienced significant clinical results from treatment with 15-20 g/day of betaine.

—U. Wendel & H.J. Bremer, "Betaine in the Treatment of Homocystinuria due to 5,10-Methylenetetrahydrofolate Reductase Deficiency," *European Journal of Pediatrics*, 142(2), June 1984, p. 147-150.

Liver Damage

Results of this study showed that 0.50% solutions of dietary betaine given to rats generated levels of SAM high enough to protect against ethanol-induced alcoholic steatosis.

—A.J. Barak, et al., "S-adenosylmethionine Generation and Prevention of Alcoholic Fatty Liver by Betaine," *Alcohol*, 11(6), November-December 1994, p. 501-503.

Results of this study showed that the administration of dietary betaine to rats elevated hepatic S-adenoyslmethionine to levels high enough to prevent fatty liver induced by ethanol.

—A.J. Barak, et al., "Dietary Betaine Promotes Generation of Hepatic S-adenosylmethionine and Protects the Liver from Ethanol-induced Fatty Infiltration," *Alcohol Clin Exp Res*, 17(3), June 1993, 552-555.

Neurological Impairment

Results of this study showed betaine to be effective in enhancing the vitamin B-12 nondependent part of methionine synthesis in bats exposed to N2O with impairment of the vitamin B-12-dependent methionine synthase reaction.

—J. van der Westhuyzen & J. Metz, "Betaine Delays the Onset of Neurological Impairment in Nitrous oxide-induced Vitamin B-12 Deficiency in Fruit Bats," *Journal of Nutrition*, 114(6), June 1984, p. 1106-1111.

This article reports on the single case of a 16-year-old Japanese girl with 5,10-methylenetetrahydrofolate reductase deficiency who was suffering from peripheral neuropathy. Treatment with betaine monohydrate led to relief from muscle weakness and gait disturbance while increasing the concentration of S-adenosylmethionine in cerebrospinal fluid to normal levels after 2 years of treatment.

 —T. Kishi, et al., "Effect of Betaine on S-adenosylmethionine Levels in the Cerebrospinal Fluid in a Patient with Mthylenetetrahydrofolate Reductase Deficiency and Peripheral Neuropathy," *Journal of Inherit Metab Disorders,* 17(5), 1994, p. 560-565.

Osmoprotective Effects

Results of this study showed betaine and urine had osmoprotective effects with 40 strains of enteric bacteria.

 —S. Chambers & C.M. Kunin, "The Osmoprotective Properties of Urine for Bacteria: The Protective Effect of Betaine and Human Urine Against Low pH and High Concentrations of Electrolytes, Sugars, and Urea," *Journal of Infectious Disease,* 152(6), December 1985, p. 1308-1316.

This review article notes studies have demonstrated proline betaine to be an osmoprotectant as effective as glycine betaine and more effective than L-proline for different strains of Staphylococcus aureus, and Staphylococcus epidermis and Staphylococcus saprophyticus.

 —U.S. Amin, et al., "Proline Betaine is a Highly Effective Osmoprotectant for Staphylococcus Aureus," *Arch Microbiol,* 163(2), February 1995, p. 138-142.

Results of this study showed that the addition of 10-25 mM-betaine to a hyperosmotic medium significantly prevented the 90% inhibition of cell proliferation that occurred in its absence. 25 mM-betaine also converted a 50% recovery of the rate of protein synthesis into 100%. and prevented a 30% decrease in cell volume while also decreasing by 73% the induction of amino acid transport via system A.

 —P.G. Petronini, et al., "Modulation by Betaine of Cellular Responses to Osmotic Stress," *Biochem Journal,* 282 (Pt 1), February 15, 1992, p. 69-73.

■ BIFIDUS

Bowel/Gastrointestinal Disorders

Results of this study showed that a multibacterial combination consisting of Lactobacillus acidophilus (10(9)) and Bifidobacterium bifidum (10(9)) administered to elderly patients with bowel disorders proved effective with respect to restoration of duodenal bacterial flora and subsidence of clinical symptoms.

 —G. Pecorella, et al., [The Effect of Lactobacillus Acidophilus and Bifidobacterium Bifidum on the Intestinal Ecosystem of the Elderly Patient], *Clin Ter,* 140(1), January 1992, p. 3-10.

This study examined the potential of a live mix of Lactobacillus acidophilus 10(9) and Bifidobacterium bifidum 10(9) to act as an ecological therapy for gastritis and duodenitis in subjects suffering from these disorders stemming from C. pylori. Results showed the treatment was effective in improving upon the results obtained through more conventional means.

—M.R. Gismondo, et al., [Competitive Activity of a Bacterial Preparation on Colonization and Pathogenicity of C. pylori. A Clinical Study], *Clin Ter,* 134(1), July 15, 1990, p. 41-46.

Results of this study showed that the administration of biopreparations containing lacto- or bifidobacteria produced a clinico-microbiological response rate above 90% in 37 patients with intestinal yersiniosis or pseudotuberculosis.

—V.F. Kuznetsov, et al., [Intestinal Dysbacteriosis in Yersiniosis Patients and the Possibility of its Correction with Biopreparations], *Ter Arkh,* 66(11), 1994, p. 17-18.

Cancer

This study examined the effects of 500 ml per day of Bifodium longum enriched yogurt and 5 g of lactulose/L colon cancer risk factors in 12 healthy subjects. Controls subjects were given standard yogurt. Results showed such a dietary approach led to stability of the human fecal flora.

—H.P. Bartram, et al., "Does Yogurt Enriched with Bifidobacterium Longum Affect Colonic Microbiology and Fecal Metabolites in Healthy Subjects?" *American Journal of Clinical Nutrition,* 59(2), February 1994, p. 428-432.

Results of this study found that dietary supplementation with Bifidobacterium inhibited chemical induced liver, colon, and mammary tumors in rats.

—B.S. Reddy & A. Rivenson, "Inhibitory Effect of Bifidobacterium Longum on Colon, Mammary, and Liver Carcinogenesis Induced by 2-amino-3-methylimidazo[4,5-f]quinoline, a Food Mutagen," *Cancer Research,* 53(17), September 1, 1993, p. 3914-3918.

Results of this study found that dietary administration of Bifidobacterium longum influences the metabolic activity some types of intestinal microflora involved in beta-glucuronidase production in rats. Results also indicate that Bifidobacterium longum inhibits aberrant crypt foci formation which can be considered an preneoplastic marker of colon cancer.

—N. Kulkarni & B.S. Reddy, "Inhibitory Effect of Bifidobacterium Longum Cultures on the Azoxymethane-induced Aberrant Crypt Foci Formation and Fecal Bacterial Beta-glucuronidase," *Proc Soc Exp Biol Med,* 207(3), December 1994, p. 278-283.

Results of this study found that Bifidobacterium strains found in fermented milk induced a significant reduction in HT-29 cell growth in vitro, suggesting fermented milk may inhibit the incidence of colon cancer in humans.

—L. Baricault, et al., "Use of HT-29, a Cultured Human Colon Cancer Cell Line, to Study the Effect of Fermented Milks on Colon Cancer Cell Growth and Differentiation," *Carcinogenesis,* 16(2), February 1995, p. 245-252.

Results of this study showed that uninoculated milk and milk cultured with Bifidobacterium or lactobacillus strains exhibited significant mutagenic effects.

—P. Cassand, et al., "Inhibitory Effect of Dairy Products on the Mutagenicities of Chemicals and Dietary Mutagens," *Journal of Dairy Research,* 61(4), November 1994, p. 545-552.

This study examined the effects of six strains of Bifidobacteria strains the procarcinogens nitrite and nitrosamines. Results showed that six strains of Bifidobacteria were responsible for nitrite elimination by a nonenzymatic mechanism and one strain metabolized nitrosamines by an intracellular mechanism.

—J.P. Grill, et al., "Effect of Bifidobacteria on Nitrites and Nitrosamines," *Letters in Applied Microbiology,* 20(5), May 1995, p. 328-330.

This study examined the effects of Bifidobacteria and bifidogenic factor Neosugar on chemical-induced colon cancer in mice. Results showed the incidence of aberrant crypts and foci were reduced significantly 38 weeks after the final carcinogen exposure in mice fed Bifidobacteria relative to controls.

—M. Koo & A.V. Rao, "Long-term Effect of Bifidobacteria and Neosugar on Precursor Lesions of Colonic Cancer in CF1 Mice," *Nutr Cancer,* 16(3-4), 1991, p. 249-257.

This study examined women diagnosed with cervical vulvar or vaginal dysplasia that were treated with vaginal recolonization treatment with Bifidobacterium bifidus, and a process of vaginal acidification. Results indicated that Bifidobacterium bifidus may be an effective new approach to the treatment of epithelial cancer.

—F.J. Gonzalez & A. Aparicio, "Regression of CIN, VIN and VaIN Dysplasias after Vaginal Recolonization with Bifidobacterium Bifidus," *Proceedings of the Annual Meeting of the American Society of Clinical Oncologists,* 13, 1994, p. A822.

Results of this study showed that the administration of intestinal bacteria including Bifodiobacterium longum, Lactobacillus acidophilus, and Eubacterium rectale in mice suppressed liver tumorigenesis which had been promoted with a bacterial mix of Escherichia coli, Streptococcus faecalis, and Clostridium paraputrificum.

—T. Mizutani & T. Mitsuoka, "Inhibitory Effect of Some Intestinal Bacteria on Liver Tumorigenesis in Gnotobiotic C3H/He Male Mice," *Cancer Letters,* 11(2), December 1980, p. 89-95.

Diarrhea

Results of this double-blind, placebo-controlled study showed that infant formula supplemented with Bifidobacterium bifidum and Streptococcus thermophilus decreased the incidence of acute diarrhea and rotavirus shedding in hospitalized infants.

—J.M. Saavedra, et al., "Feeding of Bifidobacterium Bifidum and Streptococcus Thermophilus to Infants in Hospital for Prevention of Diarrhoea and Shedding of Rotavirus," *Lancet,* 344(8929), October 15, 1994, p. 1046-1049.

In this study, human Bifidobacterium sp strain bifidum was given to lactating mice and their litters in order to assess strain's adherent properties and ability to inhibit murine rotavirus infection. Results found that following the administration of the high dose of virus, diarrhea developed in all pups. Onset of diarrhea, however, was significantly delayed in pups treated with Bifidobacterium and infected with murine rotavirus relative to litters suffering from just infection. A significant decrease in murine rotavirus shedding was seen in litters in treated with Bifidobacterium as well.

—L.C. Duffy, et al., "Effectiveness of Bifidobacterium Bifidum in Mediating the Clinical Course of Murine Rotavirus Diarrhea," *Pediatric Research,* 35(6), June 1994, p. 690-695.

Results of this literature review found that placebo-controlled studies have shown that biotherapeutic agents such as Lactobacillus caseiGG, Bifidobacterium longum, B longum with L acidophilus, and Saccharomyces boulardii have been effective in the prevention of antibiotic-associated diarrhea. Bifidobacterum bifidum with Streptococcus thermophilus can prevent acute infantile diarrhea.

> —G.W. Elmer, et al., ''Biotherapeutic Agents. A Neglected Modality for the Treatment and Prevention of Selected Intestinal and Vaginal Infections,'' *JAMA,* 275(11), March 20, 1996, p. 870-876.

General

This double-blind, placebo-controlled study administered lyophilized Bifidobacterium bifidum and Lactobacillus acidophilus capsules to 15 elderly subjects 4 times per day for a total of 28 days Results found that both Bifidobacterium bifidum and Lactobacillus acidophilus significantly reduced the colonic inflammatory infiltration, without altering T, B and Leu7 + cell percentage. Results also showed a significant increase of B cell frequency in the peripheral blood relative to controls.

> —C. De Simone, et al., ''Effect of Bifidobacterium Bifidum and Lactobacillus Acidophilus on Gut Mucosa and Peripheral Blood B Lymphocytes,'' *Immunopharmacol Immunotoxico,* 14(1-2), 1992, p. 331-340.

Results of this study found that probiotic treatment with an antibiotic-resistant strain of Bifidobacterium longum proved beneficial in treating radiation sickness, normalizing faecal flora, and inhibiting opportunistic pathogen colonization and overgrowth in men.

> —V.M. Korschunov, et al., ''Therapeutic Use of an Antibiotic-resistant Bifidobacterium Preparation in Men Exposed to High-dose Gamma-irradiation,'' *Journal of Med Microbiology,* 44(1), January 1996, p. 70-74.

This study examined the effects of Bifidobacteria and lactic acid bacteria administered orally on newborn livestock. Results showed that both proved useful, producing improved body weight gain, reduced diarrhea, improved feed conversion, and improved fecal conditions..

> —F. Abe, et al., ''Effect of Administration of Bifidobacteria and Lactic acid Bacteria to Newborn Calves and Piglets,'' *Journal of Dairy Science,* 78(12), December 1995, p. 2838-2846.

Results of this study showed the mice given peptidoglycan of Bifidobacterium thermophilum from swine experience a significantly higher survival rate against E. coli infection than controls.

> —T. Sasaki, et al., ''Enhanced Resistance of Mice to Escherichia Coli Infection Induced by Administration of Peptidoglycan Derived from Bifidobacterium Thermophilum,'' *Journal of Veterinary Medical Science,* 56(3), June 1994, p. 433-437.

Results of this study found that the oral administration of Bifidobacteria and lactobacteria following the abolition of antibiotic treatment (kanamycin or ampiox) led to the restoration of intestinal microflora in guinea pigs.

> —V.M. Korshunov, et al., [Correction of Intestinal Microflora in Chemotherapeutic Dysbacteriosis using Bifidobacterial and Lactobacterial Autologous Strains], *Zh Mikrobiol Epidemiol Immunobiol,* (9), September 1985, p. 20-25.

Results of this study showed that Bifidobacterium provided complete protection against mortality in rats consecutively infected with E. Coli.

> —J.C. Faure, et al., "Barrier Effect of Bifidobacterium Longum on a Pathogenic Escherichia Coli Strain by Gut Colonization in the Germ-free Rat," *Z Ernahrungswiss,* 23(1), March 1984, p. 41-51.

Immune Enhancement

This study examined the effects of oral intake of heat-killed Bifidobacteria, lactobacteria, enterococci and bacteroides on the resistance to experimental salmonellosis and content of immunoglobulin-synthesizing cells in the proper plate of the small intestine in mice. Results showed that resistance was increased to salmonellosis infection and induced an increase in the content of immunoglobulin-synthesizing cells in the small intestine's proper plate.

> —N.N. Mal'tseva, et al., [Immunomodulating Properties of Various Microbes—representatives of Normal Intestinal Microflora], *Antibiot Khimioter,* 37(12), December 1992, p. 41-43.

Results of this double-blind, placebo-controlled study found that regular administration of Bifidobacterium bifidum and Lactobacillus acidophilus to elderly subjects led to a modulation of the immunoglical and inflammatory response.

> —C. De Simone, et al., "Effect of Bifidobacterium Bifidum and Lactobacillus Acidophilus on Gut Mucosa and Peripheral Blood B Lymphocytes," *Immunopharmacol Immunotoxicol,* 14(1-2), 1992, p. 331-340.

Results of this murine in vivo study showed that Bifidobacteria may be a an effective immunomodulator in animal and humans intestines.

> —K. Sekine, et al., "Adjuvant Activity of the Cell Wall of Bifidobacterium Infantis for In Vivo Immune Responses in Mice," *Immunopharmacol Immunotoxicol,* 16(4), November 1994, p. 589-609.

In this case-control study, subjects consumed a fermented milk containing L. acidophilus La1 and Bifidobacteria over a three week period during which an attenuated Salmonella typhi Ty21a was administered to mimic an enteropathogenic infection. Results showed that lactic acid bacteria prevalent in the gastrointestinal tract acts as an adjuvant to the humoral immune response in man.

> —H. Link-Amster, et al., "Modulation of a Specific Humoral Immune Response and Changes in Intestinal Flora Mediated Through Fermented Milk Intake," *FEMS Immunol Med Microbiol,* 10(1), November 1994, p. 55-63.

Newborns

In this double-blind study, a fermented whey-adapted infant formula containing viable Bifidobacteria (10(6)/g of powder) fed to infants during their first 2 months was compared to a whey-adapted, nonacidified, low-phosphate infant formula. Results showed the fermented whey-adapted formula containing viable Bifidobacteria induced a prevalence of colonization with Bifidobacteria at 1 month of age similar to that of breast-fed infants but significantly greater than those fed the standard infant formula.

> —J.P. Langhendries, et al., "Effect of a Fermented Infant Formula Containing Viable Bifido-

bacteria on the Fecal Flora Composition and pH of Healthy Full-term Infants," *Journal of Pediatr Gastroenterol Nutr,* 21(2), August 1995, p. 177-181.

Ulcer

Results of this study showed that Bifidobacteria, lactobacilli and streptococci and their polysaccharides induced host repair protective systems in murine gastric ulcers.

—M. Nagaoka, et al., "Anti-ulcer Effects of Lactic Acid Bacteria and Their Cell Wall Polysaccharides," *Biol Pharm Bull,* 17(8), August 1994, p. 1012-1017.

■ BIOTIN

Brittle Nails

Results of this study showed that daily biotin supplementation over a period of six months led to clinical improvement in brittle nails.

—L.G. Hochman, et al., "Brittle Nails: Response to Daily Biotin Supplementation," *Cutis,* 51(4), April 1993, p. 303-305.

Diabetes

In this study, high doses of biotin were administered to three diabetics for 1-2 years. Results showed major improvements in symptoms of peripheral neuropathy within 4-8 weeks of treatment.

—D. Koutsikos, et al., "Biotin for Diabetic Peripheral Neuropathy," *Biomed Pharmacotherapy,* 44(10), 1990, p. 511-514.

In this study, diabetic mice received treatment for 10 weeks with either 2 mg of biotin/Kg, 4 mg of biotin/Kg, or saline which served as a control. Results showed reduced post-prandial glucose levels, and improved tolerance to glucose and insulin resistance in the mice treated with biotin relative to controls.

—A. Reddi, et al., "Biotin Supplementation Improves Glucose and Insulin Tolerances in Genetically Diabetic KK Mice," *Life Sciences,* 42(13), 1988, p. 1323-1230.

Results of this study showed that the administration of biotin over a period of 5 hours reduced hepatic phosphoenolpyruvate carboxykinase MRNA concentration in diabetic rats at the transcriptional level.

—K. Dakshinamurti & W. Li, "Transcriptional Regulation of Liver PhosphoenolpyruvateCarboxykinase by Biotin in Diabetic Rats," *Molecular Cell Biochemistry,* 132(2), March 30, 1994, p. 127-132.

General

Results of this study showed intraperitoneally administered biotin capable of regulating the glucokinase gene of starved rats at the transcriptional stage.

—J. Chauhan & K. Dakshinamurti, "Transcriptional Regulation of the Glucokinase Gene by Biotin in Starved Rats," *Journal of Biol Chem,* 266(16), June 5, 1991, p. 10035-10038.

This article reports on the case of a young woman with adult-onset myoclonus, ataxia, hearing loss, seizures, hemianopia, and hemiparesis who was treated with large doses of biotin and showed favorable results.

> —S. Bressman, et al., "Biotin-responsive Encephalopathy with Myoclonus, Ataxia, and Seizures," *Adv Neurol,* 43, 1986, p. 119-125.

Neurological Disorders

In this study, patients undergoing chronic hemodialysis for 2-10 years and suffering from encephalopathy and peripheral neuropathy, received 10 mg of biotin per day for 1-4 years. Results showed improvement in all patients within 3 months.

> —H. Yatzidis, et al., "Biotin in the Management of Uremic Neurologic Disorders," *Nephron,* 36(3), 1984, p. 183-186.

This article reports on the cases of two children with biotinidase deficiency that presented with seizures at 2 months of age due to brain atrophy. Biotin supplementation produced marked improvement in both.

> —D.P. Bousounis, et al., "Reversal of Brain Atrophy with Biotin Treatment in Biotinidase Deficiency," *Neuropediatrics,* 24(4), August 1993, p. 214-217.

This article reports on the case of a 15-year-old boy with progressive bilateral optic neuropathy of acute onset at the age of 10 years. Results showed that supplementation with 10 mg per day of biotin led to the rapid reduction of metabolic derangements which was maintained for as much as one year.

> —V.T. Ramaekers, et al., "Recovery from Neurological Deficits Following Biotin Treatment in a Biotinidase Km Variant," *Neuropediatrics,* 24(2), April 1993, p. 98-102.

Skin Conditions

Results of this study showed that supplementation with 5 mg biotin/10 kg body weight per day for 3 to 5 weeks was successful in the treatment of fur and skin conditions of dogs of various breeds.

> —M. Frigg, et al., "Clinical Study on the Effect of Biotin on Skin Conditions in Dogs," *Schweiz Arch Tierheilkd,* 131(10), 1989, p. 621-625.

■ BORAGE OIL

Atopic Dermatitis

Results of this double-blind, placebo-controlled study showed that 5 of 7 atopic dermatitis patients treated with borage oil experienced beneficial effects.

> —F.A. Bahmer & J. Schafer, "Treatment of Atopic Dermatitis with Borage Seed Oil (Glandol) — A Time Series Analytic Study," *Kinderarztl Prax,* 60(7), October 1992, p. 199-202.

Hypertension

In this study, hypertensive rats received purified diets containing evening primrose, black currant, borage or fungal oils for 7 weeks. Results found the treatment significantly reduced blood pressure.

> —M.M. Engler, "Comparative Study of Diets Enriched with Evening Primrose, Black Currant,

Borage or Fungal Oils on Blood Pressure and Pressor Responses in Spontaneously Hypertensive Rats,'' *Prostaglandins Leukot Essent Fatty Acids,* 49(4), October 1993, p. 809-814.

■ BORON

AIDS/HIV

Results of this showed boron modified peptides inhibited HIV protease.
— A.D. Pivazyan, ''Boron Modified Peptides as Inhibitors of HIV-1 Protease,'' *Int Conf AIDS,* 9(1), June 6-11, 1993, p. 230.

Arthritis

This review article cites results from placebo-controlled, double-blind studies indicating that supplementation with 6 mg per day of boron led to significant improvement in patients suffering from arthritis.
— R.E. Newnham, ''Essentially of Boron for Healthy Bones and Joints,'' *Environ Health Perspect,* 102 (Suppl 7), November 1994, p. 83-35.

Brain Function

Results of this series of studies indicate that boron supplementation improved cognitive performance and brain function in humans.
— J.G. Penland, ''Dietary Boron, Brain Function, and Cognitive Performance,'' *Environ Health Perspect,* 102 (Suppl 7), November 1994, p. 65-72.

Mineral Metabolism

Results of this study demonstrated protective and regulatory roles for boron in the mineral metabolism of STZ rats deficient in vitamin D.
— C.D. Hunt & J.L. Herbert, ''Effects of Dietary Boron on Calcium and Mineral Metabolism in the Streptozotocin-injected, Vitamin D3-deprived Rat,'' *Magnes Trace Elem,* 10(5-6), 1991-1992, p. 387-408.

■ BROMELAIN

Cancer

Results of this study found that the administration of 80 mg/kg per body weight of bromelain reduced the number of precancerous lesions in hairless mice treated with UV light relative to controls.
— N. Goldstein, et al., ''Bromelain as a Skin Cancer Preventive in Hairless Mice,'' *Hawaii Medical Journal,* 54(3), 1975, p. 91-94.

Dental Health

This double-blind, placebo-controlled study examined the effects of bromelain in patients with impacted or dislocated lower wisdom teeth. When administered in doses of 240 mg per day, results showed that bromelain reduced swelling by 7.5% one day after surgery.

—G. Hotz, et al., [Antiphlogistic Effect of Bromelaine Following Third Molar Removal], *Dtsch Zahnarztl Z,* 44(11), November 1989, p. 830-332.

General

This review article cites results from numerous studies on bromelain showing it can interfere with malignant cell growth, inhibit platelet aggregation, inhibit fibrinolytic activity, has anti-inflammatory action, modulates tumor growth and blood coagulation, debridement of third degree burns, and helps in the enhancement of absorption of drugs.

—S.J. Taussig & S. Batkin, "Bromelain, the Enzyme Complex of Pineapple (Ananas comosus) and Its Clinical Application. An Update," *Journal of Ethnopharmacology,* 22(2), February-March 1988, p. 191-203.

This review article notes that animal studies have shown bromelain to inhibit experimentally induced tumors and possess anti-inflammatory, antiedema, coagulation-inhibiting effects.

—H. Lotz-Winter, "On the Pharmacology of Bromelain: An Update with Special Regard to Animal Studies on Dose-dependent Effects," *Planta Medicine,* 56(3), June 1990, p. 249-253.

Immune Enhancement

This study examined the activation potential of CD44 T cells treated with bromelain by comparing the proliferation of sham- and bromelain-treated normal human PBMC to mitogenic CD2 mAb. Results showed that bromelain removed T cell CD44, the CD45RA isoform of CD45 as well as E2/MIC2, CD6, CD7, CD8, and Leu 8/LAM1 molecules. T cell proliferation in response to CD2 mAb increased 325% in bromelain-treated PBMC relative to controls.

—L.P. Hale & B.F. Haynes, "Bromelain Treatment of Human T Cells Removes CD44, CD45RA, E2/MIC2, CD6, CD7, CD8, and Leu 8/LAM1 Surface Molecules and Markedly Enhances CD2-mediated T Cell Activation," *Journal of Immunology,* 149(12), December 15, 1992, p. 3809-3016.

In this study, bromelain was given to patients with metastasizing cancers of the breast, ovary, lung, and bladder. Results showed that when 200-300 mg/kg of bromelain was coupled with conventional cancer therapy there was a significant reduction of malignant masses in 9/12 patients receiving the treatment. In 3/12 patients receiving 600 mg/d of bromelain alone, results showed either a total elimination or significant reduction of metastasis.

—G. Gerard, [Anticancer Therapy and Bromelain] *Agressologie,* 13(4), 1972, p. 261-274.

■ CALCIUM

Calcific Pancreatitis

This article reports on the case of a 22-year-old woman suffering from chronic calcific pancreatitis who experienced pain relief following pancreaticojejunostomy. The patient experienced steatorrhea with osteomalacia and secondary hyperparathyroidism four years later. Supplemenation with pancreatic enzyme, calcium and vitamin D led to improvements.

—N. Kaur, et al., "Chronic Calcific Pancreatitis Associated with Osteomalacia and Secondary Hyperparathryoidism," *Indian Journal of Gastroenterology,* 15(4), October 1996, p. 147-148.

Calcium Absorption

Results of this study showed that calcium citrate-malate had positive effects on bone development in weaning female rats and proved to be a more available calcium source than calcium carbonate.

—B.A. Kochanowski, "Effect of Calcium Citrate-malate on Skeletal Development in Young, Growing Rats," *Journal of Nutrition,* 120(8), August 1990, p. 876-881.

This study compared calcium absorption between calcium citrate and calcium carbonate in normal women. Results showed absorption to be significantly higher from calcium citrate than carbonate.

—J.A. Harvey, et al., "Superior Calcium Absorption from Calcium Citrate than Calcium Carbonate Using External Forearm Counting," *Journal of American College of Nutrition,* 9(6), December 1990, p. 583-587.

Cancer

Results of this study found that dietary calcium had protective effects against experimental-induced colon carcinogenesis in rats.

—B.C. Pence, et al., "Protective Effects of Calcium from Nonfat Milk Against Colon Carcinogenesis in Rats," *Nutrition and Cancer,* 25(1), 1996, p. 35-45.

This study examined the effects of calcium chemoprevention in 175 patients with adenomatous polyps on polyp recurrence. Results showed a lower rate of recurrence in those patients receiving the calcium chemoprevention relative to controls.

—I. Duris, et al., "Calcium Chemoprevention in Colorectal Cancer," *Hepatogastroenterology,* 43(7), January-February 1996, p. 152-154.

This review article discussed the results of numerous animal studies indicating that supplemental calcium can reduce mammary epithelial cell hyperplasia and hyperproliferation, as well as colonic cell hyperproliferation. Animals studies have also shown calcium reduces carcinogen-induced tumors of the colon. In humans, studies have shown calcium significantly reduced colonic epithelial cell proliferation.

—M. Lipkin & H. Newmark, "Calcium and the Prevention of Colon Cancer," *Journal of Cell Biochemistry,* 22(Suppl), 1995, p. 65-73.

Dental Health

Results of this study showed that the administration of 500 mg of ascorbic acid, 250 mg of calcium and 800 IU of vitamin D3 per day reversed clinical and dental fluorisis after 44 days in Indian children consuming water contaminated with fluoride.

—S.K. Gupta, et al., "Reversal of Clinical and Dental Fluorosis," *Indian Pediatr,* 31(4), April 1994, p. 439-443.

General

This review article notes that while excessive intracellular calcium accumulation can results in cell damage; high calcium intake may be effective in the treatment of such unrelated diseases as arterial hypertension, nephrolithiasis, colon cancer, etc.
> —G. Palmieri, "New Perspectives in Calcium Metabolism," *Medicina B. Aries,* 53(5), 1993, p. 459-466.

Hip Fracture

Results of this 3-year study found that supplementation with 1.2 g of calcium and 800 IU of vitamin D3 reduced the number of hip fractures and other non-vertebral fractures among ambulatory women living in nursing homes by 23% relative to controls.
> —P. Meunier, "Prevention of Hip Fractures by Correcting Calcium and Vitamin D Insufficiencies in Elderly People," *Scandinavian Journal of Rheumatology,* 103(Suppl), 1996, p. 75-78.

Hypertension

Results of this study found that supplementation with 2 g per day of calcium from 20 to 28 weeks of gestation up to delivery significantly reduced the rate of pregnancy induced hypertension in healthy primiparas relative to controls.
> —K. Cong, et al., "Calcium Supplementation During Pregnancy for Reducing Pregnancy Induced Hypertension," *Chinese Medical Journal,* 108(1), January 1995, p. 57-59.

Results of this study showed that daily supplementation with 1.4 g of elemental of calcium significantly reduced systolic and diastolic blood pressure in human subjects.
> —S.J. Wimalawansa, "Antihypertensive Effects of Oral Calcium Supplementation May be Mediated through the Potent Vasodilator CGRP," *American Journal of Hypertension,* 6(12), December 1993, p. 996-1002.

Osteoporosis

Results of this double-blind, placebo-controlled study examined the effects 1000 mg per day of calcium in combination with 50,000 IU per week of vitamin D on the effects of corticosteroid-induced osteoporosis. Results showed the treatment could help prevent early bone loss in the spine of such subjects.
> —J.D. Adachi, et al., "Vitamin D and Calcium in the Prevention of Corticosteroid Induced Osteoporosis: A 3 Year Follow-up," *Journal of Rheumatology,* 23(6), June 1996, p. 995-1000.

This article reports on the case of a 43-year-old male with osteoporosis who experienced healing following the administration of calcium and calcitonin.
> —M. Leyes-Vence, et al., "Transient Osteoporosis of the Hip. Presentation of a Case and Literature Review," *Acta Orthop Belg,* 62(1), March 1996, p. 56-59.

This randomized, placebo-controlled study examined the effects of increased exercise and dietary calcium in women who had been postmenopausal for longer than ten years. Results showed that calcium supplementation in the form of either 1 g per night in tablets or 1 g per night in milk powder led to bone loss cessation over a period of two years. Such effects were increased when combined with exercise.

—R. Prince, et al.., "The Effects of Calcium Supplementation (Milk Powder or Tablets) and Exercise on Bone Density in Postmodern Women," *Journal of Bone Mineral Research,* 10(7), July 1995, p. 1068-1075.

Results of this study found that supplemental calcium prevented osteopenia in ovariectomized rats.

—J. Tan, et al., "Effects of Natural Calcium Against Osteopenia in Ovariectomized Rats," *Hua Hsi I Ko Ta Hsueh Hsueh Pao,* 26(1), March 1995, p. 70-73.

Results of this study indicated that calcium supplementation can improve the bone mass of postmenopausal women using estrogen replacement therapy and with a low intake of dietary intake calcium.

—C.J. Haines, et al., "Calcium Supplementation and Bone Mineral Density in Postmenopausal Women Using Estrogen Replacement Therapy," *Bone,* 16(5), May 1995, p. 529-531.

Results of this study showed that corticosteroid treated children with rheumatic disease and osteoporoisis who were administered a minimum of 1 g per day of calcium and 400 IU of vitamin D per day for 6 months experienced significant improvements in spinal bone density.

—B.D. Warady, "Effects of Nutritional Supplementation on Bone Mineral Status of Children with Rheumatic Diseases Receiving Corticosteroid Therapy," *Journal of Rheumatology,* 21(3), March 1994, p. 530-535.

Vestibulitis

This article reports on the case of woman suffering from vulvar vestibulitis for four years who experienced significant reductions in symptoms following three months of supplementation with calcium citrate. The woman was pain free after a year of treatment.

—C.C. Solomons, et al., "Calcium Citrate for Vulvar Vestibulitis. A Case Report," *Journal of Reproductive Medicine,* 36(12), December 1991, p. 879-382.

■ CELLULASE

Phytobezoars

This study found that that cellulase was effective in breaking up phytobezoars in five patients and had no side effects.

—S.P. Lee, et al., "The Medical Dissolution of Phytobezoars Using Cellulase," *British Journal of Surgery,* 64(6), June 1977, p. 403-405.

This article reports on two cases of phytobezoar that were effectively treated with oral cellulase.

—E. Nauer & L. Filippini, [Conservative Treatment of Phytobezoars of the Stomach with Cellulase], *Dtsch Med Wochenschr,* 100(6), February 7, 1975, p. 244-246.

■ CHOLINE

Aging

Results of this study showed that treatment with choline alfoscerate treatment counteracted various anatomical changes of the rat hippocampus associated with aging.

> —A. Ricci, et al., "Oral Choline Alfoscerate Counteracts Age-dependent Loss of Mossy Fibres in the Rat Hippocampus," *Mech Ageing Dev,* 66(1), 1992, p. 81-91.

Cardiovascular/Coronary Heart Disease

Results of this study showed that intracerebroventricular choline increased blood pressure hypotensive rats

> —I.H. Ulus, et al., "Restoration of Blood Pressure by Choline Treatment in Rats Made Hypotensive by Haemorrhage," *British Journal of Pharmacology,* 116(2), September 1995, p. 1911-1917.

Results of this study indicated that intravenous CDP-choline reduced aortic wall lesions induced by a hypercholesterolic diet in rabbits.

> —G. Weber, et al., "Influence of CDP-choline Administration on the Aortic Wall Lesions in Dietically Hypercholesterolaemic Rabbits: A Morphometric Evaluation," *Drugs Exp Clin Res,* 15(6-7), 1989, p. 321-323.

Fetal Alcohol Syndrome

Results of this study showed that CDP-choline modified alcohol-induced lesions in newborn rat pups.

> —S. Patt, et al., "The Effects of CDP-choline on Newborn Rat Pups with Experimental Alcohol Fetopathy. A Golgi Study," *Histol Histopathol,* 4(4), October 1989, p. 429-434.

Head Injury

Results of this double-blind, placebo-controlled study showed that supplementation with 1 g of CDP-choline led to significant reductions in postconcussional symptoms associated with head injury relative to controls.

> —H.S. Levin, "Treatment of Postconcussional Symptoms with CDP-choline," *Journal of Neurol Sci,* 103 Suppl, July 1991, p. S39-S42.

Results of this single-blind study found that supplemental CDP-choline led to overall improvements in the outcome of patients suffering from head injury relative to controls.

> —V. Calatayud Maldonado, et al., "Effects of CDP-choline on the Recovery of Patients with Head Injury," *Journal of Neurol Sci,* 103 Suppl, July 1991, p. S15-S18.

Hemiplegia

Results of this double-blind, placebo-controlled study showed that supplemental CDP-choline in doses ranging from 250-1000 mg promoted natural recovery in cases of hemiplegia when administered over an 8 week period.

> —T. Hazama, et al., "Evaluation of the Effect of CDP-choline on Poststroke Hemiplegia

Employing a Double-blind Controlled Trial. Assessed by a New Rating Scale for Recovery in Hemiplegia,'' *International Journal of Neuroscience,* 11(3), 1980, p. 211-225.

Hepatic Steatosis

Results of this study showed that daily supplementation with 1-4 g of choline chloride over a period of 4 weeks helped prevent and ameliorate hepatic steatosis associated with parenteral nutrition.

—A.L. Buchman, et al., ''Choline Deficiency: A Cause of Hepatic Steatosis During Parenteral Nutrition that Can be Reversed with Intravenous Choline Supplementation,'' *Hepatology,* 22(5), November 1995, p. 1399-1403.

Memory

Results of this study showed that choline supplementation enhanced the spatial memory capacity of rats.

—W.H. Meck, et al., ''Pre- and Postnatal Choline Supplementation Produces Long-term Facilitation of Spatial Memory,'' *Dev Psychobiol,* 21(4), May 1988, p. 339-353.

Results of this study showed that oral choline supplementation enhanced the learning and memory capacity of rats.

—V.D. Petkov, et al., ''Effect of CDP-choline on Learning and Memory Processes in Rodents,'' *Methods Find Exp Clin Pharmacol,* 14(8), October 1992, p. 593-605.

Neurological Function

This study examined the effects of CDP-choline (6 ml per day mean dose) in 2817 patients primarily between 60-80 years old suffering from a host of different neurological conditions. Results indicated that conditions benefiting most from the treatment included dizziness, cephalea, insomnia, depression, and memory.

—R. Lozano Fernandez, ''Efficacy and Safety of Oral CDP-choline. Drug Surveillance Study in 2817 Cases,'' *Arzneimittelforschung,* 33(7A), 1983, p. 1073-1080.

Seizures

Results of this study found that oral supplementation with 12-16 g per day of choline led to a shorter length of human complex partial seizures and reduced postseizure fatigue

—J. O. McNamara, et al., ''Effects of Oral Choline on Human Complex Partial Seizures,'' *Neurology,* 30(12), 1980, p. 1334-1336.

Stroke

Results of this study showed that supplemental CDP-choline produced beneficial effects on brain dysfunction induced by cerebral ischemia-induced brain dysfunction in rats.

—M. Kakihana, et al., ''Effects of CDP-choline on Neurologic Deficits and Cerebral Glucose Metabolism in a Rat Model of Cerebral Ischemia,'' *Stroke,* 19(2), February 1988, p. 217-222.

This double-blind, placebo-controlled study examined the effects of 1000 mg of intravenous CDP-choline per day for 14 days on patients with cerebral infarction. Results showed significant improvements in level of consciousness relative to controls.

—Y. Tazaki, et al., ''Treatment of Acute Cerebral Infarction with a Choline Precursor in a

Multicenter Double-blind Placebo-controlled Study,'' *Stroke,* 19(2), February 1988, p. 211-216.

Tardive Dyskinesia

Results of this study found the oral administration of choline and lecithin to 5 male tardive dyskinesia led to improvements in all of them.

    —A.J. Gelenberg, et al., ''Choline and Lecithin in the Treatment of Tardive Dyskinesia: Preliminary Results from a Pilot Study,'' *American Journal of Psychiatry,* 136(6), June 1979, p. 772-776.

In this double-blind study, 20 patients with stable baccal-lingual-masticatory movements were administered oral choline for two weeks. Results showed that reductions in choreic movements occurred in 9 patients, worsened in 10, and remained unchanged in 1.

    —J.H. Growdon, et al., ''Oral Choline Administration to Patients with Tardive Dyskinesia,'' *New England Journal of Medicine,* 297(10), September 8, 1977, p. 524-527.

Results of this study showed that daily doses of 500-1200 mg of CDP-choline administered to elderly patients with tardive dyskinesia produced significant decreases in symptoms associated with the condition.

    —J. Arranz, & G. Ganoza, ''Treatment of Chronic Dyskinesia with CDP-choline,'' *Arzneimit-telforschung,* 33(7A), 1983, p. 1071-1073.

Results of this double-blind, crossover study showed that the administration of choline chloride to tardive dyskinesia patients produced improvements in 7 of the 11 patients treated.

    —H.A. Nasrallah, et al., ''Variable Clinical Response to Choline in Tardive Dyskinesia,'' *Psychol Med,* 14(3), August 1984, p. 697-700.

■ CHROMIUM

Cardiovascular/Coronary Heart Disease

Results of this double-blind, placebo-controlled study showed that atherosclerosis patients treated with 250 micrograms of chromium for 7-16 months experienced lower serum triglycerides relative to controls.

    —A.S. Abraham, et al., ''The Effects of Chromium Supplementation on Serum Glucose and Lipids in Patients with and without Non-insulin-dependent Diabetes,'' *Metabolism,* 41(7), July 1992, p. 768-771.

Results of this double-blind, placebo-controlled study showed that supplementation with 600 mcg per day of chromium over a period of 2 months produced beneficial increases in HDL cholesterol levels among men on beta-blockers.

    —J.R. Roeback, Jr. ''Effects of Chromium Supplementation on Serum High-density Lipoprotein Cholesterol Levels in Men Taking Beta-blockers. A Randomized, Controlled Trial,'' *Annals of Internal Medicine,* 115(12), December 15, 1991, p. 917-924.

Results of this study showed that the administration of 200 micrograms of chromium chloride and 100 mg of nicotinic acid per day over a period of several months reduced serum cholesterol levels in two hypocholestermia patients.

> —M. Urberg, et al., "Hypocholesterolemic Effects of Nicotinic Acid and Chromium Supplementation," *Journal of Family Practice,* 27(6), December 1988, p. 603-606.

Diabetes

This review article of 15 controlled studies on the relationship between supplemental chromium compounds and impaired glucose tolerance found a pattern of improvement in efficiency of insulin or the blood lipid profile of subjects treated with chromium.

> —W. Mertz, et al., "Chromium in Human Nutrition: A Review," *Journal of Nutrition,* 123(4), April 1993, p. 626-633.

Results of this double-blind, placebo-controlled study showed that the administration of 200 micrograms of chromium in healthy subjects significantly reduced 90-minute glucose concentrations and fasting glucose concentrations.

> —R.A. Anderson, et al., "Chromium Supplementation of Human Subjects: Effects on Glucose, Insulin, and Lipid Variables," *Metabolism,* 32(9), September 1983, p. 894-899.

Results of this double-blind, placebo-controlled study indicated that supplementation with 200 micrograms of chromium alleviated hypoglycemic symptoms and significantly increased minimum serum glucose levels seen 2-4 hours after a glucose load in female hypoglycemic patients. Significant improvements in insulin binding to red blood cells and insulin receptor number were seen as well.

> —R.A. Anderson, et al., "Effects of Supplemental Chromium on Patients with Symptoms of Reactive Hypoglycemia," *Metabolism,* 36(4), April 1987, p. 351-355.

This study examined the effects of oral chromic chloride on 5 elderly subjects with glucose intolerance over a 12 week period. Results showed that oral glucose tolerance curves decreased from 60 to 120 minutes with the 60-minute values being significantly reduced following supplementation.

> —J.F. Potter, et al., "Glucose Metabolism in Glucose-intolerant Older People During Chromium Supplementation," *Metabolism,* 34(3), March 1995, p. 199-204.

Results of this study found that rats fed a diet high in chromium rich barley had a modulating impact on diabetic symptoms relative to rats on a sucrose or starch-based diet. When the sucrose-based diet was supplemented with doses of trivalent inorganic chromium equivalent to that naturally occurring in barley, the differences in diabetic symptoms were eliminated.

> —G.S. Mahdi & D.J.Naismith, "Role of Chromium in Barley in Modulating the Symptoms of Diabetes," *Ann Nutr Metab,* 35(2), 1991, p. 65-70.

This article notes that chromium works to maintain normal glucose tolerance by controlling the action of insulin and that lower insulin amounts are needed when chromium intake is sufficient.

> —R.A. Anderson, "Chromium, Glucose Tolerance, and Diabetes," *Biological Trace Element Research,* 32, January-March 1992, p. 19-24.

This study examined the effects of 125 micrograms of chromium per day for 3 months on patients with clinical symptoms of hypoglycemia. Results showed a reduced negative part of the glucose tolerance curve in patients following treatment and improvements in chilliness, trembling, emotional instability, and disorientation.

—J. Clausen, "Chromium Induced Clinical Improvement in Symptomatic Hypoglycemia," *Biological Trace Element Research,* 17. September-December 1988, p. 229-236.

Results of this double-blind, placebo-controlled, crossed-over study showed that supplemental chromium picolinate administered for 2 months produced a significant reduction in serum triglycerides in patients suffering from non-insulin dependent diabetes.

—N.A. Lee & C.A. Reasner, "Beneficial Effect of Chromium Supplementation on Serum Triglyceride Levels in NIDDM," *Diabetes Care,* 17(12), December 1994, p. 1449-1452.

Results of this double-blind, placebo-controlled study, 243 diabetics were given 200 micrograms of chromium per day. Results showed the treatment led to reductions in insulin, sulfonylurea or metformin requirements in 115 patients, with such effects being greater in NIDDM than IDDM and stronger in women than men.

—A. Ravina & L. Slezack, [Chromium in the Treatment of Clinical Diabetes Mellitus], *Harefuah,* 125(5-6), September 1993, p. 142-145, 191.

This study examined the effects of chromium chloride, chromium nicotinate, and chromium picolinate on insulin internalization in cultured rat skeletal muscle cells. Results showed significant increases in insulin internalization in cells cultured in a medium that contained chromium picolinate as well as an increase glucose and leucine uptake.

—G.W. Evans & T.D. Bowman, "Chromium Picolinate Increases Membrane Fluidity and Rate of Insulin Internalization," *Journal of Inorganic Biochemisty,* 46(4), June 1992, p. 243-250.

Turner's Syndrome

Results of this study showed that the administration of 30 g of brewer's yeast containing 50 micgrograms of chromium per day for 8 weeks to Turner's syndrome patients produced a reduction in cholesterol and/or triglyceride levels and an increase in high-density lipoprotein cholesterol.

—G. Saner, et al., "Alterations of Chromium Metabolism and Effect of Chromium Supplementation in Turner's Syndrome Patients," *American Journal of Clinical Nutrition,* 38(4), October 1983, p. 574-578.

■ CITRUS BIOFLAVONOIDS

Cancer

Results of this study indicated that citrus flavonoids such nobiletin and tangeretin may be involved in cancer chemoprevention.

—M. Calomme, et al., "Inhibition of Bacterial Mutagenesis by Citrus Flavonoids," *Planta Med,* 62(3), June 1996, p. 222-226.

Results of this study showed that citrus flavonoids and catechins inhibit invasion of mouse MO4 cells into embryonic chick heart fragments in vitro.
> —M. Bracke, et al., "Effect of Catechins and Citrus Flavonoids on Invasion in Vitro," *Clin Exp Metastasis,* 9(1), January-February 1991, p. 13-25.

General

Results of this study indicated that colonic secretions can be modulated by dietary citrus flavonoids in vitro.
> —T.D. Nguyen & A.T. Canada, "Citrus Flavonoids Stimulate Secretion by Human Colonic T84 Cells," *Journal of Nutrition,* 123(2), February 1993, p. 259-268.

■ COD LIVER OIL

Cardiovascular/Coronary Heart Disease

Results of this study found that 20 ml per day of supplemental cod liver oil for 3 weeks exhibited effects on serum lipids and platelets that can decrease the tendency to thrombosis in healthy Norwegian males
> —T. Simonsen, et al., "The Effect of Cod Liver Oil in Two Populations with Low and High Intake of Dietary Fish," *Acta Med Scand,* 223(6), 1988, p. 491-498.

Results of this study showed that the daily administration of 25 ml of cod liver oil for 8 weeks in healthy subjects significantly reduced mean thromboxane B2 levels in both men and women.
> —J.B. Hansen, et al., "Effects of Dietary Supplementation with Cod Liver Oil on Monocyte Thromboplastin Synthesis, Coagulation and Fibrinolysis," *Journal of Internal Med Suppl,* 225(731), 1989, p. 133-139.

Results of this study showed that supplemental cod liver oil over a period of 6 weeks significantly reduced neutrophil chemotaxis towards both chemoattractants and monocyte chemotaxis towards N-FMLP in health males.
> —E.B. Schmidt, et al., "Cod Liver Oil Inhibits Neutrophil and Monocyte Chemotaxis in Healthy Males, *Atherosclerosis,* 77(1), May 1989, p. 53-57.

Results of this study showed that supplemental cod liver oil helped alleviate musculoskeletal pain in patients suffering from musculoskeletal disease.
> —W. Eriksen, et al., "Does Dietary Supplementation of Cod Liver Oil Mitigate Musculoskeletal Pain?" *European Journal of Clinical Nutrition,* 50(10), October 1996, p. 689-693.

Hemolytic Uremic Syndrome

This article reports on the case of a 21-month-old male severe hemolytic uremic syndrome patient who experienced a complete recovery following treatment with fresh frozen plasma, vitamin E, and cod liver oil.
> —M. Weyl, et al., "Hemolytic Uremic Syndrome; Treatment with Plasma, Vitamin E and Cod Liver Oil," *International Journal of Pediatr Nephrol,* 4(4), December 1993, p. 243-245.

■ COENZYME Q10

AIDS/HIV

This article reports on two ARC patients who have survived 4 to 5 years with no symptoms of adenopathy or infection while taking CoQ10 continuously. The authors also report results on 14 newly found normal subjects that experienced increased T4/T8 ratios in response to CoQ10 administration.

—K. Folkers, et al., "Coenzyme Q10 Increases T4/T8 Ratios of Lymphocytes in Ordinary Subjects and Relevance to Patients Having the AIDS Related Complex," *Biochem Biophys Res Commun,* 176(2), April 30, 1991, p. 786-791.

Results of this study showed that AIDS patients had a significant blood deficiency of CoQ10 relative to controls and relative to ARC patients. ARC patients showed a significant deficiency relative to controls as well, as did patients infected with HIV. Results found that CoQ10 deficiency increased with the increased severity of the disease. When 7 AIDS patients were treated with CoQ10, 5 survived and were symptomatically better after 4-7 months.

—K. Folkers, et al., "Biochemical Deficiencies of Coenzyme Q10 in HIV-infection and Exploratory treatment," *Biochem Biophys Res Commun,* 153(2), June 16, 1988, p. 888-896.

Cancer

This study examined the effects of CoQ10 on the cardiotoxicity of adriamycin in cultures of beating heart cells from neonatal rats. After 12 hours of exposure, results found that cultures treated with CoQ10 showed beating activities comparable to those of untreated controls, while adriamycin-treated cultures exhibited either arrhythmias or lacked beating activity. Cultures treated concurrently with adriamycin and CoQ10 continued to beat normally.

—A.B. Combs, et al., "Prevention by Coenzyme Q10 of the Cardiotoxicity of Adriamycin in Cultured Heart Cells," *IRCS Med Sci: Cancer,* 4(8), 1976, p. 403.

Results of this study showed that mice pretreated with CoQ10 experienced significant reductions in the lethality of antitumor antibioitc anthramycin as well as its ability to decrease ventricular weights.

—W.C. Lubawy, et al., "Protection Against Anthramycin-induced Toxicity in Mice by Coenzyme Q10," *Journal of the National Cancer Institute,* 64(1), January 1980, p. 105-109.

Results of this placebo-controlled study showed that CoQ10 treatment helped to prevent liver damage in mitomycin C-induced sarcoma 10 solid type-tumor-bearing mice.

—S. Yamada, et al., [Experimental Research on Coenzyme Q10 Treatment for Liver Damage Induced by Antibeoplastic Drugs," *Nippon Kagaku Ryoho Gakkai Zasshim,* 27(4), 1979, p. 675-680.

This article cites numerous clinical and case studies supporting the use of CoQ10 in the treatment of breast cancer. Results of one study in particular found that 390 mg per day proved effective in 3 subjects monitored over a 3-5 year period.

—K. Lockwood, et al., "Progress on Therapy of Breast Cancer with Vitamin Q10 and the Regression of Metastases," *Biochem Biophys Res Commun,* 212(1), July 6, 1995, p. 172-177.

In this study, 6 of 32 patients at high risk for breast cancer who were treated with 90 mg of CoQ10 in addition to other antioxidants and fatty acids showed partial tumor regression. When 1 of these 6 patients increased dosage to 390 mg of CoQ10 per day the tumor was no longer palpable after one month and, following another month, mammagrophy indicated an absence of tumor. When yet another case was given 300 mg of CoQ10 per day there was no residula tumor three months following the start of treatment.

> —K. Lockwood, et al., ''Partial and Complete Regression of Breast Cancer in Patients in Relation to Dosage of Coenzyme Q10,'' *Biochem Biophys Res Commun,* 199(3), March 30, 1994, p. 1504-1508.

This review article notes that studies have shown that CoQ10 can overcome adriamycin-induced inhibition in vitro when supplemented at high levels and has been shown to overcome cardiotoxicity in intact rabbits and isolated rabbit hearts.

> —T. Kishi & K. Folkers, ''Prevention by Coenzyme Q10 (NSC-140865) of the Inhibition by Adriamycin (NSC-123127) of Coenzyme Q10 Enzymes,'' *Cancer Treat Rev,* 60(3), 1976, p. 223-224.

This study examined the effects of CoQ10 administered intravenously at doses of 1 mg/kg per day on the prevention of adriamycin and dauborubicin-induced side effects in malignant lymphoma patients. Results showed the degree of alopecia, fever, nausea and vomiting, the incidences of diarrhea and stomatitis were significantly reduced in the CoQ10-treated patients relative to controls.

> —K. Tsubaki, et al., [Investigation of the Preventive Effect of CoQ10 Against the Side-effects of Anthracycline Antineoplastic agents], *Gan To Kagaku Ryoho,* 11(7), July 1984, p. 1420-1427.

Results of this study found that the administration of CoQ10 may prevent some electrocardiographic changes induce by adriamycin in humans.

> —K. Okuma, et al., [Protective Effect of Coenzyme Q10 in Cardiotoxicity Induced by Adriamycin], *Gan To Kagaku Ryoho,* 11(3), March 1984, p. 502-508.

Results of this study indicated the usefulness of CoQ10 in the enhancement of cancer immunochemotherapy in rats using masked compounds in combination with immunopotentiators and exhibited no side effects.

> —T. Kokawa, et al., [Coenzyme Q10 in Cancer Chemotherapy—experimental Studies on Augmentation of the Effects of Masked Compounds, Especially in the Combined Chemotherapy with Immunopotentiators], *Gan To Kagaku Ryoho,* 10(3), March 1983, p. 768-774.

This study examined the effects of BCG, CoQ10, or the two together on the cell-mediated immune response in tumor-bearing mice. Results found that depressed oligomycin-sensitive ATPase activity significantly recovered by treatment with BCG or coenzyme Q10.

> —I. Kawase, et al., [The Enhancing Effect of Coenzyme Q10 on Immunorecovery with BCG in Tumor Bearing Mice: In Realtion to Changes in Coeznymes Q Content and ATP-ASE Activity in Spleen Lymphocytes of Tumor-Bearing Rats,'' *Gan To Kagaku Ryoho,* 6(2), 1979, p. 281-288.

Results of this study showed that the combined treatment of CoQ10 and BCG led to improvement of depressed bioenergetic in tumor-bearing rat lymphocytes.

—H. Niitani, et al., "Combined Effect of BCG and Coenzyme Q10 on ATP-ase Activity and Coenzyme Q Content in spleen Lymphocytes of Tumor-bearing Rats," *Gann,* 70(3), June 1979, p. 315-322.

Results of this study showed that CoQ10 enhanced immunorestoration with BCG in tumor-bearing mice.

—I. Kawase, et al., "Enhancing Effect of Coenzyme, Q10 on Immunorestoration with Myco- bacterium Bovis BCG in Tumor-bearing Mice," *Gann,* 69(4), August 1978, p. 493-497.

Cardiovascular/Coronary Heart Disease

This double-blind, placebo-controlled study examined the effects of 150 mg per of CoQ10 for 4 weeks on exercise performance in middle age, stable angina pectoris patients. Results indicated CoQ10 to be an effective and safe treatment for the condition.

—T. Kamikawa, et al., "Effects of Coenzyme Q10 on Exercise Tolerance in Chronic Stable Angina Pectoris," *American Journal of Cardiology,* 56(4), August 1, 1985, p. 247-251.

Results of this study found that the administration of CoQ10 to rats significantly improved the functional recovery during reperfusion by enhancing the recovery of high-energy phosphates and preventing overload of Ca2+.

—O. Hano, et al., "Coenzyme Q10 Enhances Cardiac Functional and Metabolic Recovery and Reduces Ca2+ Overload During Postischemic Reperfusion," *American Journal of Physiology,* 266(6 Pt 2), June 1994, p. H2174-81.

Results of this case-control study found that 30-60 mg per day of CoQ10 administered orally for 6 days preoperatively significantly increased heart tolerance to ischemia during aortic clamping in humans.

—J. Tanaka, et al., "Coenzyme Q10: The Prophylactic Effect on Low Cardiac Output Follow- ing Cardiac Valve Replacement," *Annals of Thoracic Surgery,* 33(2), February 983, p. 145- 151.

Results of this case-control study found that elective coronary artery bypass patients pretreated with 150 mg per day of CoQ10 for 7 days prior to surgery showed a significantly lower incidence of ventricular arrhythmias during the recovery period than controls.

—M. Chello, et al., "Protection by Coenzyme Q10 from Myocardial Reperfusion Injury During Coronary Artery Bypass Grafting," *Annals of Thoracic Surgery,* 58(5), November 1994, p. 1427-1432.

In this study, mongrel dogs experienced an hour of carioplegic solution-induced cardiac arrest under cardiopulmonary bypass. One of three types of cardioplegic solution was used: clinical potassium cardioplegic solution (K+, 22.31 mEq/L), potassium cardioplegic solution with coenzyme Q10 added (coenzyme Q10, 30 mg/500 ml of solution), and cardioplegic solution with coenzyme Q10 solvent. Results showed that exogenous coenzyme Q10 containing solution provided significantly high myocar- dial stores of adenosine triphosphate and creatine phosphate and a low level of lactate during induced ischemia and reperfusion while recovery percentage of the aortic flow was significantly greater relative to the other two solutions as well. Results also found that CoQ10 added to potassium cardioplegia improved myocardial oxygen utilization and accelerated recovery of myocardial energy metabolism following circulation reestablishment.

> —F. Mori & H. Mohri, "Effects of Coenzyme Q10 Added to a Potassium Cardioplegic Solution for Myocardial Protection During Ischemic Cardiac Arrest," *Annals of Thoracic Surgery,* 39(1), January 1985, p. 30-36.

Results of this study showed that rabbits pretreated with CoQ10 experienced a recovery of cardiac contractile force and of myocardial ATP content upon reoxygenation, while the release of creatine phosphokinase from hearts during hypoxia and reoxygenation was totally inhibited by pretreatment. Results also showed that UV absorbance of the perfusate changes indicated that CoQ10 decreased loss of ATP metabolites from hypoxic hearts.

> —S. Takeo, et al., "Possible Mechanism by which Coenzyme Q10 Improves Reoxygenation-Induced Recovery of Cardiac Contractile Force After Hypoxia," *Journal of Pharmacol Exp Ther,* 243(3), December 1987, p. 1131-1138.

Results of this case-control study found that pretreatment with 30 mg per day CoQ10 administered for 7 days effectively decreased aortic cross clamping-induced ischemic injury in rats.

> —R. Tominaga, et al., "Effects of Pretreatment with Coenzyme Q10 on Myocardial Preservation During Aortic Cross Clamping," *Journal of Surg Res,* 34(2), February 1983, p. 111-117.

Results of this double-blind, placebo-control study found that pretreatment with CoQ10 was effective in preventing myocardial injury during preservation and subsequent reperfusion in dogs.

> —T. Matsushima, et al., "Protection by Coenzyme Q10 of Canine Myocardial Reperfusion Injury After Preservation," *Journal of Thoracic Cardiovascular Surgery,* 103(5), May 1992, p. 945-951

In this case-control study, isolated hearts from rats pretreated with either coenzyme Q10, 20 mg/kg intramuscularly and 10 mg/kg intraperitoneally 24 and 2 hours before the experiment were subjected to 15 minutes of equilibration, 25 minutes of ischemia, and 40 minutes of reperfusion. Results found that coenzyme Q10 pretreatment improved myocardial function after ischemia and reperfusion.

> —J.A. Crestanello, et al., "Elucidation of a Tripartite Mechanism Underlying the Improvement in Cardiac Tolerance to Ischemia by Coenzyme Q10 Pretreatment," *Journal of Thoracic Cardiovasc Surgery,* February 1996, 111(2), p. 443-450.

Results of this study found that the administration of CoQ10 prior to reoxygenation inhibited oxygen mediated myocardial injury in piglets caused by reoxygenation of the hypoxemic immature heart on cardiopulmonary bypass.

> —K. Morita, et al., "Studies of Hypoxemic/reoxygenation Injury: Without Aortic Clamping. VII. Counteraction of Oxidant Damage by Exogenous Antioxidants: Coenzyme Q10," *Journal of Thoracic Cardiovascular Surgery,* 110(4 Pt 2), October 1995, p. 1221-1227.

Results of this study found that CoQ10 administered to dogs intravenously prior to reperfusion enhanced the role of substrate-enriched blood cardioplegic solution in salvaging ischemic myocardium to make way for recovery.

> —F. Okamoto, et al., "Reperfusate Composition: Supplemental Role of Intravenous and

Intracoronary Coenzyme Q10 in Avoiding Reperfusion Damage,'' *Journal of Thoracic Cardiovascular Surgery,* 92(3 Pt 2), September 1986, p. 573-582.

Results of this study found that brain ischemia/reperfusion injury in dogs can result from oxygen-derived free radicals and abnormal energy metabolism and that the administration of CoQ10 can provide protection against such damage by improving cerebral metabolism
    —Z. Ren, et al., ''Mechanisms of Brain Injury with Deep Hypothermic Circulatory Arrest and Protective Effects of Coenzyme Q10,'' *Journal of Thoracic Cardiovascular Surgery,* 108(1), July 1994, p. 126-133.

Results of this double-blind, placebo-controlled study found patients pretreated with CoQ10 had less left atrial pressure, a decreased incidence of low cardiac output, a wider pulse pressure, and a better preserved right and left ventricular myocardial ultrastructure relative to controls.
    —Y.F. Chen, et al., ''Effectiveness of Coenzyme Q10 on Myocardial Preservation During Hypothermic Cardioplegic Arrest,'' *Journal of Thoracic Cardiovascular Surgery,* 107(1), January 1994, p. 242-247.

This case-control study examined the effects of CoQ10 on mice inoculated with the M variant of encephalomyocarditis virus. Results showed significantly higher rates of survival in mice receiving the CoQ10 than controls.
    —C. Kishimoto, et al., ''The Protection of Coenzyme Q10 Against Experimental Viral Myocarditis in Mice,'' *Japanese Circulatory Journal,* 48(12), December 1984, p. 1358-1361.

Results of this study found that the administration of CoQ10 for 8 weeks preserved left ventricular function and attenuated cardiomyopathy progression in hamsters.
    —S. Momomura, et al., ''Coenzyme Q10 Attenuates the Progression of Cardiomyopathy in Hamsters,'' *Japanese Heart Journal,* 32(1), January 1991, p. 101-110.

Results of this study showed that the administration of CoQ10 provided protection against chlorpromzine-induced injury in the myocardial cells of rats.
    —M. Chiba, ''A Protective Action of Coenzyme Q10 on Chlorpromazine-induced Cell Damage in the Cultured Rat Myocardial Cells,'' *Japanese Heart Journal,* 25(1), January 1984, p. 127-137.

This study examined CoQ10's electrophysiological and inotropic effects on isoproterenol or barium-induced slow responses in ventricular papillary muscle depolarized by high K+ concentration under hypoxia. Results showed significant reversing effects on hypoxia-induced deterioration of the slow response.
    —M. Arita, et al., ''Electrophysiological and Inotropic Effects of Coenzyme Q10 on Guinea Pig Ventricular Muscle Depolarized by Potassium Under Hypoxia,'' *Japanese Heart Journal,* 23(6), November 1982, p. 961-974.

Results of this study found that the combined treatment of vitamin B2-butyrate for lipid peroxidation reduction and CoQ10 for restoring deficiency can prevent adriamycin-induced cardiotoxicity in rats during cancer chemotherapy.
    —T. Katsuki, [Experimental Studies on the Combination Use of Vitamin B2-butyrate and

Coenzyme Q10 to Protect Against Adriamycin-Induced Cardiac Mitochondrial Disorders], *Kurume Igakkai Zasshi,* 44(12), 1981, p. 869-883.

Results of this study showed that Vitamin B2-butyrate and CoQ10 inhibited lipid peroxide production in Ehrlich ascites tumor cells treated with adriamycin.
  —M. Chinami, et al., "Effect of Coenzyme Q10 and Vitamin B-2 Butyrate to Anticancer Ability and Lipid Peroxidation of Adriamycin," *Kurume Igakkai Zasshi,* 44(9/10), 1981, p. 678-683.

This review article cites studies showing the CoQ10 may be an effective treatment for ischemic heart disease, congestive heart failure, toxin-induced cardiotoxicity, and hypertension.
  —S.M. Greenberg & W.H. Frishman, "Coenzyme Q10: A New Drug for Myocardial Ischemia?" *Medical Clinics of North America,* 72(1), January 1988, p. 243-258.

This article reports on the single case of a patient with mitochondrial encephalomyopathy and cytochrome c oxidase deficiency who took high doses of CoQ10 for 2 years. Results showed that such treatment led to decreases in abnormal elevation of the serum lactate per pyruvate ratio and the increased concentration of serum lactate plus pyruvate induced by exercise. Results also showed that CoQ10 improved impaired central and peripheral nerve conductivities.
  —Y. Nishikawa, et al., "Long-term Coenzyme Q10 Therapy for a Mitochondrial Encephalomyopathy with Cytochrome C Oxidase Deficiency: A 31P NMR Study," *Neurology,* 39(3), March 1989, p. 399-403.

Results of this study showed that the administration of 60 to 120 mg per day of CoQ10 for 3 months to a patient with Kearns-Sayre syndrome led to the normalization of lactate and pyruvate serum levels and improvement of occular movement and atriventricular block.
  —S. Ogasahara, et al., "Improvement of Abnormal Pyruvate Metabolism and Cardiac Conduction Defect with Coenzyme Q10 in Kearns-Sayre Syndrome," *Neurology,* 35(3), March 1985, p. 372-373.

Results of this study showed that the administration of CoQ10 led to the preservation of hepatic ischemia-induced cellular damages in rats and that such preservation was likely due to the protection of cellular and subcellular membranes from lipid peroxidation.
  —S. Marubayashi, et al., "Preservation of Ischemic Rat Liver Mitochondrial Functions and Liver Viability with CoQ10," *Surgery,* 91(6), June 1982, p. 631-637.

Results of this study showed that pretreatment of donor rats with 10 mg/kg of CoQ10 intravenously increased survival time following warm ischemic damage of rat liver grafts.
  —K. Sumimoto, et al., "Ischemic Damage Prevention by Coenzyme Q10 Treatment of the Donor Before Orthotopic Liver Transplantation: Biochemical and Histologic Findings," *Surgery,* 102(5), November 1987, p. 821-827.

Results of this study showed that CoQ10 administration exhibited protective effects on hypertrophied ischemic myocardium in dogs.
  —F. Okamoto, et al., "Effect of Coenzyme Q10 on Hypertrophied Ischemic Myocardium

During Aortic Cross Clamping for 2 Hr, from the Aspect of Energy Metabolism,'' *Adv Myocardiol,* 4, 1983, p. 559-566.

This review article cites numerous double-blind studies and case histories supporting the efficacy and safety of using CoQ10 in the treatment of heart failure.

—K. Folkers, et al., "Therapy with Coenzyme Q10 of Patients in Heart Failure Who Are Eligible or Ineligible for a Transplant," *Biochem Biophys Res Commun,* 182(1), January 15, 1992, p. 247-253.

Results of this study showed that the administration of CoQ10 can prevent or inhibit the cardiomyopathy of doxorubican in rabbits.

—N. Domae, et al., "Cardiomyopathy and Other Chronic Toxic Effects Induced in Rabbits by Doxorubicin and Possible Prevention by Coenzyme Q10," *Cancer Treat Rep,* 65(1-2), January-February 1981, p. 79-91.

Results of this study indicated that pretreatment with 5 mg/kg administered intravenously of CoQ10 was effective in the prevention of left ventricular depression in early reperfusion and in minimizing myocardial cellular injury during coronary artery bypass grafting followed by reperfusion in humans.

—M. Sunamori, et al., "Clinical Experience of Coenzyme Q10 to Enhance Intraoperative Myocardial Protection in Coronary Artery Revascularization," *Cardiovasc Drugs Ther,* 5 Suppl 2, March 1991, p. 297-300.

This study examined the effects of CoQ10 on the ischaemic myocardium following constriction of left anterior descending coronary artery in open-chest mongrel dogs. Results showed that dogs premedicated with 20 mg/kg of intravenous CoQ10 had a significantly higher ATP content in ischaemic myocardium relative to controls.

—Y. Nakamura, et al., "Protection of Ischaemic Myocardium with Coenzyme Q10," *Cardiovascular Research,* 16(3), March 1982, p. 132-137.

Results of this study found that CoQ10 improved recovery of the left ventricular peak systolic pressure and the coronary sinus flow in rats.

—T. Konishi, et al., "Improvement in Recovery of Left Ventricular Function During Reperfusion with Coenzyme Q10 in Isolated Working Rat Heart," *Cardiovascular Research,* 19(1), January 1985, p. 38-43.

Results of this study showed the administration of CoQ10 supported cardiovascular hemodynamics and prevented free radical mediated lipid peroxidation during E. coli septic shock in dogs.

—J.L. Lelli, et al., "Effects of Coenzyme Q10 on the Mediator Cascade of Sepsis," *Circ Shock,* 39(3), March 1993, p. 178-187.

This study examined the efficacy and safety of adjunctive treatment with 50-100 mg of CoQ10 per day for 3 months in congestive heart failure patients. Results showed the patient improvement rates after three months of treatment were: cyanosis 81%, edema 76.9%, pulmonary rates, 78.4%, enlargement of the liver area 49.3%, jugular reflux 81.5%, dyspnea 54.2%, palpitations 75.7%, sweating 82.4%, arrhythmia 62%, insomnia 60.2%, vertigo 73%, and nocturia 50.7%.

—E. Baggio, et al., "Italian Multicenter Study on the Safety and Efficacy of Coenzyme Q10 as Adjunctive Therapy in Heart Failure (interim analysis). The CoQ10 Drug Surveillance Investigators," *Clinical Investigations,* 71(8 Suppl), 1993, p. S145-149.

Results of this case control study of patients suffering from symptoms commonly preceding congestive heart failure showed that the administration of CoQ10 led to improvement in all patients, high blood pressure reduction in 80%, improved diastolic function all; reduction in myocardial thickness in 53% of hypertensives and 36% of the combined prolapse and fatigue syndrome groups; and reduction in fractional shortening in those high at control and an increase in those initially low.

— P.H. Langsjoen, et al., "Isolated Diastolic Dysfunction of the Myocardium and its Response to CoQ10 Treatment," *Clinical Investigations,* 71(8 Suppl), 1993, p. S140-144.

Results of this double-blind, placebo-controlled, year-long study showed that 2mg/kg per day of CoQ10 coupled with conventional therapy in chronic congestive heart failure patients significantly decreased hospitalization rates for heart failure worsening and complication incidence.

— C. Morisco, et al., "Effect of Coenzyme Q10 Therapy in Patients with Congestive Heart Failure: A Long-term Multicenter Randomized Study," *Clinical Investigations,* 71(8 Suppl), 1993, p. S134-S146.

Results of this study showed that the administration of 50 mg per day of CoQ10 for 4 weeks coupled with conventional therapy led to improvements in dyspnea at rest, exertional dyspnea, palpitation, cyanosis, hepatomegaly, pulmonary rates, ankle edema, heart rate, and both systolic and diastolic blood pressure in patients with chronic heart failure.

— M. Lampertico & S. Comis, "Italian Multicenter Study on the Efficacy and Safety of Coenzyme Q10 as Adjuvant Therapy in Heart Failure," *Clinical Investigations,* 71(8 Suppl), 1993, p. S129-S133.

This review article cites numerous studies supporting the efficacy of CoQ10 in the treatment of heart disease.

— S.A. Mortensen, "Perspectives on Therapy of Cardiovascular Diseases with Coenzyme Q10 (Ubiquinone)," *Clinical Investigations,* 71(8 Suppl), 1993, p. S116-S123.

Results of this placebo-controlled study found that pretreatment with CoQ10 provided protection of the ischemic myocardium in an open-chest swine model.

— D. Atar, et al., "Coenzyme Q10 Protects Ischemic Myocardium in an Open-chest Swine Model," *Clinical Investigations,* 71(8 Suppl), 1993, p. S103-S11.

Results of this study showed that 100 mg per day of CoQ10 proved to be an effective therapeutic agent in case of advanced chronic heart failure.

— S.A. Mortensen, et al., "Long-term Coenzyme Q10 Therapy: A Major Advance in the Management of Resistant Myocardial Failure," *Drugs Exp Clin Res,* 11(8), 1985, p. 581-593.

In this double-blind, crossover study, CoQ10 was administered to 19 chronic myocardial disease patients. Results showed that 18 experienced improved activity tolerance with replacement therapy.

Results also found significant improvements among patients in stroke volume measured by impedance cardiography, and ejection fractions calculated from systolic time intervals.

—P.H. Langsjoen, et al., "Effective Treatment with Coenzyme Q10 of Patients with Chronic Myocardial Disease," *Drugs Exp Clin Res,* 11(8), 1985, p. 577-579.

Results of this study showed that the administration of 3.0-3.4 mg per day (average) of CoQ10 was effective against cardiac dysfunction in patients with mitral valve prolapse and improved stress-induced cardiac dysfunction.

—T. Oda, "Effect of Coenzyme Q10 on Stress-induced Cardiac Dysfunction in Paediatric Patients with Mitral Valve Prolapse: A Study by Stress Echocardiography," *Drugs Exp Clin Res,* 11(8), 1985, p. 557-576.

This study examined the effects of carnitine and CoQ10 on doxorubicin cardiotoxicity in rats. Results showed that the drugs proved most effective when administered together and in doses of 200 mg/kg per day or carnitine and 10 mg/kg per day of CoQ10.

—S. Ronca-Testoni, et al., "Effect of Carnitine and Coenzyme Q10 on the Calcium Uptake in Heart Sarcoplasmic Reticulum of Rats Treated with Anthracyclines," *Drugs Exp Clin Res,* 18(10), 1992, p. 437-442.

This study examined the effects of L-carnitine, coenzyme Q10 and their combined administration on haemodynamic and metabolic variables in isolated perfused working rat hearts after 10 min of global normothermic ischaemia followed by 60 min of reperfusion. Results showed a lower purine release in the perfusate of the hearts of the rats treated with both compounds.

—A. Bertelli, et al., "L-carnitine and Coenzyme Q10 Protective Action Against Ischaemia and Reperfusion of Working Rat Heart," *Drugs Exp Clin Res,* 18(10), 1992, p. 431-436.

This study examined the relationship between CoQ10 serum levels and cardiac performance in patients suffering from either hyperthyroidism, hypothyroidism, or normal subjects. Results found a significant inverse association between thyroid hormones and Coenzyme Q10 levels. Based on their findings, the authors concluded that CoQ10 has therapeutic value for thyrotoxicosis-induced congestive heart failure

—H. Suzuki, et al., "Cardiac Performance and Coenzyme Q10 in Thyroid Disorders," *Endocrinol Jpn,* 31(6), December 1984, p. 755-761.

This study examined adriamycin-induced cardiotoxicity and the effects on it by CoQ10 in rabbits. Results showed CoQ10 injections provided protection against the cardiotoxicity.

—M. Tajima, [Chronic Cardiotoxicity of Anthracycline Derivatives and Possible Prevention by Coenzyme Q10], *Gan No Rinsho,* 30(9 Suppl), July 1984, p. 1211-1216.

Results of this study found that pretreatment with CoQ10 exhibited protection against the isolated ventricular muscle subjected to hypoxia action potential and contraction induced deterioration in guinea pigs.

—M. Aomine & M. Arita, "Pretreatment with Coenzyme Q10 Protects Guinea Pig Ventricular Muscle From Hypoxia-induced Deterioration of Action Potentials and Contraction," *Gen Pharmacol,* 16(2), 1985, p. 91-96.

Results of this study found that the administration of CoQ10 provided protection against biochemical derangements in the thyrotoxic heart in rabbits.

—C. Kotake, et al., "Protective Effect of Coenzyme Q10 on Thyrotoxic Heart in Rabbits," *Heart Vessels,* 3(2), 1987, p. 84-90.

Results of this study showed that CoQ10 administered in doses of 60 mg per day for two months reduced blood viscosity in patients with ischemic heart disease.

—T. Kato, et al., "Reduction in Blood Viscosity by Treatment with Coenzyme Q10 in Patients with Ischemic Heart Disease," *Int J Clin Pharmacol Ther Toxicol,* 28(3), March 1990, p. 123-126.

This study examined the effects of 100 mg per day of CoQ10 for 2 months on dilated cardiomyopathy patients. Results indicated that CoQ10 deficiency could be reversed through supplementation and that CoQ10 treatment may be effective when coupled with conventional treatment in patients with chronic cardiac failure.

—U. Manzoli, et al., "Coenzyme Q10 in Dilated Cardiomyopathy," *International Journal of Tissue React,* 12(3), 1990, p. 173-178.

Results of this study found that 100 mg of CoQ10 per day administered orally to be an effective treatment for chronic cardiomyopathy.

—P.H. Langsjoen, et al., "A Six-year Clinical Study of Therapy of Cardiomyopathy with Coenzyme Q10," *International Journal of Tissue React,* 12(3), 1990, p. 169-171.

Results of this study found that treatment with CoQ10 fed to highly significant increases in survival rates in patients with cardiomyopathy.

—P.H. Langsjoen, et al., "Pronounced Increase of Survival of Patients with Cardiomyopathy when Treated with Coenzyme Q10 and Conventional Therapy," *International Journal of Tissue React,* 12(3), 1990, p. 163-168.

Diabetes

This article reports on the case of a 71-year-old man diagnosed with diabetic amyotrophy who experienced relief in symptoms of the legs, fatigue, and residual urine in the bladder following the administration of CoQ10.

—Y. Suzuki, et al., "A Case of Diabetic Amyotrophy Associated with 3243 Mitochondrial tRNA(leu; UUR) Mutation and Successful Therapy with Coenzyme Q10," *Endocr Journal,* 42(2), April 1995, p. 141-145.

General

Results of this study found that a combination of CoQ10 and nicotinamide attenuated mild to moderate experimentall induced neurotoxicity.

—J.B. Schulz, et al., "Coenzyme Q10 and Nicotinamide and a Free Radical Spin Trap Protect Against MPTP Neurotoxicity," *Exp Neurol,* 132(2), April 1995, p. 279-283.

In this study, weaning rats fed a Torula yeast-based diet either unsupplemented or supplemented with 30 mg beta-carotene/kg, 30 IU vitamin E/kg, 1 mg selenium/kg or 30 mg coenzyme Q10/kg. Results showed CoQ10 and beta-carotene act as antioxidants in ways similar to selenium and vitamin E.

> —R. Zamora, et al., "Comparative Antioxidant Effectiveness of Dietary Beta-carotene, Vitamin E, Selenium and Coenzyme Q10 in Rat Erythrocytes and Plasma," *Journal of Nutrition,* 121(1), January 1991, p. 50-56.

Results of this study found that dietary CoQ10 supplementation proved active against tertbutyl hydroperoxide-induced lipid peroxidation in rats.

> —B. Leibovitz, et al., "Dietary Supplements of Vitamin E, Beta-carotene, Coenzyme Q10 and Selenium Protect Tissues Against Lipid Peroxidation in Rat Tissue Slices," *Journal of Nutrition,* 120(1), January 1990, p. 97-104.

This study examined the effects of CoQ10 on lipid peroxidation and survival time of mice treated with adriamycin. Results found that CoQ10 exhibited protective effects against a adriamycin-induced subacute toxicity, with mice administered 10 mg/kg of CoQ10 showing the most prolonged survival time.

> —S. Shinozawa, et al., "Effect of CoQ10 on the Survival Time and Lipid Peroxidation of Adriamycin (doxorubicin) Treated Mice," *Acta Med Okayama,* 38(1), February 1984, p. 57-63.

Hearing Loss

Results of this study found that CoQ10 promoted recovery auditory hair damage in guinea pigs and prevented respiratory metabolic impairment of hair cell caused by hypoxia.

> —K. Sato, "Pharmacokinetics of Coenzyme Q10 in Recovery of Acute Sensorineural Hearing Loss Due to Hypoxia," *Acta Otolaryngol Suppl,* 458, 1988, p. 95-102.

Immune Enhancement

In this study, CoQ10 and vitamin B6 were administered together and independently to three groups of subjects. Results showed that blood levels of IgG increased significantly when CoQ10 and B6 were administered together as well as when CoQ10 was administered alone. T4-lymphocyte blood levels increased significantly when CoQ10 and B6 were administered together and independently. T4/T8 lymphocytes ratio increased significantly when CoQ10 and B6 were administered together and independently.

> —K. Folkers, et al., "The Activities of Coenzyme Q10 and Vitamin B6 for Immune Responses," *Biochem Biophys Res Commun,* 193(1), May 28, 1993, p. 88-92.

This review article cites numerous studies noting the beneficial effects of CoQ10 and concludes that CoQ10 is a key factor in the optimal immune system functioning.

> —K. Folkers & A. Wolaniuk, "Research on Coenzyme Q10 in Clinical Medicine and in Immunomodulation," *Drugs Exp Clin Res,* 11(8), 1985, 539-545.

Kearns-Sayre Syndrome

Results of this study showed that the administration of 120 to 150/mg of CoQ10 per day led to an improvement in abnormal metabolism of pyruvate and NADH oxidation in the skeletal muscle of

Kearns-Sayre Syndrome patients. CoQ10 also decreased the concentration of CSF protein and CSF lactate/pyruvate ratio, while improvement were seen in neurologic symptoms and ECG abnormalities as well.

> —S. Ogasahara, et al., "Treatment of Kearns-Sayre Syndrome with Coenzyme Q10," *Neurology,* 36(1), January 1986, p. 45-53.

Liver Damage

Results of this double-blind, placebo-controlled study showed that pretreatment with CoQ10 can inhibit acetaminophen-induced hepatic injury in mice.

> —T. Amimoto, et al., "Acetaminophen-induced Hepatic Injury in Mice: The Role of Lipid Peroxidation and Effects of Pretreatment with Coenzyme Q10 and Alpha-tocopherol," *Free Radic Biol Med,* 19(2), August 1995, p. 169-176.

Results of this study indicated that CoQ10 exhibited direct antioxidative effects against CC14 hepatoxicity in rats.

> —T. Yoshikawa, et al., "The Protection of Coenzyme Q10 Against Carbon Tetrachloride Hepatotoxicity," *Gastroenterol Jpn,* 16(3), 1981, p. 281-285.

Results of this study found that the administration of CoQ10 and L-carnitine together decreased hepatic damage brought on by hyperbaric oxygen and chronic alcohol poisoning in rats.

> —A. Bertelli, et al., "Protective Action of L-carnitine and Coenzyme Q10 Against Hepatic Triglyceride Infiltration Induced by Hyperbaric Oxygen and Ethanol," *Drugs Exp Clin Res,* 19(2), 1993, p. 65-68.

Lung Disease

Results of this study showed that oral administration of 90 mg per day of CoQ10 for 8 weeks had significant beneficial effects on muscular energy metabolism in chronic lung disease patients suffering from hypoxemia either during exercise or at rest.

> —S. Fujimoto, et al., "Effects of Coenzyme Q10 Administration on Pulmonary Function and Exercise Performance in Patients with Chronic Lung Diseases," *Clinical Investigations,* 71, 1993, (8 Suppl), p. S162-S166.

Muscular Injury

This study examined the effects of CoQ10 on muscular injury due to exercise in rats. Results found that CoQ10 provided protection against exercise-induced injury in skeletal muscles.

> —Y. Shimomura, et al., "Protective Effect of Coenzyme Q10 on Exercise-induced Muscular Injury," *Biochem Biophys Res Commun,* 176(1), April 15, 1991, p. 349-355.

This study examined the effects of CoQ10 on continuous electric field stimulation-induced muscular injury in cultured cells obtained from neonatal rat femoral muscles. Results showed that administration of 5 microM CoQ10 provided protection for the cells against biochemical changes after the stimulation, indicating one of the causal mechanisms of muscular injury is an increase in [Ca2+] due to the excess entry of extracellular Ca2+, and that CoQ10 can protect skeletal muscle cells against it.

> —T. Okamoto, et al., "Protective Effect of Coenzyme Q10 on Cultured Skeletal Muscle Cell

Injury Induced by Continuous Electric Field Stimulation,'' *Biochem Biophys Res Commun,* 216(3), November 22, 1995, p. 1006-1012.

This article reports on the results from 2 double-blind, placebo-controlled studies supporting the use of CoQ10 in the treatment of Duchenne, Becker, and limb-girdle dystrophies, myotonic dystrophy, Charcot-Marie-Tooth disease, and the Welander disease.
—K. Folkers & R. Simonsen, ''Two Successful Double-blind Trials with Coenzyme Q10 (vitamin Q10) on Muscular Dystrophies and Neurogenic Atrophies,'' *Biochim Biophys Acta,* 1271(1), May 24, 1995, p. 281-286.

Stroke

This study examined the effects of long-term CoQ10 administration on membrane lipid alterations in the kidney of stroke-prone spontaneously hypertensive rats. Results found that CoQ10 attenuated the elevation of blood pressure, the membranous phospholipid degradation, and the enhanced phospholipase A2 activity.
—H. Okamoto, et al., ''Effect of CoQ10 on Structural Alterations in the Renal Membrane of Stroke-prone Spontaneously Hypertensive Rats,'' *Biochem Med Metab Biol,* 45(2), April 1991, p. 216-226.

■ CONJUGATED LINOLEIC ACID

Cancer

This review article notes that studies have shown conjugated linoleic acid to be a powerful anticarcinogen against mammary tumors on a rat model.
—C. Ip, et al., ''Conjugated Linoleic Acid. A Powerful Anticarcinogen from Animal Fat Sources,'' *Cancer,* 74(3 Suppl), August 1, 1994, p. 1050-1054.

Results of this study showed that synthetic conjugated linoleic acid inhibited DMBA-induced mammary tumors in rats.
—C. Ip, et al., ''Mammary Cancer Prevention by Conjugated Dienoic Derivative of Linoleic Acid,'' *Cancer Research,* 51(22), November 15, 1991, p. 6118-6124.

Results of this study showed that synthetic conjugated linoleic acid inhibited DMBA-induced forestomach tumors in rats.
—Y.L. Ha, et al., ''Inhibition of Benzo(a)pyrene-induced Mouse Forestomach Neoplasia by Conjugated Dienoic Derivatives of Linoleic Acid,'' *Cancer Research,* 50(4), February 15, 1990, p. 1097-1101.

Results of this study showed that conjugated linoleic acid inhibited DMBA-induced mammary tumors in rats.
—C. Ip, et al., ''Conjugated Linoleic Acid Suppresses Mammary Carcinogenesis and Proliferative Activity of the Mammary Gland in the Rat,'' *Cancer Research,* 54(5), March 1, 1994, p. 1212-1215.

Results of this study showed that synthetic conjugated linoleic acid inhibited DMBA-induced foresto-mach tumors in rats.

—H. Benjamin, et al., "TPA-Mediated Induction of Ornithine Decarboxylase Activity in Mouse Forestomach and Its Inhibition by Conjugated Dienoic Derivatives of Linoleic Acid," *FASEB Journal,* 4(3), 1990, p. A508.

Results of this study showed that dietary conjugated linoleic acid significantly suppressed subcutane-ously injected human breast cancer cell growth in mice.

—S. Visonneau, et al., "Conjugated Linoleic Acid (CLA) Suppresses Growth of Human Breast Carcinoma MDA-MB468 in SCID Mice," *FASEB Journal,* 9(4), 1995, p. A869.

Results of this study found that both linoleic acid and conjugated linoleic acid exhibited cytotoxic and cystostatic effects against human cancer cell in vitro.

—W.R. Seaman, et al., "Differential Inhibitory Response to Linoleic Acid and Conjugated Dienoic Derivatives of Linoleic Acid in Cultures of Human Cancer Cells," *FASEB Journal,* 1992, 6(4), p. A1396.

Results of this study showed that conjugated linoleic acid suppressed human cancer cell growth in vitro by inhibiting protein and nucleotide biosynthesis

—T.D. Shultz, et al., "Inhibitory Effect of Conjugated Dienoic Derivatives of Linoleic Acid and Beta-carotene on the in Vitro Growth of Human Cancer Cells," *FASEB Journal,* 6(4), 1992, p. A1396.

Results of this study showed that the oral administration of conjugated linoleic acid inhibited TPA-induced forestomach tumors in rats.

—H. Benjamin, et al., "The Effect of Conjugated Dienoic Derivatives of Linoleic Acid (CLA) on Mouse Forestomach Protein Kinase C (PKC)-like Activity," *FASEB Journal,* 6(4), 1992, p. A1396.

Results of this study found that conjugated linoleic acid exhibited cytotoxic effects against human breast cancer cells in vitro.

—T.D. Shultz, et al., "Differential Stimulatory and Inhibitory Responses of Human MCF-7 Breast Cancer Cells to Linoleic Acid and Conjugated Linoleic Acid in Culture," *Anticancer Research,* 12(6B), November-December 1992, p. 2143-2145.

Results of this study found that conjugated linoleic acid exhibited inhibitory effects against human breast, colorectal, and malignant melanoma cancer cells in vitro.

—T.D. Shultz, et al., "Inhibitory Effect of Conjugated Dienoic Derivatives of Linoleic Acid and Beta-Carotene on the in Vitro Growth of Human Cancer Cells," *Cancer Letters,* 63(2), April 15, 1992, p. 125-133.

Results of this study found that conjugated linoleic acid inhibited TPA-induced skin tumor promotion in mice.

—M.A. Belury, et al., "Dietary Conjugated Linoleic Acid Modulation of Phorbol Ester Skin Tumor Promotion," *Nutr Cancer,* 26(2), 1996, p. 149-157.

Cardiovascular/Coronary Heart Disease

Results of this study found that 12 weeks' administration of conjugated linoleic acid significantly reduced LDL cholesterol and triglyceride levels in rabbits. Significant reductions were also found in the LDL cholesterol to HDL cholesterol ratio as well total cholesterol to HDL cholesterol ratio.

> —K.N. Lee, et al., "Conjugated Linoleic Acid and Atherosclerosis in Rabbits," *Atherosclerosis,* 108(1), July 1994, p. 19-25.

■ FOLIC ACID

Anemia

The article reports on the case of a patient suffering from myelopathy associated with macrotic anemia who had experienced no benefit from treatment with vitamins B1, B6 and B12. The patient experienced a quick recovery of anemia and neurological improvement when folic acid was added to the supplemental vitamins which was maintained for as long as 10 months.

> —J.C. Raphael, et al., [Myelopathy and Macrocytic Anemia Associated with a Folate Deficiency. Cure by Folic Acid], *Ann Med Interne,* 126(5), May 1975, p. 339-348.

Arthritis

Results of this double-blind, placebo-controlled study showed folic acid at weekly doses of either 5 mg or 27.5 mg offered protection against methotrexate toxicity in rheumatoid arthritis patients without effecting the efficacy of the drug.

> —S.L. Morgan, et al., "Supplementation with Folic Acid During Methotrexate Therapy for Rheumatoid Arthritis. A Double-blind, Placebo-controlled Trial," *Annals of Internal Medicine,* 121(11), December 1, 1994, p. 833-341.

Results of this double-blind, placebo-controlled study found that the administration of 1 mg of folic acid per day significantly reduced the toxicity of methotrexate in rheumatoid arthritis patients with diminishing the drugs efficacy.

> —S.L. Morgan, et al., "The Effect of Folic Acid Supplementation on the Toxicity of Low-dose Methotrexate in Patients with Rheumatoid Arthritis," *Arthritis Rheum,* 33(1), January 1990, p. 9-18.

Results of this double-blind, placebo-controlled study showed that the daily intake of 6400 micrograms of folate plus 20 micrograms cobalamin over a period of 2 months produced beneficial effects in patients with idiopathic osteoarthritis following a ten day washout period.

> —M.A. Flynn, et al., "The Effect of Folate and Cobalamin on Osteoarthritic Hands," *Journal of American College of Nutrition,* 13(4), August 1994, p. 351-356.

Cancer

Results of this study found that supplemental folic acid suppressed epithelial hyperplasia and metaplasia of respiratory tract induced by methylcholanthrene in rats.

> —T. Kamei, et al., "Experimental Study of the Therapeutic Effects of Folate, Vitamin A,

and Vitamin B12 on Squamous Metaplasia of the Bronchial Epithelium,'' *Cancer,* 71(8), April 15, 1993, p. 2477-2483.

Results of this study showed that supplemental folic acid can enhance the antitumor selectivity of 1843U89 in mice and dogs.

—G.K. Smith, et al., ''Enhanced Antitumor Activity for the Thymidylate Synthase Inhibitor 1843U89 through Decreased Host Toxicity with Oral Folic Acid,'' *Cancer Research,* 55(24), December 15, 1995, p. 6117-6125.

Results of this study showed that the administration of supplemental folate and vitamin B12 reduced cellular atypia squamous metaplasia in heavy smokers over a period of one year.

—M. Saito, et al., ''Chemoprevention Effects on Bronchial Squamous Metaplasia by Folate and Vitamin B12 in Heavy Smokers,'' *Chest,* 106(2), August 1994, p. 496-499.

Results of this study showed that the administration of folic acid significantly suppressed carcinogen-induced ornithine decarboxylase activity in both young and old rats which, the authors argue, may contribute to its protective effects against colorectal neoplasia.

—Y.M. Nensey, et al., ''Aging. Increased Responsiveness of Colorectal Mucosa to Carcinogen Stimulation and Protective Role of Folic Acid,'' *Dig Dis Sci,* 40(2), February 1995, p. 396-401.

Results of this study showed that pretreatment with folic acid supplementation significantly improved the efficacy of the anticancer agents 5-fluorouracil, arabinosyl cytosine, and mitomycin in mice.

—M. Parchure, et al., ''Combination of Anticancer Agents with Folic Acid in the Treatment of Murine Leukaemia P388,'' *Chemotherapy,* 30(2), 1984, p. 119-124.

This review article notes that case-control studies have demonstrated increased intakes of folic acid-rich foods are associated with reduced incidence of carcinomas and that folic acid deficiencies can cause DNA damage resembling that found in cancer cells. The author therefore suggests cancer may be initiated by folic acid deficiency-induced DNA damage and argues that such deficiencies common to North American populations could responsible, in part, for the high rates of North American cancers.

—E. Jennings, ''Folic Acid as a Cancer-preventing Agent,'' *Medical Hypotheses,* 45(3), September 1995, p. 297-303.

Cardiovascular/Coronary Heart Disease

Results of this study found folic acid administered in daily doses of either 2.5 mg or 10 mg over a 6 week period reduced normal and increased plasma homocysteine concentrations in myocardial infarction patients.

—F. Landgren, et al., ''Plasma Homocysteine in Acute Myocardial Infarction: Homocysteine-lowering Effect of Folic Acid,'' *Journal of Internal Medicine,* 237(4), April, 1995, p. 381-388.

Results of this study showed that the administration of 250 mg per day of vitamin B6 and 5 mg of folic acid for 6 weeks normalized homocysteine metabolism in young patients with arterial occlusive disease.

—M. van den Berg, et al., ''Combined Vitamin B6 Plus Folic Acid Therapy in Young Patients with Arteriosclerosis and Hyperhomocysteinemia," *Journal of Vascular Surgery,* 20(6), December 1994, p. 933-940.

Results of this study found an inverse correlation between serum folate levels and the risk of fatal coronary heart disease in both men and women.
—H.I. Morrison, et al., "Serum Folate and Risk of Fatal Coronary Heart Disease," *JAMA,* 275(24), June 26, 1996, p. 1893-1896.

Results of this study found that the administration of 5 mg of folic acid per day for an average of 15 days may decrease the risk of cardiovascular disease in patients with chronic renal insufficiency.
—D.E. Wilcken, et al., "Folic Acid Lowers Elevated Plasma Homocysteine in Chronic Renal Insufficiency: Possible Implications for Prevention of Vascular Disease," *Metabolism,* 37(7), July 1988, p. 697-701.

Results of this study showed that dialysis patients administered 300 mg of pyridoxine and 5 mg of folic acid per day experienced a reduction in the risk of cardiovascular disease.
—M. Arnadottir, et al., "The Effect of High-dose Pyridoxine and Folic Acid Supplementation on Serum Lipid and Plasma Homocysteine Concentrations in Dialysis Patients," *Clinical Journal Nephrol,* 40(4), October 1993, p. 236-240.

Cervical Dysplasia

In this double-blind, placebo-controlled study, women with cervical dysplasia received 10 mg of folic acid per day for 3 months. Results showed significantly better biopsy and scores in women receiving the supplements relative to controls as well as significantly better final versus initial cytology scores.
—C.E. Butterworth, Jr., "Improvement in Cervical Dysplasia Associated with Folic Acid Therapy in Users of Oral Contraceptives," *American Journal of Clinical Nutrition,* 35(1), January 1982, p. 73-82.

Down's Syndrome

This study notes that in vitro methotrexate toxicity characteristic of Down's syndrome can be reduced by the high supplemental doses of folic acid in vivo.
—M.A. Peeters, et al., "In Vivo Folic Acid Supplementation Partially Corrects in Vitro Methotrexate Toxicity in Patients with Down Syndrome," *British of Haematology,* 89(3), March 1995, p. 678-680.

Fragile X Syndrome

This study reports on the cases of two brothers with fra(X) positive X-linked mental retardation who experienced benefits from long-term folic acid therapy. Improvements were seen with respect to decreased hyperactivity, enhanced attention span, increased motor coordination, as well as increased quantity and quality of speech.
—W.T. Brown, et al., "Folic Acid Therapy in the Fragile X Syndrome," *American Journal of Medical Genetics,* 17(1), January 1984, p. 289-297.

Results of this double-blind, placebo-controlled study showed that the administration of 10 mg per day of folic acid led to behavioral improvements in prepubertal males with fragile X syndrome.

>   —R.J. Hagerman, et al., "Oral Folic Acid Versus Placebo in the Treatment of Males with the Fragile X Syndrome," *American Journal of Medical Genetics,* 23(1-2), January-February 1986, p. 241-262.

In this study, 42 fragile X syndrome patients received 0.5 mg/kg per day of folic acid. Results showed improved behavior in most cases including improved IQ scores.

>   —J. Lejeune, et al., [Trial of Folic Acid Treatment in Fragile X Syndrome], *Ann Genet,* 27(4), 1984, p. 230-232.

Gingival Health

Results of this double-blind, placebo-controlled study found that the administration of 4 mg per day for 30 days of folic acid increased resistance of gingiva to local irritants and reduced inflammation in human subjects.

>   —R.I. Vogel, et al., "The Effect of Folic Acid on Gingival Health," *Journal of Periodontology,* 47(11), November 1976, p. 667-668.

Homocystinuria

This article reports on the case of a 15-year-old, mildly retarded boy with homocystinuria who experienced dramatic improvements following 400 mcg per day of folic acid over a period of approximately 70 days.

>   —T. Takenaka, et al., [Effect of Folic Acid for Treatment of Homocystinuria due to 5,10-methylenetetrahydrofolate Reductase Deficiency], *Rinsho Shinkeigaku,* 33(11), November 1993, p. 1140-1145.

Kidney Damage

Results of this study showed that the administration of 10 mg of folate per day for 3 months reduced elevated plasma homocysteine in patients with chronic renal failure.

>   —P. Chauveau, et al., "Long-term Folic Acid (but not pyridoxine) Supplementation Lowers Elevated Plasma Homocysteine Level in Chronic Renal Failure," *Miner Electrolyte Metab,* 22(1-3), 1996, p. 106-109.

Lithium Prophylaxis

This double-blind, placebo-controlled study examined the effects of 200 micrograms of folic acid per day on patients undergoing treatment with lithium. Results showed those patients with plasma folate increases of 13 ng/ml or higher experienced a 40% reduction in affective morbidity.

>   —A. Coppen, et al., "Folic Acid Enhances Lithium Prophylaxis," *Journal of Affective Disorders,* 10(1), January-February 1986, p. 9-13.

Multiple Sclerosis

Results of this study showed that the administration of 200-300 mcg per day of folic acid per day led to improvements in the reparative processes in the gastric mucosa and major therapeutic effects on the neurological status of patients with multiple sclerosis.

> —S.A. Kanevskaia, et al., [Folic Acid in the Combined Treatment of Patients with Disseminated Sclerosis and Chronic Gastritis], *Vrach Delo,* (4), April 1990, p. 96-97.

Pregnancy

This double-blind, placebo-controlled study examined the effects of 5 mg per day of supplemental folic acid on birth weight in normal pregnancies beginning at the 23rd week. Results showed a significant correlation between folic acid and birth weight, with folic acid infants measuring 12.7% heavier than controls.

> —J. Rolschau, et al., "Folic Acid Supplement and Intrauterine Growth," *Acta Obstet Gynecol Scand,* 58(4), 1979, p. 343-346.

In this study, 17 infants with severe or moderately severe erythroblastosis received 2-5 mg of folic acid per day from day 16 to 3-2 months. Results showed such infants experienced significant weight gain relative to controls after 4 months.

> —G. Gandy & W. Jacobson, "Influence of Folic Acid on Birthweight and Growth of the Erythroblastotic Infant. III. Effect of Folic Acid Supplementation," *Arch Dis Child,* 52(1), January 1977, p. 16-21.

Results of this literature review found an inverse correlation between serum folic acid levels and the risk of neural tube defect pregnancy.

> —N.J. Wald, et al., "Blood Folic Acid and Vitamin B12 in Relation to Neural Tube Defects," *British Journal of Obstet Gynaecol,* 103(4), April 1996, p. 319-324.

This article reports on results of recent literature reviews showing an inverse correlation between supplemental folic and the risk of neural tube defect pregnancies. The authors recommend a minimum dose of folic acid of 0.8 mg per day beginning prior to conception and continued for a minimum of 10 to 12 weeks of pregnancy.

> —M.I. Van Allen, et al., "Recommendations on the Use of Folic Acid Supplementation to Prevent the Recurrence of Neural Tube Defects. Clinical Teratology Committee, Canadian College of Medical Geneticists," *Canadian Medical Association Journal,* 149(9), November 1, 1993, p. 1239-1243.

This study examined the relationship between folic intake as part of a multivitamin and the risk of neural tube defects in 23,491 women at the 16th week of gestation. Results showed significant lower risk of defective pregnancies among women taking the supplemental folic acid relative to both straight controls and those taking a multivitamin not containing folic acid.

> —A. Milunsky, et al., "Multivitamin/folic Acid Supplementation in Early Pregnancy Reduces the Prevalence of Neural Tube Defects," *JAMA,* 262(20), November 24, 1989, p. 2847-2852.

This article notes that the United States Public Health Service recommends that all women of childbearing age in the United States who are capable of becoming pregnant should consume 0.4 mg of folic acid per day for the purpose of reducing their risk of having a pregnancy affected with spina bifida or other neural tube defects.

—"Recommendations for the Use of Folic Acid to Reduce the Number of Cases of Spina Bifida and Other Neural Tube Defects," *MMWR M,* 41(RR-14), September 11, 1992, p. 1-7.

This article reports on the results of a double-blind, placebo-controlled study which showed that 4 mg of folate per day started near conception significantly decreased the risk of neural tube defect pregnancy.

—"Folate Supplements Prevent Recurrence of Neural Tube Defects," *Nutr Rev,* 50(1), January 1992, p. 22-24.

Results of this study showed that the intake of 5 mg per day of folate significantly improved the concentration of haemoglobin in pregnant women with beta-thalassaemia minor.

—C.F. Leung, et al., "Effect of Folate Supplement on Pregnant Women with Beta-thalassaemia Minor," *European Journal of Obstet Gynecol Reprod Biol,* 33(3), December 1989, p. 209-213.

In this study, 5 mg of folic acid per day was administered to 81 women with a history of neural tube defect pregnancy for not less than one menstrual period prior to conception and up through the 10th week of pregnancy. Results showed no neural tube defect recurrence among these women or the infants of another 20 women taking supplemental folic acid at lesser doses. This contrasts with another group of 114 pregnant women studied with no supplementation and who exhibited 4 recurrences.

—R.G. Vergel, et al., "Primary Prevention of Neural Tube Defects with Folic Acid Supplementation: Cuban Experience," *Prenat Diagn,* March 1990, p. 10(3), p. 149-152.

This article argues that 70 to 100% of nerual tube defects are preventable by supplemental folic acid intake during the periconceptional period.

—O. Tonz, et al., [Folic Acid in the Prevention of Neural Tube Defects], *Schweiz Med Wochenschr,* 126(5), February 3, 1996, p. 177-187.

Results of this study indicated that the administration of folate may have preventive effects against the occurrence of neural tube defects and other signs of abnormal pregnancy in epileptic women.

—L.V. Dansky, et al., "Mechanisms of Teratogenesis: Folic Acid and Antiepileptic Therapy," *Neurology,* 42(4 Suppl 5), April 1992, p. :32-42.

Zinc Absorption

Results of this study showed that supplementation with 400 micrograms of folic acid every other day for 16 weeks had positive effects on zinc homeostasis in men.

—D.B. Milne, et al., "Effect of Oral Folic Acid Supplements on Zinc, Copper, and Iron Absorption and Excretion," *American Journal of Clinical Nutrition,* 39(4), April 1984, p. 535-539.

■ GLUTATHIONE

Aging

This study examined the association between blood glutathione levels and a host of biomedical/psychological traits among a group of 33 elderly subjects. Results showed significant positive associations between glutathione levels and fewer number of illnesses, higher levels of self-rated health, lower cholesterol lower body mass index, and lower blood pressures. Those suffering from arthritis, diabetes, or heart disease showed significantly lower glutathione levels than those without disease.

—M. Julius, et al., "Glutathione and Morbidity in a Community-based Sample of Elderly," *Journal of Clinical Epidemiology,* 47(9), September 1994, p. 1021-1026.

AIDS/HIV

This study examined the effects of glutathione and N-acetylcysteine on the replication of HIV-1 in primary monocyte/macrophages cultured in vitro. Results showed that HIV-1 infection was blocked or substantially reduced by glutathione or NAC. Reductions of 90% and higher in the amount of virus released were seen when cells were treated for 4 hours with a minimum of 10 mM of glutathione or NAC and lasted for a minimum of 35 days.

—W.Z. Ho & S.D. Douglas, "Glutathione and N-acetylcysteine Suppression of Human Immunodeficiency Virus Replication in Human Monocyte/macrophages in Vitro," *AIDS Research Human Retroviruses,* 8(7), July 1992, p. 1249-1253.

This study examined the effects of glutathione on HIV and Herpes-1 replication in vitro. Results showed that glutathione inhibited virus protein production in HIV-M/M at nontoxic concentrations with similar effects seen in herpes-1 infected VERO cells. Similar results were achieved in an RNA virus model.

—A.T. Palamara, et al., "Glutathione Directly Inhibits Late Stages of the Replication Cycle of HIV and Other Viruses," *International Conference on AIDS,* 9(1), June 6-11, 1993, p. 231Fundam .

Brain Function

Results of this study found that the intravenous injection of 1.5 g/kg of glutathione reduced decreases in local cerebral glucose utilization in rats induced by a neurotoxi and blocked neuronal loss in hippocampal CA1 and CA3 regions and prevented the development of hippocampal edema.

—A. Saija, et al., "Protective Effect of Glutathione on Kainic Acid-induced Neuropathological Changes in the Rat Brain," *Gen Pharmacol,* 25(1), January 1994, p. 97-102.

Cancer

Results of population-based, case-control study found an inverse correlation between dietary glutathione intake and the relative risk or oral cancer.

—E.W. Flagg, et al., "Dietary Glutathione Intake and the Risk of Oral and Pharyngeal Cancer," *American Journal of Epidemiology,* 139(5), March 1, 1994, p. 453-465.

Results of this double-blind, placebo-controlled study found glutathione administered at doses of 1.5 g/m2 in 100 mL of normal saline solution over a 15-minute period immediately prior to cisplatin exposure and at a dose of 600 mg by intramuscular injection on days 2 to 5 to be effective in the prevention of cisplatin-induced neuropathy without reducing the efficacy of chemotherapeutic drugs in patients with advanced gastric cancer.

   —S. Cascinu, et al., "Neuroprotective Effect of Reduced Glutathione on Cisplatin-based Chemotherapy in Advanced Gastric Cancer: A Randomized Double-blind Placebo-controlled Trial," *Journal of Clinical Oncology,* 13(1), January 1995, p. 26-32

Results of this study found that the oral administration of glutathione supplementation enhanced natural killer activity in tumor-bearing rats which led to reductions in tumor growth.

   —V.S. Klimberg, et al., "Glutamine Suppresses PGE2 Synthesis and Breast Cancer Growth," *Journal of Surg Research* 63(1), June 1996, p. 293-297.

Results of this double-blind, placebo-controlled study found that when 3 g/m2 of glutathione was added to treatment with 100 mg/m2 of cisplatin every 21 days ovarian cancer patients were able to withstand more cisplatin cycles and their overall quality of life was improved, including symptoms of depression, emesis, and neurotoxicity.

   —A. Bowman, et al., "Effect of Adding Glutathione (GSH) to Cisplatin (CDDP) in the Treatment of Stage I-IV Ovarian Cancer," *British Journal of Cancer,* 71(Suppl 24), 1994, p. 14.

Results of this study found that 1 g/kg per day of glutamine prevented chronic radiation injury and reduced complications associated with enteropathy in rats.

   —J.C. Jensen, et al., "Prevention of Chronic Radiation Enteropathy by Dietary Glutamine," *Ann Surg Oncology,* 1(2), March 1994, p. 157-163.

Results of this study showed the intravenous administration of 2.5-5 g in 100-200 ml of normal saline of glutathione over 15 minutes before cisplatin treatment to be an effective means of enhancing the drugs efficacy in patients with ovarian cancer.

   —G.B. Spatti, et al., "Cisplatin with Minimal Hydration and Glutathione Protection in the Treatment of Ovarian Carcinoma," *Anticancer Research,* 10(5B), 1990, p. 1425-1456.

Results of this study showed that the administration of glutathione significantly decreased cardiac toxicity associated with doxorubicin therapy in rats across a host of parameters.

   —F. Villani, et al., "Effect of Glutathione and N-acetylcesteine on in Vitro and in Vivo Cardiac Toxicity of Doxorubicin," *Anticancer Research,* 10(5B), 1990, p. 1421.

Results of this study found that the administration of 5 g per day of glutathione to patients suffering from hepatocellular carcinoma had beneficial effects in women, but not in men.

   —K. Dalhoff, et al., "Glutathione Treatment of Hepatocellular Carcinoma," *Liver,* 12(5), October 1992, p. 341-343.

Results of this study showed that the administration of 50 micrograms of glutathione alone as well as in combination with equivalent doses of a mixture containing the antioxidants vitamin E, ascorbic acid, and beta-carotene produced significant chemopreventive effects in hamsters with oral cancer.

   —G. Shklar, et al., "The Effectiveness of a Mixture of Beta-carotene, Alpha-tocopherol,

Glutathione, and Ascorbic Acid for Cancer Prevention,'' *Nutr Cancer,* 20(2), 1993, p. 145-151.

Results of this study showed that hamsters treated with glutathione experienced significantly fewer areas of DMBA-induced dysplastic leukoplaika relative to controls.
—D. Trickler, et al., ''Inhibition of Oral Carcinogenesis by Glutathione,'' *Nutr Cancer,* 20(2), 1993, p. 139-144.

Results of this double-blind, placebo-controlled study found that the administration of glutathione led to significant improvements in the therapeutic index of cisplatin therapy in ovarian cancer patients.
—J. Smyth, et al., ''Glutathione Improves the Therapeutic Index of Cisplatin and Quality of Life for Patients with Ovarian Cancer,'' *Procceedings of the Annual Meeting of the American Society of Clinical Oncologists,* 14, 1995, p. A761.

Cardiovascular/Coronary Heart Disease

Results of this study showed that incubation of isolated islets with glutathione boosted their secretory response to glucose stimulation and preserved their functional integrity.
—E.D. Littman, et al., ''Glutathione-mediated Preservation and Enhancement of Isolated Perifused Islet Function,'' *Journal of Surg Research,* 59(6), December 1995, p. 694-698.

Cataracts

Results of this study found that the administration of glutathione reduced and/or diminished the severity of sugar cataractogenesis in the rat lens.
—W.M. Ross, et al., ''Modelling Cortical Cataractogenesis: VI. Induction by Glucose in Vitro or in Diabetic Rats: Prevention and Reversal by Glutathione,'' *Exp Eye Research,* 37(6), December 1993, p. 559-573.

This study examined the effect of exogenous glutathione or its precursor amino acids on oxidative injury in cultured human retinal pigment epithelium. Results showed that the glutathione offered protection against oxidative injury and that glutathione synthesis mediated the protection provided by amino acid precursors.
—P. Sternberg, Jr. ''Protection of Retinal Pigment Epithelium from Oxidative Injury by Glutathione and Precursors,'' *Invest Ophthalmol Vis Sci,* 34(13), December 1993, p. 3661-3668.

Depression

Results of this study showed that the administration of glutathione and the antidepressants imipramine, maprotiline, fluvoxamine, trazodone, and alprazolam reduced and/or prevented shock-induced behavioral depression in mice.
—S.N. Pal & P.C. Dandiya, ''Glutathione as a Cerebral Substrate in Depressive Behavior,'' *Pharmacol Biochem Behavior,* 48(4), August 1994, p. 845-851.

Diabetes

Results of this double-blind, placebo-controlled study found glutathione to be somewhat effective in preventing diabetic neuropathy in diabetic rats.
—B. Bravenboer, et al., ''Potential Use of Glutathione for the Prevention and Treatment

of Diabetic Neuropathy in the Streptozotocin-induced Diabetic Rat,'' *Diabetologia,* 35(9), September 1992, p. 813-817.

Emphysema

Results of this study found glutathione capable of protecting alpha 1PI against the oxidative inactivation of alveolar inflammatory cells in an in vitro models of emphysema due to smoking.

    —B. Gressier, et al., ''Protective Role of Glutathione on Alpha 1 Proteinase Inhibitor Inactivation by the Myeloperoxidase System. Hypothetic Study for Therapeutic Strategy in the Management of Smokers' Emphysema,'' *Clin Pharmacol,* 8(6), 1994, p. 518-524.

Gastric Injury

Results of this study found that extracellular glutathione protected gastric mucosa from rats under stress.

    —M. Hirota, et al., ''Inhibition of Stress-induced Gastric Injury in the Rat by Glutathione,'' *Gastroenterology,* 97(4), October 1989, p. 853-859.

Results of this study showed glutathione provided protection against ethanol induced gastric mucosal damaged in humans.

    —C. Loguercio, et al., ''Glutathione Prevents Ethanol Induced Gastric Mucosal Damage and Depletion of Sulfhydryl Compounds in Humans,'' *Gut,* 34(2), February 1953, p. 161-165.

This study examined the of endogenous glutathione in gastric mucosal injury associated with hemorrhagic shock and reperfusion. Results showed that the glutathione protected against mucosal ischemia/reperfusion injury and prevented the ischemia/reperfusion-induced drop in mucosal glutathione.

    —H.J. Stein, et al., ''Gastric Mcosal Injury Caused by Hemorrhagic Shock and Reperfusion: Protective Role of the Antioxidant Glutathione,'' *Surgery,* 108(2), August 1990, p. 467-473.

General

Results of this study demonstrated a causal relationship between glutathione transport and protection from oxidative injury in type II cells from neonatal and fetal rats.

    —L.A. Brown, et al., ''Glutathione Protection in Alveolar Type II Cells from Fetal and Neonatal Rabbits,'' *American Journal of Physiology,* 262(3 Pt 1), March 1992, p. L305-12.

Results of this study found that reduced glutathione acted as a defense mechanism against acid-induced injury in the cultured gastric mucosal cells of rats in vitro.

    —H. Mutoh, et al., ''Reduced Glutathione Protects Cultured Gastric Mucosa Cells from Suckling Rats Against Acid,'' *American Journal of Physiologyeffects,* 261(1 Pt 1), July 1991, p. G65-70.

Results of this study showed that the supplementation of type II pulmonary cells of rabbits with glutathione's constituent amino acids and had beneficial effects.

    —N.R. Mettler, et al., ''Type II Epithelial Cells of the Lung. VII. The Effect of Ascorbic Acid and Glutathione,'' *Lab Invest,* 51(4), October 1984, p. 441-448.

Results of this study indicated the importance of glutathione in the repair of hippocampal neurons exposed to oxidative damage in vitro.

> —T.C. Pellmar, et al., "Role of Glutathione in Repair of Free Radical Damage in Hippocampus in Vitro," *Brain Research,* 583(1-2), June 26, 1992, p. 194-200.

Results of this study showed that pretreatment with glutathione reduced mortality rates in mice exposed to deadly levels of methyl bromide.

> —Y. Yamano, [Experimental Study on Methyl Bromide Poisoning in Mice. Acute Inhalation Study and the Effect of Glutathione as an Antidote], *Sangyo Igaku,* 33(1), January 1991, p. 23-30.

Herpes

This study examined the effects of glutathione in the in vitro infection and replication of human herpes 1. Results showed that the addition of glutathione inhibited the replication of the virus by as much as 99%.

> —A.T. Palamara, et al., "Evidence for Antiviral Activity of Glutathione: In Vitro Inhibition of Herpes Simplex Virus Type 1 Replication," *Antiviral Research,* 27(3), June 1995, p. 237-253.

Immune Enhancement

This study examined the effects of glutathione on the activity of interleukin-4 (IL-4) on murine cytotoxic T cells. Results showed that the glutathione regulated the binding, internalization, degradation and T-cell proliferative activity of IL-4; alteration of cellular GSH levels and affected the growth and replication of cytotoxic T cells through growth stimulating cytokines such as IL-2 and IL-4.

> —S.M. Liang, et al., "Regulation by Glutathione of Interleukin-4 Activity on Cytotoxic T Cells," *Immunology,* 75(3), March 1992, p. 435-440.

Infertility

In this study, 11 men suffering from infertility received 600 mg per day of glutathione of 2 months. Results showed the treatment to have significant beneficial effects on sperm motility patterns.

> —A. Lenzi, et al., "Glutathione Therapy for Male Infertility," *Arch Androl,* 29(1), July-August 1992, p. 65-68.

Results of this double-blind, placebo-controlled, crossover study found a statistical significant positive effect of intravenous glutathione supplementation at doses of 600 mg every other day for 2 months on sperm motility in infertile patients with dyspermia associated with unilateral varicocele or germ-free genital tract inflammation.

> —A. Lenzi, et al., "Placebo-controlled, Double-blind, Cross-over Trial of Glutathione Therapy in Male Infertility," *Human Reproduction,* 8(10), October 1993, p. 1657-1662.

Results of this double-blind, placebo-controlled study found that the administration of glutathione can partially reverse dyspermia provided structural cell membrane damage is not severe.

> —A. Lenzi, et al., "Glutathione Treatment of Dyspermia: Effect on the Lipoperoxidation Process," *Human Reproduction,* 9(11), November 1994, p. 2044-2050.

Liver Damage

Results of this study indicated that the rich hepatic supply with endogenous glutathione is central to the protection against oxygen radical injury following brief periods of total hepatic ischemia in rats.

—H.J. Stein, et al., "Oxygen Free Radicals and Glutathione in Hepatic Ischemia/reperfusion Injury," *Journal of Surgical Research,* 50(4), April 1991, p. 398-402.

Results of this study indicated that the enhanced release of hepatocellular glutathione provides protection against reactive oxygen species generated by inflammatory cells during endotoxemia and reperfusion. Such findings indicate this may be important in preventing or limiting liver damage.

—P. Liu, et al., "Beneficial Effects of Extracellular Glutathione Against Endotoxin-induced Liver Injury During Ischemia and Reperfusion," *Circ Shock,* 43(2), June 1994, p. 64-70.

Results of this study showed that the intravenous administration of high doses of glutathione for 2 weeks led to significant improvements of the enzyme patterns in the livers of chronic alcoholics.

—E.A. Nardi, et al., [High-dose Reduced Glutathione in the Therapy of Alcoholic Hepatopathy], *Clin Ter,* 136(1), January 15, 1991, p. 47-51.

Results of this study showed that high intravenous doses of glutathione administered to patients with chronic steatosic liver disease significantly improved the rate of some hepatic tests.

—P. Dentico, et al., [Glutathione in the Treatment of Chronic Fatty Liver Diseases], *Recenti Prog Med,* 86(7-8), July-August, 1995, p. 290-293.

Neuropathy

Results of this study found that the administration of glutathione reduced cisplatin-induced neurotoxicity/neuropathy in rats relative to controls.

—G. Tredici, et al., "Low-dose Glutathione Administration in the Prevention of Cisplatin-induced Peripheral Neuropathy in Rats," *Neurotoxicology,* 15(3), Fall 1994, p. 701-704.

Radiation Injury

This study examined the effects of glutathione on radiation injury in the parotid glands of rats. Results showed that glutathione administration 15 minutes prior radiation protected the parotid glands from injury.

—R. Arima & R. Shiba, "Radioprotective Effect of Exogenous Glutathione on Rat Parotid Glands," *International Journal of Radiation Biology,* 61(5), May 1992, p. 695-702.

Scurvy

Results of this study showed that the administration of glutathione ester significantly delayed the appearance of scurvy in ascorbate-deficient guinea pigs.

—J. Martensson, et al., "Glutathione Ester Delays the Onset of Scurvy in Ascorbate-deficient Guinea Pigs," *Proceedings of the National Acad Sci U S A,* 90(1), January 1, 1993, p. 317-321.

■ HESPERIDIN

Cancer

This case-control study examined the effects of hesperidin and curcumin on oral carcinogenesis in rats compared with beta-carotene. Results showed that rats fed with curcumin and beta-carotene during cancer initiation and postinitiation stage and hesperidin at the initiation stage led to a significant reduction in the frequency of tongue cancer and oral preneoplasia.

> —T. Tanaka, et al., "Chemoprevention of 4-nitroquinoline 1-oxide-induced Oral Carcinogenesis by Dietary Curcumin and Hesperidin: Comparison with the Protective Effect of Beta-carotene," *Cancer Research,* 54(17), September 1, 1994, p. 4653-4659.

Cardiovascular/Coronary Heart Disease

Results of this study showed that hesperidin taken from orange peel possessed diuretic and antihypertensive effects on both hypertensive and normotensive rats.

> —E.M. Galati, et al., "Biological Effects of Hesperidin, a Citrus flavonoid. (Note III): Antihypertensive and Diuretic Activity in Rat," *Farmaco,* 51(3), March 1996, p. 219-221.

Results of this study showed that hesperidin taken from orange peel significantly lowers cholesterol, LDL, total lipid and triglyceride while significantly increasing HDL in normolipidemic and hyperlidemia rats.

> —M.T. Monforte, "Biological Effects of Hesperidin, a Citrus Flavonoid. (note II): Hypolipidemic Activity on Experimental Hypercholesterolemia in Rat," *Farmaco,* 50(9), September 1995, p. 595-599.

This double-blind, placebo-controlled study examined the effects of a veno-active flavonoid fraction consisting of 90% micronized diosmin and 10% hesperidin in patients with symptomatic capillary fragility for 6 weeks. Results showed significant improvements in symptoms including spontaneous ecchymosis, epistaxis, purpura, petechiae, gingivorrhagia, metrorrhagia and conjunctival haemorrhage.

> —P. Galley & M. Thiollet, "A Double-blind, Placebo-controlled Trial of a New Veno-active Flavonoid Fraction (S 5682) in the Treatment of Symptomatic Capillary Fragility," *Int Angiol,* 12(1), March 1993, p. 69-72.

Results of this study showed that hesperidine methylchalcone and Ruscus extract provided protection against leakage of FITC-dextran in the hamster cheek pouch following administration of various permeability increasing substances.

> —E. Bouskela, et al., "Inhibitory Effect of the Ruscus Extract and of the Flavonoid Hesperidine Methylchalcone on Increased Microvascular Permeability Induced by Various Agents in the Hamster Cheek Pouch," *Journal of Cardiovascular Pharmacology,* 22(2), August 1993, p. 225-230.

General

Results of this study showed that hesperidin taken from orange peel possessed significant analgesic and anti-inflammatory effects.

> —E.M. Galati, et al., "Biological Effects of Hesperidin, a Citrus Flavonoid. (Note I): Antiinflammatory and Analgesic Activity," *Farmaco,* 40(11), November 1994, p. 709-712.

Results of this study showed that rats pretreated with hesperidin experienced reductions in paw oedema induced by carrageenan and by dextran. Hesperidin inhibited carrageenan-induced pleurisy as well.

—J.A. Emim, et al., ''Pharmacological Evaluation of the Anti-inflammatory Activity of a Citrus Bioflavonoid, Hesperidin, and the Isoflavonoids, Duartin and Claussequinone, in Rats and Mice,'' *Journal of Pharm Pharmacol,* 46(2), February 1994, p. 118-122.

■ INOSITOL

Cancer

This review article cites in vitro and in vivo studies which indicate the strong anticancer properties of inositol hexaphosphate

—A.M. Shamsuddin, ''Inositol Phosphates Have Novel Anticancer Function,'' *Journal of Nutrition,* 125(3 Suppl), March 1995, p. 725S-732S.

Results of this study showed that the saministration of 2% Na-InsP6 in drinking water significantly reduced experimental-induced large intestinal cancer rats.

—A.M. Shamsuddin & A. Ullah, ''Inositol Hexaphosphate Inhibits Large Intestinal Cancer in F344 Rats 5 Months after Induction by Azoxymethane,'' *Carcinogenesis,* 10(3), March 1989, p. 625-626.

Results of this study showed that the administration of INSP6+/- Ins over a period of 45 weeks inhibited experimental-induced mammary cancer in rats.

—I. Vucenik, et al., ''Inositol Hexaphosphate and Inositol Inhibit DMBA-induced Rat Mammary Cancer,'' *Carcinogenesis,* 16(5), May 1995, p. 1055-1058.

Results of this study showed myo-inositol to possess anti-tumorigenic activity in experimental-induced lung cancer in mice.

—N. Takasuka, et al., ''Prevention of Lung Carcinogenesis by Myo-inositol,'' *Japanese Journal of Cancer Research,* 7(10), 1995, p. 136.

Results of this study showed that InsP6 administered over a 45 week period provided protection against DMBA-induced mammary carcinoma in rats.

—I. Vucenik, et al., ''Inositol Phosphates Inhibit DMBA-induced Rat Mammary Cancer,'' *Proceedings of the Annual Meeting of the American Association of Cancer Researchers,* 36, 1995, p. A3527.

Results of this study showed that InsP6 administered over a 17week period provided protection against DMBA-induced mammary carcinoma in rats.

—I. Vucenik, et al., ''Mammary Carcinogenesis Inhibition by Inositol Compounds,'' *Procceedings of the Annual Meeting of American Association of Cancer Researchers,* 33, 1992, p. A993.

Cardiovascular/Coronary Heart Disease

This double-blind study compared the effects of 1.5 of pryidinolcarbamate and 1.2 g of inositol niacinate taken three times daily in patients with the ischemic ulcer due to chronic arterial occlusion over period of either 4 or 6 weeks. Results showed beneficial effects in 50% of the 4-week pyridinolcarbamate group, 57.1% of the 4-week inositol niacinate group, 68.4% of the 6-week pyridinolcarbamate group and 48.6% of the 6-week inositol niacinate group.

> —Y. Mishima, et al., "A Multiclinic Double-blind Trial of Pyridinolcarbamate and Inositol Niacinate in Ischemic Ulcer Due to Chronic Arterial Occlusion," *Angiology,* 28(2), February 1977, p. 84-94.

Results of this study showed that the intravenous administration of inositol hexasulfate inhibited clot-formation of the recalcified plasma in competition with calcium ions.

> —G. Oshima, et al., "Anticoagulant Effect of Inositol Hexasulfate as Measurable by Clotting Times of Fibrinogen and Recalcified Plasma," *Thromb Research,* 58(3), May 1, 1990, p. 243-250.

Depression

Results of this double-blind, placebo-controlled study found that the administration of 12 g per day of inositol for 4 weeks led to significant improvements in patients suffering from depression.

> —J. Levine, et al., "Double-blind, Controlled Trial of Inositol Treatment of Depression," *American Journal of Psychiatry,* 152(5), May 1995, p. 792-794.

This review article cites findings from double-blind, placebo-controlled studies supporting the efficacy of inositol as a treatment for depression.

> —J. Benjamin, et al., "Inositol Treatment in Psychiatry," *Psychopharmacol Bulletin,* 31(1), 1995, p. 167-175.

Diabetes

Results of this study found the administration of 6 g of inositol per day for 3 months to be an effective treatment for diabetic polyneuropathy.

> —F. Cai, et al., [Preliminary Report of Efficacy of Diabetic Polyneuropathy Treated with Large Dose Inositol], *Hua Hsi I Ko Ta Hsueh Hsueh Pao,* 21(2), June 1990, p. 201-203.

Obsessive Compulsive Disorder

Results of this double-blind, placebo-controlled, crossover study found that the administration of 18 g per day of inositol for 6 weeks had significant beneficial effects in patients suffering from obsessive compulsive disorder

> —M. Fux, et al., "Inositol Treatment of Obsessive-compulsive Disorder," *American Journal of Psychiatry,* 153(9), September 1996, p. 1219-1221.

Panic Disorder

In this double-blind, placebo-controlled study, panic disorder patients with or without agoraphobia received 12 g of inositol per day. Results showed a significant decline in the frequency and severity of panic attacks and agoraphobia relative to controls.

> —J. Benjamin, et al., "Double-blind, Placebo-controlled, Crossover Trial of Inositol Treatment for Panic Disorder," *American Journal of Psychiatry,* 152(7), July 1995, p. 1084-1086.

Respiratory Distress Syndrome

This double-blind, placebo-controlled study examined the effects of intravenous inositol at doses of 120-160 mg/kg per day in infants with a birth weight less than 2000 g. Results showed that the infants receiving the treatment required less mechanical ventilation during days 4-10, had less failures of indomethacin to close ductus arteriosus, and had less deaths or bronchopulmonary dysplasia relative to controls.

>   —M. Hallman, et al., "Respiratory Distress Syndrome and Inositol Supplementation in Preterm Infants," *Arch Dis Child,* 61(11), November 1986, p. 1076-1083.

Results of this double-blind, placebo-controlled study, showed that inositol supplementation at doses of 40 mg every 6 hours in preterm infants with respiratory distress syndrome produced increases in serum inositol concentration and improvement in the surfactant phospholipids.

>   —M. Hallman, et al., "Inositol Supplementation in Respiratory Distress Syndrome: Relationship Between Serum Concentration, Renal Excretion, and Lung Effluent Phospholipids," *Journal of Pediatrics,* 110(4), April 1987, p. 604-610.

Results of this double-blind, placebo-controlled study showed that supplemental inositol at doses of 70-100 mg/kg per day promotes endothelial cell growth, enhanced glucocorticoid-mediated lung epithelial cell differentiation, and acted as an antioxidant in preterm infants suffering from respiratory distress syndrome.

>   —M. Hallman, et al., "Inositol Supplementation in Respiratory Distress Syndrome," *Lung,* 168 Suppl, 1990, p. 877-882.

■ IODINE

Antibacterial Effects

In this study, women with candidal, trichomonal and nonspecific vaginitis received povidone-iodine vaginal pessaries twice per day over a period of two weeks. Results indicated the treatment to be effective and free of side effects.

>   —N.A. Darwish & M. Shaarawy, "Effect of Treatment with Povidone-iodine Vaginal Pessaries on Thyroid Function," *Postgraduate Medical Journal,* 69 (Suppl 3), 1993, p. S39-S42.

Results of this study found povidone-iodine 2.5% ophthalmic solution to be an effective and non-toxic antibacterial therapy in the treatment of conjunctiva of newborns relative to silver nitrate.

>   —S.J. Isenberg, et al., "Povidone-iodine for Pphthalmia Neonatorum Prophylaxis," *American Journal of Ophthalmology,* 118(6), December 15, 1994, p. 701-706.

Results of this study found that the incorporation of povidone-iodine into polymethylmethacrylate was inhibited growth of coagulase-positive Staphylococcus aureus in vitro.

>   —A.R. Kohlhaas & J.L. Sandrik, "The Antimicrobial Properties of Povidone-iodine Methylmethacrylate Complex. A Preliminary Report," *Clinical Orthop,* (113), November-December 1975, p. 184-186.

This study examined the effects of povidone-iodine enema on the bacterial flora of colorectal mucosa among potential colorectal surgery patients. Results showed significantly reduced total bacterial concentrations following povidone-iodine enema compared to simple water enema.

> —J.M. Hay, et al., "Povidone-iodine Enema as a Preoperative Bowel Preparation for Colorectal Surgery. A Bacteriologic Study," *Dis Colon Rectum,* 32(1), January 1989, p. 9-13.

Results of this study indicated that the combined application of iodine and sodium flouride on the molars produced antibacterial/cariostatic effects in rats.

> —P.W. Caufield, et al., "Effect of Topically-applied Solutions of Iodine, Sodium Fluoride, or Chlorhexidine on Oral Bacteria and Caries in Rats," *Journal of Dental Research,* 60(5), May 1981, p. 927-932.

Results of this study found povidone-iodine 2.5% ophthalmic solution to be an effective and non-toxic antibacterial therapy in the treatment of conjunctiva of newborns relative to silver nitrate.

> —S.J. Isenberg, et al., "A Controlled Trial of Povidone-iodine as Prophylaxis Against Ophthalmia Neonatorum," *New England Journal of Medicine,* 332(9), March 2, 1995, p. 562-566.

Results of this study found 10% povidone-iodine to be an effective killer of methicillin-resistant Staphylococcus aureus in vitro.

> —P.D. Goldenheim, "In Vitro Efficacy of Povidone-iodine Solution and Cream Against Methicillin-resistant Staphylococcus Aureus," *Postgraduate Medical Journal,* (69 Suppl 3), 1993, p. S62-S65.

This study examined the effects of one 200 mg povidone-iodine pessariy per day for 7 days on 38 women with vaginitis. Results showed a total symptomatic and microbiological recovery in 73.3% of the cases, with 16.7% experiencing a microbiological cure and improved symptoms.

> —H. Yu & M. Tak-Yin, "The Efficacy of Povidone-iodine Pessaries in a Short, Low-dose Treatment Regime on Candidal, Trichomonal and Non-specific Vaginitis," *Postgraduate Medical Journal,* 69 (Suppl 3), 1993, p. S58-S61.

This review article notes that numerous controlled studies have pointed to the efficacy of povidone-iodine on dental extraction bacteraemia.

> —R. Rahn, "Review Presentation on Povidone-iodine Antisepsis in the Oral Cavity," *Postgraduate Medical Journal,* 69(Suppl 3), 1993, p. S4-S9.

Results of this study showed that nasal application of povidone-iodine creams was an effective means of eliminating nasal methicillin-resistant Staphylococcus aureus from the nasal cavity among a population of hospital workers.

> —H. Masano, et al., "Efficacy of Intranasal Application of Povidone-iodine Cream in Eradicating Nasal Methicillin-resistant Staphylococcus Aureus in Neonatal Intensive Care Unit (NICU) Staff," *Postgraduate Medical Journal,* (69 Suppl 3), 1993, p. S122-S125.

This study examined the effects of PVP-iodine antiseptic on harmful oral bacteria. Results showed that when administered in a 5% solution, the PVP-iodine inhibited 7 of 8 bacterial strains examined.

> —R.F. Muller, et al., [Efficacy of a PVP-iodine Compound on Selected Pathogens of the Oral Cavity in Vitro], *Dtsch Zahnarztl Z,* 44(5), May 1989, p. 366-369.

Results of this study showed povidone-iodine controlled the infection and reduced the period of morbidity induced by experimentally produced staphylococcal coagulase positive corneal ulcers in rabbits relative to Gentamycin sulphate.

—L.G. Sharma, et al., "Evaluation of Topical Povidone-iodine Versus Gentamycin in Staphylococcus Coagulase Positive Corneal Ulcers—An Experimental Study," *Indian Journal of Ophthalmol,* 38(1), January-March 1990, p. 30-32.

Results of this study showed that povidone-iodine eye drops proved to be an effective treatment for conjunctivitis or keratoconjunctivitis among a group of 40 patients.

—G. Schuhman & B.Vidic, "Clinical Experience with Povidone-iodine Eye Drops in Patients with Conjunctivitis and Keratoconjunctivitis," *Journal of Hospital Infection,* 6, (Suppl A), March 1995, p. 173-175.

Results of this study found that providone-iodine solution was a safe and effective treatment for aspecific vaginitis among a group of 32 women suffering from the condition.

—R. Grio, et al., [Effectiveness of Povidone-iodine in the Treatment of Non-specific Vaginitis], *Minerva Ginecol,* 42(4), April 1990, p.129-131.

Results of this study indicated that povidone-iodine is an effective antibacterial treatment for preparing skin for surgery.

—G. Georgiade, et al., "Efficacy of Povidone-iodine in Pre-operative Skin Preparation," *Journal of Hospital Infection,* (6 Suppl A), March 1985, p. 67-71.

Results of this study found povidone-iodine ethanol solution to be an effective antibacterial agent for preoperative skin preparation.

—T. Arata, et al., "Evaluation of Povidone-iodine Alcoholic Solution for Operative Site Disinfection," *Postgraduate Medical Journal,* 69 (Suppl 3), 1993, p. S93-S96.

Antifungal Effects

In this study, povidone-Iodine Paint was administered on patients with a fungal infection: ten having pityriasis versicolor, two trichophyton rubrum, and one M. canis. Results showed that seven of the ten patients with pityriasisversicolor group experienced either complete or significant improvement.

—V.K. Manna, et al., "The Effect of Povidone-iodine Paint on Fungal Infection," *Journal of Intern Med Research,* 12(2), 1984, p. 121-123.

Empyema

Results of this study indicated that pleural washing with povidone-iodine was effective in the treatment of two patients suffering from empyema.

—K. Takayama, et al., [Pleural Washing with Povidone-iodine for Treatment of Empyema], *Kansenshogaku Zasshi,* 67(3), March 1993, p. 218-222.

General

This review article notes iodine supplementation has been shown to prevent endemic cretinism when administered prior to conception. Studies have indicated such supplementation can prevent fetal and infant death as well.

—P.O. Pharoah, ''Iodine-supplementation Trials,'' *American Journal of Clinical Nutrition,* 57(2 Suppl), February 1993, p. 276S-279S.

Herpes

Results of this study showed that a povidone-iodine solution at concentrations of 0.167% decreased end-point titers of Strain E.M. herpesvirus, type 2, by upwards of 99.99%.

—M.S. Amstey & S. Metcalf, ''Effect of Povidone-iodine on Herpesvirus Type 2, in Vitro,'' *Obstet Gynecol,* 46(5), November 1975, p. 528-529.

In this study, patients with vulvovaginal and cervical herpesvirus infections received external and intravaginal povidone-iodine preparations. Results showed a reduction in expected duration of symptoms in 9 of the 10 cases examined.

—E.G. Friedrich, Jr & T. Masukawa, ''Effect of Povidone-iodine on Herpes Genitalis,'' *Obstet Gynecol,* 45(3), March 1975, p. 337-339.

Stomatitis

This study examined the effects of a povidone-iodine gargle solution on the prevention of stomatitis in patients with acute myelogenous leukemia over a one year period, two, and three year period. Results found the therapy to be effective.

—Y. Tsuzura, et al., [Prevention of Stomatitis in Patients with Acute Myelogenous Leukemia Using PVP-iodine (Isodine) Gargle], *Gan To Kagaku Ryoho,* 19(6), June 1992, p. 817-822.

Thyroid Function

Results of this study showed that iodine inhibited thyroid cell growth in vitro at multiple loci related to both the cAMP-dependent and cAMP-independent pathways of mitogenic regulation.

—D. Tramontano, et al., ''Iodine Inhibits the Proliferation of Rat Thyroid Cells in Culture,'' *Endocrinology,* 125(2), August 1989, p. 984-992

Results of this study found that hypophysectomized rats administered diets high in iodine experienced a significantly lower increases in thyroid cyclic AMP concentration induced acutely by a single dose of TSH relative to rats fed a diet deficient in iodine.

—B. Rapoport, et al., ''Inhibitory Effect of Dietary Iodine on the Thyroid Adenylate Cyclase Response to Thyrotropin in the Hypophysectomized Rat,'' *Journal of Clinical Investigations,* 56(2), August 1975, p. 516-519.

This study examined the effects of oral iodine supplementation on goitre rate among school children between the ages of 4-16. Results showed that doses of 200mg were just as effective as 400mg for controlling and prevention iodine deficiency disorders.

—C. Abuye, et al., ''The Effect of Varying Doses of Oral Iodized Oil in the Prophylaxis of

Endemic Goitre in Elementary School Children,'' *Ethiopian Medical Journal,* 33(2), April 1995, p. 115-123.

Wound Healing

Results of this study found that the administration or povidone-iodine cream significantly reduced wound strength in murine skin incisions.

—A. Kashyap, et al., ''Effect of Povidone Iodine Dermatologic Ointment on Wound Healing,'' *American Surg,* 61(6), June 1995, p. 486-491.

Results of this study found that a 1% povidone-iodine solution reduced the incident of wound infection in traumatic lacerations among a population of 500 emergency room patients.

—A. Gravett, et al., ''A Trial of Povidone-iodine in the Prevention of Infection in Sutured Lacerations,'' *Annals of Emergency Medicine,* 16(2), February 1987, p. 167-171.

This study consisted of a retrospective analysis of the efficacy of povidone-iodine in preventing postoperative wound infections among a group of 50 patients undergoing major head and neck procedures. Results showed an infection rate of only 2%.

—D.H. Rice & D. Maceri, ''The Use of Povidone-iodine to Prevent Postoperative Wound Infection,'' *Arch Otolaryngol,* 107(5), May 1981, p. 287.

Results of this controlled study showed that povidone-iodine significantly reduced wound sepsis after gastrointestinal surgery among a group of 153 patients.

—J.G. Gray & M.J. Lee, ''The Effect of Topical Povidone Iodine on Wound Infection Following Abdominal Surgery,'' *British Journal Surgery,* 68(5), May 1981, p. 310-313.

This study examined the effects of topical povidone-iodine on infection associated with decubitus and stasis ulcers in male outpatients. Results showed statistically significant improvements in edema, pain, erythema, ulcer size, and ulcer depth within two weeks of beginning the therapy. Sixty-seven percent of the ulcers were clinically cured and 33% improved by the studies completion.

—B.Y. Lee, et al., ''Topical Application of Povidone-iodine in the Management of Decubitus and Stasis Ulcers,'' *Journal of the American Geriatric Society,* 27(7), July 1979, p. 302-306.

Results of this study showed povidone-iodine irrigation reduced wound infection in patients undergoing early repeat sternotomy following cardiac surgery.

—G.D. Angelini, et al., ''Wound Infection Following Early Repeat Sternotomy for Postoperative Bleeding. An Experience Utilizing Intraoperative Irrigation with Povidone Iodine,'' *Journal of Cardiovascular Surgery,* 31(6), November-December 1990, p. 793-795.

Results of this study showed that the preoperative bladder instillation of povidone-iodine proved effective in preventing postprostatectomy wound infection.

—S. Richter, et al., ''Single Preoperative Bladder Instillation of Povidone-iodine for the Prevention of Postprostatectomy Bacteriuria and Wound Infection,'' *Infect Control Hosp Epidemiol,* 12(10), October 1991, p. 579-582.

Results of this controlled trial involving 628 emergency unit patients indicated that povidone-iodine spray was an effective, nontoxic, antiseptic prophylactic agent for minor wounds.

> —T.C. Naunton Morgan, et al., "Prophylactic Povidone Iodine in Minor Wounds," *Injury,* 12(2), September 1980, p. 104-106.

This study compared the use of prophylactic antibiotic therapy or only local, intra-operative administration of povidone-iodine over a 6 month period in 250 patients operated on for lumbar disc prolapse. Results showed significantly less abscesses and infections in patients receiving the povidone-iodine.

> —J. Strohecker, et al., "The Intra-operative Application of Povidone-iodine in Neurosurgery," *Journal of Hospital Infection,* (6 Suppl A), March 1985, p. 123-125.

■ IRON

Anemia

Results of this double-blind, placebo-controlled study showed that supplementation with 10 mg of ferrous sulfate kg per day for 12 weeks led to significant improvements in the hematological status, growth rate, and morbidity level of anemic children.

> —L.C. Chwang, et al., "Iron Supplementation and Physical Growth of Rural Indonesian Children," *American Journal of Clinical Nutrition,* 47(3), March 1988, p. 496-501.

Results of this study showed that 60 mg of supplemental iron over a 17 week period led to a significant positive change in hemoglobin status of pregnant plantation workers in Sri Lanka, thus reducing the risk of anemia in pregnancy.

> —T.M. Atukorala, et al., "Evaluation of Effectiveness of Iron-folate Supplementation and Anthelminthic Therapy Against Anemia in Pregnancy—A Study in the Plantation Sector of Sri Lanka," *American Journal of Clinical Nutrition,* 60(2), August 1994, p. 286-292.

Results of this double-blind study found that 30 mg of Fe per day coupled with 20 mg of vitamin C for a period of 2 months led to significant improvements in the growth and hematological status of anemic preschool children in Indonesia relative to controls.

> —I.T. Angeles, et al., "Decreased Rate of Stunting Among Anemic Indonesian Preschool Children through Iron Supplementation," *American Journal of Clinical Nutrition,* 58(3), September 1993, p. 339-342.

Results of this study showed that supplementation with 200 mg of intravenous iron monthly over a period of 5 months in severe chronic renal failure patients suffering from anemia and not receiving dialysis led to significant improvements in anemia among two thirds of them.

> —D.S. Silverberg, et al., "Intravenous Iron Supplementation for the Treatment of the Anemia of Moderate to Severe Chronic Renal Failure Patients not Receiving Dialysis," *American Journal of Kidney Disease,* 27(2), February 1996, p. 234-238.

This study examined the efficacy of 100 U/kg of recombinant human erythropoietin administered subcutaneously three times per week in combination with 9 g/l human breast milk and 18 mg of iron per day for 3-8 weeks in raising haemoglobin concentrations among healthy, low birth weight infants.

Results showed significant increases in reticulocyte and haemoglobin concentrations after one week of treatment relative to controls.

—A.G. Bechensteen, et al., "Erythropoietin, Protein, and Iron Supplementation and the Prevention of Anaemia of Prematurity," *Arch Dis Child,* 69(1 Spec No), July 1993, p. 19-23.

Results of this double-blind, placebo-controlled study found that supplementation with 150 mg of sustained release ferrous sulfate per day for 14 weeks led to improvements in growth and appetite relative to controls among anemic primary school children in Kenya.

—J.W. Lawless, et al., "Iron Supplementation Improves and Growth in Anemic Kenyan Primary School Children," *Journal of Nutrition,* May 1994, p. 124(5), 645-654.

Results of this study indicated that intravenous iron saccharate may be an effective treatment for children suffering from chronic anemia who do not respond to oral iron supplementation.

—A. Martini, et al., "Intravenous Iron Therapy for Severe Anaemia in Systemic-onset Juvenile Chronic Arthritis," *Lancet,* 344(8929), October 15, 1994, p. 1052-1054.

This double-blind, placebo-controlled study examined the effects of daily supplemental iron (60 mg) and vitamin A (2.4 mg of retinol) for 8 weeks on anemic pregnant women in West Java. Results showed that 35% in the vitamin-A-supplemented group, 68% in the iron-supplemented group, 97% in the group supplemented with both, and 16% of women in the placebo group became non-amemic following treatment.

—D. Suharno, et al., "Supplementation with Vitamin A and Iron for Nutritional Anaemia in Pregnant Women in West Java, Indonesia," *Lancet,* 342(8883), November 27, 1993, p. 1325-1328.

Results of this double-blind, placebo-controlled study found that supplemental GnRH combined with iron proved effective in the treatment of anemia in patients with uterine leiomyomas, in reducing uterine-myoma volume, and in alleviating bleeding and other leiomyoma-related symptoms relative to controls.

—T.G. Stovall, et al., "GnRH Agonist and Iron Versus Placebo and Iron in the Anemic Patient Before Surgery for Leiomyomas: A Randomized Controlled Trial," *Obstet Gynecol,* 86(1), July 1995, p. 65-71.

Results of this double-blind, placebo-controlled study showed that supplementation with 40 mg per day of iron for 6 months led to significant growth increases in both anemic and normal children between the ages of 3-5.

—D. Bhatia & S. Seshadri, "Growth Performance in Anemia and Following Iron Supplementation," *Indian Pediatr,* 30(2), February 1993, p. 195-200.

Cognitive Function

This double-blind, placebo-controlled study examined the effects of 13 mg per day of supplemental iron for 8 weeks on cognitive function in adolescent girls with non-anemic iron deficiency. Results showed that girls receiving iron scored higher on verbal learning and memory tests relative to controls.

—A.B. Bruner, et al., "Randomised Study of Cognitive Effects of Iron Supplementation in

Non-anaemic Iron-deficient Adolescent Girls,'' *Lancet,* 348(9033), October 12, 1996, p. 992-996.

Kidney Damage

Results of this study showed that four months' intravenous iron administration was more effective than oral administration in the improvement of erythropoiesses among hemodialysis patients.

—S. Fishbane, et al., ''Reduction in Recombinant Human Erythropoietin Doses by the Use of Chronic Intravenous Iron Supplementation,'' *American Journal of Kidney Disease,* 26(1), July 1995, p. 41-46.

Newborns

Results of this study showed that maternal iron supplementation was effective in improving haemotolical patterns in neonates and promoting early infant growth.

—A.A. Khashaba, et al., ''Assessment of Parameters of Physical Growth of the Newborn in Relation to Maternal Supplementation with Iron Alone or with Some Biological Additives,'' *Gaz Egypt Paediatr Assoc,* 24(1-2), January-April 1976, p. 59-68.

■ LIPASE

Cystic Fibrosis

This double-blind, randomized study compared the efficacy of a high lipase preparation with a standard acid resistant microsphere pancreatic enzyme preparation in children suffering from cystic fibrosis. Results showed the lipase preparation to be superior with respect to gastrointestinal symptoms, fat absorption, and faecal fat output and energy loss.

—I.M. Bowler, et al., ''A Double Blind Lipase for Lipase Comparison of a High Lipase and Standard Pancreatic Enzyme Preparation in Cystic Fibrosis,'' *Arch Dis Child,* 68(2), February 1993, p. 227-230.

■ MAGNESIUM CITRATE

Gastrointestinal Problems

Results of this study found that magnesium citrate administered in a 6% solution reduced gastrointestinal of activated charcoal stools in children between the ages of 1 month and 6 years.

—Y.J. Sue, et al., ''Efficacy of Magnesium Citrate Cathartic in Pediatric Toxic Ingestions,'' *Ann Emerg Med,* 24(4), October 1994, p. 709-712.

Urinary Calcium Excretion

This study examined the effects of phytin and magnesium citrate on the reduction or urinary calcium excretion in rats fed a high calcium diet for four weeks. Results showed significant reductions in excretion following treatment with both agents, with stronger reductions being seen following magnesium citrate treatment.

> —N. Wu, et al., "Effects of Magnesium Citrate and Phytin on Reducing Urinary Calcium Excretion in Rats," *World J Urol,* 12(6), 1994, p. 323-328.

■ MELATONIN

Adrenal Function

This study examined the effects treatment with melatonin for 10 days on the adrenal function of male rats. Results indicated melatonin had an inhibitory action on the effect of ACTH on the adrenal gland.

> —K. Yamada, "Effects of Melatonin on Adrenal Function in Male Rats," *Research Commun Chem Pathol Pharmacol,* 69(2), August 1990, p. 241-244.

Aging

This article reviews recent findings concerning the role of melatonin in aging. Evidence is cited indicating melatonin may delay the effects of aging by attenuating negative effects associated with free radical-induced neuronal damage.

> —R. Sandyk, "Possible Role of Pineal Melatonin in the Mechanisms of Aging," *International Journal of Neuroscience,* 52(1-2), May 1990, p. 85-92.

Results of this study showed that melatonin attenuated decreases in survival rates, testosterone and brain 125I-melatonin binding sites associated with aging in rats.

> —S. Oaknin-Bendahan, et al., "Effects of Long-term Administration of Melatonin and a Putative Antagonist on the Ageing Rat," *Neuroreport,* 6(5), March 27, 1995, p. 785-788.

Antiglucocorticoid Effects

Results of this study indicated that melatonin provided significant protection from the damaging effects of a glucocorticoid in adult rats.

> —H. Aoyama, et al., "Anti-glucocorticoid Effects of Melatonin on Adult Rats," *Acta Pathol Jpn,* 37(7), July 1987, p. 1143-1148.

Cancer

In this study, 10 mg per day of oral melatonin was administered to patients with metastatic non-small cell lung cancer at 8:00 pm. Results showed that the melatonin coupled with neuroimmunotherapeutic therapy with IL-2 produced beneficial effects and was well tolerated.

> —P. Lissoni, et al., "Biological and Clinical Results of a Neuroimmunotherapy with Interleukin-2 and the Pineal Hormone mMelatonin as a First Line Treatment in Advanced Non-small Cell Lung Cancer," *British Journal of Cancer,* 66(1), July 1992, p. 155-158.

This study examined the effects of 20 mg per day of melatonin in metastatic breast cancer patients coupled with tamoxifen treatment. Results showed that the combine therapies induced objective tumor regressions.

> —P. Lissoni, et al., "Modulation of Cancer Endocrine Therapy by Melatonin: A Phase II

Study of Tamoxifen Plus Melatonin in Metastatic Breast Cancer Patients Progressing Under Tamoxifen Alone,'' *British Journal of Cancer,* 71(4), April 1995, p. 854-856.

Results of this study showed that melatonin interrupts prolactin-mediated growth signal in human breast cancer cell growth in vitro.

—A. Lemus-Wilson, et al., ''Melatonin Blocks the Stimulatory Effects of Prolactin on Human Breast Cancer Cell Growth in Culture,'' *British Journal of Cancer,* 72(6), December 1995, p. 1435-1440.

Results of this study showed that low dose IL-2 coupled with 50 mg of melatonin per day beginning seven days prior to IL-2 therapy proved to be an effective treatment for advanced digestive tract tumors.

—P. Lissoni, et al., ''Immunotherapy with Subcutaneous Low-dose Interleukin-2 and the Pineal Indole Melatonin as a New Effective Therapy in Advanced Cancers of the Digestive Tract,'' *British Journal of Cancer,* 67(6), June 1993, p. 1404-1407.

In this study, 22 renal cell carcinoma patients were monitored for the effect of a 12 month regimen of 3 mega units of intramuscular human lymphoblastoid interferon 3 times weekly and 10 mg per day of oral melatonin. Results showed 7 remissions and 9 disease stabelizations.

—B. Neri, et al., ''Modulation of Human Lymphoblastoid Interferon Activity by Melatonin in Metastatic Renal Cell Carcinoma. A Phase II Study,'' *Cancer,* 73(12), June 15, 1994, p. 3015-3019.

Results of this study showed that melatonin can improve quality of life and survival time in brain metastases patients.

—P. Lissoni, et al., ''A Randomized Study with the Pineal Hormone Melatonin Versus Supportive Care Alone in Patients with Brain Metastases Due to Solid Neoplasms,'' *Cancer,* 73(3), February 1, 1994, p. 699-701.

Results of this study showed that melatonin inhibited the development of DMBA-induced mammary tumors in rats.

—L. Tamarkin, et al., ''Melatonin Inhibition and Inhibition and Pinealectomy Enhancement of 7,12-Dimethylbenz(a)Anthracene-Induced Mammary Tumors in the Rat,'' *Cancer Research,* 41(11,part1), 1981, p. 4432-4436.

Results of this study showed that melatonin produced a direct, reversible antiproliferative effect on MCF-7 cell growth in vitro.

—S.M. Hill & D.E. Blask, ''Effects of the Pineal Hormone Melatonin on the Proliferation and Morphological Characteristics of Human Breast Cancer Cells (MCF-7) in Culture,'' *Cancer Research,* 48(21), November 1, 1988, p. 6121-6126.

Results of this study showed that melatonin significantly inhibited B16 mouse melanoma growth and led to reductions in adrenal and gonadal weights.

—T. Narita & H. Kudo, ''Effect of Melatonin on B16 Melanoma Growth in Athymic Mice,'' *Cancer Research,* 45(9), September 1985, p. 4175-4177.

This study examined the effects of melatonin on the proliferation and induction of melanogenesis in rodent melanoma cells. Results showed low concentrations of melatonin inhibited cell growth, but had not melanogenesis. High melatonin doses had the exact opposite effect.

—A. Slominski & D. Pruski, "Melatonin Inhibits Proliferation and Melanogenesis in Rodent Melanoma Cells," *Exp Cell Res,* 206(2), June 1993, p. 189-194.

Results of this study found the melatonin injections inhibited growth and increased doubling time of the R3327H Dunning prostatic adenocarcinoma in rats.

—R. Philo & A.S. Berkowitz, "Inhibition of Dunning Tumor Growth by Melatonin," *Journal of Urology,* 139(5), May 1988, p. 1099-1102.

Results of this study showed that 2 mM of melatonin inhibited the growth of ME-180 human cervical cancer cells in vitro after 48 hours of treatment.

—L.D. Chen, et al., "Melatonin's Inhibitory Effect on Growth of ME-180 Human Cervical Cancer Cells is Not Related to Intracellular Glutathione Concentrations," *Cancer Letters,* 91(2), May 8, 1995, p. 153-159.

Results of this study found melatonin antogonoized tumor-promoting actions of estradiol in a rat model of mammary tumorignesis.

—D.E. Blask, et al., "Pineal Melatonin Inhibition of Tumor Promotion in the N-nitroso-N-methylurea Model of Mammary Carcinogenesis: Potential Involvement of Antiestrogenic Mechanisms in Vivo," *Journal of Cancer Res Clin Oncol,* 117(6), 1991, p. 526-532.

Results of this study showed that melatonin modulated mammary epithelium development, thus decreasing the incidence of spontaneous mammary tumor incidence in mice.

—A. Subramanian & L. Kothari, "Melatonin, A Suppressor of Spontaneous Murine Mammary Tumors," *Journal of Pineal Research,* 10(3), April 1991, p. 136-140.

This study examined the effects of 20 mg per day of intramuscular melatonin in cancer patients with metastatic solid tumor. Treatment was followed up with 10 oral mg per day in patients experiencing remission. Results indicated that melatonin had beneficial effects in such patients with respect to PS and quality of life.

—P. Lissoni, et al., "Endocrine and Immune Effects of Melatonin Therapy in Metastatic Cancer Patients," *European Journal of Cancer Clin Oncol,* 25(5), May 1989, p. 789-795.

Results of this study indicated that 20 mg per day of oral melatonin may be a factor involved in the treatment of chemotherapy-induced myelodysplatic syndrome in cancer patients.

—S. Viviani, et al., "Preliminary Studies on Melatonin in the Treatment of Myelodysplastic Syndromes Following Cancer Chemotherapy," *Journal of Pineal Research,* 8(4), 1990, p. 347-354.

Results of this study found melatonin to have antitumor effects on MtT/F4 tumors in rats.

—S. Chatterjee & T.K. Banerji, "Effects of Melatonin on the Growth of MtT/F4 Anterior Pituitary Tumor: Evidence for Inhibition of Tumor Growth Dependent Upon the Time of Administration," *Journal of Pineal Research,* 7(4), 1989, p. 381-391.

This review article examined the effects of melatonin by itself or coupled with interleukin-2 in cancer patients in studies published between 1986-1994. The authors conclude that melatonin offers protection against interleukin-2 and the two agents synergize in their anticancer effects.

—A. Conti & G.J. Maestroni, ''The Clinical Neuroimmunotherapeutic Role of Melatonin in Oncology,'' *Journal of Pineal Research,* 19(3), October 1995, p. 103-110.

In this study, 40 advanced melanoma patients were treated with daily doses of oral melatonin ranging from 5mg/m2 to 700 mg/m2. Results showed partial responses in 6 patients and stable disease in 6 others after 5 weeks of follow-up.

—R. Gonzalez, et al., ''Melatonin Therapy of Advanced Human Malignant Melanoma,'' *Melanoma Research,* 1(4), November-December 1991, p. 237-243.

In this study, human peripheral blood cells were treated increasing concentrations of melatonin (0.5 or 1.0 or 2.0 mM) for 20 min at 37 +/- 1 degrees C and then exposed to 150 cGy gamma-radiation from a 137Cs source. Results showed that lymphocytes pretreated with melatonin exhibited a significant reduction the frequency of radiation-induced chromosome damage relative to controls.

—Vijayalaxmi, et al., ''Melatonin Protects Human Blood Lymphocytes from Radiation-induced Chromosome Damage,'' *Mutat Research,* 346(1), January 1995, p. 23-31.

This study examined the effects of 20 mg per day of intramuscular melatonin in cancer patients with metastatic solid tumor. Treatment was followed up with 10 oral mg per day in patients experiencing remission. Results indicated that melatonin had beneficial effects in such patients with respect to performance status and quality of life.

—P. Lissoni, et al., ''Clinical Results with the Pineal Hormone Melatonin in Advanced Cancer Resistant to Standard Antitumor Therapies,'' *Oncology,* 48(6), 1991, p. 448-450.

Results of this study indicated that glutathione and glutathione transferase play a direct role in the mechanisms mediating the resistance of estrogen receptor humans breast cancer cells to melatonin.

—D.E. Blask & S.T. Wilson, ''Melatonin Suppression of Human Breast Cancer Growth in Vitro Involves Glutathione,'' *Proceedings of the Annual Meeting of the American Association of Cancer Researchers,* 36, 1995, p. A1514.

Cardiovascular/Coronary Heart Disease

Results of this study showed that the administration of melatonin modulated the functional status of voltage sensitive calcium channels in the heart of rats.

—L.D. Chen, et al., ''Melatonin Reduces 3H-nitrendipine Binding in the Heart,'' *Proceedings of the Society of Exp Biol Medicine,* 207(1), October 1994, p. 34-37.

This study examined the effects of 4 mg injections of melatonin per day over a period of 10-27 days in rats fed regular and high-cholesterol diets. Results showed that the melatonin countered the effects of high-cholesterol diet on plasma lipids and lipoproteins. Melatonin reduced fatty infiltration in the liver of rats on a high-cholesterol diet as well.

—N. Mori, et al., ''Anti-hypercholesterolemic Effect of Melatonin in Rats,'' *Acta Pathol Jpn,* 39(10), October 1989, p. 613-618.

Results of this study showed that melatonin infused i.p. at a dose of 6 mg/rat per day for 5 days exhibited a antihypertensive in spontaneously hypertensive rats.

—K. Kawashima, et al., ''Antihypertensive Action of Melatonin in the Spontaneously Hypertensive Rat,'' *Clinical Exp Hypertens,* 9(7), 1987, p. 1121-1131.

Results of this study showed that melatonin produced a dose-dependent relaxation of precontracted of the isolated rat aorta and that such actions may be due in part to an interaction with perivascular nerve terminals.

—L.B. Weekley, ''Pharmacologic Studies on the Mechanism of Melatonin-induced Vasorelaxation in Rat Aorta,'' *Journal of Pineal Research,* 19(3), October 1995, p. 133-138.

Results of this study showed that the administration of melatonin produced a dose-dependent relaxation of precontracted pulmonary vein and artery.

—L. B. Weekley, ''Effects of Melatonin on Isolated Pulmonary Artery and Vein: Role of the Vascular Endothelium,'' *Pulm Pharmacol,* 6(2), June 1993, p. 149-154.

Colitis

Results of this study showed that the daily administration of intraperitoneal melatonin to mice reduced the severity of dextran sodium-induced colitis.

—P.T. Pentney & G.A. ''Melatonin Reduces the Severity of Dextran-induced Colitis in Mice,'' *Journal of Pineal Research,* 19(1), August 1995, p. 31-39.

Diabetes

Results of this study showed that melatonin supplementation decreased glucose tolerance in rabbits and most likely influenced blood glucose circadian rhythm via its impact on insulin release by pancreatic B cells.

—M. Dhar, et al., ''Effect of Melatonin on Glucose Tolerance and Blood Glucose Circadian Rhythm in Rabbits,'' *Indian Journal of Physiol Pharmacol,* 27(2), April-June 1983, p. 109-117

Encephalitis

This study examined the melatonin's effects on viral encephalitis in mice. Results showed that the daily administration of melatonin beginning 3 days prior and lasting through 10 after exposure to the virus significantly delayed disease onset and death.

—D. Ben-Nathan, et al., ''Protective Effects of Melatonin in Mice Infected with Encephalitis Viruses,'' *Arch Virol,* 140(2), 1995, p. 223-230.

Epilepsy

Results of this study showed that subcutaneous melatonin had an ameliorative effect on pinealectomy-induce seizures in gerbils.

—P.K. Rudeen, et al., ''Antiepileptic Effects of Melatonin in the Pinealectomized Mongolian Gerbil,'' *Epilepsia,* 21(2), April 1980, p. 149-154.

Gastric Lesions

Results of this study showed that prior melatonin administration produced a significant reduction in gastric ulceration in rats.

—R. Khan, et al., "The Effect of Melatonin on the Formation of Gastric Stress Lesions in Rats," *Experientia,* 46(1), January 15, 1990, p. 88-89.

Results of this study found that supplemental melatonin protected gastric mucosa from ischemia/reperfusion–induced damage in rats.

—P.C. Konturek, et al., "Melatonin Affords Protection against Gastric Lesions Induced by Ischemia-Reperfusion Possibly Due to its Antioxidant and Mucosal Microcirculatory Effects," *European Journal of Pharmacology,* 322, 1997, p. 73-77.

General

This study looked at the effects of daily melatonin administration on rats with disrupted circadian activity and drinking rhythms under constant light. Results showed that the treatment did either synchronize or at least partly synchronize disrupted circadian patterns.

—M.J. Chesworth, et al., "Effects of Daily Melatonin Injections on Activity Rhythms of Rats in Constant Light," *American Journal of Physiol,* 253(1 Pt 2), July 1987, p. R101-107.

In this study, rats received 10 mg/kg kainate i.p. which produced brain injury of the hippocampus, the amygdala, and the pyriform cortex. 2.5 mg/kg of melatonin was injected into the rats 20 minutes prior to kainate, right after, and 1-2 hours after. Results showed that the cumulative dose of 10 mg/kg of melatonin prevented kainate-induced behavioral and biochemical disturbances and neuronal death.

—P. Giusti, et al., "Neuroprotection by Melatonin from Kainate-induced Excitotoxicity in Rats," *FASEB Journal,* 10(8), June 1996, p. 891-896.

This study examined the effects of melatonin on porphyrins-induced cell damage in the Harderian gland of Syrian hamsters. Results found that melatonin produced cytoprotectives effect by inhibiting the ALA-S gene expression and by raising the mRNA levels for several antioxidant enzymes.

—I. Antolin, et al., "Neurohormone Melatonin Prevents Cell Damage: Effect on Gene Expression for Antioxidant Enzymes," *FASEB Journal,* 10(8), June 1996, p. 882-890.

This study compared the peroxyl radical scavenger ability of melatonin to that of vitamin E, vitamin C and reduced glutathione. Results showed melatonin to be twice as active as vitamin E which is though to be to be the most powerful lipophilic antioxidant.

—C. Pieri, et al., "Melatonin: A Peroxyl Radical Scavenger More Effective than Vitamin E," *Life Sci,* 55(15), 1994, p. PL271-PL276.

Results of this study showed that the administration of melatonin provided protection against H_2O_2-induced lipid peroxidation of brain homogenates in vitro.

—E. Sewerynek, et al., "H2O2-induced Lipid Peroxidation in Rat Brain Homogenates is Greatly Reduced by Melatonin," *Neurosci Lett,* 195(3), August 11, 1995, p. 203-205.

In this study, mice received intraperitoneally melatonin in doses ranging from 100 to 450 mg/kg. Results showed that such treatment proved plasma glucose increase due to alloxan-induced pancreatic toxicity.

—G. Pierrefiche, et al., "Antioxidant Activity of Melatonin in Mice," *Res Commun Chem Pathol Pharmacol,* 80(2), May 1993, p. 211-223.

Immune Enhancement

Results of this study found that exogenous melatonin totally counteracted the effects of acute anxiety-restraint stress on thymus weight and antibody response to sheep red blood cells.

—G.J. Maestroni, et al., "Role of the Pineal Gland in Immunity. III. Melatonin Antagonizes the Immunosuppressive Effect of Acute Stress via an Opiatergic Mechanism," *Immunology,* 63(3), March 1988, p. 465-469.

Results of this study showed that melatonin restored the depressed immune function following soft-tissue trauma and hemorrhagic shock in mice.

—M.W. Wichmann, et al., "Melatonin Administration Attenuates Depressed Immune Functions Trauma-Hemorrhage," *Journal of Surgical Research,* 63(1), June 1996, p. 256-262.

Results of this study showed that the chronic injection of melatonin into either young mice or those suffering from aging-induced immunodepression or immunodepression due to treatment with cyclophosphmide enhanced antibody response to a T-dependent antigen.

—M.C. Caroleo, et al., "Melatonin Restores Immunodepression in Aged and Cyclophosphamide-treated Mice," *Annals of the New York Academy of Science,* 719, May 31, 1994, p. 343-352.

Results of this study showed that the chronic injection of melatonin into young or immunodepressed mice can be an effective therapy for immunodepressive conditions.

—M.C. Caroleo, et al., "Melatonin as Immunomodulator in Immunodeficient Mice," *Immunopharmacology,* 23(2), March-April 1992, p. 81-89.

Jet Lag

Results of this double-blind, placebo-controlled study found that 5 mg of melatonin three days prior to flight, during flight, and once a day for three days after flight alleviated jet lag and fatigue in healthy volunteers.

—K. Petrie, et al., "Effect of Melatonin on Jet Lag after Long Haul Flights," *BMJ,* 298(6675), March 18, 1989, p. 705-707.

Results of this double-blind, placebo-controlled study found that 5 mg of melatonin three days prior to flight, during flight, and once a day for three days after flight alleviated jet lag and fatigue in healthy volunteers.

—K. Petrie, et al., "A Double-blind Trial of Melatonin as a Treatment for Jet Lag in International Cabin Crew," *Biological Psychiatry,* 33(7), April 1, 1993, p. 526-530.

Reproductive Function

Results of this study showed that male and female hamsters treated with melatonin experienced a prevention in reproductive organ atrophy associated with the reduced day length of winter.

> —R.J. Reiter, et al., "Prevention by Melatonin of Short Day Induced Atrophy of the Reproductive Systems of Male and Female Hamsters," *Acta Endocrinol,* 84(2), February 1977, p. 410-418.

Results of this study showed that melatonin exerted a suppressive effect on baboon dispersed luteal cell P production.

> —F.S. Khan-Dawood & M.Y. Dawood, "Baboon Corpus Luteum: The Effect of Melatonin on In Vitro Progesterone Production," *Fertil Steril,* 59(4), April 1993, p. 896-900.

Results of this study showed that melatonin administered in high doses inhibited mammary development in mice.

> —E.J. Sanchez-Barcelo, et al., "Influence of Melatonin on Mammary Gland Growth: In Vivo and In Vitro Studies," *Proc Soc Exp Biol Med,* 194(2), June 1990, p. 103-107.

Shock

Results of this study showed that a single melatonin injection protected mice treated from lethal doses of lipolysaccharide, suggesting its usefulness as a potential therapy for septic shock.

> —G.J. Maestroni, "Melatonin as a Therapeutic Agent in Experimental Endotoxic Shock," *Journal of Pineal Research,* 20(2), March 1996, p. 84-89.

This study examined the anticonvulsant effects of melatonin in male gerbils. Results showed that daily injection of 25 mg of melatonin for 10 weeks reduced both the incidence and severity of seizures associated with exposure to pentylenetetrazol.

> —T.H. Champney & J.A. Champney, "Novel Anticonvulsant Action of Chronic Melatonin in Gerbils," *Neuroreport,* 3(12), December 1992, p. 1152-1154.

Sleep

This article reports on the case of a severely mentally retarded 9-year-old boy with chronic sleep/wake disturbance. Melatonin given at 6:00 pm normalized the sleep/wake pattern and entrained the endogenous rhythm to a normalized 24-hour chronological day.

> —L. Palm, et al., "Correction of Non-24-hour Sleep/wake Cycle by Melatonin in a Blind Retarded Boy," *Ann Neurol,* 29(3), March 1991, p. 336-339.

In this double-blind, placebo-controlled study, healthy volunteers received either 0.3 or 1.0 mg of melatonin at 6, 8, or 9 PM. Results showed that either doses given at either time reduced sleep onset latency.

> —I.V. Zhdanova, et al., "Sleep-inducing Effects of Low Doses of Melatonin Ingested in the Evening," *Clin Pharmacol Therapy,* 57(5), 1995, p. 552-558.

This double-blind, placebo-controlled study examined the effects of 5 mg of melatonin for four weeks on the sleep/wake cycle in 8 patients with a delayed sleep phase syndrome. Results showed significantly earlier sleep onset time and wake time relative to controls.

    —M. Dahlitz, et al., "Delayed Sleep Phase Syndrome Response to Melatonin," *Lancet,* 337(8750), May 11, 1991, p. 1121-1124.

Results of this double-blind, placebo-controlled study showed that 2 mg per night of controlled-release melatonin for 3 weeks significantly improved sleep quality in elderly subjects.

    —D. Garfinkel, et al., "Improvement of Sleep Quality in Elderly People by Controlled-release Melatonin," *Lancet,* 346(8974), August 26, 1995, p. 541-544.

This article reports on the case of a child with a germ cell tumor involving the pineal region experiencing a melatonin secretion suppression associated with severe insomnia. Supplementation with 3 mg per night for 2 weeks normalized sleep.

    —A. Etzioni, et al., "Melatonin Replacement Corrects Sleep Disturbances in a Child with Pineal Tumor," *Neurology,* 46(1), January 1996, p. 261-263.

This double-blind, placebo-controlled study examined the effects of 75 mg per os of melatonin administered nightly at 10 PM on total sleep time and daytime alertness of chronic insomniacs. Results showed a significant increase in the subjective assessment of total sleep time and daytime alertness relative to controls.

    —J.G. MacFarlane, et al., "The Effects of Exogenous Melatonin on the Total Sleep Time and Daytime Alertness of Chronic Insomniacs: A Preliminary Study," *Biological Psychiatry,* 30(4), August 15, 1991, p. 371-376.

Results of this double-blind, placebo-controlled study showed that 5 mg per night of melatonin had positive effects with respect to sleep and alertness on police officers working successive night shifts.

    —S. Folkard, et al., "Can Melatonin Improve Shift Workers' Tolerance of the Night Shift? Some Preliminary Findings," *Chronobiol Int,* 10(5), October 1993, p. 315-320.

In this study, 15 disabled children with severe, chronic sleep disorders received 2 to 10 mg of oral melatonin. Results showed significant positive effects.

    —J.E. Jan, et al., "The Treatment of Sleep Disorders with Melatonin," *Dev Med Child Neurol,* 36(2), February 1994, p. 97-107.

In this double-blind, placebo-controlled study, 20 healthy volunteers underwent artificially-induced insomnia and were treated with melatonin. Results showed that the administration of melatonin at bedtime reduced the time the subjects were awake before sleep onset, sleep latency, and the number of awakenings during the total sleep period, while it the efficiency of sleep.

    —F. Waldhauser, et al., "Sleep Laboratory Investigations on Hypnotic Properties of Melatonin," *Psychopharmacology,* 100(2), 1990, p. 222-226.

This double-blind, placebo-controlled study examined the hypnotic effects of 5 mg of melatonin in healthy, young adults. Results showed that melatonin significantly increased sleep propensity, the spectral power in the theta, delta and spindles bands, and subjective sleepiness while significantly reducing the power in the alpha and beta bands and oral temperature.

> —O. Tzischinsky & P. Lavie, "Melatonin Possesses Time-dependent Hypnotic Effects," *Sleep,* 17(7), October 1994, p. 638-645.

This double-blind, placebo-controlled study examined the effects of melatonin replacement therapy on melatonin-deficient elderly insomniacs. Subject received 2 mg tablets of melatonin for 7 consecutive days 2 hours prior to going to bed. During another phase of the study, subjects received 1 mg of sustained-release melatonin each night at bedtime for 2 months. Results showed that 1-week treatment with 2 mg sustained-release melatonin was effective for sleep maintenance, while sleep initiation was improved by the fast-release melatonin. Such effects were increased following the 2-month 1-mg sustained-release melatonin treatment.

> —I, Haimov, et al., "Melatonin Replacement Therapy of Elderly Insomniacs," *Sleep,* 18(7), September 1995, p. 598-603.

Uterine Contraction

Results of this study showed that melatonin administration inhibited carbochol-provoked uterine contraction in rats.

> —A.G. Rillo, et al., [Uterine Contraction Induced by Carbachol is Inhibited by Melatonin], *Ginecol Obstet Mex,* 61, February 1993, p. 40-44.

Vision

This study examined the effects of 4 mg/kg per day of melatonin on the formation of cataracts in newborn rats. Results showed that the treatment led to a reduction in cataract formation.

> —M. Abe, et al., "Inhibitory Effect of Melatonin on Cataract Formation in Newborn Rats: Evidence for an Antioxidative Role for Melatonin," *Journal of Pineal Research,* 17(2), September 1994, p. 94-100.

Results of this study showed that the administration of melatonin reduced intraocular pressure in human subjects with few side effects.

> —J.R. Samples, et al., "Effect of Melatonin on Intraocular Pressure," *Current Eye Research,* 7(7), July 1988, p. 649-653.

■ MOLYBDENUM

Cancer

This study examined molybdenum and selenium sediment levels in relation to cancer mortality levels in a Japanese population. Results showed inverse correlations between molybdenum levels and rates of esophageal and rectal cancer mortality in women. No such correlations were found with selenium.

> —H. Nakadaira, et al., "Distribution of Selenium and Molybdenum and Cancer Mortality in Niigata, Japan," *Arch Environ Health,* 50(5), October-September 1995, p. 374-380.

This study examined the effects of molybdenum on esophageal cancer in rats. Results showed significant reductions in both tumor incidence and development in the esophagus of rats fed a diet high in molybdenum relative to those fed low-molybedenum diets.

> —H. Komada, et al., "Effect of Dietary Molybdenum on Esophageal Carcinogenesis in Rats Induced by N-methyl-N-benzylnitrosamine," *Cancer Research,* 50(8), April 15, 1990, p. 2418-2222.

Results of this study showed that female rats fed a diet containing 10 ppm molybdenum experienced a significantly lower rate of chemical-induced mammary carcinoma relative to controls.

> —H.J. Wei, et al., "Effects of Molybdenum and Tungsten on Mammary Carcinogenesis in SD Rats," *Journal of National Cancer Institute,* 74(2), February 1985, p. 469-473.

Results of this study showed that the dietary intake of molybdenum significantly inhibited chemical-induced cancer of the esophagus and forestomach in rats.

> —X.M. Luo, et al., "Inhibitory Effects of Molybdenum on Esophageal and Forestomach Carcinogenesis in Rats," *Journal of the National Cancer Institute,* 71(1), July 1983, p. 75-80.

Results of this study showed that the supplementation of 10 mg/L of molybdenum via drinking water led to the inhibition of mammary cancer in rats.

> —C.D. Seaborn & S.P. Yang, "Effect of Molybdenum Supplementation on N-nitroso-N-methylurea-induced Mammary Carcinogenesis and Molybdenum Excretion in Rats," *Biol Trace Elem Res,* 39(2-3), November-December 1993, p. 245-256.

Results of this study showed that molybdenum had inhibitory effects on mammary carcinogenesis and tumor growth in rats

> —H.J. Wei, et al., [Effect of Molybdenum and Tungsten on Mammary Carcinogenesis in Sprague-Dawley (SD) Rats], *Chung Hua Chung Liu Tsa Chih,* 9(3), May 1987, p. 204-207.

Results of this study indicated that molybdenum can serve as a chemopreventive agent against mammary cancer in rats.

> —R.G. Mehta, et al., "Prevention of Rat Mammary Carcinogenesis by Molybdenum," *Proceedings of the Annual Meeting of the American Association of Cancer Researchers,* 33, 1992, p. A1012.

Results of this study showed that intake of both riboflavin and molybdenum reduced esophageal and forestomach carcinoma incidence and papilloma multiplicity of the organs in rats.

> —V.G. Bespalov, et al., [The Effect of Riboflavin, Molybdenum, Selenium and Zinc on the Development of Induced Tumors of the Esophagus and Forestomach in Rats], *Vopr Onkol,* 36(5), 1990, p. 559-563.

Results of this study showed that the administration of 75 to 100 mg/kg following the injection of Ehrlich acites tumor cells in mice led to a 100% rate of inhibition for up to 30 days.

> —P. Kopf-Maier, et al., [Molybdocene Dichloride as an Antitumor Agent], Z *Naturforsch,* 34(12), December 1979, p. 1174-1176.

Lead Intoxication

Results of this study showed that sodium molybate had a significant impact on the prevention of plumbism in rats.

>—S.J. Flora, et al., "Preventive Effects of Sodium Molybdate in Lead Intoxication in Rats," *Ecotoxicol Environ Safety*, 26(2), October 1993, p. 133-137.

■ NAC

Adult Respiratory Distress Syndrome

In this double-blind, placebo-controlled study, 16 patients in the beginning phase of adult respiratory disorder syndrome received NAC. Results showed the treatment, started within eight hours of diagnosis, increased the intracellular GSH in the granulocytes without decreasing spontaneous oxidant production.

>—T. Laurent, et al., "Oxidant-antioxidant Balance in Granulocytes During ARDS. Effect of N-cetylcysteine," *Chest*, 109(1), January 1996, p. 163-166.

Results of this study found that NAC administered to sheep significantly attenuated all monitored pathophysiological changes in the endotoxin model of ARDS.

>—G.R. Bernard, et al., "Effect of N-acetylcysteine on the Pulmonary Response to Endotoxin in the Awake Sheep and Upon in Vitro Granulocyte Function," *Journal of Clinical Investigation*, 73(6), June 1984, p. 1772-1784.

Results of this series of clinical trials found that ARDS patients experienced relief in common symptoms such as depressed plasma and red cell glutathione concentrations following treatment with intravenous NAC. NAC treatment also showed measurable effects with respect to increase oxygen delivery, improved lung compliance and resolution of pulmonary oedema.

>—G.R. Bernard, "Potential of N-acetylcysteine as Treatment for the Adult Respiratory Distress Syndrome," *European Respiratory Journal Supplement*, 11, October 1990, p. 496s-498s.

Results of this study showed that NAC produced significant preventive effects in a microembolism rat model of ARDS.

>—T. Wegener, et al., "Effect of N-acetylcysteine on Pulmonary Damage Due to Microembolism in the Rat," *European Journal of Respiratory Disease*, 70(4), April 1987, p. 205-212.

Results of this study showed that the administration of NAC in vivo significantly ameliorated ARDS-like lung injury in rats.

>—C.O. Feddersen, et al., [N-acetylcysteine Decreases Functional and Structural, ARDS-typical Lung Changes in Endotoxin-treated Rats], *Med Klin*, 88(4), April 15, 1993, p. 197-206.

AIDS/HIV

Results of this study showed that the oral administration of N-acetylcysteine increased cysteine and glutathione concentrations in mononuclear cells of HIV patients.

>—B. de Quay, et al., "Glutathione Depletion in HIV-infected Patients: Role of Cysteine Deficiency and Effect of Oral N-acetylcysteine," *AIDS*, 6(8), August 1992, p. 815-819.

Results of this study indicated that the administration of NAC enhanced the number of CD4+ T cells in patients infected with HIV due to its ability to increase glutathione levels.

> —R. Kinscherf, et al., "Effect of Glutathione Depletion and Oral N-acetyl-cysteine Treatment on CD4+ and CD8+ Cells," *FASEB Journal,* 8(6), April 1, 1994, p. 448-451.

This case-control study examined the effects of NAC and glutathione on neutrophil and mononuclear cell cytotoxicity in HIV-infected patients. Results showed that 1 and 5 mM NAC partially reversed BCNU-induced intracellular glutathione depletion and antibody-dependent cellular cytotoxity of neutrophils in both controls and HIV patients.

> —R.L. Roberts, et al., "N-acetylcysteine Enhances Antibody-dependent Cellular Cytotoxicity in Neutrophils and Mononuclear Cells from Healthy Adults and Human Immunodeficiency Virus-infected Patients," *Journal of Infectious Disease,* 172(6), December 1995, p. 1492-1502.

This study examined the effects of NAC and GSH on the replication of HIV-1 primary monocyte/macrophages cultured in vitro. Results showed that both GSH and 5-20 mM of NAC significantly reduced HIV infection.

> —W.Z. Ho & S.D. Douglas, "Glutathione and N-acetylcysteine Suppression of Human Immunodeficiency Virus Replication in Human Monocyte/macrophages in Vitro," *AIDS Research Hum Retroviruses,* 8(7), July 1992, p. 1249-1253.

This review article cites studies indicating that NAC can block the expression of HIV in infection models as well as replication in normal peripheral blood mononuclear cells.

> —M. Roederer, et al., "N-acetylcysteine: A New Approach to Anti-HIV Therapy," *AIDS Research and Human Retroviruses,* 8(2), February 1992, p. 209-217.

Results of this found NAC to be a more powerful antiviral agent than oxothiazolide with respect to HIV.

> —P.A. Raju, et al., "Glutathione Precursor and Antioxidant Activities of N-acetylcysteine and Oxothiazolidine Carboxylate Compared in Vitro Studies of HIV Replication," *AIDS Research and Human Retroviruses,* 10(8), August 1994, p. 961-967.

This article reports on findings from a Stanford University double-blind, placebo-controlled study of 200 volunteers who were HIV positive. Results showed the administration of NAC increased glutathione levels and, in turn, may have enhanced survival rates.

> —J.S. James, "NAC: First Controlled Trial, Positive Results," *AIDS Treat News,* 250, July 5, 1996, p. 1-3.

This study examined the safety of NAC on patients infected with HIV over a 14 week period. Patients with under 500 CD4 cells/mm3 received either 6 weeks of NAC doses of 3.7, 11, 33 and 100 mg/kg IV tiw or 6 weeks of oral doses of 600, 1200, 2400 and 4800 mg qd. Results showed no major side effects and found NAC to be safe at the doses noted above.

> —R.E. Walker, et al., "The Safety, Pharmacokinetics, and Antiviral Activity of N-acetylcysteine in HIV-Infected Individuals," *International Conference on AIDS,* 8(1), July 19-24, 1992, Mo8.

Results of this study found that NAC enhanced T cell function and growth dramatically in culture.
>—E. ylar, et al., ''N-acetylcysteine Enhances T Cell Functions and T Cell Growth in Culture,'' *Int Immunol,* 5(1), January 1993, p. 97-101.

This review article notes that N-acetylcysteine has been shown to inhibit inflammatory stimulations such as HIV replication and replinishes glutathione depletion in vivo.
>—M. Roederer, et al., ''N-acetylcysteine: Potential for AIDS Therapy,'' *Pharmacology,* 46(3), 1993, p. 121-129.

Results of this study found that NAC inhibited the tumor necrosis factor alpha- or phorbol ester-stimulated replication of HIV in acutely infected cell cultures, while it also inhibits the cytokine-enhanced HIV long terminal repeat-directed expression of beta-galactosidase in vitro HIV model systems.
>—M. Roederer, et al., ''Cytokine-stimulated Human Immunodeficiency Virus Replication is Inhibited by N-acetyl-L-cysteine,'' *Proceedings of the National Academy of Sciences,* 87(12), June 1990, p. 4884-4888.

Brain Function

Results of this study indicated that treatment with NAC had beneficial effects on oxygen free radical-mediated brain injury in cats.
>—E.F. Ellis, et al., ''Restoration of Cerebrovascular Responsiveness to Hyperventilation by the Oxygen Radical Scavenger N-acetylcysteine Following Experimental Traumatic Brain Injury,'' *Journal of Neurosurg,* 75(5), November 1991, p. 774-749.

Cancer

Results of this study showed that NAC and ascorbic acid each demonstrated protective effects against mutagen-induced chomosomal damage in vitro.
>—Z. Trizna, et al., ''Effects of N-acetyl-L-cysteine and Ascorbic Acid on Mutagen-induced Chromosomal Sensitivity in Patients with Head and Neck Cancers,'' *American Journal of Surgery,* 162(4), October 1991, p. 294-298.

Results of this study showed that NAC administration significantly reduced mtDNA adducts in the liver and lung of rats exposed to cigarette smoke and in the liver of those treated with 2-acetylaminofluorene.
>—R. Balansky, et al., ''Induction by Carcinogens and Chemoprevention by N-acetylcysteine of Adducts to Mitochondrial DNA in Rat Organs,'' *Cancer Research,* 56(7), April 1, 1996, p. 1642-1647.

This review article discusses NAC's role as an antidote to acetaminophen poisoning as well as its chemopreventive properties.
>—N. van Zandwijk, ''N-acetylcysteine for Lung Cancer Prevention,'' *Chest,* 107(5), May 1995, p. 1437-1441.

Results of this study showed that NAC served as an effective adjunct to increase the antitumor activity of IL-2/LAK therapy in mice.
>—C.Y. Yim, et al., ''Use of N-acetyl Cysteine to Increase Intracellular Glutathione During

the Induction of Antitumor Responses by IL-2,'' *Journal of Immunology,* 152(12), June 15, 1994, p. 5796-805.

Results of this study found NAC capable of protecting against mutagenic potential of environmental clastogens/mutagens in vitro.

—R. Barale, et al., ''N-Acetylcysteine Inhibits Environmental Pollutant Gentotoxicity in Vitro,'' *Third International Conference on Mechanisms of Antimutagenesis and Anticarcinogenesis. May 5-10, 1991, Lucca, Italy, 1991,* 12, 1991.

This review article cites studies over the past decade showing NAC inhibits spontaneous mutagenicity and chemical-induced mutagenicity resulting from various sources. NAC has also been shown to significantly reduce the incidence of neoplastic and preneoplastic lesions induced by various chemical carcinogens in rodents.

—S. De Flora, et al., ''N-acetyl-Cysteine for Cancer Chemoprevention: The Experimental Background,'' *CCPC-93: Second International Cancer Chemo Prevention Conference. April 28-30, 1993, Berlin, Germany, 1993,* 32, 1993.

Results of this study showed that the administration of NAC produced significant protective effects against the cigarette smoke-induced alterations of bronchoalveolar lavage cellularity as well as the increased of miconucleated pulmonary alveolar macrophages, and bone marrow cytotoxicity in rats.

—R.B. Balansky, et al., ''Protection by N-acetylcysteine of the Histopathological and Cytogenetical Damage Produced by Exposure of Rats to Cigarette Smoke,'' *Cancer Letters,* 64(2), June 15, 1992, p. 123-131.

Results of this study found that NAC had protective effects against DMH carcinogenic activity—reducing intestinal tumor activity in rats, significantly decreasing colic tumor yield colic, and inducing a shift from distal to more proximal sites with respect to location of colon carcinomas.

—M. Wilpart, et al., ''Anti-initiation Activity of N-acetylcysteine in Experimental Colonic Carcinogenesis,'' *Cancer Letters,* 31(3), June 1986, p. 319-324.

Results of this study showed that NAC protected mice against lipopolysaccharide toxicity as well as inhibited the increase in serum tumor necrosis factor levels in mice treated with lipopolysaccarhides. Results also found NAC inhibited tumor necrosis factor production and hepatotoxicity in lipopolysaccarhides-treated mice in association with a sensitizing dose of Actinomycin D.

—P. Peristeris, et al., ''N-acetylcysteine and Glutathione as Inhibitors of Tumor Necrosis Factor Production,'' *Cell Immunology,* 140(2), April 1992, p. 390-399.

Results of this study showed that NAC administration had beneficial effects on tumor cell invasion and metastasis of malignant cells in vitro.

—A. Albini, et al., ''Inhibition of Invasion, Gelatinase Activity, Tumor Take and Metastasis of Malignant Cells by N-acetylcysteine,'' *International Journal of Cancer,* 61(1), March 29, 1995, p. 121-129.

Results of this study indicated that the administration of PZ-51 by itself or coupled with NAC moderated Adriamycin's aerobic toxicity in vitro while having no effect on its hypoxic toxicity.

—C.A. Pritsos, ''Protective Effect of N-acetylcysteine (NAC) and PZ-51 (EBSELEN) Against

Adriamycin Toxicity,'' *Proceedings of the Annual Meeting of the American Association of Cancer Researchers, 31, 1990,* p. A2406.

Results of this study showed that the administration of NAC significantly inhibited chemical-induced lung tumors in mice.

—S. De Flora, et al., "Metabolic, Desmutagenic and Anticarcinogenic Effects of N-acetylcysteine," *Respiration,* 50(Suppl 1), 1986, p. 43-49.

This study examined the protective effects of NAC on skin reaction in patients receiving radiation therapy. Results showed that those patients receiving NAC required no analgesics for pain, recovered quicker and had less severe reactions relative to controls.

—J.A. Kim, et al., "Topical Use of N-Acetylcysteine for Reduction of Skin Reaction to Radiation Therapy," *Semin Oncol,* 10(1,Suppl1), 1983, p. 86-88.

Results of this study found NAC capable of inhibiting cycylophosphamide-induced hemorrhagic cystitis without compromising antitumor or immunosuppressive activity in rats and mice.

—L. Levy & D.L. Vredevoe, "The Effect of N-acetylcysteine on Cyclophosphamide Immuno-regulation and Antitumor Activity," *Semin Oncology,* 10(1,Suppl1), 1983, p. 7-16.

Cardiovascular/Coronary Heart Disease

Results of this study found NAC elevated bovine pulmonary artery endothelial cell glutathione following in vitro incubation, prompting the authors to suggest it may be an effective agent for elevating glutathione of the pulmonary vasculature as a means of providing against oxidant stress.

—D.T. Phelps, et al., "Elevation of Glutathione Levels in Bovine Pulmonary Artery Endothe-lial Cells by N-acetylcysteine," *American Journal of Respiratory Cell Mol Biol,* 7(3), September 1992, p. 293-299.

Results of this double-blind, placebo-controlled study found that the administration of 150 mg/kg-1 of NAC significantly increased cardiac output and reduced systemic vascular resistance in patients requiring hemodynamic monitoring due to sepsis syndrome.

—K. Reinhart, et al., "N-acetylcysteine Preserves Oxygen Consumption and Gastric Mucosal pH During Hyperoxic Ventilation," *American Journal of Respiratory Critical Care Medicine,* 151(3 Pt 1), March 1995, p. 773-779.

Results of this study showed that reduced thiol NAC potentiated platelet inhibition by endothelium-derived relaxing factor in bovine aortic endothelial cells.

—J. Stamler, et al., "N-acetylcysteine Potentiates Platelet Inhibition by Endothelium-derived Relaxing Factor," *Circulatory Research,* 65(3), September 1989, p. 789-795.

Results of this study found that the intravenous administration of 2 g of NAC over 15 minutes followed by 5 mg/kg/hr coupled with intravenous isosorbide denitrate led to partial prevention of antianginal effect tolerance often associated with isosorbide treatment alone in anginal patients.

—S. Boesgaard, et al., "Preventive Administration of Intravenous N-acetylcysteine and Devel-opment of Tolerance to Isosorbide Dinitrate in Patients with Angina Pectoris," *Circulation,* 85(1), January 1992, p. 143-149.

Results of this study showed that the intravenous administration of 100 mg/kg of NAC potentiated nitroglycerin-induced vasodilater effects in patients undergoing cardiac catheterization for chest pain investigation. No such effects were seen among controls.

> —J.D. Horowitz, et al., "Potentiation of the Cardiovascular Effects of Nitroglycerin by N-acetylcysteine," *Circulation,* 68(6), December 1993, p. 1247-1253.

Results of this study found that the administration of NAC prior to reperfusion decreased myocardial stunning following reperfusion in rats.

> —M.B. Forman, et al., "Glutathione Redox Pathway and Reperfusion Injury. Effect of N-acetylcysteine on Infarct Size and Ventricular Function," *Circulation,* 78(1), July 1988, p. 202-213.

In this study, acute myocardial infarction patients were treated with either 15 g of intravenous NAC over a 24-hour period coupled with intravenous nitroglycerin. Results showed the treatment to be a safe and was associated with significant reductions in levels of oxidative controls relative to controls. Results also showed a trend toward improved preservation of the left ventricular function as well more rapid reperfusion.

> —M.A. Arstall, et al., "N-acetylcysteine in Combination with Nitroglycerin and Streptokinase for the Treatment of Evolving Acute Myocardial Infarction. Safety and Biochemical Effects," *Circulation,* 92(10), November 15, 1995, p. 2855-2862.

This double-blind, placebo-controlled study examined the effects of 0.1 microgram/kg per min intravenous nitroglycerin alone and coupled with 2 g of intravenous N-acetylcysteine followed by 5 mg/kg per hour on human veins, peripheral arteries, and microcirculation. Results showed the two agents together potentiated and preserved nitroglycerin-induced venodilation and augmented nitroglycerin's effects on small resistance vessels without influencing the response to nitroglycerin in middle-sized arteries.

> —S. Boesgaard, et al., "Altered Peripheral Vasodilator Profile of Nitroglycerin During Long-term Infusion of N-acetylcysteine," *Journal of the American College of Cardiol,* 23(1), January 1994, p. 163-169.

Results of this study showed that NAC potentiated platelet aggregation inhibition by nitroglycerin in vivo.

> —J. Loscalzo, "N-Acetylcysteine Potentiates Inhibition of Platelet Aggregation by Nitroglycerin," *Journal of Clinical Investigations,* 76(2), August 1985, p. 703-708.

Results of this study found NAC added to cardioplegic solution led to improvements in postarrest recovery of function, increasing the capacity of reperfused myocardium to handle the postischemic burst of free radical production in a rat heart model.

> —P. Menasche, et al., "Maintenance of the Myocardial Thiol Pool by N-acetylcysteine. An Effective Means of Improving Cardioplegic Protection," *Journal of Thoracic Cardiovascular Surgery,* 103(5), May 1992, p. 936-944.

This double-blind, placebo-controlled study examined the effects of pretreatment of cardiac risk patients with the 150 mg/kg NAC onVO2 and other clinical indicators of tissue oxygenation. Results showed that the NAC worked to preserve VO2, oxygen delivery, CI, LVSWI and PvaCO2 during brief hyperoxia and prevented clinical signs of myocardial ischemia.

> —C. Spies, et al., [The Effect of Prophylactically Administered N-acetylcysteine on Clinical Indicators for Tissue Oxygenation During Hyperoxic Ventilation in Cardiac Risk Patients], *Anaesthesist,* 45(4), April 1996, p. 343-350.

This study examined the effects of NAC on percutaneous transluminal angioplasty associated injury in rabbits. Results showed the treatment to be effective in the prevention of vessel damage caused by vessel damage.

> —H. Mass, et al., "N-acetylcysteine Diminishes Injury Induced by Balloon Angioplasty of the Carotid Artery in Rabbits," *Biochem Biophys Res Commun,* 215(2), October 13, 1995, p. 613-618.

This study examined the effects of NAC on vulnerability of heart arrhythmias and mechanical function during reperfusion and ischemia in rats. Results found that the incidences of ischemia-induced ventricular premature beats and ventricular tachycardia decreased from 93% and 67%, among controls to 40% and 27% with 8 microM of NAC, to 33% and 27% with 80 microM NAC, and to 40% and 13% with 2000 microM NAC. Incidence of ventricular fibrillation induced by reperfusion decreased from 93% to 60%, 67% and 47%, respectively. NAC delayed onset time of arrhthymias during ischemia and reperfusion.

> —Y. Qiu, et al., "The Influence of N-acetylcysteine on Cardiac Function and Rhythm Disorders During Ischemia and Reperfusion," *Cardioscience,* 1(1), March 1990, p. 65-74.

Results of this double-blind, placebo-controlled study found that the combination of intravenous NAC (5g 6 hourly) and nitroglycerine and unstable angina pectoris patients augmentes nitroglycerine's clinical benefits primarily by decreased acute myocardial infarction incidence.

> —J.D. Horowitz, et al., "Nitroglycerine/N-acetylcysteine in the Management of Unstable Angina Pectoris," *European Heart Journal,* 9 (Suppl A), January 1988, p. 95-100.

This study examined the effects of intravenous glutathione and NAC on the cardiotoxicity of doxorubicinkly in both in vitro and in vivo models. Results showed that both agents prevented doxorubicinkly-induced negative inotropic effects on isolated rat atria.

> —F.Villani, et al., "Effect of Glutathione and N-acetylcysteine on in Vitro and in Vivo Cardiac Toxicity of Doxorubicin.," *Free Radic Res Commun,* p. 11(1-3), 1990, p. 145-151.

This study examined the cardioprotective effects of NAC in canines. Results found NAC limited the extent of infarction and significantly decreased incidence of reperfusion ventricular arrhythmias.

> —J. Sochman, et al., "Cardioprotective Effects of N-acetylcysteine: The Reduction in the Extent of Infarction and Occurrence of Reperfusion Arrhythmias in the Dog," *International Journal of Cardiology,* 28(2), August 1990, p. 191-196.

Results of this study showed that large doses of NAC increased exercise capacity in isosorbide-5-mononitrate-treated angina pectoris patients.

> —J.H. Svendsen, et al., "N-acetylcysteine Modifies the Acute Effects of Isosorbide-5-mononitrate in Angina Pectoris Patients Evaluated by Exercise Testing," *Journal of Cardiovascular Pharmacol,* 13(2), February 1989, p. 320-323.

Results of this study indicated that in vivo NAC potentiation of nitroglycerine responses may have clinically beneficially effects on preventing or reversing the loss of hemodynamic responsiveness to nitroglycerine.

— J. Torresi, et al., "Prevention and Reversal of Tolerance to Nitroglycerine with N-acetylcysteine," *Journal of Cardiovascular Pharmacology,* 7(4), July-August 1985, p. 777-783.

This double-blind, placebo-controlled study examined the effects of a bolus of 100 mg/kg of NAC followed by a continuos infusion of 20mg/kg in the bypass circuit on oxidative response of neutrophils during cardiopulmonary bypass in adult patients. Results showed significantly lower levels of oxidative burst response of neutrophils among those receiving the NAC than controls throughout the bypass.

— L.W. Andersen, et al., "The Role of N-acetylcystein Administration on the Oxidative Response of Neutrophils During Cardiopulmonary Bypass," *Perfusion,* 10(1), 1995, p. 21-26.

Chronic Bronchitis

This double-blind, placebo-controlled study examined the clinical effects of 300 mg b.i.d of NAC on patients suffering from chronic bronchitis. Results showed a significant decrease in number or sick days taken at work following four months of NAC treatment compared to controls.

— J.B. Rasmussen & C. Glennow, "Reduction in Days of Illness after Long-term Treatment with N-acetylcysteine Controlled-release Tablets in Patients with Chronic Bronchitis," *European Respir Journal,* 1(4), April 1988, p. 351-355.

Results of this study showed that the oral administration of NAC inhibited cigarette smoke-induced mucosa cell hyperplasia and epithelial hypertrophy in rats.

— D.F. Rogers & P.K. Jeffery, "Inhibition by Oral N-acetylcysteine of Cigarette Smoke-induced 'Bronchitis' in the Rat," *Exp Lung Research,* 10(3), 1986, p. 267-283.

Results of this study found that daily treatment with 600 mg/kg of NAC of patients with chronic and acute bronchitis was effective and generally free of adverse effects.

— H.H. Gerards & U. Vits, [Therapy of Bronchitis. Successful Single-dosage Treatment with N-acetylcysteine, Results of an Administration Surveillance Study in 3,076 Patients], *Fortschr Medicine,* 109(34), November 30, 1991, p. 707-710.

In this study, atopic children with allergic rhinitis, asthma and maxillary sinusitis received 50-80 mg/kg per day of cefuroxime and 15-25 mg/kg per day of NAC over a 10 day period. Results indicated the treatment to be effective in 95.8% of the patients with 37.5% subsequently able to reduce their treatment for asthma.

— A.L. Boner, et al., "A Combination of Cefuroxime and N-acetyl-cysteine for the Treatment of Maxillary Sinusitis in Children with Respiratory Allergy," *International Journal of Clinical Pharmacol Ther Toxicol,* 22(9), September 1984, p. 511-514.

In this study, 103 children suffering from lower respiratory tract infections received a combination of cefuroxime and NAC. One hundred of the 103 experienced positive results from the treatment. In 58, a total relief of symptoms was reported, while a marked improvement was seen in 42.

— G. Santangelo, et al., "A Combination of Cefuroxime and N-acetyl-cysteine for the Treatment of Lower Respiratory Tract Infections in Children," *International Journal of Clinical Pharmacol Ther Toxicol,* 23(5), May 1985, p. 279-281.

COPD

Results of this study showed that treatment with 10 micrograms/ml of NAC enhanced the antifungal activity of peripheral blood monocyte cells from COPD patients significantly in vitro.
   —A. Vecchiarelli, et al., "Macrophage Activation by N-acetyl-cysteine in COPD Patients," *Chest,* 105(3), March 1994, p. 806-811.

Cutaneous Inflammation

Results of this study showed NAC to be an effective treatment of cutaneous inflammation mediated by tumor necrosis factor alpha in mice.
   —G. Senaldi, et al., "Protective Effect of N-acetylcysteine in Hapten-induced Irritant and Contact Hypersensitivity Reactions," *Journal Invest Dermatol,* 102(6), June 1994, p. 934-937.

Diabetes

Results of this study showed that the administration of NAC inhibited reductions in diaphragm contractility in STZ-treated rats without reductions in blood glucose levels.
   —W. Hida, et al., "N-acetylcysteine Inhibits Loss of Diaphragm Function in Streptozotocin-treated Rats," *American Journal of Respiratory Critical Care Medicine,* 153(6 Pt 1), June 1996, p. 1875-1879.

Results of this study found that the administration of NAC suppressed the enhanced tumor necrosis factor production in diabetic rats significantly, suggesting NAC may be an effective means for prevention of tumor necrosis factor mediated pathological conditions associated with the disease.
   —M Sagara, et al., "Inhibition with N-acetylcysteine of Enhanced Production of Tumor Necrosis Factor in Streptozotocin-induced Diabetic Rats," *Clin Immunol Immunopathol,* 71(3), June 1994, p. 333-337.

Results of this study found that the administration of NAC to streptozotocin-induced diabetic rats inhibited the development of functional and structural abnormalities of the peripheral nerve.
   —M. Sagara, et al., "Inhibition of Development of Peripheral Neuropathy in Streptozotocin-induced Diabetic Rats with N-acetylcysteine," *Diabetologia,* 39(3), March 1996, p. 263-269.

Diaphragmatic Function

Results of this study found that NAC exhibited direct temperature-dependent effects on diaphragm function in vitro, consistent with its known antioxidant properties.
   —P.T. Diaz, et al., "Effects of N-acetylcysteine on in Vitro Diaphragm Function are Temperature Dependent," *Journal of Applied Physiology,* 77(5), November 1994, p. 2434-2449.

This study examined the possibility of augmenting diaphragmatic stores of reduced glutathione, thus delay the development of respiratory failure during loaded breathing, via NAC administration. Results showed that the NAC blunted loading-induced decreases in diaphragmatic glutathione levels and led to a decrease in the in vitro fatigability of excised diaphragm muscle strips.

—G.S. Supinski, et al., "N-acetylcysteine Administration and Loaded Breathing," *Journal of Applied Physiology,* 79(1), July 1995, p. 340-347.

Ear Problems

Results of this study found that NAC decreases inflammation of the middle-ear mucosa and prevented the long-term fibrotic changes in patients suffering from secretory otitis media.

—T. Ovesen, et al., "Local Application of N-acetylcysteine in Secretory Otitis Media in Rabbits," *Clinical Otolaryngol,* 17(4), August 1992, p. 327-331.

Gallstones

Results of this study showed that NAC accelerated the dissolution of gallstone in vitro significantly.

—Niu & B.F. Smith, "Addition of N-acetylcysteine to Aqueous Model Bile Systems Accelerates Dissolution of Cholesterol Gallstones," *Gastroenterology,* 98(2), February 1990, p. 454-463.

General

Results of this study showed that NAC significantly prevented the immediate effects of both short-term or long-term exposure to ozone on the mucocilary functions of sheep.

—L. Allegra, et al., "Ozone-induced Impairment of Mucociliary Transport and its Prevention with N-Acetylcysteine," *American Journal of Medicine,* 91(3C), September 30, 1991, p. 67S-71S.

This study examined the effects of a 48-hour IV N-acetylcysteine treatment protocol for acute overdose of acetaminophen, consisting of 12 70 mg/kg doses every four hours and a loading dose of 140 mg/kg. Results found the protocol to be effective and equal to oral treatment over a 72-hour period.

—M.J. Smilkstein, et al., "Acetaminophen Overdose: A 48-hour Intravenous N-acetylcysteine Treatment Protocol," *Annals of Emergency Medicine,* 20(10), October 1991, p. 1058-1063.

This study examined the effects of NAC on caustic akaline injury to the esophagus in rats. Results showed that NAC as well as steroids ameliorated tissue reaction to chemical injury and tempered the degree of stenosis formation.

—A.J. Liu & M.A. Richardson, "Effects of N-acetylcysteine on Experimentally Induced Esophageal Lye Injury," *Ann Otol Rhinol Laryngol,* 94(5 Pt 1), September-October 1985, p. 477-482.

This article reports on a single case of acute methylmercury poisoning in which NAC was found to be an effective enhancer of kidney elimination of the toxin.

—M.E. Lund, et al., "Treatment of Acute Methylmercury Ingestion by Hemodialysis with N-acetylcysteine (Mucomyst) Infusion and 2,3-dimercaptopropane Sulfonate," *Journal of Toxicol Clin Toxicol,* 22(1), July 1984, p. 31-49.

This study examined the effects of a 400 mg oral dose of NAC on human blood neutrophil and monocyte function in healthy volunteers. Results showed a significant decrease in neutrophil chemiluminescene response after activation by opsonized zymosan relative to controls.

—T. Jensen, et al., ''Effect of Oral N-acetylcysteine Administration on Human Blood Neutrophil and Monocyte Function,'' *APMIS,* 96(1), January 1988, p. 62-67.

This review article reports on the efficacy of NAC in treating cases of paracetamol intoxication when administered within eight hours of intoxication.

—J. De Groote & W. Van Steenbergen, ''Paracetamol Intoxication and N-acetyl-cysteine Treatment,'' *Acta Gastroenterol Belg,* 58(3-4), May-August 1995, p. 326-334.

Results of this study showed that the administration of N-acetylcysteine before cyclophosphamide prevented hemorrhagic cystitis and lethality resulting from the drug in rats while not diminishing its immunosuppressive or antiproliferative activities.

—L. Levy & R. Harris, ''Effect of N-Acetylcysteine on Some Aspects of Cyclophophsphamide—Induced Toxicity and Immunosuppression,'' *Biochem Pharmacol,* 26(11), 1977, p. 1015-1020.

Results of this single case study indicated that the intravenous administration of N-acetylcysteine can be effective against sulphalazine-induced side effects such as hepatitis, rash, and disseminated intravascular coagulation.

—C. Gabay, et al., ''Sulphasalazine-related life-threatening Side Effects: is N-acetylcysteine of Therapeutic Value?'' *Clinical Exp Rheumatology,* 11(4), July-August 1993, p. 417-420.

Results of this double-blind, placebo-controlled study found that oral administration of N-acetylcysteine at 0.6 g per day increased mucociliary clearance rates by approximately 35% in healthy human subjects.

—T. Todisco, et al., ''Effect of N-acetylcysteine in Subjects with Slow Pulmonary Mucociliary Clearance,'' *European Journal of Respir Diseases Suppl,* 139, 1985, p. 136-141.

This study examined the effects of NAC on methyl-mercuric chloride-induced embryotoxicity in mice. Results showed that a single dose of NAC antagonized the embryolethal effects of poisoning by MMC. Palatoschisis incidence was reduced relative to the number of NAC administration. NAC administration improved body weight in fetuses from mothers poisoned with MMC back to normal ranges as well.

—F. Ornaghi, et al., ''The Protective Effects of N-acetyl-L-cysteine Against Methyl Mercury Embryotoxicity in Mice,'' *Fundam Appl Toxicol,* 20(4), May 1993, p. 437-445.

Results of this study showed that the intravenous administration of N-acetylcysteine led to significant reductions in plasma glutathione S-transferase B1 concentrations in patients suffering from severe paracetamol poisoning.

—G.J. Beckett, et al., ''Intravenous N-acetylcysteine, Hepatotoxicity and Plasma Glutathione S-Transferase in Patients with Paracetamol Overdosage,'' *Hum Exp Toxicol,* 9(3), May 1990, p. 183-186.

Results of this study showed that the administration of N-acetylcysteine 30 minutes prior to UV irradiation significantly inhibited UVB-induced immunosuppression in mice.

—L.T. van den Broeke, et al., ''Topically Applied N-acetylcysteine as a Protector Against

UVB-induced Systemic Immunosuppression,'' *J Photochem Photobiol B,* 27(1), January 1995, p. 61-65.

Results of this study found that NAC administration protected rats from the effects UVB radiation on epidermal DNA.

—L.T., van den Broeke, et al., ''The Effect of N-acetylcysteine on the UVB-induced Inhibition of Epidermal DNA Synthesis in Rat Skin,'' *J Photochem Photobiol B,* 26(3), December 1994, p. 271-276.

This review article notes recent findings indicating the ability of early administration of NAC to induce glutathione rescue and recovery, glutathione being an essential protector of biological structure and function.

—R. Ruffmann & A. Wendel, ''GSH Rescue by N-acetylcysteine,'' *Klin Wochenschr,* 69(18), November 15, 1991, p. 857-862.

Results of this study found that hyperbaric oxygen therapy induces lipid peroxidation and that the simultaneous administration of NAC provides protection against such effects.

—P. Pelaia, et al., [Assessment of Lipid Peroxidation in Hyperbaric Oxygen Therapy: Protective Role of N-acetylcysteine], *Minerva Anestesiol,* 61(4), April 6, 1995, p. 133-139.

Results of this study showed that the administration of 1000 and 2000 mg kg-1 of NAC 1 hour prior to illumination in patients treated with photodynamic therapy worked to helped ameliorate photosensitivty.

—P. Baas, et al., ''Partial Protection of Photodynamic-induced Skin Reactions in Mice by N-acetylcysteine: A Preclinical Study,'' *Photochem Photobiol,* 59(4), April 1994, p. 448-454.

This article reports on the cases of two patients with paracetamol overdose who were treated successfully with oral NAC.

—J. Brahm, et al., [Paracetamol Overdose: A New Form of Suicide in Chile and the Value of N-acetylcysteine Administration], *Rev Med Chil,* 120(4), April 1992, p. 427-499.

Results of this study showed NAC to be effective in the reversal of oligura associated with chromate and borate intoxication in rats, suggesting it to be a good potential chelation agent.

—W. Banner, Jr., et al., ''Experimental Chelation Therapy in Chromium, Lead, and Boron Intoxication with N-acetylcysteine and Other Compounds,'' *Toxicol Appl Pharmacol,* 83(1), March 30, 1986, p. 142-147.

Results of this study showed that NAC had protected paraquat-intoxicated rats against oxidative lung damage through the delay of inflammation.

—E. Hoffer, et al., ''N-acetylcysteine Delays the Infiltration of Inflammatory Cells into the Lungs of Paraquat-intoxicated Rats,'' *Toxicol Appl Pharmacol,* 120(1), May 1993, p. 8-12.

Results of this study showed that the administration of NAC to alveolar type II cells incubated with 1 mM paraquat reduced cytoxicity by enhancing glutathione content.

—E. Hoffer, et al., ''N-acetylcysteine Increases the Glutathione Content and Protects Rat

Alveolar Type II Cells Against Paraquat-induced Cytotoxicity," *Toxicol Lett,* 84(1), January 1996, p. 7-12.

Results of this study showed that the administration of NAC either 30 minutes before or 6 to 10 hours following carbon tetrachloride administration significantly prevented liver necrosis induced by the hepatotoxin..

—E.G. Valles, et al., "N-acetyl Cysteine is an Early but Also a Late Preventive Agent Against Carbon Tetrachloride-induced Liver Necrosis," *Toxicol Lett,* 71(1), March 1994, p. 87-95.

Results of this study showed that NAC protected Chinese hamster ovary cells from lead-induced oxidative stress.

—N. Ercal, et al., "N-actylcysteine Protects Chinese Hamster Ovary (CHO) Cells from Lead-Induced Oxidative Stress," *Toxicology,* 108(1-2), April 15, 1996, p. 57-64.

Glutathione Deficiency

This article reports on the case of a 45-month-old girl with 5-oxoprolinuria (pyroglutamic aciduria), hemolysis, and majorglutathione depletion due to deficiency of glutathione synthetase. Results showed that treatment with 6mmol/kg of NAC and 0.7 mmol/kg ascorbate per day for 1-2 weeks decreased turnover in patients suffering from heriditary glutathione deficiency by increasing the plasma levels of glutathione.

—A. Jan, et al., "Effect of Ascorbate or N-acetylcysteine Treatment in a Patient with Hereditary Glutathione Synthetase Deficiency," *Journal of Pediatrics,* 124(2), February 1994, p. 229-233.

Results of this study showed that the administration of 15 mg/kg per day of NAC was beneficial in increasing low intracellular concentrations and cysteine availability in patients suffering from a hereditary deficiency in glutathione deficiency.

—J. Martensson, et al., "A Therapeutic Trial with N-acetylcysteine in Subjects with Hereditary Glutathione Synthetase Deficiency (5-oxoprolinuria)," *Journal of Inherit Metab Dis,* 12(2), 1989, p. 120-130.

Hepatitis

This article reports on the case of a 54-year-old man who developed severe cholestatic jaundice and pure red cell aplasia following treatment with gold sodium thiomalate. The man experienced a complete hematologic recovery following treatment with prednisone and NAC infusions.

—R.M. Hansen, et al., "Gold Induced Hepatitis and Pure Red Cell Aplasia. Complete Recovery after Corticosteroid and N-acetylcysteine Therapy," *Journal of Rheumatology,* 18(8), August 1991, p. 1251-1253.

Liver Damage

Results of this double-blind, placebo-controlled study found that the administration of NAC to chronic liver disease patients with hepatic failure improved oxygen deliver and consumption, induced mild vasodilation, and reduced base deficit.

—P.N. Bromley, et al., "Effects of Intraoperative N-acetylcysteine in Orthotopic Liver Transplantation," *British Journal of Anaesth,* 75(3), September 1995, p. 352-354.

Results of this study showed that the injection of 150 mg/kg of NAC into rats increased L-cysteine concentrations within 15 minutes of exposure.

—H. Nakano, et al., ''Protective Effects of N-acetylcysteine on Hypothermic Ischemia-reperfusion Injury of Rat Liver,'' *Hepatology,* 22(2), August 1995, p. 539-545.

This article reports on the cases of 11 patients at risk of hepatic damage following paracetamol poisoning who received intravenous treatment with NAC. Results showed complete protection against liver failure in all cases with no reported side effects.

—T.E. Oh & G.M. Shenfield, ''Intravenous N-acetylcysteine for Paracetamol Poisoning,'' *Medical Journal of Australia,* 1(13), June 28, 1980, p. 664-665.

Results of this study showed NAC to be an effective agent for combating alcohol-induced acetaminophen toxicity in mice.

—E.A. Carter, ''Enhanced Acetaminophen Toxicity Associated with Prior Alcohol Consumption in Mice: Prevention by N-acetylcysteine,'' *Alcohol,* 4(1), January-February 1987, p. 69-71.

Results of this study demonstrated the ability of NAC to rescue mitochondrial glutathione and restore essential mitochondrial functions in rats, pointing to NAC's potential as an effective antidote to oxidative stress-related diseases.

—J. Traber, et al., ''In Vivo Modulation of Total and Mitochondrial Glutathione in Rat Liver. Depletion by Phorone and Rescue by N-acetylcysteine,'' *Biochem Pharmacol,* 43(5), March 3, 192, p. 9961-9964.

Results of this study indicated NAC coupled with cysteamine can be useful in preventing hepatic necrosis in mice following exposure to acetaminophen at toxic doses.

—T.C. Peterson and I.R. Brown, ''Cysteamine in Combination with N-acetylcysteine Prevents Acetaminophen-induced Hepatotoxicity,'' *Can J Physiol Pharmacol,* 70(1), January 1992, p. 20-28.

Results of this study showed that the pretreatment of pigs with NAC assists in the maintenance of hepatic glutathione during warm ischemia. NAC proved effective in the replenishment of depleted glutathione stores and was associated with improvements in glutathione homeostasis and bile output.

—K. Fukuzawa, et al., ''N-acetylcysteine Ameliorates Reperfusion Injury after Warm Hepatic Ischemia,'' *Transplantation,* 59(1), January 15, 1995, p. 6-9.

Results of this study showed that the administration of high doses of NAC to rats undergoing orthotopic liver transport attenuated symptoms associated with microvascular perfusion failure early following reperfusion

—T.A. Koeppel, et al., ''Impact of N-acetylcysteine on the Hepatic Microcirculation after Orthotopic Liver Transplantation,'' *Transplantation,* 61(9), May 15, 1996, p. 1397-1402.

Lung Damage

Results of this study showed that the administration of NAC prevents endotoxemia-induced release of granulocyte activating substances from the lung lymph of sheep.

—W.D. Lucht, et al., ''Prevention of Release of Granulocyte Aggregants into Sheep Lung

Lymph Following Endotoxemia by N-acetylcysteine," *American Journal of Medical Science,* 294(3), September 1987, p. 161-167.

Results of this study showed that NAC was effective in reducing lung leak, neutrophil influx into lung lavages, and defects in lung history brought on by intratracheal IL-1 administration in rats.
— J.A. Leff, et al., "Postinsult Treatment with N-acetyl-L-cysteine Decreases IL-1-induced Neutrophil Influx and Lung Leak in Rats," *American Journal of Physiol,* 265(5 Pt 1), November 1993, p. L501-L506.

In this study, intravenous NAC was administered to eight pulmonary fibrosis patients and six controls. Results showed significant increases in bronchoalveolar lavage fluid total glutathione in patients within 3 hours of 1.8 g of NAC administration. No such effects were seen in controls.
— A. Meyer, et al., "Intravenous N-acetylcysteine and Lung Glutathione of Patients with Pulmonary Fibrosis and Normals," *American Journal of Respiratory Critical Care Medicine,* 152(3), September 1995, p. 1055-1060.

Results of this double-blind, placebo-controlled study found that intravenous administration of 40 mg/kg per day over a period of 72 hours led to improvements in systemic oxygenation and decreases in the requirements for ventilatory support in acute lung injury patients.
— P.M. Suter, et al., "N-acetylcysteine Enhances Recovery from Acute Lung Injury in Man. A Randomized, Double-blind, Placebo-controlled Clinical Study," *Chest,* 105(1), January 1994, p. 190-194.

This study examined the effects of the stereoisomers of NAC on oxygen-induced lung oedema in rats. Results showed NAC, regardless of stereoconfiguration, protected lungs from oxygen toxicity.
— B. Sarnstrand, et al., "Effects of N-acetylcysteine Stereoisomers on Oxygen-induced Lung Injury in Rats," *Chem Biol Interact,* 94(2), February 1995, p. 157-164.

This study examined the effects of NAC on acute lung injury in sheep induced by endotoxins. Results indicated the treatment attenuated responses to endotoxemia, and significant reductions of the rise in pulmonary artery pressure.
— Y. Zhu, [Experimental Study of the Protective Effects of N-acetylcysteine on Endotoxin-induced Acute Lung Injury], *Chung Hua I Hsueh Tsa Chih,* 71(7), July 1991, p. 373-7, 26.

Results of this study showed that NAC offers protection against PMN mediated oxidant injury in lung cells.
— L.M. Simon & N. Suttorp, "Lung Cell Oxidant Injury: Decrease in Oxidant Mediated Cytotoxicity by N-acetylcysteine," *European Journal of Respiratory Disease Suppl,* 139, 1985, p. 132-135.

This study examined the effects of NAC on tobacco smoke toxicity in vitro. Results showed that concentrations of 1mM of NAC protected cells from toxicity and from glutathione loss.
— P. Moldeus, et al., "N-acetylcysteine Protection Against the Toxicity of Cigarette Smoke and Cigarette Smoke Condensates in Various Tissues and Cells in Vitro," *European Journal of Respiratory Disease Suppl,* 139, 1985, p. 123-129.

Results of this study showed that the administration of NAC at doses of 400 mg/kg body weight per day to mice produced significant reductions bleomcyin-induced collagen deposition in the lungs.

> —S. Shahzeidi, et al., "Oral N-acetylcysteine Reduces Bleomycin-induced Collagen Deposition in the Lungs of Mice," *European Respiratory Journal,* 4(7), July 1991, p. 845-352.

This study examined the effects of intravenous NAC on O2 toxicity in canine lungs. Results showed the treatment protects against the effects of 100% O2 when measured by both functional and structural criteria.

> —P.D. Wagner, et al., "Protection Against Pulmonary O2 Toxicity by N-acetylcysteine," *European Respiratory Journal,* 2(2), February 1989, p. 116-126.

Results of this study indicated that the administration of 200 mg t.i.d. of NAC over an 8 week period to smokers had beneficial effects on the activity of inflammatory cells in the bronchoalveolar space.

> —A. Eklund, et al., "Oral N-acetylcysteine Reduces Selected Humoral Markers of Inflammatory Cell Activity in BAL Fluid from Healthy Smokers: Correlation to Effects on Cellular Variables," *European Respir Journal,* 1(9), October 1988, p. 832-838.

Results of this study found that the administration of 200 mg t.i.d. of NAC over an 8 week period improves the function of alveolar macrophages in healthy smokers.

> —M. Linden, et al., "Effects of Oral N-acetylcysteine on Cell Content and Macrophage Function in Bronchoalveolar Lavage from Healthy Smokers," *European Respiratory Journal,* 1(7), July 1988, p. 645-650.

This study examined the effects of oral NAC on oxidant lung injury in rats using a model of acute immunological alveolitis. Results showed a single dose an hour before antigen/antibody treatment prevented pulmonary endothelial cell uptake loss induced by immune complex deposition.

> —R. Sala, et al., "Protection by N-acetylcysteine Against Pulmonary Endothelial Cell Damage Induced by Oxidant Injury," *European Respiratory Journal,* 6(3), March 1993, p. 440-446.

Results of this study showed that intratracheal NAC inhibited bleomycin lung toxicity in rats.

> —N. Berend, "Inhibition of Bleomycin Lung Toxicity by N-acetyl Cysteine in the Rat," *Pathology,* 17(1), January 1985, p. 108-110.

This review article notes that NAC has been shown to protect human bronchial fibroblasts against tobacco smoke condensates' toxic effects and tobacco smokes' glutathione depleting effects. Studies have also shown NAC can decrease the reactive oxygen intermediate hydrogen peroxide and protect against its toxic effects.

> —P. Moldeus, et al., "Lung Protection by a Thiol-containing Antioxidant: N-acetylcysteine," *Respiration,* 50 Suppl 1, 1986, p. 31-42.

This study examined the effects of NAC on the formation of pulmonary edema in isolated perfused rabbits lungs after in vivo phosgene exposure. Results showed that NAC protected against phosgene-induced lung injury by acting as an antioxidant by maintaining protective levels of glutathione, and by decreasing lipid peroxidation as well as the production of arachidonic acid metabolites.

> —A.M. Sciuto, et al., "Protective Effects of N-acetylcysteine Treatment after Phosgene

Exposure in Rabbits,'' *American Journal of Respiratory Crit Care Medicine,* 151(3 Pt 1), March 1995, p. 768-772.

Results of this study showed that NAC provided protection to mouse lungs exposed to the adverse effects bleomycin and to hyperbaric oxygen therapy.
—D.D. Jamieson, et al., ''Interaction of N-acetylcysteine and Bleomycin on Hyperbaric Oxygen-Induced Lung Damage in Mice,'' *Lung,* 165(4), 1987, p. 239-247.

Muscle Fatigue

Results of this study showed that pretreatment with 150 mg/kg of NAC improved human limb muscle performance during fatiguing exercise. Such findings, the authors argue, suggest oxidative stress may be an important factor in the fatigue process.
—M.B. Reid, et al., ''N-acetylcysteine Inhibits Muscle Fatigue in Humans,'' *Journal of Clinical Investigations,* 94(6), December 1994, p. 2468-2474.

Sjogren's Syndrome

In this double-blind, placebo-controlled study, patients suffering from primary or secondary Sjogren's syndrome received oral NAC for four weeks. Results indicated NAC had a true therapeutic effect on the ocular symptoms of such patients relative to controls.
—M.T. Walters, et al., ''A Double-blind, Cross-over, Study of Oral N-acetylcysteine in Sjogren's Syndrome,'' *Scandinavian Journal of Rheumatol Suppl,* 61, 1986, p. 253-258.

Stroke

Results of this study showed that NAC administration led to improvements in neuronal survival in rats when given before or after ischemia following cerebral ischemia.
—N.W. Knuckey, et al., ''N-acetylcysteine Enhances Hippocampal Neuronal Survival after Transient Forebrain Ischemia in Rats,'' *Stroke,* 26(2), February 1995, p. 305-311.

■ OLIVE OIL

Arthritis

Results of this study indicated that olive oil consumption exhibited protective effects against the severity of rheumatoid arthritis in patients suffering from the disease.
—A. Linos, et al., ''The Effect of Olive Oil and Fish Consumption on Rheumatoid Arthritis— A case Control Study,'' *Scandinavian Journal of Rheumatol,* 20(6), 1991, p. 419-426.

Cancer

Results of this study showed a significant inverse association between olive oil and the risk of breast cancer in a large-scale study of Greek women.
—A. Trichopoulou, et al., ''Consumption of Olive Oil and Specific Food Groups in Relation to Breast Cancer Risk in Greece,'' *Journal of the National Cancer Institute,* 87(2), January 18, 1985, 110-6

Results of this large case-control study showed an inverse association between olive oil consumption and the risk of breast cancer in Italian women.

> —C. la Vecchia, et al., "Olive Oil, Other Dietary Fats, and the Risk of Breast Cancer," *Cancer Causes Control,* 6(6), November 1995, p. 545-550.

Results of this large case-control study showed a significant inverse association between olive oil consumption and the risk of breast cancer in Spanish women.

> —J.M. Martin-Moreno, et al., "Dietary Fat, Olive Oil Intake and Breast Cancer Risk," *International Journal of Cancer,* 58(6), September 15, 1994, p. 774-780.

Cardiovascular/Coronary Heart Disease

Results of this study showed that the administration of 10% to 15% olive oil exhibited cholesterol lowering effects in rabbits.

> —P. Leth-Espensen, et al., "Antiatherogenic Effect of Olive and Corn Oils in Cholesterol-fed Rabbits with the Same Plasma Cholesterol Levels," *Arteriosclerosis,* 8(3), May-June 1988, p. 281-287.

Results of this study showed that supplementation with 50 g per day of olive oil in healthy males over a period of two weeks modified LDL lipid composition and enriched the lipoprotein with oleic acid and sitosterol.

> —M. Aviram & K. Eias, "Dietary Olive Oil Reduces Low-density Lipoprotein Uptake by Macrophages and Decreases the Susceptibility of the Lipoprotein to Undergo Lipid Peroxidation," *Ann Nutr Metab,* 37(2), 1993, p. 75-84.

Results of this study indicated that natural antioxidants found in extra-virgin olive oil prevalent in Mediterranean diets are involved in inhibiting the formation of cytotoxic products and delaying atherosclerotic damage.

> —F. Visioli, et al., "Low Density Lipoprotein Oxidation is Inhibited in Vitro by Olive Oil Constituents," *Atherosclerosis,* 117(1), September 1995, p. 25-32.

Results of this study showed that supplementation with 50 g per day of olive oil in healthy males over a period of two weeks modified LDL lipid composition and enriched the lipoprotein with oleic acid and sitosterol.

> —M. Aviram & E. Kassem, [Olive Oil Dietary Supplementation Decreases Susceptibility of LDL to Oxidation and its Uptake by Macrophages], *Harefuah,* 124(1), January 1, 1993, p. 1-4, 64.

■ OMEGA FATTY ACIDS

Arthritis

This review article notes numerous study have shown clinical benefits following ingestion of n-3 fatty acids in patients suffering from rheumatoid arthritis.

> —J.M. Kremer, "Clinical Studies of Omega-3 Fatty Acid Supplementation in Patients Who Have Rheumatoid Arthritis," *Rheum Dis Clin North Am,* 17(2), May 1991, p. 391-402.

Results of this double-blind, placebo-controlled study found that the oral intake of 2.6 g per day of omega-3 fatty acids by rheumatoid arthritis patients over a period of 12 months led to significant improvements in symptoms associated with the disease.

    —P. Geusens, et al., ''Long-term Effect of Omega-3 Fatty Acid Supplementation in Active Rheumatoid Arthritis. A 12-month, Double-blind, Controlled Study,'' *Arthritis Rheum,* 37(6), June 1994, p. 824-829.

Cancer

Results of this study showed that supplementation with arginine, RNA, and omega-3 fatty acids in the early postoperative time period improved postoperative immunologic responses in patients undergoing surgery for gastroinestinal cancer.

    —M. Kemen, et al., ''Early Postoperative Enteral Nutrition with Arginine-omega-3 Fatty Acids and Ribonucleic Acid-supplemented Diet Versus Placebo in Cancer Patients: An Immunologic Evaluation of Impact,'' *Crit Care Med,* 23(4), April 1995, p. 652-659.

Results of this double-blind, placebo-controlled study found that daily supplementation with omega-3 fatty acids (fish oil containing 4. g of eicosapentaenoic acid and 3.6 g of docosahexaenoic acid) over a period of 12 weeks had chemopreventive effects in patients suffering from sporadic adenomatous colorectal polyps.

    —M. Anti, et al., ''Effect of Omega-3 fatty Acids on Rectal Mucosal Cell Proliferation in Subjects at Risk for Colon Cancer,'' *Gastroenterology,* 103(3), September 1992, p. 883-891.

Results of this study showed that the administration of omega-3 fatty acid rich marine oil over a period of 4 weeks significantly reduced the weight and volume of experimentally-induced mammary tumors in rats.

    —R.A. Karmali, et al., ''Effect of Omega-3 Fatty Acids on Growth of a Rat Mammary Tumor,'' Journal of the National Cancer Institute, 73(2), August 1984, p. 457-461.

Results of this study found that diets in high in omega-3 fatty acids inhibited the growth and metastases of human breast cancer cells in mice.

    —D.P. Rose & J.M. Connolly, ''Effects of Dietary Omega-3 fatty Acids on Human Breast Cancer Growth and Metastases in Nude Mice,'' *Journal of the National Cancer Inst,* 85(21), November 3, 1993, p. 1743-1747.

Results of this study found that a omega-3 fatty acid rich diet of fish oil prolonged survival time of mice bearing myeloid leukemia cells.

    —L.J. Jenski, et al., ''Omega-3 Fatty Acid-containing Liposomes in Cancer Therapy,'' *Proc Soc Exp Biol Med,* 210(3), December 1995, p. 227-233.

Results of this study found that supplementation with 18 g of fish oil per day over a period of 40 days significantly increased T-helper/T-suppresser cell ratio in cancer patients with solid tumors.

    —C.A. Gogos, et al., ''The Effect of Dietary Omega-3 Polyunsaturated Fatty Acids on T-lymphocyte Subsets of Patients with Solid Tumors,'' *Cancer Detect Prev,* 19(5), 1995, p. 415-417.

Cardiovascular/Coronary Heart Disease

Results of this study found that small doses of oral omega-3 fatty acids had significant positive effects on platelet activity when administered over a period of 6 weeks in hyperlipidemic patients with preexisting, established atherothrombotic disorders.

> —P.H. Levine, et al., "Dietary Supplementation with Omega-3 Fatty Acids Prolongs Platelet Survival in Hyperlipidemic Patients with Atherosclerosis," *Arch Intern Med,* 149(5), May 1989, p. 1113-1116.

Results of this study showed that the consumption of a fish oil diet containing 24 g of omega-3 fatty acids per day for 4 weeks by healthy subjects reduced LDL plasma levels relative to controls.

> —D.R. Illingworth, et al., "Inhibition of Low Density Lipoprotein Synthesis by Dietary Omega-3 Fatty Acids in Humans," *Arteriosclerosis,* 4(3), May-June 1984, p. 270-275.

Results of this study showed that the oral administration of high levels of omega-3 fatty acids dramatically reduced VLDL triglyceride levels associated with a high-carbohydrate diet in healthy subjects.

> —W.S. Harris, et al., "Dietary Omega-3 fatty Acids Prevent Carbohydrate-induced Hypertriglyceridemia," *Metabolism,* 33(11), November 1984, p. 1016-1019.

Results of this study showed that both linoleic acid and fish oil exhibited antihypertensive effects in rats.

> —R. Hui, et al., "Antihypertensive Properties of Linoleic Acid and Fish Oil Omega-3 Fatty Acids Independent of the Prostaglandin System," *American Journal of Hypertension,* 2(8), August 1989, p. 610-617.

This review article discusses the results of numerous epidemiological studies showing dietary intake of omega-3 polyunsatured fatty acids reduced coronary artery disease and mortality.

> —C. d'Ivernois, et al., [Potential Value of Omega-3 polyunsaturated Fatty Acids in the Prevention of Atherosclerosis and Cardiovascular Diseases], *Arch Mal Coeur Vaiss,* 85(6), June 1992, p. 899-904.

Results of this study indicated that the daily ingestion of low levels of marine fish oil (900 mg f omega-3 fatty acids) over a period of 30 days had positive effects on clotting and lipid profiles in healthy male subjects.

> —C.D. Lox, "The Effects of Dietary Marine Fish Oils (Omega-3 Fatty Acids) on Coagulation Profiles in Men," *Gen Pharmacol,* 21(2), 1990, p. 241-246.

This review article cites numerous studies pointing the hypolipidemic, antihypertensive, antiatherosclerotic, anti-inflammatory, and antithrombotic effects of daily intake of omega-3 polyunsaturated fatty acids.

> —M.B. Engler, "Vascular Effects of Omega-3 fatty Acids: Possible Therapeutic Mechanisms in Cardiovascular Disease," *Journal of Cardiovascular Nurs,* 8(3), April 1994, p. 53-67.

Results of this double-blind, placebo-controlled found that daily supplementation with omega-3 fatty acids over a period of 4 weeks had antihypertensive and hypotriglceridaemic effects in hypertensive patients taking either beta blockers or diuretics for the disease.

> —Y.K. Lungershausen, et al., "Reduction of Blood Pressure and Plasma Triglycerides by

Omega-3 fatty Acids in Treated Hypertensives,'' *Journal of Hypertension,* 12(9), September 1994, p. 1041-1045.

Results of this study indicated that the administration of dietary omega-3 fatty acids inhibited onset of hypertension-induced proteinuria in rats.
>   —T.E. Rayner, et al., ''Purified Omega-3 Fatty Acids Retard the Development of Proteinuria in Salt-Loaded Hypertensive Rats,'' *Journal of Hypertension,* 13(7), July 1995, p. 771-780.

Diabetes

Results of this study found that short-term daily supplementation with omega-3 fatty acids (5.4 g eicosapentaenoic acid and 2.3 g docosahexaenoic acid) over a period of 4 weeks led to positive changes with respect to vascular risk factors common to type 1 insulin dependent diabetics.
>   —M.M. Landgraf-Leurs, et al., ''Pilot Study on Omega-3 Fatty Acids in Type I Diabetes Mellitus,'' *Diabetes,* 39(3), March 1990, p. 369-375.

Results of this study showed that supplemental omega-3 fatty acids exhibited inhibitory effects against the onset of experimental diabetic cardiomyopathy in diabetic rats.
>   —S.C. Black, et al., ''Cardiac Performance and Plasma Lipids of Omega-3 Fatty Acid-treated Streptozocin-induced Diabetic Rats,'' *Diabetes,* 38(8), August 1989, p. 969-974.

Results of this study found that supplementation with 3 g of the omega 3 fatty acids eicosapentaenoic and docosahexaenoic acid per day over a period of 8 weeks led to an increase of the membrane phospholipid unsaturation and the sphingomyelin content in NIDDM patients.
>   —C. Popp-Snijders, et al., ''Dietary Supplementation of Omega-3 Polyunsaturated Fatty Acids Improves Insulin Sensitivity in Non-insulin-dependent Diabetes,'' *Diabetes Research,* 4(3), March 1987, p. 141-147.

Dysmenorrhea

Results of this double-blind, placebo-controlled study showed that dietary fish oil (1080 mg icosapentaenoic acid, 720 mg docosahexaenoic acid, and 1.5 mg vitamin E) consumed daily over a period of 2 months had strong positive effects on symptoms associated with dysmenorrhea in adolescent girls.
>   —Z. Harel, et al., ''Supplementation with Omega-3 Polyunsaturated Fatty Acids in the Management of Dysmenorrhea in Adolescents,'' *American Journal of Obstet Gynecol,* 174(4), April 1996, p. 1335-1338.

■ PABA

Cancer

Results of this study showed that PABA administration one hour before UV light exposure protected hairless mice from tumor development relative to controls.
>   —D.S. Synder & M. May, ''Ability of PABA to Protect Mammalian Skin from Ultraviolet Light-induced Skin Tumors and Actinic Damage,'' *Journal of Invest Dermatol,* 65(6), December 1975, p. 543-546.

Results of this study showed that the administration of PABA significantly inhibited the proccess of photocarcinogenesis in hairless mice exposed to UV light radiation relative to controls.

> —H. Flindt-Hansen, et al., ''The Effect of Short-term Application of PABA on Photocarcino-genesis,'' *Acta Derm Venereol,* 70(1), 1990, p. 72-75.

Results of this study showed that a 5% solution of PABA inhibited tumor induction time significantly while decreasing carcinoma and tumor yield in hairless mice exposed to UV light.

> —H. Flindt-Hansen, et al., ''The Inhibiting Effect of PABA on Photocarcinogenesis,'' *Arch Dermatol Research,* 282(1), 1990, p. 38-41.

Results of this study showed that the use of a PABA/alcohol sunscreen reduced the incidence of skin cancer in an 11-year-old patient with pigmentosum who received chronic sunlight exposure.

> —N. Goldstein & V. Hay-Roe, ''Prevention of Skin Cancer with a PABA in Alcohol Sunscreen in Xeroderma Pigmentosum,'' *Cutis,* 15(1), 1975, p. 61-64.

■ PAPAIN

Lung Abscess

Results of this study showed that the transthoracal injection of a 0.5% solution of papain in patients with lung abscess boosted the effects of anti-inflammatory therapy.

> —V.M. Udod, et al., ''Treatment of Patients with Lung Abscess by Local Administration of Papain,'' *Vestn Khir,* 142(3), March 1989, p. 24-27.

Wound Healing

This study examined the effects of papain on visceral irrigation in patients with severe infections. Results showed a marked decrease in purulent secretion 72 hours following treatment.

> —N.M. Rogensk, et al., ''Use of Papain in Visceral Infections,'' *Rev Bras Enferm,* 48(2), April-June 1995, p. 140-143.

Results of this study involving 123 surgical patients found that the administration of papain shortened the purification period of purulent wounds of the lactating mammary gland and produced quicker healing.

> —V.T. Storozhuk, et al., ''Immobilized Papain in the Treatment of Acute Destructive Lactation Mastitis,'' *Vestn Khir,* 135(10), October 1985, p. 42-46.

■ PANTOTHENIC ACID

Acne

In this article, the author puts forth the idea that a deficiency in pantothenic acid availability contributes to the onset of acne and that the condition can be cured through liberal supplementation.

> —L.H. Leung, ''Pantothenic Acid Deficiency as the Pathogenesis of Acne Vulgaris,'' *Medical Hypotheses,* 44(6), June 1995, p. 490-492.

Alcohol Consumption

Results of this study showed that the intravenous administration of 200 mg/kg of pantothenic acid prior to the administration of 1.0 gm/kg of ethanol totally counteracted the normal ethanol-induced motor skill disturbances in squirrel monkeys that occurred in the absence of pantothenic acid exposure.

—M.C. Newland, et al., "Interactions between Ethanol and Pantothenic Acid on Tremor and Behavior in Squirrel Monkeys," *Journal of Studies on Alcohol,* 53(1), January 1993, p. 80-85.

Cancer

Results of this study found that pantothenic acid and its related compounds provided significant protection for the plasma membrane of Ehrlich ascites tumor cells against oxygen free radical damage due to increasing cellular level of CoA.

—V.S. Slyshenkov, et al., "Pantothenic Acid and its Derivatives Protect Ehrlich Ascites Tumor Cells Against Lipid Peroxidation," *Free Radic Biol Med,* 19(6), December 1995, p. 767-772.

Cardiovascular/Coronary Heart Disease

This article reports on the single case of a young boy with dilated cardiomyopathy who showed initial improvement following dioxin treatment which was not maintained over time. Large doses of pantothenic acid were administered once the boy reached a moribund stage which resulted in marked and lasting improvements in myocardial growth and function, neutrophil cell count, hypocholesterolaemia and hyperuricaemia. At 13 months, clinical improvement was being sustained with the boy's myocardial function being close to normal.

—I. Ostman-Smith, et al., "Dilated Cardiomyopathy due to Type II X-linked 3-methylgluta-conicAciduria: Successful Treatment with Pantothenic Acid," *British Heart Journal,* 72(4), October 1994, p. 349-353.

Results of the study demonstrated that a mild deficiency in pantothenate had noticeable effects in vivo on triglyceride metabolism in rats prior to significant weight loss due to more pronounced deficiency.

—C.T. Wittwer, et al., "Mild Pantothenate Deficiency in Rats Elevates Serum Triglyceride and Free Fatty Acid Levels," *Journal of Nutrition,* 120(7), July 1990, p. 719-725.

Results of this study of an isolated heart model with experiment-induced reperfusion and ischemia found that derivatives of pantothenic acid acted as cardioprotectors.

—A.O. Kumerova, et al., [Study of Pantothenic Acid Derivatives as Cardiac Protectors in a Model of Experimental Ischemia and Reperfusion of the Isolated Heart], *Biull Eksp Biol Med,* 113(4), April 1992, p. 373-375.

General

This study compared changes in mouse fuel metabolism during exercise and fasting to CoA tissue levels in mice receiving pantothenate-deficient and pantothenate-supplemented diets. Results showed significantly lower tissue levels in nonexercised, pantothenic-deficient mice relative to controls.

—C.M. Smith, et al., "The Effect of Pantothenate Deficiency in Mice on their Metabolic Response to Fast and Exercise," *Metabolism,* 36(2), February 1987, p. 115-121.

This review article argues that deficiency in pantothenic acid leads to a generalized clinical malaise despite its not having been linked with any diseases specifically.

—A.G. Tahiliani and C.J. Beinlich, ''Pantothenic Acid in Health and Disease,'' *Vitam Horm,* 46, 1991, p. 165-228.

Hepatitis

Results of this study found that daily doses of 300 and 600 mg of calcium pantothemate and 90 mg and 180 mg of pantethein taken for 3-4 weeks had positive immunomodulatory action and effects on blood serum levels of immunoglobulins and phagocytic activity of peripheral blood neutrophils in hepatitis patients.

—V.I. Komar, [The Use of Pantothenic Acid Preparations in Treating Patients with Viral Hepatitis A], *Ter Arkh,* 63(11), 1991, p. 58-60.

Liver Damage

Results of this study showed that daily administration of 500 mg/kg of pantethine, 100 mg/kg of pantothenic acid or 50 mg/kg for 5 days led to significant protection against experimental hepatotoxic and peroxidative action in rats.

—I. Nagiel-Ostaszewski & C.A. Lau-Cam, ''Protection by Pantethine, Pantothenic Acid and Cystamine against Carbon Tetrachloride-induced Hepatotoxicity in the Rat,'' *Res Commun Chem Pathol Pharmacol,* 67(2), February 1990, p. 289-292.

Pregnancy

This case-control study evaluated the pantothenic acid nutritional status in 26 pregnant women during their third trimester of pregnancy and at 2 weeks and 3 months postpartum. Results found that pregnant and lactating women may required a higher consumption of pantothenate in order to maintain a sufficient blood level of the vitamin.

—W.O. Song, et al., ''Pantothenic Acid Status of Pregnant and Lactating Women,'' *Journal of the American Dietetic Association,* 85(2), February 1985, p. 192-198.

Weight Loss

In this article, the author proposed the idea that supplementation with pantothenic acid can facilitate complete catabolism of fatty acid and therefore circumvent the formation of ketone bodies during periods of weight loss.

—L.H. Leung, ''Pantothenic Acid as a Weight-reducing Agent: Fasting without Hunger, Weakness and Ketosis,'' *Medical Hypotheses,* 44(5), May 1995, p. 403-405.

Wound Healing

This study examined the modulating effect of Ca-pantothenic acid to subsequent stimulation with a variety of stimuli was on isolated human PMN using functional assay systems: Lucigenin-dependent chemiluminescence (CL), release of myeloperoxidase (MPO). Results showed that Ca-panthotenate significantly inhibited the CL response of PMN upon stimulation with the chemotactic petide f-met-leu-phe, the tumor promotor PMA, and the granulocyte activating cytokines GM-CSF and TNF alpha.

—A. Kapp and G. Zeck-Kapp, ''Effect of Ca-panthotenate on Human Granulocyte Oxidative Metabolism,'' *Allerg Immunol,* 37(3-4), 1991, p. 145-150.

■ PHOSPHATIDYLSERINE

Aging

Results of this study showed that chronic phosphatidylserine treatment can improve the release of acetylccholine in aging rats.

>—F. Casamenti, et al., "Phosphatidylserine Reverses the Age-dependent Decrease in Cortical Acetylcholine Release: A Microdialysis Study," *European Journal of Pharmacology*, 194(1), February 26, 1991, p. 11-16.

Results of this study showed that the administration of phosphatidylserine balanced age-altered enzymatic functions in rats.

>—C. Gatti, et al., "Effect of Chronic Treatment with Phosphatidyl Serine on Phospholipase A1 and A2 Activities in Different Brain Areas of 4 Month and 24 Month Old Rats," *Farmaco*, 40(7), July 1985, p. 493-500.

Results of this study showed that phosphatidylserine administered to aging rats can restore acetylcholine by maintaining a sufficient level in the cortical slices.

>—M.G. Vannucchi & G. Pepeu, "Effect of Phosphatidylserine on Acetylcholine Release and Content in Cortical Slices from Aging Rats," *Neurobiol Aging*, 8(5), September-October 1987, p. 403-407.

This study examined the effects of phosphatidylserine in aged rats. Results showed the treatment decreased the number of seizures due to spontaneous EEG bursts by 65% and the length of seizure duration by 70%.

>—F. Aporti, et al., "Age-dependent Spontaneous EEG Bursts in Rats: Effects of Brain Phosphatidylserine," *Neurobiol Aging*, 7(2), March-April 1986, p. 115-120.

Results of this study showed that the administration of phosphatidylserine to rats led to a reduction in decreases in acetylcholine release due to age by influencing mechanism of stimulus-secretion coupling.

>—F. Pedata, et al., "Phosphatidylserine Increases Acetylcholine Release from Cortical Slices in Aged Rats," *Neurobiol Aging*, 6(4), Winter 1985, p. 337-339.

Allergic Neuritis

Results of this study found that phosphatidylserine administered in daily intraperitoneal 30 mg/kg injections for a period of 14 days led to a marked reduction in clinical severity and mortality in allergic neuritis rats relative to controls.

>—Y. Maeda, et al., "Phosphatidylserine Suppresses Myelin-induced Experimental allergic Neuritis (EAN) in Lewis Rats," *Journal of Neuropathology Exp Neurol*, 53(6), November 1994, p. 672-677.

Alzheimer's Disease

Results of this study showed that phosphatidylserine administered in doses of 400 mg per day led to significant, short-term neuropsychological improvements in patients with Alzheimer's disease relative to controls.

>—W.D. Heiss, et al., "Long-term Effects of Phosphatidylserine, Pyritinol, and Cognitive

Training in Alzheimer's Disease. A Neuropsychological, EEG, and PET Investigation,'' *Dementia,* 5(2), March-April 1994, p. 88-98.

Results of this double-blind, placebo-controlled study showed that the administration of 300 mg per day of phosphatidylserine for 8 weeks led to significant clinical improvements in patients with mild primary degenerative dementia relative to controls.

—R.R. Engel, et al., ''Double-blind Cross-over Study of Phosphatidylserine vs. Placebo in Patients with Early Dementia of the Alzheimer Type,'' *Eur Neuropsychopharmacol,* 2(2), June 1992, p. 149-155.

In this double-blind, placebo-controlled study, Alzheimer's patients received 100 mg per day of bovine cortex phosphatidylserine for 12 weeks. Results showed the treatment improved several cognitive measures relative to controls.

—T. Crook, et al., ''Effects of Phosphatidylserine in Alzheimer's Disease,'' *Psychopharmacol Bulletin,* 28(1), 1992, p. 61-66.

Antiviral Effects

Results of this study showed that phosphatidylserine binds directly to vesicular stomatitis virus and inhibits its attachment and infectivity on the surface of vero cells.

—R. Schlegel, et al., ''Inhibition of VSV Binding and Infectivity by Phosphatidylserine: Is Phosphatidylserine a VSV-binding Site?,'' *Cell,* 32(2), February 1983, p. 639-646.

Behavioral Effects

This study examined the effects of phosphatidylserine administered for 5 days on the behavior of aged rats. Results showed the treatment led to a facilitated acquisition of active avoidance behavior and an improved retention of passive avoidance responses.

—F. Drago, et al., ''Behavioral Effects of Phosphatidylserine in Aged Rats,'' *Neurobiol Aging,* 2(3), Fall 1981, p. 209-213.

This set of studies examined the effects of phosphatidylserine on the behavior of aged rats. Results showed significant dose-related effects on retention of passive avoidance responses.

—J. Corwin, et al., ''Behavioral Effects of Phosphatidylserine in the Aged Fischer 344 Rat: Amelioration of Passive Avoidance Deficits without Changes in Psychomotor Task Performance,'' *Neurobiol Aging,* 6(1), Spring 1985, p. 11-15.

Results of this study showed that the administration of 15 mg/kg ip of phosphatidylserine for 30 days led to significant increases in the avoidance performances of rats.

—A. Zanotti, et al., ''Effects of Phosphatidylserine on Avoidance Relearning in Rats,'' *Pharmacol Res Commun,* 16(5), May 1984, p. 485-493.

Results of this study showed that the administration of phosphatidylserine to mice during the first sixty days of life led to the improvement of cognitive abilities in adulthood.

—F. Ammassari-Teule, et al., ''Chronic Administration of Phosphatidylserine During Ontogeny Enhances Subject-environment Interactions and Radial Maze Performance in C57BL/6 Mice,'' *Physiol Behav,* 47(4), April 1990, p. 755-760.

Brain Function

Results of this study showed that patients suffering from chronic cerebral decomponensation experienced improvements in mnesic and neuropsychic symtpomatology following phosphatidylserine administration for 60 days.

> —G.F. Lombardi, [Pharmacological Treatment with Phosphatidyl Serine of 40 Ambulatory Patients with Senile Dementia Syndrome], *Minerva Med*, 80(6), June 1989, p. 599-602.

Results of this study showed that the administration of phosphatidlyserine for 21 days led to partial restoration of decreased density of muscarinic cholinergic receptors in age mouse brains in a dose-dependent manner.

> —C.M. Gelbmann & W.E. Muller, "Chronic Treatment with Phosphatidylserine Restores Muscarinic Cholinergic Receptor Deficits in the Aged Mouse Brain," *Neurobiol Aging*, 13(1), January-February 1992, p. 45-50.

Results of this double-blind, placebo-controlled study showed that age-associated memory impairment patients treated with 100 mg of phosphatidylserine for 12 weeks experienced clinical improvement relevant to controls.

> —T.H. Crook, et al., "Effects of Phosphatidylserine in Age-associated Memory Impairment," *Neurology*, 41(5), May 1991, p. 644-649.

This double-blind, placebo-controlled study examined the effects of 3 x 100 mg of phosphatidylserine on patients hospitalized with dementia. Results showed a significant improvement in the patients receiving phosphatidylserine relative to controls.

> —P.J. Delwaide, et al., "Double-blind Randomized Controlled Study of Phosphatidylserine in Senile Demented Patients," *Acta Neurol Scand*, 73(2), February 1986, p. 136-140.

This double-blind, placebo-controlled study examined the effects of 300 mg per day of phosphatidylserine for 30 days on cognitive, affective and behavioral symptoms of elderly women with depressive disorders. Results showed that patients receiving phosphatidylserine experienced improvements with respect to memory, behavior, and depressive symptoms relative to controls.

> —M. Maggioni, et al., "Effects of Phosphatidylserine Therapy in Geriatric Patients with Depressive Disorders," *Acta Psychiatr Scand*, 81(3), March 1990, p. 265-270.

This double-blind, placebo-controlled study examined the effects of 300 mg per day of phosphatidylserine in cognitive impaired geriatric patients. Results showed the treatment had significant positive cognitive and behavioral effects relative to controls.

> —T. Cenacchi, et al., "Cognitive Decline in the Elderly: A Double-blind, Placebo-controlled Multicenter Study on Efficacy of Phosphatidylserine Administration," *Aging*, 5(2), April 1993, p. 123-133.

Results of this study found that the aged mice treated with 20 mg/kg ip per day of phosphatidylserine over a period of three weeks totally normalized enhanced efficacy and affinity of L-glutamate and glycine and elevated NMDA receptor density by approximately 25%.

> —S.A. Cohen & W.E. Muller, "Age-related Alterations of NMDA-receptor Properties in

the Mouse Forebrain: Partial Restoration by Chronic Phosphatidylserine Treatment," *Brain Research*, 584(1-2), July 3, 1992, p. 174-180.

Results of this study indicated that the oral administration of 300 mg per day of soybean transphosphatidylated phosphatidylserine can improve and/or prevent senile dementia in humans.
—M. Sakai, et al., "Pharmacological Effects of Phosphatidylserine Enzymatically Synthesized from Soybean Lecithin on Brain Functions in Rodents," *Journal of Nutr Sci Vitaminol*, 42(1), February 1996, p. 47-54.

Results of this study showed definite improvements in memory performance in mice treated with bovine brain phosphatidylserine relative to controls.
—L. Valzelli, et al., "Activity of Phosphatidylserine on Memory Retrieval and on Exploration in Mice," *Methods Find Exp Clin Pharmacol*, 9(10), October 1987, p. 657-660.

Results of this study showed that the postnatal administration of an aqueous suspension of phosphatidylserine led to improvements of memory processes in mice.
—S. Fagioli, et al., "Phosphatidylserine Administration During Postnatal Development Improves Memory in Adult Mice," *Neurosci Letters*, 101(2), June 19, 1989, p. 229-233.

Results of this study showed that oral administration of 50 mg/kg per day of phosphatidylserine for 12 weeks improved spatial memory and passive avoidance retention of aged impaired rats.
—A. Zanotti, et al., "Chronic Phosphatidylserine Treatment Improves Spatial Memory and Passive Avoidance in Aged Rats," *Psychopharmacology*, 99(3), 1989, p. 316-321.

Cancer

Results of this study showed that bovine cortex phosphatidylserine significantly reduced experimental autoimmune encephalomyelitis in mice while not inhibiting effector T cells.
—G. Monastra, et al., "Phosphatidylserine, a Putative Inhibitor of Tumor Necrosis factor, Prevents Autoimmune Demyelination," *Neurology*, 43(1), January 1993, p. 153-163.

Results of this study showed that parental administration of liposomes containing the aminophospholipids phosphatidylserine, and phosphatidylethanolamine is an efficient mode to decrease the endotoxin-induced production of tumor necrosis factor in mice and rabbits.
—G. Monastra & A. Bruni, "Decreased Serum Level of Tumor Necrosis Factor in Animals Treated with Lipopolysaccharide and Liposomes Containing Phosphatidylserine," *Lymphokine Cytokine Res*, 11(1), February 1992, p. 39-43.

Cardiovascular/Coronary Heart Disease

Results of this study showed that smooth muscle cells expressed phosphatidylserine during apoptosis which partly mediated binding and phagocytosis of dead cells. The authors suggest that these effects could be important in promoting rapid cell removal in the vessel wall.
—M.R. Bennett, et al., "Binding and Phagocytosis of Apoptotic Vascular Smooth Muscle Cells is Mediated in Part by Exposure of Phosphatidylserine," *Circ Research*, 77(6), December 1995, p. 1136-1142.

Results of this study showed that an anticoagulant containing heparin and phosphatidylserine enhanced rat tolerance to thromboplastin administration to the blood flow. Such effects led to a major decrease in death rate and fibrinogen consumption decrease due to thromboplastin.
— A. Byshevskii & S.R. Sokolovskii, [Protective Effect of Heparin and Phosphatidylserine in Exogenous Thromboplastinemia], *Biull Eksp Biol Med,* 94(12), December 1982, p. 23-25.

Results of this study found that the intravenous administration of phosphatidylethanol amine-and sphyngomyelin-stabilized phosphatidylserine emulsion produced hypocoagulemia in white mice in a dose dependent manner.
— M.K. Chabanov, et al., [Effect of an Intravenously Administered Phosphatidylserine Emulsion on Blood Coagulation and Blood System Indices], *Farmakol Toksikol,* 42(3), May-June 1979, p. 257-261.

Results of this study showed that the administration of phosphatidylserine into the circulation of rats reduced fibrinogen consumption which was provoked by simultaneous thrombin injection, indicating phosphatidylserine works as an anticoagulant.
— A. Byshevskii, et al., [Effect of Phosphatidyl Serine on Conversion of Fibrinogen to Fibrin], *Vopr Med Khim,* 29(4), July-August 1983, p. 16-22.

Results of this study showed that phosphatidylserine containing anticoagulant and heparin mutually increased their anticoagulating activity under conditions of simultaneous treatment both in vitro as well as in vivo.
— A. Byshevskii & S.R. Sokolovskii, [Potentiation of the Anticoagulant Effects of a Phosphatidylserine-Containing Anticoagulant and Heparin], *Vopr Med Khim,* 28(2), March-April 1982, p. 30-34.

Results of this study found that the intravenous administration 30 and 60 mg of phosphatidylserine emulsion led to a rapid reduction in blood coagulation activity in a dose dependent manner.
— O.A. Tersenov & M.K. Chabanov, [Anticoagulant Effect of Phosphatidylserine], *Vopr Med Khim* (1981 Sep-Oct) 27(5), September-October 1981, p. 619-623.

Epilepsy

This study examined the effect of gamma-aminobutyric and phosphatidylserine administered together to drug resistant epilepsy patients. Results showed a dramatic decrease in absence seizures following treatment.
— C. Loeb, et al., "Preliminary Evaluation of the Effect of GABA and Phosphatidylserine in Epileptic Patients," *Epilepsy Research,* 1(3), May 1987, p. 209-212.

General

Results of this study found that both saturated and unsaturated phosphatidylserine inhibited lipid peroxidation induced by ferrous-ascorbate system in the presence of phosphatidylcholine hydroperoxides.
— K. Yoshida, et al., "Inhibitory Effect of Phosphatidylserine on Iron-dependent Lipid Peroxidation," *Biochem Biophys Res Commun,* 179(2), September 16, 1991, p. 1077-1081.

Immune Function

Results of this study showed that phosphatidylserine can upregulate contact hypersensitivy by stimulating the function of APC of epidermal Langerhans cells in mice.

—G. Girolomoni G, et al, "Phosphatidylserine Enhances the Ability of Epidermal Langerhans Cells to Induce Contact Hypersensitivity," *Journal of Immunology,* 150(10), May 15, 1993, p. 4236-4243.

Results of this study showed that phosphatidylserine administered to rats reversed age-induced physiological decline of the humoral immune response. In addition, the same treatment reversed the pharmacological associated depression of specific antibody production in young rats.

—V. Guarcello, et al., "Phosphatidylserine Counteracts Physiological and Pharmacological Suppression of Humoral Immune Response," *Immunopharmacology,* 19(3), May-June 1990, p. 185-195.

Parkinson's Disease

This article notes that clinical and experimental research indicates phosphatidylserine prepared from cow's brain can have positive effects on cerebral changes involved in the symptoms of Alzheimer's type senile dementia among patients with Parkinson's disease.

—E.W. Funfgeld, et al., "Double-blind Study with Phosphatidylserine (PS) in Parkinsonian Patients with Senile Dementia of Alzheimer's Type," *Prog Clin Biol Res,* 317, 1989, p. 1235-1246.

Schizophrenia

This case-control study examined the effects of phosphatidylserine on platelet B-type monoamine oxidase in schizophrenics. Results supported the idea of phosphatidylserine as an allosteric regulator of platelet B-type monoamine oxidase in vivo.

—K.H. Tachik, et al., "Phosphatidylserine Inhibition of Monoamine Oxidase in Platelets of Schizophrenics," *Biological Psychiatry,* 21(1), January 1986, p. 59-68.

Stress

This double-blind, placebo-controlled study examined the effects of the administration of 800 mg per day of phosphatidylserine for 10 days on neuroendocrine responses to physical stress in healthy males. Results showed that treatment counteracted activation of the hypothalamo-pituitary-adrenal axis induced by stress.

—P. Monteleone, et al., "Blunting by Chronic Phosphatidylserine Administration of the Stress-induced Activation of the Hypothalamo-pituitary-adrenal Axis in Healthy Men," *European Journal of Clinical Pharmacology,* 42(4), 1992, p. 385-388.

Results of this study showed that old rats subjected to various stresses that received 20 mg/kg per day of phosphatidlyserine for 20 days experienced a normalization of core body temperature relative to controls.

—F. Drago, et al., "Protective Action of Phosphatidylserine on Stress-induced Behavioral and Autonomic Changes in Aged Rats," *Neurobiol Aging,* 12(5), September-October 1991, p. 437-440.

Results of this double-blind, placebo-controlled study showed that healthy males pretreated with both 50 and 75 mg per day of brain cortex-derived phosphatidylserine experienced a significant blunting of the ACTH and cortisol responses to physical stress.

—P. Monteleone, et al., ''Effects of Phosphatidylserine on the Neuroendocrine Response to Physical Stress in Humans,'' *Neuroendocrinolgy*, 52(3), September 1990. p. 243-248.

■ POTASSIUM

Cardiovascular/Coronary Heart Disease

This double-blind, placebo-controlled study examined the effects of 80 mmol per day of supplemental potassium on blood pressure among middle-aged African Americans on a low-potassium diet. Results showed a significant net decline in systolic blood pressure and a decline in diastolic blood pressure in the treatment group relative to controls.

—F.L. Brancati, et al., ''Effect of Potassium Supplementation on Blood Pressure in African Americans on a Low-potassium Diet. A Randomized, Double-blind, Placebo-controlled Trial,'' *Archives of Internal Medicine*, 156(1), January 8, 1996, p. 61-67.

Results of this study showed that the administration of a 1% (w/v) KCl solution significantly attenuated the blood pressure rise generally associated with age in spontaneously hypertensive rats.

—A. Barden, et al., ''Effect of Potassium Supplementation on Blood Pressure and Vasodilator Mechanisms in Spontaneously Hypertensive Rats,'' *Clin Sci*, 75(5), November 1988, p. 527-534.

Results of this double-blind, placebo-controlled study showed that moderate restriction of dietary sodium coupled with 60 mmol per day of supplemental potassium for 2 months led to the reduction of supine blood pressure in patients with moderate to mild essential hypertension.

—G.A. MacGregor, et al., ''Moderate Potassium Supplementation in Essential Hypertension,'' *Lancet*, 2(8298), September 11, 1982, p. 567-570.

Results of this double-blind, placebo-controlled study showed that supplementation with 60 mmol per day of potassium chloride for 6 weeks ameliorated diuretic-induced hypokalemia and led to a decrease in blood pressure in hypertension patients as well.

—N.M. Kaplan, et al., ''Potassium Supplementation in Hypertensive Patients with Diuretic-induced Hypokalemia,'' *New England Journal of Medicine*, 312(12), March 21, 1985, p. 746-749.

This double-blind, placebo-controlled study examined the effects of 60 mmol per day of potassium supplementation on postural blood-pressure in elderly patients with symptomatic idiopathic postural hypotension. Results showed a significant reduction in the orthostatic fall in systolic blood pressure and supine blood pressure potassium and control phases.

—D. Heseltine, et al., ''Potassium Supplementation in the Treatment of Idiopathic Postural Hypotension,'' *Age Ageing*, 19(6), November 1990, p. 409-414.

Results of this study showed that the supplementation with potassium significantly reduced systolic blood pressure in healthy, normotensive children.

—J.Z. Miller, et al., "Blood Pressure Response to Sodium Restriction and Potassium Supplementation in Healthy Normotensive," *Clin Exp Hypertens,* 8(4-5), 1986, p. 823-827.

Results of this study indicated that 2 mg per day of supplemental potassium hydrochloride or a combination of 2 g per day of potassium hydrochloride and 1000 mg per day of magnesium hydroxide added to 24 weeks of diuretic therapy after the 8th week suppressed ventricular ectopic activity in mild hypertensives.

—J.A. Lumme & A.J. Jounela, "The Effect of Potassium and Potassium Plus Magnesium Supplementation on Ventricular Extrasystoles in Mild Hypertensives Treated with Hydrochlorothiazide," *International Journal of Cardiology,* 25(1), October 1989, p. 93-97.

This double-blind study compared the effects of 64 mmol per day of supplemental potassium with 10 mg per day of bendrofulazide in black patients suffering from untreated hypertension. Results showed the two treatments to be equally effective in reducing diastolic blood pressure over a 28 week period, with those receiving potassium exhibiting fewer side effects.

—A.O. Obel & D.K. Koech, "Potassium Supplementation Versus Bendrofluazide in Mildly to Moderately Hypertensive Kenyans," *Journal of Cardiovascular Pharmacol,* 17(3), March 1991, p. 504-507.

In this study, essential hypertension patients received either low sodium diet, high sodium diet, or high sodium diet combined with KCl supplementation. Results showed that blood pressure increased during NaCl loading and decreased during KCl supplementation.

—Y. Tabuchi, et al., "Hypotensive Mechanism of Potassium Supplementation in Salt-loaded Patients with Essential Hypertension," *Journal of Clinical Hypertension,* 1(2), June 1985, p. 145-152.

In this double-blind, crossover study, untreated essential hypertensive patients received 64 mmol KCl or placebo during two 4 week periods. By the 4th week of the potassium supplementation period, significant reductions were seen in diastolic blood pressure.

—G. Valdes, et al., "Potassium Supplementation Lowers Blood Pressure and Increases Urinary Kallikrein in Essential Hypertensives," *Journal of Human Hypertension,* 5(2), April 1991, p. 91-96.

Results of this meta-analysis involving 19 clinical trials found that oral potassium supplements significantly lowered systolic and diastolic blood pressure. Results indicated that such effects were greatest in patients with high blood pressure.

—F.P. Cappuccio & G.A. MacGregor, "Does Potassium Supplementation Lower Blood Pressure? A Meta-analysis of Published Trials," *Journal of Hypertension,* 9(5), May 1991, p. 465-473.

Results of this double-blind study found a mild hypotensive effect of high potassium intake (72 mmol/day) coupled with moderate sodium restriction over a period of six weeks in young patients with hypertension.

—D.E. Grobbee, et al., "Sodium Restriction and Potassium Supplementation in Young People with Mildly Elevated Blood Pressure,'' *Journal of Hypertension,* 5(1), February 1987, p. 115-119.

Results of this double-blind, placebo-controlled, crossover study showed that daily supplementation with 65 mmol of potassium chloride salt over a 6 week period significantly reduced systolic and diastolic blood pressure in hyptertensive black females.
> —S.M. Matlou, et al., ''Potassium Supplementation in Blacks with Mild to Moderate Essential Hypertension,'' *Journal of Hypertension,* 4(1), February 1986, p. 61-64.

This double-blind, placebo-controlled, crossover study examined the effects of 60 mmol per day of potassium chloride on blood pressure in untreated elderly hypertensives. Results showed the treatment reduced 24-hour ambulatory blood pressure after a period of 4 weeks.
> —M.D. Fotherby & J.F. Potter, ''Potassium Supplementation Reduces Clinic and Ambulatory Blood Pressure in Elderly Hypertensive Patients,'' *Journal of Hypertension,* 10(11), November 1992, p. 1403-1408.

Results of this study found that 100 mmol per day of supplemental potassium administered over a period of ten days can modify noradrenergic blood pressure regulation in hypertensives.
> —M.G. Bianchetti, et al., ''Correction of Cardiovascular Hypersensitivity to Norepinephrine by Potassium Supplementation in Normotensive Members of Hypertensive Families and Patients with Essential Hypertension,'' *Journal of Hypertension Suppl,* 2(3), December 1984, p. S445-S448.

Results of this study found that essential hypertensive patients experienced reductions in blood pressure following long-term but not short-term supplementation with potassium.
> —A. Overlack, et al., ''Hemodynamic, Renal, and Hormonal Responses to Changes in Dietary Potassium in Normotensive and Hypertensive Man: Long-term Antihypertensive Effect of Potassium Supplementation in Essential Hypertension,'' *Klin Wochenschr,* 63(8), April 15, 1985, p. 352-360.

Results of this study indicated that 0.5 meq/kg intravenous potassium chloride administered over a 2-hour period was effective and without side effects in pediatric postoperative cardiac patients.
> —D.E. Schaber, et al., ''Intravenous KCl Supplementation in Pediatric Cardiac Surgical Patients,'' *Pediatric Cardiology,* 6(1), 1985, p. 25-28.

■ PYCNOGENOL

Cancer

Results of this study showed that procyanidol oligomers injected into rabbits bind to skin elastic fibers making them more resistant to hydrolytic action of human leukocyte elastase and porcine pancreatic elastase also injected into the rabbits.
> —J.M. Tixier, et al., ''Evidence by in Vivo and in Vitro Studies that Binding of Pycnogenols

to Elastin Affects its Rate of Degradation by Elastases," *Biochem Pharmacol,* 33(24), December 15, 1984, p. 3933-3939.

Cardiovascular/Coronary Heart Disease

Results of this study found that the administration of 150 mg of a procyanidol oligomers had beneficial effects on capillary resistance disorders in diabetic and hypertension patients.

—G. Lagrua, et al., "A Study of the Effects of Procyanidol Oligomers on Capillary Resistance in Hypertension and in Certain Nephropathies," *Sem Hop,* 57, 1981, p. 1399-1401.

Results of this double-blind study found that procyanidolic oligomers were significantly more effective in treating peripheral venous insufficiency than semi-synthetic diosmin.

—P. Delacrois, "Double-blind Study of Endotelon in Chronic Venous Insuffiency," *La Revue De Med,* 27, 1981, p. 28-31.

General

Results of this study found that pycnogenol protected vascular endothelial cells from oxidant injury in vitro.

—Y. Rong, et al., "Pycnogenol Protects Vascular Endothelial Cells from t-butyl Hydroperoxide Induced Oxidant Injury," *Biotechnol Ther,* 5(3-4), 1994-1995, p. 117-26

This study examined pycnogenol's effects on immune dysfunction in normal mice and ethanol mice or mice infected with the murine retrovirus LP-BM5. Results showed that pycnogenol enhanced in vitro IL-2 production by mitogen-stimulated splenocytes if its production was suppressed in ethanol-fed or retrovirus-infected mice. Pycnogenol decreased the elevated levels of interleukin-6 produced in vitro by cells from retrovirus infected mice and IL-10 secreted by spleen cells from mice consuming ethanol, and increased natural killer cell cytotoxicity.

—J.E. Cheshier, et al., "Immunomodulation by Pycnogenol in Retrovirus-infected or Ethanol-fed Mice," *Life Sciences,* 58(5), 1996, PL 87-96.

PMS

Results of this study found that endotelon improved or eliminated symptoms in 60.8% after 2 cycles of treatment and 78.8% after 4 cycles of treatment in 165 women receiving ambulatory treatment for PMS. Conditions improved included mammary symptoms, abdominal swelling, pelvic pain, weight variations, and venous problems of the legs.

—M. Amsellem, et al., "Endotelon in the Treatment of Venolymphatic Problems in Premenstrual Syndrome, Multicenter Study on 165 Patients," *Tempo Medical,* 282, 1987.

Postoperative Edema

Results of this double-blind, placebo-controlled study showed that endotelon significantly increased the speed of postoperative edema disappearance in patients following face-lifting.

—J. Baruch, "Effect of Endotelon in Postoperative Edema. Results of a Double-blind Study with Placebo on a Group of Thirty-two Patients," *Ann Chir Plast Esthet,* 4, 1984.

Vision

Results of this study showed that the administration of 4 tablets containing 50 mg of procyanidolic oligomers per day for 5 weeks had significant beneficial effects relative to controls with respect to various conditions associated with light vision in human subjects.

> —C. Corbe, et al., "Light Vision and Chorioretinal Circulation. Study of the Effect of Procyanidolic Oligomers (Endotelon)," *Journal of Fr Ophtalmol,* 11, 1988, p. 453-460.

■ QUERCETIN

Cancer

Results of this study found that quercetin and cisplatin in combination and alone inhibited the proliferation of ovarian cancer cells in vitro.

> —G. Scambia, et al., "Synergistic Antiproliferative Activity of Quercetin and Cisplatin on Ovarian Cancer Cell Growth," *Anticancer Drugs,* 1, 1990, p. 45-48.

Results of this study found that quercetin and cisplatin in combination and alone inhibited the proliferation of ovarian and endothelial cancer cells in vitro.

> —G. Scambia, et al., "Inhibitory Effect of Quercetin (Q) on Primary Ovarian and Endometrial Cancer and Synergistic Activity with Cis -Diamminedichloroplatinum(II) (CDDP)," *Proc Annu Meet Am Soc Clin Oncol,* 11, 1992, p. A760.

Results of this study showed that quercetin inhibited leukaemic cell growth in vitro.

> —L.M. Larocca, et al., "Antiproliferative Activity of Quercetin on Normal Bone Marrow and Leukaemic Progenitors," *British Journal of Haematology,* 79, 1991, p. 562-566.

Results of this study showed that quercetin inhibited the enhanced capacity for operation of signal transduction in human carcinoma cells in vitro.

> —N. Prajda, et al., "Linkage of Reduction in 1-phosphatidylinositol 4-kinase Activity and Inositol 1,4,5 Trisphosphate Concentration in Human Ovarian Carcinoma Cells Treated with Quercetin," *Life Sci,* 56(19), 195, p. 1587-1593.

Results of this study showed that quercetin inhibited the growth of human breast cancer cell in vitro.

> —R.L. Singhal, et al., "Quercetin: Inhibition of Signal Transduction Activity in Human Breast Carcinoma MDA-MB-435 Cell Line," *Proc Annu Meet Am Assoc Cancer Res,* 36, 1995, p. A2610.

Cardiovascular/Coronary Heart Disease

Results of this study showed that quercetin exhibited protective effects against reperfusion-induced arrhythmias in rats.

> —D. Xiao, et al., "Effects of Quercetin on Platelet and Reperfusion-induced Arrhythmias in Rats," *Chung Kuo Yao Li Hsueh Pao,* 14(6), November 1993, p. 505-508.

Diabetes

Results of this study found that the continuos oral administration of quercetin delayed the onset of cataract in diabetic rats.

—S.D. Varma, et al., "Diabetic Cataracts and Flavonoids," *Science,* 195(4274), January 14, 1977, p. 205-206.

Results of this study showed that doses of 10 mg/kg and 50 mg/kg of quercetin administered to diabetic rats promoted normalization of the level of glycemia and blood coagulation, increased liver glycogen content, decreased high blood serum concentrations of cholesterol and low density lipoproteins.

—IuN Nuraliev & G.A. Avezov, "The Efficacy of Quercetin in Alloxan Diabetes," *Eksp Klin Farmakol,* 55(1), January-February 1992, p. 42-44.

Flexner's Dysentery

Results of this study showed that the intravenous administration of quercetin and tocopherol acetate for 7 days enhanced normalization of clinical indices and restoration of the immune homeostasis in patients suffering from Flexner's dysentery.

—V.M. Frolov, et al., [The Efficacy of Quercetin and Tocopherol Acetate in Treating Patients with Flexner's Dysentery], *Vrach Delo,* (4), April 1993, p. 84-86.

Hypoxia

Results of this study showed that 100 mg/kg of quercetin administered 3 hours prior to acute systemic hypoxia combined with hyperthermia prevented drastic activation of lipid peroxidation and arachidonic acid metabolism.

—V.D. Lukianchuk & L.V. Savchenkova, "The Effect of Quercetin on the Metabolic Processes in Combined Body Exposure to Hypoxia and Hyperthermia," *Eksp Klin Farmakol,* 56(1), January-February 1993, p. 44-47.

Pollinosis

Results of this study indicated quercetin was an effective treatment for correcting metabolic problems involving lymphocyte membrane lipids in children with pollinosis.

—I.I. Balabolkin, et al., "Use of Vitamins in Allergic Illnesses in Children," *Vopr Med Khim,* 38(5), September-October 1992, p. 36-40.

Ulcer

Results of this study showed that the administration of quercetin inhibited experimentally-induced gastric ulcers in rodents.

—C. Alarcon de la Lastra, et al., "Antiulcer and Gastoprotective Effects of Quercetin: A Gross and Histologic Study," *Pharmacology,* 48, 1994, p. 1994.

■ RUTIN

Cancer

Results of this case-control study showed that quercetin and rutin suppressed chemical-induced colonic tumor multiplicity and development in female mice.
—E.E. Deschner, et al., "Quercetin and Rutin as Inhibitors of Azoxymethanol-induced Colonic Neoplasia," *Carcinogenesis,* 12(7), July 1991, p. 1193-1196.

Cardiovascular/Coronary Heart Disease

Results of this study found that rutin delayed the development of hypercholesterinemia and peroxidation syndrome as well aortal atherosclerotic affection in rabbits.
—O.N. Voskresenskii, et al., [Effect of Ascorbic Acid and Rutin on the Development of Experimental Peroxide Atherosclerosis], *Farmakol Toksikol,* 42(4), July-August 1979, p. 378-382.

General

Results of this study found both quercetin and rutin could suppress free radical activity at the point of superoxide ion formation, the generation of hydroxyl radicals in Fenton reaction, as well as the formation of lipid peroxy radicals in rat liver microsomes.
—I.B. Afanas'ev, et al., "Chelating and Free Radical Scavenging Mechanisms of Inhibitory Action of Rutin and Quercetin in Lipid Peroxidation," *Biochem Pharmacol,* 38(11), June 1, 1989, p. 1763-1769.

Results of this study found that rutin inhibited oxidative damage in pathological human red blood cells.
—L.N. Grinberg, et al., "Protective Effects of Rutin Against Hemoglobin Oxidation," *Biochem Pharmacol,* 48(4), August 17, 1994, p. 643-649.

Results of this study showed that rutin in addition to alpha-tocopherol and ascorbic acid provided protection against injury from oxidation of LDL in cultured endothelial cells.
—A. Negre-Salvayre, et al., "Alpha-Tocopherol, Ascorbic Acid, and Rutin Inhibit Synergistically the Copper-promoted LDL Oxidation and the Cytotoxicity of Oxidized LDL to Cultured Endothelial Cells," *Biol Trace Elem Research,* 47(1-3), January-March 1995, p. 81-91.

This study examined the effects of rutin, ascorbic acid, and alpha-tocopherol on peroxidative processes in xanthine-xanthine oxidase system, linoleic acid ufasomes and human erythrocyte membranes. Results showed rutin to be the most effective radical scavenger and enhance the potency of the other two when administered in combinations.
—A. Negre-Salvayre, et al., "Additional Antilipoperoxidant Activities of Alpha-tocopherol and Ascorbic Acid on Membrane-like Systems are Potentiated by Rutin," *Pharmacology,* 42(5), 1991, p. 262-272.

Peritonitis

Results of this study showed that the rutin administered subcutaneously inhibited silver nitrate-induced peritonitis in rats.

  —P.N. Aleksandrov, et al., [Effect of Rutin and Esculamine on Models of Aseptic Inflammation] *Farmakol Toksikol,* 49(1), January-February 1986, p. 84-86.

Results of this study showed that the administration of 100 mg/kg of rutin offered protection against ethanol-induced gastric injury in rats.

  —C. Perez Guerrero, et al., "Prevention by Rutin of Gastric Lesions Induced by Ethanol in Rats: Role of Endogenous Prostaglandins," *Gen Pharmacol,* 25(3), May 1994, p. 575-580.

■ SELENIUM

Aging

Results of this study found that supplemental beta-carotene and selenium enhanced the immune function among a group of healthy elderly subjects.

  —S.M. Wood, "Effects of Beta-carotene and Selenium Supplementation in Aged Humans," *Dissertation Abstracts International,* 55(4), 1994, p. 1387.

Results of this study showed that supplemental selenium restored cell proliferation defects associated with aging in mice by increasing the number of high-affinity IL-2 receptors.

  —M. Roy, et al., "Supplementation with Selenium Restores Age-related Decline in Immune Cell Function," *Proc Soc Exp Biol Med,* 209(4), September 1995, p. 369-375.

Cancer

This study examined selenium's inhibitory effects on DMH-induced colon carcinogenesis in rats. Results showed significant reductions in the incidence, total number, and total number of tumors per rat in those animals receiving selenium relative to controls.

  —M.M. Jacobs, "Selenium Inhibition of 1,2-dimethylhydrazine-induced Colon Carcinogenesis," *Cancer Research,* 43(4), April 1983, p. 1646-1649.

Results of this study showed selenium to have significant inhibitory effects on DMH-induced colon tumorigenesis in rats.

  —M.M. Jacobs, "Inhibitory Effects of Selenium on 1,2-Dimethylhydrazine and Methylazoxymethanol Colon Carcinogenesis. Correlative Studies on Selenium Effects on the Mutagenicity and Sister Chromatid Exchange Rates of Selected Carcinogens," *Cancer,* 40(5, Suppl), 1977, p. 2557-2564.

This study examined selenium's potential chemoprotective effects in a murine model of mammary tumorigenesis. Results showed it significantly decreased tumor incidence under numerous experimental conditions.

  —D. Medina, "Selenium and Murine Mammary Tumorigenesis," *Cancer Bulletin,* 34(4), 1982, p. 162-165.

Results of this study found supplemental selenium to be an effective chemopreventive agent against DMBA-induced mammary cancer in rats fed a high-fat diet.

> —C. Ip, ''Prophylaxis of Mammary Neoplasia by Selenium Supplementation in the Initiation and Promotion Phases of Chemical Carcinogenesis,'' *Cancer Research,* 41(11 Pt 1), November 1981, p. 4386-4390.

Results of this study showed that 11210 leukemic cell-treated mice treated with a combination therapy of selenium and methotrexate experienced a significantly longer life span than mice administered either agent alone.

> —J.A. Milner & C.Y. Hsu, ''Inhibitory Effects of Selenium on the Growth of L1210 Leukemic Cells,'' *Cancer Research,* 41(5), May 1981, p. 1652-1656.

This study examined the effects of selenium on cis-diamminedichloroplatinum nephrotoxicity in mice and rats. Results showed that selenium exhibited protective effects, but only when administered prior to c-DDP.

> —G.S. Baldew, et al., ''Selenium-induced Protection Against Cis-diamminedichloroplatinum(II) Nephrotoxicity in Mice and Rats,'' *Cancer Research,* 49(11), June 1, 1989, p. 3020-3023.

Results of this study showed an inverse association between selenium status and the risk of lung cancer in a large-scale, three year study of Dutch men and women between the ages of 55-69.

> —P.A. van den Brandt, et al., ''A Prospective Cohort Study on Selenium Status and the Risk of Lung Cancer,'' *Cancer Research,* 53(20), October 15, 1993, p. 4860-4865.

Results of this study showed that supplemental selenium reduced bis(2-oxopropyl)nitrosamine-induced colon and lung adenocarcinoma yield in male rats relative to controls.

> —D.F. Birt, et al., ''Inhibition By Dietary Selenium of Colon Cancer Induced in the Rat By Bis(2-oxopropyl)nitrosamine,'' *Cancer Research,* 42(11), 1982, p. 4455-4459.

Results of this study found that supplemental selenium exhibited significant preventive effects against DMH-induced intestinal cancer in rats.

> —S.W. Jao, et al., ''Effect of Selenium on 1,2-dimethylhydrazine-induced Intestinal Cancer in Rats,'' *Dis Colon Rectum,* 39(6), June 1996, p. 628-631.

Results of this study showed that supplemental selenium administered daily over a period of 18 days totally inhibited tumor growth in mice inoculated with 5 x 10(5) Ehrlich ascites tumor cells.

> —K.A. Poirier, ''Selenium: An Inhibitor of Tumor Growth in Vitro and in Vivo,'' *Dissertation Abstracts International,* 45(1), 1984, p. 133-B.

Results of this study showed that supplemental selenium and retinoic acid inhibited development of DMBA-induced squamous cell carcinoma of the hamster tongue.

> —W.J. Goodwin, Jr., et al., ''Inhibition of Hamster Tongue Carcinogenesis by Selenium and Retinoic Acid,'' *Ann Otol Rhinol Laryngol,* 95(2 Pt 1), March-April 1986, p. 162-166.

Results of this 43 week study showed that supplemental selenium significantly inhibited the initiation phase of DMBA-induced carcinogenesis in female rats.

—J. Milner, et al., "Selenite Inhibition of Mammary Tumors Induced by 7,12-Dimethylbenz(A)anthracene (DMBA)," *FASEB Journal,* 4(4), 1990, p. A1042.

Results of this double-blind, placebo-controlled study showed that the combined supplementation with selenium and retinyl acid reduced the rate of N-methyl-N-nitrosourea-induced mammary carcinogenesis in rats.

—H.J. Thompson, et al., "Effect of Combined Selenium and Retinyl Acetate Treatment on Mammary Carcinogenesis," *Cancer Research,* 41(4), April 1981, p. 1413-1416.

This study examined the effects of supplemental selenium on N-methyl-N-nitrosourea (MNU)-induced mammary carcinogenesis in rats. Results showed the treatment prolonged the latency of mammary cancer appearance and decreased the average number of cancers per rat.

—H.J. Thompson & P.J. Becci, "Selenium Inhibition of N-Methyl-N-Nitrosourea-Induced Mammary Carcinogenesis in the Rat," *Journal of the National Cancer Institute,* 65(6), 1980, p. 1299-1301.

This study examined the effects of supplemental selenium on DMBA-induced sqaumous cell carcinoma of the tongue in hamsters. Results showed the treatment produced modest inhibitory effects.

—W.J. Goodwin, et al., "Selenium Inhibition of Chemical Carcinogenesis in the Upper Aerodigestive Tract of Hamsters," *Otolaryngol Head Neck Surg,* 93(3), June 1985, p. 373-379.

Results of this study showed that supplemental selenium inhibited rat mammary tumor cell proliferation, the synthesis of protein synthesis, and DNA replication in vitro.

—W.M. Lewko & K.P. McConnell, "Influence of Selenium on the Growth of N-nitrosomethylurea-induced Mammary Tumor Cells in Culture," *Proc Soc Exp Biol Med,* 180(1), October 1985, p. 33-38.

Results of this study showed that supplemental selenium inhibited Ehrlich ascites tumors in mice.

—G.A. Greeder & J.A. Milner, "Factors Influencing the Inhibitory Effect of Selenium on Mice Inoculated with Ehrlich Ascites Tumor Cells," *Science,* 209(4458), 1980, p. 825-827.

This review article examined the role of selenium in carcinogenesis with respect to epidemiological cancer data, chemical carcinogenesis, virally-induced tumors and selenium, human tumors and selenium intakes, experimentally transplanted tumors and selenium inhibition, and forms of selenium. Studies have shown that selenium inhibits the growth of various neoplastic cells in vitro and in vivo and can reduced the incidence of chemically and virally induced tumors.

—J.A. Milner, "Selenium and Carcinogenesis," *ACS Symp Ser,* (277), 1985, p. 267-282.

Results of this study showed that selenium exhibited a dose-dependent protective against UV light-induced skin cancer in hairless mice.

—E.B. Thorling, et al., "Oral Selenium Inhibits Skin Reactions to UV Light in Hairless Mice," *Acta Pathol Microbiol Scand,* 91(1), 1983, p. 81-83.

This review article cites results from numerous studies indicating selenium exhibits anticarcinogenic and antitumorigenic properties.

 —J.A. Milner, ''Inhibition of Chemical Carcinogenesis and Tumorigenesis by Selenium,'' *Adv Exp Med Biol,* 206, 1986, p. 449-463.

Results of this study showed supplemental selenium inhibited viral and chemical-induced mammary carcinogenesis in mice.

 —D. Medina, et al., ''Effects of Selenium on Mouse Mammary Tumorigenesis and Glutathione Peroxidase Activity,'' *Anticancer Research,* 1(6), 1981, p. 377-382.

Results of this study showed that supplemental selenium inhibited the growth of DU-145 human prostate carcinoma cells in vitro.

 —M.M. Webber, et al., ''Inhibitory Effects of Selenium on the Growth of DU-145 Human Prostate Carcinoma Cells in Vitro,'' *Biochem Biophys Res Commun,* 130(2), July 31, 1985, p. 603-609.

This review article cites studies indicating that the administration of selenium via water supply significantly reduces the incidence of spontaneous mammary tumors in female mice. Findings from epidemiological studies indicate cancer mortality in humans is lower in areas providing an adequate dietary intake of selenium.

 —G.N. Schrauzer, ''Selenium and Cancer: A Review,'' *Bioinorganic Chemistry,* 5(3), 1976, p. 275-281.

Results of this study showed that selenium supplemented via drinking water significantly prevented spontaneous mammary tumors from developing in mice relative to controls.

 —G.N. Schrauzer, et al., ''Inhibition of the Genesis of Spontaneous Mammary Tumors in C3H Mice: Effects of Selenium and of Selenium-Antagonistic Elements and their Possible Role in Human Breast Cancer,'' *Bioinorg Chem,* 6(3), 1976, p. 265-270.

Results of this study showed significant reductions in the incidence of DMH-induced colon carcinogenesis in rats receiving supplemental selenium both alone and in combination with other antioxidants.

 —M.M. Jacobs & A.C. Griffin, ''Effects of Selenium on Chemical Carcinogenesis. Comparitive Effects of Antioxidants,'' *Biological Trace Element Research,* 1(1), 1979, p. 1-13.

Results of this study showed that the selenium supplementation inhibited the viability of human breast cancer cells in vitro in a dose-dependent manner. Results also found that parenteral administration of sodium selenite significantly inhibited the growth of the cancerous cell lines transplanted into nude mice.

 —A.M. Watrach, et al., ''Inhibition of Human Breast Cancer Cells by Selenium,'' *Cancer Letters,* 25(1), November 1984, p. 41-47.

Results of this study indicated that supplemental selenium reduced the incidence and total number of colon tumors induced by DMH and/or MAM in rats.

 —M.M. Jacobs, et al., ''Inhibitory Effects of Selenium on 1,2-dimethylhydrazine and Methylazoxymethanol Acetate Induction of Colon Tumors,'' *Cancer Letters,* 2(3), January 1977, p. 133-137.

Results of this study showed a marked suppression of DMBA-induced mammary tumorigenesis in rats following selenium and retinyl acetate supplementation.

—C. Ip & M.M. Ip, "Chemoprevention of Mammary Tumorigenesis by a Combined Regimen of Selenium and Vitamin A," *Carcinogenesis,* 2(9), 1981, p. 915-918.

Results of this study found that supplemental selenium inhibited the formation of DMBA-induced mammary tumors, ductal hyperplasias, and mammary tumor virus-induced alveolar hyperplasias in mice.

—D. Medina & F. Shepherd, "Selenium-Mediated Inhibition of 7,12-Dimethylbenz(a)Anthracene-Induced Mouse Mammary Tumorigenesis," *Carcinogenesis,* 2(5), 1981, p. 451-455.

Results of this study showed that supplemental selenium reduced DMBA-induced mammary neoplasia in rats fed high-saturated fat diet.

—C. Ip & D. Sinha, "Anticarcinogenic Effect of Selenium in Rats Treated with Dimethylbenz(A)anthracene and Fed Different Levels and Types of Fat," *Carcinogenesis,* 2(5), 1981, p. 435-438.

Results of this study indicated that the combined supplementation of selenium, vitamin A, and BHT inhibited the growth of human tongue cancer cell lines in vitro.

—I. Inoue, et al., "Inhibitory Effects of Selenium, Vitamin A and Butylated Hydroxytoluene on in Vitro Growth of Human Tongue Cancer Cells," *Eur Arch Otorhinolaryngol,* 252(8), 1995, p. 509-512.

These review article makes the following observations with respect to cancer and selenium: selenium intake protects organisms from various carcinogens. Human and animal studies have demonstrated an inverse association between serum selenium levels and cancer risk. Selenium's chemopreventive effects are the likely results of its antioxidant properties.

—G. Hocman, "Chemoprevention of Cancer: Selenium," *International Journal of Biochem,* 20(2), 1988, 123-132.

Results of this study showed that selenium supplementation prevented the development of benzpyrene-induced sarcoma in mice relative to controls.

—C. Witting, et al., "The Tumor-protective Effect of Selenium in an Experimental Model," *Journal of Cancer Research and Clinical Oncology,* 104(1-2), 1982, p. 109-113.

This study examined the chemopreventive effects of sodium selenite, magnesium chloride, ascorbic acid and retinyl acetate on DMBA-induced mammary carcinogenesis in female rats. Results showed the treatment to have significant chemopreventive effects, especially when administered together.

—A. Ramesha, et al., "Chemoprevention of 7,12-dimethylbenz[a]nthracene-induced Mammary Carcinogenesis in Rat by the Combined Actions of Selenium, Magnesium, Ascorbic Acid and Retinyl Acetate," *Japanese Journal of Cancer Research,* 81(12), December 1990, p. 1239-1246.

This review article cites numerous epidemiological studies indicating a significant inverse association between selenium intake and the risk of cancer in humans.

—A. Bruce, [Selenium and Tumors], *Lakartidningen,* 78(8), 1981, p. 658.

Results of this study indicated the selenium supplementation significantly inhibited MCA-induced hyperplasia and dysplasia in adult mice.

> —S.P. Hussain & A.R. Rao, ''Chemopreventive Action of Selenium on Methylcholanthrene-induced Carcinogenesis in the Uterine Cervix of Mouse,'' *Oncology*, 49(3), 1992, p. 237-240.

Results of this study showed that selenium supplementation enhanced the generation of cytotoxic lymphoyctes and the host's ability to destroy malignant cells in mice.

> —M. Roy, et al., ''Selenium and Immune Cell Functions. II. Effect on Lymphocyte-mediated Cytotoxicity,'' *Proc Soc Exp Biol Med*, 193(2), February 1990, p. 143-148.

Cardiovascular/Coronary Heart Disease

In this controlled study, 6 mcg per day of sodium selenite was added to the drinking water of rats for 4 weeks. Results showed such treatment had protective effects against experimentally-induced cardiac ischemia and reperfusion.

> —R. Poltronieri, et al., ''Protective Effect of Selenium in Cardiac Ischemia and Reperfusion,'' *Cardioscience*, 3(3), September 1992, p. 155-160.

Results of this study found that selenium and vitamin E administered together protected rabbits against heart muscle changes associated with a high-fat diet.

> —L. Rozewicka, et al., ''Protective Effect of Selenium and Vitamin E Against Changes Induced in Heart Vessels of Rabbits Fed Chronically on a High-fat Diet,'' *Kitasato Arch Exp Med*, 64(4), December 1991, p. 183-192.

Results of this study showed that selenium supplementation reduced adriamycin-induced cardiotoxicity in isolated rat hearts undergoing a sequence of ischemia/reperfusion.

> —F. Boucher, et al., ''Oral Selenium Supplementation in Rats Reduces Cardiac Toxicity of Adriamycin During Ischemia and Reperfusion,'' *Nutrition*, 11(5 Suppl), September-October 1995, p. 708-711.

Dental Health

This study examined the effects of selenium on dental caries in pregnant rats. Rats received distilled drinking water or water containing 0.8 ppm or 2.4 ppm selenium, as sodium selenite or selenomethionine, until the pups were weaned. Results showed that moderate levels of developmental selenium significantly reduced caries in male rats relative to both control rats and to animals receiving high levels of selenium.

> —J.L. Britton, et al., ''Cariostasis by Moderate Doses of Selenium in the Rat Model,'' *Arch Environ Health*, 35(2), March-April 1980, p. 74-76.

This letter notes that the conditions of children's teeth has shown marked improvement in Finland since the beginning of selenium supplementation to foodstuffs and water.

> —A. Parko, ''Has the Increase in Selenium Intake Led to a Decrease in Caries Among Children and the Young in Finland,'' *Proceedings of the Finnish Dental Society*, 88(1-2), 1992, p. 57-60.

Diabetes

Results of this study showed that supplemental selenium coupled with supplemental vitamin E led to the protection of kidneys from glumerular lesions in diabetic rats.

> —C. Douillet, et al., "A Selenium Supplement Associated or not with Vitamin E Delays Early Renal Lesions in Experimental Diabetes in Rats," *Proceedings of the Soc Exp Biol Med,* 211(4), April 1996, p. 323-331.

Results of this study showed that supplemental selenium exhibited insulin-like effects in diabetic mice.

> —R. Ghosh, et al., "A Novel Effect of Selenium on Streptozotocin-induced Diabetic Mice," *Diabetes Research,* 25(4), 1994, p. 165-171.

Results of this study indicated that supplemental selenium decreased elevated serum glucose leves in experimentally-induced diabetic rats.

> —Y. Iizuka, et al., [Effects of Selenium on the Serum Glucose and Insulin Levels in Diabetic Rats], *Nippon Yakurigaku Zasshi,* 100(2), August 1992, p. 151-156.

General

Results of this study indicated that selenium supplementation reduced injury to human hepatocytes brought on by lipid peroxidation in vitro.

> —S. He, et al., [Preliminary Studies on Protective Effects of Selenium on Human Fetal Hepatocyte in Vitro Injured by Lipid Peroxidation], *Chung Hua Yu Fang I Hsueh Tsa Chih,* 29(3), May 1995, p. 165-167.

Immune Function

This study examined the effects of selenium via dietary and in vitro supplementation on the activity of spleen natural killer cells and plastic-adherent lymphokine-activated killer cells from mice. Results showed that dietary supplementation produced a significant increase in the lytic activity of activated NK cells.

> —L. Kiremidjian-Schumacher, et al., "Supplementation with Selenium Augments the Functions of Natural Killer and Lymphokine-activated Killer Cells," *Biological Trace Element Research,* 52(3), June 1996, p. 227-239.

This double-blind, placebo-controlled study examined the effects of 3 months of selenium supplementation at thrice weekly doses of 500 micrograms followed by three months at 200 micrograms on the immune parameters in haemodialysis patients. Results showed an improvement in T-cell response to phytohaemoagglutinin and a significant progressive increase in delayed-type hypersensitivity relative to controls.

> —M. Bonomini, et al., "Effects of Selenium Supplementation on Immune Parameters in Chronic Uraemic Patients on Haemodialysis," *Nephrol Dial Transplant,* 10(9), 1995, p. 1654-1661.

Results of this study showed that supplementation with 200 micrograms of selenium per day for 2-4 months led to enhanced immune response in patients suffering from short-bowel syndrome.

> —A. Peretz, et al., "Effects of Selenium Supplementation on Immune Parameters in Gut Failure Patients on Home Parenteral Nutrition," *Nutrition,* 7(3), May-June 1991, p. 215-221.

Keshan Disease

This study found that supplemental selenium and vitamin E protected the myocardial mitochondria from lipid peroxidation-induced damage in rats fed grains from areas with high rates of Keshan disease.

—S.Y. Liu, [Protective Effects of Vitamin E and Selenium on Myocardial Mitochondria in Rats—a Study on the Pathogenic Factors and Pathogenesis of Keshan Disease], *Chung Hua Yu Fang I Hsueh Tsa Chih,* 24(4), July 1990, p. 214-216.

Kidney Damage

The present study examined selenium's ability to protect against gentamicin-induced renal damage in rats. Results indicated that rats treated with selenium experienced fewer negative effects relative to controls.

—E.O. Ngaha, et al., "Protection by Selenium Against Gentamicin-induced Acute Renal Damage in the Rat," *Journal of Biochemistry,* 95(3), March 1984, p. 831-837.

Lupus

Results of this study showed that selenium supplementation produced significant improvements in survival rates among autoimmune mice with lupus-like disease.

—J.R. O'Dell, et al., "Improved Survival in Murine Lupus as the Result of Selenium Supplementation," *Clin Exp Immunol,* 73(2), August 1988, p. 322-327.

Mood

Results of this double-blind, placebo-controlled study showed that supplementation with 100 mcg of selenium per day for 5 weeks led to measurable improvements in mood scores.

—D. Benton & R. Cook, "The Impact of Selenium Supplementation on Mood," *Biological Psychiatry,* 29(11), June 1, 1991, p. 1092-1098.

Myotonic Dystrophy

This article reports on the case of a myotonic dystrophy patient who received supplemental vitamin E and selenium for two years. The treatment produced a dramatic recovery with respect to objective and subjective improvements.

—G. Orndahl, et al., "Selenium Therapy of Myotonic Dystrophy," *Acta Med Scand,* 213(3), 1983, p. 237-239.

Ulcer

This study examined the effects of supplemental selenium and vitamin E on chemical and stress-induced gastric ulcers in rats. Results showed that the treatment led to significant decreases in basal gastric acid secretions and offered significant protection gastric mucosa from lesions produced by hypothermic restraint stress and chemicals.

—A.R. al-Moutairy & M. Tariq, "Effect of Vitamin E and Selenium on Hypothermic Restraint Stress and Chemically-induced Ulcers," *Dig Dis Sci,* 41(6), June 1996, p. 1165-1171.

This study examined the protective effects of selenium in the gastric mucosa of rats against injuries induced by hypothermic restraint stress, aspirin, indomethacin, reserpine, dimaprit, and a host of other gastric mucosal-damaging agents in rats. Results showed selenium exhibited significant antiulcer effects against such agents.

—N.S. Parmar, et al., 'Gastric Anti-ulcer and Cytoprotective Effect of Selenium in Rats,'' *Toxicol Appl Pharmacol,* 92(1), January 1988, p. 122-130.

■ SILICON

Cancer

This study examined the antitumor effects of the silicon compounds 2-trimethylsilylethylthioethylamine(KAS-010) and its conjugate with 5-FU (KAS-011). Results showed that the oral administration of both KAS-010 and KAS-011 to be on B 16 melanoma, Meth A sarcoma and MM 46 mammary carcinoma in vivo while KAS-011 also demonstrated a marked antitumor activity against L 1210 leukemia-bearing mice. Results showed these compounds significantly inhibited metastases to the lymph nodes and lung of Lewis lung carcinoma implanted id into the right ear of BDF1 mice.

—K. Fukushima, [Characteristics in Antitumor Effects of Organic Silicon Related Compounds], *Gan To Kagaku Ryoho,* 16(6), June 1989, p. 2173-2181.

Wound Healing

Results of this study showed that application of silicon organic sorbents in burn patients led to a decrease in activity of proteolytic enzymes in wound discharge, increase in the activity of microbial systems of neutrophilic leukocytes, and the formation of phagocytic type of local resistance of an organism. In addition, results found patients experienced a decrease in the area of deep wound burns following treatment.

—G.P. Kozinets, et al., [The Use of Silicon Organic Sorbents for the Local Treatment of Burn Wounds], *Klin Khir,* (3), 1989, p. 25-27.

■ SUPEROXIDE DISMUTASE

Arthritis

Results of this study showed that recombinant human superoxide dismutase exhibited inhibitory effects on the articular cartilage tissue damage associated with osteoarthritis.

—S. Hoedt-Schmidt, et al., "Histomorphological Studies on the Effect of Recombinant Human Superoxide Dismutase in Biochemically Induced Osteoarthritis," *Pharmacology,* 47(4), October 1993, p. 252-260.

Behcet's Disease

Results of this study showed that treatment with CuZn superoxide dismutase significantly improved clinical symptoms associated with Behcet's syndrome.

—J. Emerit, et al., "Preliminary Study of the Therapeutic Effect of Superoxide Dismutase in 7 Cases of Behcet's Disease," *C R Acad Sci III,* 302(7), 1986, p. 243-246.

Brain Injury

Results of this study showed that superoxide radicals inhibited vasogenic brain edema onset following brain injury.

—P.H. Chan, et al., "Protective Effects of Liposome-entrapped Superoxide Dismutase on Posttraumatic Brain Edema," *Ann Neurol*, 21(6), January 1987, p. 540-547.

Bronchopulmonary Dysplasia

Results of this study found that the administration of superoxide dismutase reduced the severity of bronchopulmonary dysplasia in infants suffering from respiratory distress syndrome.

—W. Rosenfeld, et al., "Prevention of Bronchopulmonary Dysplasia by Administration of Bovine Superoxide Dismutase in Preterm Infants with Respiratory Distress Syndrome," *Journal of Pediatr*, 105(5), November 1984, p. 781-785.

Cancer

Results of this study showed that superoxide dismutase was effective in reducing radioinduced cystitis in patients suffering from bladder cancer.

—F. Sanchiz, et al., "Prevention of Radioinduced Cystitis by Orgotein: A Randomized Study," *Anticancer Research*, 16(4A), July-August 1996, p. 2025-2058.

Cardiovascular/Coronary Heart Disease

Results of this study showed that superoxide dismutase protected rabbit hearts against functional and structural alterations due to ischemia and reflow.

—K.P. Burton, "Superoxide Dismutase Enhances Recovery Following Myocardial Ischemia," *American Journal of Physiol*, 248(5 Pt 2), May 1985, p. H637-H643.

Results of this study found that superoxide dismutase modified reperfusion-induced impaired coronary vasodilator reserve in dogs when administered prior to reperfusion.

—J.L. Mehta, et al., "Protection by Superoxide Dismutase from Myocardial Dysfunction and Attenuation of Vasodilator Reserve after Coronary Occlusion and Reperfusion in Dog," *Circulatory Research*, 65(5), November 1989, p. 1283-1295.

Results of this study showed that the infusion of superoxide dismutase + catalase significantly reduced blood pressure during reperfusion in dogs.

—K. Przyklenk & R.A. Kloner, "Superoxide Dismutase Plus Catalase Improve Contractile Function in the Canine Model of the Stunned Myocardium," *Circulatory Research*, 58(1), January 1986, p. 148-156.

Results of this study showed that superoxide dismutase decreased infarct size in dogs during reperfusion.

—G. Ambrosio, et al., "Reduction in Experimental Infarct Size by Recombinant Human Superoxide Dismutase: Insights into the Pathophysiology of Reperfusion Injury," *Circulation*, 74(6), December 1986, p. 1424-1433.

Results of this study showed that superoxide dismutase attenuated platelet thrombus formation in damaged rabbit hearts.

> —Y.Y. Meng, et al., "Potentiation of Endogenous Nitric Oxide with Superoxide Dismutase Inhibits Platelet-mediated Thrombosis in Injured and Stenotic Arteries," *Journal of American College Cardiol* 25(1), January 1995, p. 269-275.

Results of this study found that superoxide dismutase combined with catalase protected ischemic dog hearts from reperfusion injury.

> —H. Otani, et al., "Protection Against Oxygen-induced Reperfusion Injury of the Isolated Canine Heart by Superoxide Dismutase and Catalase," *Journal of Surg Res,* 41(2), August 1986, p. 126-133.

Results of this study found that superoxide dismutase and catalase significantly enhanced myocardial protection against normothermic ischemia/reperfusion injury in rats.

> —D.T. Greenfield, et al., "Enhancement of Crystalloid Cardioplegic Protection Against Global Normothermic Ischemia by Superoxide Dismutase Plus Catalase but not Diltiazem in the Isolated, Working Rat Heart," *Journal of Thorac Cardiovasc Surg,* 95(5), May 1988, p. 799-813.

Results of this study showed that superoxide dismutase reduced norepinephrine-induced mortality in rats as well as decreasing blood pressure in hypertensive rats.

> —X.M. Zhang & E.F. Ellis, "Superoxide Dismutase Decreases Mortality, Blood Pressure, and Cerebral Blood Flow Responses Induced by Acute Hypertension in Rats," *Stroke,* 22(4), April 1991, p. 489-494.

Results of this study found that superoxide dismutase inhibited myocardial injury caused by ischemic reperfusion in rat hearts.

> —M.F. Xu, et al., "Effects of Superoxide Dismutase on Ischemic Reperfusion Injury in Isolated Working Heart and Cultured Myocardial Cells of Rats," *Chung Kuo Yao Li Hsueh Pao,* 11(4), July 1990, p. 324-328.

Results of this study found that superoxide dismutase administered to rats undergoing superior mesenteric artery occlusion shock protected cells against lipid peroxidation injury and extended rats survival time.

> —J.H. Wang, et al., "Oxygen-derived Free Radicals Induced Cellular Injury in Superior Mesenteric Artery Occlusion Shock: Protective Effect of Superoxide Dismutase," *Circ Shock,* 32(1), September 1990, p. 31-41.

Results of this study found that the administration of superoxide dismutase and catalase reduced damaging effects associated with heart transplantation in rats.

> —J. Bergsland, et al., "Allopurinol in Prevention of Reperfusion Injury of Hypoxically Stored Rat Hearts," *Journal of Heart Transplant,* 6(3), May-June 1987, p. 137-140.

Results of this study showed that the combination of superoxide dismutase and catalase added to cardioplegic solution or reperfusion fluid had protective effects on the myocardium against ischemic or reperfusion injury in isolated rat hearts.

> —Y. Nishikawa, et al., "The Effect of Superoxide Dismutase and Catalase on Myocardial

Reperfusion Injury in the Isolated Rat Heart," *Japanese Journal of Surgery,* 21(4), July 1991, p. 423-432.

This review article notes that the most promising use for superoxide dismutase with respect to humans involves protecting against ischaemia and post-ischaemic reperfusion damage of various organs and tissues.

—R. Ferrari, et al., "Superoxide Dismutase: Possible Therapeutic Use in Cardiovascular Disease," *Pharmacol Research,* 21(Suppl 2), November-December 1989, p. 57-65.

Cochlear Damage

Results of this study found that pretreatment with superoxide dismutase or allopurinol attenuated ischemia and reperfusion-induced cochlear damage in rats.

—M.D. Seidman, et al., "The Protective Effects of Allopurinol and Superoxide Dismutase-polyethylene Glycol on Ischemic and Reperfusion-induced Cochlear Damage," *Otolaryngol Head Neck Surg,* 105(3), September 1991, p. 457-463.

Results of this study found that treatment with superoxide dismutase or allopurinol had protective effects against noise-induced cochlear damage in rats.

—.S.D. Seidman, et al., "The Protective Effects of Allopurinol and Superoxide Dismutase on Noise-Induced Cochlear Damage," *Otolaryngol Head Neck Surg,* 109(6), December 1993, p. 1052-1056.

Fanconi Anaemia

In this study, 4 fanconi anaemia patients received 25 mg/kg per day of human superoxide dismutase for 2 weeks. Results showed the treatment reduced lymphocyte chromosomal aberrations induced by diepoxybutane in 2 patients increased bone marrow progenitors in another.

—J.M. Liu, et al., "A Trial of Recombinant Human Superoxide Dismutase in Patients with Fanconi Anaemia," *British Journal of Haematol,* 85(2), October 1993, p. 406-408.

Flu

Results of this study found that mice treated with superoxide dismutase at the late period of influenza infection increased survival rate by between 30-50%.

—B.P. Sharonov, et al., "The Effective Use of Superoxide Dismutase from Human Erythrocytes in the Late Stages of Experimental Influenza Infection," *Vopr Virusol,* 36(6), November-December 1991, p. 477-480.

Gastric Mucosal Lesions

Results of this study found that the intravenous administration of superoxide dismutase normalized systemic circulation and vascular permeability of gastric mucosa while also preventing stress-induced gastric injury in rats.

—M. Hirota, et al., "Inhibition of Stress-induced Gastric Mucosal Injury by a Long Acting Superoxide Dismutase that Circulates Bound to Albumin," *Arch Biochem Biophys,* 280(2), August 1, 1990, p. 269-273.

Results of this study showed that the administration of Cu, Zn-superoxide dismutase exhibited protective effects against emotional-stress-induced gastric mucosa damage in rats.

> —F.A. Zvershkhanovskii, et al., "Protective Effect of Superoxide Dismutase against the Damage of the Rat Gastric Mucosa During Emotional and Pain Stress," *Vopr Med Khim,* 33(3), May-June 1987, p. 49-53.

Hemorrhagic Shock

Results of this study found that the administration of superoxide dismutase enhanced the lifespan of rats exposed to hemorrhagic shock.

> —L.R. Tan, et al., "Superoxide Dismutase and Allopurinol Improve Survival in an Animal Model of Hemorrhagic Shock," *Am Surg,* 59(12), December 2993, p. 797-800.

Ischemic Spinal Cord Injury

Results of this study showed that treatment with superoxide dismutase reduced motor dysfunction and spinal infarcts a week following ischemia in rabbits.

> —P. Cuevas, et al., "Ischemic Reperfusion Injury in Rabbit Spinal Cord: Protective Effect of Superoxide Dismutase on Neurological Recovery and Spinal Infarction," *Acta Anat,* 137(4), 1990, p. 303-310.

Kidney Damage

Results of this study showed that superoxide dismutase had significant protective effects against kidney damage induced by ischemia and reperfusion in dogs.

> —K. Ouriel, et al., "Protection of the Kidney after Temporary Ischemia: Free Radical Scavengers," *Journal of Vascular Surgery,* 2(1), January 1985, p. 49-53.

Results of this study showed that intravenous superoxide dismutase had significant protective effects against ischemia-induced kidney damage in rats.

> —A. Bayati, et al., "Prevention of Ischaemic Acute Renal Failure with Superoxide Dismutase and Sucrose," *Acta Physiol Scand,* 130(3), July 1987, p. 367-372.

Liver Damage

Results of this study found that the glycosulated superoxide dismutase derivates, galactosylated and mannosylated, prevented ischemia/reperfusion-induced liver damage in rats.

> —T. Fujita, et al., "Therapeutic Effects of Superoxide Dismutase Derivatives Modified with Mono-or Polysaccharides on Hepatic Injury Induced by Ischemia/reperfusion," *Biochem Biophys Res Commun,* 189(1), November 30, 1992, p. 191-196.

Lung Damage

Results of this study found that the elevated enzyme levels in rats' lungs treated with liposome-encapsulated superoxide dismutase or catalase led to significant improvements in survival rates following hyperoxic exposure for 72 hours as well as a reduced rate of lung injury relative to controls.

> —R.V. Padmanabhan, et al., "Protection Against Pulmonary Oxygen Toxicity in Rats by the

Intratracheal Administration of Liposome-encapsulated Superoxide Dismutase or Catalase,'' *American Rev Respir Disease,* 132(1), July 1985, p. 164-167.

Results of this study showed that prophylactice intratraceal administration of superoxide dismutase significantly ameliorated acute lung injury caused from hyperoxia and hyperventilation in piglets.
—J.M. Davis, et al., ''Prophylactic Effects of Recombinant Human Superoxide Dismutase in Neonatal Lung Injury,'' *Journal of Applied Physiology,* 74(5), May 1993, p. 2234-2241.

Results of this study found that superoxide dismutase protected hamsters against radiation-induced pulmonary injury.
—R. Breuer, et al., ''Superoxide Dismutase Inhibits Radiation-induced Lung Injury in Hamsters,'' *Lung,* 170(1), 1992, p. 19-29.

Results of this study showed that superoxide dismutase reduced the severity of radiation-induced lesions in rat lungs.
—K. Malaker & R.M. Das, ''Effect of Superoxide Dismutase on Early Radiation Injury of Lungs in the Rat,'' *Mol Cell Biochem,* 84(2), December 1988, p. 141-145.

Results of this study showed that superoxide dismutase protected dogs undergoing lung transplant from lung edema.
—H. Date, ''Experimental Studies on Reimplantation Response after Lung Transplantation,'' *Nippon Kyobu Geka Gakkai Zasshi,* 37(3), March 1989, p. 510-521.

Multiple Organ Failure

Results of this placebo-controlled study showed that 3000 mg per day of intravenous recombinant human superoxide dismutase administered over a period of 5 days following multiple injuries attenuated multiple organ failure with respect to cardiovascular and pulmonary functions in human patients.
—I. Marzi, et al., ''Value of Superoxide Dismutase for Prevention of Multiple Organ Failure after Multiple Trauma,'' *Journal of Trauma,* 35(1), July 1993, p. 110-119.

Muscle Injury

Results of this study found that superoxide dismutase protected against muscle injury induced by ischemia/reperfusion in rats.
—R. Giardino, et al., ''Biopolymeric Modification of Superoxide Dismutase (mPEG-SOD) to Prevent Muscular Ischemia-reperfusion Damage,'' *Int J Artif Organs,* 18(3), March 1995, p. 167-172.

Paraquat Toxicity

Results of this study found that superoxide dismutase protected rats from acute paraquat toxicity.
—B. Wasserman & E.R. Block, ''Prevention of Acute Paraquat Toxicity in Rats by Superoxide Dismutase,'' *Aviat Space Environ Med,* 49(6), June 1978, p. 805-809.

Penis Plastica

Results of this study found that superoxide dismutase exhibited beneficial effects in patients suffering from plastic penile induration.

> —S. Pastorini, et al., "The Therapy of Plastic Penile Induration Using Superoxide Dismutase Per os and Injection Combined with Vasoactive Intracavernous Pharmacotherapy," *Minerva Urol Nefro,* 43(2), April-June 1991, p. 75-78.

Respiratory Distress Syndrome

Results of this placebo-controlled study showed that a single intratracheal dose of recombinant human superoxide dismutase had protective effects against lung injury in preterm infants suffering from respiratory distress syndrome.

> —W.N. Rosenfeld, et al., "Safety and Pharmacokinetics of Recombinant Human Superoxide Dismutase Administered Intratracheally to Premature Neonates with Respiratory Distress Syndrome," *Pediatrics,* 97(6 Pt 1), June 1996, p. 811-817.

Skin Lesions

Results of this study found topical superoxide dismutase to be an effective treatment against burn-induced skin lesions in human patients.

> —Y. Niwa, "Lipid Peroxides and Superoxide Dismutase (SOD) Induction in Skin Inflammatory Diseases, and Treatment with SOD Preparations," *Dermatologica,* 179(Suppl 1), 1989, p. 101-106.

Results of this study found superoxide dismutase cream to be an effective therapy against skin and mucosal lesions associated with a variety of different diseases including progressive systemic sclerosis, lupus, burns, Behcet's disease, and herpes simplex.

> —Y. Mizushima, et al., "Topical Application of Superoxide Dismutase Cream," *Drugs Exp Clin Res,* 17(2), 1991, p. 127-131.

Stroke

Results of this study found that the administration of human recombinant superoxide dismutase protected against ischemic neuronal damage in gerbils.

> —O. Uyama, et al., "Protective Effects of Human Recombinant Superoxide Dismutase on Transient Ischemic Injury of CA1 Neurons in Gerbils," *Stroke,* 23(1), January 1992, p. 75-81.

TMJ

Results of this study found that intra-articular injection of superoxide dismutase was an effective treatment for TMJ patients not responsive to traditional therapy.

> —Y. Lin, et al., "Use of Superoxide Dismutase (SOD) in Patients with Temporomandibular Joint Dysfunction—A Preliminary Study," *International Journal of Oral Maxillofac Surg,* 23(6 Pt 2), December 1994, p. 428-429.

Ulcer

Results of this study showed that superoxide dismutase exhibited protective effects against indomethacin-induced intestinal ulcers in rats.

> —I. Zahavi, et al., "Oxygen Radical Scavengers are Protective Against Indomethacin-induced Intestinal Ulceration in the Rat," *Journal of Pediatric Gastroenterol Nutrition,* 21(2), August 1995, p. 154-157.

Results of this study showed that superoxide dismutase injected into the bladderwall was an effective treatment for ulcus simples vesicae and irradiation bladder ulcer in female patients.

> —K. Reuss & P. Carl, "Treatment of Ulcus Simplex of the Bladder and Ulcerating Radiogenic Cystitis with Superoxide Dismutase," *Urologe,* 22(5), September 1983, p. 290-293.

Wound Healing

Results of this study found that superoxide dismutase treatment coupled with wound excision had therapeutic effects on severe burn injury in rats.

> —D. Saitoh, et al., "Prevention of Ongoing Lipid Peroxidation by Wound Excision and Superoxide Dismutase Treatment in the Burned Rat," *American Journal of Emergency Medicine,* 12(2), March 1994, p. 142-146.

Results of this study found that superoxide radical scavenging agents were an effective therapy for ocular alkali burns in rabbits.

> —V.S. Nirankari, et al., "Superoxide Radical Scavenging Agents in Treatment of Alkali Burns. An Experimental Study," *Arch Ophthalmol,* 99(5), May 1981, p. 886-887.

Results of this study found that the intravenous administration of 1000 units per kg of polyethylene glycol- conjugated superoxide dismutase within 6 hours of injury was an effective treatment for patients suffering from burns.

> —P.D. Thomson, et al., "Superoxide Dismutase Prevents Lipid Peroxidation in Burned Patients," *Burns,* 16(6), December 1990, p. 406-408.

Results of this study indicated that superoxide dismutase exhibited curative effects on periodontal wound healing in rats.

> —H. Misaki, et al., "The Effect of Superoxide Dismutase on the Inflammation Induced by Periodontal Pathogenic Bacteria and Wound Healing of Gingival Incision," *Nippon Shishubyo Gakkai Kaishi,* 32(1), March 1990, p. 93-110.

■ VITAMIN A/BETA-CAROTENE

Abetalipoproteinemia

This study reports on the cases of one child and one adult with abetalipoproteinemia who were maintained on a high doses of vitamins A and E. Five years of such supplementation resulted in a halt of neurological disease progression in the adult patient.

> —D.R. Illingworth, et al., "Abetalipoproteinemia: Report of Two Cases and Review of Therapy," *Arch Neurol,* 37(10), October 1980, p. 659-662.

In this study, 8 abetalipoproteinaemia patients were treated with a combination of supplemental vitamins A and E over a period of 2-6 years. Results showed the therapy halted the progression of visual function disturbance in all patients, prompting the authors to suggest vitamins A and E could be an effective means of arresting retinal deterioration caused by this condition.

—S. Bishara, et al., "Combined Vitamin A and E Therapy Prevents Retinal Electrophysiological Deterioration in Abetalipoproteinaemia," *British Journal of Ophthalmology,* 66(12), December 1992, p. 767-770.

Acne

Results of this study found that the treatment of 30 acne vulgaris patients with 0.025% vitamin A acid in gel form for 12 weeks reduced the amount of papules, pustules, and comedones in 25 of the patients.

—L. Juhlin, "Topical Vitamin A Acid in Acne Vulgaris," *Acta Derm Venereol Suppl,* 74, January 27-29, 1975, p. 133-134.

This review article reports the results of one study showing the efficacy of retinol in doses of 300,000 IU and 400,000 IU in women and men, respectively, for the treatment of acne vulgaris. The authors argue that the risk of hypervitaminosis A for such levels of treatment has been overblown and that retinol is an effective drug for treating this condition. Treatment usually takes 3-4 months with dosages being gradually reduced in accordance with reduction of symptoms.

—A.M. Kligman, et al., "Oral Vitamin A in Acne Vulgaris: Preliminary Report," *International Journal of Dermatology,* 20(4), May 1981, p. 278-285.

Aging

This placebo-controlled study examined whether or not the immune systems of elderly subjects could be enhanced by supplemental beta-carotene and selenium. Results found that beta-carotene administered by itself and in combination with selenium enhanced natural killer activity.

—S.M. Wood, "Effects of Beta-Carotene and Selenium Supplementation in Aged Humans," *Dissertation Abstracts International,* 55(4), 1994, p. 1387

Results of this study found that the median life span of Drosophilla could be increased by up to 17.5% following an increase in dietary vitamin A to adequate from inadequate levels during the various stages of development. Maximum life span was reduced when vitamin A was administered in amounts exceeding the optimal value.

—H.R. Massie, et al., "Effect of Vitamin A on Longevity," *Exp Gerontol,* 28(6), November-December 1993, p. 601-610.

AIDS/HIV

This placebo-controlled study examined the effects of supplemental vitamin A (50,000 IU at 1 and 3 months; 100,000 IU at 6 and 9 months; 200,000 IU at 12 and 15 months) on children born to women infected with HIV. Results found that children receiving supplements had a lower overall morbidity than controls and that diarrhea in HIV-infected children was significantly reduced.

—A. Coutsoudis, et al., "The Effects of Vitamin A Supplementation on the Morbidity of

Children Born to HIV-infected Women," *American Journal of Public Health,* 85(8 Pt 1), August 1995, p. 1076-1081.

This study looked at the effects of vitamin A plasma levels on immunologic status and clinical outcome in patients infected with HIV-1. Results found that a deficiency in vitamin A was associated with lower CD4 levels among both seronegative individuals and seropositive individuals as well as increased mortality in seropositive individuals. The authors conclude that vitamin A deficiency is a serious risk factor for the progression of disease in those infected with HIV-1.

> —R.D. Semba, et al., "Increased Mortality Associated with Vitamin A Deficiency During Human Immunodeficiency Virus Type 1 Infection," *Archives of Internal Medicine,* 153(18), September 27, 1993, p. 2149-2154.

This study examined the effects of vitamin deficiency on the rate of mother-to-child transmission of HIV. Results showed that approximately 70% of pregnant women with HIV were deficient in serum vitamin A. Women with lowest levels showed the highest rates of HIV transmission to their infants and infant mortality rates were also highest among the babies born to vitamin A deficient mothers. The vitamin A deficient mothers themselves had an increased risk of nearly twice that of non-deficient mothers.

> —R.D. Semba, et al., "Vitamin A Deficiency, Infant Mortality, and Mother-to-child Transmission of HIV," *Lancet,* 343(8913), June 25, 1994, p. 1593-1597.

This double-blind, placebo-controlled study examined the effects of 180 mg per day of beta-carotene for 4 weeks on the CD4 counts in HIV-infected patients. Results showed that supplementation of beta-carotene significantly increased total WBC count, % change in CD4 count, and % change in CD4/CD8 ratios relative to controls.

> —G.O. Coodley, et al., "Beta-carotene in HIV Infection," *Journal of Acquired Immune Deficiency Syndrome,* 6(3), March 1993, p. 272-276.

In this study, 50 adult injection drug users who died from AIDS were matched to 235 controls who survived. Results found that vitamin A deficiency and wasting were associated with mortality and common during HIV infections. Both were shown to be independent predictors or mortality among injection drug users infected with HIV.

> —R.D. Semba, et al. "Vitamin A Deficiency and Wasting as Predictors of Mortality in Human Immunodeficiency Virus-infected Injection Drug Users," *Journal of Infectious Disease,* 171(5), May 1995, p. 1196-1202.

Results of this study found that a severe deficiency in vitamin A was found to be associated with a 20-fold increase in the risk of having HIV-1 DNA in breast milk among women with 400 CD4 cells/mm3. Such women may be at an increased risk of transmitting HIV-1 through breast milk to their infants.

> —R.W. Nduati, et al., "Human Immunodeficiency Virus Type 1-infected Cells in Breast Milk: Association with Immunosuppression and Vitamin A Deficiency," *Journal of Infectious Disease,* 172(6), December 1995, p. 1461-1481.

In this study, 11 HIV-infected patients received 60 mg of beta-carotene per day for 4 months. Increases were found in the percent of natural killer cells, Ia antigrm and transferrin receptor were observed following treatment for 3 months.

> —H.S. Garewal, et al., "A Preliminary Trial of Beta-carotene in Subjects Infected with the

Human Immunodeficiency Virus,'' *Journal of Nutrition,* 122(3 Suppl), March 1992, p. 728-732.

In this pilot study, 10 patients infected with HIV who had just discontinued use of either AZT or DDI received 1 session of whole body hyperthermia with a noninvasive procedure at 42 degrees C core temperature for one hour, and subsequently supplemented with 120 mg per day of beta-carotene. Results showed the treatment was tolerated well by all patients aside from one who died within 4 months. The remaining 9 experienced an HIV burden diminution, clinical improvement and amelioration of laboratory data, and reported subjective improvements in overall quality of life.

—P. Pontiggia, et al., ''Whole Body Hyperthermia Associated with Beta-carotene Supplementation in Patients with AIDS,'' *Biomed Pharmacotherapy,* 49(5), 1995, p. 263-265.

In this study, 7 AIDS patients on AZT received 60 mg of beta-carotene twice a day along with one daily multivitamin for 4 weeks. Results found that the beta-carotene was well tolerated with no side effects. Half the patients experienced increases in CD4 counts during supplementation with a return to baseline levels once the trial was over.

—D.A. Fryburg, et al., ''The Immunostimulatory Effects and Safety of Beta-carotene in Patients with AIDS,'' *International Conference on AIDS,* 8(2), July 19-24, 1992, p. B163.

This study examined the effects of 30 mg per day of beta-carotene for 4 months on the lymphocytes of 11 AIDS patients. Results showed significant increases in the number of cells with NK markers and markers of activation after 3 months.

—R.R. Watson, et al., ''Immunostimulatory Effects of Beta-carotene on T-cell Activation Markers and NK Cells in HIV Infected Patients,'' *International Conference on AIDS,* 5, June 4-9, 1989, p. 663.

Results of this study showed that high dietary vitamin A was associated with a retarded death rate in mice infected with LP-BM5 murine leukemia, an AIDS-like condition, relative to controls.

—R.R. Watson, et al., ''Enhanced Survival by Vitamin A Supplementation During a Retrovirus Infection Causing Murine AIDS,'' *Life Science,* 43(6), 1988, p. xiii-xviii.

In this single-blind, pilot study, ARC patients supplemented with beta-carotene experienced a decrease in the progress towards AIDS, as well as recoveries from asthenia, fever, nocturnal sweating, diarrhea, and weight loss.

—A. Bianchi-Santamaria, et al., ''Short Communication: Possible Activity of Beta-Carotene in Patients with the AIDS Related Complex: A Pilot Study,'' *Medical Oncology Tumor Pharmacotherapy,* 9(3), 1992, p. 151-153.

Alzheimer's Disease

In examining Alzheimer's patients and those with multi-infarct dementia, this study found that both had significantly lower levels of vitamin E and beta-carotene than controls. Alzheimer's patients were shown to have significantly reduced levels of vitamin A as well.

—Z. Zaman, et al., ''Plasma Concentrations of Vitamins A and E and Carotenoids in Alzheimer's Disease,'' *Age Ageing,* 21(2), March 1992, p. 91-94.

Anemia

This double-blind, placebo-controlled study examined the influence of vitamin A (2.4 mg retinol) and iron (60 mg elemental iron) supplementation in anemic pregnant women between the ages of 17-35 years. Results found that the proportion of women who became non-anemic after supplementation was 35% in those receiving just vitamin A, 68% in those receiving just iron, 97% in those receiving both, and 16% among controls.

> —D. Suharno, et al., "Supplementation with Vitamin A and Iron for Nutritional Anemia in Pregnant Women in West Java, Indonesia," *Lancet,* 342(8883), November 27, 1993, p. 1325-1328.

Arthritis

Results of this study found that rats with experimentally-induced arthritis experienced a toxicity free decrease in clinical disease following the oral administration of retinoids. The authors suggest retinoids should be considered as possible therapeutic agents in treating rheumatoid arthritis.

> —C.E. Brinckerhoff, et al., "Effect of Retinoids on Rheumatoid Arthritis, a Proliferative and Invasive Non-malignant Disease," *Ciba Found Sympathy,* 113, 1985, p. 191-211.

Bitot's Spots

This study examined the effects of treatment with either a 100,000 IU or 200,000 IU dose of vitamin A on Bitot's spots in Indonesian children. Results showed that either dose proved effective, with the key factor in respect to treatment being the baseline serum retinol concentration. After six months, those receiving the higher dose of vitamin A were 82% less likely to have a relapse relative to those receiving the lower dose.

> —I. Sovani, et al., "Response of Bitot's Spots to a Single Oral 100,000- or 200,000-IU Dose of Vitamin A," *American Journal of Ophthalmology,* 118(6), December 15, 1994, p. 792-796.

Blindness

Results of this study found that the central cause of severe visual impairment and blindness among children in India is a deficiency in vitamin A.

> —J.S. Rahi, et al., "Childhood Blindness Due to Vitamin A Deficiency in India: Regional Variations," *Archives Dis Child,* 72(4), April 1995, p. 330-333.

In this study, 50,000 poor preschool children in India were administered 200,000 IU of vitamin A once every 6 months. Results showed that in areas of the country effected by the study the incidence of keratomalacia decreased by 80% relative to a 20% reduction in control areas.

> —K. Vijayaraghavan, et al., "Impact of Massive Doses of Vitamin A on Incidence of Nutritional Blindness," *Lancet,* 2(8395), July 21, 1984, p. 149-151.

Results of this case-control study found a significant inverse association between the consumption of carotenoid rich foods and the risk of exudative age-related macular degeneration, the leading cause of irreversible blindness in adults.

> —J.M. Seddon, et al., "Dietary Carotenoids, Vitamins A, C, and E, and Advanced Age-

related Macular Degeneration: Eye Disease Case-Control Study Group,'' *JAMA,* 272(18), November 9, 1994, p. 1413-1420.

In this study, the risk of night blindness was cut in half in preschool-aged children from Bangladesh who were orally administered 200,000 IU of vitamin A with 40 IU of vitamin E relative to controls. Data also showed that the risk of corneal ulcers or keratomalacia (X3A/B) was 2.7 times higher in controls.

    —N. Cohen, et al., ''Impact of Massive Doses of Vitamin A on Nutritional Blindness in Bangladesh,'' *American Journal of Clinical Nutrition,* 45(5), May 1987, p. 970-976.

Results of this study found that vitamin A deficiency may be considered a risk factor for developing night blindness among children in Bangladesh.

    —B.F. Stanton, et al., ''Risk Factors for Developing Mild Nutritional Blindness in Urban Bangladesh,'' *American Journal of Disea Child,* 140(6), June 1986, p. 584-588.

This study describes the case of a single patient with cystic fibrosis and hepatic involvement who developed vitamin A deficiency, night blindness, and a characteristic fundus picture. The oral supplementation with vitamin A was shown to reverse all such abnormalities.

    —M. O'Donnell and J.F. Talbot, ''Vitamin A Deficiency in Treated Cystic Fibrosis: Case Report,'' *British Journal of Ophthalmology,* 71(10), October 1987, p. 787-790.

This study reports on the cases of three patients with late stage primary biliary cirrhosis who were suffering from appreciable night blindness and low serum concentrations of vitamin. Each of the three patients responded well to high dose oral supplementation of vitamin A, demonstrating a full recovery of adaptation to dark and visual fields.

    —R.P. Walt, et al., ''Vitamin A Treatment for Night Blindness in Primary Biliary Cirrhosis,'' *British Medical Journal,* 288(6423), April 7, 1984, p. 1030-1031.

Cancer

Results of this study found that supplementation with 60 mg of vitamin A a week for 6 months produced a total remission of leukoplakias in 57% of the betal quid tobacco chewing fishermen from India examined. A reduction of micronucleated cells was seen in 96% of the subjects. Doses of 2.2 mmol per week of beta-carotene produced remission of leukoplakia in 14.8% and a reduction of micronucleated cells in 98%. The formation of new leukoplakia was completely suppressed by vitamin A and repressed by 50% as a result of beta-carotene with 6 months. Withdrawal of either beta-carotene or vitamin A supplementation resulted in the reappearance of leukoplakias and an increase in the frequency of micronuclei in oral mucosa. Lower doses of both agents prolonged the effect of the original treatment by a minimum of 8 additional months.

    —H.F. Stich, et al., ''Remission of Precancerous Lesions in the Oral Cavity of Tobacco Chewers and Maintenance of the Protective Effect of Beta-carotene or Vitamin A,'' *American Journal of Clinical Nutrition,* 53(1 Suppl), January 1991, p. 298S-304S.

This review article notes that beta-carotene is a promising agent for chemoprevention, especially due to its lack of toxicity. Beta-carotene suppresses micronuclei in exfoliated oral mucosal cells from those at risk for oral cancer and has been shown to reverse leukoplakia. The article also discusses the anti-cancer effects of retinoids, but points out their limitations with respect to toxicity.

—H.S. Garewal, ''Potential Role of Beta-carotene in Prevention of Oral Cancer,'' *American Journal of Clinical Nutrition,* 53(1 Suppl), January 1991, p. 294S-297S.

Results of this follow-up phase of the large scale Basel Study, which was begun in 1959, found that low carotene levels showed significant correlations for an increased risk of lung cancer among men. Increased risks for all cancers studied were found in cases where both carotene and retinol levels were low.

—H.B. Stahelin, et al., ''Beta-carotene and Cancer Prevention: The Basel Study,'' *American Journal of Clinical Nutrition,* 53(1 Suppl), January 1991, p. 265S-269S.

This review article notes that studies have consistently shown an increased risk of lung cancer among those with a low intake of vegetables, fruits, carotenoids, and beta-carotene. Studies also suggest that increasing their intake may lead to a reduction in the risk of the following cancers: mouth, cervix, bladder, rectum, pharynx, larynx, esophagus, colon, and stomach.

—R.G. Ziegler, et al., ''Vegetables, Fruits, and Carotenoids and the Risk of Cancer,'' *American Journal of Clinical Nutrition,* 53(1 Suppl), January 1991, p. 251S-259S.

Results of this case-control study of 83 breast cancer patients found that low plasma beta-carotene levels were associated with an increased risk of the disease.

—N. Potischman, et al., ''Breast Cancer and Dietary and Plasma Concentrations of Carotenoids and Vitamin A,'' *American Journal of Clinical Nutrition,* 52(5), November 1990, p. 909-915.

Results of this study showed that 10 mumol/L of beta-carotene produced significant retardation of growth in three cervical dysplasia cell lines.

—Y. Muto, et al., ''Growth Retardation in Human Cervical Dysplasia-derived Cell Lines by Beta-carotene through Down-regulation of Epidermal Growth Factor Receptor,'' *American Journal of Clinical Nutrition,* 62(6 Suppl), December 1995, p. 1535S-1540S.

This review article reports on the results of a large study of locally applied beta-trans retinoic acid which showed it to be an effective agent in reversing moderate cases of cervical intraepithelial neoplasia. Results from another study showed that beta-carotene suppressed cervical intraepithelial neoplasia.

—F.L. Meyskens, Jr. and A. Manetta, ''Prevention of Cervical Intraepithelial Neoplasia and Cervical Cancer,'' *American Journal of Clinical Nutrition,* 62(6 Suppl), December 1995, p. 1417S-1419S.

Results of this double-blind, placebo-controlled study showed that moderate presupplementation with beta-carotene (30 mg per day) can prevent beta-carotene depletion in the skin caused by ultraviolet radiation and in turn extend the prevention of free radical damage due to such radiation.

—C.F. Hemmes, et al., ''Effect of Beta-carotene Supplementation on Sun-induced Biochemical Alterations of the Skin in Normal Young Females,'' *Melanoma Research,* 3, 1993, p. 20-21.

In this article, the author presents evidence from laboratory studies, animals model systems, epidemiologic surveys, and intervention trials involving reversal of premalignant changes, and prevention of malignancies in particularly high-risk subjects, supporting the use of beta-carotene and vitamin E in the prevention of cancer of the oral cavity.

—H. Garewal, "Antioxidants in Oral Cancer Prevention," *American Journal of Clinical Nutrition,* 62(6 Suppl), December 1995, p. 1410S-1416S.

This review article notes that results from both cohort and case-control studies have shown consistent associations between a low intake of dietary and plasma beta-carotene and an increased risk of lung cancer. Similar, although less strong, associations have been found for stomach cancer and colorectal cancer.

—G. van Poppel and R.A. Goldbohm, "Epidemiologic Evidence for Beta-carotene and Cancer Prevention," *American Journal of Clinical Nutrition,* 62(6 Suppl), December 1995, p. 1393S-1402S.

Results of this study found a significant association between dietary intake of carotene-containing vegetables and a reduced risk of cancer mortality in elderly individuals.

—G.A. Colditz, et al., "Increased Green and Yellow Vegetable Intake and Lowered Cancer Deaths in an Elderly Population," *American Journal of Clinical Nutrition,* 41(1), January 1985, p. 32-36.

This placebo-controlled study examined the effects of beta-carotene and ascorbic acid on spontaneous and x-ray-induced appearance of micronuclei in human lymphocytes in healthy volunteers. Results found a significant inverse correlation between the frequency of irradiated lymphocytes and plasma beta-carotene levels, prompting the authors to conclude that beta-carotene may protect human lymphocytes from genetic damage caused by x-rays.

—K. Umegaki, et al., "Beta-carotene Prevents X-ray Induction of Micronuclei in Human Lymphocytes," *American Journal of Clinical Nutrition,* 59(2), February 1994, p. 409-412.

Results of this study showed that the administration of vitamin A palmitate to hamsters inhibited the 3,4-benzpyrene induction of squamous metaplasia and squamous cell carcinoma in the tracheobronchial mucosa and squamous cell papillomas of the forestomach.

—U. Saffiotti, "Role of Vitamin A in Carcinogenesis," *American Journal of Clinical Nutrition,* 22(8), 1969, p. 1088.

Results of this third examination phase of the large-scale Basel Study found that low carotene levels showed significant correlations for an increased risk of a host of different cancers among men.

—H.B. Stahelin, et al., "Plasma Antioxidant Vitamins and Subsequent Cancer Mortality in the 12-year Follow-up of the Prospective Basel Study," *American Journal of Epidemiology,* 133(8), April 15, 1991, p. 766-775.

This case-control study examined the relationship between serum beta-carotene levels and cancer. Low beta-carotene levels were found in subjects as well as the relatives of subjects with cancers of the lung, uterus, cervix, stomach, small intestine, and esophagus. Correlations proved to be the strongest among subjects and their relatives with respect to lung cancer.

—A.H. Smith and K.D. Waller, "Serum Beta-carotene in Persons with Cancer and their Immediate Families," *American Journal of Epidemiology,* 133(7), April 1, 1991, p. 661-671.

Results of this study on 427 male lung cancer patients found a negative association between dietary vitamin A and the risk of squamous cell and small cell carcinoma of the lung.

> —T. Byers, et al., "Dietary Vitamin A and Lung Cancer Risk: An Analysis by Histologic Subtypes," *American Journal of Epidemiology,* 120(5), November 1984, p. 769-776.

Results of this case-control study found evidence suggesting a high intake of beta-carotene may protect women against developing ovarian cancer.

> —M.L. Slattery, et al., "Nutrient Intake and Ovarian Cancer," *American Journal of Epidemiology,* 130(3), September 1989, p. 497-502.

Results of this study found a significant association between intake of vitamin A from fruits and vegetables and a reduced risk of lung cancer in men.

> —T.E. Byers, et al., "Diet and Lung Cancer Risk: Findings from the Western New York Diet Study," *American Journal of Epidemiology,* 125(3), March 1987, p. 351-363.

This study examined the beta-carotene levels in tissue samples of uterine leiomyomas and adjacent normal myometrium obtained at hysterectomy from the uteri of 18 patients. Beta-carotene levels were also taken from tissue samples of cancers of the breast, colon, lung, liver, rectum, cervix, endometrium, and ovary. Results showed that beta-carotene levels were significantly less in fibroid tissue than in normal myometrium. Levels also proved to be lower in all cancer tissue when compared to tissue taken from normal adjacent sites.

> —P.R. Palan, et al., "Decreased Beta-carotene Tissue Levels in Uterine Leiomyomas and Cancers of Reproductive and Nonreproductive Organs," *American Journal of Obstetrics and Gynecology,* 161(6 Pt 1), December 1989, p. 1649-1652.

Results of this study found that plasma beta-carotene levels and cervicovaginal cells were significantly lower in women with cervical intraepithelial cancer neoplasia and cervical cancer relative to controls. Oral supplementation with beta-carotene increased beta-carotene levels in cervicovaginal cells in 79% of the patients studied.

> —P.R. Palan, et al., "Beta-carotene Levels in Exfoliated Cervicovaginal Epithelial Cells in Cervical Intraepithelial Neoplasia and Cervical Cancer," *American Journal of Obstetrics and Gynecology,* 167(6), December 1992, p. 1899-1903.

Results of this study showed that pretreatment with vitamin A or vitamin A coupled with vitamin E protected rats against the dimethylbenzanthracene's carcinogenic action.

> —K.H. Calhoun, et al., "Vitamins A and E Do Protect Against Oral Carcinoma," *Arch Otolaryngol Head Neck Surg,* 115(4), April 1989, p. 484-488.

This review article notes that beta-carotene and other antioxidants have been shown to inhibit oral carcinogenesis in animal models. Epidemiologic studies have provided similar results. The authors also discuss the findings of eight clinical studies which have demonstrated the ability of beta-carotene and vitamin E to cause a regression of oral leukoplakia.

> —H.S. Garewal and S. Schantz, "Emerging Role of Beta-carotene and Antioxidant Nutrients in Prevention of Oral Cancer," *Arch Otolaryngol Head Neck Surg,* 121(2), February 1995, p. 141-144.

Results of this study showed that the administration of vitamin A to rats in high doses (greater than 100 IU/bw for 4 days) increased the tumoricidal and phagocytic activities of alveolar macrophages.

    —K. Tachibana, et al., "Stimulatory Effect of Vitamin A on Tumoricidal Activity of Rat Alveolar Macrophages," *British Journal of Cancer,* 49(3), March 1984, p. 343-348.

In this study, serum beta-carotene levels taken from 271 men prior to their diagnosis with cancer were compared to matched controls. Results showed significantly lower levels in the cancer patients, with men in the top two quintiles of serum beta-carotene having only about 60% of the risk of developing cancer compared with those in the bottom quintile.

    —N.J. Wald, et al., "Serum Beta-carotene and Subsequent Risk of Cancer: Results from the BUPA Study," *British Journal of Cancer,* 57(4), April 1988, p. 428-433.

Results of this study of colon and rectal cancer patients found independent inverse associations between these conditions and the intake of beta-carotene, ascorbic acid, vitamin E, and folate.

    —M. Ferraroni, et al., "Selected Micronutrient Intake and the Risk of Colorectal Cancer," *British Journal of Cancer,* 70(6), December 1994, p. 1150-1155.

In this placebo-controlled study, patients who had endoscopic removal of polyps received either a combination of 30,000 U of vitamin A, 70 mg of vitamin E and 1 g of vitamin C daily; 20-40 g per day of lactulose; or no treatment. Results showed a significantly lower level of polyp reappearance in the vitamin group relative to the other two.

    —M. Ponz de Leon, et al., "Antioxidant Vitamins (A, E and C) and Lactulose in the Prevention of the Recurrence of Adenomatous Polyps: Preliminary Results of a Controlled Study," *British Journal of Cancer,* 62(3), 1990, p. 496.

Results of this study showed that rats fed a diet deficient in vitamin A experienced a greater incidence of benzo(a)pyrene-induced lung tumors compared to those maintained on a control diet.

    —S.C. Dogra, et al., "The Effect of Vitamin A Deficiency on the Initiation and Postinitiation Phases of Benzo(a)pyrene-induced Lung Tumourigenesis in Rats," *British Journal of Cancer,* 52(6), December 1985, p. 931-935.

Results of this study showed that beta-carotene proved to be the most important dietary variable in improving survival in breast cancer patients.

    —D. Ingram, "Diet and Subsequent Survival in Women with Breast Cancer," *British Journal of Cancer,* 69(3), March 1994, p. 592-595.

This double-blind study examined the effects of supplementation with 20 mg of beta-carotene per day of a period of 14 weeks on the frequency of micronuclei in sputum in 114 heavy smokers. Results showed that beta-carotene levels in the treatment groups increased 13-fold during intervention. A 47% decrease in micronuclei counts was recorded in the treatment groups during intervention compare to just a 16% decrease among controls.

    —G. van Poppel, et al., "Beta-carotene Supplementation in Smokers Reduces the Frequency of Micronuclei in Sputum," *British Journal of Cancer,* 66(6), December 1992, p. 1164-1168.

In this letter, the author argues that vitamin A and its analogs are likely involved in the prevention of cancer. The author makes the point that vitamin A is involved in the synthesis of glycoproteins and that derangements in mucus glycoproteins have been found to present in gastric, colonic and bronchoalveolar cancer. Thus the role of analogs in cancer prevention may be mediated through mucus glycoprotein synthesis normalization.

> —M. Guslandi, "Vitamin A, Retinol, Carotene, and Cancer Prevention," *British Medical Journal,* 281(6251), 1980, p. 1352.

Results of this 12-14 year study of a population of approximately 3000 in one Georgia county found an inverse relationship between serum retinol levels and the risk of cancer.

> —J.D. Kark, et al., "Serum Retinol and the Inverse Relationship Between Serum Cholesterol and Cancer," *British Medical Journal,* 284(6310), January 16, 1982, p. 152-154.

This case-control study examined the relationship between serum selenium, vitamin A and vitamin E levels and cancer mortality risk. With respect to vitamin A, results showed that serum retinol concentrations were 26% lower in smoking men with cancer than in smoking controls.

> —J.T. Salonen, et al., "Risk of Cancer in Relation to Serum Concentrations of Selenium and Vitamins A and E: Matched Case-Control Analysis of Prospective Data," *British Medical Journal,* 290(6466), February 9, 1985, p. 417-420.

This article reviews the existing literature on the antineoplastic effects of retinoids. Based on the results of in vitro studies, the author makes the following observations: hyperplastic and metaplastic response to chemical carcinogens of mouse prostate cultures is suppressed by the addition of retinoids to the culture medium. Retinoids partially inhibit the morphologic transformation of 10T 1/2 cells by physical or chemical carcinogens. The growth of some non-neoplastic and some neoplastic cell lines can be inhibited by retinoids. With respect to the findings of in vivo studies, the author notes that retinoids can suppress papilloma and carcinoma development (the promotion phase) in the two-stage skin carcinogenesis assay. They inhibit mammary and bladder carcinogenesis in mice and rats. They can inhibit the growth of some transplantable tumor lines. In conclusion, the author argues that practically all synthetic retinoids have been seen to have a higher therapeutic index than natural retinoids with respect to cancer treatment.

> —P. Nettesheim, "Inhibition of Carcinogenesis by Retinoids," *Canadian Medical Association Journal,* 122(7), April 5, 1980, p. 757-765.

This review article notes that retinoids have been shown to control some proliferative skin tumors and that there is early evidence to suggest that 13-cis-retinoic acid can modify oral cavity leukoplakia.

> —J.J. DeCosse, "Potential for Chemoprevention," *Cancer,* 50(11 Suppl), December 1, 1982, p. 2550-2553.

This study examined the effects of vitamin A on cancer of the colon in rats. Results showed that in rats exposed to dimethylhydrazine, 100% of animals deficient in vitamin A developed colon tumors compared to just 60% of those receiving vitamin A supplementation. In another line of experiments, rats were fed 25 ug aflatoxin B1 (AFB1) per day for 15 days or AFB1 was added to the diet at 1 ppm, a significant incidence of colon tumors was noted in rats fed only 0.3 ug/g vitamin A. Rats fed 30 ug/g vitamin A showed a decreased incidence of colon cancer.

> —P.M. Newberne and V. Suphakarn, "Preventive Role of Vitamin A in Colon Carcinogenesis in Rats," *Cancer,* 40(5, Suppl), 1977, p. 2553-2556.

Results of this case-controlled study found a significant inverse association between both beta-carotene and total carotenoid levels and the risk of lung cancer in men.

> —J.E. Connett, et al., "Relationship Between Carotenoids and Cancer: The Multiple Risk Factor Intervention Trial (MRFIT) Study," *Cancer,* 64(1), July 1, 1989, p. 126-134.

This review article notes that studies have suggested a deficiency in vitamin A may lead to squamous cell metaplasia and be related to cancers of the nasopharynx, lower respiratory tract, endocervix and stomach. Vitamin A has also been shown to be a key factor in the control of growth, differentiation, and function of epithelial tissues.

> —R.J. Shamberger, "Vitamins and Cancer: Current Controversies," *Cancer Bulletin,* 34(4), 1982, p. 150-155.

Results of this study showed that rats receiving concentrations of either 0.6 or 1.0mM per kg of diet of retinyl acetate three days following exposure to 7,12-dimethylbenzathracene experienced a significant reduction in the incidence of experimentally-induced mammary carcinomas.

> —C.W. Welsch and J.V. DeHoog, "Retinoid Feeding, Hormone Inhibition, and/or Immune Stimulation and the Genesis of Carcinogen-induced Rat Mammary Carcinomas," *Cancer Research,* 43(2), February 1983, p. 585-591.

Results of this placebo-controlled study showed that the administration of 328 mg of retinyl acetate starting 7 days after carcinogen treatment inhibited DMBA-induced mammary tumorigenesis in mice.

> —H.J. Thompson, et al., "Effect of Retinyl Acetate on the Occurrence of Ovarian Hormone-responsive and -nonresponsive Mammary Cancers in the Rat," *Cancer Research,* 42(3), March 1982, p. 903-905.

Results of this placebo-controlled study showed that rats supplemented with either 300 mg of retinyl acetate and/or the retinyl acetate combined 4 mg of selenium per kg diet suffered from a lower mammary tumor incidence following exposure to N-methyl-N-nitrosourea than controls.

> —H.J. Thompson, et al., "Effect of Combined Selenium and Retinyl Acetate Treatment on Mammary Carcinogenesis," *Cancer Research,* 41(4), April 1981, p. 1413-1416.

Results of this study showed that certain retinoids reduce the ability of fresh human melanoma cells taken from ten patients with metastatic melanoma to form colonies in soft agar.

> —F.L. Meyskens, Jr. and S.E. Salmon, "Inhibition of Human Melanoma Colony Formation by Retinoids," *Cancer Research,* 39(10), October 1979, p. 4055-4057.

Results of this placebo-controlled study found that mice fed 200 mg of 13-cis-retinoic acid per kg 7 days after exposure to OH-BBN experienced a reduced incidence of carcinomas, noninvasive papillomas, and neoplastic development in the urinary bladder relative to controls.

> —P.J. Becci, et al., "Inhibitory Effect of 13-cis-retinoic Acid on Urinary Bladder Carcinogenesis Induced in C57BL/6 Mice by N-butyl-N-(4-hydroxybutyl)-nitrosamine," *Cancer Research,* 38(12), December 1978, p. 4463-4466.

Results of this study showed that the daily feeding of retinyl methyl ether to rats starting a week after exposure to 7,12-dimethylbenz(a)anthracene led to the inhibition of mammary cancer and reduction in the number of mammary tumors caused by the carcinogen. The latency period of cancer appearance was also increased. This retinoid proved superior to the use of retinyl acetate and produced no evident toxicity.

> —C.J. Gurbbs, et al., "Inhibition of Mammary Cancer by Retinyl Methyl Ether," *Cancer Research,* 37(2), February 1977, p. 599-602.

Results of this study found treatment with retinoic acid significantly reduced growth in vivo of the human mammary carcinoma cell line MDA-MB-231.

> —S.A. Halter, et al., "Effect of Retinoids on Xenotransplanted Human Mammary Carcinoma Cells in Athymic Mice," *Cancer Research,* 48(13), July 1, 1988, p. 3733-3736.

Results of this study on the relationship between dietary intake of beta-carotene and risk of prostate cancer in Japan found that risk reduction by beta-carotene and vitamin A was significant in men between the ages of 70-79.

> —Y. Ohno, et al., "Dietary Beta-carotene and Cancer of the Prostate: A Case-control Study in Kyoto, Japan," *Cancer Research,* 48(5), March 1, 1988, p. 1331-1336.

This study examined the effects of dietary vitamin A on mammary tumorigenesis in rats exposed to 7,12-dimethylbenz(a)anthracene. The following results were obtained: mammary tumors were significantly (P reduced relative to controls (10 micrograms per day of vitamin A) if rats were fed either 30 micrograms (moderate increase) or 3 micrograms per day (marginal amount) of vitamin A prior to and during initiation with 7,12-dimethylbenz(a)anthracene. Tumors also decreased significantly when a moderately increased or marginal amount of vitamin A was provided during the phase of tumor promotion.

> —M.H. Zile, et al., "Effect of Moderate Vitamin A Supplementation and Lack of Dietary Vitamin A on the Development of Mammary Tumors in Female Rats Treated with Low Carcinogenic Dose Levels of 7,12-dimethylbenz(a)anthracene," *Cancer Research,* 46(7), July 1986, p. 3495-3503.

Results of this study found a significant inverse association between serum levels of beta-carotene and the risk of lung cancer in Hawaiian men.

> —A.M. Nomura, et al., "Serum Vitamin Levels and the Risk of Cancer of Specific Sites in Men of Japanese Ancestry in Hawaii," *Cancer Research,* 45(5), May 1985, p. 2369-2372.

This study examined the effects of 30 mg of oral beta-carotene per day for 6 months on 20 male subjects who had previously undergone resection of colonic adenocarcinoma. Results showed that mucosal ornithine decarboxylase activity was inhibited by 44% after 2 weeks of beta-carotene administration and 57% after 9 weeks, remaining low for up to 6 months following discontinuation.

> —R.W. Phillips, et al., "Beta-Carotene Inhibits Rectal Mucosal Ornithine Decarboxylase Activity in Colon Cancer Patients," *Cancer Research,* 53(16), August 15, 1993, p. 3723-3725.

In this nested case-control study, the serum level nutrients of 28 subjects who developed oral and pharyngeal cancer during 1975-1990 were compared to controls. Results showed that serum levels of beta-carotene as well as all individual carotenes were lower in the cancer subjects.

> —W. Zheng, et al., "Serum Micronutrients and the Subsequent Risk of Oral and Pharyngeal Cancer," *Cancer Research,* 53(4), February 15, 1993, p. 795-798.

Results of this study found an inverse association between vitamin A and esophageal cancer as well as vitamin A and alcoholic hepatitis.

—B.A. Cuccherini, "The Association of Vitamin A with Esophageal Cancer," *Dissertation Abstracts International,* 48(5), 1987, p. 1319.

Results of this study showed associations between the risk of breast cancer and low beta-carotene and alpha-tocopherol and high triglyceride values. Associations were also seen between the risk of benign breast disease and low plasma beta-carotene and high triglycerides.

—N.A. Potischman, "The Associations Between Breast Cacncer and Biochemical and Dietary Indicators of Nutrient Status," *Dissertation Abstracts International,* 50(3), 1989, p. 909.

Results of this study showed that smokeless tobacco using, oral lesion patients who received 30 mg per day of beta-carotene experienced a dramatic improvement of the oral mucosa.

—R.B. Brandt, et al., "Beta-Carotene Treatment of Oral Lesions," *FASEB Journal,* 4(4), 1990, p. A1174.

In this study, patients with premalignant lesions of the oral cavity were given daily doses of 30 mg of beta-carotene, 1000 mg of ascorbic acid and 800 IU of alpha tocopherol for 9 months. Results found that 55.6% of subjects showed either partial or complete clinical resolution of their oral lesions.

—G. Kaugars, et al., "Serum and Tissue Antioxidant Levels in Supplemented Patients with Premalignant Oral Lesions," *FASEB Journal* 7(4), 1993, p. A519.

This review article notes that studies have shown mammary tumorigenesis in rodents to be suppressed by the combined administration of 250 mg/kg of retinly acetate and 4 mg/kg of selenium. The promise of vitamin A in protecting against tumorigenesis is also stressed.

—F.H. Nielsen, "Effect of Trace Minerals and Vitamins on Tumor Formation," *Food Technology,* 37(3), 1983, p. 63-67.

This study examined the therapeutic activity of 3000 IU of vitamin A and/or 0.2 mg of BCG in mice inoculated with Lewis Lung Tumor. Results showed a major decrease in the incidence of lung metastases and primary tumor development when vitamin A and BCG were administered together relative to controls.

—T. Kurata and M. Micksche, "Immumoprophylasxis in Lewis Lung Tumor with Vitamin A + BCG," *IRCS Med Sci: Cancer,* 5(6), 1977, p. 277.

This study examined the effects of retinoids on the in vitro clonal growth of myeloid leukemia cells. Results showed that retinoic acid inhibited growth of KG-1, acute myeloblastic leukemia, and the HL-60, acute promyelocytic leukemia, human cell lines. The KG-1 cells were sensitive to retinoic acid, with 50% of the colonies inhibited by 2.4-nM concentrations of the drug. A 50% growth inhibition of HL-60 was achieved by 25 nM retinoic acid. Complete inhibition of growth of both leukemia cell lines was seen with 1 microM retinoic acid. Exposure of KG-1 cells to retinoic acid for only 3-5 d was sufficient to inhibit all clonal growth. The all-trans and 13-cis forms of retinoic acid were equally effective in inhibiting proliferation. Retinoic acid also inhibited the clonal growth of leukemia cells from five of seven patients with acute myeloid leukemia. Retinoic acid at concentrations of 5 nM to 0.3 microM inhibited 50% clonal growth, and 1 microM retinoic acid inhibited 64- 98% of the leukemic colonies. Based on these findings, the authors suggest retinoic acid may be an effective means of treating human myeloid leukemia.

> —D. Douer and H.P. Koeffler, ''Retinoic Acid: Inhibition of the Clonal Growth of Human Myeloid Leukemia Cells,'' *Journal of Clinical Investigations,* 69(2), February 1982, p. 277-283.

Results of this study showed that retinoids may be a central factor in the treatment and regulation of breast cancer in humans by using human breast cancer cell lines as useful model to study their potential role in the disease.

> —A. Lacroix and M.E. Lippman, ''Binding of Retinoids to Human Breast Cacner Cell Lines and their Effects on Cell Growth,'' *Journal of Clinical Investigations,* 65(3), 1980, p. 586-591.

This review article argues that retinoids play important roles during normal fetal development and induce differentiation and/or growth inhibition in a variety of tumor-cell lines. The authors state that retinoid effects appear to result from changes in gene expression mediated via specific nuclear receptors (termed retinoic acid receptors, RAR- alpha, -beta, and -gamma), and a specific chromosomal translocation involving the RAR-alpha gene occurs in APL patients. They also point out that in addition to the very high clinical response rate for RA in patients with APL, significant clinical responses have been observed for patients with cutaneous T-cell malignancies, juvenile chronic myelogenous leukemia, and dermatologic malignancies.

> —M.A. Smith, et al., ''Retinoids in Cancer Therapy,'' *Journal of Clinical Oncology,* 10(5), May 1992, p. 839-864.

Results of this study found that the administration of beta-carotene in doses of 30 mg per day had marked protective activity against oral premalignancy and is an ideal means of treatment due to its lack of toxicity.

> —H.S. Garewal, et al., ''Response of Oral Leukoplakia to Beta-carotene,'' *Journal of Clinical Oncology,* 8(10), October 1990, p. 1715-1720.

This placebo-controlled study showed that the daily oral administration of 300,000 IU of vitamin A for 12 months significantly reduced the number of tobacco-related new primary tumors in lung cancer patients relative to controls.

> —U. Pastorino, et al., ''Adjuvant Treatment of Stage I Lung Cancer with High-dose Vitamin A,'' *Journal of Clinical Oncology,* 11(7), July 1993, p. 1216-1222.

This placebo-controlled study examined the effects of supplementation with vitamins A, C, and E in patients with colorectal adenomas 6 months after complete polypectomy. Results found that the supplementation lead to a reduction in abnormalities in cell kinetics that may indicate a precancerous condition.

> —G.M. Paganelli, et al., ''Effect of Vitamin A, C, and E Supplementation on Rectal Cell Proliferation in Patients with Colorectal Adenomas,'' *Journal of the National Cancer Institute,* 84(1), January 1, 1992, p. 47-51.

Results of this study showed a decreased tumor incidence, increased latent period, and increased survival time in C3H/HeJ mice fed supplemental beta-carotene for 3 days prior to being injected with 10(4) C3HBA tumor cells. Mice fed beta-carotene after inducoulation with 2 X 10(5) C3HBA tumor cells, also showed decreased tumor growth and increased survival time. Mice already possessing palpable tumors showed a slowed tumor growth and extended time following beta-carotene supplementation as well.

> —G. Rettura, et al., "Prophylactic and Therapeutic Actions of Supplemental Beta-carotene in Mice Inoculated with C3HBA Adenocarcinoma Cells: Lack of Therapeutic Action of Supplemental Ascorbic Acid," *Journal of the National Cancer Institute,* 69(1), July 1982, p. 73-77.

Results of this study showed CBA/J mice fed supplemental beta-carotene before and/or after injection with Moloney sarcoma virus experienced a decreased tumor frequency, increased latent period, and increased rate of tumor regression.. Beta-carotene also increased the rate of tumor regression when administered after tumors were already present and was shown to minimize the virus-induced thymus gland involution that accompanies tumor growth.

> —E. Seifter, et al., "Moloney Murine Sarcoma Virus Tumors in CBA/J Mice: Chemopreventive and Chemotherapeutic Actions of Supplemental Beta-carotene," *Journal of the National Cancer Institute,* 68(5), May 1982, p. 835-840.

Results of this study showed that when mice exposed to C3HBA tumors were fed supplemental vitamin A, resistance to the tumor was dramatically increased.

> —E. Selfter, et al., "Decreased Resistance of C3H/HeHa Mice to C3HBA Tumor Transplants; Increased Resistance Due to Supplemental Vitamin A," *Journal of the National Cancer Institute,* 67(2), August 1981, p. 467-472.

Results of this study found that the administration of a 250-ppm retinyl acetate dietary supplement significantly inhibited the induction of mammary cancers in rats exposed to 50 mg of benzo(a)pyrene.

> —D.L. McCormick, et al., "Inhibition of Benz[a]pyrene-induced Mammary Carcinogenesis by Retinyl Acetate," *Journal of the National Cancer Institute,* 66(3), March 1981, p. 559-564.

Results of this study of male lung cancer patients and controls with nonrespiratory, nonneoplastic disease showed an inverse association between vitamin A and risk of lung cancer among heavy smokers.

> —C. Mettlin, et al., "Vitamin A and Lung Cancer," *Journal of the National Cancer Institute,* 62(6), June 1979, p. 1435-1438.

This study examined the effects of either 2 or 22 mg/kg of dietary beta-carotene on 1,2-dimethylhydrazine-induced colon cancer in mice. Results showed that the incidence and multiplicity of colon tumors were reduced by half in mice receiving the 22 mg/kg dose of beta-carotene compared to controls, as was the mortality rate.

> —N.J. Temple and T.K. Basu, "Protective Effect of Beta-carotene Against Colon Tumors in Mice," *Journal of the National Cancer Institute,* 78(6), June 1987, p. 1211-1244.

Results of this study showed that the oral administration of 120 mg per day of beta-carotene for 9 days starting on the day of inoculation with sc with 10(7) syngeneic BALB/c Meth A fibrosarcoma cells (Meth A) led to a marked rejection against rechallenged Meth A implanted sc on day 10 in mice.

> —Y. Tomita, et al., "Augmentation of Tumor Immunity Against Syngeneic Tumors in Mice by Beta-Carotene," *Journal of the National Cancer Institute,* 78(4), April 1987, p. 679-681.

Results of this study showed that vitamin A exerted anticarcinogenic effects in mice exposed to chemically-induced carcinomas by inhibiting DNA synthesis, disrupting cell surfaces, and possibly interfering with MCA metabolism in epidermal cells.

> —A. Lupulescu, "Inhibition of DNA Synthesis and Neoplastic Cell Growth by Vitamin A," *Journal of the National Cancer Institute,* 77(1), July 1986, p. 149-156.

Results of this study showed that mice supplemented with beta-carotene and vitamin A received far more benefit from local irradiation against 2 X 10(5) C3HBA-induced carcinogenesis than controls. Beta-carotene proved to be more powerful than vitamin A in this respect.

> —E. Seifter, et al., "Regression of C3HBA Mouse Tumor Due to X-ray Therapy Combined with Supplemental Beta-Carotene or Vitamin A," *Journal of the National Cancer Institute,* 71(2), August 1983, p. 409-417.

Results of this case-control study found an inverse association between dietary intake of beta-carotene, vitamin E supplements, raw fruits and vegetables and the risk of lung cancer in nonsmokers of both sexes.

> —S.T. Mayne, et al., "Dietary Beta Carotene and Lung Cancer Risk in U.S. Nonsmokers," *Journal of the National Cancer Institute,* 86(1), January 5, 1994, p. 33-38.

This study examined the effects of vitamin A on tumor establishment, growth and metastasis in rats with N-2-fluorenylacetamide-induced solid tumors. Results found that tumor growth was similar in both rats fed both deficient and adequate levels of vitamin A when supplementation was started at the same time as carcinogen exposure. Tumors were reduced when supplementation was started 2 weeks prior to exposure in rats fed either a diet deficient in vitamin A or with vitamin A in excess levels.

> —D.M. Morre, et al., "Chemoprevention of Tumor Development and Metastasis of Transplantable Hepatocellular Carcinomas in Rats by Vitamin A," *Journal of Nutrition,* 110(8), August 1980, p. 1629-1234.

Results of this study showed an inverse association between the intake of beta-carotene and rate of lung cancer in middle-aged men.

> —R.B. Shekelle, et al., "Dietary Vitamin A and Risk of Cancer in the Western Electric Study," *Lancet,* 2(8257), 1981, p. 1185-1190.

Results of this study found that serum retinol levels in the lowest quintile of the 16,000 men studied were associated with a 2.2 times greater risk of cancer compared to men whose serum retinol levels measured in the highest quintile.

> —N. Wald, et al., "Low Serum-vitamin-A and Subsequent Risk of Cancer: Preliminary Results of a Prospective Study," *Lancet,* 2(8199), October 18, 1980, p. 813-815.

This study reports on the cases of two cutaneous metastatic melanoma patients who were treated topically with beta-all-trans-retinoic acid. One patient experienced a complete regression of the treated lesions while the other experienced partial regression.

   —N. Levine and F.L. Meyskens, "Topical Vitamin-A-acid Therapy for Cutaneous Metastatic Melanoma," *Lancet,* 2(8188), August 2, 1980, p. 224-226.

Results of this study found that 3 months of supplementing the diet of 40 rural Filipino betel chewers with sealed capsules of retinol (100 000 IU/week) and beta-carotene (300 000 IU/week) was associated with a threefold decrease in the mean proportion of cells with micronuclei inside the cheekpouch. Such effects were seen in 37 of the 40 subjects who received supplementation compared to no changes seen in any of the controls. The authors suggest such findings indicate that the dietary intake of beta-carotene and retinol may reduce the risk of oral cancer.

   —H.F. Stich, et al., "Reduction with Vitamin A and Beta-carotene Administration of Proportion of Micronucleated Buccal Mucosal Cells in Asian Betal Nut and Tobacco Chewers," *Lancet,* 1(8388), June 2, 1984, p. 1204-1206.

After reviewing the existing literature, this article notes that vitamin A and its derivatives most likely is a key component in the treatment skin malignancies as well as in the treatment of several bronchial dysplasias and prevention of recurring bladder tumors.

   —M. Clerici, et al., [Current Status of the Use of Vitamins (A, E, C, D), Folates and Selenium in the Chemoprevention and Treatment of Malignant Tumors], *Minerva Med,* 78(6), March 31, 1987, p. 377-386.

Results of this case-control study showed a strong inverse association between serum beta-carotene levels and the risk of lung cancer.

   —M.S. Menkes, et al., "Serum Beta-carotene, Vitamins A and E, Selenium, and the Risk of Lung Cancer," *New England Journal of Medicine,* 315(20), November 13, 1986, p. 1250-1254.

In this study, 9 males with metastatic unresectable squamous cell carcinoma of the lung were treated with up to 7 treatment courses of either 13-cis vitamin A acid or vitamin A palmitate over a period of 60 weeks. Results showed the vitamin A treatment to have an immune potentiating effect as was evident from a significant increase of lymphocyte blastogenesis response to phytochemagglutinin relative to pretreatment values, and increases in delayed cutaneous hypersensitivity reactions seen in all patients.

   —M. Micksche, et al., [Immune Stimulation for Lung Cancer Patients Using Vitamin A Therapy], *Oesterr Z Onkol,* 1(2), 1978, p. 57-62.

In this study, 79 oral leukoplakia patients were given 30 mg of beta-carotene, 1000 mg of ascorbic acid, and 800 IU of alpha-tocopherol per day for 9 months. Results found that 55.7% of the patients showed an improvement, particularly in those who reduced their use of tobacco and alcohol.

   —G.E. Kaugars, et al., "A Clinical Trial of Antioxidant Supplements in the Treatment of Oral Leukoplakia," *Oral Surg Oral Med Oral Pathology,* 78(4), October 1994, p. 462-468.

Results of this study showed that 13-cis-retinoic acid administration inhibited the incidence and degree of N-methyl-N- nitrosourea-induced bladder cancer in rats.

—M.B. Sporn, et al., "13-cis-retinoic Acid: Inhibition of Bladder Carcinogenesis in the Rat," *Science,* 195(4277), February 4, 1977, p. 487-489.

This study examined the effects of topical beta-trans retinoic acid applied for three four-day periods three months apart on cervical intraepithelial neoplasia. Results showed that treatment had favorable effects on patients with moderate cervical dysplasia, but not on those suffering from severe cervical dysplasia.

—T.E. Moon, et al., "The Evaluation of Topically Applied Retinoic Acid in the Regression of Cervical Intraepithelial Neoplasia," *American Society of Preventive Oncology, 17th Annual Meeting, March 20-23, 1993, Tucson, AZ.*

This review article makes the following observations with respect to beta-carotene and cancer of the oral cavity: Low dietary intake is associated with an increased risk of cancer. The use of tobacco results in lower beta-carotene levels in buccal mucosal cells which have been associated with more premalignant changes. Animal models have shown such agents inhibit the formation of oral cancer. At least five clinical trials have shown that they produce regression of oral leukoplakia.

—H.S. Garewal, "Carotenoids in Oral Cancer Prevention," *Carotenoids in Human Health.* February 6-9, 1993, San Diego, CA, p. A16.

This study examined the relationships of beta-carotene, vitamin A and vitamin E serum levels in head and neck cancer patients with primary tumors. Results found that patients with single head and neck cancer had lowered levels of beta-carotene and also suggest that low levels of vitamins A and E may be involved in the etiology of second tumors among such patients.

—N. de Vries and G.B. Snow, "Vitamin A, Vitamin E and Beta-carotene Serum Levels in Head and Neck Cancer Patients with andwithout Second Primary Tumors," *Third International Head and Neck Oncology Research Conference, September 26-28, 1990, Las Vegas, NV, The American Society for Head and Neck Surgery,* A3.1, 1990.

This review article makes the following observations with respect to antioxidants and oral cancer prevention: laboratory and animal models have demonstrated beta-carotene and other antioxidant nutrients strongly inhibit oral carcinogenesis. Smokers have lower beta-carotene levels in plasma and oral mucosal cells than nonsmokers, thus increasing their risk for oral cancer. Clinical trials have shown beta-carotene and vitamin E produce regression of oral leukoplakia.

—H. Garewal, "Evidence for Oral Cancer Prevention: An Update," *Second International Conference: Antioxidant Vitamins and Beta-Carotene in Disease Prevention, October 10-12, 1994, Berlin, Germany,* 26.

This review article makes the case for beta-carotene as a potential chemoprevention drug. The following data taken from specific studies are cited: beta-carotene at $10(-2)$ to $10(-4)$ g/kg suppressed and at $10(-5)$ to $10(-8)$ g/kg stimulated a 3- to 6-fold increase in antibody formation. The beta-carotene effect on interleukin II secretion is proven to be dose-dependent, as well as on activity of cytolytic T lymphocytes and natural killers, functional activity of murine peritoneal macrophages. In normal donors, high (2000 mg) doses of beta-carotene induced short-term reversible leukopenia without changing other characteristics; 650 mg and lower doses provided increase in the leukocyte and lymphocyte counts and recovery on day 7. In colonic cancer patient administration of beta-carotene at 250 mg for 10 days led to increase in the peripheral blood lymphocyte relative count, the relative and absolute counts of T cells forming active rosettes. Under stimulation with mitogen PWM the lymphocyte proliferative activity showed a statistically significant rise, while under the effect of ConA and alloantigens the response did not change.

> —A.B. Syrkin, et al., "Immunopharmacology of Beta-carotene," CCPC-93: *Second International Cancer Chemo Prevention Conference. April 28-30, 1993, Berlin, Germany, 1993*, 127.

Results of this study found that supplementation with beta-carotene rich foods was able to counteract the cancer-causing effects of smoke from cigarettes by maintaining vitamin A levels in smokers.

> —W.P. Mulloy, "Counteracting Carcinogenic Effects of Cigarette Smoking with Beta Carotene," CCPC-93: *Second International Cancer Chemo Prevention Conference. April 28-30, 1993, Berlin, Germany, 1993*, 122.

In this study, chronic myelogenous leukemia patients pulse oral busulfan either with or without daily oral doses of 50,000 IU of vitamin A. Results showed that the risk of death or clinical progression was 33% higher in the busulfan alone group compared to those also taking vitamin A.

> —F. Meyskens and K. Kopecky, "Phase III Randomized Trial of Oral Vitamin A in Chronic Myelogenous Leukemia (CML): Prevention of Progression to Blast Crisis and Increased Survival," CCPC-93: *Second International Cancer Chemo Prevention Conference. April 28-30, 1993, Berlin, Germany, 1993*, 87.

This article comments on early results of an ongoing study showing a response rate of 56% in subjects being treated for oral leukoplakia with beta-carotene supplementation for 6 months.

> —H. Garewal, et al., "Beta-carotene and Other Antioxidant Nutritional Agents in Oral Leukoplakia," CCPC-93: *Second International Cancer Chemo Prevention Conference, April 28-30, 1993, Berlin, Germany, 1993*, 52.

Results of this study found an inverse association between plasma beta-carotene levels and the risk of cervical intraepithelial neoplasia.

> —P.R. Palan, et al., "Antioxidant Beta-carotene Levels in Exfoliated Cervicovaginal Epithelial Cells in Cervical Intraepithelial Neoplasia," *Society of Gynecologic Oncologists Twenty-third Annual Meeting. March 15-18, 1992, San Antonio, TX, 1992*, 40.

Results of this study showed that the oral administration of beta-carotene to mice produced a decrease in angiogenesis evoked by HPV-transformed tumorigenic cell lines.

> —A. Szmurlo, et al., "Beta-carotene in Prevention of Cutaneous Carcinogenesis," *Acta Derm Venereol*, 71(6), 1991, p. 528-530.

This review article notes the prophylactic and therapeutic effects of vitamin A acid on chemically-induced benign and malignant epithelial tumors in mice; while also pointing out that the oral administration of vitamin A can cause skin papilloma regression.

> —W. Bollag and F. Ott, "Vitamin A Acid in Benign and Malignant Epithelial Tumors of the Skin," *Acta Derm Venereol Suppl*, 74, January 27-29, 1975, p. 163-166.

Results of this study found that doses of 100,000 IU per day of vitamin A for 2 weeks produced an enhancement of antibody-dependent cell-mediated cytotoxicity, natural killer cell activity and blastogenic response to plant mitogens in patients with chronic lymphocytic leukemia.

> —P. Gergely, et al., "Effect of Vitamin A Treatment on Cellular Immune Reactivity in Patients with CLL," *Acta Med Hung,* 45(3-4), 1988, p. 307-311.

This review article notes epidemiological studies have shown an inverse association between low serum levels of vitamin A or beta-carotenoids and the risk epithelial cancer. Clinical studies have dealt primarily with the importance of vitamin A in chemoprevention of risk conditions and in preventing the recurrence of cancer.

> —S. Toma, et al., [Biological Aspects and Perspectives Applicable to the Chemoprevention of Cancer of the Upper Respiratory-digestive Tract], *Acta Otorhinolaryngol Ital,* 10 Suppl 27, 1990, p. 41-54.

This review article notes studies have found retinoic acid has been shown to be an effective treatment for chemically-induced tumors. In one particular study, its use resulted in either complete or partial bladder papilloma regression in 33 patients.

> —C.F. Lopes, [Retinoids in Dermatology and Oncology], *An Bras Dermatology,* 57(3), 1982, p. 155-159.

In this double-blind, placebo-controlled study, middle-aged men from an area of the former Soviet Union with a high incidence of oral and esophageal cancer were randomly allocated into groups receiving either 80 mg per week of riboflavin; or a combination of 100,000 IU per week of retinol, 80 mg per week of vitamin E, and 40 mg per day of beta-carotene; or both. Results showed a significant decrease in the prevalence odds ratio of oral leukoplakia after 6 months in the men receiving the combination of supplements. Results also showed that men with medium and high blood concentrations of beta-carotene after 20 months had a lower risk of chronic esophagitis progression.

> —D. Zaridze, et al., "Chemoprevention of Oral Leukoplakia and Chronic Esophagitis in an Area of High Incidence of Oral and Esophageal Cancer," *Ann Epidemiology,* 3(3), May 1993, p. 225-234.

Results of this study found that a diet with excess retinyl acetate fed to rats before being injected with a metastatic line of transplantable hepatoma prevented establishment of secondary tumor foci. 75% of the rats fed a diet containing adequate retinyl acetate showed pulmonary metastases.

> —D.J. Morre, et al., "Glycosylation Reactions and Tumor Establishment: Modulation by Vitamin A," *Annals of the New York Academy of Sciences,* 359, February 27, 1981, p. 367-382.

Data from this study demonstrated that beta-carotene and canthaxanthine helped to prevent benzo[a]pyrene (BP)-induced skin carcinogenesis in the dark and BP photocarcinogenesis (UV 300-400 nm) when administered orally to mice. The two carotenoids were shown to be strong antitumorgenics when the same experimental procedure was adapted to 8-methoxypsoralen (8-MOP) photoinduction of mammary carcinomas in mice. According to the authors, such findings suggest that supplemental carotenoids can be used by outdoor workers in place of sunscreen to prevent skin cancer. They add that such natural antioxidants may be effective chemoprevention agents against neoplasias of the lung, breast, urinary bladder, and colon and rectum in humans as well.

—L. Santamaria, et al., "Chemoprevention of Indirect and Direct Chemical Carcinogenesis by Carotenoids as Oxygen Radical Quenchers," *Annals of the New York Academy Sciences,* 534, 1988, p. 584-596.

This study examined the effects of Dunaliella, a beta-rich algae, on spontaneous mammary tumourigenesis in mice. Results showed significant inhibition in the rats fed diets supplemented with spray dried powder of D. bardawil and oily solution of D. salina Teod. extract relative to controls.

—H. Nagasawa, et al., "Inhibition by Beta-carotene-rich Algae Dunaliella of Spontaneous Mammary Tumourigenesis in Mice," *Anticancer Research,* 9(1), January-February 1989, p. 71-75.

This review article argues that, despite studies pointing in both directions, the cancer preventive effects of vitamin A should be attributed primarily to carotenoids rather than retinol.

—H.C. De Vet, "The Puzzling Role of Vitamin A in Cancer Prevention," *Anticancer Research,* 9(1), January-February 1989, p. 145-151.

This article reviews the potential role of retinoids in treating cancer and cites one study in particular in which all-trans retinoic acid alone achieved complete remission in 80% of acute promyelcytic leukemia patients treated.

—M. Cornic, et al., "Retinoids and Differentiation Treatment: A Strategy for Treatment in Cancer," *Anticancer Research,* 14(6A), November-December 1994, p. 2339-2346.

This study examined the effects of the beta-carotene rich algae Dunaliella Bardawil on mammary tumors in mice. Results found that the progression of tumors was inhibited by Dunaliella Bardawil due to its increasing the homeostatic potential of the host animal as well as the antioxidant activity beta-carotene.

—H. Nagasawa, et al., "Suppression by Beta-carotene-rich Algae Dunaliella Bardawil of the Progression, but not the Development, of Spontaneous Mammary Tumors in SHN Virgin Mice," *Anticancer Research,* 11(2), March-April 1991, p. 713-717.

Results of this study showed that mice given daily doses of 170,000 IU/kg experienced a reduction in ethylnitrosourea-induced leukomogenesis as high as 50%.

—H. Wrba, et al., "Influence of Vitamin A on the Formation of Ethylnitrosourea (ENU)-induced Leukemias," *Arch Geschwulstforsch,* 53(2), 1983, p. 89-92.

In this study of 88 women with gynecological cancer, results showed a significant inverse association between serum levels of vitamin A and the risk of ovarian cancer.

—P.K. Heinonen, et al., "Serum Vitamins A and E and Carotene in Patients with Gynecologic Cancer," *Arch Gynecol Obstet,* 241(3), 1987, p. 151-156.

This article reviewed the role of vitamin A and retinoids as potential therapeutic agents in treating cancer. The author makes the following observations: animals experiments indicate retinoids increase cell-mediated cytotoxicity. Other studies showed that retinoids can restore lymphocyte phytohemagglutinin-responsiveness in terminal cancer patients. In vitro and in vivo data have indicated that retinoids may function as natural antipromoters of transformation and may be useful in reversing preneoplastic lesions of diverse origin. Studies of animal systems both in vitro and in vivo have shown that the growth of established epithelial tumors and cell lines can be inhibited by retinoids and that the phenotypic expression of carcinogen-induced tumors can be suppressed in the constant presence of retinoid. Retinoids have been shown to inhibit proliferation in cultured human melanoma cell lines and can reduce melanoma colony formation from fresh biopsies of human melanoma tissue.

—F.L. Meyskens, ''Vitamin A and Cancer,'' *Ariz Med,* 37(2), 1980, p. 84-86.

In this study, 250 mg/ml of beta-carotene dissolved in mineral and either applied topically or injected locally (190 mg/ml dissolved in media) into a DMBA-induced or HCPC-1 cell line-produced cancer of the hamster buccal pouch lead to tumor regression.

—J. Schwartz, et al., ''Beta-carotene is Associated with the Regression of Hamster Buccal Pouch Carcinoma and the Induction of Tumor Necrosis Factor in Macrophages,'' *Biochem Biophys Res Commun,* 136(3), May 14, 1986, p. 1130-1135.

Results of this study found an inverse relationship between the incidence of ovarian cancer and serum levels of both vitamin A and total cholesterol concentrations in Singaporian women.

—N.P. Das, et al., ''The Relationship of Serum Vitamin A, Cholesterol, and Triglycerides to the Incidence of Ovarian Cancer,'' *Biochem Med Metab Biol,* 37(2), April 1987, p. 213-219.

Results of this study found that the administration of beta-carotene partially inhibited Cyclophosphamide metabolism via hepatic mixed function oxidase enzymes to mutagenic species both in vitro and in vivo.

—M.A. Belisario, et al., ''Inhibition of Cyclophosphamide Mutagenicity by Beta-carotene,'' *Biomed Pharmacotherapy,* 39(8), 1985, p. 445-448.

This study examined the effects of beta-carotene and canthaxanthine against the benzo(a)pyrene carcinogenesis and its photocarcinogenic activity in mice. Results showed that the peroral administration of both carotenoids was preventive of the photocarcinogenic activity up to rates as high as 79% with respect to beta-carotene and 66% for canthaxanthine.

—L. Santamaria, et al., ''Prevention of the Benzo(alpha)pyrene Photoocarcinogenic Effect by Beta-Carotene and Canthanxanthin: Preliminary Study,'' *Boll Chim Farm,* 119(12), 1980, p. 745-748.

Results of this case-control study showed an inverse association between intake of beta-carotene and colon cancer risk among younger men and women.

—M.L. Slattery, et al., ''Age and Risk Factors for Colon Cancer (United States and Australia): Are there Implications for Understanding Differences in Case-control and Cohort Studies?'' *Cancer Causes Control,* 5(6), November 1994, p. 557-563.

Results of this study found a significant inverse association between beta-carotene intake and the risk of esophageal cancer in nonsmokers.

—A. Tavani, et al., ''Risk Factors for Esophageal Cancer in Lifelong Nonsmokers,'' *Cancer Epidemiol Biomarkers Prev,* 3(5), July-August 1994, p. 387-392.

Results of this case-control study showed a significant inverse association between the risk of cervical dysplasia and the intake of vitamin A.

—T. Liu, et al., "A Case Control Study of Nutritional Factors and Cervical Dysplasia," *Cancer Epidemiol Biomarkers Prev,* 2(6), November-December 1993, p. 525-530.

Results of this large, nested case-control study found a significant inverse association between the risk of cervical cancer and serum levels of total carotenoids, alpha-carotene, and beta-carotene.

—A.M. Batieha, et al., "Serum Micronutrients and the Subsequent Risk of Cervical Cancer in a Population-based Nested Case-control Study," *Cancer Epidemiol Biomarkers Prev,* 2(4), July-August 1993, p. 335-339.

Results of this study show that beta-carotene reversed the human tumor-induced inhibition of IFN in vitro.

—J. Rhodes, et al., "Human Tumor-induced Inhibition of Interferon Action in Vitro: Reversal of Inhibition by Beta-carotene," *Cancer Immunol Immunotherapy,* 16(3), 1984, p. 189-192.

Results of this study found that beta-carotene inhibited MCF-7 breast cancer cells in vitro.

—T.D. Shultz, et al., "Inhibitory Effect of Conjugated Dienoic Derivatives of Linoleic Acid and Beta-Carotene on the in Vitro Growth of Human Cancer Cells," *Cancer Letters,* 63(2), April 15, 1992, p. 125-133.

In this study, mice given 100 IU of vitamin A experienced an inhibition of Ehrlic ascites tumor by close to 50% while mice given a dose of 250 IU experienced enhanced growth of the same tumor by 60%.

—S. Saha and A. Ghosh, "Changes in Plasma Gangliosides in Relation to Tumor Growth Modified by Vitamin A," *Cancer Letters,* 56(3), March 1991, p. 251-258.

This study examined the effects of vitamin A on the development of lung tumors in mice exposed to radiation. Results showed that mice fed a diet low in vitamin A 100 IU/100 g experienced significantly less tumors than those fed a diet high in vitamin A (800 IU/100 g diet) 40 weeks after irradiation.

—T.A. Mian, et al., "Effect of Vitamin A on Lung Tumorigenesis in Irradiated and Unirradiated Strain A Mice," *Cancer Letters,* 22(1), February 1984, p. 103-112.

Results of this study showed that mice fed dietary beta-carotene from 3 weeks of age experienced a suppression of DMBA-induced papilloma growth relative to animals fed a normal diet.

—H.H. Steinel and R.S. Baker, "Effects of Beta-carotene on Chemically-induced Skin Tumors in HRA/Skh Hairless Mice," *Cancer Letters,* 51(2), May 30, 1990, p. 163-168.

This study examined the modulating effects of beta-carotene and selenium on the development of azaserine and N-nitrosobis(2-oxopropyl)amine (BOP)—induced putative preneoplastic foci in the exocrine pancreas of rats and hamsters. Results showed that both beta-carotene and selenium inhibited the growth of basophilic foci in the rat pancreas and caused a significant decrease in the number of early ductal complexes in the hamster pancreas.

—R.A. Woutersen, et al., "Inhibition of Dietary Fat Promoted Development of (pre)neoplastic Lesions in Exocrine Pancreas of Rats and Hamsters by Supplemental Selenium and Beta-carotene," *Cancer Letters,* 42(1-2), September-October 1988, p. 79-85.

This placebo-controlled study examined the effects of supplementation with 200,000 IU of vitamin A per week for 6 months on tobacco/betal nut chewers with oral leukoplakias. Results found that vitamin A lead to total remission in 57.1% of participants and total remission of the development of new leukoplakias in all subjects taking vitamin A. By contrast, the corresponding rates in controls were 3% and 21%, respectively.

> —H.F. Stich, et al., "Response of Oral Leukoplakias to the Administration of Vitamin A," *Cancer Letters,* 40(1), May 1988, 93-101.

Results of this study found that beta-carotene and vitamin E inhibited the growth of colonic aberrant crypt foci in rats exposed to azoxymethane and a high-fat, low-fiber diet for 10 weeks.

> —N. Shivapurkar, et al., "Inhibition of Progression of Aberrant Crypt Foci and Colon Tumor Development by Vitamin E and Beta-carotene in Rats on a High-risk Diet," *Cancer Letters,* 91(1), May 4, 1995, p. 125-132.

In this study, rats exposed to 1,2-dimethylhydrazine were fed a diet consisting of either 0.005% beta-carotene, 0.02% sodium ascorbate or 1.5% cellulose for 14 weeks. Results showed a significantly lower incidence of carcinomas in the rats given beta-carotene when compared to controls.

> —I. Yamamoto, et al., "Effect of Beta-carotene, Sodium Ascorbate and Cellulose on 1,2-dimethylhydrazine-induced Intestinal Carcinogenesis in Rats," *Cancer Letters,* 86(1), October 28, 1994, p. 5-9.

This review article notes that evidence from dietary and serum studies suggests there to be a long-term inverse association between the risk of cancer and beta-carotene.

> —N. Wald, "Retinol, Beta-carotene and Cancer," *Cancer Surv,* 6(4), 1987, p. 635-651.

This study examined the effects of the administration of beta-carotene during the DMBA-induced transformation of the epithelial cells in organ culture of the whole mammary glands of mice. Results showed that treatment with beta-carotene during days 3 and 4 of DMBA exposure lead to a 68% inhibition in the number of glands with NLAL. When beta-carotene treatment took place 4-10 days after exposure there was an inhibition of 49%.

> —S. Som, et al., "Beta-carotene Inhibition of 7,12-dimethylbenz[a]anthracene-induced Transformation of Murine Mammary Cells in Vitro," *Carcinogenesis,* 5(7), July 1984, p. 937-940.

In this study, 7,12-dimethylbenz[a]anthracene-induced mammary tumorigenesis in mice was suppressed by supplementation with a combination of retinyl acetate and sodium selenite. Results showed a reduction in the final tumor yield to 8% of control as compared with 51% and 36%, respectively, for selenium and retinyl acetate by themselves.

> —C. Ip and M.M. Ip, "Chemoprevention of Mammary Tumorigenesis by a Combined Regimen of Selenium and Vitamin A," *Carcinogenesis,* 2(9), 1981, p. 915-918.

Results of this study found dietary beta-carotene and wheat bran, both in combination and alone, provided protection against chemically-induced benign or malignant tumor formation and aberrant crypt foci in the colon of rats fed high-fat diets.

> —O. Alabaster, et al., "Effect of Beta-carotene and Wheat Bran Fiber on Colonic Aberrant Crypt and Tumor Formation in Rats Exposed to Azoxymethane and High Dietary Fat," *Carcinogenesis,* 16(1), January 1995, p. 127-132.

Results of this series of studies found that beta-carotene exerted antimutagenic effects against chemically-induced carcinogenesis in rats.

> —A. Aidoo, et al., "In Vivo Antimutagenic Activity of Beta-carotene in Rat Spleen Lymphocytes," *Carcinogenesis,* 16(9), September 1995, p. 2237-2241.

Results of this study showed that the topical application of beta-carotene significantly inhibited the formation of DMBA-induced cancer of the hamster buccal pouch relative to controls.

> —D. Suda, et al., "Inhibition of Experimental Oral Carcinogenesis by Topical Beta Carotene," *Carcinogenesis,* 7(5), May 1986, p. 711-715.

Results of this study showed that hamsters fed a diet high in beta-carotene had only a 2% mortality rate 69 weeks after exposure to benzo(a)pryene compared to a rate of 25% in controls. Lipid peroxidation was reduced by 40% in the livers of the rats fed beta-carotenes as well.

> —A.P. Wolterbeek, et al., "High Survival Rate of Hamsters Given Intratracheal Instillations of Benzo[a]pyrene and Ferric Oxide and Kept on a High Beta-carotene Diet," *Carcinogenesis,* 15(1), January 1994, p. 133-136.

Results of this study showed that beta-carotene modified the DNA damaging effects of DMBA and DENA in mouse mammary cells and thus inhibited the carcinogenic process from getting underway.

> —K. Manoharan and M.R. Banerjee, "Beta-Carotene Reduces Sister Chromatid Exchanges Induced by Chemical Carcinogens in Mouse Mammary Cells in Organ Culture," *Cell Biol Int Rep,* 9(9), September 1985, p. 783-789.

Results of this study showed that vitamin A checked the progression of tumor growth and increased the effectiveness of chemotherapy in mice.

> —J. Ghosh and S. Das, "Role of Vitamin A in Prevention and Treatment of Sarcoma 180 in Mice," *Chemotherapy,* 33(3), 1987, p. 211-218.

Results of this study found that beta-carotene at concentrations of 6.25 micrograms/ml significantly inhibited the colony forming efficiency of cultured human lung cancer 801 cell line and completely inhibited colony forming efficiency at 12.5 micrograms/ml. When mice were fed 25 mg/100 g diet of beta-carotene, results showed a 42-68% decrease in spontaneous lung metastasis of LA795 murine pulmonary adenocarcinoma.

> —B.T. Lai, [Effects of Beta-Carotene on Lung Cancer], *Chung Hua Chung Liu Tsa Chih,* 15(5), September 1993, p. 351-354.

Results of this case-control study found an inverse association between the risk of lung cancer and the dietary intake of beta-carotene.

> —A.J. Tan, et al., [A Matched Case-control Study on the Relations Between Beta-carotene and Lung Cancer], *Chung Hua Liu Hsing Ping Hsueh Tsa Chih,* 16(4), August 1995, p. 199-202.

Results of this case-control study found an inverse association between the risk of lung cancer and the serum levels of beta-carotene.

> —G.G. Li and A.J. Tan, [A Case-control Study of Serum Beta-carotene and Lung Cancer], *Chung Hua Yu Fang I Hsueh Tsa Chih,* 28(2), March 1994, p. 81-83.

This study examined the relationship between serum micronutrients and precancerous gastric lesions among subjects in an area at high risk for gastric cancer in China. Results found strong protective effects for beta-carotene and vitamin C against precancerous gastric lesions.

—L. Zhang, et al., [Relationship Between Serum Micronutrients and Precancerous Gastric Lesions], *Chung Hua Yu Fang I Hsueh Tsa Chih,* 29(4), July 1995, p. 198-201.

Results of this study found that rats deficient in vitamin A had an increased susceptibility to chemically-induced lung cancers compared to those animals fed a vitamin A adequate diet.

—P. Nettesheim, et al., "Vitamin A and the Susceptibility of Respiratory Tract Tissues to Carcinogenic Insult," *Environmental Health Perspect,* 29 April 1979, p. 89-93.

Results of this study showed that the topical application of beta-carotene inhibited carcinogensis and reduced gamma glutamyl transpeptidase activity in the puccal pouches of hamsters exposed to DMBA relative to controls.

—D. Suda, et al., "GGT Reduction in Beta Carotene-inhibition of Hamster Buccal Pouch Carcinogenesis," *European Journal of Cancer and Clinical Oncology,* 23(1), January 1987, p. 43-46.

This review article notes in vitro experiments have shown beta-carotene can inhibit carcinogenesis through an antigenotoxic action, particularly in the early stages. Data from animals studies have demonstrated beta-carotene's ability to inhibit cancer development. Clinical studies suggest beta-carotene is an ideal chemopreventive agent due to its lack of toxicity; and human intervention studies have produced positive findings with respect to beta-carotene's effectiveness in treating cancers of the oral cavity, colon, and head and neck.

—S. Toma, et al., "Effectiveness of Beta-carotene in Cancer Chemoprevention," *European Journal of Cancer Prevention,* 4(3), June 1995, p. 213-224.

Results of this study showed that daily supplementation of gastric mucosa patients with 20 mg of beta-carotene for 3 weeks produced a significant decrease of ornithine decarboxylase activity which has been associated with cell proliferation and tumor promotion.

—Y.V. Buki, et al., "Effect of Beta-carotene Supplementation on the Activity of Ornithine Decarboxylase (ODC) in Stomach Mucosa of Patients with Chronic Atrophic Gastritis," *European Journal of Cancer Prevention,* 2(1), January 1993, p. 61-68.

Results of this study found significant, independent inverse associations between dietary beta-carotene and vitamin A and the risk of epidermoid lung cancer in humans.

—J.F. Dartigues, et al., "Dietary Vitamin A, Beta Carotene and Risk of Epidermoid Lung Cancer in Southwestern France," *European Journal of Epidemiology,* 6(3), September 1990, p. 261-265.

Results of this study showed that mice supplemented with 5 or 10 mg of vitamin A-palmitate twice a week either topically or orally for 3 months lead to a reduction in tumors induced from black pepper extract.

—M.H. Shwaireb, et al., "Carcinogenesis Induced by Black Pepper (Piper nigrum) and Modulated by Vitamin A," *Exp Pathol,* 40(4), 1990, p. 233-238.

Results of this study showed that beta-carotene and canthaxanthine prevented the enhancement of benzo(a)pyrene-induced photocarcinogenisis in mice.

>—L. Santamaria, et al., "Dietary Carotenoids Block Photocarcinogenic Enhancement by Benzo(a)pyrene and Inhibit its Carcinogenesis in the Dark," *Experientia,* 39(9), September 15, 1983, p. 1043-1045.

This study examined the effects of retinoic acid on DMBA-induced papilloma and carcinoma in mice. Results showed that biweekly gastric intubation of retinoic acid produced a decrease in mean number of papillomas and mean papilloma volume per rat over time whereas such values increased in controls. At 288 days following initial DMBA exposure, 50% of surviving rats given retinoic acid were tumor free compared to just 16% of controls.

>—W. Bollag, "Prophylasis of Chemically Induced Papillomas and Carcinomas of Mouse Skin by Vitamin A-Acid," *Experientia,* 28(10), 1972, p. 1219-1220.

In this study, mice with established papillomas induced by 7,12- dimethylbenz(a)anthracene and croton oil showed significant tumor regression after 4-5 d of treatment with 20-400 mg/d day or week po 100-400 mg/wk ip of vitamin A alcohol or vitamin A palmitate in doses of 40-800 mg/d or wk po.

>—W. Bollag, "Therapy of Chemically Induced Skin Tumors of Mice with Vitamin A Palmitate and Vitamin A Acid," *Experientia,* 27(1), 1971, p. 90-92.

This article reports on the findings of two studies examining the effects of beta-carotene on cancer. Results of both showed that beta-carotene had protective effects against chemically-induced carcinogeneis in mice.

>—A. Kornhauser, et al., "beta-Carotene Inhibition of Chemically Induced Toxicity in Vivo and in Vitro," *Food Chem Toxicol,* 32(2), February 1994, p. 149-154.

Results of this study showed that the inhibition of HeLa cell growth in culture by 6- mercaptopurine was greatly enhanced in combination with retinol, retinal or retinol. Retinol pamitate was shown to enhance the antitumor effect of 6-mercaptopurine against murine L1210 leukemia to a significant extent, increasing the lifespan by 69%.

>—S. Akiyama, et al., "Enhancement of the Antitumor Effect of 6-mercaptopurine by Vitamin A," *Gann,* 72(5), October 1981, p. 742-746.

Results of this study showed that hypervitaminosis A inhibited keratinization and squamous metaplasia in bladder lesions induced by N-butyl-N-(4-hydroxybutyl)nitrosamine in mice. Results also found that the incidence of transitional cell carcinoma of papilloma of the urinary bladder was reduced significantly at a dose greater than 100 IU/g diet.

>—Y. Miyata, et al., "Effect of Vitamin A Acetate on Urinary Bladder Carcinogenesis Induced by N-butyl-N-(4-hydroxybutyl)nitrosamine in Rats," *Gann,* 69(6), December 1978, p. 845-848.

Results of this study found inverse associations between tissue levels of beta-carotene and the risk of cervical and endometrial cancer.

>—P.R. Palan, et al., "Lipid-soluble Antioxidants: Beta-carotene and Alpha-tocopherol Levels in Breast and Gynecologic Cancers," *Gynecol Oncol,* 55(1), October 1994, p. 72-77.

Results of this study showed inverse associations between serum vitamin A levels and the risk of oral leukoplakia and oral cancer.

> —P.N. Wahi, et al., "Serum Vitamin A Studies in Leukoplakia and Carcinoma of the Oral Cavity," *Indian Journal of Pathol Bacteriol,* 5(1), 1962, p. 10-16.

Results of this placebo-controlled study showed that supplementation with 180 mg per week of beta-carotene and beta-carotene combined with 100,000 IU of vitamin A per week lead to the remission and inhibition of new oral leukoplakia in subjects who chewed tobacco containing betel quids on a daily basis.

> —H.F. Stich, "Remission of Oral Leukoplakias and Micronuclei in Tobacco/betel Quid Chewers Treated with Beta-carotene and with Beta-carotene Plus Vitamin A," *International Journal of Cancer,* 42(2), August 15, 1988, p. 195-199.

Results of this study found that dietary beta-carotene effectively reduced hepatocarcinogenesis rats fed 3'-methyl-4-dimethylaminoazobenzene (3'-Met- DAB).

> —A. Sarkar, et al., "Inhibition of 3'-methyl-4-dimethylaminoazobenzene-induced Hepatocarcinogenesis in Rat by Dietary Beta-carotene: Changes in Hepatic Anti-oxidant Defense Enzyme Levels," *International Journal of Cancer,* 61(6), June 9, 1995, p. 799-805.

Results of this study found an inverse association between dietary vitamin A and lung cancer among male smokers at all levels.

> —E. Bjelke, "Dietary Vitamin A and Human Lung Cancer," *International Journal of Cancer,* 15(4), April 15, 1975, p. 561-565.

In this placebo-controlled study of Inuits in northwestern Canada, beta-carotene supplemenation (180 mg/week, given twice weekly in 6 capsules of 30 mg each) proved to be an efficient inhibitor of exfoliated cells with micronuclei in the oral mucosa of smokeless tobacco chewers not already deficient in vitamin A.

> —H.F. Stich, et al., "A Pilot Beta-carotene Intervention Trial with Inuits Using Smokeless Tobacco," *International Journal of Cancer,* 36(3), September 15, 1985, p. 321-327.

This study compared the serum levels of retinol, beta-carotene, alpha-tocopherol, zinc, and selenium in children with newly diagnosed malignancy to cancer-free controls. Results showed that age- and sex-adjusted serum concentrations of retinol, beta-carotene and alpha-tocopherol were significantly inversely associated with cancer. The cancer sites that were associated with serum beta-carotene included leukemia, lymphoma, central nervous system, bone and renal tumors. Leukemia was also associated with low mean serum levels of retinol, selenium and zinc. Subjects with lymphoma, bone and renal tumors also had lower mean retinol and alpha-tocopherol levels than controls.

> —D.J. Malvy, et al., "Serum Beta-carotene and Antioxidant Micronutrients in Children with Cancer: The Cancer in Children and Antioxidant Micronutrients' French Study Group," *International Journal of Epidemiology,* 22(5), October 1993, p. 761-771.

This study examined the effects of dietary beta-carotene intake on changes in leukocyte numbers in peripheral rat blood. Results showed a significantly positive correlation between beta-carotene intake and monocyte numbers, prompting the authors to suggest that beta-carotene may be an effective means of cancer prevention.

—P.B. Brevard, ''beta-Carotene Increases Monocyte Numbers in Peripheral Rat Blood,'' *International Journal of Vitamin and Nutrition Research,* 64(1), 1994, p. 21-25.

Results of this study showed that the administration of 600 IU per kg of feed of retinyl acetate significantly inhibited chemically-induced transitional cell carcinoma in mice.

—W.D. Dawson, et al., ''Retinyl Acetate Prophylaxis in Cancer of the Urinary Bladder,'' *Invest Urol,* 16(5), March 1979, p. 376-377.

This review article argues that beta-carotene and vitamin E both fulfill all the criteria for suitable chemopreventive agents since several lines of evidence point toward preventive roles for them in oral cancer. With respect to beta-carotene, the author notes that findings from epidemiologic studies have shown that low intake of beta-carotene has been associated with higher cancer risk and that smokers, whose habit is a major risk factor, have lower beta-carotene levels in oral mucosal cells compared with nonsmokers. Animal studies have produced findings that both agents strongly inhibit oral cavity carcinogenesis. Five clinical trials have found beta-carotene capable of producing a regression of oral leukoplakia.

—H.S. Garewal, ''Beta-carotene and Vitamin E in Oral Cancer Prevention,'' *Journal of Cell Biochem Suppl,* 17F, 1993, p. 262-269.

This review article makes the following observations with respect to vitamin A and cancer of epithelial origin: animal studies have demonstrated an association between vitamin A and such cancers and that vitamin A and its analogues delay tumor appearance, retard tumor growth and regress tumors induced by carcinogenic polycyclic aromatic hydrocarbons. In human studies, data indicate that such cancers may be associated with vitamin A deficiency.

—T.K. Basu, ''Vitamin A and Cancer of Epithelial Origin,'' *Journal of Human Nutrition,* 33(1), February 1979, p. 24-31.

This study examined the effects of beta-carotene on cytokine production by human peripheral blood leukocytes. Results showed that beta-carotene stimulated the secretion of a novel cytotoxic cytokine when peripheral blood cells were exposed to carotenoid concentrations between $10(-6)$ and $10(-10)$ M. Such findings indicate beta-carotene can prompt human leukocytes to secrete one or more cytokines which can manifest cytotoxic activity against human tumor cells in vitro.

—E.R. Abril, et al., ''Beta-carotene Stimulates Human Leukocytes to Secrete a Novel Cytokine,'' *Journal of Leukoc Biol,* 45(3), March 1989, p. 255-261.

This study examined the pharmokinetics of retinol palmitate in patients with acute non-lymphocytic leukemia. Results pointed to retinol palmitate's potential to function as a salvage therapy by inducing maturation and slowing proliferation, clearing out the residual leukemic cells following conventional chemotherapy as a result.

—H. Tsutani, et al., ''Pharmacological Studies of Retinol Palmitate and its Clinical Effect in Patients with Acute Non-lymphocytic Leukemia,'' *Leukemia Research,* 15(6), 1991, p. 463-471.

This study examined the antiproliferative effects of vitamin A analogs and difluoromethyl ornithine in cultured neuroblastoma and glioma cells. Results showed that retinol and retinoic acid arrested the proliferation of neuroblastoma at concentrations of 50 uM, with retinol being effective at concentrations of 5 uM.

> —S.K. Chapman, "Antitumor Effects of Vitamin A and Inhibutirs of Ornithine Decarboxylase in Cultured Neuroblastoma and Gliona Cells," *Life Science,* 26(16), 1980, p. 1359-1366.

Results of this study showed that HL 60 cells incubated with a water soluble beta-carotene (5 um) demonstrated beta-carotene's ability to inhibit growth and induce differentiation not unlike retinoic acid. Beta-carotene, however, is much less toxic which the authors suggest may make it a useful alternative promyelocytic leukemia.

> —H. Schafer and H.K. Biesalski, "Beta-carotene Induced Differentiation and Reduced Growth in a Promyelocytic Leukemia Cell Line (HL 60)," *Melanoma Research,* 3, 1993, p. 40.

This extensive review article notes that early results with beta-carotene have been very promising especially in lesions of the oral cavity. The authors make a strong case for the use of beta-carotene in place of retinoids due to its relative lack of toxicity.

> —H. Garewal and G.J. Shamdas, "Intervention Trials with Beta-carotene in Precancerous Conditions of the Upper Aerodigestive Tract," in A. Bendich and C.E. Butterworth, Jr. (eds.), *Micronutrients in Health and in Disease Prevention,* New York, Marcel Dekker, 1991, p. 127-140.

Results of this study showed that beta-carotene produced significant protection against cyclophosphamide-induced genotoxicity and chromosomal damage in mice.

> —D.M. Salvadori, et al., "The Protective Effect of Beta-carotene on Genotoxicity Induced by Cyclophosphamide," *Mutation Research,* 265(2), February 1992, p. 237-244.

Results of this study showed a significant decrease in the frequency of micronuclei induced by cyclophosphamide in human hepatoma cells when the cells were treated with beta-carotene.

> —D.M. Salvadori, et al., "The Anticlastogenicity of Beta-carotene Evaluated on Human Hepatoma Cells," *Mutation Research,* 303(4), December 1993, p. 151-156.

In this study, the anticlastogenic activity of beta-carotene against cyclophosphamide was studied in bone marrow cells of mice in vivo. Results showed that seven days' oral priming with 2.7 and 27 mg/kg of beta-carotene followed by an acute treatment with cyclophosphamide inhibited clastogenicity.

> —A. Mukherjee, et al., "Anticlastogenic Activity of Beta-carotene Against Cyclophosphamide in Mice in Vivo," *Mutation Research,* 263(1), May 1991, p. 41-46.

In this ongoing study, preliminary results indicate vitamin A has a protective effect against lung cancer in males and bladder cancer in both sexes.

> —LAN. Kolonel, et al., "Relationship of Dietary Vitamin A and Ascorbic Acid Intake to the Risk for Cancers of the Lung, Bladder, and Prostate in Hawaii," *National Cancer Institute Monograph,* 69, December 1985, p. 137-142.

This review article notes that studies have consistently shown inverse associations between vitamin A and lung cancer. Evidence is also discussed with respect to the protective effects of vitamin A and carotene in cancer at other sites.

—A.H. Smith, ''Relationship Between Vitamin A and Lung Cancer,'' *National Cancer Institute Monograph,* 62(62), 1982, p. 165-166.

Results of this study found that vitamin A levels in liver samples obtained in autopsy of cancer patients were significantly lower than controls, suggesting a true vitamin A deficiency in cancer patients.

—J. Ostrowski, et al., ''Liver Vitamin A Concentration in Patients Who Died of Cancer,'' *Neoplasma,* 36(3), 1989, p. 353-355.

In this study, an oral combination of beta-carotene and alpha-tocopherol mixed in vegetable oil was proven effective in regressing DMBA-induced epidermoid carcinomas of the hamster buccal pouch.

—G. Shklar, et al., ''Regression of Experimental Cancer by Oral Administration of Combined Alpha-tocopherol and Beta-carotene,'' *Nutr Cancer,* 12(4), 1989, p. 321-325.

Results of this study showed that hamsters exposed to DMBA which were supplemented with 10 mg of retinyl acetate 3 times/week in a 5% solution in peanut oil for 12-20 weeks suffered fewer tumors and the tumors they did have were smaller than controls.

—A. Burge-Bottenbley and G. Shklar, ''Retardation of Experimental Oral Cancer Development by Retinyl Acetate,'' *Nutrit Cancer,* 5(3-4), 1983, p. 121-129.

In this study, mice exposed to DMBA and TPA were fed either a 3% beta-carotene diet or control diet, beginning 11 weeks prior to chemical exposure. Results found that rats fed a beta-carotene diet showed a decrease in the number of cumulative tumors relative to controls.

—L.A. Lambert, et al., ''Antitumor Activity in Skin of Skh and Sencar Mice by Two Dietary Beta-Carotene Formulations,'' *Nutr Cancer,* 13(4), 1990, p. 213-221.

Results of this study showed that local injections of beta-carotene produced a significant regression in DMBA-induced epidermoid carcinomas in the buccal pouch of hamsters relative to hamsters injected with canthaxanthin as well as controls.

—J. Schwartz and G. Shklar, ''Regression of Experimental Oral Carcinomas by Local Injection of Beta-Carotene and Canthaxanthin,'' *Nutr Cancer,* 11(1), 1988, p. 35-40.

Results of this study found that the concentration of beta-carotene in the colon, rectum, and tumor tissue of cancer patients was significantly lower than that in tissue samples from polyp patients and controls.

—G. Maiani, et al., ''Accumulation of Beta-carotene in Normal Colorectal Mucosa and Colonic Neoplastic Lesions in Humans,'' *Nutr Cancer,* 24(1), 1995, p. 23-31.

Results of this study showed a significant inverse association between plamsa beta-carotene levels and the risk of lung cancer in women. Inverse associations were also seen between dietary retinol and beta-carotene and lung cancer risk.

—U. Pastorino, et al., ''Vitamin A and Female Lung Cancer: A Case-control Study on Plasma and Diet,'' *Nutr Cancer,* 10(4), 1987, p. 171-179.

Results of this study showed that rats supplemented with 25 mg/kg or more of beta-carotene experienced less DMBA-salivary tumor incidence than rats receiving lower doses of beta-carotene.

—B.S. Alam and S.Q Alam, ''The Effect of Different Levels of Dietary Beta-carotene on DMBA-induced Salivary Gland Tumors,'' *Nutr Cancer,* 9(2-3), 1987, p. 93-101.

Results of this study showed a clear inhibition of DMBA-induced mutagenesis in a human epithelial-like cell line by vitamin A.

—A.M. Ferreri, et al., ''Effect of Antioxidants on Mutagenesis Induced by DMBA in Human Cells,'' *Nutr Cancer,* 8(4), 1986, p. 267-272.

Results of this retrospective case-control study found that vitamin A was associated with lower risk for cancers of the tongue, floor, and other mouth, pharynx, larynx, esophagus, and lung in males. In females, only an association was detected for a lower risk in bladder cancer.

—B. Middleton, et al., ''Dietary Vitamin A and Cancer—A Multisite Case-control Study,'' *Nutr Cancer,* 8(2), 1986, p. 107-116.

Results of this case-control study found that women with low intakes of vitamin A or beta-carotene were 3 times more likely to suffer from severe dysplasia or carcinoma in situ than controls.

—J.A. Wylie-Rosett, et al., ''Influence of Vitamin A on Cervical Dysplasia and Carcinoma in Situ,'' *Nutr Cancer,* 6(1), 1984, p. 49-57.

Results of this study showed that 50 micrograms of beta-carotene administered either alone or in combination with other antioxidants significantly reduced DMBA-induced oral tumor burden in hamsters relative to controls.

—G. Shklar, et al., ''The Effectiveness of a Mixture of Beta-carotene, Alpha-tocopherol, Glutathione, and Ascorbic Acid for Cancer Prevention,'' *Nutr Cancer,* 20(2), 1993, p. 145-151.

Results of this study showed that mice supplemented with beta-carotene beginning 5 weeks prior to exposure to N-butyl-N-(4-hydroxybutyl)nitrosamine developed significantly fewer bladder tumors than controls.

—M.M. Mathews-Roth, et al., ''Effects of Carotenoid Administration on Bladder Cancer Prevention,'' *Oncology,* 48(3), 1991, p. 177-179.

Results of this study showed that the administration of vitamin A caused a reduction of transplacentally-induced leukemias. It was also observed that subsequent to a transplacental application of ENU, addition of vitamin A as a suspension to drinking water lead to a reduction of leukemia incidence to 50% as well as to a corresponding decrease of this disease as a cause of death.

—H. Wrba, et al., ''Prevention of Transplacentally Induced Malignant Diseases,'' *Oncology,* 41(1), 1984, p. 33-35.

Results of this study showed that mice supplemented with beta-carotene experienced significantly less DMBA-induced tumors than controls. Similar findings were seen in mice exposed to UV-B.

—M.M. Mathews-Roth, ''Antitumor Activity of Beta-carotene, Canthaxanthin and Phytoene,'' *Oncology,* 39(1), 1982, p. 33-37.

In this study, 9 male patients with metastatic unresectable squamous cell carcinoma of the lung were treated with vitamin A palmitate or 13-cis vitamin A acid over a period of 60 weeks. Results showed a significant increase of lymphocyte blastogenesis response to PHA in all but one of the patients and all patients showed and increased delayed cutaneous hypersensitivity reaction.

> —M. Micksche, et al., "Stimulation of Immune Response in Lung Cancer Patients by Vitamin A Therapy," *Oncology,* 34(5), 1977, p. 234-238.

This study examined the therapeutic activity of 3000 IU of vitamin A and/or 0.2 mg of BCG in mice inoculated with Lewis Lung Tumor. Results showed a major decrease in the incidence of lung metastases and primary tumor development when vitamin A and BCG were administered together relative to controls.

> —T. Kurata and M. Micksche, "Suppressed Tumor Growth and Metastasis by Vitamin A + BCG in Lewis Lung Tumor Bearing Mice," *Oncology,* 34(5), 1977, p. 212-215.

This review article notes that studies have shown vitamin A and its analogs can enhance the effects of radiation therapy, chemotherapy, and surgery in treating patients with epithelial cancer.

> —L. Israel and J. Aguilera, [Vitamin A and Cancer], *Pathol Biol,* 28(4), April 1980, p. 253-259.

Results of this study showed supplemental beta-carotene increased survival time of mice transplanted with Dalton's lymphoma relative to controls. Tumor cell-count, body weight pattern, and various hematological parameters all were positively altered in a dose-responsive manner.

> —B. Ghosh, et al., "Physiological Potential of Beta-carotene in Prolonging the Survival of the Host Bearing Transplantable Murine Lymphoma," *Planta Med,* 61(4), August 1995, p. 317-320.

In this study, 12 benign breast disease patients were orally administered 150,000 IU of vitamin A per day. Results showed that, after 3 months, 5 patients experienced complete or partial remissions and marked pain reductions were experienced by 9 patients.

> —P.R. Band, et al., "Treatment of Benign Breast Disease with Vitamin A," *Prev Medicine,* 13(5), September 1984, p. 549-554.

Results of this study showed that chewers of betel quids in Kerala, India administered 180 mg/week of beta-carotene plus 100,000 IU/week of vitamin A or 200,000 IU/week of vitamin A alone led to a reduction in the frequency of micronucleated buccal mucosal cells, a remission of oral leukoplakia, and an inhibition of the development of new leukoplakias.

> —H.F. Stich, et al., "Chemopreventive Trials with Vitamin A and Beta-carotene: Some Unresolved Issues," *Prev Medicine,* 18(5), September 1989, p. 732-739.

Results of this study showed that high doses of dietary vitamin A protected rats against PCP-induced preneoplasitc and pathological changes.

> —L.W. Robertson, et al., "Effect of Vitamin A on the Promotion of Diethyl-Nitrosamine (DEN)-Induced Hepatocarcinogenesis by Two Polychlorinated Biphenyl (PCB) Congeners," *Proceedings of the Annual Meeting of the American Association of Cancer Researchers,* 32, 1991, p. A959.

Results of this study demonstrated beta-carotene's ability to induce apoptic changes in human oral squamous carcinoma cells in vitro.

—J.L. Schwartz, "Beta-carotene Cytotoxicity in Human Oral Carcinoma: Induction of Apoptosis," *Proceedings of the Annual Meeting of the American Association of Cancer Researchers,* 35, 1994, p. A3760.

Results of this study showed that beta-carotene in conjunction with melphalan significantly enhanced the capacity of melphalan to inhibit the survival and proliferation of human oral carcinoma SCC-25 cells in vitro.

—J.L. Schwartz, et al., "Injectable Beta-carotene-enhanced Chemotherapeutic Tumor Growth Delay in Vivo," *Proceedings of the Annual Meeting of the American Association of Cancer Researchers,* 34, 1993, p. A1595.

This study examined the effects of orally administered 250 IU per day of retinoic acid on the prevention of certain characteristics of chemically-induced tumors, specifically tumor growth, metastatic spread, and suppression of T-lymphocyte proliferation in mice. Results showed that retinoic acid prevented the growth of primary tumors, the development of spontaneous lung metastases, and aberrations in lymphocytes.

—D.D. Taylor, et al., "Inhibition of Tumor Growth and Malignant Progression by Retinoids," *Proceedings of the Annual Meeting of the American Society of Clinical Oncologists,* 9, 1990, p. A381.

Results of this study showed that the local application of vitamin A acid had beneficial effects on women with moderate cervical dysplasia.

—F.L. Meyskens, Jr., et al., "A Placebo-controlled, Randomized Phase III Trial of Locally Applied Beta-trans-retinoic acid (vitamin A acid, RA) in Cervical Intraepithelial Neoplasia (CIN): Favorable Effect on CIN II (Moderate Dysplasia)," *Proceedings of the Annual Meeting of the American Society of Clinical Oncologists,* 12, 1993, p. A465.

Results of this study showed that vitamin A inhibited the growth of immunogenic melanoma in immunosuppressed mice. The direct injection of vitamin A into existing tumors produced a 50% regression of transplanted tumors as opposed to the control tumors in which 100% progressed.

—E.L. Felix, "Vitamin A: Inhibition of Murine Melanoma: A Possible Mechanism," *Proceedings of the Institute of Med Chic,* 31(3), 1976, p. 74.

Results of this study found that hamsters exposed to cigarette smoke who were fed a diet deficient in vitamin A were at increased risk of tumor development than those exposed to smoke maintained on a diet containing adequate vitamin A levels.

—P.D. Meade, et al., "Influence of Vitamin A on the Laryngeal Response of Hamsters Exposed to Cigarette Smoke," *Prog Exp TumorResearch,* 24, 1979, p. 320-329.

Results of this case-control study found a significant inverse association between daily intake of beta-carotene and vitamin A and the risk of prostatic cancer.

—K. Oishi, et al., "A Case-control Study of Prostatic Cancer with Reference to Dietary Habits," *Prostate,* 12(2), 1988, p. 179-190.

Results of this third phase of the well-known Basel Study found strong inverse associations between dietary beta-carotene and all cancers examined, particularly cancers of the lung and stomach. Similar inverse associations were seen with respect to vitamin A and cancer, although not as strong as those for beta-carotene.

—H.B. Stahelin, [Vitamins and Cancer: Results of a Basel Study], *Soz Praventivmed,* 34(2), 1989, p. 75-77.

Results of this study showed that supplemenation with high doses of vitamin A significantly reduced the incidence of benzo(a)pyrene-induced forestomach tumorigenesis in mice.

—T. Yamada, et al., "Effect of Dietary Vitamin A on Forestomach Tumorigenesis During the Total and Postinitiation Stages in Mice Treated with High- or Low-dose Benzo(a)pyrene," *Surgery Today,* 25(8), 1995, p. 729-736.

Results of this study showed that both retinol and retinoic acid inhibited AFB1-induced mutagenesis in S. typhimurium TA- 98 by up to 50% and that retinol inhibited mutagenesis in TA-100 by up to 75%.

—V. Raina and H.L. Gurtoo, "Effects of Vitamins A, C, and E on Aflatoxin B1-induced Mutagenesis in Salmonella Typhimurium TA-98 and TA-100," *Teratog Carcinog Mutagen,* 5(1), 1985, p. 29-40.

Results of this study suggest that high doses of vitamin A may prevent the carcinogen-induced increase in adhesion between mature cells in the rat epidermis and murine colon.

—A.G. Melikiants, et al., [Vitamin A Prevents an Increase in Epitheliocyte Adhesion Induced by Carcinogens in the Epidermis of Rats and the Large Intestine of Mice], *Tsitologiia,* 30(10), October 1988, p. 1260-1263.

This study examined the effects of 6 days of vitamin A supplementation at doses of 200,000 IU on the lipid levels and their fractions in RBC membranes in rats with transplanted Guerin's carcinoma. Results showed the supplementation had protective effects.

—E.N. Liubovych and M.N. [Level of Lipids and their Fractions in Membranes of Erythrocytes of Rats with Guerin's Carcinoma, Deficiency of Vitamin A, and in Rats Exposed to Elevated Doses of Vitamin A], *Ukr Biokhim Zh,* 51(5), 1979, p. 463-466.

This study examined the effects of beta-carotene on the content of some metabolites of lipid peroxidation and activity of ornithine decarboxylase in rat gastric mucosal membrane during MNNG-induced gastric carcinogenesis. Results showed that the repeated administration of beta-carotene significantly reduced the constitution-dependent enzymatic activation in the gastric mucosal membrane and to the inhibition of locus formation with abnormally high activity of ornithine decarboxylase. According to the authors, such findings indicate the anticarcinogenic effect beta-carotene may take place at the stage of carcinogenesis promotion.

—V.A. Draudin-Krylenko, et al., [Potential Cancer-protective Effect of Beta-carotene in Experimental Stomach Carcinogenesis], *Vopr Med Khim,* 38(6), November-December 1992, p. 36-39.

Results of this study showed that rats fed a diet containing 2.5 mg beta-carotene for 10 weeks following exposure to DMBA experienced a decrease in adenocarcinoma, increases in latent period of neoplasm development and rate of tumor differentiation, and an inhibition of metastatic spreading into the regional lymph nodes.

> —T.I. Sergeeva, et al., [Preventive Effect of Domestic, Synthetic Beta-carotene on the Development of Rat Mammary Tumors Induced by DMBA], *Vopr Med Khim,* 38(6), November-December 1992, p. 14-16.

This review article notes that data from both experimental and clinical studies have demonstrated an association between a deficiency in vitamin A and malignant tumor incidence. Studies have also shown such deficiencies to enhance the carcinogenic effect of benzo(a)pyrene and that the administration of vitamin A or its derivatives inhibited the growth of carcinogen-induced tumors.

> —K.D. Pletsityi, [Oncogenesis and Vitamin A], *Vopr Onkol,* 24(10), 1978, p. 85-92.

Cardiovascular/Coronary Heart Disease

Results of this study found significant, independent inverse associations between plasma levels of vitamins A, C, E, and beta-carotene and the risk of coronary artery disease among middle-aged to elderly subjects in an urban population of India.

> —R.B. Singh, et al., "Dietary Intake, Plasma Levels of Antioxidant Vitamins, and Oxidative Stress in Relation to Coronary Artery Disease in Elderly Subjects," *American Journal of Cardiology,* 76(17), December 15, 1995, p. 1233-1288.

Results of this study found significant, independent inverse associations between plasma levels of vitamins C, E, and beta-carotene and the risk of coronary artery disease among subjects 26-65 years of age in an urban population of India.

> —R.B. Singh, et al., "Diet, Antioxidant Vitamins, Oxidative Stress and Risk of Coronary Artery Disease: The Peerzada Prospective Study," *Acta Cardiol,* 49(5), 1994, p. 453-467.

In this study, patients undergoing carotid endarterectomy were pretreated with low-dose, oral beta carotene to determine whether the carotenoid content of plaque could be increased in vivo. Beta-carotene-treated patients had a 50-fold increase in their plaque beta-carotene level and the plaque from beta-carotene-treated patients had higher carotenoid levels and higher absorption compared with controls. Such findings of increased preferential absorption by plaque, the authors argue, suggest that selective ablation of atherosclerotic plaque may be enhanced by pretreating patients with oral beta-carotene.

> —M.R. Prince, et al., "Increased Preferential Absorption in Human Atherosclerotic Plaque with Oral Beta Carotene: Implications for Laser Endarterectomy," *Circulation,* 78(2), August 1988, p. 338-344.

Results of this study found that all-trans beta-carotene-derived metabolites inhibited atherosclerosis in hypercholesterolemic rabbits.

> —A. Shaish, et al., "Beta-carotene Inhibits Atherosclerosis in Hypercholesterolemic Rabbits," *Journal of Clinical Investigations,* 96(4), October 1995, p. 2075-2082.

This study examined the effects of dietary beta-carotene (0, 125, 250 or 500 mg/kg for 44 days) on serum lipid concentrations in spontaneously hypertensive rats. Results showed that supplementation caused significant dose-related decreases in serum total, LDL and HDL cholesterol concentrations and serum total, VLDL and LDL triacylglycerol concentrations.

—A.C. Tsai, et al., "Dietary Beta-carotene Reduces Serum Lipid Concentrations in Spontaneously Hypertensive Rats Fed a Vitamin A-fortified and Cholesterol-enriched Diet," *Journal of Nutrition,* 122(9), September 1992, p. 1768-1771.

This study examined the effects of 150 IU/ g diet of vitamin A palmitate supplementation on the healing of aortas in rats. Results found no significant effects of vitamin A in non-operated rats on aortic hydroxyproline content or collagenase activity. However, in rats that underwent longitudinal aortotomy and suture, a significant increase in hydroxyproline content at both the healing arteriotomy and at the adjacent non-wounded aorta in the vitamin A-supplemented group as well as a significant increase in bursting strength of the healing aortic anastomosis.

—X.T. Niu, et al., "Effect of Dietary Supplementation with Vitamin A on Arterial Healing in Rats," *Journal of Surg Research,* 42(1), January 1987, p. 61-65.

Results of this case-control study found that high beta-carotene concentrations within the normal range reduced the risk of first myocardial infarction.

—A.F. Kardinaal, et al., "Antioxidants in Adipose Tissue and Risk of Myocardial Infarction: The EURAMIC Study," *Lancet,* 342(8884), December 4, 1993, p. 1379-1384.

Results of this case-control study found an independent, significant inverse associations between mean plasma levels of vitamins A, C, E and beta-carotene and the risk of acute myocardial infarction. Such associations were strongest with respect to beta-carotene and vitamin C.

—R.B. Singh, et al., "Plasma Levels of Antioxidant Vitamins and Oxidative Stress in Patients with Acute Myocardial Infarction," *Acta Cardiol,* 49(5), 1994, p. 441-452.

Results from this series of studies showed strong, independent inverse associations between plasma levels of vitamins A and E and the risk of ischemic heart disease.

—K.F. Gey and P. Puska, "Plasma Vitamins E and A Inversely Correlated to Mortality from Ischemic Heart Disease in Cross-cultural Epidemiology," *Annals of the New York Academy of Sciences,* 570, 1989, p. 268-282.

Results of this study showed that 2 microM of beta-carotene proved more potent than 40 microM of alpha-tocopherol in inhibiting LDL oxidation and thus could be a key factor in atherosclerosis prevention.

—I. Jialal, et al., "beta-Carotene Inhibits the Oxidative Modification of Low-density Lipoprotein," *Biochim Biophys Acta,* 1086(1), October 15, 1991, p. 134-138.

Results of this study found that the administration of vitamins A, E, C, P for 12 days reduced the death rates of rats with exogenous thromboplastinemia and reduced hemocoagulative changes, microcirculation disorders, destructive changes of functionally active elements of inner organs. Such effects were promoted by hypoactivity of platelet aggregation, by low thromboplastic activity of erythrocytes, by limited destruction of vascular endothelium.

—ASh Byshevskii, et al., [Effects of Vitamins A, E, C and P on Intensity of Blood Coagulation in Experimental Animals], *Biull Eksp Biol Med,* 114(9), September 1992, p. 262-265.

Results of this study showed that supplementation with beta-carotene and alpha-tocopherol had beneficial effects on the excessive myocardial ischaemia/reperfusion injury of smoke exposed rats.
—H. Van Jaarsveld, et al., "Antioxidant Vitamin Supplementation of Smoke-exposed Rats Partially Protects Against Myocardial Ischaemic/reperfusion injury," *Free Radic Res Commun,* 17(4), 1992, p. 263-269.

Results of this case-control study found a significant inverse association between serum beta-carotene levels and the risk for cardiovascular disease.
—M. Torun, et al., "Evaluation of Serum Beta-carotene Levels in Patients with Cardiovascular Diseases," *Journal of Clinical Pharm Therapy,* 19(1), February 1994, p. 61-63.

Results of this study found that rabbits treated with 400 IU/kg of vitamin A and 0.4 mg/kg of vitamin E with experimental myocardial infarction showed a pronounced reduction of cardiac contractility relative to untreated rabbits with induced infarction or those treated with much higher doses.
—V.A. Frolov and V.A. Kapustin, [Effect of Vitamins A and E on the Contractile Function of the Heart in Experimental Myocardial Infarction], *Kardiologiia,* 23(7), July 1983, p. 93-95.

Cataracts

Results of this case-control study showed that low serum concentrations of beta-carotene and alpha-tocopherol increased the risk for developing end stage senile cataracts among Finnish subjects ranging in age from 40-83.
—P. Knekt, et al., "Serum Antioxidant Vitamins and Risk of Cataract," *British Medical Journal,* 305(6866), December 5, 1992, p. 1392-1394.

This review article notes that both epidemiological and animals studies have shown an inverse association between dietary beta-carotene and the risk of cataract development.
—H. Heseker, [Antioxidative Vitamins and Cataracts in the Elderly], *Z Ernahrungswiss,* 34(3), September 1995, p. 167-176.

Cholestasis

This study examined the effects of vitamin A injections on liver and blood concentrations in 9 children with chronic cholestasis over a period of one year. Results showed the treatment to be well tolerated and effective.
—O. Amedee-Manesme, et al., "Short-and Long-term Vitamin A Treatment in Children with Cholestasis," *American Journal of Clinical Nutrition,* 47(4), April 1988, p. 690-693.

Colonic Injury

Results of this study showed that supplemental vitamin A at doses of 662 IU/kg and sodium meclogenamate prevented radiation injury to the colon of rats being treated for pelvic malignancies.
—J.S. Wiseman, et al., "Methods to Prevent Colonic Injury in Pelvic Radiation," *Diseases of the Colon and Rectum,* 37(11), November 1994, p. 1090-1094.

Cystic Fibrosis

Results of this study showed that 3 months of oral beta-carotene supplementation effectively normalized excess lipid peroxidation in vitamin A deficient cystic fibrosis patients.
—B.M. Winklhofer-Roob, et al., "Enhanced Resistance to Oxidation of Low Density Lipoproteins and Decreased Lipid Peroxide Formation During Beta-Carotene Supplementation in Cystic Fibrosis," *Free Radic Biol Med,* 18(5), May 1995, 849-859.

Darier's Disease

In this study, 3 Darier's disease patients received 1 X 10(6) IU of oral vitamin A daily for 14 days. Results showed 50% to 80% improvement in the skin lesions of all patients.
—J.R. Thomas, 3d, et al., "High-dose Vitamin A Therapy for Darier's Disease," *Arch Dermatol,* 118(11), November 1982, p. 891-894.

Diabetes

This study examined the effects of vitamins C, E, and beta-carotene in preventing nerve conduction and nutritive blood flow deficits in streptozotocin-diabetic rats. Results showed that one month of diabetes caused a 19.1% reduction in sciatic motor conduction velocity and that this was approximately prevented 80-90% by high-dose (1000 mg.kg-1.day-1) vitamin E and beta-carotene treatments.
—M.A. Cotter, et al., "Effects of Natural Free Radical Scavengers on Peripheral Nerve and Neurovascular Function in Diabetic Rats," *Diabetologia,* 38(11), November 1995, p. 1285-1294.

Results of this study showed that supplementation with vitamins C, E and beta-carotene improved the antioxidative status of kidneys of rats with streptozotocin-induced diabetes.
—D. Mekinova, et al., "Effect of Intake of Exogenous Vitamins C, E and Beta-carotene on the Antioxidative Status in Kidneys of Rats with Streptozotocin-induced Diabetes," *Nahrung,* 39(4), 1995, p. 257-261.

Results of this study showed that a deficiency in vitamin A contributed to a greater incidence of abnormalities in experimental animals with alloxan-induced insulin-dependent diabetes relative to animals maintained on a diet adequate in the vitamin.
—B.A. Kudriashov, et al., [Prophylactic Effect of Vitamin A, Neutralizing the Development of Experimental Insulin-dependent Diabetes in Animals], *Vopr Med Khim,* 39(1), January-February 1993, p. 20-22.

Erythropoietic Protoporphyria

Results of this study found that 84% of erythropoietic protoporphyria patients treated with 180 mg/day of oral beta-carotene showed a 3-fold increase in their ability to tolerate sunlight.
—M.M. Mathews-Roth, et al., "Beta-carotene Therapy for Erythropoietic Protoporphyria and Other Photosensitivity Diseases," *Arch Dermatol,* 113(9), September 1977, p. 1229-1232.

In this study, the photoprotective effects of beta-carotene were compared with those of alpha-tocopherol. Both agents showed partial protection in the photohemolysis model. In hematoporphyrin-photosensitized mice, beta-carotene showed greater protection at low concentrations and tocopherol showed some protection at high doses. Such findings suggest that photoprotective was due to free radical scavenging or singlet oxygen quenching, properties common to both agents.

> —A.N. Moshell and L. Bjornson, ''Photoprotection in Erythropoietic Protoporphyria: Mechanism of Photoprotection by Beta-carotene,'' *Journal of Invest Dermatology,* 68(3), March 1977, p. 157-160.

General

Results of this study found a noticeable decrease in mortality relative to controls among preschool-age Sumatran children receiving supplementation with one capsule containing 200,000 IU of vitamin A every 6 months.

> —I. Tarwotjo, et al., ''Influence of Participation on Mortality in a Randomized Trial of Vitamin A Prophylaxis,'' *American Journal of Clinical Nutrition,* 45(6), June 1987, p. 1466-1471.

Results of this study found a strong inverse association between the risk of childhood mortality and total dietary intake of vitamin A among Sudanese children ages 6 months to 6 years.

> —W.W. Fawzi, et al., ''Dietary Vitamin A Intake and the Risk of Mortality Among Children,'' *American Journal of Clinical Nutrition,* 59(2), February 1994, p. 401-408.

This cross-sectional study examined the association between mild vitamin A deficiency and the occurrence of diarrhea and respiratory disease in Thai children 1-8 years of age. Results found a negative association between serum retinol and both diarrhea and respiratory. Three month follow-up data showed that serum retinol deficient children had a fourfold greater risk of respiratory disease than controls. Vitamin A supplementation led to a reduction in the incidence of both diarrhea and respiratory disease for a minimum of 2 months.

> —M.W. Bloem, et al., ''Mild Vitamin A Deficiency and Risk of Respiratory Tract Diseases and Diarrhea in Preschool and School Children in Northeastern Thailand,'' *American Journal of Epidemiology,* 131(2), February 1990, p. 332-339.

This double-blind, placebo-controlled study examined the effects of vitamin A supplementation on diarrhea and acute lower-respiratory-tract infections in children aged 6-48 months. Results found that the overall incidence of diarrhea episodes was significantly lower in the vitamin A-supplemented group than controls. No significant effects were seen with respect to acute lower-respiratory-tract infections.

> —M.L. Barreto, et al., ''Effect of Vitamin A Supplementation on Diarrhea and Acute Lower-respiratory-tract Infections in Young Children in Brazil,'' *Lancet,* 344(8917), July 23, 1994, p. 228-231.

Results of this study found that beta-carotene offered protection against oxidative stress in primary cultures of chicken embryo fibroblasts exposed to paraquat in vitro.

> —S.M. Lawlor and N.M. O'Brien, ''Modulation of Oxidative Stress by Beta-carotene in Chicken Embryo Fibroblasts,'' *British Journal of Nutrition,* 73(6), June 1995, p. 841-850.

This meta-analysis pooled the results of 12 previous studies on the relationship between vitamin A supplementation and childhood mortality. Results found a significant association between supplementation and a reduced risk of mortality.

    —W.W. Fawzi, et al., "Vitamin A Supplementation and Child Mortality: A Meta-Analysis," *JAMA,* 269(7), February 17, 1993, p. 898-903.

Results of this study found a noticeable decrease in mortality relative to controls among preschool-age Sumatran children receiving supplementation with one capsule containing 200,000 IU of vitamin A every 6 months. Data showed a 49% greater rate of mortality among controls than children receiving supplements and that boys experienced more impact from the treatment than did girls.

    —A. Sommer, et al., "Impact of Vitamin A Supplementation on Childhood Mortality: A Randomized Controlled Community Trial," *Lancet,* 1(8491), May 24, 1986, p. 1169-1173.

Results of this case-control, randomized study of Indian preschool-age children found that those receiving supplementation with 8333 IU of vitamin A led to a mean reduction in the mortality rate of 54% relative to controls. The effects of supplementation were strongest among children under age 3 and already malnourished.

    —L. Rahmathullah, et al., "Reduced Mortality Among Children in Southern India Receiving a Small Weekly Dose of Vitamin A," *New England Journal of Medicine,* 323(14), October 4, 1990, p. 929-935.

Results of this study showed that the combination of beta-carotene and alpha-tocopherol produced an inhibition of lipid perpoxidation which significantly exceeded the sum of each agent's individual inhibitions.

    —P. Palozza and N.I. Krinsky, "beta-Carotene and Alpha-Tocopherol are Synergistic Antioxidants," *Arch Biochem Biophys,* 297(1), August 15, 1992, p. 184-187.

Results of this double-blind study found that supplementation with 200,000 IU of vitamin A and 40 IU of vitamin E significantly reduced the incidence and severity of diarrhea and respiratory disease in one-year-old children in northern China over a 12 month period.

    —C. Lie, et al., "Impact of Large-dose Vitamin A Supplementation on Childhood Diarrhoea, Respiratory Disease and Growth," *European Journal of Clinical Nutrition,* 47(2), February 1993, p. 88-96.

Results of this study found that supplementation with the beta-carotene rich algae led to improvements in the reproduction and body growth of mice relative to controls.

    —H. Nagasawa, et al., "Effects of Beta-carotene-rich Algae Dunaliella on Reproduction and Body Growth in Mice," *In Vivo,* 3(2), March-April 1989, p. 79-81.

In this study, vitamin A exhibited varying degrees of inhibition on induced iron and ascorbic acid lipid peroxidation of rat brain mitochondria. The fat-soluble vitamins retinol, retinol acetate, retinoic acid, retinol palmitate, and retinal at concentrations between 0.1 and 10.0 mmol/L inhibited brain lipid peroxidation, with retinol and retinol acetate proving to be most effective.

    —N.P. Das, "Effects of Vitamin A and its Analogs on Nonenzymatic Lipid Peroxidation in Rat Brain Mitochondria," *Journal of Neurochemistry,* 52(2), February 1989, p. 585-588.

In this study, iron-dependent peroxidation of rat liver microsomes, enhanced by adriamycin, was measured in the presence of increasing concentrations of alpha-tocopherol, beta-carotene and retinol at low and high pO2. Results found that beta-carotene and alpha-tocopherol inhibited lipid peroxidation by more than 60% when present at concentrations greater than 50 nmol/mg microsomal protein at both high and low pO2. Retinol inhibited peroxidation by 39% at concentrations greater than 100 nmol/mg microsomal protein.

> —G.F. Vile and C.C. Winterbourn, "Inhibition of Adriamycin-promoted Microsomal Lipid Peroxidation by Beta-carotene, Alpha-tocopherol and Retinol at High and Low Oxygen Partial Pressures," *FEBS Letters,* 238(2), October 10, 1988, p. 353-356.

Hair Loss

Results of this double-blind, placebo-controlled study found that long-term oral therapy with daily doses of 18,000 IE retinol, 70 mg L-cystine and 700 mg gelatin led to an improvement of diffuse hair loss relative to controls.

> —H. Hertel, et al., [Low Dosage Retinol and L-cystine Combination Improve Alopecia of the Diffuse Type Following Long-term Oral Administration], *Hautarzt,* 40(8), August 1989, p. 490-495.

Hearing Loss

Results of this showed that treatment with vitamins A and E for 28-48 days improved symptoms in 40 middle age to elderly patients affected by presbycusis.

> —G. Romeo and M. Giorgetti, [Therapeutic Effects of Vitamin A Associated with Vitamin E in Perceptual Hearing Loss], *Acta Vitaminol Enzymol,* 7(1-2), 1985, p. 139-143.

Herpes

This study examined ocular infections with herpes simplex virus-1 in vitamin A deficient rats and pair-fed controls. Results found that the onset of herpetic keratitis was more rapid and the clinical effects more severe in rats deficient in vitamin A than in controls. Mild vitamin A deficiency increased the severity of experimental corneal HSV infections and lead to a high incidence of epithelial ulceration and necrosis.

> —K.M. Nauss, et al., "Ocular Infection with Herpes Simplex Virus (HSV-1) in Vitamin A-deficient and Control Rats," *Journal of Nutrition,* 115(10), October 1985, p. 1300-1315.

Results of this study found that topical treatment of primary herpetic keratitis with 0.25% of retinoic acid significantly reduced the severity of epithelial lesions in rabbits. Topical instillation of retinoic acid into the eyes of rabbits at the same dose also reduced the rate of incorporation of thymide into DNA by 27%.

> —J.L. Taylor and W.J. O'Brien, "The Effects of Retinoids on the Replication of Herpes Simplex Virus Type 1," *Current Eye Research,* 3(3), March 1984, p. 481-488.

Ichthyosiform Erythroderma

This article reports on the cases of three patients with congenital ichthyosiform erythroderma who benefited from treatment with oral retinoic acid. Response to therapy proved to be slow but definite with suppression of scale formation, marked reduction of painful cracking of the underlying epidermis and disappearance of skin irritation.

—L. Eriksen and R.H. Cormane, "Oral Retinoic Acid as Therapy for Congenital Ichthyosiform Erythroderma," *British Journal of Dermatology,* 92(3), March 1975, p. 343-345.

Immune Enhancement

Results of this study showed both 13-cis-retinoic acid and beta-carotene had positive in vivo effects on the immune system. 13-cis-Retinoic acid resulted in an increase in the percentage of peripheral blood lymphoid cells expressing surface markers for T-helper cells and beta-carotene produced an increase in the percentage of cells expressing natural killer cell markers.

—R.H. Prabhala, et al., "The Effects of 13-cis-retinoic Acid and Beta-carotene on Cellular Immunity in Humans," *Cancer,* 67(6), March 15, 1991, p. 1556-1560.

This placebo-controlled study examined the effects of 30 mg of beta-carotene per day on immunosuppression seen with long-wave ultraviolet-light against exposure in healthy young men. Results showed that such suppression was inversely associated with plasma beta-carotene concentrations.

—C.J. Fuller, et al., "Effect of Beta-carotene Supplementation on Photosuppression of Delayed-type Hypersensitivity in Normal young Men," *American Journal of Clinical Nutrition,* 56(4), October 1992, p. 684-690.

In this study, rats were fed diets containing either 2 g/kg (0.2%) beta-carotene, canthaxanthin or basal diet for up to 66 wk. Results showed that T- and B-lymphocyte responses were enhanced in the groups fed beta-carotene or canthaxanthin.

—A. Bendich and S.S. Shapiro, "Effect of Beta-carotene and Canthaxanthin on the Immune Responses of the Rat," *Journal of Nutrition,* 116(11), November 1986, p. 2254-2262.

This double-blind, placebo-controlled study examined the effects of vitamin A deficiency and supplementation on the T-cell subsets of Indonesian children between the ages of 3-6 years. Results found that children deficient in vitamin A had underlying immune abnormalities in T-cell subsets which proved to be reversible with supplementation of vitamin A.

—R.D. Semba, et al., "Abnormal T-cell Subset Proportions in Vitamin-A-deficient Children," *Lancet,* 341(8836), January 2, 1993, p. 5-8.

This study examined the effects of vitamin A therapy on immune responsiveness following extensive surgical treatment in vitro. Results showed that pharmacological doses of vitamin A prevented depression of total lymphocyte count, prompting the authors to conclude that vitamin A seems to be an immunostimulant in humans.

—B.E. Cohen, et al., "Reversal of Postoperative Immunosuppression in Man by Vitamin A," *Surg Gynecol Obstet,* 149(5), November 1979, p. 658-662.

This study examined the effects of 30 mg per day of oral beta-carotene in oral leukemia patients. Results showed increased plasma levels of TNF-alpha in patients who responded positively to the treatment.

—R.H. Prabhala, et al., "Influence of Beta-carotene on Immune Functions," *Annals of the New York Academy of Sciences,* 691, December 31, 1993, p. 262-263.

Results of this study found that the long-term feeding of mice with beta-carotene microgranules led to enhanced T-cell proliferative response to ConA. Beta-carotene oil solution given mice previously immunized with alloantigens (0.17-0.34 mg of beta-carotene per mouse) enhanced T-cell cytotoxicity against L-929 and YAC-1 cells and macrophage cytotoxicity against L- 929 cells. Such supplementation also reduced T-suppresser activity.

> —I.F. Abronina, et al., [The Beta-carotene Stimulation of Cellular Immunity Reactions in Mice], *Biull Eksp Biol Med,* 116(9), September 1993, p. 295-298.

This review article notes that at least 12 clinical studies have shown that supplementation with vitamin A can reduce severe morbidity and mortality from infectious diseases among children with acute endemic deficiencies in vitamin A or who have measles. The author goes on to make the following observations: vitamin A deficiency is an immunodeficiency disorder characterized by widespread alterations in immunity, including pathological alterations in mucosal surfaces, impaired antibody responses to challenge with protein antigens, changes in lymphocyte subpopulations, and altered T- and B-cell function. Vitamin A and its metabolites are immune enhancers that have been shown to potentiate antibody responses to T cell-dependent antigens, increase lymphocyte proliferation responses to antigens and mitogens, inhibit apoptosis, and restore the integrity and function of mucosal surfaces.

> —R.D. Semba, "Vitamin A, Immunity, and Infection," *Clinical Infectious Disease,* 19(3), September 1994, p. 489-499.

This study examined the effects of vitamin A alcohol on cell-mediated immunity in vitro as well as its capacity to prevent the immunosuppressive effects of prednisolone and cyclophosphadmie in vivo in mice. Results showed a significant enhancement of spleen lymphocyte transformation in the vitamin A supplemented mice in the PDD-sensitive cells and the T-cells at large. Vitamin A normalized cellular and humoral forms of immunity in prednisolone and cyclophosphamide-treated animals as well.

> —N. Nuwayri-Salti and T. Murad, "Immunologic and Anti-immunosuppressive Effects of Vitamin A," *Pharmacology,* 30(4), 1985, p. 181-187.

Results of this study found that supplementation with vitamin A for one week in human subjects produced increases in the content of peripheral blood lymphocytes, the relative and absolute content of B lymphocytes, and the number of T cells in the peripheral blood. Data also demonstrated an increase in the complementary activity of the blood serum and an increase in IgA content.

> —K.D. Pletsityi, et al., [Further Study of the Role of Vitamin A in Immunologic Reactions], *Vopr Pitan,* (1), January-February 1984, p. 26-29.

Results of this study showed that 3 days of supplementation with 30,000 IU of vitamin A produced partial normalization of alcohol suppressed immunological parameters in guinea pigs.

> —T.V. Davydova, et al., [Further Study of Immuno-correcting Properties of Vitamins A and E in Experimental Chronic Alcoholic Intoxication], *Vopr Pitan,* (3), May-June 1988, p. 45-48.

In this study, the 3 days of oral administration with vitamin A or E oil solution in doses 3000 and 5 IU/day, respectively, led to a correction of the immune response to sheep red blood cells disordered as a result of alcoholic intoxication.

> —T.V. Davydova, et al., [The Use of Vitamins A and E for the Correction of Immunologic Disorders in Chronic Alcoholic Intoxication], *Vopr Pitan,* (4), July-August, 1987, p. 50-52.

Results of this meta-analysis of 12 studies showed that the adequate levels of vitamin A is a key factor in the prevention of mortality and morbidity of children in developing countries, particularly with respect to deadly infectious disease such as measles.

> —P.P. Glasziou and D.E. Mackerras, "Vitamin A Supplementation in Infectious Diseases: A Meta-Analysis," *British Medical Journal,* 306(6874), February 6, 1993, p. 366-370.

Results of this double-blind, placebo-controlled study found that supplementation with 20 mg of beta-carotene per day for 2 weeks moderately enhanced certain aspects of immune response in healthy male cigarette smokers.

> —G. van Poppel, et al., "Effect of Beta-carotene on Immunological Indexes in Healthy Male Smokers," *American Journal of Clinical Nutrition,* 57(3), March 1993, p. 402-407.

Intestinal Anastomoses

This study examined the effects of vitamin A supplementation for 2 weeks at doses of either 1000 IU/kg per day or 10,000 IU/kg per day on experimentally-induced intestinal anastomosis in rabbits. Results showed that high doses of vitamin A showed positive effects.

> —J.D. Phillips, et al., "Effects of Chronic Corticosteroids and Vitamin A on the Healing of Intestinal Anastomoses," *American Journal of Surg,* 163(1), January 1992, p. 71-77.

Kyrle's Disease

This study presents the case of a 60-year-old man with a twelve-year history of Kyrle's disease that had not responded to numerous topical and systemic medications. Megadoses of oral vitamin A resulted in the resolution of most of the lesions. The amount of vitamin A was gradually reduced, and therapy was continued with a combination of vitamin A and vitamin E.

> —H. Aram, et al., "Kyrle's Disease: Response to High-dose Vitamin A," *Cutis,* 30(6), December 1982, p. 753-755, 759.

Liver Damage/Disease

This study examined the effects of vitamin A on pig serum and carbon tetrachloride-induced hepatic fibrosis in rats. Results showed that vitamin A suppressed hepatic fibrogenesis with such effects possibly being mediated by an action on stellate cells rather than hepatocytes.

> —H. Senoo and K. Wake, "Suppression of Experimental Hepatic Fibrosis by Administration of Vitamin A," *Laboratory Investigations,* 52(2), February 1985, p. 182-194.

Results of this study found that vitamin A levels in the liver of rats proved to be a key factor in hepatic fibrogenesis, with low levels being a risk factor for liver fibrosis development.

> —W.F. Seifert, et al., "Vitamin A Deficiency Potentiates Carbon Tetrachloride-induced Liver Fibrosis in Rats," *Hepatology,* 19(1), January 1994, p. 193-201.

This study examined the effects of beta-carotene on CC14-related general and hepatic toxicity in rats. Results found that oral supplementation with beta-carotene during CC14-treatment led to a significantly lower increase hydroxyproline liver content and in less severe liver fibrosis relative to controls. Beta-carotene prevented the long-term loss of rentinoids from the CC14-injured liver as well.

> —W.F. Seifert, et al., "Beta-carotene Decreases the Severity of CCl4-induced Hepatic Inflammation and Fibrosis in Rats," *Liver,* 15(1), February 1995, p. 1-8.

Results of this study showed a serum vitamin A deficiency and abnormal dark adaption in 9 of 11 patients with primary biliary cirrhosis Seven patients who received supplementation with 25,000 to 50,000 IU of vitamin A per day for 4 to 12 weeks experienced normalization of serum vitamin A levels and subsequent significant improvements in dark adaptation.

> —H.F. Herlong, et al., "Vitamin A and Zinc Therapy in Primary Biliary Cirrhosis," *Hepatology*, (4), July-August 1981, p. 348-351.

Lupus

Results of this study showed that systemic lupus erythematosus patients treated with 100,000 IU daily of vitamin A for 2 weeks led to an enhancement of antibody-dependent cell-mediated cytotoxicity, natural killer cell activity and blastogenic response to plant mitogens and interleukin-2.

> —C.V. Vien, et al., "Effect of Vitamin A Treatment on the Immune Reactivity of Patients with Systemic Lupus Erythematosus," *Journal of Clinical Laboratory Immunology*, 26(1), May 1988, p. 33-35.

Mastitis

Results of this study found that vitamin A-deficient mice showed a reduction in mammary development and an increased pathological damage to the mammary gland following intrammary challenge with staphylococcus relative to mice sufficient in vitamin A.

> —B.P. Chew, et al., "Effect of Vitamin A Deficiency on Mammary Gland Development and Susceptibility to Mastitis through Intramammary Infusion with Staphylococcus Aureus in Mice," *American Journal of Veterinary Research*, 46(1), January 1985, p. 287-293.

Measles

Results of this placebo-controlled study showed that mortality rates were significantly reduced in children aged 4-24 months hospitalized from measles following supplementation with vitamin A.

> —A. Coutsoudis, et al., "Vitamin A Supplementation Reduces Measles Morbidity in Young African Children: A Randomized, Placebo-controlled, Double-blind Trial," *American Journal of Clinical Nutrition*, 54(5), November 1991, p. 890-895.

Results of this double-blind, placebo-controlled study found that oral supplementation with 400,000 IU vitamin A led to a reduction or morbidity and mortality in children hospitalized with measles. Data showed that children taking vitamin A had significantly faster recovery times with respect to pneumonia and diarrhea, the had less croup, spent less time in the hospital, and had a death rate during hospitalization of half that of controls.

> —G.D. Hussey and M. Klein, "A Randomized, Controlled Trial of Vitamin A in Children with Severe Measles," *New England Journal of Medicine*, 323(3), July 19, 1990, p. 160-164.

Results of this study found an inverse association between serum retinol levels and the incidence and severity of measles cases among children under the age of 5 in an urban American population.

> —J.C. Butler, et al., "Measles Severity and Serum Retinol Concentration among Children in the United States," *Pediatrics*, 91(6), June 1993, p. 1176-1181.

This review article notes that mortality and susceptibility to infection and diarrhea have been shown to be greater in vitamin A deficient children, particularly with respect to measles. Studies have shown vitamin A supplementation reduced mortality and complications resulting from measles.

—M.M. Rumore, "Vitamin A as an Immunomodulating Agent," *Clinical Pharmacology,* 12(7), July 1993, p. 506-514.

This review article notes the findings from numerous studies linking a deficiency of vitamin A to increased incidence of childhood respiratory and diarrheal infection. Studies have also shown that supplementation with vitamin A could reduce the rate of childhood mortality by a mean of 35% and the rate of childhood mortality from measles specifically by a minimum of 50%. The authors cite estimates that vitamin A supplementation of deficient children could prevent as many as 1-3 million death each year worldwide.

—A. Sommer, "Vitamin A, Infectious Disease, and Childhood Mortality: A 2 Solution?" *Journal of Infectious Disease,* 167(5), May 1993, p. 1003-1007.

Menorrhagia

Results of this study found that hypovitaminosis A was shown to be an important cause of menorrhagia, with a significant difference demonstrated between the fasting serum vitamin A values of menorrhagia patients and healthy controls. Data also showed the level of endogenous 17 beta-oestradiol appeared to be elevated with vitamin A therapy and menorrhagia was alleviated in more than 92% of patients treated.

—D.M. Lithgow and W.M. Politzer, "Vitamin A in the Treatment of Menorrhagia," *South African Medical Journal,* 51(7), February 12, 1977, p. 191-193.

Papillomas

This study examined the effects of vitamin A acid on skin papillomas induced in rabbits by the bite of bed bugs pre-irradiated with gamma rays. Results showed that painting the papillomas with an oily 13-cis-retinoic acid suspension twice a week in a dose of 25 mg/kg body weight led to significant regression of these structures.

—S.A. Sakr, "Effect of Vitamin A Acid on Papillomas Induced by Irradiated Bed Bugs in Rabbit Skin," *Folia Morphol,* 38(4), 1990, p. 339-343.

Pneumonia

This study reports on the case of a 29-year-old woman who experienced overwhelming rubeola pneumonia requiring endotracheal intubation and mechanical ventilation. High dose treatment with corticosteroids and vitamin A produced immediate clinical recovery.

—M.E. Rupp, et al., "Measles Pneumonia: Treatment of a Near-fatal Case with Corticosteroids and Vitamin A," *Chest,* 103(5), May 1993, p. 1625-1626.

This study examined the effects of daily doses of 500,000 IU of vitamin A for one week on immunity patterns in chronic pneumonia patients. Results showed that supplementation stimulated the content of T- and B lymphocytes in peripheral circulation as well as IgG and IgM blood serum. Cellular immunity was also stimulated which involved the activation of lymphocyte blast transformation with PHA and the increase in exhibition of skin reaction towards PHA.

—K.D. Pletsitnyi, et al., [Effect of Vitamin A on Immunological Status of Patients with Chronic Pneumonia], *Vopr Med Khim,* 28(5), September-October 1982, p. 119-122.

Polyoma Virus Inhibition

Results of this study showed that vitamin A inhibited polyoma virus replication in confluent mouse embryo cells. A significant, dose dependent inhibition occurred following the pretreated of monolayer cells with concentrations of vitamin A (10(-8) to 10(-6) M) thought to approximate those found in vivo. Growth curves of polyoma virus in the presence and absence of vitamin A suggested that vitamin A actually inhibited, and did not simply delay, virus replication. Data also showed that vitamin A caused a significant decrease in overall DNA synthesis.

—J.K. Russell and J.E. Blalock, "Vitamin A Inhibition of Polyoma Virus Replication," *Biochem Biophys Res Commun,* 122(2), July 31, 1984, p. 851-858.

PROM

Results of this study showed beta-carotene and ascorbic-acid may act together to prevent preterm rupture of fetal membrane (PROM) in smokers.

—B.M. Barrett, et al., "Potential Role of Ascorbic Acid and Beta-carotene in the Prevention of Preterm Rupture of Fetal Membranes," *International Journal of Vitamin and Nutrition Research,* 64(3), 1994, p. 192-197.

Pulmonary Health

In this study, plasma concentrations of retinol and retinol-binding protein were measured at birth in 91 preterm infants. Results found that 64% of these babies had retinol values less than 20 micrograms/dl which indicates deficiency. Babies with respiratory distress syndrome had retinol binding protein levels on the third day of life than did controls. Babies with bronchopulmonary dysplaisa had significantly lower retinol levels at birth and 21 days of age than those without bronchopulmonary dysplasia.

—V.A. Hustead, et al., "Relationship of Vitamin A Status to Lung Disease in the Preterm Infant," *Journal of Pediatrics,* 105(4), October 1984, p. 610-615.

This study examined the vitamin A levels of infants born at less than 32 weeks gestational age with and without chronic lung disease. Results showed that infants with chronic lung disease had significantly lower vitamin A levels on days 21 to and days 31 to 40; and levels were less than 60% of the lowest acceptable levels.

—V. Chan, et al., "Vitamin A Levels and Feeding Practice in Neonates With and Without Chronic Lung Disease," *Journal of Perinat Medicine,* 21(3), 1993, p. 205-210.

Radiation Injury

This study examined the influence of supplemental vitamin A on certain aspects of experimentally-induced radiation injury in mice. Results found that supplemented mice experienced less weight loss after irradiation relative to controls. Supplementation significantly diminished adrenal enlargement following irradiation, prevented radiation-induced thymic involution, and significantly increased white blood cell count.

> —E. Seifter, et al., ''Vitamin A Inhibits Some Aspects of Systemic Disease Due to Local X-irradiation,'' *JPEN J Parenter Enteral Nutrition,* 5(4), 1981, p. 288-294.

Retinitis Pigmentosa

Results of this study showed that supplementation with 15,000 IU per day of vitamin A proved to have beneficial effects on the course of retinitis pigementosa.

> —E.L. Berson, et al., ''A Randomized Trial of Vitamin A and Vitamin E Supplementation for Retinitis Pigmentosa,'' *Arch Ophthalmol,* 111(6), June 1993, p. 761-772.

Stress

This review article notes that studies on mice have found that oral vitamin A administration prevents stress-induced immunological disorders: depression of antibody-forming cell production, decrease in natural killer cell activity and T-lymphocyte mitogenic response. Data have also demonstrated that vitamin A prevents the development of thymus atrophy, lymphopenia and depression of phagocytic activity of peritoneal macrophages.

> —K.D. Pletsityi, et al., [Immuno-correcting Activity of Vitamin A in Stress], *Biull Eksp Biol Medicine,* 104(11), November 1987, p. 609-611.

Ulcers

This study examined the effect of vitamin A on restraint stress ulcer formation in rats. Results showed that rats administered i.m. injections of 1000 or 2000 IU vitamin A, respectively, every 6 h after 19 h of immobilisation had significantly fewer and smaller ulcers than controls.

> —V. Schumpelick and E. Farthmann, [Study on the Protective Effect of Vitamin A on Stress Ulcer of the Rat], *Arzneimittelforschung,* 26(3), 1976, p. 386-388.

Results of this study found that the oral administration of water-soluble beta-carotene in combined treatment of patients with duodenal ulcers induced more significant reduction of inflammatory and atrophic lesions, faster healing compared to controls.

> —V.V. Neliubin, et al., [The Use of Water-soluble Beta-carotene in the Combined Treatment of Patients with Duodenal Peptic Ulcer and Chronic Proctosigmoiditis at Krainka General Health Resort], *Vopr Kurortol Fizioter Lech Fiz Kult,* (4), July-August 1994, p. 20-22.

Vaginal Candidiasis

Results of this case-control study showed that a decrease in beta-carotene levels along with other antioxidants can alter the local immune response in women, creating disturbances in vaginal flora, candida overgrowth, and vaginal candidiasis development.

> —M.S. Mikhail, et al., ''Decreased Beta-carotene Levels in Exfoliated Vaginal Epithelial Cells in Women with Vaginal Candidiasis,'' *American Journal of Reproductive Immunology,* 32(3), October 1994, p. 221-225.

Warts

Result of this study showed that the administration of vitamin A acid (2% in petrolatum, 1 x day, topically) to patients suffering from plantar wars produced good results in 9 of 17 after 4 weeks, completely curing 2.

> —J. De Bersaques, "Vitamin A Acid in the Topic Treatment of Warts," *Acta Derm Venereol Suppl,* 55(74), 1975, p. 169-170.

Wound Healing

Results of this study showed that vitamin A was an effective agent for reversing the inhibition of cell-mediated immunity in burned mice.

> —S.F. Pang, [The Effect of Vitamin A and Astragalus on the Splenic T lymphocyte-CFU of Burned Mice], *Chung Hua Cheng Hsing Shao Shang Wai Ko Tsa Chih,* 5(2), June 1989, p. 122-124, 159.

Results of this study showed that rabbits with corneal epithelial wounds treated with 0.1% all-trans-retinoic acid three times per day experienced a 21% increase in the healing rate relative to controls. Treatment five times a day resulted in an increase of 35%.

> —J.L. Ubels, et al., "Healing of Experimental Corneal Wounds Treated with Topically Applied Retinoids," *American Journal of Ophthalmology,* 95(3), March 1983, p. 353-358.

This study examined the effects of feeding vitamin A deficient rats various levels and combinations of retinyl acetate, beta-carotene, or retinoic acid on skin wound healing. Results found that supplemental retinyl acetate, beta-carotene, or in some cases all-trans-retinoic acid effectively enhanced wound healing following surgery.

> —L.E. Gerber and J.W. Erdman, Jr., "Effect of Dietary Retinyl Acetate, Beta-carotene and Retinoic Acid on Wound Healing in Rats," *Journal of Nutrition,* 112(8), August 1982, p. 1555-1564.

Results of this study showed that supplementation with 150,000 IU per day of vitamin A prevented impaired wound healing and lessened the weight loss, leukopenia, thrombocytopenia, thymic involution, adrenal enlargement, decrease in splenic weight, and gastric ulceration of radiation-induced wounded rats.

> —S.M. Levenson, et al., "Supplemental Vitamin A Prevents the Acute Radiation-induced Defect in Wound Healing," *Ann Surg,* 200(4), October 1984, p. 494-512.

This study examined the effects of daily injections of either 3000 IU of vitamin A or an equal volume of 0.9 N saline on the suppression of cellular immunity after a 30% body surface area experimental burn in mice. Results showed that the vitamin A treated mice had a significant improvement rate of 52% relative to controls compared to 21% of saline treated mice relative to controls.

> —S. Fusi, et al., "Reversal of Postburn Immunosuppression by the Administration of Vitamin A," *Surgery,* 96(2), August 1984, p. 330-335.

Results of this study showed that retinol palmitate 0.1% ointment applied to the right eyes of nine incised rabbits doubled wound strength at 13 days.

> —P.R. Kastl, et al., "Topical Vitamin A Ointment Increases Healing of Cataract Incisions," *Ann Ophthalmology,* 19(5), May 1987, p. 175-177, 180.

Xerophthalmia

This study examined the effects of supplementation with 60 mg of vitamin A every 6 months on xerophthalmia rates among preschool children. Results showed that although supplementation with vitamin A only led to a moderate reduction in the risk of xerophthalmia, total dietary vitamin A intake showed a strong association with risk reduction.

> —W.W. Fawzi, et al., "Vitamin A Supplementation and Dietary Vitamin A in Relation to the Risk of Xerophthalmia," *American Journal of Clinical Nutrition,* 58(3), September 1993, p. 385-391.

Results of this study showed that retinoic acid 0.1% in arachis oil applied to the eye of patients with corneal xerophthalmia was associated with an increased rate of healing of corneal lesions relative to treatment with only arachis oil alone.

> —A. Sommer, "Treatment of Corneal Xerophthalmia with Topical Retinoic Acid," *American Journal of Ophthalmology,* 95(3), March 1983, p. 349-352.

This study examined the effects of biannual distribution of 200,000 IU of vitamin A in preventing xerophthalmia in 25,000 Sumatran preschool children. Results found that distribution was associated with a major decline in xerophthalmia prevalence.

> —E. Djunaedi, et al., "Impact of Vitamin A Supplementation on Xerophthalmia: A Randomized Controlled Community Trial," *Arch Ophthalmology,* 106(2), February 1988, p. 218-222.

This study examined the effects of supplementation of 50,000 IU-200,000 IU (depending on age) of vitamin A every 4 months on the prevalence and incidence of xerophthalmia among preschool-age children in Nepal. Results showed the vitamin A supplementation reduced the prevalence of xerophthalmia by 63%.

> —J. Katz, et al., "Impact of Vitamin A Supplementation on Prevalence and Incidence of Xerophthalmia in Nepal," *Invest Ophthalmol Vis Sci,* 36(13), December 1995, p. 2577-2583.

■ VITAMIN B1

AIDS/HIV

Results of this study showed that thiamine possessed anti-HIV-Tat activity and inhibited the production of progeny HIV-1 in chronic and acute HIV-1-infected CEM at nontoxic concentrations of 500-1000 microM. Results also found that 500 microM of thiamine disulfide blocked 99.7% of HIV-1 production after 96 hour culture in acute HIV-1 infection and inhibited 90-98% of HIV-1 production in chronic-infected cells.

> —S. Shoji, et al., "Thiamine Disulfide as a Potent Inhibitor of Human Immunodeficiency Virus (type-1) Production," *Biochem Biophys Res Commun,* 205(1), November 30, 1994, p. 967-975.

Alzheimer's Disease

Results of this double-blind, placebo-controlled, 12 week study found that 100 mg per day of the thiamine derivative fursultiamine had positive effects on Alzheimer's patients.

> —Y. Mimori, et al., "Thiamine Therapy in Alzheimer's Disease," *Metab Brain Disease,* 11(1), March 1966, p. 89-94.

Cardiovascular/Coronary Heart Disease

This double-blind, placebo-controlled study examined the effect of 200 mg per day of thiamine repletion on thiamine status, functional capacity, and left ventricular ejection fraction in CHF patients who had taken a minimum of 80 mg per day of furosemide over a period of 3 months or more. Results showed the treatment led to improvements in left ventricular function relative to controls.

> —I. Shimon, et al., "Improved Left Ventricular Function after Thiamine Supplementation in Patients with Congestive Heart Failure Receiving Long-term Furosemide Therapy," *American Journal of Medicine,* 98(5), May 1995, p. 485-490.

In this study, B1 was injected into patients with pulmonary and myocardial insufficiency in incremental doses during the postoperative period. Results showed that, relative to controls, 50 mg/kg of thiamine produced an increase in blood pressure of 20 mmHg with an elevation of central venous pressure by 3 mmHg.

> —E. Freye & E. Hartung, "The Potential Use of Thiamine in Patients with Cardiac Insufficiency," *Acta Vitaminol Enzymol,* 4(4), 1982, p. 285-290.

This study examined the cardiovascular reactions following the administration of 2.4 g/kg in dogs. Results indicated the following with respect to the thiamine: It decreased mean peripheral pressure as much as 25%. It reduced LEVDP, left ventricular pressure, and LV dP/dtmax as much as 10%, 15%, and 20% respectively. It reduced pulse rate up to 25%. It decreased coronary sinus blood flow up to 31%. And it decreased myocardial oxygen consumption as much as 45%.

> —E. Freye, "Cardiovascular Effects of High Doses of Thiamine (vit B1) in the Dog with Special Reference to Myocardial Oxygen Consumption," *Basic Research in Cardiology,* 71(2), March-April 1976, p. 192-198.

This study examined the effects of vitamins B1 and PP on ischemic heart damage. Results showed that a single dose of thiamine led to significant cytoprotective effects.

> —A.B. Shneider, [Anti-ischemic Heart Protection Using Thiamine and Nicotinamide], *Patol Fiziol Eksp Ter,* (1), January-February 1991, p. 9-10.

Epilepsy

Results of this study found that treatment with PHT, thiamine produced improvements in neuropsychological functions among epileptics including visuo-spatial analysis, visuo-motor speed and verbal abstracting ability.

> —M.I. Botez, et al., "Thiamine and Folate Treatment of Chronic Epileptic Patients: A Controlled Study with the Wechsler IQ Scale," *Epilepsy Research,* 16(2), October 1993, p. 157-163.

Fatigue

In this double-blind, placebo-controlled study, male athletes with varying blood levels of thiamine exercised on a bicycle ergometer and were then examined for the effects of thiamine supplementation relative to controls. Results found that supplementation with thiamine significantly suppressed blood glucose increases in subjects with normal thiamine levels while significantly decreasing the number of fatigue complaints.

—M. Suzuki & Y. Itokawa, "Effects of Thiamine Supplementation on Exercise-induced Fatigue," *Metabalic Pr Brain Dis,* 11(1), March 1996, p. 95-106.

Febrile Lymphadenopathy

This article reports on two cases of children with recurrent episodes of fever and cervical lymphadenopathy who experienced rapid improvement following the administration of large doses of thiamine hydrochloride after failed attempts at conventional therapy.

—D. Lonsdale, "Recurrent Febrile Lymphadenopathy Treated with Large Doses of Vitamin B1: Report of Two Cases," *Dev Pharmacol Ther,* 1(4), 1980, p. 254-564.

General

Results of this double-blind, placebo-controlled study showed the administration of thiamine to have a cholinomimetic effect on the central nervous system of healthy young adults.

—K.J. Meador, et al., "Evidence for a Central Cholinergic Effect of High-dose Thiamine," *Ann Neurol,* 34(5), November 1993, p. 724-726.

This double-blind, placebo-controlled study examined the effects of 10 mg of thiamine per day on the health and general well-being of healthy elderly Irish women. Results showed that the women receiving thiamine had significant increases in energy intake, appetite, body weight, and general well-being. Fatigue and daytime sleep were decreased by supplementation as well.

—L.J. Smidt, et al., "Influence of Thiamin Supplementation on the Health and General Well-being of an Elderly Irish Population with Marginal Thiamin Deficiency," *Journal of Gerontology,* 46(1), January 1991, p. M16-22.

Lactic Acidosis

This article reports on the cases of two middle-age patients who developed severe metabolic acidosis following abdominal surgery which was not helped by conventional treatment. The administration of two 400 mg doses of thiamine immediately eliminated the lactic acidosis in both patients.

—G. Klein, et al., [Life-threatening Lactic Acidosis During Total Parenteral Nutrition. Successful Therapy with Thiamine], *Dtsch Med Wochenschr,* 115(7), February 16, 1990, p. 254-256.

Lead Intoxication

This study examined the effects of thiamine and ascorbic acid on experimentally-induced lead intoxication in rats. Results showed that administration of the two together proved most effective in reducing the detrimental effects as compared to either vitamin administered alone.

—S.J. Flora & S.K. Tandon, "Preventive and Therapeutic Effects of Thiamine, Ascorbic Acid and their Combination in Lead Intoxication," *Acta Pharmacol Toxicol,* 58(5), May 1996, p. 374-378.

Liver Disease

Results of this study showed that thiamine administered in doses of 50 mg per capita per day for 30 days significantly reduced blood glucose levels in patients with liver cirrhosis.

—R. Hassan, et al., "Effect of Thiamine on Glucose Utilization in Hepatic Cirrhosis," *Journal of Gastroenterology Hepatology,* 6(1), January-February 1991, p. 59-60.

Results of this study found that supplementation with 200 mg per day of thiamine over a one week period restored levels of thiamine pyrophosphate, an essential co-factor in intermediary metabolism, to normal levels in chronic liver disease patients.

—J.E. Rossouw, et al., "Red Blood Cell Transketolase Activity and the Effect of Thiamine Supplementation in Patients with Chronic Liver Disease," *Scandinavian Journal of Gastroenterology,* 13(2), 1978, p. 133-138.

Seasonal Ataxia

Results of this double-blind, placebo-controlled study found thiamine supplementation significantly improved the condition of Nigerian patients suffering from seasonal ataxia relative to controls.

—B. Adamolekun, et al., "A Double-blind, Placebo-controlled Study of the Efficacy of Thiamine Hydrochloride in a Seasonal Ataxia in Nigerians," *Neurology,* 44(3 Pt 1), March 1994, p. 549-551.

Surgical Stress

In this study, the effects of thiamine on blood 11-HOCS, hydrocortisone and corticosterone levels were examined in patients subjected to herniotomy or appendectomy under local anesthesia. Results showed that IV administration of 0.12 g one day and 1.5 to 2 hours prior to surgery decreased the corticosteroid reaction prior to the operation and at the height of the surgery. Results also showed that thiamine administration following surgery prevented decreased blood corticosteroid levels during the postoperative period.

—V.V. Vinogradov, et al., [Thiamine Prevention of the Corticosteroid Reaction after Surgery], *Probl Endokrinol,* 27(3), May-June 1981, p. 11-16.

VITAMIN B2

Antibacterial Effects

Results of this study showed that the intramuscular administration of 6.25 mg/kg—100 mg/kg of vitamin B2 to mice strengthened host resistance to E. coli in a dose-dependent manner. Treatment also provided protection against Pseudomonas aeruginosa, Klebsiella pneumoniae, Staphylococcus aureus, and Actinobacillus pleuropneumoniae.

—S. Araki, et al., "Enhancement of Resistance to Bacterial Infection in Mice by Vitamin B2," *Journal of Veterinary Medical Science,* 57(4), August 1995, p. 599-602.

Brain Function

This study examined the effects of vitamin B2 pretreatment the formation of brain edema during focal ischemia in rats. Results showed that vitamin B2 pretreatment reduced total hemisphere edema formation by 48%.

—A.L. Betz, et al., ''Riboflavin Reduces Edema in Focal Cerebral Ischemia,'' *Acta Neurochir Suppl,* 60, 1994, p. 314-317.

Results of this study showed that riboflavin and its derivatives FAD, FMN, and lumichrome exhibited protective effects against ischemia-reperfusion injury in vitro to a rat myocardium.

—M. Kotegawa, et al., ''Protective Effects of Riboflavin and its Derivatives Against Ischemic Reperfused Damage of Rat Heart,'' *Biochem Mol Biol Int,* 34(4), October 1994, p. 685-691.

Cancer

Results of this study showed that riboflavin 2',3',4',5'-tetrabutyrate (B2-But4) suppressed chemical-induced skin tumors in mice when administered locally.

—M. Ohkoshi, et al., ''Effect of Vitamin B2 on Tumorigenesis of 3-Methylcholanthrene in the Mouse Skin,'' *Gan,* 73(1), 1982, p. 105-107.

Results of this study showed that the administration of vitamin B2-butyrate and CoQ10 inhibited lipid peroxide production in Ehrlich ascites tumor cells treated with ADM.

—M. Chinami, et al., [Effect of Coenzyme Q10 and Vitamin B2-Butyrate to Anticancer Ability and Lipind Peroxidation of Adriamycin,'' *Kurume Igakkai Zasshi,* 44(9/10), 1981, p. 678-683.

Results of this study found that a deficiency in riboflavin can increase cancer risk in rats, and that such risks can be reversed through supplementation.

—J. Pangrekar, et al., ''Effects of Riboflavin Deficiency and Riboflavin Administration on Carcinogen-DNA Binding,'' *Food Chem Toxicol,* 31(10), October 1993, p. 745-750.

Cardiovascular/Coronary Heart Disease

Results of this study showed that the administration of vitamin B2 and CoQ10 prevented lipid peroxidation and ADM-induced cardiotoxicity in rats during chemotherapy.

—T. Katsuki, [Experimental Studies on the Combination Use of Vitamin B2-Butyrate and Coenzyme Q10 (COQ(10)) To Protect Against Adriamycin-induced Cardiac Mitochondrial Disorders,'' *Kurume Igakkai Zasshi,* 44(12), 1981, p. 869-883.

Congenital Methaemoglobinaemia

This article reports on the case of a Japanese family with congenital methaemoglobinaemia who experienced positive results from oral treatment with 120 mg per day of riboflavin.

—M. Hirano, et al., ''Congenital Methaemoglobinaemia Due to NADH Methaemoglobin Reductase Deficiency: Successful Treatment with Oral Riboflavin,'' *British Journal of Haematology,* 47(3), March 1981, p. 353-359.

Depression

This double-blind, placebo-controlled study examined the efficacy of augmenting open tricyclic antidepressant treatment with vitamins B1, B2, and B6 at doses of 10 mg each in geriatric depression inpatients. Results showed those taking vitamins exhibited significantly stronger B2 and B6 status on enzyme activity coefficients and trends toward improved depressed and cognitive function scores relative to controls.

> —I.R. Bell, et al., "Brief Communication. Vitamin B1, B2, and B6 Augmentation of Tricyclic Antidepressant Treatment in Geriatric Depression with Cognitive Dysfunction," *Journal of the American College of Nutrition,* 11(2), April 1992, p. 159-163.

General

This review article notes that studies have found elevated riboflavin levels can provide protection against oxidative damage due to oxidized forms of hemeproteins.

> —H.N. Christensen, "Riboflavin Can Protect Tissue from Oxidative Injury," *Nutr Rev,* 51(5), May 1993, p. 149-150.

This review article notes that studies have found low concentrations of riboflavin can protect isolated rabbit hearts reoxygenation injury, rat lung from injury due to systemic activation of complement, and rat brain from damage due to four hours of ischemia.

> —D.E. Hultquist, et al., "Evidence that NADPH-dependent Methemoglobin Reductase and Administered Riboflavin Protect Tissues from Oxidative Injury," *American Journal of Hematology,* 42(1), January 1993, p. 13-18.

This study examined the effects of 5 mg of vitamin B2/100 g b.wt. on the nephrotoxic effect of 1 or 2 mg $Na_2Cr_2O_7$/100 g b.wt. in rats. Results showed that vitamin B2 administered 3 hours after NaCr207 significantly diminished nephrotoxicity in 55- and 10-day-old rats.

> —D. Appenroth, et al., "Riboflavin Can Decrease the Nephrotoxic Effect of Chromate in Young and Adult Rats," *Toxicol Letters,* 87(1), September 1996, p. 47-52.

Migraine

In this study, migraine patients received 400 mg of riboflavin in a single oral dose for at least 3 months. Results showed a 68.2% global improvement following treatment.

> —J. Schoenen, et al., "High-dose Riboflavin as a Prophylactic Treatment of Migraine: Results of an Open Pilot Study," *Cephalalgia,* 14(5), October 1994, p. 328-329.

Sickle Cell Disease

This case-control study examined the effects of 5 mg of riboflavin taken twice a day for 8 weeks on reduced blood glutathione and iron status in patients with sickle cell disease. Results showed that the treatment significantly increased serum iron and TS.

> —O.A. Ajayi, et al., "Clinical Trial of Riboflavin in Sickle Cell Disease," *East African Medical Journal,* 70(7), July 1993, p. 418-421.

Spontaneous Gonarthrosis

Results of this case-controlled study found that 1 mg/kg body weight of riboflavin administered daily for 4 months via drinking water decreased the incidence of gonarthrosis by half relative to controls.

> —G. Wilhelmi & K. Tanner, "Effect of Riboflavin (vitamin B2) on Spontaneous Gonarthrosis in the Mouse," *Z Rheumatol,* 47(3), May-June 1988, p. 166-172.

■ VITAMIN B6

AIDS/HIV

Results of this study showed that normalization of vitamin B6 levels in HIV-infected patients suffering from a deficiency led to significant improvements in CD4 cell number as well as other functional parameters of immunity.

> —E. Mantero-Atienza, et al., "Vitamin B6 and Immune Function in HIV Infection," *International Conference on AIDS,* 6(2), June 20-23, 1990, p. 432.

Anemia

This study examined the effects of the oral administration of vitamin B6 on hemodialysis patients suffering from microscopic and hypochromic anemia. Results showed the greatest improvement in patients receiving both 180 mg of vitamin B6 for 20 weeks and 40 mg of iron for 12 consecutive dialysis treatments.

> —T. Toriyama, et al., "Effects of High-dose Vitamin B6 Therapy on Microcytic and Hypochromic Anemia in Hemodialysis Patients," *Nippon Jinzo Gakkai Shi,* 35(8), August 1993, p. 975-980.

Asthma

Results of this double-blind, placebo-controlled study found the administration of 200 mg per day of pyridoxine for five months led to significant improvement in children suffering from bronchial asthma.

> —P.J. Collipp, et al., "Pyridoxine Treatment of Childhood Bronchial Asthma," *Ann Allergy,* 35(2), August 1975, p. 93-97.

Autism

This non-blind, placebo-controlled study reports on findings from a previous study showing the efficacy of vitamin B6 treatment in 16 autistic children.

> —B. Rimland, et al., "The Effect of High Doses of Vitamin B6 on Autistic Children: A Double-blind Crossover Study," *American Journal of Psychiatry,* 135(4), April 1978, p. 472-475.

Cancer

Results of this study showed that high vitamin B6 intake suppressed the development of experimentally-induced tumors in mice by regulating PLP growth or by immune enhancement.

> —D.S. Gridley, et al., "Suppression of Tumor Growth and Enhancement of Immune Status

with High Levels of Dietary Vitamin B6 in BALB/c Mice," *Journal of the National Cancer Institute,* 78(5), May 1987, p. 951-959.

This study examined the effects of supplementation with vitamin B-6 on the growth of a human malignant melanoma cell line in vitro. Results showed that pyridoxine or pyridoxal may regulate melanoma cell growth.

—T.D. Shultz TD, et al., "Effect of Pyridoxine and Pyridoxal on the in Vitro Growth of Human Malignant Melanoma," *Anticancer Research,* 8(6), November-December 1988, p. 1313-1318.

Results of this in vitro study indicated that tumor necrosis factor coupled with pyridoxine may be a more effective cancer treatment than the administration of tumor necrosis factor by itself.

—E. Hofsli & A. Waage, "Effect of Pyridoxine on Tumor Necrosis Factor Activities in Vitro," *Biotherapy,* 5(4), 1992, p. 285-290.

This article cites results from numerous in vitro studies indicating vitamin B6 can kill hepatoma cells and may be an effective antineoplastic agent.

—D.M. DiSorbo & G. Litwack, "Vitamin B6 Kills Hepatoma Cells in Culture," *Nutr Cancer,* 3(4), 1982, p. 216-222.

This study examined the effects of vitamin B6 on B16 melanoma cell growth both in vitro and in vivo. Results showed that high doses of the vitamin inhibited growth in vivo and in vitro.

—D.M. DiSorbo, et al., "In Vivo and in Vitro Inhibition of B16 Melanoma Growth by Vitamin B6," *Nutr Cancer,* 7(1-2), 1985, p. 43-52.

Cardiovascular/Coronary Heart Disease

This study examined the effects of 6 weeks worth of treatment with 250 mg of vitamin B6 and 5 mg of folic acid in patients with mild hyperhomocystinemia and cardiovascular disease. Results showed that the treatment normalized postload homocysteine concentration in 92% of patients and fasting homoscyteimenia was normalized in 91%.

—M. van den Berg, et al., "Combined Vitamin B6 Plus Folic Acid Therapy in Young Patients with Arteriosclerosis and Hyperhomocysteinemia," *Journal of Vascular Surgery,* 20(6), December 1994, p. 933-940.

Results of this study showed that patients taking vitamin B6 for carpal tunnel syndrome and other degenerative diseases exhibited a risk of developing acute cardiac chest pain or myocardial infarction which was 27% compared to patients who had not taken vitamin B6. Results also showed a lifespan 8 years longer among elderly patients who died from myocardial infarction relative to those who had not taken vitamin B6.

—J.M. Ellis & K.S. McCully, "Prevention of Myocardial Infarction by Vitamin B6," *Research in Commun Mol Pathol Pharmac,* 89(2), August 1995, p. 208-220.

Carpal Tunnel Syndrome

Results of this double-blind, placebo-controlled study found that supplementation with 100 mg of vitamin B6 per day corrected deficiencies in patients suffering from carpal tunnel syndrome as well as produced improvements in symptoms associated with the syndrome itself.

—J. Ellis, et al., "Clinical Results of a Cross-over Treatment with Pyridoxine and Placebo of the Carpal Tunnel Syndrome," *American Journal of Clinical Nutrition,* 32(10), October 1979, p. 2040-2046.

Results of this 12-year study found that 68% of a group of 494 patients treated with 100 mg per day of vitamin B6 experienced improvement in symptoms associated with carpal tunnel syndrome.
> —M.L. Kasdan & C. Janes, "Carpal Tunnel Syndrome and Vitamin B6," *Plastic Reconstructive Surgery,* 79(3), March 1987, p. 456-462.

Results of this double-blind, placebo-controlled study showed that 10 of 15 patients receiving vitamin B6 over a ten week period experienced improvements in symptoms associated with carpal tunnel syndrome.
> —M. Stransky, et al., "Treatment of Carpal Tunnel Syndrome with Vitamin B6: A Double-blind Study," *Southern Medical Journal,* 82(7), July 1989, p. 841-842.

In this article, a physician in private practice discussed the positive results he has experienced using vitamin B6 in doses of 100 mg to 200 mg per day for 12 weeks in patients suffering from carpal tunnel syndrome.
> —J.M. Ellis, "Treatment of Carpal Tunnel Syndrome with Vitamin B6," *Southern Medical Journal,* 80(7), July 1987, p. 882-884.

Results of this study found that carpal tunnel syndrome patients experienced benefits from treatment with 150 mg of pyridoxine per day for 3 months despite having no initial deficiencies in the vitamin.
> —F.J. Laso Guzman, et al., "Carpal Tunnel Syndrome and Vitamin B6," *Klin Wochenschr,* 67(1), January 4, 1989, p. 38-41.

Results of this study showed that 12 weeks of treatment with vitamin B6 proved to be effective in 4 patients suffering from carpal tunnel syndrome.
> —J. Ellis, et al., "Therapy with Vitamin B6 With and Without Surgery for Treatment of Patients having the Idiopathic Carpal Tunnel Syndrome," *Res Commun Chem Pathol Pharmacol,* 33(2), August 1981, p. 331-344.

Dental Health

Results of this study showed that the administration of cariogenic diets supplemented with vitamin B6 and zinc led to a reduction in the number of dental caries in rats relative to controls.
> —E. Rapisarda & A. Longo, [Effects of Zinc and Vitamin B6 in Experimental Caries in Rats], *Minerva Stomatol,* 30(4), July-August 1981, p. 317-320.

Diabetes

Results of this study indicated that gestational diabetes can be caused by increased xanthurenic-acid synthesis during pregnancy and that vitamin B6 supplementation can normalize the production of xanthurenic-acid by restoring tryptophan metabolism and thus improve oral glucose tolerance in such patients.
> —H.J. Bennink & W.H. Schreurs, "Improvement of Oral Glucose Tolerance in Gestational Diabetes by Pyridoxine," *British Medical Journal,* 3(5974), July 5, 1975, p. 13-15.

Hyperkinetic Syndrome

Results of this double-blind, placebo-controlled study found that pyridoxine and methlyphenidate were more effective than controls in reducing symptoms associate with hyperkinesis in six patients.

> —M. Coleman, et al., "A Preliminary Study of the Effect of Pyridoxine Administration in a Subgroup of Hyperkinetic Children: A Double-blind Crossover Comparison with Methylphenidate," *Biological Psychiatry,* 14(5), October 1979, p. 741-751.

Immune Function

In this study, male patients undergoing hemodialysis were examined to determine the effects of supplemental pyridoxine hydrochloride at doses of 50 mg per over a 3 to 5 week period on immune function. Results showed improvement in numerous parameters of immune function following the treatment.

> —D.A. Casciato, et al., "Immunologic Abnormalities in Hemodialysis Patients: Improvement after Pyridoxine Therapy," *Nephron,* 38(1), 1984, p. 9-16.

Infantile Spasms

This article reports on three cases studies in which a dose of 0.2-0.4 g.kg-1 pyridoxine stopped infantile spasms with hypsarrhythmia within five to six days.

> —G. Blennow & L. Starck, "High Dose B6 Treatment in Infantile Spasms," *Neuropediatrics,* 17(1), February 1986, p. 7-10.

Results of this study showed high doses of vitamin B6 coupled with valproic acid to be an effective treatment for infantile spasms.

> —M. Ito, et al., "Vitamin B6 and Valproic Acid in Treatment of Infantile Spasms," *Pediatr Neurol,* 7(2), March-April 1991, p. 91-96.

Results of this study showed that 300 mg/kg per day of vitamin B6 administered orally to children suffering from infantile spasms led to an elimination of seizure after 4 weeks in all 17 patients receiving the treatment.

> —J. Pietz, et al., "Treatment of Infantile Spasms with High-dosage Vitamin B6," *Epilepsia,* 34(4), July-August, 1993, p. 757-763.

Memory

Results of this double-blind, placebo-controlled study showed that vitamin B6 supplementation improved memory in healthy elderly men when administered in doses of 20 mg pyridoxine HCL per day for 3 months.

> —J.B. Deijen, et al., "Vitamin B-6 Supplementation in Elderly Men: Effects on Mood, Memory, Performance and Mental Effort," *Psychopharmacology,* 109(4), 1992, p. 489-496.

PMS

This study examined the effects of vitamin B6 supplementation in 630 PMS patients over a seven year period beginning in 1976. Women received daily doses of pyridoxine hydrochloride in doses ranging between 40 to 100 mg early in the study and 120 to 200 mg towards its later stages. Results showed the treatment to be effective in 65-68 per cent of patients at the lower doses and 70-88 per cent at higher doses.

> —M.G. Brush, et al., "Pyridoxine in the Treatment of Premenstrual Syndrome: A Retrospective Survey in 630 Patients," *British Journal of Clinical Practice,* 42(11), November 1988, p. 448-452.

Results of this double-blind, placebo-controlled study found that the administration of pyridoxine to 434 women with PMS led to improvements in 7 of 9 symptoms measured and a significant improvement in overall global assessment.

> —M.J. Williams, et al., "Controlled Trial of Pyridoxine in the Premenstrual Syndrome," *Journal of Internal Medicine Research,* 13(3), 1985, p. 174-179.

This double-blind, placebo-controlled, crossover study examined the effects of 50 mg per day of pyridoxine on PMS symptoms in women between the ages of 14-89. Results showed the treatment had significant beneficial effects on emotional symptoms such as fatigue, depression, and irritability.

> —H. Doll, et al., "Pyridoxine (Vitamin B6) and the Premenstrual Syndrome: A Randomized Crossover Trial," *J R Coll Gen Pract,* 39(326), September 1989, p. 364-368.

Pregnancy

Results of this double-blind, placebo-controlled study showed that patients receiving 25 mg tablets of vitamin B6 every 8 hours for 72 hours experienced a significant reduction in nausea and vomiting associated with pregnancy.

> —V. Sahakian, et al., "Vitamin B6 is Effective Therapy for Nausea and Vomiting of Pregnancy: A Randomized, Double-blind Placebo-controlled Study," *Obstet Gynecol,* 78(1), July 1991, p. 33-36.

Primary Hyperoxaluria

This study examined the effects of therapy with orthophosphate and pyridoxine in primary hyperoxaluria patients who were treated for an average of 10 years. Results showed the therapy reduced urinary calcium oxalate crystallization and preserved renal function.

> —D.S. Milliner, et al., "Results of Long-term Treatment with Orthophosphate and Pyridoxine in Patients with Primary Hyperoxaluria," *New England Journal of Medicine,* 331(23), December 8, 1994, p. 1553-1558.

■ VITAMIN B12

AIDS/HIV

Results of this study found that normalizing the status of vitamin B12 by supplementation of 250 mg/ml in HIV-infected patients produced significant improvements in cognitive function.

> —M.K. Baum, et al., "Vitamin B12 and Cognitive Function in HIV Infection," *International Conference on AIDS,* 6(2), June 20-23, 1990, p. 97.

Anemia

Results of this study showed that vitamin B12 supplementation reversed previous increases levels of ineffective erythropoieses in pernicious anemia patients within 24 hours of administration.

—D. Samson, et al., "Reversal of Ineffective Erythropoiesis in Pernicious Anaemia Following Vitamin B12 Therapy," *British Journal Haematology,* 35(2), February 1977, p. 217-224.

This article reports on the cases of two elderly patients deficient in vitamin B12 and having low immunoglubulin levels. Supplementation with vitamin B12 returned the immunoglobulin levels.

—K. Kafetz, "Immunoglobulin Deficiency Responding to Vitamin B12 in Two Elderly Patients with Megaloblastic Anaemia," *Postgraduate Medical Journal,* 61(722), December 1985, p. 1065-1056.

This article reports on the case of a patient with pernicious anemia with a severely decreased percentage of OKT8-positive blood cells which led to increased OKT4/OKT 8 ratio. Vitamin B12 supplementation returned the levels of OKT8-positive blood cells to normal.

—K. Kubota, et al., "Restoration of Decreased Suppressor Cells by Vitamin B12 Therapy in a Patient with Pernicious Anemia," *American Journal of Hematol,* 24(2), February 1987, p. 221-223.

This article reports on the case of a patient with post-gastrectomy megaloblastic anemia with abnormally high ratio of CD4/CD8 ration of blood cells and low level of natural killer cell activity. Treatment with vitamin B12 corrected these levels.

—K. Kubota, et al., "Restoration of Abnormally High CD4/CD8 Ratio and Low Natural Killer Cell Activity by Vitamin B12 Therapy in a Patient with post-gastrectomy Megaloblastic Anemia," *Internal Medicine,* 31(1), January 1992, p. 125-126.

Apthae

Results of this case control study found that supplementation with vitamin B12 led to marked improvements in outpatients suffering from recurrent aphthous initially deficient in vitamin B12.

—D. Wray, et al., "Recurrent Aphthae: Treatment with Vitamin B12, Folic Acid, and Iron," *British Medical Journal,* 2(5969), May 31, 1975, p. 490-493.

Bronchial Squamous Metaplasia

In this double-blind, placebo-controlled study, 73 male smokers with a 20 or more pack-year history and metaplasia on one or more sputnam samples were given 10 mg of folate coupled with 500 micrograms of hydroxocobalamin for 4 months. Results showed significantly more reduction of atypia in the treatment group relative to controls.

—D.C. Heimburger, et al., "Improvement in Bronchial Squamous Metaplasia in Smokers Treated with Folate and Vitamin B12. Report of a Preliminary Randomized, Double-blind Intervention Trial," *JAMA,* 259(10), March 11, 1988, p. 1525-1530.

Cancer

Results of this study found that treatment with a mixture of vitamin B12 and vitamin C inhibited mitotic activity of the transplantable mouse tumors, Sarcoma 37, Krebs-2, and Ehrlich carcinomas, in the ascites form.

> —M.E. Poydock, et al., "Inhibiting Effect of Vitamins C and B12 on the Mitotic Activity of Ascites Tumors," *Exp Cell Biol,* 47(3), 1979, p. 210-217.

This study examined vitamin B12's antitumor effects in mice, MH134 hepatoma ascites cells, Lewis lung cancer cells, and Ehrlich ascites tumor cells. Results showed that 1.0-10 micrograms/ml doses of vitamin B12 enhanced PHA- and Con-A-induced lymphocyte blastoformation of mice and that 7 days of 50 or 100 micrograms per day ip of vitamin B12 suppressed the growth of MH134 tumors on their backs as well as increased survival time relative to controls. Results also showed that the administration of 50 micrograms per day ip of vitamin B12 increased survival time relative to controls and reduced the growth of Ehrlich ascites tumor cells inoculated into mice 17 and 19 days following inoculation.

> —N. Shimizu, et al., "Experimental Study of Antitumor Effect of Methyl-B12," *Oncology,* 44(3), 1987, p. 169-173.

Cognitive Function

This study examined the effects of vitamin B12 on cognitive disturbance in rats. Results indicated that vitamin B12 potentiates learning in an acetylcholine-deprived brain.

> —H. Sasaki, et al., "Vitamin B12 Improves Cognitive Disturbance in Rodents Fed a Choline-deficient Diet," *Pharmacol Biochem Behav,* 43(2), October 1992, p. 635-639.

Dementia

In this study, platelet monoamine oxidase activity was examined in patients with senile dementia of the Alzheimer type experiencing low serum levels of vitamin B12 and some with pernicious anemia. Results showed that vitamin B12 therapy significantly decreased platelet monoamine oxidase activity in both groups of patients relative to controls.

> —B. Regland, et al., "Vitamin B12-induced Reduction of Platelet Monoamine Oxidase Activity in Patients with Dementia and Pernicious Anaemia," *Eur Arch Psychiatry Clin Neurosci,* 240(4-5), 1991, p. 288-291.

Dental Health

This article notes that vitamin B12 supplements have the potential to reverse some of the negative effects of chronic exposure to nitro oxide inhalation common to dental settings.

> —D.S. Ostreicher, "Vitamin B12 Supplements as Protection Against Nitrous Oxide Inhalation," *New York State Dental Journal,* 60(3), March 1994, p. 47-49.

General

Results of this study showed that subjects with normal vitamin B12 levels who received supplements via injection scored better on the MMPI relative to subjects not receiving the supplements.

> —H.L. Newbold, "Vitamin B-12: Placebo or Neglected Therapeutic Tool?" *Medical Hypotheses,* 28(3), May 1989, p. 155-164.

This article recommends parental regimens use 1000 micrograms cyanocobalamin: 5 or 6 biweekly injections for loading, and once-a-month for maintenance. The authors also notes that oral intake of 300-1000 micrograms per day may be therapeutically equivalent to parenteral therapy.

> —D.T. Watts, "Vitamin B12 Replacement Therapy: How Much is Enough?" *Wisconsin Medical Journal,* 93(5), May 1994, p. 203-205.

Hepatitis

In this study, two sets of patients taken from the same hepatitis A epidemic were given either coenzyme-B12 or cyanocobalamin. Results showed a quicker return of serum aminotransferase (S-ALAT) levels to normal in those receiving the coenzyme-B12.

> —S. Iwarson & J. Lindberg, "Coenzyme-B12 Therapy in Acute Viral Hepatitis," *Scandinavian Journal of Infectious Disease,* 9(2), 1977, p. 157-158.

Results of this study showed that the intravenous administration of 100 micrograms of cyanocobalamin to hepatitis patients every other day produced a significant normalizing effect on the level of unbound vitamin B12, bilirubin, the thymol test, aldolase and alanine aminotransferase of the blood relative to treatment with 200 microgram doses.

> —I.V. Komar , [Use of Vitamin B12 in the Combined Therapy of Viral Hepatitis], *Vopr Pitan,* (1), February 1982, p. 26-29.

Imerslund-Grasbeck Syndrome

This article reports on the case of a Saudi child with spasticity, truncal ataxia, cerebral atrophy, megaloblastic anemia and proteinuria who experienced a total resolution of his neurological findings and brain atrophy following parental vitamin B12 therapy.

> —M.M. Salameh, et al., "Reversal of Severe Neurological Abnormalities after Vitamin B12 Replacement in the Imerslund-Grasbeck Syndrome," *Journal of Neurology,* 238(6), September 1991, p. 349-350.

Immune Enhancements

Results of this study indicated that methyl-B12 modulated human lymphocyte function by augmenting regulatory T-cell activities in vitro.

> —T. Sakane, et al., "Effects of Methyl-B12 on the in Vitro Immune Functions of Human T Lymphocytes," *Journal of Clinical Immunology,* 2(2), April 1982, p. 101-109.

Methylmalonic Acidemia

This article reports on the case of a 3-month-old male infant who had experienced two episodes of fever, projectile vomiting, dehydration, generalized fine tremors and severe metabolic ketoacidosis. High concentrations of methylmalonic acid were found in both serum and urine. Results showed that the administration of vitamin B12 produced a marked reduction in methylmalonic aciduria. Continuous intramuscular vitamin B12 supplements in doses of 1 mg on alternate days followed by 15 mg per day taken orally led to normal progression of physical and intellectual development and has helped the patient survive acute respiratory tract infections without metabolic acidosis recurring.

> —B.A. Gordon & R.A. Carson, "Methylmalonic Acidemia Controlled with Oral Administra-

tion of Vitamin B12," *Canadian Medical Association Journal,* 115(3), August 7, 1976, p. 233-236.

Multiple Sclerosis

In this study, 60 mg of vitamin B12 was administered to chronic multiple sclerosis patients every day for 6 months. Results showed improvement in both abnormalities of the visual and brainstem auditory evoked potentials relative to controls.

> —J. Kira, et al., "Vitamin B12 Metabolism and Massive-dose Methyl Vitamin B12 Therapy in Japanese Patients with Multiple Sclerosis," *Internal Medicine,* 33(2), February 1994, p. 82-86.

Sleep

Results of this double-blind, placebo-controlled study indicated that vitamin B12 supplementation at doses of 3 mg per day may advance human circadian rhythm by increasing circadian clock light sensitivity in healthy subjects.

> —K. Honma, et al., "Effects of Vitamin B12 on Plasma Melatonin Rhythm in Humans: Increased Light Sensitivity Phase-advances the Circadian Clock?" *Experientia,* 48(8), August 15, 1992, p. 716-720.

This article reports on the cases of two adolescent patients with sleep-wake schedule disorders that responded positively to vitamin B12 supplementation at doses of 3000 micrograms per day.

> —T. Ohta, et al., "Treatment of Persistent Sleep-wake Schedule Disorders in Adolescents with Methylcobalamin (Vitamin B12)," *Sleep,* 14(5), October 1991, p. 414-418.

This article reports on the cases of two patients with long-time, differing sleep-wake rhythm disorders who received vitamin B12 therapy. The first patient was a blind, 15-year-old girl with hypernychthermal syndrome which had persisted for approximately 13 years. 1.5 mg per day t.i.d. of vitamin B12 was administered to her beginning at 14. Her sleep-wake rhythm was entrained to the environmental 24-h rhythm shortly thereafter. The second patient was a 55-year-old male suffering from delayed sleep phase syndrome, a condition which had persisted since age 18. Daily doses of 1.5 mg of vitamin B12 improved his sleep-wake rhythm disorder for the entire 6 month time was receiving the treatment.

> —M. Okawa, et al., "Vitamin B12 Treatment for Sleep-wake Rhythm Disorders," *Sleep,* 13(1), February 1990, p. 15-23.

Vitiligo

Results of this study found that the oral administration of folic acid coupled with parenteral treatment with vitamin B12 and oral ascorbic acid produced repigmentation without side effects in eight patients suffering from vitiligo.

> —L.F. Montes, et al., "Folic Acid and Vitamin B12 in Vitiligo: A Nutritional Approach," *Cutis,* 50(1), July 1992, p. 39-42.

■ VITAMIN C

Adrenal Function

Ascorbate's effects on the regulation of 11 beta-hydroxylase in culture were studied. In the absence of ACTH, 11 beta-hydroxylase activity declined with a half-time of approximately 40 hours. With the addition of 50 microM cortisol, the half-time was reduced to approximately 6 hours. The rate of loss of 11 beta-hydroxylase activity in the presence of cortisol was greatly reduced with the addition of 5 mM of ascorbate. 5mM of ascorbate coupled with a lowered concentration of oxygen (2%) proved to be synergistic in their protective action, preventing the loss of 11 beta-hydroxylase activity in the presence of 50 microM cortisol..

> —P.J. Hornsby, et al., "The Role of Ascorbic Acid in the Function of the Adrenal Cortex: Studies in Adrenocortical Cells in Culture," *Endocrinology,* 117(3), September 1985, p. 1264-1271.

Aging

This study examined the effects of ascorbic acid on cell proliferation and collagen expression in dermal fibroblasts from young children (ages 3-8) and the elderly (ages 78-93). The presence of ascorbic acid in both age groups resulted in a faster rate of cell proliferation and reached higher densities than controls. Collagen biosynthesis was found to be inversely related to age, while the stimulation by ascorbic acid appeared to be age independent.

> —C.L. Phillips, et al., "Effects of Ascorbic Acid on Proliferation and Collagen Synthesis in Relation to the Donor age of Human Dermal Fibroblasts," *Journal of Invest Dermatol,* 103(2), August 1994, p. 228-232.

Vitamins E, C, and beta-carotene were studied to determine if they induce an increase of singlet oxygen protection of erythrocytes' subjects. Beta-carotene (15-30 mg/day), vitamin E (15 mg/day) and vitamin C (30 mg/day) were all shown to produce an increase of singlet oxygen protection of erythrocytes of subjects after just 15 days of treatment.

> —E. Postaire, et al., "Increase of Singlet Oxygen Protection of Erythrocytes by Vitamin E, Vitamin C, and Beta Carotene Intakes," *Biochem Mol Biol Int,* 35(2), February, 1995, p. 371-374.

Dietary ascorbic acid intake and serum lipid concentration intake was studied in the aged (65 and older). Significant positive correlations were found between dietary ascorbic acid and HDLC, the intake of carbohydrates and protein and total fat. Significant negative correlations were found between dietary ascorbic acid and LDLC and LDLC/HDLC. The authors suggest that their results point to a preventive role of ascorbic acid in atherogenic diseases.

> —K. Okamoto, et al., [The Relationship Between Dietary Ascorbic Acid Intake and Serum Lipid Concentration in the Aged], *Nippon Ronen Igakkai Zasshi,* 29(12), December 1992, p. 908-911.

In this study a relationship was demonstrated between serum concentrations of vitamin and cortisone stimulated blood glucose responses. High vitamin C concentrations resulted in lower blood glucose response in subjects of all ages. A similar relationship was found between vitamin E consumption and serum. Daily ingestion of less than 100 mg of ascorbic acid resulted in the highest number of nonspecific clinical signs and symptoms. Daily ingestion of 200 mg or more of ascorbic acid resulted in the least for all ages. Those who ingested the most vitamin C (50 years of age or older) were clinically similar to the 40-year-olds who ingested the least. Subjects ingesting 22 I.U. of vitamin E per day increased in serum cholesterol far more than subjects ingesting 158 I.U.

> —E. Cheraskin, "Chronologic Versus Biologic Age," *Journal of Advancement in Medicine,* 7(1), Spring 1994, p. 31-41.

This article reviews data suggesting that insufficient intake of antioxidants have a higher risk of cancer. One large study cited demonstrated a significant relationship between low vitamin C intake and higher risks of heart disease mortality and overall mortality over the following ten year time period. Additional studies are cited that demonstrate connections between vitamin C and other antioxidants and cataracts. Vitamin C has also been shown to be essential as a scavenger of free radicals which is important in collagen formation, and hormone and neurotransmitter synthesis.

> —"Vitamin C, Cancer and Aging," *Age,* 16, 1993, p. 55-58.

The effects of vitamin C on immunity the elderly were studied. Elderly lymphocytes cultured in the presence of 10 micrograms/ml of vitamin C and pre-incubated overnight, resulted in mitogen-stimulated lymphocyte proliferation which was similar to that from younger controls without vitamin C in culture. Oral ingestion of 2 g of vitamin C daily on certain in vitro and in vivo immunologic parameters in the elderly was also examined and proved to be beneficial. These results coupled with related findings in the study point to vitamin C as a potentially effective agent in enhancing immune functions in the elderly.

> —J.C. Delafuente, et al, "Immunologic Modulation by Vitamin C in the Elderly," *International Journal of Immunopharmacology,* 8(2), 1986, p. 205-211.

AIDS/HIV

This study demonstrated Ca-ascorbate's ability to reduce HIV reverse transcriptase activity at approximately the same levels as ascorbic acid administered at equivalent doses. Previous studies have found that ascorbate was essential for the suppression of HIV. When tested at the same time with ascorbic acid, NAC (10 mmol/L) caused less than twofold inhibition of HIV RT and produced a synergistic effect. Nonesterified GSH (less than or equal to 1.838 mmol/L) did not have an effect on RT concentrations nor did it potentiate the anti-HIV effect of ascorbic acid. The authors argue that their results add additional support to ascorbate's reported antiviral activity and suggest it be used, in combination with thiols, in treating HIV infection.

> —S. Harakeh and R.J. Jariwalla, "Comparative Study of the Anti-HIV Activities of Ascorbate and Thiol-Containing Reducing Agents in Chronically HIV-Infected Cells," *American Journal of Clinical Nutrition,* 54(6 Suppl), December 1991, p. 1231S-1235S.

This study examined cell-free human immunodeficiency (CFHIV) inactivation by the treatment of blood products with ascorbic acid. Results demonstrated that 500 micrograms/ml of ascorbic acid in replication-competent virions with aliquots of a culture medium, whole blood, or leukocyte depleted blood, inactivated CFHIV in vitro.

> —B.D. Rawal, et al., "In Vitro Inactivation of Human Immunodeficiency Virus by Ascorbic Acid," *Biologicals,* 23(1), March 1995, p. 75-81.

This study looked at the molecular basis of the inhibitory effect of ascorbate on HIV expression in unstimulated chronically infected and reporter cell lines. No significant differences were found in the synthesis or processing of individual viral RNA and polypeptides, which indicates ascorbate's inhibitory effect is not focused on steps of viral transcription or translation. Enzyme assays on cell abstracts found the activity of an HIV LTR-directed reporter protein made in ascorbate-treated cells was reduced to about 11% in relation to controls. Such findings are in line with a mechanism of action where ascorbate exerts a posttranslational inhibitory effect on HIV by causing impairment of enzymatic activity.

—S. Harakeh, et al., "Mechanistic Aspects of Ascorbate Inhibition of Human Immunodeficiency Virus," *Chem Biol Interact,* 91(2-3), June 1994, p. 207-215.

Noting the frequency of GSH of deficiency in AIDS patients and persons infected with HIV, this study compared the effectiveness of ascorbate N-acetylcysteine (NAC), a GSH precursor, against HIV replication in an infected T cell line. Non cytoxic concentrations of ascorbate (0.43-0.85 mmol/L) or NAC (10 mmol/L), with the addition of antioxidants solutions daily, to a growing HXB cell line. Extracellular RT activity was lowered by greater than 99% and p24 HIV core antigen was reduced by approximately 90% in HXB cells exposed to the highest amounts of ascorbate (0.85mM) at 37 degrees for 4 days. A nontoxic dose of NAC (10 mM) by itself, caused approximately 46% inhibition of HIV RT activity and approximately 90% reduction in the p24 antigen level in the culture supernatant. The authors argue that their results add additional support to ascorbate's reported antiviral activity and suggest it be used, in combination with thiols, in treating HIV infection.

—R.J. Jariwalla and S. Harakeh, "HIV Suppression by Ascorbate and its Enhancement by a Glutathione Precursor," *International Conference on AIDS,* 8(2):B207 (abstract no. PoB 3697), July 19-24, 1992.

The author hypothesizes, based on his clinical experience, that ascorbate would be useful in the treatment of AIDS. He cites preliminary clinical evidence that large doses of ascorbate (50-200 grams per 24 hours) can suppress AIDS symptoms and can reduce secondary infections. Ascorbate, when used with standard treatments for secondary infections, can lead to a clinical remission which evidence suggests of being prolonged if treatment is continued, despite evidence of helper T-cell suppression.

—R.F. Cathcart RF, III, "Vitamin C in the Treatment of Acquired Immune Deficiency Syndrome (AIDS)," *Medical Hypotheses,* 14(4), August 1985, p. 423-433.

The authors have demonstrated ascorbate's ability to suppress virus production and cell fusion in T-lymphocytic cell lines infected with HIV. Ascorbate reduced extracellular reverse transcriptase (RT) activity by greater than 99% and of p24 antigen by 90% in the culture supernatant in chronically infected cells expressing HIV at peak levels. Ascorbate also inhibited the formation of giant-cell syncytia by 93% in newly infected CD4+ cells. Cell-free virus exposure to ascorbate for 1 day at 37 degrees C had no effect on its RT activity or syncytium-forming ability; however, exposure at the same temperature for 4 days, in the presence 100-150 micrograms/ml of ascorbate produced a drop by a factor of 3-14 in RT activity as compared to a reduction by a factor of 25-172 in extracellular RT released from chronically infected cells. The authors suggest such results indicate ascorbate mediates an anti-HIV effect by diminishing viral protein production in infected cells and RT stability in extracellular virions.

—S. Harakeh, et al., "Suppression of Human Immunodeficiency Virus Replication by Ascorbate in Chronically and Acutely Infected Cells," *Proc Natl Acad Sci U S A,* 87(18), September 1990, p. 7245-7249.

108 seropositive AIDS homosexual or bisexual males were studied for daily micronutrient intake relative to the progression rate to AIDS over a period of 6.8 years. Progression rates for those with highest total intake of vitamins C and B1 and niacin were significantly slower than those ingesting lower doses.

—A.M. Tang, et al., "Dietary Micronutrient Intake and Risk of Progression to Acquired Immunodeficiency Syndrome (AIDS) in Human Immunodeficiency Virus Type 1 (HIV-1)-Infected Homosexual Men," *American Journal of Epidemiology,* 1993, 138(11), p. 937-951.

Continued exposure of T lymphocyte cell culture lines infected with HIV to vitamin C resulted in significant inhibition of viral replication in chronically infected cells and multinucleated giant cell formation in cells acutely infected at doses of 75, 100, and 150 ug/ml, suggesting a virus specific action of ascorbate. The authors suggest ascorbate may inhibit the reverse transcriptase required for HIV replication.

—S. Davies, et al., "Suppression of Human Immunodeficiency Virus Replication by Ascorbate in Chronically and Acutely Infected Cells," *Journal of Nutritional Medicine,* 1, 1990, p. 345-346.

Alcohol Toxicity

Ascorbic acid pretreatment on ethanol clearance, toxicity, and behavioral impairment after an acute dose of ethanol in humans was studied. Ascorbic acid or a placebo was given to 20 healthy males before ethanol consumption (0.95 gm/kg body weight over 2.5 hour period)for 2 weeks. Pretreatment with ascorbic acid improved motor coordination and color discrimination in half the subjects after ethanol consumption. It also resulted in significant enhancement in blood ethanol clearance and an increase in serum triglyceride levels after ethanol consumption in half of the subjects. Intellectual function was not improved nor did ascorbic acid pretreatment influence elevated blood lactate/pyruvate ratios or impaired intellectual function.

—R.L. Susick, Jr. and V.G. Zannoni, "Effect of Ascorbic Acid on the Consequences of Acute Alcohol Consumption in Humans," *Clin Pharmacol Ther,* 41(5), May 1987, p. 502-509.

Alcohol consumption has been shown to lead to non-dialysis cytotoxic activity against A9 cells. In this study, seven healthy subjects consumed 84 g of ethanol following pretreatment with 1 g vitamin C daily for 3 days. 8 hours after the ethanol and vitamin C consumption, the cytotoxicity developing in serum albumin was abolished. The authors argue such results suggest vitamin C may play a part in limiting those elements of alcohol toxicity that are mediated by circulating acetaldehyde.

—S.N. Wickramasinghe and R. Hasan, "In Vivo Effects of Vitamin C on the Cytotoxicity of Post-Ethanol Serum," *Biochem Pharmacol,* 48(3), August 3, 1994, p. 621-624.

Ascorbic acid supplementation was found to significantly enhance the clearance of plasma alcohol in 13 clinically healthy male subjects tested at alcohol doses of both 0.5 and 0.8 g/kg body weight.

—M.F. Chen, et al., "Effect of Ascorbic Acid on Plasma Alcohol Clearance," *Journal of American College of Nutrition,* 9(3), June 1990, p. 185-189.

Allergic Rhinititis

Synthetic ascorbic acid solution decreased symptoms in 74% of patients suffering from perennial allergic rhinitis. In addition, the pH of nasal secretion decreased to normal limits.

—L. Podoshin, et al., "Treatment of Perennial Allergic Rhinitis with Ascorbic Acid Solution [letter]," *Ear Nose Throat Journal,* 70(1), January 1991, p. 54-55.

Anti-Histamine Effects

This study of 437 human blood samples demonstrated that when the plasma-reduced ascorbic acid level falls below 1 mg/100 ml, the whole blood histamine level increases exponentially as the ascorbic acid level decreases. When the ascorbic acid level falls below 0.7 mg/100 ml, blood histamine levels increase significantly. Oral administration of 1 g daily of ascorbic acid for 3 days resulted in a reduction of the blood histamine level in 11/11 subjects.

—C.A. Clemetson, "Histamine and Ascorbic Acid in Human Blood," *Journal of Nutrition,* 110(4), April 1980, p. 662-668.

Anti-Psychotic Effects

Ascorbic acid (1000 milligrams per kilogram of body weight) enhanced the antiamphetamine and cataleptogenic effects of haloperidol in rats. The authors conclude that their results, coupled with similar biochemical evidence, suggest that ascorbic acid has a key role to play in modulating the effects of anti-psychotic drugs such as haloperidol.

—G.V. Rebec, et al., "Ascorbic Acid and the Behavioral Response to Haloperidol: Implications for the Action of Antipsychotic Drugs," *Science,* 227(4685), January 25, 1985, p. 438-440.

This study examined individual behaviors produced by ascorbic acid in combination with typical and atypical antipsychotic drugs. The combination of antipsychotic drugs with ascorbic acid 250 mg/kg i.p. led to a decrease in open-field parameters when compared with controls. Such in vivo results provide more evidence for ascorbic acids antidopaminergic effects, particularly when combined with antipsychotic drugs.

—L. de Angelis, "Ascorbic Acid and Atypical Antipsychotic Drugs: Modulation of Amineptine-Induced Behavior in Mice," *Brain Research,* 670(2), January 30, 1995, p. 303-307.

Arthritis

Treatment with vitamin C supplements resulted in the resolution of significant cutaneous hemorrhages in three elderly rheumatoid patients, all of which were ascorbic-acid deficient.

—K.G. Oldroyd KG and P.T. Dawes, "Clinically Significant Vitamin C Deficiency in Rheumatoid Arthritis," *British Journal of Rheumatology,* 24(4), November 1985, p. 362-363.

The treatment with a daily dose of 150 mg/kg of subcutaneous vitamin C over a period of 20 days reduced arthritic swelling, increased pain tolerance, and decreased polymorphonuclear leukocyte infiltration in rat paws, with no significant change in surface temperature. Such findings suggest that vitamin C may be explored as a treatment for patients with rheumatoid arthritis.

—R.H. Davis, et al., "Vitamin C Influence on Localized Adjuvant Arthritis," *Journal of American Podiatry Medical Association,* 80(8), August 1990, p. 414-418.

The addition of ascorbic acid (0.57 mM) reduced growth inhibition of rabbit and human articular chondrocytes and human fibroblasts produced by increasing concentrations homogentisic acid (HGA) and prevented the morphologic changes that results from such inhibition.

—A.P. Angeles, et al., "Chondrocyte Growth Inhibition Induced by Homogentisic Acid and its Partial Prevention with Ascorbic Acid," *Journal of Rheumatology,* 16(4), April 1989, p. 512-517.

This study examined the effect of vitamin C when taken in a 50 mg/kg daily dose for 4 and 21 days in arthritic rats. When administered for 21 days, vitamin C increased the lowered serum sulphydryl (SH-groups) to prearthritic values and decreased the elevated level of blood glutathione (GSH). Vitamin C administered over 21-day and 7-day periods also improved the lowered A/G ratio in the rats. Such results point to vitamin C as a potentially effective therapy for the treatment of arthritis.

—A.A. Eldin, et al., "Effect of Vitamin C Administration in Modulating Some Biochemical Changes in Arthritic Rats," *Pharmacol Research,* 26(4), December 1992, p. 357-366.

Asthma

This is a review article looking at the relationship between asthma and vitamin C. Studies show that vitamin C intake in the general population correlates with the incidence of asthma. Asthma symptoms in adults have been shown to decrease following vitamin C supplementation.

—G.E. Hatch, "Asthma, Inhaled Oxidants, and Dietary Antioxidants," *American Journal of Clinical Nutrition,* 61(3 Suppl), March 1995, p. 625S-630S.

Standard anti-asthma chemoprophylaxis (SAC) supplemented with 1 g ascorbic acid (Redoxon) given as a single daily dose for a 6-month period significantly improved polymorphonuclear leucocyte (PMNL) motility and decreased antistreptolysin O (ASO) levels in children with bronchial asthma.

—R. Anderson, et al., "Ascorbic Acid in Bronchial Asthma," *South African Medical Journal,* 63(17), April 23, 1983, p. 649-652.

Ten children suffering from bronchial asthma and exercise induced bronchoconstriction supplemented their standard therapy with 1 g/d of ascorbate. Results indicated that after 6 months of ascorbate supplemented therapy, functions in the following case all normalized: 2 children with depressed neutrophil motility, 4 children with depressed lymphocyte transformation, and 7 with elevated levels of ASO. The 6 months of ascorbate therapy also reduced serum total Ige levels but not specific IgE levels.

—R. Anderson, et al., "The Effect of Ascorbate on Cellular Humoral Immunity in Asthmatic Children," *South African Medical Journal,* 58(24), December 13, 1980, p. 974-977.

This study examined 41 asthmatics in remission in which half were administered 1 g of ascorbic acid daily and the other half a placebo. Asthmatics taking ascorbic acid experienced less severe and fewer asthma attacks when assessed after 14 weeks of treatment. When those in the experimental group stopped taking ascorbic acid, attack rates increased.

—C.O. Anah, et al., "High Dose Ascorbic Acid in Nigerian Asthmatics," *Trop Geogr Med,* 32(2), June 1980, p. 132-137.

124 patients with bronchial asthma were studied, 96.8% of which were found to be deficient in ascorbic acid. Treatment that did not include vitamin C was ineffective. Administering doses of 275-300 mg of vitamin C, in combination with other vitamins, over many days proved more successful. The authors suggest that vitamin treatment of asthmatics intensifies therapy effectiveness and reduces the terms of inpatient treatment.

> —E.M. Rozanov, et al., [Vitamin PP and C Allowances and Their Correction in the Treatment of Bronchial Asthma Patients], *Vopr Pitan*, (6):21-4, November-December, 1987, p. 21-24.

Autism

The administration of 8 g/70 kg/day of ascorbic acid to autistic treatment was examined in this 30 week, double-blind, placebo-controlled study. The results showed a reduction in symptom severity and proved to be consistent with the theory of a dopaminergic mechanism of action for ascorbic acid.

> —M.C. Dolske, et al., "A Preliminary Trial of Ascorbic Acid as Supplemental Therapy for Autism," *Prog Neuropsychopharmacol Biol Psychiatry*, 17(5), September 1993, p. 765-774.

Blunt Trauma

This placebo controlled study examined whether supplementation with ascorbic acid and alpha-tocopherol improves neutrophil (PMN) locomotroy defect, as is often found in patients with serious trauma. Both antioxidants were found to significantly improve PMN locomotion compared to placebo, prompting the authors to suggest the use of antioxidant replacement therapy in patients suffering from PMN locomotory abnormality as a result of blunt trauma.

> —E.G. Maderazo, et al., "A Randomized Trial of Replacement Antioxidant Vitamin Therapy for Neutrophil Locomotory Dysfunction in Blunt Trauma," *Journal of Trauma*, 31(8), August 1991, p. 1142-1150.

Candida

Ascorbic acid enhanced the lethal but not the permeabilizing effects of amphotericin B on Candida albicans and Cryptococcus neoformans cells. Two other ene-diol acids, D-erythorbate and dihydroxyfumarate, also enhanced the lethal action of amphotericin B on Can. albicans. It is believed that ascorbic acid and the two other ene-diol acids acting as pro-oxidants augmented the oxidation-dependent killing of fungal cells induced by amphotericin B.

> —J. Brajtburg, et al., "Effects of Ascorbic Acid on the Antifungal Action of Amphotericin B," *Journal of Antimicrobial Chemotherapy*, 24(3), September 1989, p. 333-337.

Cancer

This review article notes that approximately 90 studies have been done on the role of vitamin C in cancer prevention, with most finding statistically significant effects. Protective effects have been shown for cancers of the pancreas, oral cavity, stomach, esophagus, cervix, rectum, breast, and lung.

> —G. Block, et al., "Epidemiologic Evidence Regarding Vitamin C and Cancer," *American Journal of Clinical Nutrition*, 54(6 Suppl), December 1991, p. 1310S-1314S.

Daily supplementation of 1 g of vitamin C decreased the amount of chromosome damage induced in lymphocytes by an exposure to bleomycin during the last 5 h of cell culture. The authors suggest a similar assay for genetic instability might be helpful in detecting heterozygotes for chromosome-breakage syndromes and recommend considering dietary and lifestyle factors when interpreting results from this bleomycin assay and related assays for genetic instability.

—H. Pohl and J.A. Reidy, ''Vitamin C Intake Influences the Bleomycin-induced Chromosome Damage Assay: Implications for Detection of Cancer Susceptibility and Chromosome Breakage Syndromes,'' *Mutat Research,* 224(2), October 1989, p. 247-252.

A ternary antioxidant vitamin mix consisting of ascorbic acid, alpha-tocopherol and lecithin as well as a rosemary extract with carnosic acid and carnosol as the two major active ingredients were shown to exhibit strong antimutagenic effects in Ames tester strain TA102. Ascorbic acid was held responsible for this inhibitory property in the vitamin mix, while carnosic acid was identified as the antimutagenic agent in the rosemary extract. The authors conclude that these antioxidants might exhibit anticarcinogenic properties.

—M. Minnunni, et al., ''Natural Antioxidants as Inhibitors of Oxygen Species Induced Mutagenicity,'' *Mutat Research,* 269(2), October 1992, p. 193-200.

A mixture of ascorbic acid and cupric sulfate significantly inhibited human mammary tumor growth in mice when administered orally, while the administration of either alone did not. The activity of D-isoascorbic acid was similar to that of ascorbic acid. The authors suggest ascorbic acid's antitumor activity was due to its chemical properties rather than the metabolism of ascorbic acid as a vitamin.

—C.S. Tsao, ''Inhibiting Effect of Ascorbic Acid on the Growth of Human Mammary Tumor Xenografts,'' *American Journal of Clinical Nutrition,* 54(6 Suppl), December 1991, p. 1274S-1280S.

In this study, vitamin C was shown to decrease kidney tumor incidence by approximately 50% in Syrian hamsters, lower the concentration of diethylstilbestrol-4',4"-quinone, the genotoxic metabolite of diethylstilbestrol, in vitro and in hamsters treated with stilbene, and decreases the levels in hamsters of DES-DNA adducts formed by the quinone metabolite. Noting that estrogens may spawn tumors by their metabolic oxidation to corresponding quionone metabolites, the authors argue that vitamin C may inhibit the formation of tumors by decreasing concentrations of quinone metabolites and their DNA adducts.

—J.G. Liehr, ''Vitamin C Reduces the Incidence and Severity of Renal Tumors Induced by Estradiol or Diethylstilbestrol,'' *American Journal of Clinical Nutrition,* 54(6 Suppl), December 1991, p. 1256S-1260S.

This paper reports on the results of two large-scale studies of L-ascorbic acid in the food on tumor-free survival in mice. The first found that increasing ascorbic acid in the diet significantly delayed the development of spontaneous mammary tumors, with the median age at first tumor at 124.9 weeks in the highest-dose ascorbate group and 82.5 wk in ad libitum controls. The proportion of mice with tumors was also reduced. The second discovered a significant effect of ascorbate in delaying the onset and reducing the incidence of malignant lesions. Approximately five times the number of mice developed lesions in the zero-ascorbate as in the high-ascorbate group after 20 weeks of administration.

—L. Pauling, ''Effect of Ascorbic Acid on Incidence of Spontaneous Mammary Tumors and UV-Light-Induced Skin Tumors in Mice,'' *American Journal of Clinical Nutrition,* 54(6 Suppl), December 1991, p. 1252S-1255S.

Ascorbate stabilizes the normal state of the avian tendon cell by reducing Rous sarcoma virus production and promoting the synthesis of differentiated proteins which allows the virus to coexist within the cell rather than completely take it over.

> —R.I. Schwarz, "Ascorbate Stabilizes the Differentiated State and Reduces the Ability of Rous Sarcoma Virus to Replicate and to Uniformly Transform Cell Cultures," *American Journal of Clinical Nutrition,* 54(6 Suppl), December 1991, p. 1247S-1251S.

Noting theories that ascorbic acid might lower the risk of gastric cancer by preventing their formation within gastric juice, the authors measured both gastric juice ascorbic and total vitamin C in subjects and found that ascorbic acid is secreted into the gastric lumen so that gastric juices are frequently higher than concentrations in plasma. Gastric pathology affects this secretion, leading to values in gastric juice that are lower than plasma levels.

> —C.J. Schorah, et al., "Gastric Juice Ascorbic Acid: Effects of Disease and Implications for Gastric Carcinogenesis," *American Journal of Clinical Nutrition,* 53(1 Suppl), January 1991, p. 287S-293S.

This case-control study evaluated the association between specific substances of the diet and invasive cervical cancer in four Latin American countries. Vitamin C was shown to significantly decrease the risk of invasive cervical cancer, as was the case with beta-carotene and other carotenoids. These results are consistent with those from other studies suggesting a protective role for vitamin C in the development of invasive cervical cancer.

> —R. Herrero, et al., "A Case-Control Study of Nutrient Status and Invasive Cervical Cancer: I. Dietary Indicators," *American Journal of Epidemiology,* 134(11), December 1, 1991, p. 1335-1346.

2,974 men participating in the third examination of the prospective Basel Study in 1971-1973 were measured for plasma antioxidant vitamins A, C, and E, and carotene. Low mean plasma levels of carotene adjusted for cholesterol and of vitamin C was associated with overall mortality from cancer. Lower mean vitamin C levels were found to increase the risks of stomach cancer and gastrointestinal cancer in older subjects. In light of these results for vitamin C, in combination with those of the other vitamins studied, the authors conclude that low levels of antioxidants are associated with an increased risk of mortality from numerous cancers.

> —H.B. Stahelin, et al., "Plasma Antioxidant Vitamins and Subsequent Cancer Mortality in the 12-year Follow-up of the Prospective Basel Study," *American Journal of Epidemiology,* 133(8), April 15, 1991, p. 766-775.

Inverse relationships were found between intake of carotenoids, vitamin E, and vitamin C and the incidence of lung cancer among nonsmokers in a 20 year follow-up study of 4,538 initially cancer-free Finnish men. The authors suggest that increased intake of these nutrients may protect against the development of lung cancer among nonsmokers.

> —P. Knekt, et al., "Dietary Antioxidants and the Risk of Lung Cancer," *American Journal of Epidemiology,* 134(5), September 1, 1991, p. 471-479.

NAC administered in doses from 0.1 to 10 mmol/L reduced the number of mutagenic-induced breaks per cell in a range from 23% to 73%. In a dose range from 0.01 to 1 mmol/L, ascorbic acid reduced chromosomal breakage by 21% to 58%. These results illustrate NAC and ascorbic acid's protective effects mediated in vitro against mutagen induced chromosomal damage. The difference in occurrence of head and neck cancer between population with varying diets may be explained by related in vivo phenomenon.

> —Z. Trizna, et al., "Effects of N-acetyl-L-cysteine and Ascorbic Acid on Mutagen-induced Chromosomal Sensitivity in Patients with Head and Neck Cancers," *American Journal of Surgery* 162(4), October 1991, p. 294-298.

Results of this placebo-controlled study found that powdered chow supplemented with 7%/wt ascorbic acid significantly reduced 1,2-dimethylhydrazine-induced tumor formation significantly in rats.

> —T.A. Colacchio and V.A. Memoli, "Chemoprevention of Colorectal Neoplasms: Ascorbic Acid and Beta-Carotene," *Arch Surg* (1986 Dec) 121(12), December 1986, p. 1421-1444.

158 samples from 139 lung-cancer patients were examined with respect to levels of plasma and buffy-coat vitamin C. Diet dependent hypovitaminosis C tended to be present in the majority of samples and proved capable of being increased by oral supplementation. Assays demonstrated that tumors had a greater vitamin C content that normal lung tissue.

> —H.M. Anthony and C.J. Schorah, "Severe Hypovitaminosis C in Lung-Cancer Patients: The Utilization of Vitamin C in Surgical Repair and Lymphocyte-Related Host Resistance," *British Journal of Cancer,* 46(3), September 1982, p. 354-367.

Beta carotene and ascorbic acid were shown to persistently protect against colorectal cancer in this case-controlled study of 828 patients with colon cancer and 498 patients with rectal cancer in Northern Italy.

> —M. Ferraroni, et al., "Selected Micronutrient Intake and the Risk of Colorectal Cancer," *British Journal of Cancer,* 70(6), December 1994, p. 1150-1155.

Vitamin C supplement use was shown to be inversely related to bladder and colon cancer in women in an 8 year follow-up study beginning in 1981 of 11,580 residents of a retirement community initially free from cancer.

> —A. Shibata, et al., "Intake of Vegetables, Fruits, Beta-Carotene, Vitamin C and Vitamin Supplements and Cancer Incidence Among the Elderly: A Prospective Study," *British Journal of Cancer* (1992 Oct) 66(4), October 1992, p. 673-679.

This double-blind, placebo-controlled study examined the relationship between ascorbic acid and large bowel adenomas. 3 g/day of ascorbic acid reduced polyp area in the treatment group at nine months of follow-up and resulted in a trend toward the decrease in both area and number of rectal polyps midway through the trial.

> —H.J. Bussey, et al., "A Randomized Trial of Ascorbic Acid in Polyposis Coli," *Cancer,* 50(7), October 1, 1982, p. 1434-1439.

Human neoplastic cell lines MCF-7 (breast carcinoma), KB (oral epidermal carcinoma), and AN3-CA (endometrial adenocarcinoma) were studied relative to the effects of in vivo administration either in combination or alone of sodium ascorbate (vitamin C) and 2-methyl-1,4-napthoquinone (vitamin K3). When administered separately, vitamin C or K3 showed a growth inhibiting effect but only at high concentrations (5.10(3) mumol/1 and 10(5) nmol/l, respectively). When administered in combination both vitamins showed a synergistic inhibition of cell growth at 10 to 50 times lower concentrations.

The addition of catalase to the culture medium containing vitamins C and K3 totally suppressed this tumor cell growth inhibitory effect. The authors argue this suggests an excessive production of hydrogen peroxide as being implied in mechanisms responsible for the tumor cell growth inhibitory effects.

> —V. Noto, et al., "Effects of Sodium Ascorbate (Vitamin C) and 2-methyl-1,4-Naphthoquinone (Vitamin K3) Treatment on Human Tumor Cell Growth in Vitro. I. Synergism of Combined Vitamin C and K3 Action," *Cancer,* 63(5), March 1, 1989, p. 901-906.

In this hospital based, case-control study of lung cancer, a strong protective effect for squamous and small cell carcinoma was associated with dietary vitamin C intake based on data obtained from food frequency questionnaires

> —E.T. Fontham, et al., "Dietary Vitamins A and C and Lung Cancer Risk in Louisiana," *Cancer,* 62(10), November 15, 1988, p. 2267-2273.

The effects of 6-hydroxydopamine (6-OHDA) and H2O2 on metabolic parameters critical for cell survival were examined in cells with low and high ferritin content in the presence and absence of ascorbate in this study. Human neuroblastoma SK-N-SH cells were pretreated with 100 microM FeSO4 and 10 microM desferrioxamine, respectively, for 24 hours yielding cells with different ferritin contents. The most pronounced effects were in ferritin-rich cells and in the presence of ascorbic acid. Using isolated CCC PM2 DNA, 6-OHDA and ascorbic acid caused strand breaks that were prevented in the presence of mannitol or desferrithiocine. H2O2-mediated strand breaks were observed only in the presence of ascorbic acid. The authors suggest their data along with the results of previous studies suggests that high dosages of ascorbic acid continuously applied may be an effective new approach in neuroblastoma therapy.

> —G. Bruchelt, et al., "Ascorbic Acid Enhances the Effects of 6-Hydroxydopamine and H2O2 on Iron-Dependent DNA Strand Breaks and Related Processes in the Neuroblastoma Cell Line SK-N-SH," *Cancer Research,* 51(22), November 15, 1991, p. 6066-6072.

In this study, mice were fed one of three diets both with and without sodium ascorbate (30 mg/ml) in the drinking water starting 2 weeks before inoculation of 10(6) melanoma cells. Mice fed the purified diet experienced inhibited tumor growth in some cases, while it had no effect on others in the commercial diet group, ascorbate stimulated tumor growth. In mice fed the deficient diet, ascorbate inhibited tumor growth and survival was increased by 82%. Unlike mice fed the commercial diet, drug treatment reduced growth significantly in mice fed the purified diet and moderately increased their survival. Drug activity was enhanced and the survival of tumor-bearing mice increased by 73% as well in the deficient diet group. Drug and ascorbate therapy combined resulted in mice fed the purified diet experiencing smaller tumors and living 55% longer than controls. Deficient diet fed mice who were administered the same combination experienced slowed tumor growth and their survival time was increased 123%.

> —H.F. Pierson and G.G. Meadows, "Sodium Ascorbate Enhancement OF Carbidopa-Leveodopa Methyl Ester Antitumor Activity Against Pigmented B16 Melanoma," *Cancer Res,* 43(5), 1983, p. 2047-2051.

This study involving patients with acute nonlymphocytic leukemia found that the numbers of leukemic bone marrow cell colonies grown in culture were decreased 21% of control in 7/28 patients by adding 0.3 milliM of L-ascorbic acid to the culture medium. Concentrations of L-ascorbic acid as low as 0.1 milliM was capable of suppressing the leukemic cell colony in cultures of both leukemic and normal marrow cells. However, 1 milliM of L-ascorbic acid was required for suppression of normal myeloid colonies. Based on their results, the authors argue that the achieved suppression was a specific effect of L-ascorbic acid and was not due to its oxidation-reduction potential or pH change since normal hemopoietic cells were not suppressed while leukemic cells were selectively affected at an L-ascorbic acid concentration attainable in vivo.

—C.H. Park, et al., "Growth Suppression of Human Leukemic Cells in Vitro by L-Ascorbic Acid," *Cancer Research,* 40(4), 1980, p. 1062-1065.

This in vitro study on the effects of L-ascorbic acid (LAA) on the growth of human leukemic colony-forming cells (L-CFC) demonstrated that L-CFC growth suppression by LAA is observed in one-sixth of leukemic patients, L-CFC enhancement in one-third of patients, and that L-CFC growth enhancement is a significant discovery with a biological mechanism as the basis.

—C.H. Park, "Biological Nature of the Effect of Ascorbic Acids on the Growth of Human Leukemic Cells," *Cancer Research,* 45(8), August 1985, p. 3969-3973.

81 patients with premalignant lesions of the oral cavity were given 30 mg of beta-carotene, 1000 mg of ascorbic acid, and 800 IU of alpha tocopherol daily for nine months. 55.6% experienced either complete or partial clinical resolution of their lesions. Based on these findings, the authors recommend the use of antioxidant supplements as a treatment for oral premalignant lesions.

—G. Kaugars, et al., "Serum and Tissue Antioxidant Levels in Supplemented Patients With Premalignant Oral Lesions (Meeting abstract)," *FASEB Journal,* 7(4), 1993, A519.

This study examined levels of vitamin C and ascorbic acid in the gastric juice of 77 patients suffering from dyspepsia. Gastric concentrations of vitamin C and ascorbic acid were significantly lower in chronic gastritis patients and patients with hypochlorhydia were found to have particularly low levels of ascorbic acid concentrations.

—G.M. Sobala, et al., "Ascorbic Acid in the Human Stomach," *Gastroenterology,* 97(2), August 1989, p. 357-363.

In this placebo-controlled study, vitamin supplementation was examined in relation to its effects on cell kinetics in uninvolved rectal mucosa patients with colorectal adenomas. Vitamins A, C, and E were administered to twenty subjects 6 months after complete polypectomy. Results indicate that supplementation was successful in reducing abnormalities in cell kinetics that may indicate a precancerous condition.

—G.M. Paganelli, et al., "Effect of Vitamin A, C, and E Supplementation on Rectal Cell Proliferation in Patients with Colorectal Adenomas," *Journal of the National Cancer Institute,* 84(1), January 1, 1992, p. 47-51.

In this case-control study of 117 in situ cervical patients, plasma vitamin C was found to reduce the risk of cancer by 60%.

—K.E. Brock, et al., "Nutrients in Diet and Plasma and Risk of in Situ Cervical Cancer," *Journal of the National Cancer Institute,* 80(8), June 15, 1988, p. 580-585.

This case-control study of 419 colon and rectal cancer patients found that dietary vitamin C intake resulted in reduced risk of rectal cancer in women.

—J.D. Potter and A.J. McMichael, "Diet and Cancer of the Colon and Rectum: A Case-Control Study," *Journal of the National Cancer Institute,* 76(4), April 1986, p. 557-569.

Noting that the use of ascorbate to treat cancer began in 1971, this case-control study involved over 300 patients with cancer who received 2.5 g of vitamin C four times a day in combination with standard surgical treatment and radiotherapy (a few cases of chemotherapy). Of 266 patients with incurable cancer were found to benefit significantly from the vitamin C therapy was shown to have significant benefits for those suffering from cancer of the stomach and colon, while there was a similar trend for those with cancer of the bladder. Based on their results, the authors conclude that ascorbate in high doses can improve survival in certain types of cancer.

> —L. Moffat, et al., "High Dose Ascorbate Therapy and Cancer," *NFCR Cancer Research Association Symposium,* (2), 1983, p. 243-256.

This study found that large amounts of vitamin C administered in drinking water reduced benzo(a)pyrene (BP) induced tumors in mice, resulting in an extended survival time for those animals exposed to the carcinogen.

> —G. Kallistratos, et al., "The Prophylactic and Therapeutic Effect of Vitamin C on Experimental Malignant Tumors," *NFCR Cancer Research Association Symposium,* (2), 1983, p. 221-242.

This review article on the effects of vitamins A, C, E, and selenium on cancer cites research pointing to ascorbic acid's ability to prevent formation of nitrosamine and other N-nitroso compounds. Studies also show supplementation with vitamin C can inhibit skin, nose, kidney, lung and tracheal cancer.

> —D.F. Birt, "Update on the Effects of Vitamins A, C, and E and Selenium on Carcinogenesis," *Proc Soc Exp Biol Med,* 183(3), December 1986, p. 311-320.

The administration of ascorbic acid (0.1-20 micrograms/ml for the first week) was found to suppress x-ray induced transformation of C3H10T1/2 cells in a concentration-dependent manner after irradiation.Cells initiated by radiation remained vulnerable to ascorbic acid up until the moment of morphological phenotype expression. Based on these findings, the authors postulate that expression of the neoplastically transformed phenotype is promoted by reactive oxygen species and peroxy radicals generated in cells during the whole assay period and they suggest their data might be helpful as a guide for chemopreventive efforts against radiation carcinogenesis.

> —M. Yasukawa, et al., "Radiation-induced Neoplastic Transformation of C3H10T1/2 Cells is Suppressed by Ascorbic Acid," *Radiation Research,* 120(3), December 1989, p. 456-467.

This study found that pretreatment of tumor target cells in vitro with a combination of interferon and ascorbate resulted in a 71% increase in growth inhibition of target cells compared to inhibition with interferon by itself. Administration of ascorbate alone showed minimal effect on tumor target cell growth in human monocytes.

> —M.J. Skeen, et al., "Synergy of Interferon and Ascorbic Acid in Stimulating Human Monocyte Cytostasis Against Tumor Target Cells," *Rev Latinoam Oncology Clin,* 13(4), 1981, p. 9-14.

This study found that a 4 mg/kg body wt/week dose of cisplatin supplemented with a 200 mg/alternated day dose of vitamin E and a 200 mg/day dose of vitamin C given to rats increased cisplatin's therapeutic potential in the treatment of oral cancer compared to the administration of cisplatin alone.

> —D.K. Sharma, "Amylase Activity of the Malignant Rat Salivary Gland after Cisplatin,

Vitamin E and C Treatment,'' *Third International Congress on Engineered Oral Cancer,* January 22-25, 1994, Madras, India, 1994.

Vitamin C (35 mg/kg) ingestion has been shown to result in a reduction in DNA single strand breaks induced by ionizing radiation in human lymphocytes, as indicated by a significant decrease in overall comet length in both unirradiated control and the dose response to ionizing radiation damage. The effect was found to persist for up to six hours.
    —C.F. Arlett, et al., ''The Modulation of DNA damage in Human Lymphocytes by Dietary Vitamin C Supplementation,'' *Molecular Mechanisms in Radiation Mutagenesis and Carcinogenesis.* April 19-22, 1993, Doorwerth, The Netherlands.

Patients with oral leukoplakia were administered 30 mg of beta-carotene, 1000 mg of ascorbic acid, and 800 IU of alpha-tocopherol per day for 9 months. 55.6% of the 81 patients who completed the study showed either partial or complete clinical resolution of their oral lesions.
    —G. Kaugars, et al., ''The Role of Antioxidants in the Treatment of Oral Leukoplakia,'' *CCPC-93: Second International Cancer Chemo Prevention Conference,* April 28-30, 1993, Berlin, Germany, p. 65

24 lung cancer and 35 bladder cancer patients were treated with doses of 5 g/day of ascorbic acid. Results suggest that such high doses are useful in correcting low haematic levels of vitamin C and in increasing the defense reactions in patients suffering from these types of cancer.
    —A.M. Greco, et al., ''Study of Blood Vitamin C in Lung and Bladder Cancer Patients Before and After Treatment with Ascorbic Acid: A Preliminary Report,'' *Acta Vitaminol Enzymol,* 4(1-2), 1982, p. 155-162.

This review article points out that vitamin C's role in preventing cancer has been discussed in the literature for over fifty years and cites studies which suggest that foods rich in vitamin C are associated with lower risks of stomach cancer and cancer of the esophagus. Ascorbic acid had been demonstrated to interact with a number of tumor-inducing compounds, such as precursors of N-nitroso compounds to prevent tumors. Animal and in vivo studies have also shown ascorbic acid disrupts tumor promotion. Based on a review of the existing evidence, the authors conclude that vitamin C can inhibit the formation of some types of cancer.
    —B.E. Glatthaar, et al., ''The Role of Ascorbic Acid in Carcinogenesis,'' *Adv Exp Med Biol,* 206, 1986, p. 357-377.

The administration of flavone, quercetin and fisetin either alone, or in combination with ascorbic acid, were studied for their effects on the growth of a human squamous cell carcinoma cell line (HTB 43) in vitro. When combined with ascorbic acid (2 micrograms/ml), fisetin and quercetin (2 micrograms/ml of either) impaired cell growth in 72 hours significantly. Ascorbic acid administered alone had no effect, nor did it when in combination with flavone.
    —C. Kandaswami, et al., ''Ascorbic Acid-enhanced Antiproliferative Effect of Flavonoids on Squamous Cell Carcinoma in Vitro,'' *Anticancer Drugs,* 4(1), February 1993, p. 91-96.

This review article on the relationship between vitamin C, vitamin E, and cancer cites studies which suggest that the consumption of foods containing vitamin C is related to a reduced risk of esophageal and stomach cancer. Supplementation with vitamin C has been shown to inhibit nerve, lung, kidney and skin cancer. Studies have also shown vitamin C is capable of inhibiting tumor cell growth and carcinogen-induced DNA damage. In vitro and animals studies have demonstrated that vitamin C inhibits the formation of carcinogenic nitrosamines.

> —L.H. Chen, et al., "Vitamin C, Vitamin E and Cancer," *Anticancer Research,* 8(4), July-August 1988, p. 739-748.

Previous research has shown ascorbic acid to be cytotoxic to neuroblastoma cells in vitro and in vivo. In this study, ascorbic acid proved to be more cytotoxic than dehydroascorbic acid in neuroblastoma SK-N-SH cells. It was also discovered that uptake of [14C] ascorbic acid and [14C] dehydroascorbic acid was impaired by gluthathione and diethiothreitol. [14C] Dehydroascorbic acid was partially reduced to [14C] ascorbic acid once inside the cell. The authors argue that their results add support to previous beliefs that ascorbic acid acts as a pro-oxidant inside neuroblastoma cells and they recommend the use of ascorbic acid in treating neurobastoma.

> —S.L. Baader, et al., "Uptake and Cytotoxicity of Ascorbic Acid and Dehydroascorbic Acid in Neuroblastoma (SK-N-SH) and Neuroectodermal (SK-N-LO) Cells," *Anticancer,* 14(1A), January-February 1994, p. 221-227.

L-ascorbate and its oxidative product dehydroascorbate have been shown to be lethal or cytoxic to fast-growing malignant cells while being less toxic to nonmalignant cells. Similar effects were seen with D-ascorbate and D-isoascorbate. Additional studies on the viability of treated cells have found that the effect on cell growth was a result of ascorbate's direct killing action rather than being cytostatic in nature.

> —P.Y. Leung, et al., "Cytotoxic Effect of Ascorbate and its Derivatives on Cultured Malignant and Nonmalignant Cell Lines," *Anticancer Research,* 13(2), March-April 1993, p. 475-480.

Sodium benzylideneascorbate (SBA) dose dependently induced degeneration of 3'-methly-4-dimethy-lamioazobenzene-induced hepatocellular carcinoma in rats. At the same time, it did not significantly induce fibrosis in the liver, lymphocyte infiltration, nor damage the gross morphology of spleen and kidney cells. The authors suggest such findings may point to an antitumor action of SBA by way of induction of apoptosis in the tumor.

> —H. Sakagami, et al., "Effect of Sodium Benzylideneascorbate on Chemically-Induced Tumors in Rats," *Anticancer Research,* 13(1), January-February 1993, p. 65-71.

This long-term study found that ascorbic acid (administered via drinking water) resulted in the suppression of gastric tumor development in rats.

> —S. Dittrich, et al., [Effects of Nitrate and Ascorbic Acid on Carcinogenesis in the Operated Rat Stomach], *Arch Geschwulstforsch,* 58(4), 1988, p. 235-242.

Noting the radioprotective effect of ascorbic acid patients with head and neck cancer, this paper recommends the oral administration of ascorbic acid for patients suffering from these conditions.

> —R. Garcia-Alejo Hernandez, et al., [Radioprotective Effect of Ascorbic Acid on Oral Structures in Patients with Cancer of the Head and Neck], *Av Odontoestomatol,* 5(7), September 1989, p. 469-472.

This study found that doses of 2mM of ascorbic acid had a strong cytotoxic effect on neuroblastoma, osteosarcoma, rhabdomyosarcoma and reinoblastoma cells cultured in vitro. Ascorbic acid administered at 0.2 2mM continue to be cytotoxic for neuroblastoma, osteosarcoma and retinoblastoma cells, but stimulates the growth of rhabdomyosarcoma cells.

  —M.A. Medina, et al., "Ascorbic Acid is Cytotoxic for Pediatric Tumor Cells Cultured in Vitro," *Biochem Mol Biol Int,* 34(5), November 1994, p. 871-874.

The administration of parahydroxyphenyllactic acid (5 mg, sc 2x/wk) in combination with ascorbic acid (250 mg/100 ml in drinking water) increased the latent period of tumor development in C57BL mice exposed to tyroxine metabolites. Animals administered the same dose of parahydrophenyllactic acid without ascorbic acid developed bladder precancer and experienced no antitumor effects.

  —N.A. Khar'kovskaia, et al., [Effect of Ascorbic Acid on the Carcinogenic Activity of P-Hydroxyphenyllactic Acid], *Bull Eksp Biol Med,* 92(1), 1982, p. 64-66.

10 micrograms/ml of L-ascorbic acid increased alkaline phosphatase activity in the osteoblast-like rat osteosarcoma cell line, UMR-106, 6 hours after the addition of 100 micrograms/ml of ascorbic acid to the medium. The response of cAMP to both PTH and PGE1 was potentiated by 100 micrograms/ml ascorbic acid treatment of the cells. The increasing concentrations of ascorbic acid also inhibited cell growth, and significantly reduced the number of colonies formed by the cell grown in soft agar. Such results suggest the differentiation of osteoblasts may be effected by the presence of ascorbic acid.

  —T. Sugimoto, et al., "Effects of Ascorbic Acid on Alkaline Phosphatase Activity and Hormone Responsiveness in the Osteoblastic Osteosarcoma Cell Line UMR-106," *Calcif Tissue Int,* 39(3), September 1986, p. 171-174.

This study examined the relationship between hyperthermia and ascorbic acid on DNA synthesis in Ehrlich ascites tumor cells. When 75 microM of ascorbic acid was administered to cells at a low density of 5 x 10(3)/ml for 1 hour, DNA synthesis was inhibited at 37 degrees C. Treatment at 42% degrees significantly enhanced the inhibition. In the absence of ascorbic acid, DNA synthesis failed to be inhibited. Treatment with 75 microM ascorbic acid and hyperthermia at 42 degrees C in cells transplanted into mice also prolonged the survival time relative to untreated cells. Based on these findings, the authors recommend the ascorbic acid and hyperthermia be considered for the treatment of cancer.

  —K. Kageyama, et al., "Enhanced Inhibitory Effects of Hyperthermia Combined with Ascorbic Acid on DNA synthesis in Ehrlich Ascites Tumor cells Grown at a Low cell Density," *Cancer Biochem Biophys,* 14(4), January 1995, p. 273-280.

In this case-control study of 723 gastric cancer patients, significant protective effects were found between ascorbic acid and the risk of developing the disease.

  —C. La Vecchia, et al., "Selected Micronutrient Intake and the Risk of Gastric Cancer," *Cancer Epidemiol Biomarkers Prevention,* 3(5), July-August 1994, p. 393-398.

An inverse association was found between dietary vitamin C and cervical intraepithelial neoplasia (CIN) in this case-control study of biopsy confirmed CIN patients.

  —J. VanEenwyk, et al., "Folate, Vitamin C, and Cervical Intraepithelial Neoplasia," *Cancer Epidemiol Biomarkers Prevention,* 1(2), January-February 1992, p. 119-124.

In examining the effects of ascorbic acid on in vitro multiplication of ascites tumor cells (ATP C+), of fibroblast-like cells and hepatocytes from chick embryos, the authors found that ATP C+ cells were the most vulnerable to ascorbic acid's toxic effects and hepatocytes the least. Catalase greatly decreased the damage ATP C+ cells suffered from exposure to ascorbic acid. These findings led the authors to propose that the inhibition of cell multiplication by ascorbic acid is the result of the H202 formed by its oxidation and that those cells most resistant to its toxic effects have the greatest amount of catalase.

    —F.S. Liotti, et al., "Antagonism Between Catalase and Ascorbic Acid in Control of Normal and Neoplastic Cell Multiplication," *Cancer Letters,* 33(1), October 1986, p. 99-106.

This study examined the effects of nitric oxided and ascorbate on the control human brain tumor cells. Results indicated that combining nitroprusside and ascorbate may be an effective approach for treating brain tumors.

    —Y.S. Lee and R.D. Wurster, "Potentiation of Anti-Proliferative Effect of Nitroprusside by Ascorbate in Human Brain Tumor Cells," *Cancer Letters,* 78(1-3), April 1, 1994, p. 19-23.

This study found that daily doses of 2 mg/ml of ascorbic acid administered over a period of 16 weeks significantly inhibited cervical cancer induced by methythlcholanthrene in mice.

    —P. Das, et al., "Influence of Ascorbic Acid on MCA-induced Carcinogenesis in the Uterine Cervix of Mice," *Cancer Letters,* 72(1-2), August 16, 1993, p. 121-125.

This study found that the cytotoxic effects of ascorbic acid on two sensitive lymphocyte tumor and cell lines were time and dose dependent. The authors suggest that the existence of lymphocyte lines with differing sensitivities to ascorbic acid might be considered a useful model in the study of vitamin C's action on cancer cells.

    —T.L. Kao, et al., "Inhibitory Effects of Ascorbic Acid on Growth of Leukemic and Lymphoma Cell Lines," *Cancer Letters,* 70(1-2), June 15, 1993, p. 101-106.

Noting that DES or estradiol-treated male Syrian hamsters supplemented with vitamin C have been shown to inhibit renal carcinogenesis, the effects of administered vitamin C on a series of biochemical markers of kidney carcinogenesis was studied. Results indicate that vitamin C inhibits estrogen-induced carcinogenesis by decreasing concentrations of estrogen quinone metabolites and their DNA adducts.

    —J.G. Liehr, et al., "Mechanism of Inhibition of Estrogen-Induced Renal Carcinogenesis in Male Syrian Hamsters by Vitamin C," *Carcinogenesis,* 10(11), November 1989, p. 1983-1988.

43 patients were treated with oral supplementation of vitamin C. Treatment with vitamin C in patients with normal gastric mucosa resulted in elevation of intragastric ascorbate levels in all cases. Vitamin C supplementation decreased gastric mucosal DNA damage in 28 or the 43 patients which suggests that it may provide a protective role against the onset of gastric cancer.

    —G.W. Dyke, et al., "Effect of Vitamin C Supplementation on Gastric Mucosal DNA Damage," *Carcinogenesis,* 15(2), p. 291-295.

Noting that chromium metal salts are thought to be human carcinogens, and that lead chromate has been shown to be tumorigenic, genotoxic and clastogenic; this study demonstrated that a nontoxic dose of vitamin C blocked uptake of ionic chromium and eliminated the clastogenic activity of particles in cells treated with lead chromate particles.

—J.P. Wise, et al., "Inhibition of Lead Chromate Clastogenesis by Ascorbate: Relationship to Particle Dissolution and Uptake," *Carcinogenesis,* 14(3), March 1993, p. 429-434.

This study found a positive relationship between human exposure to nitrosamines and the risk of esophageal cancer mortality. Vitamin C reduced the amount of gastric N-nitroxamines in the stomach and thus may be considered of potential value in the prevention of esophageal cancer.

—W.X. Yang, [Exposure Level of N-nitrosamines in the Gastric Juice and its Inhibition by Vitamin C in High Risk Areas of Esophageal Cancer], *Chung Hua Chung Liu Tsa Chih,* 14(6), November 1992, p. 407-410.

This study found vitamin C to have a distinct inhibitory effect on the mutational specificity of 6 antineoplastic drugs. Such results, the authors argue, are significant with respect to the clinical prevention of tumors.

—Z.Z. Zhao and M.T. Huang, [A Study of Vitamin Inhibition on the Mutagenicity of the Antineoplastic Drugs], *Chung Hua Yu Fang I Hsueh Tsa Chih,* 26(5), September 1992, p. 291-293.

Rats fed a diet including vitamins A, C, E, and selenium compounds followed by aflatoxin B treatment for a period of 24 months remained free of cancer whereas the majority of controls not fed the vitamins developed liver during the same period. Based on these results, the authors suggest liver cancer can be inhibited with the intake of vitamins by inducing hepatic microsomal enzyme that metabolize aflatoxins to noncarcinogenic products.

—H.S. Nyandieka and J. Wakhisis, "The Impact of Vitamins A,C,E, and Selenium Compound on Prevention of Liver Cancer in Rats," *East African Medical Journal,* 70(3), March 1993, p. 151-153.

This study found that ascorbic administered in drinking water (0.3%) inhibited the promoting effect of estradiol dipropionate on the 1,2-dimthylhydrazine-induced uterine sarcogenesis in CBA mice.

—L.S. Trukhanova, [Modifying Effect of Ascorbic Acid and Sodium Ascorbate on Uterine Carcomogenesis Induced by 1,2-dimethylhydrazine in CBA Mice], *Eksp Onkol,* 10(5), 1988, p. 65-66.

This study found that ascorbic acid intake affects in vivo N-ethyl-N-nitrosourea (ENU) mutagenicity in rats. The authors suggest that previously reported antioxidant inhibitory effects on carcinogenesis could be partially mediated by its effects on mutagenesis.

—A. Aidoo, et al., "Ascorbic Acid (vitamin C) Modulates the Mutagenic Effects Produced by an Alkylating Agent in Vivo," *Environ Mol Mutagen,* 24(3), 1994, p. 220-228.

This case-control, population-based study found vitamin C intake, attenuated by age, level of education, and lifetime cigarette use, offers protective effects against developing cervical cancer.

—M.L. Slattery, et al., "Dietary Vitamins A, C, and E and Selenium as Risk Factors for Cervical Cancer," *Epidemiology,* 1(1), January 1990, p. 8-15.

This paper reports the discovery of a new malignant human T-cell line-labeled PFI-285 in a boy with malignant lymphoma. One of the striking characteristics of this new T-cell line was its sensitivity to ascorbic acid, evidence by the fact that concentrations as low as 50 mumuol/l resulted in cell death within hours.

—J. Helgestad, et al., "Characterization of a New Malignant Human T-cell Line (PFI-285) Sensitive to Ascorbic Acid," *European Journal of Haematology,* 44(1), January 1990, p. 9-17.

This study found that oral administration of vitamin C can retard the onset of N-nitrosodiethylamine induced liver cancer in rats.

—H. Kessler, et al., "Potential Protective Effect of Vitamin C on Carcinogenesis Caused by Nitrosamine in Drinking Water: An Experimental Study on Wistar Rats," *European Journal of Surgery and Oncology,* 18(3), June 1992, p. 275-281.

The survival rate of mice bearing P388 leukemia and Ehrlich carcinoma was increased after treatment with a mixture of vitamins C and B12. All the mice receiving the vitamins outlived the control group. At the termination of the experiment 30 days later, 50% of the treated mice appeared normal and healthy, whereas the remainder showed signs of tumor distention.

—M.E. Poydock, et al., "Influence of Vitamins C and B12 on the Survival Rate of Mice Bearing Ascites Tumor," *Exp Cell Biol,* 50(2), 1982, p. 88-91.

This study found that a daily dose of 50 mg/kg of vitamin C in combination with methylcholanthrene (MCA) over 9 months significantly reduced MCA-induced squamous cell carcinomas in mice and basal cell carcinomas in rats over a period of nine months. The authors conclude that vitamin C's antineoplastic effects are the result of increasing autophagic and cytolytic activity, increased collagen synthesis, and cell membrane disruption.

—A. Lupulescu, "Ultrastructure and Cell Surface Studies of Cancer Cells Following Vitamin C Administration," *Exp Toxicol Pathol,* 44(1), March 1992, p. 3-9.

This study found that vitamin C reduced the incidence of DMBA induced epithelial tumor in the hamster cheek pouch.

—P.D. Potdar, et al., "Modulation by Vitamin C of Tumor Incidence and Inhibition in Oral Carcinogenesis," *Funct Dev Morphol,* 2(3), 1992, p. 167-172.

Previous studies have found that nitrosation can be decreased by the administration of ascorbic acid in vivo and that vitamin C rich foods are inversely related to gastric cancer. This study treated 62 high-risk patients for gastric cancer with 1 g of ascorbic acid taken 4 times a day for four weeks. Results found that ascorbic acid given in high doses can reduce the intragastric formation of nitrite and N-nitroso compounds.

—P.I. Reed, et al., "Effect of Ascorbic Acid on the Intragastric Environment in Patients at Increased Risk of Developing Gastric Cancer," *IARC Sci Publ,* (105), 1991, p.139-142.

1000 mg/kg of ascorbic acid in combination with mitomycin and 5-fluorouracil significantly inhibited tumor growth in mice implanted with Lewis lung carcinoma cells relative to mice treated with mitomycin and 5-fluorouracil in the absence of ascorbic acid or animal that received only ascorbic acid alone.

> —K. Nakano, et al., "Antitumor Activity of Ascorbic Acid in Combination with Antitumor Agents Against Lewis Lung Carcinoma," *In Vivo,* 2(3-4), May-August 1988, p. 247-252.

This study found that 1 or 5 g/liter of ascorbic acid in the drinking water significantly inhibited the growth of human mammary tumor fragments implanted beneath the renal capsule of immunocompetent mice. Mice fed a diet including 50g/kg ascorbic acid and 18 or 90 mg/liter of cupric sulfate in the drinking water also experienced inhibited tumor growth. The authors conclude ascorbic acid contains specific oxidation and degradation products that serve as antineoplastic agents for human mammary carcinoma.

> —C.S. Tsao, et al., "In Vivo Antineoplastic Activity of Ascorbic Acid for Human Mammary Tumor," *In Vivo,* 2(2), March-April 1988, p. 147-150.

This study found that administration of 500 mg/kg of L-ascorbic acid to athymic nude mice bearing human mammary carcinoma inhibited tumor cell growth. Treatment with L-ascorbic acid was also found to induce cellular DNA strand breaks and DNA cross links. When L-ascorbic acid was removed from cell cultures, researchers witnessed an immediate onset of spontaneous repair of single or double stranded DNA breaks. Reintroduction of L-ascorbic acid reversed this process.

> —K. Pavelic, et al., "Antimetabolic Activity of L-ascorbic Acid in Human and Animal Tumors," *International Journal of Biochemistry,* 21(8), 1989, p. 931-935.

This population-based dietary study found inverse relationship between vitamin C consumption in women and the risk of developing cancer in the lower urinary tract.

> —A.M. Nomura, et al, "Dietary Factors in Cancer of the Lower Urinary Tract," *International Journal of Cancer,* 48(2), May 10, 1991, p. 199-205.

An inverse relationship was found in this population-based, case-control study between the intake of vitamin C and invasive cervical cancer.

> —R. Verreault, et al., "A Case-Control Study of Diet and Invasive Cervical Cancer," *International Journal of Cancer,* 43(6), June 15, 1989, p. 1050-1054.

This study found that guinea pigs fed high vitamin C diets experienced a significantly less mutagenic effect after being injected with $K_2Cr_2O_7$ than those fed a vitamin C deficient diet. Vitamin C deficient animals also suffered greater mutagenic and toxic effects from hexavelent chromium. High vitamin C guinea pigs experienced no mutagenic effects in the bone marrow or changes in microsomal enzymes in the liver following exposure to bichromate. In interpreting their results, the authors suggest that vitamin C's protective effects likely consist in the enhanced extracellular and intracellular reduction of hexavelnt chromium in the less toxic and less mutagenic trivalent chromium.

> —E. Ginter, et al., "Vitamin C Lowers Mutagenic and Toxic Effect of Hexavalent Chromium in Guinea Pigs," *International Journal of Vitamin and Nutritional Research,* 59(2), 1989, p. 161-166.

In this study, ascorbic acid deficiencies in guinea pig were found to change leukocyte morphology and significantly interfere the bactericidal effectiveness of circulating leukocytes against ingested, cell-associated, and extracellular bacterial cells of Acitonyces viscous. Adding vitamin C can reverse this activity.

> —M.C. Goldschmidt, et al., "The Effect of Ascorbic Acid Deficiency on Leukocyte Phagocytosis and Killing of Actinomyces Viscosus," *International Journal of Vitamin and Nutrition Research,* 58(3), 1988, p. 326-334.

This review article points out the importance of vitamin C, as well as vitamins A and E, as regulators of cancer cell differentiation, cell regression, membrane biogenesis, DNA, RNA, protein, and collagen synthesis, as well as transformation of precancer cells into cancer cells. Vitamins C, A, and E can reverse the cancer cell to the normal phenotype and possess cytotoxic and cytostatic effects.

> —A. Lupulescu, "The Role of Vitamins A, Beta-carotene, E and C in Cancer Cell Biology," *International Journal of Vitamin and Nutrition Research,* 64(1), 1994, p. 3-14.

This study found that mice consuming distilled water suffered from tumor growth after being injected with Ehrlich ascites tumor cells at a rate significantly faster than those consuming 0.1% ascorbic acid in distilled water.

> —F.A. Tewfik, et al., "The Influence of Ascorbic Acid on the Growth of Solid Tumors in Mice and on Tumor Control by X-Irradiation," *International Journal of Vitamin and Nutrition Research Suppl,* 23, 1982, p. 257-263.

This comprehensive review article cites numerous studies supporting ascorbic acid's protective effects against cancer and recommends that it be used in treatment. Clinical trials over the last ten years are summarized, with the majority of them supporting this view. The authors predict that supplemental ascorbate will soon secure an established place in all full-scale therapeutic programs for cancer.

> —E. Cameron, "Vitamin C and Cancer: An Overview," *International Journal of Vitamin and Nutrition Research Suppl,* 23, 1982, p. 115-127.

This study reported on two sets of Japanese clinical trials involving the use of supplemental ascorbate to treat terminal cancer patients. The first trial found average survival time of high ascorbate patients was 246 compared to 43 days for low ascorbate patients. Results of the second trial were similar, with high ascorbate patients surviving an average of 115 days compared to 48 days for those in the low ascorbate group.

> —A. Murata, et al., "Prolongation of Survival Times of Terminal Cancer Patients by Administration of Large Doses of Ascorbate," *International Journal of Vitamin and Nutrition Research Suppl,* 23, 1982, p. 103-113.

This study demonstrated the effectiveness of ascorbic acid as a blocking agent in vivo and in vitro to N-Nitroso compounds, which can lead to cancer of the stomach.

> —S.R. Tannenbaum, "Preventive Action of Vitamin C on Nitrosamine Formation," *International Journal of Vitamin and Nutrition Research Suppl,* 30, 1989, p. 109-113.

Ascorbic acid and dehydroascorbic acid have both been shown to favor ATP C+ cell multiplication in vitro at low doses and inhibit it at high doses. Ascorbic acid was found to be more effective in determining both sets of effects than dehydroascorbic acid. Fractioned rather than single administration of both substance proved to the most efficient method for inhibiting cell multiplication.

> —F.S. Liotti, et al., "Effects of Ascorbic and Dehydroascorbic Acid on the Multiplication

of Tumor Ascites Cells in Vitro,'' *Journal of Cancer Research and Clinical Oncology,* 108(2), 1984, p. 230-232.

In this study, the oral administration of 525 mg/day of vitamin C greatly inhibited benzo(a)pyrene induced local malignant tumors in rats relative to controls.
—G. Kallistratos and E. Fasske, ''Inhibition of Benzo(a)pyrene Carcinogenesis in Rats with Vitamin C,'' *Journal of Cancer Research and Clinical Oncology,* 97(1), 1980, p. 91-96.

This study found that catecholamine-positive neuroblastoma cell line SK-N-SH was inhibited by high doses of ascorbic acid as were LS cells and catechoalime-negative SK-N-LO, all be to a smaller extent.
—S.L. Baader, et al., ''Ascorbic-acid-mediated Iron Release from Cellular Ferritin and its Relation to the Formation of DNA Strand Breaks in Neuroblastoma Cells,'' *Journal of Cancer Research and Clinical Oncology,* 120(7), 1994, p. 415-421.

This study examined the effects of vitamin C on the efficacy and adverse effects of drug 864T in Ehrlich ascites carcinoma (EAC) cells in vivo. Results demonstrated that vitamin C both potentiates the anticancer effect of 864T as well as helps to counteract the drug's adverse effects.
—M.M. el-Merzabani MM, et al., ''Potentiation of Therapeutic Effect of Methanesulphonate and Protection Against its organ Cytotoxicity by Vitamin C in Ehrlich Ascites Carcinoma Bearing Mice,'' *Journal of Pharm Belg,* 44(2), March-April 1989, p. 109-116.

This study documents the case of one patient given large doses of ascorbic acid with indomethacin who consequently experienced a slow tumor resolution that has continued for 14 months. Similar effects were seen in a second patient receiving the same treatment.
—W.R. Waddell and R.E. Gerner, ''Indomethacin and Ascorbate Inhibit Desmoid Tumors,'' *Journal of Surg Oncol,* 15(1), 1980, p. 85-90.

This comparative study of normal and malignant conditions in humans and in mice found that serum levels of vitamin C were lower in all human malignant cases relative to controls. With respect to mice, results showed that vitamin C and vitamin A supplementation administered at the start of tumor development reduced both tumor take and rate of growth and prolonged host survival relative to controls.
—J. Ghosh and S. Das, ''Evaluation of Vitamin A and C Status in Normal and Malignant Conditions and their Possible Role in Cancer Prevention,'' *Japanese Journal of Cancer Research,* 76(12), December 1995, p. 1174-1178.

This study compared 294 incurable patients treated with supplemental ascorbate with 1,532 untreated patients who served as controls over a 4.5 year period. The median survival time of the ascorbate group was 343 days compared to 180 days for the controls.
—E. Cameron and A. Campbell, ''Innovation vs. Quality Control: An 'Unpublishable' Clinical Trial on Supplemental Ascorbate in Incurable Cancer,'' *Medical Hypotheses,* 36(3), November 1991, p. 185-189.

Noting that previous studies have found ascorbic acid and its salts to be toxic to tumor cells in vitro and in vivo, this study presents data showing that ascorbic acid plasma levels can be sustained above levels toxic to tumor cells in vitro. The authors argue that ascorbic acid's cytoxic properties should qualify it for consideration as a chemotherapeutic agent.

> —N.H. Riordan, et al., "Intravenous Ascorbate as a Tumor Cytotoxic Chemotherapeutic Agent," *Medical Hypotheses*, 44(3), March 1995, p. 207-213.

This article examined the results and methodology of a controversial case-control study involving the treatment of 100 incurable patients with 10 g a day of vitamin C. The study has received criticism for not being conducted on a randomized, double-blind basis out of ethical considerations. Instead, test cases were studied against historical controls. Results found that patients receiving vitamin C outlived controls by an average of 255 days (671%). This author considers the various criticisms the study has received, yet concludes that vitamin C is likely to have increased survival time an average of 100% in cancer patients who had failed to respond to previous treatments.

> —M. Jaffey, "Vitamin C and Cancer: Examination of the Value of Leven Trial Results Using Broad Inductive Reasoning," *Medical Hypotheses*, 8(1), 1982, p. 49-84.

This paper reports on the case of a 42-year-old man suffering from reticulum cell sarcoma who experienced two complete spontaneous regressions following the intravenous administration of high doses of ascorbate in 1975.

> —A. Campbell, et al., "Reticulum Cell Sarcoma: Two Complete Spontaneous' Regressions, in Response to High-Dose Ascorbic Acid Therapy. A Report on Subsequent Progress," *Oncology* (1991) 48(6), 1991, p. 495-497.

This study looked at vitamin C's effects on methylcholanthrene induced local malignant sarcomas in mice. Results found that doses of 6, 25, and 35 mg/day of vitamin C five times weekly for 20 weeks offered significant prevention against the induction of sarcomas relative to controls.

> —M. Abdel-Galil, "Preventive Effect of Vitamin C (L-ascorbic acid) on Methylcholanthrene-induced Soft Tissue Sarcomas in Mice," *Oncology*, 43(5), 1986, p. 335-337.

This 12-year mortality follow-up study reports that vitamin C is inversely associated with overall mortality from cancer and cardiovascular disease.

> —M. Eichholzer, et al., "Inverse Correlation Between Essential Antioxidants in Plasma and Subsequent Risk to Develop Cancer, Ischemic Heart Disease and Stroke Respectively: 12-Year Follow-up of the Prospective Basel Study," *EXS*, 62, 1992, p. 398-410.

This double-blind, randomized, crossover study found that ascorbic acid significantly reduced muscle soreness in subjects following strenuous use of posterior calf muscles relative to subjects taking a lactose placebo.

> —M. Kaminski and R. Boal, "An Effect of Ascorbic Acid on Delayed-onset Muscle Soreness," *Pain*, 50(3), September 1992, p. 317-321.

This review article cites immunological studies documenting ascorbic acid's ability to induce immunity in mice against certain types of cancer. The authors argue that ascorbate works as an effective thiolprive in oxygenated cancer tissues which is primarily responsible for its immunological effects.

> —F.E. Knock, et al., "Ascorbic Acid as a Thiolprive: Ability to Induce Immunity Against Some Cancers in Mice," *Physiol Chem Phys*, 13(4), 1981, p. 325-333.

This study found that combinations of vitamin C and cisplatin lead to the regression of Dalton's lymphoma tumor activity in mice, which resulted in significantly increased host survival.
　　—S.B. Prasad, et al., "Use of Subtherapeutical Dose of Cisplatin and Vitamin C Against Murine Dalton's Lymphoma," *Pol J Pharmacol Pharm*, 44(4), July-August 1992, p. 383-391.

This study found that the administration of 8 g/day over 8-10 days before starting chemotherapy with cytostatics decreased p-hydroxyphenl lactic acid (pHPLA) excretion in leukemia patients. Mice given 5 mg, 2x/wk, sc, 5wk of pHPLA with 250 mg/100 ml of ascorbic acid were also found to experience a reduction in the incidences of hepatoma, leukemia and bladder cancer. Based on these results, the authors argue that pHPLA carcinogenesis is inhibited by ascorbic acid.
　　—M.O. Raushenbakh, et al., [Effect of Ascorbic Acid on Formation and Leukemogenic Activity of P-Hydroxyphenyllactic Acid], *Probl Gematol Pereliv Krovi*, 27(7), 1982, p.3-6.

This study showed that treatment with vitamin C and chlorophyllin significantly reduced cytotoxicity and the rate of 6-sulfooxymethyl benzo[a]pyrene (SMBP) induced mutagenicity in animal and bacterial cell cultures.
　　—A.S. Chung and Y.S. Cho, "Antimutagenicity of Vitamin C and Chlorophyllin on 6-sulfooxymethyl benzo[a]pyrene in Salmonella Typhimurium and V79 Cell Line," *Proceedings of the Annual Meeting of the American Association of Cancer Researchers*, 36, 1995, A755.

Rat liver carcinogenesis was found to be inhibited by vitamin C and vitamin E derivatives in this study when administered at concentrations of 0.01, 0.05 or 0.10% for 12 weeks. Among the four vitamin derivatives administered, 2-O-octadecylascorbic acid (CV3611) proved to be the most effective.
　　—D. Nakae, et al., "Inhibitory Effects of Vitamin C and E Derivatives on Rat Liver Carcinogenesis Induced by a Choline-Deficient L-Amino Acid (CDAA)-Defined Diet," *Proceedings of the Annual Meeting of the American Association of Cancer Researchers*, 34, 1993, A729.

In this study, MethA tumor cell proliferation was found to be inhibited in vitro after simultaneous exposure to diethyldithiocarbamate (DDC) (1 to approx $2 \times 10(-7)$) and ascorbic acid (1 to approx $5 \times 10(-5)$M). The two substances were able to inhibit tumor proliferation at slightly lower doses when cells were pretreated at 37 degrees C for one hour. In a mouse injected with 2 million tumor cells, 25 mg or 50 mg of ascorbic acid and 10 mg of DDC was also observed to inhibit tumor growth.
　　—H. Mashiba and K. Matsunaga, "Inhibition of Metha Tumor Cell Proliferation In Vitro and Tumor Inhibition of Metha Tumor Cell Proliferation in Vitro and Tumor Growth in Combined Use of Diethyldithiocarbamate with Ascorbic Acid," *Proceedings of the Annual Meeting of the American Association of Cancer Researchers*, 33, 1992, A2649.

This study of ultraviolet light induced malignant skin tumors and other lesions in hairless mice found that animals fed a standard diet including L-ascorbic acid experienced significantly less malignant lesions as well as significant delays in those that did develop relevant to controls.
　　—W.B.Dunham, et al., "Effects of Intake of L-ascorbic Acid on the Incidence of Dermal Neoplasms Induced in Mice by Ultraviolet Light," *Proceedings of the National Academy of Sciences*, 79(23), December 1982, p. 7532-7536.

This study found that vitamin C prevented cigarette smoke induced leukocyte adhesion to micro and macrovascular endothelium and leukocyte-platelet aggregate formation in mice.

> —H.A. Lehr, et al., "Vitamin C Prevents Cigarette Smoke-Induced Leukocyte Aggregation and Adhesion to Endothelium in Vivo," *Proceedings of the National Academy of Sciences,* 91(16), August 2, 1994, p. 7688-7692.

Percentages of L-ascorbic acid contained in food ranging from 0.076% to 8.3% were studied for their effects on spontaneous mammary tumors in mice. Results showed that as ascorbic acid dosages were increased significant decreases occurred in the first-order appearance tumors after lag time detection by palpitation when compared to controls.

> —L. Pauling, et al., "Effect of Dietary Ascorbic Acid on the Incidence of Spontaneous Mammary Tumors in RIII Mice," *Proceedings of the National Academy of Sciences,* 82(15), August 1985, p. 5185-5189.

In this study, 6-deoxy-6-bromo-ascorbic acid (6-Br-AA) in concentrations 10(-1) to 10(-8)M and incubated for periods of 2, 18, 24 and 72 hours was found to greatly inhibit the growth and DNA synthesis of melanoma cells in mice and was confirmed by in vivo experiments. Mice given 9 mg of 6-Br-AA three times daily for 16 days experienced tumor suppressing effects on solid melanoma.

> —M. Osmak, et al., "6-Deoxy-6-bromo-ascorbic Acid Inhibits Growth of Mouse Melanoma Cells," *Res Exp Med* (Berl), 190(6), 1990, p. 443-449.

In this seven year follow-up study of 2974 men, average vitamin C levels were found to be lower in stomach cancer death cases relative to controls.

> —H.B. Stahelin, [Vitamins and Cancer: Results of a Basel Study], *Soz Praventivmed,* 34(2), 1989, p. 75-77.

This study found that ascorbic acid incubation in cultured stomach cancer surgery specimens resulted in a 50-90% increase in the rate of 5-fluorouracil incorporation into RNA of 5-fluorouracil-sensitive stomach tumors and in an approximately 50% increase of the rate of 5-fluorouracil-resistant tumors.

> —M.P. Shlemkevich, [Effect of Ascorbic Acid on In Vitro (6-3H)-5-Fluorouracil Incorporation into RNA of Stomach Cancer Tissue, Normal Gastric Mucosa, and Normal Small Intestine Mucosa], *Vopr Med Khim,* 29(1), 1983, p. 17-19.

This study demonstrated that a 3% solution of ascorbic acid in drinking water added to estradiol propionate (carcinogen) decreased the incidence of uterine sarcoma tumors in mice by 35%.

> —L.S. Trukhanova, et al., [The Inhibitory Effect of Ascorbic Acid on the Estrogen-Stimulated Promotion of Uterine Sarcoma Development in Mice] *Vopr Onkol,* 36(5), 1990, p. 563-567.

This study showed that injections of ascorbic acid before onset and at the start of tumor development decreased blood and urine 3-oxyanthranilic acid-antigen levels down to its eventual elimination from the body in rats and mice. Such activity was found to prevent the subsequent development of hepatoma.

> —T.A. Korosteleva, et al., [Effects of the Administration of Ascorbic Acid on 3-OAA-antigen Levels Formed During Chemical Hepatocarcinogenesis], *Vopr Onkol,* 35(12), 1989, p. 1455-1461.

In this randomized study, postoperative treatment of 95 stomach cancer patients with vitamins C,E and A following resulted in a decreased rate of postoperative complications from 30.9% to 1.9%.

—V.N. Sukolinskii and T.S. Morozkina, [Prevention of Postoperative Complications in Patients with Stomach Cancer Using an Antioxidant Complex], *Vopr Onkol*, 35(10), 1989, p. 1242-1245.

This study found that cancer patients suffered from a decreased level of ascorbic acid relative to non-cancer patients in addition to showing that such decreases correlated with an increase in blood concentrations of malonic and pyruvic acids. When cancer patients were given 1.5 g of ascorbic acid daily over a period of 7 days, blood levels of ascorbic acid returned to almost normal and lactate and pyruvate levels exhibited a decrease. In addition to these changes, ascorbic acid deficiencies were found to result in an increased risk of postoperative complications. This risk was decreased by increasing the levels of ascorbic acid in the blood of deficient patients.

—E.G. Gorozhanskaia, et al., [The Role of Ascorbic Acid in the Combined Preoperative Preparation of Cancer Patients], *Vopr Onkol*, 35(4), 1989, p. 436-441.

This study showed that mice treated with doses of 1.5, 0.25, and 0.025% of ascorbic acid in drinking water all experienced decreases in the frequency of N-nitroso compound induced tumors.

—N.L. Vlasenko, et al., [Effect of Different Doses of Ascorbic Acid on the Induction of Tumors with N-Nitroso Compound Precursors in Mice], *Vopr Onkol*, 34(7), 1988, p. 839-843.

Doses of 0.3, 0.75 or 1.5% of ascorbic acid administered in drinking water inhibited the growth of 1,2 dimethylhydrazine and estradiol-dipropionate induced uterine sarcomas in mice.

—L.S. Trukhanova, [Effect of Ascorbic Acid on the Induction of Uterine Sarcomas in Mice], *Vopr Onkol*, 33(11), 1987, p. 53-57.

The effect of high doses of ascorbic acid (100 mg/kg daily) on tyrosine metabolism and clinical course of acute lymphoblastic leukemia was studied in nine children. Ascorbic acid administration was shown to prevent or to considerably lower the excretion of a blastogenic metabolites of tyrosine - p-hydroxyphenylpyruvic acid. The treatment improved clinical blood count indexes, prevented hemorrhage and was followed by an earlier onset of complete remission after chemotherapy. Although chemotherapy suppressed p-hydroxyphenylpyruvic acid excretion, its level was inordinately high as late as on day 12. It is concluded that although the effects of ascorbic acid and cytostatic drugs on p-hydroxyphenylpyruvate hydroxylase level are similar, that of ascorbic acid is more specific and is followed by a complete recovery of tyrosine metabolism.

—V.N. Baikova, et al., [The Effect of Large Doses of Ascorbic Acid on Tyrosine Metabolism and Hemoblastosis Course in Children], *Vopr Onkol*, 28(9), 1982, p. 28-34.

This case-control study of diet and breast cancer in 2 Chinese populations found a strong inverse association between breast cancer and the intake of vitamin C, carotene, and crude fiber.

—J.M. Yuan, et al., ''Diet and Breast Cancer in Shanghai and Tianjin, China,'' *British Journal of Cancer*, 71, 1995, p. 1353-1358.

This review article looked at 12 case-control studies on the relationship between breast cancer and diet. The most consistently significant inverse association found was between vitamin C and breast cancer risk.

 —G.R. Howe, et al., "Dietary Factors and the Risk of Breast Cancer: Combined Analysis of 12 Case-Controlled Studies," *Journal of the National Cancer Institute,* 82 1990, p. 561-569.

This review article cites results from several studies documenting the protective effects of vitamin C in reducing the risk of cervical cancer. One, in particular, found that women with the highest levels of dietary vitamin C decreased their chances of developing cervical cancer by 4-5 times compared to those with the lowest levels.

 —J. VanEenwyk, "The Role of Vitamins in the Development of Cervical Cancer," *The Nutrition Report,* 11(1), January 1993, p. 1-8.

Dietary vitamin C was found to be protective against cervical intraepithelial neoplasia in this case-control study.

 —C.F. Amburgey, et al., "Undernutrition as a Risk Factor for Cervical Intraepithelial Neoplasia: A Case-control Analysis," *Nutrition and Cancer,* 20(1), 1993, p. 51-60.

Cardiovascular/Coronary Heart Disease

This randomized, double-blind, placebo-controlled study found that men possessing low antioxidant status supplemented with 600 mg of ascorbic acid, 300 mg of alpha-tocopherol, 27 mg of beta-carotene, and 75 mg of selenium daily experienced reductions in lipid peroxidation, platelet aggregation, platelet production of thromboxone A2, and platelet activation in vivo.

 —J.T. Salonen, et al., "Effects of Antioxidant Supplementation on Platelet Function: A Randomized Pair-Matched, Placebo-Controlled, Double-Blind Trial in Men with Low Antioxidant Status," *American Journal of Clinical Nutrition,* 53(5), May 1991, p. 1222-1229.

In reviewing the evidence on the possible link between vitamin C and cardiovascular risk factors, this article comments on a recent placebo-controlled, double-blind study which showed that 6 weeks of ascorbic acid supplementation lowered pulse and systolic pressure in subjects suffering from borderline hypertension.

 —D.L. Trout, Vitamin C and Cardiovascular Risk Factors," *American Journal of Clinical Nutrition,* 53(1 Suppl), January 1991, p. 322S-325S.

This study found that ascorbic acid deficiency in guinea pigs causes intracellular oxidative damage to the cardiac tissues. Evidence of this damage can be seen through lipid peroxidation, loss of structural integrity of the microsomal membranes and the formation of fluorescent pigment. Treatment with ascorbic acid was seen to reverse each of these conditions leading the authors to conclude that such results, when considered in the context of human beings, suggest that ascorbic acid deficiency may lead to permanent heart disease as a result of progressive oxidative damage.

 —S. Chakrabarty, et al., "Protective Role of Ascorbic Acid Against Lipid Peroxidation and Myocardial Injury," *Mol Cell Biochem,* 111(1-2), April 1992, p. 41-47.

This study found that 3.0 g of ascorbic acid and 2.0 g of Trolox, both antioxidants, infused into the ascending aorta 30 seconds before and four minutes after repurfusion proved to be effective in reducing myocardial necrosis after ischemia in a canine model.

> —D.A. Mickle, et al., "Myocardial Salvage with Trolox and Ascorbic Acid for an Acute Evolving Infarction," *Ann Thorac Surg,* 47(4), April 1989, p. 553-557.

Results of this in vitro study demonstrated that ascorbic acid was capable of preventing superoxide-initiated lipid peroxidation and protein changes in guinea pig cardiac microsomes. Ascorbic acid remained effective when superoxide was replaced with NADPH as the initiating agent.

> —M. Mukhopadhyay, et al., "Protective Effect of Ascorbic Acid Against Lipid Peroxidation and Oxidative Damage in Cardiac Microsomes," *Mol Cell Biochem,* 126(1), September 8, 1993, p. 69-75.

This randomized study of 81 patients with coronary artery disease found that both unstable patients as well as patients with stable coronary artery disease requiring coronary artery bypass grafting benefited from treatment with vitamin E, vitamin C and perioperative allopurinol.

> —T. Sisto, et al., "Pretreatment with Antioxidants and Allopurinol Diminishes Cardiac Onset Events in Coronary Artery Bypass Grafting," *Ann Thorac Surg,* 59(6), June 1995, p. 1519-1523.

This study found a strong inverse correlation between the concentration of serum ascorbate and haemostatic factors fibrinogen, factor VIIC, and to acute phase proteins. A positive relationship was observed between serum ascorbate concentrations and forced expiratory volume in one second. Increasing vitamin C in the diet by 60 mg resulted in a reduction of the risk of ischaemic heart disease by approximately 10%.

> —K.T. Khaw and P. Woodhouse, "Interrelation of Vitamin C, Infection, Haemostatic Factors, and Cardiovascular Disease," *British Medical Journal,* 310(6994), June 17, 1995, p. 1559-1563.

This study found that treatment of idopathic thrombocytopenic purpura with ascorbate was successful in 7/11 patients, improving both the intravascular survival of platelets as well as platelet count.

> —A.G. Brox, et al., "Treatment of Idiopathic Thrombocytopenic Purpura with Ascorbate," *British Journal of Haematology* 70(3), November 1988, p. 341-344.

Pretreatment with dietary or intravenous vitamin C showed protective effects on oxLDL-induced leukocyte adhesion and aggregate formation in hamsters in this study which, the authors argue, suggests that similar therapeutic benefits can be expected in humans considering that the vitamin C plasma levels used in this study can also be reached in humans either through diet or supplementation.

> —H.A.Lehr, et al., "Protection from Oxidized LDL-induced Leukocyte Adhesion to Microvascular and Macrovascular Endothelium in Vivo by Vitamin C but not by Vitamin E," *Circulation,* 91(5), March 1, 1995, p. 1525-1532.

This study found that vitamin C and vitamin E supplementation for 10 days prior to donating blood resulted in a significant decrease in lipid peroxidation in stored red cells in both irradiated and non-irradiated samples relative to controls.

> —J.A. Knight, et al., "The Effect of Vitamins C and E on Lipid Peroxidation in Stored

Erythrocytes,'' *Annals of Clinical Laboratory Science,* 23(1), January-February 1993, p. 51-56.

This randomized, single-blind, controlled study examined the effectiveness of dietary modification aimed at increasing plasma ascorbic acid levels one week following acute myocardial infarction. Results suggest that an antioxidant-rich diet increases the plasma level of ascorbic acid and can decrease the plasma levels of lipid peroxide and cardiac enzyme. Myocardial necrosis and reperfusion injury induced by oxygen free radicals may also be reduced by foods rich in antioxidants.

 —R.B. Singh, et al., ''Effect of Antioxidant-Rich Foods on Pasma Ascorbic Acid, Cardiac Enzyme, and Lipid Peroxide Levels in Patients Hospitalized with Acute Myocardial Infarction,'' *Journal of the American Dietetic Association,* 95(7), July 1995, p. 775-780.

Results of this study demonstrated that LDL is protected against atherogenic modification by vitamin C due to ascorbic acid's free scavenging which keeps aqueous oxidants from oxidizing LDL and stable modification of LDL by DHA or decomposition products thereof imparts increased resistance to metal ion-dependent oxidation.

 —K.L. Retsky, et al., ''Ascorbic Acid Oxidation Product(s) Protect Human Low Density Lipoprotein Against Atherogenic Modification. Anti-rather than Prooxidant Activity of Vitamin C in the Presence of Transition Metal Ions,'' *Journal of Biol Chem,* 268(2), January 15, 1993, p. 1304-1309.

This case-control study found that mean levels of vitamins C, E, A and beta-carotene were significantly lower and lipid peroxides significantly higher in patients with suspected acute myocardial infarction (AMI) than controls. Based on these findings, the authors conclude that one risk factor for acute myocardial infarction may be vitamin deficiency and recommend antioxidant supplementation for the prevention of coronary artery disease.

 —R.B. Singh, et al., ''Plasma Levels of Antioxidant Vitamins and Oxidative Stress in Patients with Acute Myocardial Infarction,'' *Acta Cardiol,* 49(5), 1994, p. 441-452.

In this case-control study of 125 cases of angina in Scottish men, plasma vitamin C levels were found to be lower in cases of angina than controls and it is believed that smoking may be a major causative factor responsible for this deficiency.

 —R.A. Riemersma, et al., ''Low Plasma Vitamins E and C. Increased Risk of Angina in Scottish Men,'' *Annals of the New York Academy of Science,* 570, 1989, p. 291-295.

Epidemiological results from this study support the findings of previous studies suggesting that less than 23 microM = 0.4mg/dl of vitamin C in the plasma may be considered a risk factor for ischemic heart disease.

 —K.F. Gey, et al., ''Relationship of Plasma Level of Vitamin C to Mortality from Ischemic Heart Disease,'' *Annals of the New York Academy of Science,* 498, 1987, p. 110-123.

This study showed that intravenous infusion of 2 g of ascorbic acid in 10 healthy volunteers resulted in a reduction of malondialdehyde concentrations and platelet aggregation inhibition.

 —C. Cordova, et al., ''Influence of Ascorbic Acid on Platelet Aggregation in Vitro and in Vivo,'' *Atherosclerosis,* 41(1), January 1982, p. 15-19.

In this case-control study, patients with a history of myocardial infarction that were treated with 2 g of vitamin C daily experienced an increase of approximately 96% in serum ascorbate acid while their fibrinolytic activity increased by 45% and platelet adhesive index decreased by 27%. A 12% drop was seen in their serum cholesterol level, beta lipoproteins were reduced significantly, and an increase occurred in the alpha fraction. Similar results were seen in a second placebo-controlled group of acute myocardial infarction patients given 2 g daily of vitamin C for 20 days. Fibrinolytic activity rose 62.5% and serum ascorbic acid 94% after 40 days.

> —A.K. Bordia, "The Effect of Vitamin C on Blood Lipids, Fibrinolytic Activity and Platelet Adhesiveness in Patients with Coronary Artery Disease," *Atherosclerosis,* 35(2), February 1980, p. 181-187.

This study found that low micromolar concentrations of L-ascorbic acid (AA) and dehydro-L-ascorbic acid (DHA) protect LDL from oxidation induced by $Cu2+$ or be hemin and hydrogen peroxide. Both AA and DHA prevented initiation of lipid peroxidation in a dose dependent manner and also preserved the LDL-associated antioxidants, alpha-tocopherol, beta-carotene, and lycopene.

> —K.L. Retsky and B. Frei, "Vitamin C Prevents Metal ion-Dependent Initiation and Propagation of Lipid Peroxidation in Human Low-Density Lipoprotein," *Biochim Biophys Acta,* 1257(3), August 3, 1995, p. 279-287.

In this study, white rats given vitamins A, E, C and P over a 12 day period showed decreases in death rate from exogenous thromboplastinemia, and reductions in hemocoagulative changes, microcircuculation disorders, and destructive changes of functionally active elements of inner organs. The authors argue that the protective effect of the vitamins studied in thromboplastinemia is promoted by hypoactivity of platelet aggregation, by low thromboplastic activity of erythrocytes, and by limited destruction of vascular endothelium.

> —Ash, Byshevskii, et al., [Effects of Vitamins A, E, C and P on Intensity of Blood Coagulation in Experimental Animals], *Biull Eksp Biol Med,* 114(9), September 1992, p. 262-265.

This study compared 10 patients who received 250 mg/kg of vitamin C prior to undergoing open heart surgery to 10 similar patients receiving no vitamin C. MDA and CPK-MB concentrations differed significantly between the two groups from 2 to 12 hours following the operation. It is the author's view that vitamin C's effect in reducing CPK-MB and MDA release after the surgery was the result of its oxygen free radical scavenging activity.

> —C.C. Li, [Changes of Creatine Phosphokinase and Malondialdehyde in the Serum and Clinical Use of Large Doses of Vitamin C Following Open Heart Surgery], *Chung Hua Wai Ko Tsa Chih,* 28(1), January 1990, p. 16-17, 60-61.

In this study, 1 g of vitamin C was shown to prevent platelet adhesiveness and platelet aggregation induced by feeding healthy males 75 g of butter. The administration of 1g of vitamin C every 8 hours over 10 days in coronary artery disease patients significantly reduced platelet adhesiveness and platelet aggregation as well.

> —A. Bordia and S.K.Verma, "Effect of Vitamin C on Platelet Adhesiveness and Platelet Aggregation in Coronary Artery Disease Patients," *Clinical Cardiology,* 8(10), October 1985, p. 552-554.

This is a general review article on the preventative role of antioxidants in atherosclerosis. The author cites studies reporting the effectiveness of antioxidants, specifically vitamin C, in reducing the susceptibility of LDL to oxidation.

    —W.S. Harris, "The Prevention of Atherosclerosis with Antioxidants," *Clinical Cardiology,* 15(9), September 1992, p. 636-640.

This study showed that ascorbic acid modified the serum levels of apo B in total serum an in lipoprotein classes of density less than 1.050 g/ml in rats fed a cholesterol enriched diet and reduced cholesterol and triglycerides in all lipoprotein classes tested.

    —M. Santillo, et al., "Effect of Ascorbic Acid Administration on B and E Apoproteins in Rats Fed a Cholesterol Enriched Diet," *Horm Metab Res,* 25(3), March 1993, p. 156-159.

Results of this correlational study indicate systolic blood pressure was inversely associated with serum ascorbic acid levels in healthy adults between the ages of 30-39 years old. Increases in ascorbic acid levels decreased the prevalence of hypertension.

    —M. Yoshioka, et al., "Inverse Association of Serum Ascorbic Acid Level and Blood Pressure or Rate of Hypertension in Male Adults Aged 30-39 Years," *International Journal of Vitamin and Nutrition Research,* 54(4), 1984, p. 343-347.

Noting recent evidence linking vitamin C to regulation of cholesterol and blood pressure, results of this study demonstrated that with every 30 mumol/L increase in plasma ascorbic acid 3.7-9.5% higher levels of HDL-C, 4.1% lower levels of LDL-C, and 1.9-5.5% lower levels of blood pressure were observed in a large, randomized field trial of subjects receiving vitamin C supplementation.

    —P.F. Jacques, "Effects of Vitamin C on High-Density Lipoprotein Cholesterol and Blood Pressure," *Journal of the American College of Nutrition,* 11(2), April 1992, p. 139-144.

This article reviews the existing literature on vitamin C's relationship to cardiovascular disease. The author cites correlational human studies showing an inverse relationship between cardiovascular disease mortality and vitamin C intake as well as observational and experimental studies suggesting vitamin C may work to stabilize levels of total cholesterol. Studies documenting vitamin C's influence on lipid peroxidation are also looked at. Evidence is reviewed regarding high risk groups such as smokers, oral estrogen contraceptive users, diabetics and hypertensives and their reported low levels of plasma vitamin C. The author concludes by stating that data attributing vitamin C to cardiovascular disease in human is primarily circumstantial, yet is suggestive in its entirety of a possible association.

    —J.A. Simon, "Vitamin C and Cardiovascular Disease: A Review," *Journal of the American College of Nutrition,* 11(2), April 1992, p. 107-125.

In this placebo-controlled study examining the effects of vitamin C on cardiovascular diseases, subjects given a dose of 500 mg/day of vitamin C experienced significant reductions in body fat, systolic blood pressure, pulse and a significant increase in high density lipoprotein relative to controls.

    —S. Mostafa, et al., "Beneficial Effects of Vitamin C on Risk Factors of Cardiovascular Diseases," *Journal of Egyptian Public Health Association* 64(1-2), 1989, p. 123-133.

Plasma ascorbic acid concentration was found to have a moderate inverse association with blood pressure that was independent of other factors in this study of middle-aged Finnish men free of hypertension and cerebrovascular disease.

    —J.T. Salonen, et al., "Vitamin C Deficiency and Low Linolenate Intake Associated with

Elevated Blood Pressure: The Kuopio Ischaemic Heart Disease Risk Factor Study," *Journal of Hypertension Suppl,* 5(5), 1987, p. S521-S524.

In this study, experimentally-induced hypertension in rats was reduced 4% by the intake of 0.3% ascorbate solution with a low-fat diet and by 14% with a high-fat diet. Ascorbate also lowered blood pressure in rats on a NaCl free high-fat diet and diminished urine calcium output.
—S. Ziemlanski, et al., "Effect of Exogenous Ascorbic Acid on Experimental Hypertension and Mineral Balance in Rats Fed Low- and High-Fat Diets," *Nutrition,* 7(2), March-April 1991, p.131-135.

Rabbits fed a 150 mg/day combined with a cholesterol-rich diet in this study experienced a reduction in lipid infiltration and intimal thickening in the thoracic aorta. A higher dose of 600 mg/day kept the intimal prostacylcin production levels normal for a minimum of 8 weeks.
—J.R. Beetens, et al., "Vitamin C Increases the Prostacyclin Production and Decreases the Vascular Lesions in Experimental Atherosclerosis in Rabbits," *Prostaglandins,* 32(3), September 1986, p. 335-352.

This study found a significant difference between dietary ascorbic acid levels in patients with normal blood levels of cholesterol versus those with hypercholesterolemia, with those patients suffering from hypercholesterolemia reporting a lower ingestion of ascorbic acid than patients with normal cholesterol.
—I. Fujimura, et al., [Correlation Between Hypercholesterolemia and Vitamin C Deficient Diet]," *Rev Hosp Clin Fac Med Sao Paulo,* 46(1), January-February 1991, p. 14-18.

This study found that a group of healthy young people randomly administered 1 g of ascorbic acid experienced a subsequent significant 16% fall in serum cholesterol within 2 months. A group of healthy older people recorded a 14% fall following a similar supplement within 6-12 months. Seasonal fluctuations of 16% in serum cholesterol were found in a mixed age group of healthy subjects, with the highest levels being recorded in the winter and lowest levels in summer. An inverse relationship was observed between such fluctuations and serum ascorbic acid and leucocytes. Winter elevations of serum cholesterol was stopped by treatment with 1 g of ascorbic acid per day over the course of a year.
—H.M. Dobson, et al., "The Effect of Ascorbic Acid on the Seasonal Variations in Serum Cholesterol Levels," *Scottish Medical Journal,* 29(3), July 1984, p. 176-182.

This is a general review article stressing the importance of antioxidants, including vitamin C, in the prevention of cardiovascular disease and citing various studies of European populations that support this view
—K.F. Gey, et al., [Essential Antioxidants in Cardiovascular Diseases—Lessons for Europe], *Ther Umsch,* 51(7), July 1994, p. 475-482.

85 patients undergoing Cariopulmonary Bypass were studied for the effects of 250 mg/kg of ascorbic acid on the myocardium. Ascorbic acid was shown to decrease lipid peroxidation in the cell membrane and protect the myocardium from ischemia-repurfusion injury during and after the operation by removing radicals.
—H. Dingchao, et al., "The Protective Effects of High-Dose Ascorbic Acid on Myocardium

Against Reperfusion Injury During and After Cardiopulmonary Bypass,'' *Thorac Cardiovasc Surg,* 42(5), October 1994, p. 276-278.

In this study an inverse relationship was found between the consumption of vitamin C, arterial hypertension, hyperlipoproteinemia, overweight, and coronary heart disease in a male based population.
—N.V. Davydenko and V.I. Kolchinskii, [Relation Between Vitamin C Consumption and Risk of Ischemic Heart Disease], *Vopr Pitan,* (6), November-December, 1983, p. 17-19.

This study found that in white rats fed a combination of vitamins A, E, P, and C over a period of 12 days hypocoagulemia, induced by either surgery or exogenic thromboplastinemia, was prevented.
—Ash, Bysheskii, et al., [The Effect of Vitamins A, E, C, P and PP on Blood Coagulation in Experimental Thromboplastinemia], *Vopr Pitan,* (6), November-December 1989, p. 50-52.

This placebo-controlled study investigated the effects of supplemental ascorbic acid on red blood cell glutathione. Results showed that reduced blood concentrations of glutathione were maintained by 500 mg/d of vitamin C and that higher dosages of ascorbic acid did not have a significantly greater effect.
—C.S. Johnston, et al., ''Vitamin C Elevates Red Blood Cell Glutathione in Healthy Adults,'' *American Journal of Clinical Nutrition,* 58(1), July 1993, p. 103-105.

Cataracts

This study examined the relationship between cataracts and antioxidant status. Low vitamin C intake and consuming less than 3.5 servings of fruit and vegetables per day were found to be associated with an increased risk of cortical cataracts.
—P.F. Jacques and L.T. Chylack, Jr., ''Epidemiologic Evidence of a Role for the Antioxidant Vitamins and Carotenoids in Cataract Prevention,'' *American Journal of Clinical Nutrition,* 53(1 Suppl), January 1991, p. 352S-355S.

This study of 175 cataract patients compared with 175 individually matched, cataract free, controls found that consumption of supplementary vitamin C and E was significantly higher in the control group.
—J.M. Robertson, et al., ''A Possible Role for Vitamins C and E in Cataract Prevention,'' *American Journal of Clinical Nutrition,* 53(1 Suppl), January 1991, p. 346S-351S.

High levels of two of the three vitamins examined in this study (vitamin E, C, or carotenoids) were found to be associated with a reduced cataract risk when compared to subjects with low levels of at least one of the vitamins.
—P.F. Jacques, et al., ''Antioxidant Status in Persons with and without Senile Cataract,'' *Arch Ophthalmol,* 106(3), March 1988, p. 337-340.

This study found ascorbate significantly prevented selenite-induced cataracts in rat pups.
—P.S. Devamanoharan, et al., ''Prevention of Selenite Cataract by Vitamin C,'' *Exp Eye Res,* 52(5), May 1991, p. 563-568.

This review article discusses the findings of previous in vitro and in vivo studies which found that sugar, steroid, and light-induced cataracts to be significantly prevented by vitamins C and E. Previous epidemiological research has also demonstrated that high intakes or blood levels of antioxidants reduce the risk of cataracts in humans.

—H. Gerster, ''Antioxidant Vitamins in Cataract Prevention,'' *Z Ernahrungswiss,* 28(1), March 1989, p. 56-75.

Cervical Dysplasia

Noting that approximately 35% of reproductive age women in the United States consume less than 30 mg of vitamin C while 68% consume less than 88 mg, this case-control study found that the intake of vitamin C is an independent risk factor for cervical dysplasia when other variables such as age and sexual activity are controlled.

—S. Wassertheil-Smoller, et al., ''Dietary Vitamin C and Uterine Cervical Dysplasia,'' *American Journal of Epidemiology,* 114(5), November 1981, p. 714-724.

This case-control study found that mean plasma concentration of vitamin C was significantly lower in women with cervical dysplasia than controls.

—S.L. Romney, et al., ''Plasma Vitamin C and Uterine Cervical Dysplasia,'' *American Journal of Obstetrics and Gynecology,* 151(7), April 1, 1985, p. 976-980.

This case-control study examined the relationship between cervical dysplasia and nutrition. Controlling for high risk variables such as sexual activity, HPV infection, and smoking; the results showed that an insufficient intake of ascorbate as well as vitamin A, riboflavin and folate were all associated with an increased risk of cervical dysplasia.

—T. Liu, et. al., ''A Case Control Study of Nutritional Factors and Cervical Dysplasia,'' *Cancer Epidemiol Biomarkers Prev,* 2(6), Nov-Dec 1993, p. 525-530.

Common Cold

In reviewing the existing literature on the relationship between vitamin C and the common cold, this paper points out that while there is no evidence to date suggesting supplemental vitamin C decreases the incidence of the common cold, studies do exists documenting its efficacy in decreasing the length of colds as well as the severity of cold symptoms.

—H. Hemila, ''Vitamin C and the Common Cold,'' *British Journal of Nutrition,* 67(1), January 1992, p. 3-16.

This article reviews the 21 placebo-controlled studies done since 1971 examining what effects if any 1 g of vitamin C a day has on the common cold. No evidence exists linking vitamin C to a reduction of cold incidence, yet each of the studies reviewed reported that vitamin C decreased the length of colds and cold symptoms by an average of 23%.

—H. Hemila, ''Does Vitamin C Alleviate the Symptoms of the Common Cold?—A Review of Current Evidence,'' *Scandanavian Journal of Infectious Disease,* 26(1), 1994, p. 1-6.

Crohn's Disease

This study found that in patients with active or inactive Crohn's disease low leukocyte or serum levels of ascorbate are relatively common and are partially the result of low intake of dietary ascorbate.

Results demonstrated that increasing vitamin C intake with the help of diet counseling can significantly improve ascorbate status.

> —S. Imes, et al., "Vitamin C Status in 137 Outpatients with Crohn's Disease: Effect of Diet Counseling," *Journal of Clinical Gastroenterology,* 8(4), August 1986, p. 443-446.

Dermatitis

This study reports on a single case of a worker with a severe chromium sensitivity who was required to handle inks containing chromium which eventually led to a severe case of hand dermatitis. A 10% ascorbic acid solution applied to the hands at his worksite produced a speedy recovery after various other treatments and preventative attempts had failed.

> —J.E. Milner, "Ascorbic Acid in the Prevention of Chromium Dermatitis," *Journal of Occupational Medicine,* 22(1), January 1980, p. 51-52.

Diabetes

This double-blind, placebo-controlled study found that 2 g/d of ascorbic acid taken for 2 weeks delayed the insulin response to a glucose challenge in nonglycemic adults and subsequently prolonged the postprandial hyperglycemia.

> —C.S. Johnston and M.F. Yen, "Megadose of Vitamin C Delays Insulin Response to a Glucose Challenge in Normoglycemic Adults," *American Journal of Clinical Nutrition,* 60(5), November 1994, p. 735-738.

In a case-control study of aged healthy subjects and type II diabetics, vitamin C infusion rates of 0.9 mmol/minm were shown to improve Conard's K values and the disposal of whole body glucose in the diabetics and healthy subjects alike due to an improvement in nonoxidative glucose metabolism.

> —G. Paolisso, et al., "Plasma Vitamin C Affects Glucose Homeostasis in Healthy Subjects and in Non-Insulin-Dependent Diabetics," *American Journal of Physiology,* 266(2 Pt 1), February 1994, p. E261-8.

This paper reports the case of a 58-year-old man affected with malignant external otitis who was healed by taking ascorbic acid for one month after all previous treatments had failed.

> —J. Corberand, et al., "Malignant External Otitis and Polymorphonuclear Leukocyte Migration Impairment: Improvement with Ascorbic Acid," *Arch Otolaryngol,* 108(2), February 1982, p. 122-124.

In this study, nondiabetic subjects took 1 g/d of vitamin C for 3 months. Plasma and intraerthrocyte glucose, vitamin C, glycosylated hemoglobin and glycosylated albumin were measured at the end of each month. Results suggest glycosylation of proteins in vivo may be inhibited by the oral intake of vitamin C.

> —S.J. Davie, et al., "Effect of Vitamin C on Glycosylation of Proteins," *Diabetes,* 41(2), February 1992, p. 167-73

In this study 10 normoglycemics were given 500 mg/d of ascorbic acid alone or in a citrus fruit medium for 2 weeks followed by a washout period of 10 days. Ascorbic acid administered via the citrus fruit medium resulted in a significantly higher increase in erythrocyte ascorbic acid than did ascorbic acid administered by itself. Erythrocyte sorbitol was decreased 12.6% when ascorbic acid was given alone compared to 27.2% in the citrus fruit medium. Erythrocyte sorbitol was reduced by 56.1% when the dosage of ascorbic acid was increased to 2000 mg/d in another set of normaglycemic subjects, and 44% when given to a set of diabetic subjects either by itself or in the citrus fruit medium.

—J.A. Vinson, et al., "In Vitro and in Vivo Reduction of Erythrocyte Sorbitol by Ascorbic Acid," *Diabetes*, 38(8), August 1989, p. 1036-1041.

This study found that treatment of diabetic rats with 20-40 mg/d of ascorbic acid prevented the decrease in activity of granulation tissue prolyl hydroxylase, prompting the authors to conclude that ascorbic acid can prevent diabetic complications involving collagen abnormalities.

—S. McLennan, et al., "Deficiency of Ascorbic Acid in Experimental Diabetes: Relationship with Collagen and Polyol Pathway Abnormalities," *Diabetes*, 37(3), March 1988, p. 359-361.

In this study, ascorbic acid reduced the ratio of sorbitol to glucose in erythrocyte and erythrocyte sorbitol in vitro.

—H. Wang, et al., [Reduction of Erythrocyte Sorbitol by Ascorbic Acid in Patients with Diabetes Mellitus] *Chung Hua I Hsueh Tsa Chih*, 74(9), September 1994, p. 548-551, 583.

This study of diabetic patients found an inverse correlation between plasma ascorbic acid and its urinary excretion and glycosylate hemoglobin levels.

—D.K. Yue, et al., "Abnormalities of Ascorbic Acid Metabolism and Diabetic Control: Differences Between Diabetic Patients and Diabetic Rats," *Diabetes Res Clin Pract* (1990 Jul) 9(3), July 1990, p. 239-244.

This study examined the association between vitamin C, glucose, and insulin in the plasma of a non-diabetic male who received intravenous vitamin C. A follow-up study was done in 3 diabetic patients in which the effect of intravenous vitamin C was recorded. Results indicated that vitamin C was best administered via the drip infusion method, insulin concentrations in the plasma followed a bimodal curve, and vitamin C benefited all three diabetic patients.

—M. Kodama, et al., "Diabetes Mellitus is Controlled by Vitamin C Treatment," *In Vivo*, 7(6A), November-December 1993, p. 535-542.

This study found that vitamin C supplements of 100-600 mg daily taken for 58 days were effective in decreasing the accumulation of sorbitol in the erythrocytes of young insulin dependent diabetics.

—J.J. Cunningham, et al., "Vitamin C: An Aldose Reductase Inhibitor that Normalizes Erythrocyte Sorbitol in Insulin-Dependent Diabetes Mellitus," *Journal of the American College of Nutrition*, 13(4), August 1994, p. 344-350.

This study found that adult insulin-dependent diabetics' levels of vitamin C in mononuclear leukocytes was 33% below average, indicating the possibility of an approximately 50% storage deficit in diabetic patients.

—J.J.Cunningham, et al., "Reduced Mononuclear Leukocyte Ascorbic Acid Content in Adults with Insulin-Dependent Diabetes Mellitus Consuming Adequate Dietary Vitamin C," *Metabolism*, 40, 1991, p. 146-149.

Fatigue

Oral supplementation of 30 mg of vitamin C per day for thirty days prolonged contraction time in the gastrocnemius muscle of the rat by 19% which delayed fatigue but did not decrease muscle strength.

—J.H. Richardson and R.B. Allen, "Dietary Supplementation with Vitamin C Delays the Onset of Fatigue in Isolated Striated Muscle of Rats," *Canadian Journal of Applied Sport Sciences*, 8(3), September 1983, p. 140-142.

This survey study found a significant inverse relationship between vitamin consumption of vitamin C and fatigue among dentists and their wives. Those with lowest intake of vitamin C reported twice as many fatigue symptoms as those with the highest vitamin C consumption levels.

—E. Cheraskin, et al., "Daily Vitamin C Consumption and Fatigability," *Journal of the American Geriatric Society*, 24(3), 1976, p. 136-137.

Fertility

This placebo-controlled study of men between 20-35 years old found that heavy smokers who consumed more than 200 mg/d of supplemental ascorbic acid experienced improvements in sperm quality relative to fertility.

—E.B. Dawson, et al., "Effect of Ascorbic Acid Supplementation on the Sperm Quality of Smokers," *Fertil Steril*, 58(5), November 1992, p. 1034-1049.

This is a general review of the literature pertaining the relationship between ascorbic and both male and female fertility. Three main function of ascorbic acid the article is primarily concerned with as a function of enhanced fertility are its promotion of collagen synthesis, role in hormone production, and its ability to shield cells from free radicals. The author concludes that ascorbic acid is an essential compound in gonad physiology.

—M.R. Luck, et al., "Ascorbic Acid and Fertility," *Biol Reprod*, 52(2), February 1995, p. 262-266.

In this study, rats fed 100 mg of ascorbic acid daily for days prior to being subjected to simulated altitude of 6060 m and 7576 m for 6 h/day for 7 days did not experience the same loss of weight or atrophy of reproductive organs nor did they suffer from an increase in alkaline and acid phosphatase, and decrease in protein, sialic acid and glyceryl phophorycholine content in reproductive tissue to the same degree that rats not fed ascorbic acid did. The authors conclude that supplementation with ascorbic acid may protect the male reproductive system from the effects of hypoxia.

—G. Ilavazhagan, et al., "Effects of Ascorbic acid Supplementation on Male Reproductive System During Exposure to Hypoxia," *International Journal of Biometeorol*, 33(3), October 1989, p. 165-172.

Gallbladder Disease

This article notes guinea pigs deficient in ascorbic acid frequently suffer from cholesterol gallstones. In humans, risk factors include diabetes, pregnancy, obesity, aging, and estrogen treatment: all groups for which ascorbic acid levels are often reduced. Vegetarian diets are normally high in ascorbic acid and offer protection against gallstones. Factors such as these have lead the author to suggest gallbladder disease may be prevented by increased intake of ascorbic acid.

—J.A. Simon, "Ascorbic Acid and Cholesterol Gallstones," *Medical Hypotheses,* 40(2), February 1993, p. 81-84.

General

This study indicates that ascorbate induces the expression of type X collagen, stimulates phosphatase activity of maturing chondrocytes, and regulates the energy status of maturing chondrocyte. Results point to the fact ascorbate's presence produces a change in oxidative activity. Lactate formation is therefore inhibited, the charge ratio of adenylate energy increases, and there is an elevation in the activity of isocitrate dehydgorenase. Such results indicate multiple effects of vitamin C on chondrocyte maturation involving changes in protein synthesis and energy metabolism.

—I.M. Shapiro, et al., "Ascorbic Acid Regulates Multiple Metabolic Activities of Cartilage Cells," *American Journal of Clinical Nutrition,* 54(6 Suppl), December 1991, p. 1209S-1213S.

This is a lengthy review on the existing literature concerning vitamin C and health in humans, animals, and cell cultures. Studies are discussed linking vitamin C to iron absorption, folic acid metabolism, aging, cancer, cardiovascular disease, and cataract formation. The author also addresses the debate concerning the optimal daily levels of vitamin C, coming down on the side that the current RDA are insufficient.

—S.N. Gershoff, "Vitamin C (Ascorbic Acid): New Roles, New Requirements?" *Nutr Rev,* 51(11), November 1993, p. 313-326.

Results of this study suggest ascorbate supplementation can prevent pathologically relevant lipid hydroperoxide formation consequent to acute or chronic leukocyte activation. For this reason, the authors argue, ascorbate should prove to be useful in the prevention and treatment of oxidative stress-induced diseases and degenerative processes.

—B. Frei, et al., "Ascorbate: The Most Effective Antioxidant in Human Blood Plasma," *Adv Exp Med Biol,* 264, 1990, p. 155-163.

This study found that 2 g/d of vitamin C resulted in a decrease in ApoB in men and women. Women were found to receive more overall benefits from vitamin C therapy than men.

—J.A. Munoz, et al., "Effect of Vitamin C on Lipoproteins in Healthy Adults," *Ann Med Intern,* 145(1), 1994, p. 13-19.

Results of this study, First National Health and Nutrition Examination Survey (NHANES I) Follow-up Study cohort, showed that vitamin C intake has a strong inverse association with the standard mortality ration for all causes of death in males, but is only weakly inverse in females.

—J.E. Enstrom, et al., "Vitamin C Intake and Mortality Among a Sample of the United States Population," *Epidemiology,* 3(3), May 1992, p. 194-202.

This study found that guinea pigs fed a diet including 660 mg of vitamin C a day (40 times the daily requirement) over a period of five weeks boosted the global antioxidant capacity of the animals and provided protection against endogenous lipid and protein oxidation in the liver.

—G. Barja, et al., "Dietary Vitamin C Decreases Endogenous Protein Oxidative Damage,

Malondialdehyde, and Lipid Peroxidation and Maintains Fatty Acid Unsaturation in the Guinea Pig Liver,'' *Free Radic Biol Med,* 17(2), August 1994, p. 105-115.

This study showed that mice fed 1% ascorbic acid in drinking water daily over the course of their lives increased the average life span by 8.6% with some mice increasing it as much as 20.4%.
—H.R. Massie, et al., ''Dietary Vitamin C Improves the Survival of Mice,'' *Gerontology,* 30(6), 1984, p. 371-375.

This review article cites data indicating that populations that vitamin C consumption levels higher than current RDAs show reduced risks of cancer, cardiovascular diseases, and cataracts. Eight placebo-controlled, double-blind studies are cited along with six non-placebo clinical trials supporting the safety of higher than RDA levels of vitamin C.
—A. Bendich and L. Langseth, ''The Health Effects of Vitamin C Supplementation: A Review,'' *Journal of the American College of Nutrition,* 14(2), April 1995, p. 124-13.

This review article on vitamin C and chiropractic cites studies documenting vitamin C's positive influences on wound healing, respiratory distress, immune enhancement, and osteoarthritis. The author concluded that supplementation with vitamin C might be utilized for numerous conditions commonly seen by chiropractors.
—D.R. Dryburgh, ''Vitamin C and Chiropractic,'' *Journal of Manipulative Physiol Ther,* 8(2), 1985. p. 95-103.

This general article summarizes some of the better known health effects of antioxidants, including vitamin C, such as immune enhancement, anticarcinogenic, anti-inflammatory, etc.. The authors argue that high dose supplementation with antioxidants may gain a significant role in the prevention and treatment of many of todays most common major ailments in the future.
—E.J. Crary and M.F. McCarty, ''Potential Clinical Applications for High-Dose Nutritional Antioxidants,'' *Medical Hypotheses,* 13(1), January 1984, p. 77-98.

This paper addresses several key issues important to the use of very high doses of vitamin C in the treatment of disease. One is the question of bowel tolerance. The author notes that the amount a person can tolerate without diarrhea increases somewhat proportionally to the toxicity of his or her disease. He also stresses the importance of the need to use very high doses in the treatment of existing diseases.
—R.F. Cathcart, III ''Vitamin C: The Nontoxic, Nonrate-Limited, Antioxidant Free Radical Scavenger,'' *Medical Hypotheses,* 18(1), September 1985, p. 61-77.

Glaucoma

This study examined whether or not high concentration of ascorbic acid normally present in aqueous humor inhibits wound healing after filtration surgery. Results found that 1.1mmol/L of ascorbic acid decreased the plating efficiency of cell suspension of human Tenon's capsule fibroblasts by a mean of 40%. Ascorbic acid decreased the cell number by 90% when added to a low-density monolayer culture of fibroblasts, and effect prevented by catalase. Ascorbic acid decreased cell number 14% when added to confluent cultures. Based on these results, the author suggests that ascorbic acid may contribute to incomplete wound healing that is necessary of successful glaucoma surgery if similar effects on fibroblasts are seen in vivo.

—H.D. Jampel, "Ascorbic Acid is Cytotoxic to Dividing Human Tenon's Capsule Fibroblasts: A Possible Contributing Factor in Glaucoma Filtration Surgery Success," *Arch Ophthalmol*, 108(9), September 1990, p. 1323-1325.

Glutathione Deficiency

The results of this single case study found that 0.7 mmol/kg per day of ascorbate or 0.6 mmol/kg per day of N-acetylcysteine administered for 1-2 weeks to a 45-month-old girl with 5-oxoprolinuria (pyroglutamic aciduria), hemolysis, and marked glutathione depletion caused by deficiency of glutathione synthetase decreased erythrocyte turnover by successful increasing glutathione levels to a normal state.

—A. Jain, et al., "Effect of Ascorbate or N-acetylcysteine Treatment in a Patient with Hereditary Glutathione Synthetase Deficiency," *Journal of Pediatrics*, 124(2), February 1994, p. 229-233.

Hepatitis

Results from this study found that ascorbic acid significantly reduced iproniazid-induced hepatitic injury in rats.

—Y. Matsuki, et al., "Effects of Ascorbic Acid on Iproniazid-Induced Hepatitis in Phenobarbital-Treated Rats," *Biol Pharm Bull*, 17(8), August 1994, p. 1078-1082.

This study found that patients with virus hepatitis tend to suffer more from C-hypovitaminosis in the winter-spring period. Results suggest that 300 mg of ascorbic acid for 1.5 g of galascorbin/day appears to be the best dose for reversing a deficiency in vitamin C in these patients. Ascorbic acid supplements resulted in T-Lymphocyte content recovery in the patients suffering from suppression during acute periods of virus hepatitis A.

—V.S. Vasil'ev and V.I. Komar, [Ascorbic Acid Level and the Indicators of Cellular Immunity in Patients with Hepatitis A During Pathogenetic Therapy], *Vopr Pitan*, (4), July-August 1988, p. 31-34.

Herpes

This study showed the administration of 100 mg of zinc sulfate and 250 mg of vitamin C twice daily for 6 weeks to patients with recurrent herpes simplex type I resulted in either total suppression of the eruption, a local tingling sensation, but no eruptions or local swelling and limited vesiculation which receded within 24 hours, or one violent eruption that was not repeated as long as vitamin supplementation was not stopped.

—J. Fitzherbert, "Genital Herpes and Zinc," *Medical Journal Aust*, 1, 1979, p. 399.

This study found significant differences between herpes patients treated with 200 mg of vitamin C and 200 mg of bioflavonoids 3 or 5 times daily for 3 days beginning 48 hours after the onset of symptoms and controls. Those treated with vitamin C and bioflavonoids experience complete remission in an average of 4.2 days versus 9.7 days in the placebo group.

—G.T. Terezhalmy, et. al., "The Use of Water-Soluble Bioflavonoid-Ascorbic Acid Complex in the Treatment of Recurrent Herpes Labialis," *Oral Surgery*, 45, 1978, p. 56-62.

HTLV-I Associated Myelopathy (HAM)

This study documented the effectiveness of high doses of vitamin C as a therapy in patients with HTLV-I associated myelopathy (HAM). Seven patients received oral doses between 1.5 to 3.0 g/d of vitamin C for 3 to 5 days followed by two weeks without vitamin C. All patients responded well to the therapy, indicating a successful clinical outcome.

    —A. Kataoka, et al., [Intermittent High-Dose Vitamin C Therapy in Patients with HTLV-I-Associated Myelopathy], *Rinsho Shinkeigaku,* 33(3), March 1993, p. 282-288.

Immune Enhancement

This study reports normal adult volunteers who ingested 2 to 3 g of ascorbate daily experienced enhanced neutrophil motility to a chemotactic stimulus of endotoxin-activated authologous serum. Stimulation of lymphocyte transformation to phytohaemagglutinin and concanavalin A was also detected in volunteers after the ingestion of 2 and 3 g of daily ascorbate.

    —R. Anderson, et al., "The Effects of Increasing Weekly Doses of Ascorbate on Certain Cellular and Humoral Immune Functions in Normal Volunteers," *American Journal of Clinical Nutrition,* 33(1), January 1980, p. 71-76.

This placebo-controlled study of elderly long-stay patients found dietary supplementation with vitamins A, C, and E resulted in improved cell-mediated immune function indicated by significant increases in total number of T cells, T4 subsets, T4 to T8 ratio, and the proliferation of lymphocytes in response to phytohaemagagglutinin. No such changes were experienced in the placebo group.

    —N.D. Penn, et al., "The Effect of Dietary Supplementation with Vitamins A, C and E on Cell-Mediated Immune Function in Elderly Long-Stay Patients: A Randomized Controlled Trial," *Age Ageing,* 20(3), May 1991, p. 169-174.

This review article notes the effectiveness of vitamins A, C, E, and carotenoids in promoting cellular and tissular physiological behavior, immune response, and protecting tissues against reactive oxygen species.

    —M. Nicol, [Vitamins and Immunity], *Allerg Immunol,* 25(2), February 1993, p. 70-73.

This study found that ascorbate acid inhibits human natural killer cell activity in a dose-dependent manner while no effecting effector/target cell binding nor interferon or interlekin-2-induced increases of NK activity. The authors suggest ascorbic acid's noted effects are likely the result of its radical scavenging activity.

    —T. Huwyler, et al., "Effect of Ascorbic Acid on Human Natural Killer Cells," *Immunology Letters,* 10(3-4), 1985, p. 173-176.

In the first half of this study the effect of vitamin C injection treatment on the eosinophil count and 5 plasma steroids in plasma on the one hand, and on diuresis and 17-hydroxycorticoids excretion on the other hand was examined in a healthy male volunteer. The second half of the study looked at vitamin C's effect on 4 patients with autoimmune disease. Results indicated that vitamin C induced an increase of plasma glucocorticoid activity with a 2 hour delay. Two hours after the treatment with vitamin C plasma cortisol declined with a change in eosinophil count, suggesting a cortisol absorber presence. Diuresis and 17 hydroxychorticoids were also accelerated by the vitamin C treatments.

    —M. Kodama, et al., "Autoimmune Disease and Allergy are Controlled by Vitamin C Treatment," *In Vivo,* 8(2), March-April 1994, p. 251-257.

In this placebo-controlled study, vitamin C supplementation's effect on immune enhancement was examined among a group of elderly subjects both in vitro (10 micrograms/ml) and in vivo (2 g/d for 3 weeks). Results suggest that vitamin C may be an important factor in correcting faulty immunologic functions in the elderly.

—J.C. Delafuente, et al., "Immunologic Modulation by Vitamin C in the Elderly," *International Journal Immunopharmacology,* 8(2), 1986, p. 205-211.

This extensive review of the literature on immunostimulation by vitamin C cites evidence regarding the following positive effects: resistance against infections, increases chemotaxis of granulocytes and of magrophages, increases phagocytic activity of granulocytes and macrophages, necessary for induction of hypersensitivity, and increases the efficiency of rabies vaccine in guinea pigs.

—S. Banic, "Immunostimulation by Vitamin C," *International Journal of Vitamin and Nutrition Research Supp,* 23, 1982, p. 49-52.

In pointing out that allergic and sensitivity reaction are frequently ameliorated and sometimes completely blocked by massive doses of ascorbate, this author proposes the theory that one mechanism allergic symptom blocking is the reduction of disulfide bonds between the chains in antibody molecules making the bonding antigen impossible. He suggests that antibodies seek to match antigens only in areas where stray free radicals or a relatively oxidizing redox potential exists.

—R.F. Cathcart, III, "The Vitamin C Treatment of Allergy and the Normally Unprimed State of Antibodies," *Medical Hypotheses,* 21(3), November 1986, p. 307-321.

Iron Absorption

Eleven premenopausal women who were depleted of storage iron were given a diet containing 13.7 mg Fe/2000 kcal in addition to either 1500 mg of ascorbic acid daily or placebo with meals for 5.5 weeks. The ascorbic acid group showed improvements in the absorption of iron and hemoglobin, serum iron and erythrocyte protoporphyrins.

—J.R. Hunt, et al., "Ascorbic Acid: Effect on Ongoing Iron Absorption and Status in Iron-Depleted Young Women," *American Journal of Clinical Nutrition,* 51(4), April 1990, p. 649-655.

This review article notes the generally recognized fact that ascorbic acid is importance in dietary nonheme iron absorption and states two main reasons for its effectiveness. The first is the prevention of the formation of insoluble and unabsorbable iron compound and the second is the reduction of ferric to ferrous iron, which, she suggests, seems to be a requirement for the uptake of iron into the mucusal cells.

—L. Hallberg, et al., "The Role of Vitamin C in Iron Absorption," *International Journal of Vitamin and Nutrition Research Suppl,* 30, 1989, p. 103-108.

Liver Disease

This study demonstrated that ascorbic acid suppressed lipid peroxidation of reoxgenated rat liver tissue in a dose-dependent manner in vivo. Results suggest it functions as an antioxidant by being oxidized to dehydroascorbic acid right after reoxygenation.

—M. Ozaki, et al., "The in Vivo Cytoprotection of Ascorbic Acid Against Ischemia/Reoxygenation Injury of Rat Liver," *Arch Biochem Biophys,* 318(2), April 20, 1995, p. 439-445.

Menkes' Disease

This paper reports on a single Menkes' disease patient successfully treated with oral intake of vitamin C. Vitamin C improved bone changes, and resulted in a rise of plasma copper and ceruplasmin.

>—Y. Ueki, et al., ''Menkes' Disease: Is Vitamin C Treatment Effective?'' *Brain Development,* 7(5), 1985, p. 519-522.

Menopause

This study treated 40 menopausal women suffering from a variety of symptoms with 200 mg of hesperidin and 200 mg of vitamin C following each meal at bedtime for 2 weeks plus another 100 mg of both 4 times a day for four weeks. Dosages were reduced to 200 mg of each a day and eventually discontinued once menopausal symptoms had disappeared. Results found that 4/14 women noted a decrease in nocturnal leg cramps within 2 weeks, 11/15 patients recovered from easy bruising after eight weeks followed by another 4 in 16 weeks, 8/11 women stopped having nosebleeds after 6-11 weeks.

>—A. Horoschak, ''Nocturnal Leg Cramps, Easy Bruisability and Epistaxis in Menopausal Patients: Treated with Hesperidin and Ascorbic Acid,'' *Delaware State Medical Journal,* January 1959, p. 19-22.

Neutrophil Dysfunction

This study documented the cases of three patients suffering from impairment of neutrophil function who were successfully treated with ascorbic acid.

>—A. Rebora, et al., ''Neutrophil Dysfunction and Repeated Infections: Influence of Levamisole and Ascorbic Acid,'' *British Journal of Dermatology,* 102(1), January 1980, p. 49-56.

This paper reports on the case of a patient with a history of recurrent furunculosis who suffered from altered neutrophil functions. Treatment with 500 mg/d of vitamin C for 30 days resulted in a significant improvement of neutrophil function.

>—R. Levy and F. Schlaeffer, ''Successful Treatment of a Patient with Recurrent Furunculosis by Vitamin C: Improvement of Clinical Course and of Impaired Neutrophil Functions,'' *International Journal of Dermatology,* 32(11), November 1993, p. 832-834.

Obesity

This double-blind, placebo-controlled study found that 19 severely obese subjects given 3 g/day of ascorbic acid over a six week period lost significantly more weight than controls.

>—G.J. Naylor, et al., ''A Double Blind Placebo Controlled Trial of Ascorbic Acid in Obesity,'' *Nutr Health,* 4(1), 1985, p. 25-28.

Ocular Inflammation

This study found that a decrease in the ascorbic acid concentration within the aqueous humor of a rabbit eye was associated with an experimentally induced inflammatory response. Other in vivo studies have shown activated leukocytes diminished the amount of ascorbic acid in the eye. Based on these findings, the authors suggest ascorbic acid offers extracelluar protection for the ocular tissues against oxygen radicals and metabolites released by infiltrating leukocytes during ocular inflammation when present in the aqueous humor in large amounts.

—R.N. Williams and C.A. Paterson, "A Protective Role for Ascorbic Acid During Inflammatory Episodes in the Eye," *Exp Eye Res,* 42(3), March 1986, p. 211-218.

This study found that myeloperoxidase was inhibited from isolated rabbit leukocytes by ascorbic acid, suggesting that ascorbic acid might be considered as an endogenous anti-inflammatory agent in the eye.

—R.N. Williams, et al., "Ascorbic Acid Inhibits the Activity of Polymorphonuclear Leukocytes in Inflamed Ocular Tissues," *Exp Eye Res,* 39(3), September 1984, p. 261-265.

Opiate Addiction

This study demonstrated the administration of 1g/l of ascorbic acid in drinking water for 3 days or in a dose of 200 mg/kg 3 times daily for 3 days greatly decreased the withdrawal effects in guinea-pigs given 15 mg/kg s.c. 2 hours following a single dose of 15 mg/kg s.c. of morphine sulphate.

—P.A. Johnston and L.A. Chahl, "Chronic Treatment with Ascorbic Acid Inhibits the Morphine Withdrawal Response in Guinea-Pigs," *Neuroscience Letters,* 135(1), January 20, 1992, p. 23-27.

Paget's Disease

In this study, Paget's disease patients were either treated for 2 weeks with ascorbic acid and calcitonin together or calcitonin alone. 73% of patients receiving the combined treatment reported pain relief compared with 85% taking calcitonin alone. Yet 62% of the combined treatment patients claimed major pain relief compared to only 36% to the calcitonin only patients.

—M. Smethurst, et al., "Combined Therapy with Ascorbic Acid and Calcitonin for the Relief of Bone Pain in Paget's Disease," *Acta Vitaminol Enzymol,* 3(1), 1981, p. 8-11.

Pancreatitis

This study examined vitamin C and ascorbic acid levels in the fasting plasma samples of 29 pancreatitis patients, 27 patients with other acute abdominal crisis, and 30 healthy controls. Results indicated that abdominal crisis is associated with low plasma levels of vitamin C. Pancreatitis makes the problem worse since as oxidative stress that accompanies the condition denatures the available vitamin. In light of these findings, the authors suggest that pancreatitis patients may benefit from large doses of ascorbic acid as a way of enhancing antioxidant defense.

—P. Scott, et al., "Vitamin C Status in Patients with Acute Pancreatitis," *British Journal of Surgery,* 80(6), June 1993, p. 750-754.

Parkinson's Disease

This study examined the effects of ascorbate and alpha-tocopherol administered to Parkinson's disease patients in high doses. Results indicate that intake of both substances may retard the progression of the disease.

—S. Fahn, "A Pilot Trial of High-Dose Alpha-Tocopherol and Ascorbate in Early Parkinson's Disease," *Annals of Neurology,* 32 Suppl, 1992, p. S128-S132.

This double-blind, crossover study found that ascorbic acid administered to six patients with Parkinson's disease resulted in a modest improvement in the performance of motor functions.

—D.K. Reilly, et al., "On-off Effects in Parkinson's Disease: A Controlled Investigation of Ascorbic Acid Therapy," *Advanc Neurol,* 37, 1983, p. 51-60.

This review article on anti-Parkinsonian therapies notes that vitamin C as well as deprenyl have been shown to prevent the inhibitory effect of dopamine and levodopa on brain mitochondrial complex I activity.

—S. Przedborski, et al., "Antiparkinsonian Therapies and Brain Mitochondrial Complex I Activity," *Movement Disorder,* 10(3), May 1995, p. 312-317.

Results of this study showed that levodopa toxicity was prevented in a human neuroblastoma cell line by the administration of 10(-3)M of ascorbic acid and 10(-4) M of deprenyl. The authors do not believe the mechanisms by which each functions are related.

—B. Pardo, et al., "Ascorbic Acid Protects Against Levodopa-induced Neurotoxicity on a Catecholamine-rich Human Neuroblastoma Cell Line," *Movement Disorders,* 8(3), July 1993, p. 278-284.

In this study, 21 Parkinsonian patients suffering from motor complications were given a solution of levodopa-carbidopa and ascorbic acid (LCASS). The number of hours with good functional capacity improved in eight patients who stayed on the therapy for 16.8 months and symptoms like dystonia and akathisia ceased in cases where they had been present prior to LCAAS treatment. Patients who continued the LSAAS treatment also reduced their reliance on other anti-Parkinsonian drugs.

—G. Linazasoro and A. Gorospe, [Treatment of Complicated Parkinson Disease with a Solution of Levodopa-Carbidopa and Ascorbic Acid], *Neurologia,* 10(6), June-July, 1995, p. 220-223.

This study found a significant association between vitamin C deficiency and Parkinson's disease when new residents were medically screened prior to admission in a nursing home.

—S.C. Yapa, "Detection of Subclinical Ascorbate Deficiency in Early Parkinson's Disease," *Public Health,* 106(5), September 1992, p. 393-395.

Periodontal Disease

This study found that gingival bleeding increased significantly during a period of experimental depletion of ascorbic acid and returned to baseline values following its repletion in healthy men aged 25 to 43 years old.

—P.J. Leggott, et al., "Effects of Ascorbic Acid Depletion and Supplementation on Periodontal Health and Subgingival Microflora in Humans," *Journal of Dental Research,* 70(12), December 1991, p. 1531-1536.

In this general review article on the role of vitamin C and oral health, the author notes that vitamin C's role in maintaining healthy teeth and gingivae remains unchallenged.

—A.B. Rubinoff, et al., "Vitamin C and Oral Health," *Journal of the Canadian Dental Association,* 55(9), September 1989, p. 705-707.

This study found a direct relationship between low ascorbic acid status and gingival inflammation in healthy young men between the ages of 19-28 whose ascorbic acid intake was carefully controlled over a 3 month period.

—P.J. Leggott, et al., "The Effect of Controlled Ascorbic Acid Depletion and Supplementation on Periodontal Health," *Journal of Periodontology,* 57(8), August 1986, p. 480-485.

Pulmonary Function

This study, part of the first National Health and Nutrition Examination Survey (NHANES 1), found a positively significant relationship between dietary vitamin C intake the level of pulmonary function as measured in forced expiratory volume in 1 s.

—J. Schwartz and S.T Weiss, "Relationship Between Dietary Vitamin C Intake and Pulmonary Function in the First National Health and Nutrition Examination Survey (NHANES I)," *American Journal of Clinical Nutrition,* 59(1), January 1994, p. 110-114.

Respiration

This randomized, placebo-controlled study examined the effect of 600 mg of vitamin C a day on incidence of symptoms of upper-respiratory-tract (URT) infections in ultramarathoners. 14 days after the target race, 33% of supplemented subjects reported URT symptoms compared to 68% of the controls, a significant difference.

—E.M. Peters, et al., "Vitamin C Supplementation Reduces the Incidence of Postrace Symptoms of Upper-Respiratory-Tract Infection in Ultramarathon Runners," *American Journal of Clinical Nutrition,* (2), February 1993, p.170-174.

This double-blind, randomized study found that pretreatment with 500 mg 4 times a day of ascorbic acid for 3 days totally prevented NO2-induced airway hyperresponsiveness in normal subjects.

—V. Mohsenin, "Effect of Vitamin C on NO2-induced Airway Hyperresponsiveness in Normal Subjects: A Randomized Double-blind Experiment.," *American Review of Respiratory Disease,* 136(6), December 1987, p. 1408-1411.

In this study, mice were given 200 mg/kg/d vitamin C and then exposed to 3 Streptococcus pneumonia intratracheally to assess the effects of vitamin C on pulmonary antibacterial mechanisms. Results indicate that the pulmonary defense mechanisms were altered by high amounts of vitamin C, yet they did not offer a significant advantage to the host.

—A.L. Esposito, "Ascorbate Modulates Antibacterial Mechanisms in Experimental Pneumococcal Pneumonia," *American Review of Respiratory Disease,* 133(4), April 1986, p. 643-647.

This double-blind, crossover study found that 2 g of vitamin C administered to patients with allergic rhinititis produced a significant positive effect one hour after treatment on bronchial responsiveness to inhaled histamine relative to controls.

—C. Bucca, et al., "Effect of Vitamin C on Histamine Bronchial Responsiveness of Patients with Allergic Rhinitis," *Annals of Allergy,* 65(4), October 1990, p. 311-314.

Results of this double-blind study suggest that chronic ascorbate deficiency may attenuate histamine bronchial responsiveness in heavy smokers. Under such conditions, short-term treatment with 2 g of vitamin C can heighten the bronchoconstrictive response to inhaled histamine.

    —C. Bucca, et al., ''Effects of Vitamin C on Airway Responsiveness to Inhaled Histamine in Heavy Smokers,'' *European Respir Journal,* 2(3), March 1989, p. 229-233.

Retinal Light Damage

This study compared ascorbate treated rats exposed to various cycles of intermittent light to untreated rats. Exposure to 2 or 3 hours of intermittent light caused a five to sixfold increase in phagosome density in untreated rats compared to unexposed controls. Ascorbate treated rats experienced no increase in phagosome density under the same conditions. Based on these results, the authors argue that ascorbate's protective effect could be the result of its ability to prevent rod outer segment shedding and phagocytosis under severe light.

    —J.C. Blanks, et al., ''Ascorbate Treatment Prevents Accumulation of Phagosomes in RPE in Light Damage,'' *Invest Ophthalmol Vis Sci,* 33(10), September 1992, p. 2814-2821.

This study examined dark-reared rats supplemented with ascorbic acid and exposed to multiple doses of intermittent light for retinal damage compared with dark-reared and cyclic-light-reared rats not receiving ascorbic acid. Results indicated that ascorbic acid had a protective effect on the eye of dark-reared rats by decreasing the irreversible Type I form of light damage. The authors suggest that ascorbate appears to shift light damage to the Type II form typical of cyclic-light-reared animals.

    —D.T. Organisciak, et al., ''The Protective Effect of Ascorbic Acid in Retinal Light Damage of Rats Exposed to Intermittent Light,'' *Invest Ophthalmol Vis Sci,* 31(7), July 1990, p. 1195-1202.

This study compared the light damaged retinas of rats supplemented with ascorbate against those that weren't. Retinas of supplemented rats had significantly less damage that unsupplemented rats when examined 6-13 days after hours of light exposure.

    —Z.Y. Li, et al., ''Amelioration of Photic Injury in Rat Retina by Ascorbic Acid: A Histopathologic Study,'' *Invest Ophthalmol Vis Sci,* 26(11), November 1985, p. 1589-1598.

This study found that dark-reared and cyclic-light-reacted rats supplemented with L-ascorbic acid, sodium ascorbate, and dehydroascorbate suffered less loss of rhodopsin and photoreceptor cell nuclei following exposure to intense light than unsupplemented animals. Supplementation proved to be effective only prior to light exposure.

    —D.T. Organisciak, et al., ''The Protective Effect of Ascorbate in Retinal Light Damage of Rats,'' *Invest Ophthalmol Vis Sci,* November 1985, p. 1580-1588

Schizophrenia

This paper reports on a single case of 37-year-old schizophrenic who was observed to have benefited from ascorbic acid supplementation to his ongoing neuropleptic medication.

    —R. Sandyk and J.D. Kanofsky, ''Vitamin C in the Treatment of Schizophrenia,'' *International Journal of Neuroscience,* 68(1-2), January 1993, p. 67-71.

Sickle Cell Anemia

This study found that concentrations of ascorbic acid and alpha-tocopherol were significantly depressed in sickle cell anemia. The author argues that such depleted antioxidant levels might be a factor in sickle cell anemia manifestations such as haemolysis and increased susceptibility of infection.

—E.U. Essien, "Plasma Levels of Retinol, Ascorbic Acid and Alpha-Tocopherol in Sickle Cell Anaemia," *Central African Journal of Medicine,* 41(2), February 1995, p. 48-50.

This study found that not only did sickle cell patients suffer from low levels of plasma ascorbic acid, but that sickle cell pretreatment with ascorbic acid offers membrane protection against hydrogen peroxide induced lipid peroxidation

—S.K. Jain, et al., "Reduced Levels of Plasma Ascorbic Acid (Vitamin C) in Sickle Cell Disease Patients: its Possible Role in the Oxidant Damage to Sickle Cells in Vivo," *Clin Chim Acta,* 149(2-3), July 15, 1985, p. 257-261.

Smoking Cessation

This study involved two clinical smoking cessation trials using ascorbic acid aerosol in a dose of approximately 1 mg a puff up to a maximum of 300 mg/day. In the first trial users of the ascorbic acid device who also received counseling showed significantly greater abstinence rates versus those only receiving counseling 3 weeks into the study. Trial 2 compared the effectiveness of different ascorbic acid delivery systems and found little difference between them. Based on their findings, the authors suggest that such uses of ascorbic acid may be an effective and novel way to promote smoking cessation.

—E.D. Levin, et al., "Clinical Trials Using Ascorbic Acid Aerosol to Aid Smoking Cessation," *Drug Alcohol Depend,* 33(3), October 1993, p. 211-223.

Stress

This study examined the effects of 100 mg/kg of ascorbic acid on the stress response in chickens. One day following administration of ascorbic acid chickens were chilled at 6 degree C for one hour and compared to a group of unsupplemented chickens receiving the same exposure. The ascorbic acid chickens had significantly lower Heterophil:lymphocyte ratios than controls. Chickens fed the ascorbic acid diet also showed increased resistance to virus Mycoplasma gallisepticum infection, a secondary Escherichia coli infection, and to primary E. coli infection.

—W.B. Gross, "Effects of Ascorbic Acid on Stress and Disease in Chickens," *Avian Disease,* 36(3), July-September, p. 688-692.

Stroke

This randomized, 20-year follow-up study found a significant relationship between risk of death from stroke but not coronary heart disease and vitamin C in people over the age of 65.

—C.R. Gale, et al., "Vitamin C and Risk of Death from Stroke and Coronary Heart Disease in Cohort of Elderly People," *British Medical Journal,* 310(6994), June 17, 1995, p. 1563-1566.

Tetanus

This study examined the effect of 1000 mg/d intravenous intake of ascorbic acid in tetanus patients ranging from 1-30 years old. Thirty one patient in the 1-12 year age group received ascorbic acid treatment along with conventional antitetanus therapy and none died compared to a 74.2% mortality rate among patients taking conventional antitetanus therapy, but not ascorbic acid. Mortality rates in 13-30 year old group between patients taking ascorbic acids and those not were 37% and 67.8% respectively.

> —J.K. Jahan, et al., "Effect of Ascorbic Acid in the Treatment of Tetanus," *Bangladesh Medical Research Council Bulletin,* 10(1), June 1985, p. 24-28

Ultraviolet Radiation

This article notes that topical application of vitamin C has been reported to significantly increase cutaneous vitamin C levels in pigs. Evidence is also presented that UV radiation can deplete skin vitamin C levels, thus weakening the skin's ability to protect the body as a whole.

> —D. Darr, et al., Topical Vitamin C Protects Porcine Skin from Ultraviolet Radiation-induced Damage," *British Journal of Dermatology,* 127(3), September 1992, p. 247-253.

Vitamin B-12 Deficiency

This study found that diets containing up to 150 mg of ascorbic significantly raised B-12 values significantly in vitamin B-12 deficient rats.

> —S. W. Thenen, "Megadose Effects of Vitamin C on Vitamin B-12 Status in the Rat," *Journal of Nutrition,* 119(8), August, 1989, p. 1107-114.

Wound Healing

In this study, the authors report success in wound healing using doses of vitamin C between 500 to 3000 mg a day in subjects recovering from surgery, decubital ulcers, leg ulcers, and other unspecified injuries. Mention is made of a previous study showing that genetic impairment of collagen synthesis was treated by the administration of 4 g of ascorbic acid in an 8-year-old boy with type VI Ehler-Danlos syndrome

> —W.M. Ringsdorf, Jr. and E. Cheraskin, "Vitamin C and Human Wound Healing," *Oral Surg Oral Med Oral Pathol,* 53(3), March 1982, p. 231-236.

This study found that pressure sores in elderly patients suffering from femoral neck fractures were associated with deficiencies of leucocyte vitamin C.

> —H.F. Goode, et al., "Vitamin C Depletion and Pressure Sores in Elderly Patients with Femoral Neck Fractures," *British Medical Journal,* 305(6859), October 17, 1992, p. 925-927.

Results of this study demonstrated that levels of ascorbic acid ranging from 50-300 mg/ml were necessary for optimal flexor tendon repair in animals in vivo.

> —J.E. Russell and P.R. Manske, "Ascorbic Acid Requirement for Optimal Flexor Tendon Repair in Vitro," *Journal of Orthop Res,* 9(5), September 1991, p. 714-719.

This study demonstrated that a 500 mg/kg dose per day of ascorbic acid given for 3 days significantly enhanced the decline in peroxidase activity provoked by inflammatory agents in the feet of mice.

> —D. Nowak, et al., "Ascorbic Acid Enhances the Decrease in Peroxidase Activity in Inflamed Tissues of Mice," *Arch Immunol Ther Exp,* 41(5-6), 1993, p. 321-326.

This study used burned guinea pigs to investigate vitamin C's effects on metabolic and immune response trauma. Results found that vitamin C administered in large amounts had positive effects on the maintenance of metabolism and body weight following burn trauma.

>   —J.L. Nelson, et al., "Metabolic and Immune Effects of Enteral Ascorbic Acid after Burn Trauma," *Burns,* 18(2), April 1992, p. 92-97.

In studying burn injuries in the hind paws of dogs, this study found that the administration of 14 mg/kg/hr of ascorbic acid on the site of burn injury decreased early postburn microvascular leakage of fluid and protein.

>   —T. Matsuda, et al., "Effects of High-dose Vitamin C Administration on Postburn Microvascular Fluid and Protein Flux," *Journal of Burn Care Rehabilitation,* 13(5), September-October 1992, p. 560-566.

■ VITAMIN D

Bone Loss

This double-blind, placebo-controlled study examined the effects of 15,000 IU of vitamin D on corctical bone loss in elderly women. Results showed that the treatment significantly reduced the rate of bone loss relative to controls.

>   —B.E. Nordin, et al., "A Prospective Trial of the Effect of Vitamin D Supplementation on Metacarpal Bone Loss in Elderly Women," *American Journal of Clinical Nutrition,* 42(3), September 1985, p. 470-474.

Results of this double-blind, placebo-controlled study showed that the administration of 500 IU daily of vitamin D led to significant reductions in wintertime bone loss and improved net bone density in women with a normal intake of 100 IU daily.

>   —B. Dawson-Hughes, et al., "Effect of Vitamin D Supplementation on Wintertime and Overall Bone Loss in Healthy Postmenopausal Women," *Annals of Internal Medicine,* 115(7), October 1, 1991, p. 505-512.

Results of this study found that vitamin D supplementation at doses of 4000 IU/m2 body surface area/day for 6 months led to improvements in disabled youth bone status.

>   —M.H. Fischer, et al., "Bone Status in Nonambulant, Epileptic, Institutionalized Youth. Improvement with Vitamin D Therapy," *Clinical Pediatrics,* 27(10), October 1988, p. 499-505.

This double-blind, placebo-controlled study examined the effects of 400 IU of vitamin D on bone loss and turnover in elderly women over a two year period. Results showed that the supplementation decreased PTH secretion slightly and led to increased bone mineral density at the femoral neck.

>   —M.E. Ooms, et al., "Prevention of Bone Loss by Vitamin D Supplementation in Elderly Women: A Randomized Double-blind Trial," *Journal of Clinical Endocrinol Metab,* 80(4), April 1995, p. 1052-1058.

Cancer

This article reports on results from a 19-year-long study of 1954 Chicago men which showed that an intake of greater than 3.75 micrograms per day of vitamin D was associated with a 50% reduction of colorectal cancer. Another large study found that moderately elevated concentrations of 25-hydroxyvitamin D ranging in dosage from 65-100 nmol/L showed even stronger association with reduction in incidence of the disease among a population of 25,620 individuals.

> —C.F. Garland, et al., "Can Colon Cancer Incidence and Death Rates be Reduced with Calcium and Vitamin D?" *American Journal of Clinical Nutrition,* 54(1 Suppl), July 1991, p. 193S-201S.

Results of this study showed that vitamin D analogues coupled with retinoids inhibit human pancreatic cancer cell growth.

> —G. Zugmaier, et al., "Growth-inhibitory Effects of Vitamin D Analogues and Retinoids on Human Pancreatic Cancer Cells," *British Journal of Cancer,* 73(11), June 1996, 1341-1346.

Results of this in vitro study indicated that vitamin D may reduce the risk of prostate cancer in humans.

> —R.J. Skowronski, et al., "Vitamin D and Prostate Cancer: 1,25 Dihydroxyvitamin D3 Receptors and Actions in Human Prostate Cancer Cell Lines," *Endocrinology,* 132(5), May 1993, p. 1952-1960.

Results of this study found that increasing dietary vitamin D and calcium levels in DMH exposed rats can reduce the number of colon tumors.

> —M.M. Beaty, et al., "The Effects of Dietary Calcium and Vitamin D on Colon Carcinogenesis Induced by 1,2-Dimethylhydrazine, *FASEB Journal,* 5(5), 1991, p. A926.

Results of this study found that vitamin D inhibited cell proliferation in normal and premalignant rectal epithelium as well as suppressed growth in vitro of a colorectal cancer cell line.

> —M.G. Thomas, et al., "Vitamin D and its Metabolites Inhibit Cell Proliferation in Human Rectal Mucosa and a Colon Cancer Cell Line," *Gut,* 33(12), December 1992, p. 1660-1663.

Results of this study showed that vitamin D inhibited the growth of human retinoblastoma in transgenic mice.

> —D.M. Albert, et al., "The Antineoplastic Effect of Vitamin D in Transgenic Mice with Retinoblastoma," *Invest Ophthalmol Vis Sci,* 33(8), July 1992, p. 2354-2364.

This study examined the effects of dietary vitamin D and calcium on chemical-induced colon cancer in rats. Results showed a 45% lower total tumor incidence and tumor incidence in the distal colon for rats receiving highest doses of vitamin D and calcium relative to controls.

> —M.M. Beaty, et al., "Influence of Dietary Calcium and Vitamin D on Colon Epithelial Cell Proliferation and 1,2-dimethylhydrazine-induced Colon Carcinogenesis in Rats Fed High Fat Diets," *Journal of Nutrition,* 123(1), January 1993, p. 144-152.

This review article argues that the present data support the view that vitamin D may be effective in the treatment of prostate cancer.

> —D. Feldman, et al., "Vitamin D and Prostate Cancer," *Adv Exp Med Biol,* 375, 1995, p. 53-63.

This review article notes that in vitro and in vivo studies have found that vitamin D analogs can inhibit breast cancer cell growth.

> —S. Christakos, "Vitamin D and Breast Cancer," *Adv Exp Med Biol*, 364, 1994, p. 115-118.

Cardiovascular/Coronary Heart Disease

This double-blind, placebo-controlled study examined the effects of the vitamin D analog, alphacalcidol, on patients with marginal, intermittent hypercalcaemia. Results showed that the administration of 1 microgram alphacalcidol raised serum calcium by 0.07 mmol/l significantly reduced diastolic blood pressure over a 6 month period.

> —L. Lind, et al., "Blood Pressure is Lowered by Vitamin D (alphacalcidol) During Long-term Treatment of Patients with Intermittent Hypercalcaemia. A Double-blind, Placebo-controlled Study," *Acta Med Scand*, 222(5), 1987, p. 423-427.

Results of this double-blind, placebo-controlled study showed that 1 microgram per day of vitamin D taken for 6 months reduced blood pressure in hypercalcemic patients.

> —L. Lind, et al., "Hypertension in Primary Hyperparathyroidism—reduction of Blood Pressure by Long-term Treatment with Vitamin D (alphacalcidol). A Double-blind, Placebo-controlled Study," *American Journal of Hypertension*, 1(4 Pt 1), October 1988, p. 397-402.

In this study, serum levels of 1,25-(OH)2-vitamin D, 25-OH- vitamin D, and blood pressure were examined in 34 middle-aged men and metabolic cardiovascular risk factors were evaluated. Results found an inverse correlation between blood pressure, VLDL triglycerides, and to triglyceride removal at the intravenous fat tolerance test

> —L. Lind, et al., "Vitamin D is Related to Blood Pressure and Other Cardiovascular Risk Factors in Middle-aged Men," *American Journal of Hypertension*, 8(9), September 1995, p. 894-901.

Crohn's Disease

Results of this study showed that supplementation with 1000 IU per day of vitamin D over a period of one year prevented bone loss in Crohn's disease patients.

> —H. Vogelsang, et al., "Prevention of Bone Mineral Loss in Patients with Crohn's Disease by Long-term Oral Vitamin D Supplementation," *European Journal of Gastroenterol Hepatol*, 7(7), July 1995, p. 609-614.

Diabetes

In this study, 61 diabetics with associated osteomalacia received vitamin D in daily doses between 42,000 to 85,000 i.u. and 470-700 mg of calcium. Results showed an average rise in the calcium level of 0.15 mmol/l and decline in blood sugar level of 1.69 mmol/l after 6 weeks of treatment.

> —J. Kocian, [Diabetic Osteopathy. Favorable Effect of Treatment of Osteomalacia with Vitamin D and Calcium on High Blood Glucose Levels], *Vnitr Lek*, 38(4), April 1992, p. 352-356.

Migraine

This article reports on the cases of two postmenopausal women suffering from severe migraines who experienced dramatic improvements following supplementation with vitamin D and calcium.
        —S. Thys-Jacobs, "Alleviation of Migraines with Therapeutic Vitamin D and Calcium," *Headache,* 34(10), November-December 1994, p. 590-592.

Nephrotic Syndrome

Results of this study showed that low levels of vitamin D in patients with nephrotic syndrome were normalized following long-term supplementation with daily doses of 25 micrograms of vitamin D3 per os.
        —B. Haldimann & U. Trechsel, "Vitamin D Replacement Therapy in Patients with the Nephrotic Syndrome," *Miner Electrolyte Metab,* 9(3), 1983, p. 154-156.

Osteoporosis

Results of this study indicated that the primary effect of oral supplementation with vitamin D and of calcium per day in patients with osteoporosis was a decrease in bone turnover.
        —B.L. Riggs, et al., "Effects of Oral Therapy with Calcium and Vitamin D in Primary Osteoporosis," *Journal of Clinical Endocrinol Metab,* 42(6), June 1976, p. 1139-1144.

This review article argues that RDA levels of 200 IU of vitamin D may be too low in the elderly, noting that doses of 800 IU per day have been found to lower the incidence of osteoporotic fractures.
        —J.C. Gallagher, "Vitamin D Metabolism and Therapy in Elderly Subjects," *Southern Medical Journal,* 85(8), August 1992, p. 2S43-2S47.

Pregnancy

Results of this double-blind, placebo-controlled study found that pregnant women receiving supplements of 1000 IU per day of vitamin D experienced more rapid weight gain than controls and demonstrated better protein-calorie nutrition. Results also showed maternal weight gain correlated with postpartum levels of both retinol binding protein and thyroid binding prealbumin. Close to twice the number of infants of mother not receiving supplements weighed less than 2500 g at birth and had significantly lower retinol binding protein levels than infants of the mothers who received the supplements.
        —J.D. Maxwell, et al., "Vitamin D Supplements Enhance Weight Gain and Nutritional Status in Pregnant Asians," *British Journal of Obstet Gynaecol,* 88(10), October 1981, p. 987-991.

Results of this study showed that fetal birth weight was significantly increased for women receiving two large doses of 600,000 U each in months 7 and 8 of pregnancy relative to controls.
        —R.K. Marya, et al., "Effects of Vitamin D Supplementation in Pregnancy," *Gynecol Obstet Invest,* 12(3), 1981, p. 155-161.

Psoriasis

This review article cites studies showing the efficacy of vitamin D3 analogs in providing significant improvements of psoriatic lesions in humans.
        —O.E. Araugo, et al., "Vitamin D Therapy in Psoriasis," *DICP,* 25(7-8), July-August, 1991, p. 835-839.

This review article cites studies showing the efficacy of vitamin D3 analogs in the treatment of psoriasis in humans.

—T. Menne & K. Larsen, "Psoriasis Treatment with Vitamin D Derivatives," *Semin Dermatol,* 11(4), December 1992, p. 278-283.

Rickets

This article reports on the cases of two sibings with absent vitamin D receptors who experienced a healing of severe rickets with long-term supplementation of high doses of vitamin D.

—K. Kruse & E. Feldmann, "Healing of Rickets During Vitamin D Therapy Despite Defective Vitamin D Receptors in Two Siblings with Vitamin D-dependent Rickets Type II," *Journal of Pediatrics,* 126(1), January 1995, p. 145-148.

In this study, 42 rickets patients deficient in vitamin D received a single-day large dose vitamin D supplement. The treatment proved to safe and effective, producing a response within 4 to 7 days of administration.

—B.R. Shah & L. Finberg, "Single-day Therapy for Nutritional Vitamin D-deficiency Rickets: A Preferred Method," *Journal of Pediatrics,* 125(3), September 1994, p. 487-490.

■ VITAMIN E

Abetalipoproteinemia

This study reported on the cases of two male patients, one adult and one child, suffering from abetalipoproteinemia who were successfully maintained using high doses of vitamins A and E.

—D.R. Illingworth, et al., "Abetalipoproteinemia. Report of Two Cases and Review of Therapy," *Arch Neurol,* 37(10), October 1980, p. 659-662.

This study documented the cases of eight patients with abetalipoproteinaemia whom were kept from progressing upon the administration of vitamin A and E therapy.

—S. Bishara, et al., "Combined Vitamin A and E Therapy Prevents Retinal Electrophysiological Deterioration in Abetalipoproteinaemia," *British Journal of Ophthalmology,* 66(12), December 1982, p. 767-770.

This study found that early therapy with vitamin E may prevent and delays the onset of neurological complications in patients with abetalipoproteinaemia and that vitamin E can reverse the neuropathy associated with established lesions. Neurological manifestations similar to those that result from untreated abetalipoproteinaemia have also been shown to benefit from vitamin E supplementation as have chronic fat absorption disorders.

—D.P. Muller, et al., "Vitamin E and Neurological Function: Abetalipoproteinaemia and Other Disorders of Fat Absorption," *Ciba Found Symp,* 101, 1983, p. 106-121.

This article notes that studies in vitamin E-deficient humans, monkeys, and rats have demonstrated the importance of vitamin E in optimal neurological function. Studies on abetalipoproteinaemia and other chronic fat malabsorptive states have also found vitamin E has provided similar findings.

—D.P. Muller, et al., "The Role of Vitamin E in the Treatment of the Neurological Features of Abetalipoproteinaemia and Other Disorders of Fat Absorption," *Journal of Inherit Metab Dis,* 8(Suppl) , 1985, p. 88-92.

This study reports on a single case of a 16-year-old girl successfully treated for the progressive neuropathy and myopathy associated with abetalipoproteinemia using oral doses as high as 3200 mg per day of vitamin E over 7 years.

—R.A. Hegele and A. Angel, "Arrest of Neuropathy and Myopathy in Abetalipoproteinemia with High-Dose Vitamin E Therapy," *Canadian Medical Association Journal,* 132(1), January 1, 1985, p. 41-44.

Acne

This study found that acne patients treated with 0.2mg of selenium and 10 mg of tocopheryl succinate twice daily for 6-12 weeks experienced positive results.

—G. Michaelsson and L.E. Edqvist, "Erythrocyte Glutathione Peroxidase Activity in Acne Vulgaris and the Effect of Selenium and Vitamin E Treatment," *Acta Derm Venereol,* 64(1), 1984, p. 9-14.

Aging

This study examined the relationship between aging and the concentration of vitamin E in the sciatic nerves of rats. Results suggest a relationship between vitamin E and (n-6) PUFA in the Peripheral Nervous System membranes throughout development and aging.

—M. Clement and J.M. Bourre, "Alteration of Alpha-Tocopherol Content in the Developing and Aging Peripheral Nervous System: Persistence of High Correlations with Total and Specific (n-6) Polyunsaturated Fatty Acids," *Journal of Neurochemistry,* 54(6), June 1990, p. 2110-2117.

This study found that rats fed a diet enriched with 0.1 ppm of sodium selenite per 100 g of diet and 6 mg of alpha-tocopherol per 100 g of diet over 12 months experienced a reduction in the production of lipid peroxides in the serum and liver. Such findings prompted the authors to conclude that selenium and vitamin E inhibit the aging process in rats.

—B. Panczenko-Kresowska and S. Ziemlanski, "The Effect of Long-Term Selenium and Vitamin E-Enriched Diet on the Content of Lipid Peroxides and Cholesterol in Rats," *Acta Physiol Pol,* 38(4), July 1987, p. 346-352.

This review article notes the many positive aspects of vitamin E with respect to the aging process, including its ability to modify free radicals, deficiency of protein synthesis, ameliorate the functionality of important body organs, help maintain bone matrix trophysm.

—M. Passeri and D. Provvedini, [Vitamin E in Geriatric Physiopathology], *Acta Vitaminol Enzymol,* 5(1), 1983, p. 53-63.

This review article notes the role of oxidative damage to cell membranes as a key element in the aging process and stresses the importance of vitamin E as means of combating it.

—F. Pentimone, et al., [Vitamin E in the Aged], *Clin Ter,* 144(6), June 1994, p. 521-525.

This study examined the effects of dietary selenium and vitamin E on the age pigment accumulation in the rat superior cervical ganglion, vagal ganglion and dorsal root ganglion. In the dorsal root ganglion, vitamin E was found to regulate age pigment content and a deficiency in vitamin E resulted in a 3-times increase in age pigment content at 8 months old.

> —J. Koistinaho, et al., "Effect of Vitamin E and Selenium Supplement on the Aging Peripheral, Neurons of the Male Sprague-Dawley Rat," *Mech Ageing Dev,* 51(1), January 1990, p. 63-72.

This study begins by pointing out that choline acetyltransferase (ChAT) is reduced in the hippocampus and neocortex of patients with Alzheimer's disease and other problems related to aging brains. Researchers then tested the effects of d-alpha-Tocopherol supplementation on cholinergic hypofunction in aging rats. Results showed that when given 24 hours and 15 minutes before AF84A administration, vitamin E significantly decreased the lesion-inducing effects of AF64A in hippocampal choline acetyltransferase activity. Vitamin E administered to aging rats in doses of 50 mg/kg over 30 days also significantly restored enzyme activity in the striatum.

> —Y. Maneesub, et al., "Partial Restoration of Choline Acetyltransferase Activities in Aging and AF64A-Lesioned Rat Brains by Vitamin E," *Neurochem Int,* 22(5), May 1993, p. 487-491.

Results of this study showed that vitamin E, manntiol, and dexamethasone have significant cerebral protective effects in dogs and that such effects are multiplied when administered together and with PFC, an artificial blood substitute.

> —K. Mizoi, et al., "Development of New Cerebral Protective Agents: The Free Radical Scavengers," *Neurol Res,* 8(2), June 1986, p. 75-80.

Results of this study found that the administration of an antioxidant medicamentous combination made from vitamin E, vitamin C and Rutin to aged and sick patients modified lipoperoxidation and enzymatic protection system.

> —A. Courtiere, et al., [Lipid Peroxidation in Aged Patients. Influence of an Antioxidant Combination (vitamin C-vitamin E-rutin)], *Therapie,* 44(1), January-February 1989, p. 13-17.

AIDS/HIV

This study examined the effects of vitamin E on LP-BM5 retrovirus-induced murine AIDS. Results found that a 15-fold dietary vitamin E increase had the following effects: restored concentrations of vitamins A, E, zinc, and copper in the liver, serum, and thymus. Partially restored production of IL-2 and IFN-gamma by splenocytes. Normalized elevated production levels of IL-4, IL-5, and IL-6 by splenocytes in vitro. Normalized elevated release of TNF-alpha, IgA and IgG produced by splenocytes in vitro. Prevented suppression of splenocyte proliferation and natural killer cell activity.

> —Y. Wang, et al., "Nutritional Status and Immune Responses in Mice with Murine AIDS are Normalized by Vitamin E Supplementation," *Journal of Nutrition,* 124(10), October 1994, p. 2024-2032.

This study examined the ability of vitamin E to stimulate erythroid progenitor cells and to inhibit replication of HIV. Results showed that the administration of 50 mg/kg per day of vitamin E over 5 days or 0.4 U per day of Epo over 5 days to CD-1 mice fed AZT protected their bone marrow by 75% and 86%, respectively, relative to controls. Vitamin E inhibited HIV replication in MT4 cells with an ED50 of 15 ug/ml in vitro. 15 ug/ml of vitamin E potentiated the anti-HIV activity of AZT 8-fold by lowering the ED95 from 0.5 uM to 0.06 uM.

 —S.R. Gogu, et al., "Protection of Zidovudine (AZT)-Induced Bone Marrow Toxicity and Potentiation of Anti-HIV Activity with Vitamin E," *90th Annual Meeting of the American Society for Microbiology May13-17, 1990,* Anaheim, CA, 1990, 338, 1990.

Results of this study showed that the addition of alpha-D-tocopherol acid succinate (ATS) (doses of 5 to 15 micrograms/ml) to MT4 cells and murine hemotopoietic progenitor cells treated with AZT resulted in increased anti-HIV activity relative to the use of AZT alone.

 —S.R. Gogu, et al., "Increased Therapeutic Efficacy of Zidovudine in Combination with Vitamin E," *Biochem Biophys Res Commun,* 165(1), November 30, 1989, p. 401-407.

Results of this study showed that incubation of human Jurkat T cells with vitamin E acetate or alpha-tocopheryl succinate (10 microM to 1mM) exhibited a concentration dependent inhibition of NF-kappa B activation. Such findings support the possible use of vitamin E derivites as a treatment for AIDS.

 —Y.J. Suzuki and L. Packer, "Inhibition of NF-kappa B Activation by Vitamin E Derivatives," *Biochem Biophys Res Commun,* 193(1), May 28, 1993, p. 277-283.

This study demonstrated that increasing dietary vitamin E 15-fold (160 IU/liter) normalized hepatic and serum vitamin E levels normally reduced by infection with retrovirus. Vitamin E supplementation restored significantly the release of interleukin-2 (IL) and interferon-gamma by splenocytes which are suppressed by infection and significantly slowed the development of splenomegaly and hypergammaglobulinemia induced by infection. Vitamin E also inhibited infection-induced elevated production of IL-4 and IL-6 by splenoyctes, and increased levels of IL-6 and tumor necrosis factor-alpha produced by splenocytes during progression to murine AIDS.

 —Y. Wang, et al., "Long-term Dietary Vitamin E Retards Development of Retrovirus-induced Disregulation in Cytokine Production," *Clin Immunol Immunopathol,* 72(1), July 1994, p. 70-75.

Data from this study showed that 1-100 mumol/l of vitamin E significantly increased the growth BFU-E and colony-forming units granulocyte monocyte from patients infected with HIV, as did 5-10 U/ml of EPO. Compared to healthy controls, tocopherol equally ameliorated the growth of BFU-E and CFU-GM from the HIV-positive subjects in the presence of AZT.

 —R.G. Geissler, et al., "In Vitro Improvement of Bone Marrow-Derived Hematopoietic Colony Formation in HIV-Positive Patients by Alpha-D-Tocopherol and Erythropoietin," *European Journal of Haematology,* 53(4), October 1994, p. 201-206.

This study on the effects of vitamin E in a murine AIDS model made the following observations: A 15-fold increase in vitamin E (160 IU/l) modulated the production of interleukin-2 (IL) in both uninfected mice and retrovirus-infected mice. Vitamin E significantly reduced the level of IL-4 secretion in the uninfected mice at 4 and 8 weeks, but not at 12 and 16 weeks. Vitamin E significantly reduced IL-4 production, elevated by retrovirus infection and significantly reduced IL-6. Vitamin E significantly increased thymic and serum vitamin E concentration previously reduced by retrovirus infection.

 —Y. Wang, et al., "Vitamin E Supplementation Modulates Cytokine Production by Thymocytes During Murine AIDS," *Immunol Res,* 12(4), 1993, p. 358-366.

This article summarized the literature involving vitamin E and immune problems resulting from AIDS. The authors note that the immune abnormalities surrounding AIDS are not unlike those stimulated or restored by high intake of vitamin E. Studies are cited linking vitamin E intake with an increased therapeutic efficiency of drugs such as AZT. Vitamin E supplementation has also been shown to result in a decrease in the progression of disease to AIDS.

—O.E. Odeleye and R.R. Watson, "The Potential Role of Vitamin E in the Treatment of Immunologic Abnormalities During Acquired Immune Deficiency Syndrome," *Prog Food Nutr Sci*, 15(1-2), 1991, p. 1-19.

This review article argues that nutritional agents low in toxicity and with immunoenhancing, antioxidant activities like vitamin E may slow the progression of AIDS by helping to normalize retrovirus-induced immune dysfunctions, malnutrition, and various other symptoms.

—Y. Wang and R.R. Watson, "Is Vitamin E Supplementation a Useful Agent in AIDS Therapy?" *Prog Food Nutr Sci*, 17(4), October-December 1993, p. 351-375.

Alcoholism

This review article argues that, based on studies supporting the positive effects of vitamin E on the numerous immune problems involved with AIDS, vitamin E may also be an effective treatment for alcohol-related immunosuppression.

—Y. Wang and R.R. Watson, "Ethanol, Immune Responses, and Murine AIDS: The Role of Vitamin E as an Immunostimulant and Antioxidant," *Alcohol*, 11(2), March-April 1994, p. 75-84.

Results of this study showed that daily doses of 50 IU of vitamin E given to alcohol poisoned guinea pigs over a 3 day period completely normalized suppression of the T-system immunity. Daily 30,000 IU doses of vitamin A had similar yet weaker effects.

—T.V. Davydova, et al., [Further Study of Immuno-Correcting Properties of Vitamins A and E in Experimental Chronic Alcoholic Intoxication], *Vopr Pitan*, (3), May-June 1988, p. 45-48.

In this study, 3000 IU of vitamin A and 5 IU of vitamin E oil solution per day administered orally over 3 days resulted in a normalization of immune responses to the disordered red blood cells of sheep caused by chronic alcohol intoxication.

—T.V. Davydova and K.D. Pletsityi, [The Use of Vitamins A and E for the Correction of Immunologic Disorders in Chronic Alcoholic Intoxication], *Vopr Pitan* (1987 Jul-Aug)(4), July-August 1987, p. 50-52.

Alzheimer's Disease

This review article notes that vitamin E inhibits amyloid beta protein induced cell death, a key factor in Alzheimer's disease.

—C. Behl, et al., "Vitamin E Protects Nerve Cells from Amyloid Beta Protein Toxicity," *Biochem Biophys Res Commun*, 186(2), July 31, 1992, p. 944-950.

This article notes that Down's syndrome patients are at high risk for Alzheimer's disease. Vitamin E has been shown to protect against oxidative damage caused by gene coding of superoxide dismutase-/

on chromosome 21 resulting in excess activity of the enzyme, thus suggesting its potential as a preventive approach to Alzheimer's.

> —C.V. Jackson, et al., "Vitamin E and Alzheimer's Disease in Subjects with Down's Syndrome," *Journal of Mental Deficit Research,* 32(Pt 6), December 1988, p. 479-484.

This study found that vitamin E levels were twice as high in the midbrain of Alzheimer's patients and Alzheimer's patients with signs of Parkinson's disease relative to controls. Such findings, the authors argue, suggest that compensatory increases in vitamin E levels occur in such patients after specific regions of the brain have been damaged.

> —J.D. Adams, Jr., et al., "Alzheimer's and Parkinson's Disease. Brain Levels of Glutathione, Glutathione Disulfide, and Vitamin E," *Mol Chem Neuropathol,* 14(3), June 1991, p. 213-226.

Anemia

This study measured vitamin E levels in dialysis patients before and after oral supplementation with 600 mg daily of vitamin E for 30 days. Results showed that while plasma vitamin E levels were normal, red blood cell levels in packed red cells were significantly lower than controls. Supplementation increased levels in both plasma and red blood cells. Mean osmolarities at the beginning and end of hemolysis significantly decreased in patients receiving vitamin E supplementation from 102.8 +/- 0.9 to 98.9 +/- 0.7 and 72.1 +/-1.1 to 67.4 +/- 0.8 mosm/l, respectively. Hematocrit increased significantly in these patients from 26.1 +/- 1.0 to 28.1 +/- 1.2%. Based on such findings, the author concludes that vitamin E supplementation could be effective in reversing anemia by reducing the fragility of red blood cells in regular dialysis patients.

> —K. Ono, "Effects of Large Dose Vitamin E Supplementation on Anemia in Hemodialysis Patients," *Nephron,* 40(4), 1985, p. 440-445.

Anoxic Damage

Using the hippocampal slice method, this study examined the effect of alpha tocopherol on irreversible transmission loss subsequent to anoxia. Results showed that free radicals are partially responsible for irreversible anoxic damage and that alpha-tocopherol might be an effective means of protecting the brain against anoxic damage.

> —D. Acosta, et al., "Effect of Alpha-Tocopherol and Free Radicals on Anoxic Damage in the Rat Hippocampal Slice," *Exp Neurol,* 97(3), September 1987, p. 607-614.

Arthritis

Results of this study showed that oral daily doses of 147 mg/kg body wt of vitamin E for one week to arthritic rats before and after adjuvant inoculation increased the lowered serum-SH group in arthritic rats to pre-arthritic values.

> —A.A. Kheir-Eldin, et al., "Biochemical Changes in Arthritic Rats Under the Influence of Vitamin E," *Agents Actions,* 36(3-4), July 1992, p. 300-305.

This study examined the effects of vitamin E supplementation and deficiency in rats with induced adjuvant arthritis. Results showed that rats deficient in vitamin E suffered more from arthritis than those in the supplemented group. Researchers also made the following observations: A/G ratios were depressed in vitamin E deficient rats, while those supplemented with vitamin E experienced a fast recovery. Rats in the vitamin E deficient group showed a dramatic increase in the serum levels of lysosomal enzymes, while levels were inhibited in the supplemented rats. Elevated levels of thiobarbutic acid (TBA) reactants in the synovia resulting from adjunvant exposure were inhibited in the supplemented rats. Such findings led the authors to conclude that vitamin E, being an antioxidant, may benefit those suffering from arthritis since the disease may be associated with lipid peroxidation.

> —T. Yoshikawa, et al., "Effect of Vitamin E on Adjuvant Arthritis in Rats," *Biochem Med,* 29(2), April 1983, p. 227-234.

This study demonstrated that the oral administration of vitamin E starting one day after the onset of arthritis resulted in the inhibition of the development and generalization of the disease.

> —K.D. Pletsityi, et al., [Inhibition of the Development of Adjuvant Arthritis in Rats as Affected by Vitamin E], *Biull Eksp Biol Med,* 103(1), January 1987, p. 43-45.

This study examined total cholesterol levels and levels of vitamins A and E in 125 juvenile chronic arthritis patients. Results showed that cholesterol and vitamin E were significantly lower in the children with arthritis compared to healthy controls. The authors suggest that low levels of vitamin E and damaged antioxidant protection influence low serum cholesterol levels in children with juvenile chronic arthritis.

> —V.E. Honkanen, et al., "Serum Cholesterol and Vitamins A and E in Juvenile Chronic Arthritis," *Clin Exp Rheumatol,* 8(2), March-April 1990, p. 187-191.

This study found that serum levels of vitamins A and E were lower in rheumatoid arthritis patients (RA) than controls. Such deficiencies, the authors argue, can result in a highly decreased antioxidant capacity and enhanced eicosanoid production in RA.

> —V. Honkanen, et al., "Vitamins A and E, Retinol Binding Protein and Zinc in Rheumatoid Arthritis," *Clin Exp Rheumatol,* 7(5), September-October 1989, p. 465-469.

This study examined the effects of different combination of DL-alpha-tocopherol (TOC) and acetylsalicylic acid (ASS) on adjuvant-induced arthritis in rats. Six experimental groups of adjuvans arthritis rats were treated with the following combinations: ASS/TOC (mg/kg BW/d each) 250/-, 250/250, 167/250, 83/250, 167/167 and 167/83. The ASS/TOC combination of 250 mg/kg BW each, the produced the greatest anti-inflammatory effects compared to all other groups.

> —K. Brandt, et al., [Effect of Various Combinations of DL-alpha-tocopherol and Acetylsalicylic Acid on Adjuvant Arthritis in the Rat], *Z Rheumatol,* 47(6), November-December 1988, p. 381-387.

Ataxia

In this case study of progressive spinocerebellar syndrome due to isolated vitamin E deficiency, the authors argue that replacement treatment in patients deficient in vitamin E can halt or improve the associated neurological disorder.

> —R.J. Rayner, et al., "Isolated Vitamin E Deficiency and Progressive Ataxia," *Arch Dis Child,* 69(5), November 1993, p. 602-603.

Brain Edema

The effects of vitamin E supplementation on regional cerebral blood flow in a murine model of focal epidural brain compression was examined in this study. Reductions in rCBF in the previously compressed cortex and hyperemia were witnessed in the mice with normal vitamin E levels and in those suffering from vitamin E deficiency. An increased flow in the previously compressed cortex was seen in vitamin E supplemented rats and there was a tendency to eliminate rCBF gradients between subjacent zones as well.

> —R. Busto, et al., "Regional Blood Flow in Compression-Induced Brain Edema in Rats: Effect of Dietary Vitamin E," *Ann Neurol,* 15(5), May 1984, p. 441-448.

This study examined the degree of edema resulting from focal brain compression in rats fed vitamin E-deficient, -normal, or -supplemented diets. Results showed that the amount of swelling and sodium increase in areas previously compressed were most apparent in the rats deficient in vitamin E and least apparent in the supplemented group.

> —S. Yoshida, et al., "Compression-induced Brain Edema: Modification by Prior Depletion and Supplementation of Vitamin E," *Neurology,* 33(2), February 1993, p. 166-172.

Results of this study found that the cerebral content of fatty acids in epidurial brain compression regions were reduced by 19-22% in vitamin E deficient rats relative to controls. Fatty acid levels were reduced by 4-13% in vitamin E normal rats relative to controls and by 0-7% in vitamin E supplemented rats relative to controls. Based on these findings, the authors suggest that vitamin E may stabilize membranes following brain edema.

> —S. Yoshida, et al., "Compression-induced Brain Edema in Rats: Effect of Dietary Vitamin E on Membrane Damage in the Brain," *Neurology,* 35(1), January 1985, p. 126-130.

Brain Injury

In this study either intracerebral infusion or phosphatidylcholine liposomes or D-alpha-tocopherol-enriched liposomes delivered for 7 days was administered by subcutaneous osmotic pumps to the damaged cortex regions of adult rats with bilateral frontal cortex lesions. Results found that the rats receiving alpha-tocopherol treatment were less impaired than rats receiving liposome treatment and that alpha-tocopherol reduced some of the injury-induced, secondary reactive changes that frequently follow frontal cortex damage.

> —D.G. Stein, et al., "Intracerebral Administration of Alpha-tocopherol-containing Liposomes Facilitates Behavioral Recovery in Rats with Bilateral Lesions of the Frontal Cortex," *Journal of Neurotrauma,* 8(4), Winter 1991, p. 281-292.

In this study, lipid peroxidation was measured after 3 microliters of 100 mM FeC12 focal injection into rat amygdala. The quantity of peroxidation products generated was limited by acutre parenteral administration of [dl]-alpha-tocopheral. Such findings, the authors argue, suggest brain injury responses may be limited by the administration of alpha-tocopherol.

> —W.J. Triggs and L.J. Willmore," Effect of [dl]-alpha-tocopherol on FeCl2-induced Lipid Peroxidation in Rat Amygdala," *Neurosci Lett,* 180(1), October 10, 1994, p. 33-36.

This study examined the effects of vitamin E on cerebral ischemia in dogs. Results found that recovery time was statistically reduced in dogs administered 30 mg/kg of vitamin E compared to controls.
  —S. Fujimoto, et al., "The Protective Effect of Vitamin E on Cerebral Ischemia," *Surg Neurol,* 22(5), November 1984, p. 449-454.

This study found that a dose of 300 mg/kg body weight of vitamin E administered intraperitoneally to rats resulted in a protective effect against 5xg positive radial acceleration-induced stagnant hypoxia.
  —S. Trojan, "Protective Effect of Vitamin E in Stagnant Hypoxia of the Brain," *Physiol Res,* 40(6), 1991, p. 595-597.

This study of alpha-tocopherol acetate and selenium in the treatment of patients with small ischemic insult and middle severity ischemic insult found that such treatment decreased the content of diene conjugates and malonic dialdehyde and increased the activity of superoxide dismutase, catalase, glutathione peroxidase and reductase.
  —T.G. Dzhandzhgava and R.R. Shakarishvili, [Effect of Alpha-tocopherol and Selenium on the Activity of Antioxidant Enzymes and Level of Lipid Peroxidation Products in Erythrocytes of Patients with Cerebral Ischemia], *Vopr Med Khim,* 37(5), September-October 1991, p. 79-82.

Breast Implants

This article suggests that vitamin E may be a safe and inexpensive way of decreasing the amount of postoperative capsular contractures following breast augmentation. The author notes that no side effects have been witnessed and that synthetic vitamin E in the form of alpha-tocopherol is best with ideal doses being 1000 IU, b.i.d. beginning a week after surgery and lasting up to 2 years.
  —J.L. Baker, Jr., "The Effectiveness of Alpha-tocopherol (vitamin E) in Reducing the Incidence of Spherical Contracture Around Breast Implants," *Plast Reconstr Surg,* 68(5), November 1981, p. 696-699.

Brown Bowel Syndrome

This review article argues that brown bowel syndrome is caused from vitamin E deficiency and that vitamin E deficiency is probably at least partly to blame for the high rates of malignancy in patients with chronic pancreatis and celiac sprue.
  —H. Reynaert, et al., "The Brown Bowel Syndrome and Gastrointestinal Adenocarcinoma: Two Complications of Vitamin E Deficiency in Celiac Sprue and Chronic Pancreatitis?" *Journal of Clinical Gastroenterology,* 16(1), January 1993, p. 48-51.

Cadmium Intoxication

This study examined the effects of vitamin E on cadmium intoxication in rats. Results showed that exposure to 1mg/kg of Cd as $CdCl_2.2H_2O$, intraperitoneally for 7 days led to a reduction in the activity of hepatic and renal glutamic oxalacetic and glutamic pyruvic transaminases, and alkaline phosphatase. The administration of 5 mg/kg of vitamin E intramuscularly for 7 days at the same time was found to reduce the Cd induced changes noted above. Vitamin E exposure also significantly reduced the accumulation of Cd in the liver, kidney, and blood.

> —S.K. Tandon, et al., "Preventive Effect of Vitamin E in Cadmium Intoxication," *Biomed Environ Science,* 5(1), March 1992, p. 39-45.

Cancer

In this 8 year follow-up study, alpha-tocopherol serum concentrations was studied in 36,265 Finnish adults as a cancer predictor. Results showed a 1.5 times greater risk of cancer in those with low alpha-tocopherol levels compared to those with higher levels. The strongest such correlations were seen in the cases of gastrointestinal cancers and the combined group cancers that were not related to smoking.

> —P. Knekt, et al., "Vitamin E and Cancer Prevention," *American Journal of Clinical Nutrition,* 53(1 Suppl), January 1991, p. 283S-286S.

This review article concludes that while the relationships between cancer and vitamin E are yet to completely understood, research has shown vitamin E to be capable of protecting against tumor growth and carcinogenesis. Studies have also suggested vitamin E can reduce the toxicity of several anticancer therapies. In summary, the author states that vitamin E might be useful as a cancer chemopreventive agent.

> —S. Das, "Vitamin E in the Genesis and Prevention of Cancer: A Review," *Acta Oncol* (1994) 33(6), 1994, p. 615-619.

Results of this study showed that doses of 5, 25, or 50 mg/100 g per body wt of tocopherol significantly enhanced the retardation of irradiation-induced growth of a transplanted rat sarcoma.

> —A. Kagerud and H.I. Peterson, "Tocopherol in Irradiation of Experimental Neoplasms: Influence of Dose and Administration," *Acta Radiol Oncol,* 20(2), 1981, p. 97-100.

Results of this 10 year follow-up study of 21,172 Finnish men found that a high serum level of alpha-tocopherol was associated with a reduced cancer risk. The association was strongest for cancers unrelated to smoking.

> —P. Knekt, et al., "Serum Vitamin E and Risk of Cancer Among Finnish Men During a 10-year Follow-up," *American Journal of Epidemiology,* 127(1), January 1988, p. 28-41.

This 20 year follow-up study examined the relationship between intake of vitamin E, vitamin C, retionoids, carotenoids, and selenium and the subsequent risk of lung cancer in 4,538 Finnish men initially free of cancer. Results demonstrated inverse gradients between vitamin E, vitamin C, and carotenoids and the rate of lung cancer in nonsmokers.

> —P. Knekt, et al., "Dietary Antioxidants and the Risk of Lung Cancer," *American Journal of Epidemiology,* 134(5), September 1, 1991, p. 471-479.

Results of this study allowed the authors to conclude that pretreatment with vitamins A, or A and E together offers protection against the carcinogenic action of dimethylbenzanthracene, and that the mechanism of this protection is early truncation of the ornithine decarboxylase response to dimethylbenzanthracene.

> —K.H. Calhoun, et al., "Vitamins A and E Do Protect Against Oral Carcinoma," *Arch Otolaryngol Head Neck Surg,* 115(4), April 1989, p. 484-488.

This review article notes that results from eight clinical trials have shown beta-carotene and vitamin E produce regression of oral leukoplakia and that all available evidence points to a major role for antioxidant nutrients in the prevention of oral cancer.

—H.S. Garewal and S. Schantz, ''Emerging Role of Beta-carotene and Antioxidant Nutrients in Prevention of Oral Cancer,'' *Arch Otolaryngol Head Neck Surg,* 121(2), February 1995, p. 141-144.

In this study, an organospecific, 1,2-dimethylhydrazine-induced murine tumor model was incorporated to test the effects of the following supplements on tumor formation: ascorbic acid, 7% per weight; alpha-tocopherol, 1% per weight; beta-carotene, 1% per weight; and canthazanthin, 1% per weight. After a period involving four weeks of dietary acclimation, 16 weeks of 1,2-dimethylhydrazine induction, and a four-week hiatus; the animals were killed and autopsies were conducted to record the formation of tumors. Results found that only alpha-tocopherol and ascorbic acid resulted in significant reductions in tumor formation relative to controls.

—T.A. Colacchio, et al., ''Antioxidants vs Carotenoids: Inhibitors or Promoters of Experimental Colorectal Cancers,'' *Arch Surg,* 124(2), February 1989, p. 217-221.

In this prospective study of 5,004 women in Guernsey, a strong association was demonstrated between low plasma levels of vitamin E and an increased risk of breast cancer. The actual risk of breast cancer in women with the lowest levels of vitamin E proved to be 5 times greater than in those with the highest levels.

—N.J. Wald, et al., ''Plasma Retinol, Beta-Carotene and Vitamin E Levels in Relation to the Future Risk of Breast Cancer,'' *British Journal of Cancer,* 49(3), March 1984, p. 321-324.

Serum samples taken from 22,000 men attending a cancer screening center were collected and stored in this study. In 271 men who were subsequently identified as having cancer, the concentration of vitamin E was measured and compared to cancer free controls. Results showed cancer subjects diagnosed as having the disease prior to the elapse of one year from the time of initial blood collection had significantly lower concentrations of vitamin E than controls. The authors argue that such findings are likely a result of the cancer rather than a factor influencing its development.

—N.J. Wald, et al., ''Serum Vitamin E and Subsequent Risk of Cancer,'' *British Journal of Cancer,* 56(1), July 1987, p. 69-72.

This case-control study examined the associations of vitamin E, vitamin A, and selenium concentrations with the risk cancer mortality. Results showed an 11.4 fold adjusted risk for subjects with both low vitamin E and low selenium serum concentrations.

—J.T. Salonen, et al., ''Risk of Cancer in Relation to Serum Concentrations of Selenium and Vitamins A and E: Matched Case-control Analysis of Prospective Data,'' *British Medical Journal,* 290(6466), February 9, 1985, p. 417-420.

Results of this study found that 1000 mg/kg of vitamin E was capable of potentiating selenium's (2.5 mg/kg) ability to inhibit dimethylbenza(a)anthracene-induced mammary tumor development in rats. The administration of vitamin E alone did not produce similar results.

—P.M. Horvath and C. Ip, ''Synergistic Effect of Vitamin E and Selenium in the Chemoprevention of Mammary Carcinogenesis in Rats,'' *Cancer Research,* 43(11), November 1983, p. 5335-5341.

This study examined the effects of different forms of vitamin E on mouse melanoma (B-16) and mouse fibroblasts (L-cells) cells in culture. The following results were observed: for the criterion of growth inhibition, melanoma cells were approximately twice as sensitive to vitamin E succinate as fibroblasts. D-alpha-tocopherol acid succinate induced morphological alterations and growth inhibition in melanoma cells and when vitamin E acid succinate was removed 4 days after treatment, the above changes remained irreversible for 24 hours, after which resistant cells and partially affected cells renewed cell division and eventually reached confluency. Vitamin E acid succinate-induced morphological changes and growth inhibition in melanoma cells were expressed in hormone-supplemented serum-free medium, but the concentration requirement was about 5 times less than that needed in serum-supplemented medium.

—K.N. Prasad and J. Edwards-Prasad, "Effects of Tocopherol (vitamin E) Acid Succinate on Morphological Alterations and Growth Inhibition in Melanoma Cells in Culture," *Cancer Research,* 42(2), 1982, p. 550-555.

In this double-blind study, mammary dysplasia patients were given 600 units per day of alpha-tocopherol. Results showed that 88% responded clinically and that the progesterone to estradiol ratio, abnormal in mammary dysplasia patients, increased from 30 +/- 7 (S.E.) to 53 +/- 11 in patients after alpha-tocopherol therapy. No such significant changes were observed in controls. These findings, according to the authors, suggest numerous implications for reducing malignant breast disease through alpha-tocopherol therapy.

—R.S. London, et al., "Endocrine Parameters and Alpha-tocopherol Therapy of Patients with Mammary Dysplasia," *Cancer Research,* 41(9 Pt 2), September 1981, p. 3811-3813.

This study used a rat skin model to examine what protective effects, if any, dimethyl sulfoxide and alpha-tocopherol have against Adriamycin-induced skin necrosis. Results showed that 1 ml of 10% topical alpha-tocopherol succinate in dimethyl sulfoxide applied daily for 2 days brought on a dramatic reduction in ulcer diameter of up to 68% after 2 weeks. Slightly less activity was seen with the use of alpha-tocopherol acetate, but both it and alpha-tocopherol succinate were much more active than alpha-tocopherol alcohol. In light of these findings, the authors conclude that alpha-tocopherol and dimethly sulfoxide might be useful for the treatment of accidentally extravasated Adriamycin in people with cancer.

—B.A. Svingen, et al., "Protection Against Adriamycin-induced Skin Necrosis in the Rat by Dimethyl Sulfoxide and Alpha-Tocopherol," *Cancer Research,* 41(9 Pt 1), September 1981, p. 3395-3399.

This study examined the effects of dietary vitamin E on dimethylhydrazine-induced colonic tumors in mice. When mice receiving 10 mg/kg of vitamin E were compared to those receiving 600 mg/kg, results showed that 42 and 51 mice survived, respectively. In addition, significantly more adenomas and invasive carcinomas were seen in 10 mg/kg supplemented vitamin E mice than in those supplemented with 600 mg/kg.

—M.G. Cook and P. McNamara, "Effect of Dietary Vitamin E on Dimethylhydrazine-induced Colonic Tumors in Mice," *Cancer Research,* 40(4), April 1980, p. 1329-1331.

This set of two randomized, placebo-controlled studies examined the effects of vitamin and mineral supplementation in lowering esophageal and gastric cancer rates among high risk Chinese populations. Results found that following 5.25 years of supplementation at levels of 1-2 times USRDA levels, subjects receiving vitamin E, beta-carotene, and selenium experienced a 42% reduction in esophageal cancer prevalence as well as a significant reduction in overall cancer mortality.

—P.R. Taylor, et al., ''Prevention of Esophageal Cancer: The Nutrition Intervention Trials in Linxian, China: Linxian Nutrition Intervention Trials Study Group,'' *Cancer Research,* 54(7 Suppl), April 1, 1994, p. 2029s-2031s.

This study examined the effects of high antioxidant intakes on the incidence of colon cancer using data obtained via food questionnaire from 35,215 Iowa women in their mid fifties to late sixties. Results showed an inverse association between vitamin E intake and colon cancer risk.

—R.M. Bostick, et al., ''Reduced Risk of Colon Cancer with High Intake of Vitamin E: The Iowa Women's Health Study,'' *Cancer Research,* 53(18), September 15, 1993, p. 4230-4237.

This study examined the relationship between the risk of oral and pharyngeal cancer and serum micronutrient levels using data obtained from 25,802 adults. Results showed that high serum levels of alpha-tocopherol were associated to a decreased risk of oral cancer in later life relative to controls.

—W. Zheng, et al., ''Serum Micronutrients and the Subsequent Risk of Oral and Pharyngeal Cancer,'' *Cancer Research,* 53(4), February 15, 1993, p. 795-798.

This study examined the effects of high levels of vitamin E on transplanted syngeneric murine sarcoma cells. The results enabled the author to summarize his findings by putting forth the following postulations relative to the protective mechanisms of vitamin E: (1) stimulation of host immune responses probably by increased antibody synthesis which participates in ADCC reactions with FcR+ NK cells and macrophages, (2) inhibition of tumor-induced immunosuppression and (3) decreased tumor cell surface sialic acid which may result in increased antigenicity and susceptibility to immune killing.

—I.N. Mbawuike, ''Mechanisms of Vitamin E Protection Against Transplanted Murine Sarcoma Cells,'' *Dissertaition Abstracts International,* 44(10), 1984, p. 3036-B.

This study examined the effects of a semi-purified low selenium diet with or without adequate vitamin E on 6-8 week old hamsters. The following results were observed: vitamin E deficient hamsters experienced weight loss, an increase in erythrocyte hemolysis, a decrease in plasma vitamin E, the development of testicular atrophy muscle degeneration, mild liver necrosis/hypertrophy, and atrophy of the exocrine pancreas. Vitamin E supplementation resulted in the prevention of acinar cell loss in the pancreas, the repair of injury to the testes and muscle, the return of erythrocyte hemolysis and plasma vitamin E to control levels, and a reversal of the trend towards growth reduction.

—M.A. Banks, ''Vitamin E and Bop-Induced Pancreatic Cancer in Hamsters,'' *Dissertation Abstracts International,* 47(6), 1986, p. 2409.

Results of this population-based, case-control study showed an inverse correlation between serum vitamin E levels and the risk of lung cancer.

—M.J. Menkes, ''Vitamin A, E, Selenium and Risk of Lung Cancer,'' *Dissertation Abstracts International,* 46(11), 1986, p. 3807.

This study examined the role of increased lipid peroxidation in the various stages of cancer and alcoholic liver injuries. Results found that vitamin E supplementation decreased the indices of lipid peroxidation as well as the frequency and size of preneoplastic tumors. The author concludes that increased lipid peroxdiation, attenuated by vitamin E in the diet, is a key factor in the process of carcinogenesis induced by a chemical carcinogen, and promoted by ethanol, retrovirus infection, and protein malnutrition.

> —O.E. Odeleye, "Lipid Peroxidation in the Etiology of Alcohol Liver Injury and Cancer: Modulatory Role of Vitamin E," *Dissertation Abstracts International,* 52(7), 1992, p. 3538.

This study examined the effects of alpha-tocopherol on the proliferation of human osteosarcoma cells, fibroblasts, vascular smooth muscle cells, and neuroblastoma cells. Results showed that physiologically relevant concentrations of alpha-tocopherol inhibited the proliferation of vascular smooth muscle cells.

> —D. Boscoboinik, et al., "Inhibition of Cell Proliferation by Alpha-Tocopherol: Role of Protein Kinase C," *Journal of Biol Chem,* 266(10), April 5, 1991, p. 6188-6194.

Results of this study showed that hamsters treated orally with 10 mg or vitamin E twice weekly and who had the left buccal pouch painted three times weekly with DMBA (0.5% solution of 7,12 dimethylbenz(a)anthracene in heavy mineral oil) experienced a less dramatic reduction in Langerhans cells after 8 weeks then hamsters treated with either substance alone or those not receiving any treatment. Based on these findings and those of previous studies, the authors suggest that vitamin E may slow carcinogenesis by maintaining the amount of Langerhans cells.

> —J. Schwartz, et al., "Alpha Tocopherol alters the Distribution of Langerhans Cells in DMBA-Treated Hamster Cheek Pouch Epithelium," *Journal of Dental Research,* 64(2), February 1985, p. 117-121.

This article pooled the results of five previous studies on the relationship between serum alpha-tocopherol concentrations and the risk of colon cancer. Results showed evidence of a possible inverse relationship between the two.

> —M.P. Longnecker, et al., "Serum Alpha-tocopherol Concentration in Relation to Subsequent Colorectal Cancer: Pooled Data from Five Cohorts," *Journal of the National Cancer Institute,* 84(6), March 18, 1992, p. 430-435.

Results of this study showed that hamsters treated orally with 10 mg or vitamin E twice weekly experienced a significant reduction in the number and size of oral tumors compared to hamsters who had the left buccal pouch painted three times weekly with DMBA (0.5% solution of 7,12 dimethylbenz(a)anthracene in heavy mineral oil) without vitamin E treatment.

> —G. Shklar, et al., "Oral Mucosal Carcinogenesis in Hamsters: Inhibition by Vitamin E," *Journal of the National Cancer Institute,* 68(5), May 1982, p. 791-797.

In this study, the injection of 250 micrograms of vitamin E injected into the tumor-bearing buccal pouch twice a week for 4 weeks of hamsters was found to regress established epidermoid carcinomas following tumor induction by the application 3 times weekly of 0.5% 7,12-dimethylbenz[a]anthracene (CAS: 57-97-6) in mineral oil for a total of 13 weeks.

> —G. Shklar, et al., "Regression by Vitamin E of Experimental Oral Cancer," *Journal of the National Cancer Institute,* 78(5), May 1987, p. 987-992.

Results of this study showed that 10 mg of alpha-tocopherol on alternate days inhibited 0.5% solution of 7,12-dimethylbenz[a]anthracene [(DMBA) CAS: 57-97-6 induced carcinogenesis in the hamster buccal pouch.

> —D. Trickler, et al., "Prevention by Vitamin E of Experimental Oral Carcinogenesis," *Journal of the National Cancer Institute,* 78(1), January 1987, p. 165-169.

Results of this set of studies showed that alpha-tocopherol and carotenoids exhibited a selective cytotoxic effect on the growth of human tumor cells in vitro. The malignant cell lines studied included two lines of oral carcinoma, two lines of lung carcinoma, two cell lines of breast cancer, and malignant melanoma.

—J. Schwartz and G. Shklar, "The Selective Cytotoxic Effect of Carotenoids and Alpha-tocopherol on Human Cancer Cell Lines in Vitro," *Journal of Oral Maxillofac Surgery,* 50(4), April 1992, p. 367-373.

This study examined the role of vitamin E acid succinate in adjuvant chemotherapy with ADR in DU-145 human prostatic carcinoma cells in culture. Results showed that vitamin E succinate inhibited carcinoma cell growth in a dose-dependent manner, achieving as much as 50% inhibition relative to controls in the clonal and cell count assays. Vitamin E succinate also increased adriamycin's tumor cell cytotoxicity. Such findings prompted the authors to conclude that vitamin E, as an adjuvant agent to adriamycin, might play a role in treating prostatic cancer.

—E.A. Ripoll, et al., "Vitamin E Enhances the Chemotherapeutic Effects of Adriamycin on Human Prostatic Carcinoma Cells in Vitro," *Journal of Urology,* 136(2), August 1986, p. 529-531.

Results of this population-based, case-control study showed an inverse correlation between serum vitamin E levels and the risk of lung cancer.

—M.S. Menkes, et al., "Serum Beta-Carotene, Vitamins A and E, Selenium, and the Risk of Lung Cancer," *New England Journal of Medicine,* 315(20), November 13, 1986, p. 1250-1254.

This study found that d- and dl-alpha-tocopheryl succinate produced morphological changes and inhibited growth in mouse melanoma (B-16), mouse neuroblastoma (NBP2), and rat glioma (C-6) cells in culture.

—B.N. Rama and K.N. Prasad, "Study on the Specificity of Alpha-tocopheryl (vitamin E) Acid Succinate Effects on Melanoma, Glioma and Neuroblastoma cells in Culture," *Proc Soc Exp Biol Med,* 174(2), November 1983, p. 302-307.

This review article makes the following observations with respect to vitamin E and cancer: it can inhibit nitrosation, inhibit skin, cheek pouch, and forestomach carcinogenesis, inhibit colon carcinogenesis, and inhibit mammary gland carcinogenesis.

—D.F. Birt, "Update on the Effects of Vitamins A, C, and E and Selenium on Carcinogenesis," *Proc Soc Exp Biol Med,* 183(3), December 1986, p. 311-320.

In this study, malignancy induced rats were given 4 mg/kg body weight per week of cisplatin or cisplatin with 200 mg of vitamin E on alternate days 200 mg every day of vitamin C. Autopsies performed after 60 days produced results demonstrating the efficacy of the vitamins' ability to enhance the therapeutic potential of cisplatin in treating oral cancer.

—D.K. Sharma, "Amylase Activity of the Malignant Rat Salivary Gland after Cisplatin, Vitamin E and C Treatment," *Third International Congress on Engineered Oral Cancer,* January 22-25, 1994, Madras, India, 1994, 31, 1994.

This case-control, clinic-based study examined the association between basal cell carcinoma and vitamin supplementation. Results showed a significant inverse relationship between intake of vitamins E (greater than 100 IU/day), and A (greater than 5000 IU/day) and cancer risk.

> —Q. Wei, et al., "Vitamin Supplementation has a Protective Effect on Basal Cell Carcinoma," *American Society of Preventive Oncology, 17th Annual Meeting, March 20-23, 1993, Tucson, AZ, 1993.*

In this study, oral leukoplakia patients were given a daily antioxidant combination including 30 mg of beta-carotene, 1000 mg of ascorbic acid, 800 IU of alpha-tocopherol for 9 months. Results found that 55.6% of the 81 patients who completed the protocol experienced partial or complete clinical resolution of their oral lesions. Results also showed that the antioxidant supplementation was most effective in those who abstained from the use of alcohol and tobacco during the study.

> —G. Kaugars, et al., "The Role of Antioxidants in the Treatment of Oral Leukoplakia," *CCPC-93: Second International Cancer Chemo Prevention Conference. April 28-30, 1993, Berlin, Germany, 1993, 65, 1993.*

This review article notes that studies continue to suggest antioxidants, most noticeably alpha-tocopherol and beta-carotene, play a role in preventing cancer of the oral cavity.

> —H. Garewal, et al., "Beta-carotene and Other Antioxidant Nutritional Agents in Oral Leukoplakia," *CCPC-93: Second International Cancer Chemo Prevention Conference. April 28-30, 1993, Berlin, Germany, 1993, 52, 1993.*

This study examined the effects of vitamin E on the mutagenic activities of adriamycin and aflatoxin. Results found vitamin E to only show antimutagenic activity towards aflatoxin B1 when homogenized with liver tissue.

> —B. Chlopkiewicz, et al., "An Evaluation of Antimutagenic Properties of Vitamin E," *Acta Pol Pharm,* 48(3-4), 1991, p. 33-34.

Results from this study show that diets including high levels of vitamin E suppressed the promotion of cancer by ethanol in mice.

> —C.D. Eskelson, et al., "Modulation of Cancer Growth by Vitamin E and Alcohol," *Alcohol,* 28(1), January 1993, p. 117-125.

This study examined the role of vitamin E in treating chemotherapy-induced mucositis. Results found that vitamin E may play a role in prevention, particularly during inductions therapy for acute myelogenous leukemia.

> —I. Lopez, et al., [Treatment of Mucositis with Vitamin E During Administration of Neutropenic Antineoplastic Agents], *Ann Med Interne,* 145(6), 1994, p. 405-408.

This study examined the relationship between vitamin E, smoking, and lung cancer in a large population of Finnish men over the age of 15. Results showed a significant inverse association between vitamin E status and the occurrence of lung cancer occurrence in nonsmokers but not smokers. A 12-fold greater risk of lung cancer was reported in nonsmokers with low serum vitamin E levels compared to those with sufficient levels.

> —P. Knekt, "Vitamin E and Smoking and the Risk of Lung Cancer," *Annals of the New York Academy of Sciences,* 686, May 28, 1993, p. 280-287.

This study examined the effects of alpha-tocopherol acid and alpha-tocopherol acid succinate on mutagen-induced gentoxicicty in human lymphoblastoid cell lines and lymphocytes from cultures of peripheral blood. Results found that both alpha-tocopherol acid and alpha-tocopherol acid succinate led to a dose-dependent protection in the cell lines and lymphocytes of patients with cancers of the head and neck.

—Z. Trizna, et al., "Protective Effects of Vitamin E Against Bleomycin-induced Genotoxicity in Head and Neck Cancer Patients in Vitro," *Anticancer Research,* 12(2), March-April 1992, p. 325-327.

Results of this study found that 5-fluorouracil treated rats that received supplements of vitamin E showed significantly lower levels liver and plasma lipoperoxide than rats only receiving the anticancer drug.

—I.D. Capel, et al., "Vitamin E Retards the Lipoperoxidation Resulting from Anticancer Drug Administration," *Anticancer Research,* 3(1), January-February 1983, p. 59-62.

While stressing that the existing research in general is inconclusive, this review article note that vitamin E has been shown in some studies to inhibit skin, liver, oral, ear duct, and forestomach carcinogenesis; and to inhibit mammary gland or colon carcinogenesis.

—L.H. Chen, et al., "Vitamin C, Vitamin E and Cancer," *Anticancer Research,* 8(4), July-August 1988, p. 739-748.

Results from this case-control of postmenopausal women showed that the risk for breast cancer was inversely related to the intake of high amounts of vitamin E from food sources.

—S.J. London, et al., "Carotenoids, Retinol, and Vitamin E and Risk of Proliferative Benign Breast Disease and Breast Cancer," *Cancer Causes Control,* 3(6), November 1992, p. 503-512.

In this study, the administration of 400 IU of alpha-tocopherol was administered to oral leukoplakia patients resulted in a significant reduction in micronuclei frequencies in specimens from visible lesions and normal appearing mucosa. Such findings indicate alpha-tocopherol has a beneficial effect in oral carcinogenesis.

—S.E. Benner, et al., "Reduction in Oral Mucosa Micronuclei Frequency Following Alpha-tocopherol Treatment of Oral Leukoplakia," *Cancer Epidemiol Biomarkers Prev,* 3(1), January-February 1994, p. 73-76.

Results of this study showed that the oral administration of 100 mg/kg per day of vitamin E for 4 days significantly inhibited the formation of 8-OH-dG in the liver nuclear DNA of rats injected with 2-NP (100 mg/kg BW, i.p., killed 6 h later).

—A. Takagi, et al., "Inhibitory Effects of Vitamin E and Ellagic Acid on 8-hydroxydeoxyguanosine Formation in Liver Nuclear DNA of Rats Treated with 2-nitropropane," *Cancer Letters,* 91(1), May 4, 1995, p. 139-144.

Results of this study found that dietary vitamin E and beta-carotene supplementation significantly decreased the number of colonic aberrant crypt foci of different multiplicities when compared to the effects of a low-fat high-fiber diet alone in rats.

—N. Shivapurkar, et al., "Inhibition of Progression of Aberrant Crypt Foci and Colon Tumor

Development by Vitamin E and Beta-carotene in Rats on a High-risk Diet," *Cancer Letters,* 91(1), May 4, 1995, p. 125-132.

Results of this study found that a vitamin E supplemented diet significantly reduced the rate of spontaneous lung tumorigenesis in mice relative to controls.
    —T. Yano, et al., "Vitamin E Acts as a Useful Chemopreventive Agent to Reduce Spontaneous Lung Tumorigenesis in Mice," *Cancer Letters,* 87(2), December 9, 1994, p. 205-210.

Results of this study found that high doses of vitamin E reduced glycerol-enhanced lung tumorigenesis in mice treated with 4NQO plus glycerol.
    —T. Yano, et al., "Is Vitamin E a Useful Agent to Protect Against Oxy Radical-Promoted Lung Tumorigenesis in ddY Mice?" *Carcinogenesis,* 14(6), June 1993, p. 1133-1136.

This study examined the role of retroviral immunosuppression on N-nitrosomethylbenzylamine (NMBzA)-induced esophageal cancer in mice and the effects of dietary vitamin E (30 IU or 172 IU/kg of diet) on this cancer. Results found that vitamin E retarded the incidence of esophageal cancers through its antioxidant activities.
    —O.E. Odeleye, et al., "Vitamin E Protection Against Nitrosamine-induced Esophageal Tumor Incidence in Mice Immunocompromised by Retroviral Infection," *Carcinogenesis,* 13(10), October 1992, p. 1811-1816.

This study examined the effects of vitamins A, C, E, and selenium compound on liver cancer in rats. Results showed that rats deprived of these vitamins in their diets developed liver cancer at rates higher than controls. The authors argue the liver cancer inhibiting effects of vitamins may be the results of their inducing hepatic microsomal enzymes that metabolize aflatoxins to noncarcinogenic products.
    —H.S. Nyandieka and J. Wakhisi, "The Impact of Vitamins A,C,E, and Selenium Compound on Prevention of Liver Cancer in Rats," *East African Medical Journal,* 70(3), March 1993, p. 151-153.

Results of this study suggest that low serum levels of vitamin E and vitamin A are involved in the etiology of seond tumors in head and neck cancer patients.
    —N. de Vries and G.B. Snow, "Relationships of Vitamins A and E and Beta-carotene Serum Levels to Head and Neck Cancer Patients with and without Second Primary Tumors," *Eur Arch Otorhinolaryngol,* 247(6), 1990, p. 368-370.

This review article argues that vitamin E and beta-carotene meet the criteria for an effective chemopreventive agent of oral cancer and it points to the results of eight clinical trials to support this view:
    —H. Garewal, "Chemoprevention of Oral Cancer: Beta-Carotene and Vitamin E in Leukoplakia," *European Journal of Cancer Prevention,* 3(2), March 1994, p. 101-107.

Results of this study found that 100 micrograms/ml of DL-alpha-tocopherol significantly reduced the percentage of benzo(a)pyrene induced chromosomal aberrations in vitro.
    —E. Smalls and R.M. Patterson, "Reduction of Benzo(a)pyrene Induced Chromosomal Aberrations by DL-Alpha-tocopherol," *European Journal of Cell Biology,* 28(1), August 1982, p. 92-97.

This study examined if any differences in specific tissue antioxidant levels were measurable in randomly selected human breast and gynecologic malignant neoplasms and nonneoplastic tissue samples obtained from the same patient. With respect to alpha-tocopherol, results showed that concentrations were significantly higher in cancer tissues of the cervix and endometrium than those in adjacent noninvolved tissue sites. Comparable tissue concentrations were found in malignant and adjacent normal sites in the vulva, breast, and ovary.

—P.R. Palan, et al., "Lipid-soluble Antioxidants: Beta-carotene and Alpha-tocopherol Levels in Breast and Gynecologic Cancers," *Gynecol Oncol,* 55(1), October 1994, p. 72-77.

In this study, 20 units per 200 g/bw of vitamin E in combination with chemotherapy was given to rats. Results found that the vitamin E reduced Adriamycin toxicity and assisted in tumor reduction decreases in metastasis. The efficacy of Cyclophosphamide, Adriamycin and Methotrexate also appeared to be enhanced by the vitamin E treatment.

—J.R. Drago, et al., "Chemotherapy and Vitamin E in Treatment of Nb Rat Prostate Tumors," *In Vivo,* 2(6), November-December 1988, p. 399-401.

Results of this longitudinal study of 36,265 Finnish men found an inverse relationship between alpha-tocopherol serum levels and the risk of upper gastrointestinal tract cancer as well as colorectal cancer.

—P. Knekt, et al., "Serum Vitamin E, Serum Selenium and the Risk of Gastrointestinal Cancer," *International Journal of Cancer,* 42(6), December 15, 1988, p. 846-850.

Results of this 8-year follow-up study of 15,093 women found an inverse association between serum alpha-tocopherol levels and the risk of many forms of cancer. A particularly strong relationship was seen between low serum alpha-tocopherol levels and epithelial cancers.

—P. Knekt, "Serum Vitamin E Level and Risk of Female Cancers," *International Journal of Epidemiology,* 17(2), June 1988, p. 281-286.

This study examined the effects of vitamin E on 4-nitroquinoline 1-oxide (4NQO)-induced oxidative damage on pulmonary nuclei and lung tumorigenesis in mice. Results indicated that vitamin E may partially suppress 4NQO-induced lung tumorigenesis.

—T. Yano, et al., "Effect of Vitamin E on 4-nitroquinoline 1-oxide-induced Lung Tumorigenesis in Mice," *International Journal of Vitam Nutr Res,* 64(3), 1994, p. 181-184.

This review article notes that autoradiographic, ultrastructural and cell surface studies have demonstrated that vitamins A, E and C are important regulator factors of cancer cell differentiation, cell regression, membrane biogenesis, DNA, RNA, protein, and collagen synthesis, as well as transformation of precancer cells into cancer cells. Studies have also found these vitamins to exhibit cytotoxic and cytostatic effects, and may reverse the cancer cell to the normal phenotype.

—A. Lupulescu, "The Role of Vitamins A, Beta-carotene, E and C in Cancer Cell Biology," *International Journal of Vitam Nutr Research,* 64(1), 1994, p. 3-14.

This review article highlights the effectiveness of vitamin E in preventing the nitrosation of amino substrates under physiological conditions. It also notes that the combination of vitamins E and C have an even greater inhibiting effect on the formation of N-Nitrosamine. The authors conclude that when taken at the same time as food, vitamin E can reduce the exposure of humans to carcinogenic N-Nitrosamine.

> —D. Lathia and A. Blum, "Role of Vitamin E as Nitrite Scavenger and N-nitrosamine Inhibitor: A Review," *International Journal of Vitam Nutr Research,* 59(4), 1989, p. 430-438.

This review article cites numerous in vitro studies showing that vitamin E supplementation reduces the risk of chemical and radiation induced cancers in both human and animals cells. Alpha-tocopherol succinate has proven to be the most effective form of vitamin E in such studies.

> —K.N. Prasad and J. Edwards-Prasad, "Vitamin E and Cancer Prevention: Recent Advances and Future Potentials," *Journal of the American College of Nutrition,* 11(5), October 1992, p. 487-500.

Results of this study found that vitamin E may be effective in preventing oxy radical-enhanced lung tumorigenesis in mice.

> —T. Ichikawa, et al., "The Prevention of Oxy Radical-Mediated Lung Tumorigenesis in Mice by Vitamin E," *Journal of Nutr Sci Vitaminol,* 39(Suppl), 1993, p. S49-55.

This study examined the effects of vitamin E succinate and prostaglandin E2 on human tongue squamous carcinoma cells in vitro. Results showed that, when administered independently, vitamin E succinate and prostaglandin E2 at doses of 10(-9)-10(-6) M, produced significant dose-dependent inhibition in DNA synthesis. In combination, doses of 10(-5) M resulted in significant additive inhibition averaging 43.53%.

> —T.M. ElAttar and H.S Lin, "Inhibition of Human Oral Squamous Carcinoma Cell (SCC-25) Proliferation by Prostaglandin E2 and Vitamin E Succinate," *Journal of Oral Pathol Med,* 22(9), October 1993, p. 425-427.

Results of this study found that vitamin E levels in patients with breast cancer were significantly lower than controls, with the mean levels being 0.44mg/100ml vs. 1.108mg/100ml respectively.

> —M. Torun, et al., "Serum Vitamin E Level in Patients with Breast Cancer," *Journal of Clin Pharm Ther,* 20(3), June 1995, p. 173-178.

Results of this study found that heat (41 degrees-40 degrees) in combination with 5 micrograms/ml of vitamin E succinate proved effective in inhibiting the growth of neuroblastoma cells in mice.

> —B.N. Rama and K.N. Prasad, "Effect of Hyperthermia in Combination with Vitamin E and Cyclic AMP on Neuroblastoma Cells in Culture," *Life Sci,* 34(21), May 21, 1984, p. 2089-2097.

In this study, 32 high risk breast cancer patients were given a combination of antioxidants which included 2500 IU of vitamin E, 32.5 IU of beta-carotene, 2850 mg of vitamin C, 387 micrograms of selenium, 90 mg of CoQ10, 1.2 g of gamma linolenic acid, 3.5 g n-3 fatty acids, and a host of secondary vitamins and minerals. Results found that none of the patients taking the antioxidants died during treatment or showed signs of further distant metastases. The use of painkillers was reduced and six patients experienced partial remission.

> —K. Lockwood, et al., "Apparent Partial Remission of Breast Cancer in 'High Risk' Patients

Supplemented with Nutritional Antioxidants, Essential Fatty Acids and Coenzyme Q10,'' *Mol Aspects Med,* 15(Suppl), p. 231-240.

This review article makes the following observations with respect to vitamin E and cancer: in vitro proliferation of vascular smooth muscle cells, Balb c/3T3 fibroblasts, retinal neuroepithelial cells and neuroblastoma cells is inhibited by d-alpha-tocopherol. PDGF-BB activated proliferation is highly d-alpha-tocopherol sensitive. D-alpha-tocopherol inhibits protein kinase C activity as well a activation of the transcription activation complex AP-1.

    —A. Azzi, et al., ''D-alpha-tocopherol Control of Cell Proliferation,'' *Mol Aspects Med,* 14(3), 1993, p. 265-271.

Results of this study found that n-3 PUFA may offer protection against colon cancer in high-risk subjects by a mechanism involving vitamin E modulation.

    —G.M. Bartoli, et al., ''N-3 PUFA and Alpha-tocopherol Control of Tumor Cell Proliferation,'' *Mol Aspects Med,* 14(3), 1993, p. 247-252.

This study examined the effects of vitamin E on tumor take, tumor growth, and host survival in a transplantable lymphoma in mice as well as its relationship to immunofunction in normal and malignant conditions in murine and human systems. Results found vitamin E serum levels to be lower in human and animal cases of lymphoma and leukemia relative to controls. Vitamin E supplementation beginning at the initial developmental phase of lymphomas in mice resulted in a reduced rate of tumor growth and improvement in host survival. Supplementation activated specific mitogen induced blastogenesis of peripheral blood lymphocytes and elevated serum IgC levels as well.

    —J. Dasgupta, et al., ''Vitamin E—Its Status and Role in Leukemia and Lymphoma,'' *Neoplasma,* 40(4), 1993, p. 235-240.

Results of this study found the doses of vitamin E in excess of 80 IU/kg per day suppressed lymphoproliferative responses and inhibited Meth-A tumor cell growth in mice.

    —T. Yasunaga, et al., [Vitamin E and Cancer Therapy - Experimental Study in Mice], *Nippon Gan Chiryo Gakkai Shi,* 17(8), 1982, p. 2074-2083.

This study examined the effects of vitamin E supplementation and a mild increase in selenium levels on short-term lipid peroxidation induced by on 7,12- dimethylbenz[a]anthracene (DMBA) and the long term development of mammary tumors in rats. Results showed that supplementation with 235 mg/kg vitamin E and 0.6 mg/kg selenium administered up to three week after DMBA or the end of the experiment significantly inhibited tumors relative to the control group. Significant inhibition of elevated lipid peroxidation in both mammary fat pads and livers of animals was also seen.

    —H. Takada, et al., ''Inhibition of 7,12-Dimethylbenz[a]anthracene-induced Lipid Peroxidation and Mammary Tumor Development in Rats by Vitamin E in Conjunction with Selenium,'' *Nutr Cancer,* 17(2), 1992, p. 115-122.

Results of this study showed that rats fed normal vitamin E diets (26-50 ppm) for 30-34 weeks had a 30% lower incidence of tumors and 25%-50% lower burden than rats fed a diet low in vitamin E (1-5 ppm). Results also found that rats fed diets low in vitamin E (5 ppm) and high in calcium (1.0%)

produced a larger reduction in tumor incidence and burden compared to rats fed diets of 50 ppm vitamin E and 0.2% calcium.

 —G.H. McIntosh, "The Influence of Dietary Vitamin E and Calcium Status on Intestinal Tumors in Rats," *Nutr Cancer,* 17(1), 1992, p. 47-55.

Results of this study found women with cervical dysplasias or cancer had significantly reduced plasma levels of beta-carotene and alpha-tocopherol. The effects of these antioxidants appeared to be independent of one another in relation to the pathogenesis of cervical cancer and cervical intraepithelial lesions.

 —R.R. Palan, et al., "Plasma Levels of Antioxidant Beta-carotene and Alpha-tocopherol in Uterine Cervix Dysplasias and Cancer," *Nutr Cancer,* 15(1), 1991, p. 13-20.

Results of this case-control study of 59 newly diagnosed lung cancer patients found a possible inverse association between vitamin E levels and the risk of lung cancer.

 —B.Y LeGardeur, et al., "A Case-control Study of Serum Vitamins A, E, and C in Lung Cancer Patients," *Nutr Cancer,* 14(2), 1990, p. 133-140.

This study found that the oral administration of 200 mg of alpha-tocopherol in combination with 200 mg of beta-carotene in vegetable oil was effective in regressing epidermoid carcinomas of the buccal pouch in hamsters.

 —G. Shklar, et al., "Regression of Experimental Cancer by Oral Administration of Combined Alpha-Tocopherol and Beta-carotene," *Nutr Cancer,* 12(4), 1989, p. 321-325.

Results of this study showed mice fed 0.5 g of DL-alpha-tocopheryl acetate/kg diet experienced a reduced rate and incidence of tumors produced by transplantable sarcoma cells relative to controls. Such effects proved to be dependent on the level of unsaturation of dietary fat. It was also seen that in vitro treatment of the K3T3 cells with vitamin E enhanced its cytotoxic effects, suggesting that vitamin E acts directly on the tumor cell instead of the immune system.

 —M.P. Kurek and L.M. Corwin, "Vitamin E Protection Against Tumor Formation by Transplanted Murine Sarcoma Cells," *Nutr Cancer,* 4(2), 1982, p. 128-139.

Results of this study found that dietary supplementation with vitamin E led to significant reductions in the size and frequency of N-nitrosomethylbenzylamine-induced esophageal tumors in mice.

 —O.E Odeleye, et al., "Vitamin E Inhibition of Lipid Peroxidation and Ethanol-mediated Promotion of Esophageal Tumorigenesis," *Nutr Cancer,* 17(3), 1992, p. 223-234.

This studied examined the ability of topical vitamin E to prevent photocarcinogenesis in mice. Results showed that mice given 25 mg of vitamin E three times weekly for three weeks significantly reduced UV induced skin cancer.

 —H.L. Gensler and M. Magdaleno, "Topical Vitamin E Inhibition of Immunosuppression and Tumorigenesis Induced by Ultraviolet Irradiation," *Nutr Cancer,* 15(2), 1991, p. 97-106.

Results of this study found that rats fed a vitamin E and selenium deficient diet suffered from more DMBA induced palpable mammary tumors relative to rats fed a diet adequate in both nutrients.

 —H.J. Thompson, "Effects of Combined Deficiencies of Selenium (SE) and Vitamin E (VIT

E) on the Initiation and Promotion Phases of 7,12-Dimethyl[A]anthracene (DMBA)-Induced Mammary Tumorigenesis," *Proc Annu Meet Am Assoc Cancer Res,* 32, 1991, p. A877.

Results of this study found that the use of vitamin E in combination with low levels of vitamin D3 significantly enhanced the differentiation markers in HL-60 leukemia relative to controls.

—J.A. Sokoloski, et al., "Induction of the Differentiation of HL-60 Leukemia Cells by Vitamin E and other Antioxidants in Combination with Vitamin D3," *Proceeding of the Annual Meeting of the American Association of Cancer Researchers,* 36, 1995, p. A2073.

This study demonstrated that the in vitro proliferation of estrogen receptor positive (ER+) MCF-7 and (ER-) MDA-MB-435 breast cancer cells is inhibited by RRR-alpha-tocopheryl succinate by approximately 25%, 40%, and 60% at 1, 2, and 3 days after treatment, respectively.

—K. Kline, et al., "In Vitro Treatment of Human Breast Cancer Cells with RRR-alpha-tocopheryl Succinate (Vitamin E Succinate) Inhibits Proliferation and Enhances the Secretion of Biologically Active Transforming Growth Factor-Beta (TGF-beta) (Meeting Abstract)," *Proceedings of the Annual Meeting of the American Association of Cancer,* 35, 1994, p. A1641.

This study examined the potential of alpha-D-tocopherol succinate to protect bone marrow from anticancer drug-induced toxicity in vitro. Results showed that treatment offered protection of up to 43%. When 50 mg/kg po of alpha-D-Tocopherol was used in combination with Melphalan of Erythroid Progenitor Cells.

—S.R. Gogu, et al., "Selective Protection of Murine Erythroid Progenitor Cells with Vitamin E from Drug-induced Toxicity," *Proceedings of the Annual Meeting of the American Association of Cancer,* 31, 1990, p. A2400.

This study examined the effects of the derivatives of vitamins C and E, 2-O-octadecylascorbic acid (CV3611), L-ascorbic acid, DL-alpha-tocopherol and 6-hydroxy-2,5,7,8-tetramethylchroman-2-carboxylic acid, on carcinogenesis of the liver in rats. Following 12 weeks of a diet containing concentrations with or without one of the four vitamin derivitives at a concentration of 0.01, 0.05 or 0.10%, results showed that the greatest overall inhibition in a dose-dependent manner was accomplished by CV3611.

—D. Nakae, et al., "Inhibitory Effects of Vitamin C and E Derivatives on Rat Liver Carcinogenesis Induced by a Choline-Deficient L-Amino Acid (CDAA)-Defined Diet (Meeting abstract)," *Proceedings of the Annual Meeting of the American Association of Cancer Researchers,* 34, 1993, p. A729

Results of this study showed that gamma-tocopherol was found to react with NO2 to regenerate NO and inhibit N-nitrosamine formation and that gamma-tocopherol proved to be a more effective inhibitor of neoplastic transformation in C3H/10T1/2 fibroblasts than alpha-tocopherol, exhibiting a dose-dependent decrease in transformation between 0.3 uM and 30 uM.

—R.V. Cooney, et al., "Gamma-tocopherol Inhibition of Nitrogen Oxide-Mediated Nitrosation and its Role in Cancer Chemoprevention (Meeting abstract)," *Proceedings of the Annual Meeting of the American Association of Cancer Researchers,* 34, 1993, p. A3324.

This double-blind, placebo-controlled study examined the effects of 400 mg/ml in oil form of vitamin E topically applied to lesions for one week in patients receiving chemotherapy for oral musositis. Results showed the treatment to be significantly effective relative to controls.

> —R. Wadleigh, et al., "Vitamin E in the Treatment of Chemotherapy-Induced Mucosisitis," *Proceedings of the Annual Meeting of the American Society of Clinical Oncologists,* 9, 1990, p. A1237.

Results of this study found that the administration of alpha-tocopherol in an escalating dose schedule of 800, 1200, 1600, and 2000 IU per day for each subsequent 4-wk cycle until disease progression or unacceptable toxicity occurred reduced the level of major toxicities of high dose 13-cRA in patient suffering from skin, head and neck, or lung cancer.

> —I. Dimery, et al., "Reduction in Toxicity of High Dose 13-CIS-Retinoic Acid (13-CRA) with Alpha-Tocerphorl," *Proceedings of the Annual Meeting of the American Society of Clinical Oncologists,* 11, 1992, p. A399.

This review article notes that earlier studies have shown that vitamin E succinate along with prostaglandin E2 may act to inhibit human oral squamous carcinoma cell proliferation. It adds that more recent studies have seen similar anticancer results with antineoplastic PGs, delta 12-PG2 and PG12.

> —T.M. elAttar and H.S Lin, "Vitamin E Succinate Potentiates the Inhibitory Effect of Prostaglandins on Oral Squamous Carcinoma Cell Proliferation," *Prostaglandins Leukot Essent Fatty Acids,* 52(1), January 1995, p. 69-73.

Results of this study showed that the rate of postoperative complications in a group of gastric cancer patients taking a complex administration of vitamin C, E, and A preoperatively dropped from 30.9% to 1.9%.

> —V.N. Sukolinskii and T.S. Morozkina, [Prevention of Postoperative Complications in Patients with Stomach Cancer Using an Antioxidant Complex], *Vopr Onkol,* 35(10), 1989, p. 1242-1245.

Results of this study of 28 liver cancer patients found that treatment with 600 mg of alpha-tocopherol, 100,000 MU of retinol and 1.5 g of ascorbic acid for 7days prior to surgery was shown to significantly reduce the level of dialdehyde in the liver and increase the level of catalase. Following antioxidant treatment, purulent and septic complications were 1.6 times less as well.

> —E.G. Gorozhanskaia, et al., [The Role of Alpha-Tocopherol and Retinol in Correcting Disorders of Lipid Peroxidation in Patients with Malignant Liver Neoplasms], *Vopr Onkol,* 41(1), 1995, p. 47-51.

Cardiovascular/Coronary Heart Disease

This placebo-controlled, double-blind study examined the effects on platelet function in low antioxidant men of supplementation with 600 mg ascorbic acid, 300 mg alpha-tocopherol, 27 mg beta-carotene, and 75 micrograms of selenium in yeast daily for 5 months. Results showed that relative to controls, men taking the antioxidants experienced 20% reductions in serum lipid peroxides, 24% reductions in ADP-induced platelet aggregation, 42% reductions in the rate of ATP release during aggregation,

51% reductions in serum thromboxane B2, and 29% reductions in plasma beta-thromboglobulin concentration.

—J.T. Salonen, et al., "Effects of Antioxidant Supplementation on Platelet Function: A Randomized Pair-Matched, Placebo-controlled, Double-blind Trial in Men with Low Antioxidant Status," *American Journal of Clinical Nutrition,* 53(5), May 1991, p. 1222-1229.

Results of this large-scale, longitudinal study of coronary heart disease mortality among men in 17 western European countries found that vitamin E intake specifically rather than the consumption of wine is most likely the best explanation of what has been come to be called the "European Paradox": that is the paradoxically low rates of CHD in several European countries which have a relatively high intake of saturated fatty acids.

—M.C. Bellizz, et al., "Vitamin E and Coronary Heart Disease: The European Paradox," *European Journal of Clinical Nutrition,* 48(11), November 1994, p. 822-831.

Results of this study showed that the consumption of one palmvitee capsule per day (containing approximately 18 mg of tocopherols, 42 mg of tocotrienols, and 240 mg of palm olein) for 30 days lowered both serum total cholesterol (ranging from 5% to 35.9%) and low-density-lipoprotein cholesterol (ranging from 0.9% to 37%) concentrations in all subjects.

—D.T. Tan, et al., "Effect of a Palm-oil-vitamin E Concentrate on the Serum and Lipoprotein Lipids in Humans," *American Journal of Clinical Nutrition,* 53(4 Suppl), April 1991, p. 1027S-1030S.

This double-blind, crossover study compared the effects on the serum lipids of hypercholesterolemic human subjects of the tocotrienol-enriched fraction of palm oil in the form of 200 mg palmvitee capsules per day with those of 300 mg of corn oil per day. In the case of the 15 subjects taking the palmvitee, results showed significant reductions in the concentrations of serum total cholesterol (-%15), LDL cholesterol (-8%), Apo B (-10%), thromboxane (-25%), platelet factor 4 (-16%), and glucose (-12%). In 7 hypercholesterolemic subjects, results showed a 31% mean reduction in serum cholesterol concentrations over a 4 week period while they were taking 200 mg of gamma-tocotrienol/d, suggesting it could be the strongest inhibitor of cholesterol in the palmvitee capsules.

—A.A. Qureshi, et al., "Lowering of Serum Cholesterol in Hypercholesterolemic Humans by Tocotrienols (Palmvitee)," *American Journal of Clinical Nutrition,* 53(4 Suppl), April 1991, p. 1021S-1026S.

Results of this study showed supplementing plasma with vitamin E increased the alpha-tocopherol content of LDL as well as the oxidative resistance in linear proportion with the increases in alpha-tocopherol content.

—H. Esterbauer, et al., "Role of Vitamin E in Preventing the Oxidation of Low-Density Lipoprotein," *American Journal of Clinical Nutrition,* 53(1 Suppl), January 1991, p. 314S-321S.

Results of this double-blind, placebo-controlled study found that the intake of 900 mg per day for 4 months of vitamin E by elderly insulin-resistant nondiabetics proved to be a useful therapy for coronary heart disease.

—G. Paolisso, et al., "Chronic Intake of Pharmacological Doses of Vitamin E Might be

Useful in the Therapy of Elderly Patients with Coronary Heart Disease," *American Journal of Clinical Nutrition,* 61(4), April 1995, p. 848-852.

Results of this study showed that significant reductions in the indexes of oxidative stress in both smokers and nonsmokers as well as reductions in serum platelet numbers following the intake of 280 mg per day for 10 weeks of dl-alpha-tocopherol acetate. The authors conclude that such findings may suggest the efficacy of vitamin E in preventing the lipid peroxidation associated with atherosclerosis and fibrinolysis.

—K.M. Brown, et al., "Vitamin E Supplementation Suppresses Indexes of Lipid Peroxidation and Platelet Counts in Blood of Smokers and Nonsmokers but Plasma Lipoprotein Concentrations Remain Unchanged," *American Journal of Clinical Nutrition,* 60(3), September 1994, p. 383-387.

Results of this study showed that alpha-tocopherol specifically inhibited aorta smooth muscle cell proliferation and protein kinase C activity, findings which may be relevant to the development of atherosclerosis and related diseases.

—D. Boscoboinik, et al., "Alpha-tocopherol (Vitamin E) Regulates Vascular Smooth Muscle Cell Proliferation and Protein Kinase C Activity," *Arch Biochem Biophys,* 286(1), April 1991, p. 264-269.

This double-blind study of 100 patients with transient ischemic attacks, minor strokes, or residual ischemic neurologic deficits compared the effects of aspirin plus 400 IU per day of vitamin E with aspirin alone (325 mg) for up to 2 years. Results showed patients in the vitamin E plus aspirin group experienced a significant reduction in the rate of ischemic events relative to patients taking just the aspirin. Significant reductions were also seen in platelet adhesiveness in patients taking the vitamin E plus aspirin relative to those taking aspirin only. Based on these findings, the authors conclude that vitamin E plus aspirin is an effective preventive therapy for transient ischemic attacks and related cerebrovascular disorders.

—M. Steiner, et al., "Vitamin E Plus Aspirin Compared with Aspirin Alone in Patients with Transient Ischemic Attacks," *American Journal of Clinical Nutrition,* 62(6 Suppl), December 1995, p. 1381S-1384S

In this study, healthy subjects were given 400 IU per day of either 268 mg of D-alpha-tocopherol or 364 mg of DL-alpha-tocopherol for 4 weeks. Results showed that vitamin E exerted a differential effect on peroxidase activities and platelet lipooxygenase.

—A.C. Chan, et al., "Transitory Stimulation of Human Platelet 12-lipooxygenase by Vitamin E Supplementation," *American Journal of Clinical Nutrition,* 44(2), August 1986, p. 278-282.

Results of this study showed that combined treatment with 12 g of vitamin E acetate intravenously 3 times for one week prior to ischemic and 4.4 g of intravenous vitamin C before reperfusion in one group and treatment with 12 g of vitamin E intraarterially and 4.4 g of intravenous vitamin C during ischemia each reduced the size of infarct in porcine hearts.

—H.H. Klein, et al., "Combined Treatment with Vitamins E and C in Experimental Myocardial Infarction in Pigs," *American Heart Journal,* 118(4), October 1989, p. 667-673.

Results of this study found that the administration of vitamin E in rabbits was associated with a reduction in blood and aortic tissue malondialdehyde concentration despite hypercholesterolemia.

—K. Prasad and J. Kalra, "Oxygen Free Radicals and Hypercholesterolemic Atherosclerosis: Effect of Vitamin E," *American Heart Journal,* 125(4), April 1993, p. 958-973.

Results of this study found that the combined administration of vitamin E and 17 beta-estradiol provides protection for LDL against oxidation in postmenopausal women.

—V. Guetta, et al., "Effect of Combined 17 Beta-estradiol and Vitamin E on Low-density Lipoprotein Oxidation in Postmenopausal Women," *American Journal of Cardiology,* 75(17), June 15, 1995, p. 1274-1276.

This study examined the relationship between dietary intake of vitamin C, vitamin E, and carotene and the risk of coronary mortality in a group of 5,133 Finnish adults initially heart disease free. Results showed an inverse association between vitamin E intake and coronary mortality in both sexes.

—P. Knekt, et al., "Antioxidant Vitamin Intake and Coronary Mortality in a Longitudinal Population Study," *American Journal of Epidemiology,* 139(12), June 15, 1994, p. 1180-1189.

Results of this study found that alpha-tocopherol was effective in the attenuation of ischemia and reperfusion damage in rats. The authors argue that such findings suggest that the reduction of lipid alterations could be protect against membrane damage subsequent to ischemia and reperfusion.

—K.D. Massey, et al., "Alpha-Tocopherol Attenuates Myocardial Membrane-Related Alterations Resulting from Ischemia and Reperfusion," *American Journal of Physiology,* 256(4 Pt 2), April 1989, p. H1192-1199.

This study examined the effects of oral vitamin E and vitamin C supplementation in patients with coronary artery disease. Results showed that patients receiving supplementation either immediately before or after coronary artery bypass suffered fewer ischemic electrocardiographic events and needed less dopamine perioperatively relative to controls.

—T. Sisto, et al., "Pretreatment with Antioxidants and Allopurinol Diminishes Cardiac Onset Events in Coronary Artery Bypass Grafting," *Ann Thorac Surg,* 59(6), June 1995, p. 1519-1523.

This study examined the effects of D,L-alpha-tocopherol, beta-carotene and smoking on LDL's resistance against copper-mediated oxidation. Results found that ingestion of 1000 IU per day of D,L-alpha-tocopheral acetate for 7 days by 6 nonsmoking subjects increased plasma and LDL levels of alpha-tocopherol 3.0 and 2.4 fold, respectively. In addition, the rate of oxidation showed significant decreases of 19% and significant elevations of LDL oxidation resistance by 41%.

—H.M. Princen, et al., "Supplementation with Vitamin E but Not Beta-carotene in Vivo Protects Low Density Lipoprotein from Lipid Peroxidation in Vitro: Effect of Cigarette Smoking," *Arteriosclerosis Thrombosis,* 12(5), May 1992, 554-562.

This study supplemented the diet of Watanabe heritable hyperlipidemic rabbits with either a low dose 0.025% wt/wt of vitamin E or probucol for 6 months. Results showed that vitamin E proved to be the more effective antioxidant at low doses.

—H.A. Kleinveld, et al., "Comparative Study on the Effect of Low-dose Vitamin E and

Probucol on the Susceptibility of LDL to Oxidation and the Progression of Atherosclerosis in Watanabe Heritable Hyperlipidemic Rabbits,'' *Arterioscler Thromb,* 14(8), August 1994, p. 1386-1391.

This study examined the effects of a 1% cholesterol plus 0.2% vitamin E diet in preparations of isolated carotoid from cholesterol-fed rabbits for 4 weeks. Results showed that relaxant responses to acetylcholine were enhanced in the rabbits fed both cholesterol and vitamin E in raised-tone preparations, reversing the reduction in responses measured in preparations from cholesterol-fed rabbits. Similar results were seen with respect to relaxant responses to the calcium ionophore A23187. In rabbits fed a cholesterol plus vitamin E diet, the copper-induced oxidation of beta-very-low-density lipoproteins showed close to complete inhibition relative to the oxidation of beta VLDL from rabbits fed only cholesterol. Based on these findings, the authors suggest that vitamin E may play a role in preventing functional impairment associated with atherosclerosis.

—A.L. Stewart-Lee, et al., ''Vitamin E Protects Against Impairment of Endothelium-Mediated Relaxations in Cholesterol-fed Rabbits,'' *Arterioscler Thromb,* 14(3), March 1994, p. 494-999.

Results of this study found that vitamin E fed guinea pigs experienced significant reductions in intimal atheromatous lesions of the aorta when compared to guinea pigs fed a cholesterol diet and to controls. Vitamin E was also shown to inhibit lipid deposition and development associated with an irregular distribution of proteoglycan. According to the authors, such findings suggest that vitamin E may play a role in inhibiting atherogenesis in cholesterol-fed guinea pigs by preserving the morphological and functional integrity of the vascular wall.

—Y. Qiao, et al., ''Effect of Vitamin E on Vascular Integrity in Cholesterol-fed Guinea Pigs,'' *Arterioscler Thromb,* 13(12), December 1993, p. 1885-1892.

Results of this study showed that oral supplementation with vitamin E led to increases in LDL alpha-tocopherol content, increases in LDL resistance to oxidation, and reductions in the cytotoxicity of oxidized LDL to cultured vascular endothelial cells.

—J.D. Belcher, et al., ''Vitamin E, LDL, and Endothelium: Brief Oral Vitamin Supplementation Prevents Oxidized LDL-Mediated Vascular Injury in Vitro,'' *Arterioscler Thromb,* 13(12), December 1993, p. 1779-1789.

This study compared the effects of 8 weeks of supplementation with 1600 mg per day of either RRR-alpha-tocopherol or the synthetic racemic form of alpha-tocopherol on the susceptibility of isolated lipoproteins to oxidation. Results showed that supplementation with either form of vitamin E resulted in the same level of antioxidant protection to LDL.

—P.D. Reaven and J.L. Witztum, ''Comparison of Supplementation of RRR-alpha-tocopherol and Racemic Alpha-tocopherol in Humans. Effects on Lipid Levels and Lipoprotein Susceptibility to Oxidation,'' *Arterioscler Thromb,* 13(4), April 1993, p. 601-608.

Results of this study showed that long-term supplementation with large doses of vitamin E alone, but not beta-carotene, produced an increase in protection to LDL in vitro assays of oxidation.

—P.D. Reaven, et al., ''Effect of Dietary Antioxidant Combinations in Humans: Protection of LDL by Vitamin E but not by Beta-carotene,'' *Arterioscler Thromb,* 13(4), April 1993, p. 590-600.

This review article outlines the many positive aspects of the natural metabolite of vitamin E, vitamin E quinone, and notes that its greater potency in suppressing platelet function relative to vitamin E suggest it might be a more effective antithrombotic agent and may well be responsible for the in vivo effects previously attributed to vitamin E.

> —A.C. Cox, et al., "The Influence of Vitamin E Quinone on Platelet Structure, Function, and Biochemistry," *Blood,* 55(6), June 1980, p. 907-914.

Results of this study showed that platelet adherence decreased an average of 75% after 2 weeks of supplementation of 200 IU of vitamin E per day in normal individuals. An 82% reduction occurred following 2 weeks of supplementation with 400 IU per day.

> —J. Jandak, et al., "Alpha-tocopherol, an Effective Inhibitor of Platelet Adhesion," *Blood,* 73(1), January 1989, p. 141-149.

This study examined the relationship between the intake of supplemental and dietary vitamin C, alpha-tocopherol, and provitamin A carotenoids and average carotid artery wall thickness in approximately 11,000 middle-age adults. With respect to vitamin E, results showed an inverse relationship with wall thickness, but only in women.

> —S.B. Kritchevsky, et al., "Dietary Antioxidants and Carotid Artery Wall Thickness: The ARIC Study. Atherosclerosis Risk in Communities Study," *Circulation,* 92(8), October 15, 1995, p. 2142-2150.

This placebo-controlled study examined the effects of combined supplementation with 800 IU per day of alpha-tocopherol, 1 g per day of ascorbate and 30 mg per day of carotene over a 3 month period on copper-catalyzed LDL oxidation in 12 men. Results showed that the antioxidant therapy produced a twofold prolongation of the lag phased and reduced the oxidation rate by 40%. Subjects receiving just 800 IU of alpha-tocopherol experienced no significant differences with the combined antioxidant subjects with respect to LDL oxidation kinetics, thus the authors argue alpha-tocopherol should be favored in future trials on coronary prevention.

> —I. Jialal and S.M. Grundy, "Effect of Combined Supplementation with Alpha-tocopherol, Ascorbate, and Beta-carotene on Low-density Lipoprotein Oxidation," *Circulation,* 88(6), December 1993, p. 2780-2786.

This study examined the effects of supplementation with 500 mg daily of alpha-tocopherol on lethal ventricular arrhythmias and infarct size in dogs. Results suggested that supplementation prevented lethal ventricular arrhythmias associated with ischemia and reperfusion.

> —L. Sebbag, et al., "Effects of Dietary Supplementation with Alpha-tocopherol on Myocardial Infarct Size and Ventricular Arrhythmias in a Dog Model of Ischemia-Reperfusion," *Journal of the American College of Cardiology,* 24(6), November 15, 1994, p. 1580-1585.

Results of this study showed the aerobic incubation of brain after a period of ischemia-induced lipid peroxidation was greatest in rats deficient in vitamin E, intermediate in rats normal in vitamin E, and least in rats receiving vitamin E supplementation.

> —S. Yoshida, et al., "Brain Lipid Peroxidation Induced by Postischemic Reoxygenation in Vitro: Effect of Vitamin E," *Journal of Cerebral Blood Flow Metabolism,* 4(3), September 1984, p. 466-469.

Results of this study demonstrated the ability of alpha-tocopherol to reduce restenosis after angioplasty in a rabbit model in which angioplasty was performed on established atherosclerotic lesions.

> —A.M. Lafont, et al., "Effect of Alpha-tocopherol on Restenosis After Angioplasty in a Model of Experimental Atherosclerosis," *Journal of Clinical Investigations,* 95(3), March 1995, p. 1018-1025.

This study examined the effects of alpha-tocopherol on endothelium-dependent arterial relaxation in rabbits fed diets containing either no additive, 1% cholesterol, or 1% cholesterol with either 1000 IU/kg chow of alpha-tocopherol or 10,000 IU/kg chow of alpha-tocopherol. Results showed that compared to control (no additive) and cholesterol groups, vessels in the groups taking 10,000 IU/kg of alpha-tocopherol showed significant impairment of arterial relaxation and significantly more intimal proliferation than other groups. In addition to these findings, it was observed that LDL from both dosage groups of alpha-tocopherol was more resistant to oxidation than LDL from controls.

> —J.F. Keaney, Jr., et al., "Low-dose Alpha-tocopherol Improves and High-Dose Alpha-tocopherol Worsens Endothelial Vasodilator Function in Cholesterol-Fed Rabbits," *Journal of Clinical Investigations,* 93(2), February 1994, p. 844-851.

This study examined the levels of serum cholesterol, alpha-tocopherol, retinol, albumin, selenium, and other major risk factors in male subjects living in Northern Finland. Results showed that subjects living in the lowest coronary mortality areas showed higher levels of serum-lipid-adjusted alpha-tocopherol, albumin, selenium, cholesterol, and LDL cholesterol relative to those in a reference area. Based on these findings, the authors conclude alpha-tocopherol, albumin, and selenium may be a factor in the low coronary heart disease mortality rates in northermost Finland.

> —P.V. Luoma, et al., "High Serum Alpha-tocopherol, Albumin, Selenium and Cholesterol, and Low Mortality from Coronary Heart Disease in Northern Finland," *Journal of Internal Medicine,* 237(1), January 1995, p. 49-54.

In this double-blind, crossover study, 12 healthy volunteers were administered 30 ml/day of either fish oils supplemented with 0.3 IU/g or 1.5 IU/g for 3 weeks. Results showed that the intake of the vitamin E-rich fish oil produced a 48% decrease in serum triglycerides and an 11% decrease in fibrinogen. Smaller effects were seen with respect to serum triglycerides after supplementation with low-vitamin E fish oil and there were no reductions of fibrinogen.

> —O. Haglund, et al., "The Effects of Fish Oil on Triglycerides, Cholesterol, Fibrinogen and Malondialdehyde in Humans Supplemented with Vitamin E," *Journal of Nutrition,* 121(2), February 1991, p. 165-169.

Results of this study showed that mice fed a diet deficient in vitamin E increased pathology in hearts infected with a myocarditic coxsackievirus B3 (CVB3/20).

> —M.A. Beck, et al., "Vitamin E Deficiency Intensifies the Myocardial Injury of Coxsackievirus B3 Infection of Mice," *Journal of Nutrition,* 124(3), March 1994, p. 345-358.

Results of this study showed that alpha-tocopherol in doses of 10, 20, and 40 microM significantly reduced the toxicity of 30 microM of the antidysrhthmic drug amiodarone in vitro.

> —D.L. Kachel, et al., "Amiodarone-induced Injury of Human Pulmonary Artery Endothelial cells: Protection by Alpha-Tocopherol," *Journal of Pharmacol Exp Ther,* 254(3), September 1990, p. 1107-1112.

Results of this study suggest that systemic lipid peroxidation takes place during bypass and that, by attenuating the degree of peroxidative damage, vitamin E might offer protection during normal bypass grafting.

—J.G. Coghlan, et al., "Lipid Peroxidation and Changes in Vitamin E Levels During Coronary Artery Bypass Grafting," *Journal of Thorac Cardiovasc Surg,* 106(2), August 1993, p. 268-274.

Results of this study are consistent with earlier data demonstrating that some of alcohol's toxic effects may be mediated through free radical mechanisms leading to lipid peroxidation. Further, alpha tocopherol's ameliorating effects may correspond to its role as a free radical scavenger and antioxidant.

—J.E. Redetzki, et al., "Amelioration of Cardiotoxic Effects of Alcohol by Vitamin E," *Journal of Toxicol Clin Toxicol,* 20(4), June 1983, p. 319-331.

This placebo-controlled study examined the relationship between dietary vitamin E and C with coronary heart disease progression in men. Results showed that those taking 100 IU per day or more of vitamin E had less coronary artery lesion progression than subjects taking less than this amount and such benefits were seen in all lesions.

—H.N. Hodis, et al., "Serial Coronary Angiographic Evidence that Antioxidant Vitamin Intake Reduces Progression of Coronary Artery Atherosclerosis," *JAMA,* 273(23), June 21, 1995, p. 1849-1854.

This placebo-controlled study examined the effects of intravenous vitamin E on ventricular fibrillation threshold in an experimental model of acute myocardial ischemia in rats. Results found that vitamin E prevented ventricular fibrillation.

—A.J. Fuenmayor, et al., "Vitamin E and Ventricular Fibrillation Threshold in Myocardial Ischemia," *Japanese Circulation Journal,* 53(10), October 1989, p. 1229-1232.

This study examined the relationship between plasma concentrations of vitamins A, C, E, and carotene and the risk of angina pectoris. Results found that after smoking was controlled for only plasma concentrations of vitamin E showed a significant inverse relationship with angina risk.

—R.A. Riemersma, et al., "Risk of Angina Pectoris and Plasma Concentrations of Vitamins A, C, and E and Carotene," *Lancet,* 337(8732), January 5, 1991, p. 1-5.

This study measured alpha-tocopherol and beta-carotene concentrations in the adipose-tissue samples of patients with acute myocardial infarction. Results supported previous findings suggesting that reductions of risk from vitamin E intake come with supplementation only.

—A.F. Kardinaal, et al., "Antioxidants in Adipose Tissue and Risk of Myocardial Infarction: The EURAMIC Study," *Lancet,* 342(8884), December 4, 1993, p. 1379-1384.

This study examined the effect of vitamin E on the production of PG12 and other prostaglandins (prostaglandin E2 [PGE2], thromboxane A2 [TXA2], and 15-hydroxyeicosatetraenoic acid [15-HETE]) by bovine aortic endothelial cells cultured in a high concentration of glucose. Results suggest that vitamin E can increase to normal reduced levels of PGI2, PGE2, or TXA2 production.

—M. Kunisaki, et al., "Vitamin E Restores Reduced Prostacyclin Synthesis in Aortic Endothelial Cells Cultured with a High Concentration of Glucose," *Metabolism,* 41(6), June 1992, p. 613-621.

Results of this study found an association between a high intake of vitamin E (60 IU per day or more) and a reduced risk of coronary heat disease in middle-aged men.

—E.B. Rimm, et al., "Vitamin E Consumption and the Risk of Coronary Heart Disease in Men," *New England Journal of Medicine,* 328(20), May 20, 1993, p. 1450-1456.

Results of this study found an association between vitamin E supplementation and a reduced risk of coronary heart disease in middle-age women.

—M.J. Stampfer, et al., "Vitamin E Consumption and the Risk of Coronary Disease in Women," *New England Journal of Medicine,* 328(20), May 20, 1993, p. 1444-1449.

This review article notes that vitamin E is the most effective chain-breaking antioxidant that exists and that evidence points to the potency of vitamin E as an antioxidant both in vitro and to it protective actions against lipid peroxidation in vivo. Studies are cited on erythrocyte ghosts and blood plasma demonstrating vitamin E to most likely be the only, lipid soluble, chain-breaking antioxidant in human blood.

—G.W. Burton and K.U. Ingold, "Mechanisms of Antioxidant Action. Studies on Vitamin E and Related Antioxidants in Biological Systems," *NFCR Cancer Res Assoc Symp,* (2), 1983, p. 81-99.

Results of this study found that spontaneously hypertensive rats had significantly lower tissue vitamin E levels than normotensive, genetically related ones. Such differences continued in the presence of identical supplementation with vitamin E.

—A. Bendich, et al., "Differences in Vitamin E Levels in Tissues of the Spontaneously Hypertensive and Wistar-Kyoto Rats," *Proc Soc Exp Biol Med,* 172(3), March 1983, p. 297-300.

The study examined the dietary intakes of antioxidants relative to prevalence of coronary artery disease in an Indian suburban population. Results found that plasma vitamin C, E, and beta-carotene were significantly lower and lipid peroxides higher in coronary artery disease patients compared to controls.

—R.B. Singh, et al., "Diet, Antioxidant Vitamins, Oxidative Stress and Risk of Coronary Artery Disease: The Peerzada Prospective Study," *Acta Cardiol,* 49(5), 1994, p. 453-467.

This study examined the effects of short-term vitamin E deficiency on lipid peroxidative properties in mouse skeletal and cardiac muscles. Results showed there to be significant negative correlations between vitamin E concentrations and in vitro lipid peroxidation in skeletal and cardiac muscles and may expose them to peroxidative injuries.

—A. Salminen, et al., "Vitamin E Deficiency and the Susceptibility to Lipid Peroxidation of Mouse Cardiac and Skeletal Muscles," *Acta Physiol Scand,* 122(4), December 1984, p. 565-570.

This study examined the lipid peroxidation products and the phospholipid fatty acid concentrations in the hearts of rats consuming chronic amounts of ethanol supplemented with high doses of vitamin E. Results showed increases in cardiac phospholipid level in rats chronically consuming excess vitamin E and/or alcohol. By preventing changes in their fatty acid composition and peroxidative deterioration, vitamin E was seen to have a stabilizing effect on heart phospholipids.

—S.V Pirozhkov, et al., "Effect of Chronic Consumption of Ethanol and Vitamin E on Fatty

Acid Composition and Lipid Peroxidation in Rat Heart Tissue," *Alcohol* (1992 Jul-Aug) 9(4), July-August 1992, p. 329-334.

This review article on vitamin E notes that it may have the ability to prevent the initiation/progression of spontaneous atheroscerlosis based on the findings of in vitro studies which have found that vitamin E influences the responses of vascular endothelial cells, leukocytes, vascular smooth muscle cells and the modification of lipoproteins.

> —A. Cogny, et al., [Vitamin E: Metabolism and Role in Atherosclerosis], *Ann Biol Clin,* 52(7-8), 1994, p. 515-522.

Results of this study showed that supplementation with vitamins E and C for 10 days before blood donation reduced LP stored in red blood cells significantly in both irradiated and non-irradiated samples relative to pre-vitamin red cell LP.

> —J.A. Knight, et al., "The Effect of Vitamins C and E on Lipid Peroxidation in Stored Erythrocytes," *Ann Clin Lab Sci* , 23(1), January-February 1993, p. 51-56.

This review article on antioxidants notes that studies have suggested vitamin E reduces platelet aggregability.

> —J.T. Salonen, "Antioxidants and Platelets," *Ann Med,* 21(1), February 1989, p. 59-62.

This study examined the effects of alpha-tocopherol nicotinate, alpha-tocopherol and dodecanoic acid on the positive inotropic action of ouabain and digoxin and on cardiac glycoside induced arrhythmias has in isolated guinea-pig left atria and in anaesthetized guinea-pigs. Results showed that alpha-tocopherol nicotinate and dodecanoic acid reduced significantly diogoxin's positive inotropic action in isolated guinea-pig atria. The authors note that Ouabain and digoxin induced arrhythmias are suppressed by the three compounds in isolated guinea-pig atria and in anaesthetized guinea-pigs: alpha-tocopherol nicotinate has the highest antiarrhythmic activity followed by dodecanoic acid and alpha-tocopherol.

> —P. Schlieper and H. Tawfik, "Antiarrhythmic Activity of Alpha-tocopherol Nicotinate and Related Compounds and their Physico-Chemical Properties," *Arzneimittelforschung,* 37(8), August 1987, p. 920-923.

Results of this study found that the supplementation with 0.5% wt/wt of vitamin E for 10-12 weeks in rabbits produced a significant hypocholesterolemic responses as well as offered significant protection on LDL from oxidative modification. One, the other, or both played a role in the inhibition of early aortic lesion development.

> —R.J. Williams, et al., "Dietary Vitamin E and the Attenuation of Early Lesion Development in Modified Watanabe Rabbits," *Atherosclerosis,* 94(2-3), June 1992, p. 153-159.

Results of this study found that selenium and vitamin E when supplemented together enhanced the improvement of metabolic processes as well as on atherosclerotic plaque formation reduction in rabbits.

> —J. Wojcicki, et al., "Effect of Selenium and Vitamin E on the Development of Experimental Atherosclerosis in Rabbits," *Atherosclerosis,* 87(1), March 1991, p. 9-16.

Results of this study showed that high levels of vitamins E and C protect plasma lipoproteins from the oxidative stress caused by smoking.

> —D. Harats, et al., ''Effect of Vitamin C and E Supplementation on Susceptibility of Plasma Lipoproteins to Peroxidation Induced by Acute Smoking,'' *Atherosclerosis,* 85(1), November 1990, 47-54.

Results of this study found that doses as low as 50-100 microM of vitamin E, when combined with an inhibitor of the arachidonate pathway, inhibit cyclooxygenase-independent platelet aggregation.

> —F. Violi, et al., ''Inhibition of Cyclooxygenase-independent Platelet Aggregation by Low Vitamin E Concentration,'' *Atherosclerosis,* 82(3), June 1990, p. 247-252.

Results of this study found that the oral administration of alpha-tocopherol for 2 weeks reduced the number of age related spontaneous injuries in rats which occurred in the aortic endothelium of ICR.

> —M. Masuda, ''Spontaneous Injuries in the Aortic Endothelium of the Inherited Cataract Rats and their Prevention by Tocopherol: A Study by Scanning Electron Microscopy,'' *Atherosclerosis,* 75(1), January 1989, p. 23-30.

Results of this study found that supplementation with vitamin E offers protection for LDL against copper-induced and macrophage-mediated oxidation. It was also shown to inhibit oxidation-dependent accumulation of LDL in macrophages and prevent stimulation of cholesteryl ester formation in macrophages. Intra-cellular vitamin E enrichment was observed to prevent LDL oxidative modification by macrophages as well.

> —M. Suzukawa, et al., ''Effects of Supplementing with Vitamin E on the Uptake of Low Density Lipoprotein and the Stimulation of Cholesteryl Ester Formation in Macrophages,'' *Atherosclerosis,* 110(1), September 30, 1994, p. 77-86.

Results of this study on rabbits showed that vitamin E proved effective in decreasing oxidative injury with the potential of leading to the impairment of nitric oxide-mediated responses in early hypercholesterolaemia.

> —J. Matz, et al., ''Dietary Vitamin E Increases the Resistance to Lipoprotein Oxidation and Attenuates Endothelial Dysfunction in the Cholesterol-fed Rabbit,'' *Atherosclerosis,* 110(2), October 1994, p. 241-249.

This study examined the effects of vitamin E on cholesterol-induced endothelial dysfunction in the coronary circulation of rabbits. Results found that cholesterol feeding for 4 and 8 weeks induced an endothelial dysfunction in coronary circulation and that protection against such effects was obtained from vitamin E. Vitamin E was also shown to prevent additional deterioration of the endothelial function in rabbit hearts and reverse the negative effects of hypercholesterolaemia.

> —T.L. Andersson, et al., ''Vitamin E Reverses Cholesterol-induced Endothelial Dysfunction in the Rabbit Coronary Circulation,'' *Atherosclerosis,* 111(1), November 1994, p. 39-45.

Results of this study found that a myocardium deficiency in vitamin E of cardiomyopathic hamsters in addition to oxidative stress together are important factors in initiating the pathogenesis of myocardial lesions. Ten days of vitamin E supplementation was seen to restore creatine kinase activity and restore myocardium lipid peroxide content levels to normal.

> —T. Sakanashi, et al., ''Vitamin E Deficiency has a Pathological Role in Myocytolysis

in Cardiomyopathic Syrian Hamster (BIO14.6)," *Biochem Biophys Res Commun,* 181(1), November 27, 1991, p. 145-150.

In this study, hamsters supplemented with vitamin E 10, 15, and 25 mg three-week slow release pellets were found to experience significant reductions in myocardial lesions caused by magnesium deficiency.
> —A.M. Freedman, et al., "Magnesium Deficiency-induced Cardiomyopathy: Protection by Vitamin E," *Biochem Biophys Res Commun,* 170(3), August 16, 1990, p. 1102-1106.

Results of this study found that high endogenous vitamin E combined with exogenous dihydrolipoic acid can create synergistic protective effects on ischemia recovery during reperfusion in rats.
> —N. Haramaki, et al., "Cardiac Recovery During Post-ischemic Reperfusion is Improved by Combination of Vitamin E with Dihydrolipoic Acid," *Biochem Biophys Res Commun,* 196(3), November 15, 1993, p. 1101-1107.

Results of this study obtained the following results: diabetic rats supplemented with vitamin E experienced a reduction in Schiff bases and anti-protein-MDA adduct antibodies and restored the fatty acid profile to that similar to controls. Vitamin E supplementation reduced stearic acid in free fatty acids, cholesterol esters, and phospholipids as well as canceled the decrease in low molecular triglycerides observed in diabetic rats. In addition to these findings, vitamin E maintained the ratio of monounsaturated and polyunsaturated fatty acids, especially in the cases of oleic acid (C18:1), dihomo-gamma-linolenic acid (C20:3 n-6), eicosapentaenoic (C20:5 n-3), and docosapentaenoic acid (C22:5 n-3), in serum phospholipids.
> —C. Douillet, et al., "High Dosage Vitamin E Effect on Oxidative Status and Serum Lipids Distribution in Streptozotocin-induced Diabetic Rats," *Biochem Med Metab Biol,* 50(3), December 1993, p. 265-76.

Results of this study showed that a combination of 15 or 30 mg/day of beta-carotene, 15 mg/day of vitamin E, and 30 mg/day of vitamin C involves an increase of singlet oxygen protection of erythrocytes of subjects which shows up quickly following treatment for 15 days.
> —E. Postaire, et al., "Increase of Singlet Oxygen Protection of Erythrocytes by Vitamin E, Vitamin C, and Beta-carotene Intakes," *Biochem Mol Biol Int,* 35(2), February 1995, p. 371-374.

Results of this study found that the central explanatory factor in cross-cultural differences of mortality from ischaemic heart disease is the plasma status of vitamin E.
> —K.F. Gey, "The Antioxidant Hypothesis of Cardiovascular Disease: Epidemiology and Mechanisms," *Biochem Soc Trans,* 18(6), December 1990, p. 1041-1045.

Results of this study found that dialdehyde content in the myocardium of rats deprived for 2 months of vitamin E was increased 53% relative to controls. It was also shown that the incidence of ventricular fibrillation, tachycardia, extrasystoles and the additive duration of arrhythmias were increased significantly in vitamin E deficient ischemic rats relative to controls.
> —L.M. Belkina, [Effect of Vitamin E Deficiency on the Development of Cardiac Arrhythmias as Affected by Acute Ischemia], *Biull Eksp Biol Med,* 102(11), November 1986, p. 530-532.

This study examined the effects of vitamin E on adrenaline-induced arrhythmias in rats with chronic heart hypertrophy subsequent to narrowing of the abdominal aorta. Results showed that the administration of two 50 mg/kg doses of vitamin E given 24 hours and 1 hour prior to adrenaline infusion, significantly increased the adrenaline amount required to produce pathological arrhythmias, thus allowing for a higher therapeutic dose in the treatment of failing hearts.

    —L.A. Kirshenbaum, et al., "Antioxidant Protection Against Adrenaline-induced Arrhythmias in Rats with Chronic Heart Hypertrophy," *Canadian Journal of Cardiology*, 6(2), March 1990, p. 71-74.

Results of this study found that rabbits given 10 days of supplemental vitamin E (200 IU/day) or a single oral dose of 2000 IU 72 hours before ischemia reduced myocardial infarct size, suggesting its potential as a preventive agent against reperfusion injury and myocardial ischemia.

    —R.A. Axford-Gately and G.J. Wilson, "Myocardial Infarct Size Reduction by Single High Dose or Repeated Low Dose Vitamin E Supplementation in Rabbits," *Canadian Journal of Cardiology*, 9(1), January-February 1993, p. 94-98.

This review article notes that recent studies have indicated modified vitamin E analogues may be more efficacious than natural vitamin E and may permit myocardial salvage from acute myocardial ischemic injury.

    —D.A. Mickle and R.D. Weisel, "Future Directions of Vitamin E and its Analogues in Minimizing Myocardial Ischemia-reperfusion Injury," *Canadian Journal of Cardiology*, 9(1), January-February 1993, p. 89-93.

Results of this study found that high dose dietary supplements with vitamin E (200 IU/kg per day) improved myocardial tolerance to ischemia and reperfusion by decreasing myocardial infarct size significantly.

    —R.A. Axford-Gatley and G.J. Wilson, "Reduction of Experimental Myocardial Infarct Size by Oral Administration of Alpha-tocopherol," *Cardiovascular Research*, 25(2), February 1991, p. 89-92.

Results of this study found that vitamin E supplementation restored reduced vascular response to acetylcholine in rabbits fed cholesterol.

    —T.O. Klemsdal, et al., "Vitamin E Restores Endothelium Dependent Vasodilatation in Cholesterol Fed Rabbits: In Vivo Measurements by Photoplethysmography," *Cardiovasc Res*, 28(9), September 1994, p. 1397-1402.

Results of this study found that the intravenous infusion of MDL 74,405, a hydrophilic cardioselective alpha tocopherol analogue, produced an attenuation of myocardial stunning in dogs comparable to that previously observed with intracoronary administration of additional antioxidants. Such findings indicate than an effective treatment for postischemic dysfunction may be the systemic administration of hydrophilic, cardioselective alpha tocopherol analogues.

    —M.E. Zughaib, et al., "Beneficial Effects of MDL 74,405, a Cardioselective Water Soluble Alpha-tocopherol Analogue, on the Recovery of Function of Stunned Myocardium in Intact Dogs," *Cardiovascular Research*, 28(2), February 1994, p. 235-241.

This study examined the effects of a single PGE2 dose in combination with vitamin E and with estradiol on experimental atherosclerosis. Results found those subjects receiving the combination treatment showed more coordinative inhibition on aortic and coronary atherosclerotic lesions, as well as on platelet aggregation, smooth muscle cell proliferation and lipid peroxidation than subjects receiving only PGE2 alone.

> —J. Qiu, et al., "Experimental Study on Antiatherosclerotic Treatment by PGE2 Combined with Vitamin E and Estradiol," *Chinese Medical Journal,* 108(1), January 1995, p. 33-36.

Results of this study found that the antioxidants vitamin E, selenium, and SOD may be a key factor in retarding atherogenesis through their protective effects on endothelial cells.

> —X.H. Yang and T.Z. Chen, [Protective Effect of the Antioxidants Selenium, Vitamin E, and Superoxide Dismutase on Cultured Human Endothelial Cells (ECs) Injured by Lipid Peroxidation], *Chung-hua Ping Li Hsueh Tsa Chih,* 19(1), March 1990, p. 8-11.

Results of this study found that doses of 400 IU per day of vitamin E inhibited platelet adhesion to a variety of adhesive proteins by more than 75%. Such effects, the authors suggest, may be related to decreases in the number and size of pseudopia upon platelet activation.

> —M. Steiner, "Vitamin E: More than an Antioxidant," *Clin Cardiol,* 16(4 Suppl 1), April 1993, p. I16-118.

This review article notes that the antioxidants vitamin E, C, beta-carotene, and monosaturated fatty acids can reduce the susceptibility of LDL to oxidation.

> —W.S. Harris, "The Prevention of Atherosclerosis with Antioxidants," *Clin Cardiol,* 15(9), September 1992, p. 636-640.

Results of these in vivo and in vitro studies found that most of estrogen's negative effects on blood platelets in rats was neutralized by the administration of alpha-tocopherol.

> —M. Ciavatti, et al., "Vitamin E Prevents the Platelet Abnormalities Induced by Estrogen in Rat," *Contraception,* 30(3), September 1984, p. 279-287.

This study examined platelet functions, platelet lipid biosynthesis, sterol composition and phospholipid fatty acid relative to plasma lipids, fatty acids, and dietary habits at day 5 and 21 of the menstrual cycle in female contraceptive users. Results showed platelet hyperactivity in long-term hormonal contraceptive users is possibly dependent upon a low platelet alpha-tocopherol level which can be corrected with supplementation of 200 IU per day.

> —S. Renaud, et al., "Influence of Vitamin E Administration on Platelet Functions in Hormonal Contraceptive Users," *Contraception,* 36(3), September 1987, 347-358.

This study examined the molecular events responsible for cell proliferation inhibition by alpha-tocopherol. In vitro results showed smooth cells to inhibited by alpha-tocopherol and a concomitant inhibition of protein kinase C activity. Results also showed alpha-tocopherol was responsible for the stimulation of protein kinase C biosynthesis in the S and G2 phases of the cell cycle in smooth muscle cells.

> —D. Boscoboinik, et al., "Molecular Basis of Alpha-tocopherol Inhibition of Smooth Muscle Cell Proliferation in Vitro," *EXS,* 62, 1992, p. 164-177.

This study evaluated the alpha-tocopherol analogue MDL 73404 for its effects on infarct size in an anaesthetized rat model of coronary artery ligation and reperfusion. Results showed that 0.3-3 mg/kg per hour intravenous infusing beginning 10 minutes before occlusion up until the end of reperfusion reduced infarct size as did 3 mg/kg per hour infusion beginning 30 minutes before reperfusion until the end. With respect to the isolated rat heart subjected to 30 min no-flow global ischaemia, pretreatment with 0.03 and 0.1 mM MDL 73404 in the perfusion buffer and during 30 min of reperfusion produced a significant increase in the maximal pressure development (+dP/dt max) and relaxation (-dP/dt max), left ventricular systolic pressure and heart rate during reperfusion. Diastolic pressure in the left ventricle was decreased significantly.

> —M.A. Petty, et al., ''Protective Effects of an Alpha-tocopherol Analogue Against Myocardial Reperfusion Injury in Rats,'' *European Journal Pharmacology,* 210(1), January 7, 1992, p. 85-90.

This study evaluated the alpha-tocopherol analogue MDL 73404 for its effects on infarct size in an anaesthetized rat model of coronary artery ligation and reperfusion. Results showed that 0.3-3 mg/kg per hour intravenous infusing beginning 10 minutes before occlusion up until the end of reperfusion reduced infarct size as did 3 mg/kg per hour infusion beginning 30 minutes before reperfusion until the end. Such findings prompted the authors to suggest that MDL 74270 has potential for cardioprotective use in conditions of acute reperfusion.

> —M.A. Petty, et al., ''Effect of a Cardioselective Alpha-tocopherol Analogue on Reperfusion Injury in Rats Induced by Myocardial Ischaemia,'' *European Journal of Pharmacology,* 192(3), January 17, 1991, p. 383-388.

Results of this study showed that the supplementation of 200 mg/kg of vitamin E in albino rats before ischemia produced changes in energy support of the ischemic myocardium leading to prolonged maintenance of synthesis process. These factors, the authors conclude, are likely to determine the anti-ischemic effect of vitamin E providing adequate restoration of the myocardial function in the postischemic period.

> —S.D. Artamonov, et al., [Effect of Vitamin E on the Energy Allowance of Functional and Plastic Processes in the Myocardium During Ischemia and Reoxygenation], *Farmakol Toksikol,* 51(3), May-June 1988, p. 27-30.

This review article reports that studies have shown vitamin E's antiatherogenic activity may be a reflection of its activities as a regulator of endothelial, smooth muscle, or monocyte-macrophage function, an inhibitor of endothelial membrane lipid peroxidation, a modulator of plasma lipid levels and lipid distribution among circulating lipoproteins, and a preventor of lipoprotein oxidative modification.

> —D.R. Janero, ''Therapeutic Potential of Vitamin E in the Pathogenesis of Spontaneous Atherosclerosis,'' *Free Radic Biol Med,* 11(1), 1991, p. 129-144.

This review article discusses the positive effects of vitamin E on oxidative heart damage, the inverse epidemiological correlations between vitamin E plasma level and anginal pain or mortality due to ischemic heart disease, and the fact that these things combined point to the therapeutic and protective roles vitamin E may play against myocardial ischemic reperfusion injury.

> —D.R. Janero, ''Therapeutic Potential of Vitamin E Against Myocardial Ischemic-reperfusion Injury,'' *Free Radic Biol Med,* 10(5), 1991, p. 315-324.

Results of this study found that a deficiency in magnesium predisposed postischemic rat hearts to increased functional loss and oxidative injury. Vitamin E, among other antioxidants, provided significant protection against such effects.

> —J.H. Kramer, et al., ''Magnesium-deficiency Potentiates Free Radical Production Associated with Postischemic Injury to Rat Hearts: Vitamin E Affords Protection,'' *Free Radic Biol Med,* 16(6), June 1994, p. 713-723.

This review article notes that studies involving 125I-low density lipoprotein have demonstrated 10 microM of probucol and 100 microM of alpha-tocopherol inhibit protein degradation in LDL exposed to Cu (II) in vitro. Alpha-tocopherol's inhibitory effect on protein fragmentation was greater than that of probucol.

> —J.V. Hunt, ''Differing Effects of Probucol and Vitamin E on the Oxidation of Lipoproteins, Ceroid Accumulation and Protein Uptake by Macrophages,'' *Free Radic Res,* 20(3), March 1994, p. 189-201.

Results of this study found that supplementing acetaminophen treated rats with vitamin E was effective in increasing the GSH content, and brought the (Na+, K+)-ATPase activity and O.F. back to almost normal.

> —M. Suhail and I. Ahmad, ''In Vivo Effects of Acetaminophen on Rat RBC and Role of Vitamin E,'' *Indian Journal of Exp Biol,* 33(4), April 1995, p. 269-271.

Results of this study found supplementation with 400 mg/kg of vitamin E per day for 60 days prevented plasma lipid level elevations, reduced LDLc/HDLc ratio, lipid peroxide levels, and elevated the level of reduced glutathione in hyperlipidemic rats fed high fat diets.

> —R. Manimegalai, et al., ''Effect of Vitamin-E on High Fat Diet Induced Hyperlipidemia in Rats,'' *Indian Journal of Exp Biology,* 31(8), August 1993, p. 704-707.

Results of this study found that cholesterol-fed rabbits supplemented with 2100 IU of vitamin E weekly experienced a hypocholesterolemic effect after four weeks and a 50% reduction by week 8.

> —C. Phonpanichrasamee, et al., ''Hypocholesterolemic Effect of Vitamin E on Cholesterol-fed Rabbit,'' *International Journal of Vitam Nutr Res,* 60(3), 1990, p. 240-244.

Results of this study demonstrated the protective effects of vitamin E with respect to oxidant-mediated vascular injury in endothelial cells, suggesting its potential as an effective therapy for atherosclerosis.

> —B. Hennig, ''Protective Effects of Vitamin E in Age-related Endothelial Cell Injury,'' *International Journal of Vitam Nutr Research,* 59(3), 1989, p. 273-279.

Results of this study found that daily oral supplementation with doses of either 5 mg or 20 mg/100 g body weight of alpha-tocopherol for two weeks normalized the altered lipid profile of atherogenesis and decreased infarction risk in experimental atherogenic rats.

> —J. Paul, et al., ''Effect of Vitamin E on Lipid Components of Atherogenic Rats,'' *International Journal of Vitam Nutr Research,* 59(1), 1989, p. 35-39.

Results of this study showed that 50 mg/kg IP injections of dl-alpha-tocopheryl acetate daily for 4 days in rats significantly reduced platelet aggregation relative to controls. Platelet-rich plasma and platelet-poor plasma-thromboelastograms had thromboplastine-formation times significantly higher than controls as well. According to the authors, such findings suggest the efficacy of vitamin E as a potential therapy of several hyperaggregable or hypercoagulable states.

> —M.L. Diez Marques, et al., "Dl-alpha-Tocopheryl Acetate Induces Hypocoagulability and Platelet Hypoaggregability in Rats," *International Journal of Vitam Nutr Research,* 57(4), 1987, p. 375-379.

This review article concludes, based on the available clinical data, that vitamin E is likely to have beneficial effects on cardiovascular disease, especially in intermittent claudication.

> —J. Kleijnen, et al., "Vitamin E and Cardiovascular Disease," *European Journal of Clinical Pharmacology,* 37(6), 1989, p. 541-544.

Results of this study showed that plasma vitamin E levels, more than any other antioxidant, were significantly inversely related to the risk of ichaemic heart disease.

> —K.F. Gey, "Inverse Correlation of Vitamin E and Ischemic Heart Disease," *International Journal of Vitam Nutr Research Suppl,* 30, 1989, p. 224-231.

This study examined platelet activity and function in chronic haemodialysis treatment patients both prior and during antiplatelet therapy with alpha-tocopherol and sulphinpyrazone. Results showed significant reductions of spontaneous and ADP-induced aggravation with respect to both treatments.

> —A. Dmoszynska-Giannopoulou, et al., "The Effect of Sulphinpyrazone and Alpha-tocopherol on Platelet Activation and Function in Haemodialysed Patients," *International Urol Nephrol,* 22(6), 1990, p. 561-566.

This placebo-controlled study found that supplementation with 500 IU per day of vitamin E for 3 months proved effective in hyperlipoproteinemia and may be considered a useful agent for combatting the risk of coronary heart disease.

> —M.J. Cloarec, et al., "Alpha-tocopherol: Effect on Plasma Lipoproteins in Hypercholesterolemic Patients," *Israeli Journal of Medical Science,* 23(8), August 1987, p. 869-872.

This study examined the effects of d-alpha-tocopherol on the prevention and regression of induced atherosclerosis in primates. Results showed d-alpha-tocopherol to have both therapeutic and phophylactic benefits.

> —A.J. Verlangieri and M.J. Bush, "Effects of D-alpha-tocopherol Supplementation on Experimentally Induced Primate Atherosclerosis," *Journal of the American College of Nutrition,* 11(2), April 1992, p. 131-138.

This review article on vitamin E and human platelet function makes the following observations: vitamin E inhibits platelet aggregation and release when tested in vitro, an effect which is believed to be the result of reduced platelet cyclooxygenase activity and lipid peroxide formation inhibition. Doses as low as 200 IU per day of vitamin E have been shown to inhibit platelet adhesion.

> —M. Steiner, "Influence of Vitamin E on Platelet Function in Humans," *Journal of the American College of Nutrition,* 10(5), October 1991, p. 466-473.

Results of this study found that supplementation with 150 mg per day for 1 week, followed by 300 mg per day for 3 weeks of vitamin E in vitro offered protection against oxidative modification as well as significantly reduced the HDL oxidation propagation rate. Such findings, the authors suggest, speak to the potential benefits for ameliorating atherosclerosis of vitamin E in low doses.

> —M. Suzukawa, et al., "Effect of in-vivo Supplementation with Low-dose Vitamin E on susceptibility of Low-density Lipoprotein and High-density Lipoprotein to Oxidative Modification," *Journal of the American College of Nutrition,* 14(1), February 1995, p. 46-52.

In this study, 800 IU per day of vitamin E and 1g per day of vitamin C were given to healthy subjects. When the two were given together for 10 days, results showed a 57% reduction in Cu-catalyzed production of thiobarbituric acid reactive substances (TBARS). Reductions in electophoretic mobility, production of conjugated dienes and modification of amino groups were seen as well, and the susceptibility of lipoproteins to MC-mediated oxidation decreased by 78%. Subjects supplemented with vitamin E only experienced a TBARS reduction of 52%.

> —V.A. Rifici and A.K. Khachadurian, "Dietary Supplementation with Vitamins C and E Inhibits in Vitro Oxidation of Lipoproteins," *Journal of the American College of Nutrition,* 12(6), December 1993, p. 631-637.

Results of this study demonstrated that the combined pretreatment with tocopherol and nifeipine pretreatment prevented acute cardiac reactions as seen by changes in STI values in women with breast cancer.

> —R. Lenzhofer, et al., "Acute Cardiac Toxicity in Patients after Doxorubicin Treatment and the Effect of Combined Tocopherol and Nifedipine Pretreatment," *Journal of Cancer Res Clin Oncol,* 106(2), 1983, p. 143-147.

Results of this study found that the administration of vitamin E protected the skeletal muscle and hyperthyroid heart from lipid peroxidation in rats, independently of oxidative enzymes and antioxidant enzymes changes.

> —K. Asayama, et al., "Vitamin E Protects Against Thyroxine-Induced Acceleration of Lipid Peroxidation in Cardiac and Skeletal Muscles in Rats," *Journal of Nutr Sci Vitaminol,* 35(5), October 1989, p. 407-418.

Results of this study found that the administration of vitamin E significantly prevented in vivo platelet activation, an increase of lipid peroxides, and renal dysfunction in rats resulting from hypertension.

> —K. Umegaki and T. Ichikawa, "Vitamin E Did Not Prevent Platelet Activation, but Prevented Increase of Lipid Peroxides and Renal Dysfunction in DOCA-salt Hypertensive Rats," *Journal of Nutr Sci Vitaminol,* 39(5), October 1993, p. 437-449.

This study examined the effects of vitamin E on atherosclerosis in hemodialysis patients. Results found that long term supplementation with vitamin E suppressed the progress of the disease.

> —S. Yukawa, et al., "Prevention of Aortic Calcification in Patients on Hemodialysis by Long-term Administration of Vitamin E," *Journal of Nutr Sci Vitaminol,* Spec No:187-90, 1992.

Results of this study showed that the administration of vitamin E together with selenium protected rabbits fed a high-fat diet from changes evoked in the heart muscle.

> —L. Rozewicka, et al., "Protective Effect of Selenium and Vitamin E Against Changes

Induced in Heart Vessels of Rabbits fed Chronically on a High-fat Diet," *Kitasato Arch Exp Med,* 64(4), December 1991, p. 183-192.

Results of this study showed that spontaneously hypertensive rat myocardium and myocardial membrane contained more than 3 times less the alpha-tocopherol of normotensive heart muscle and cardiac membrane.

—D.R. Janero and B. Burghardt, "Cardiac Membrane Vitamin E and Malondialdehyde Levels in Heart Muscle of Normotensive and Spontaneously-hypertensive Rats," *Lipids,* 24(1), January 1989, p. 33-38.

Results of this study found that two months of dietary supplementation with vitamin E on a daily basis protected rats from oxidative damages brought on by endurance exercise.

—C.T. Kumar, et al., "Dietary Supplementation of Vitamin E Protects Heart Tissue from Exercise-Induced Oxidant Stress," *Mol Cell Biochem,* 111(1-2), April 1992, p. 109-115.

This study examined the effects alpha-tocopherol on the in vitro and in vivo metabolism MDA-LDL occurring in chronic haemodialysis patients. Results showed that, depending upon the degree of return to normal MDA concentrations in LDL, doses of 600 mg per day of alpha-tocopherol for 2 weeks produced improvements.

—S. Yukawa, et al., "Effect of Alpha-tocopherol on In Vitro and In Vivo Metabolism of Low-Density Lipoproteins in Haemodialysis Patients," *Nephrol Dial Transplant,* 10(Suppl 3), 1995, p. 1-3.

This review article notes that antioxidants such as vitamin E, vitamin C, beta-carotene, and monunsaturate fatty acids reduce LDL's susceptibility to oxidation.

—A. Jendryczko, [Prevention of Atherosclerosis with the Help of Antioxidants (editorial)], *Pol Tyg Lek,* 49(20-22), May 16-30, 1994, p. 456-458.

This review article notes that while alpha-tocopherol shows modes anticlotting activity, vitamin E quinone is a strong anticoagulant and inhibitor of the vitamin K-dependent carboxylase that controls clotting.

—P. Dowd and Z.B. Zheng, "On the Mechanism of the Anticlotting Action of Vitamin E Quinone," *Proc Natl Acad Sci U S A,* 92(18), August 29, 1995, p. 8171-8175.

Results of this study found that a deficiency can be prothrombogenic by increasing platelet arcachidonate, lipid peroxidation and serum TXA2 levels while supplementation with vitamin E may lead to reductions of such effects.

—H.W. Chen, et al., "Vitamin E Deficiency Increases Serum Thromboxane A2, Platelet Arachidonate and Lipid Peroxidation in Male Sprague-Dawley Rats," *Prostaglandins Leukot Essent Fatty Acids,* 51(1), July 1994, p. 11-17.

Results of this study showed that alpha-tocopherol and tocopherol acetate produced a small increase in the amount of thromboxane in treated compared to untreated platelets, and significantly more lipoxygenase products were produced in tocopherol acetate-treated platelets.

—K.C. Srivastava, "Vitamin E Exerts Antiaggregatory Effects without Inhibiting the Enzymes of the Arachidonic Acid Cascade in Platelets,'' *Prostaglandins Leukot Med,* 21(2), February 1986, p 177-185.

This review article notes that simultaneous correction of low antioxidant levels, including vitamin E, may be an effective approach to the prevention of cardiovascular disease as witnessed from studies in Northern Europe. American data shows that risk of the disease can be reduced by daily supplements of 140 mg of vitamin C, 100 mg of vitamin E and 8.6 mg of gamma-carotene.
—K.F. Gey, et al., [Essential Antioxidants in Cardiovascular Diseases—Lessons for Europe], *Ther Umsch,* 51(7), July 1994, p. 475-482.

This study examined the effects of vitamin E on platelet function on a group of healthy adults. Results found that administration of vitamin E alone (400 IU to 1200 IU) over six weeks or in combination with aspirin had positive effects in patients with arterial thromboembolic diseases.
—M. Steiner, ''Effect of Alpha-tocopherol Administration on Platelet Function in Man,'' *Thromb Haemost,* 49(2), April 28, 1993, p. 73-77.

Results of this study found that the vitamin E dose of between 20-200 micrograms/ml inhibited platelet aggregation in whole blood and that such effects are possibly due PAF synthesis inhibition, rather than related to thromboxane A2 or adenosine diphosphate.
—E. Kakishita, et al., ''Inhibitory Effect of Vitamin E (alpha-tocopherol) on Spontaneous Platelet Aggregation in Whole Blood,'' *Thromb Research* (1990 Dec 15) 60(6), December 15, 1990, p. 489-499.

This study examined platelet adhesion ex vivo in normal adults on doses of vitamin E ranging from 400 IU per day to 1600 IU per day. Results found that 400 IU per day appeared to be the optimal dose for platelet adhesivity reduction.
—J. Jandak, et al., ''Reduction of Platelet Adhesiveness by Vitamin E Supplementation in Humans,'' *Thromb Res,* 49(4), February 15, 1988, p. 393-404.

This study found that the administration of alpha-tocopherol in combination with sodium nucleinate lead to normalization of qualitative and quantitative content of phospholipids in rabbit myocardiums that have been experimentally induced with myocardial infarction. Results also showed that accompanying such changes were the simultaneous limitation of lipid peroxidation activity the normalization of phospholipid-phospholipid interrelations.
—A.A. Engibarian and K.G. Karagezian, [Role of Combined Administration of Alpha-tocopherol and Sodium Nucleinate in Normalizing the Phospholipid Composition of Cardiac Muscle in a Model of Myocardial Infarction], *Ukr Biokhim Zh,* 56(2), March-April 1984, p. 146-152.

Results of this study showed that 45 IU of DL-alpha-tocopherol acetate administered daily for 3 weeks significantly increased decreased neutrophil chemotaxis from 15 +/- 3 to 4 +/- 1 micron/h. Based on these findings, the authors suggest vitamin E could be beneficial in pathological conditions like ischaemic heart disease, which activate neutrophils.
—R. Luostarinen, et al., ''Effects of Dietary Supplementation with Vitamin E on Human Neutrophil Chemotaxis and Generation of LTB4,'' *Ups Journal of Med Sci,* 96(2), 1991, p. 103-111.

Results of this study found that vitamin E and its derivitives were effective in correcting deteriorations of the oxidative metabolism of rats suffering from experimentally induced impairments of heart tissue.
—IuV Khmelevskii, et al., [Vitamin E and its Synthetic Analogs in Experimental Cardiovascular Pathology], *Vopr Med Khim,* 38(5), September-October 1992, p. 30-33.

Results of this study showed that the administration of alpha-tocopherol and thiamine normalized elevated lipid peroxidation levels and induced the elevation of glutathione reductase activity in rats with experimentally induced cardiac hypertrophy.
—O.I. Tolsty and IuV Khmelevskii, [The Role of Alpha-tocopherol and Thiamine in the Direction of Lipid Peroxidation in Compensatory Myocardial Hypertrophy], *Vopr Pitan,* 3, May-June 1991, p. 38-42.

This study examined the effects of alpha-tocopherol alone and in combination with nicotinic acid in patients with ischemic heart disease. Results showed that tocopherol coupled with nicotinic acid normalized the process of blood coagulation, favoured activation of fibrinolysis and led to an improvement of the microcirculatory bed.
—N.N. Chernomorets, et al., [The Effect of Tocopherol and Nicotinic Acid on the Microcirculation and Blood Coagulability in Patients with Ischemic Heart Disease], *Vrach Delo,* (12), December 1990, p. 6-8.

Results of this study showed that treatment with alpha-tocopherol had a beneficial effect on normalization of the reduced stroke volume of the heart and increased peripheral resistance close to the middle of the acute and beginning of subacute periods in myocardial infarction patients.
—I.A. Shekhunova, [The effect of Alpha-tocopherol on the Hemodynamic Indices of Myocardial Infarct Patients], *Vrach Delo,* (11), November 1989, p. 47-49.

Cataracts

This study found that antioxidant such as vitamin E, vitamin C, and pyruvate can thwart the cataractogenic effect of oxyradicals and may be effective in cataract treatment or prevention.
—S.D Varma, ''Scientific Basis for Medical Therapy of Cataracts by Antioxidants,'' *American Journal of Clinical Nutrition,* 53(1 Suppl), January 1991, p. 335S-345S.

Results of this study showed that adults with high levels of two or more of either vitamin E, C, or carotenoids had a decrease in the risk of cataracts compared to those with low levels or one or more.
—P.F. Jacques, et al., ''Antioxidant Status in Persons with and without Senile Cataract,'' *Arch Ophthalmol,* 106(3), March 1988, p. 337-340.

This study examined the relationship between serum concentrations of alpha-tocopherol, beta-carotene, retinol, and selenium and cataracts. Results showed that low serum levels of alpha-tocopherol and beta-carotene proved to be risk factors for end stage senile cataracts.
—P. Knekt, et al., ''Serum Antioxidant Vitamins and Risk of Cataract,'' *British Medical Journal,* 305(6866), December 5, 1992, p. 1392-1394.

This review article notes the results of a study showing that patients with cataracts had low levels of vitamins E, C, or carotenoids relative to controls and that those with less cataracts used significantly more supplements of vitamins E and C.

> —J.M. Robertson, et al., "Vitamin E Intake and Risk of Cataracts in Humans," *Annals of the New York Academy of Sciences,* 570, 1989, p. 372-382.

Results of this study found that vitamin E-containing liposome was effective in significantly preventing the formation of experimental rat sugar cataracts in vitro.

> —H. Hattori, et al., [Effect of Vitamin E-containing Liposome on Experimental Sugar Cataract], *Nippon Ganka Gakkai Zasshi,* 93(1), January 1989, p. 97-102.

This review article notes that vitamin E has been shown to protect cell membranes from both animal and plants from light-induced damage.

> —M.J. Fryer, "Evidence for the Photoprotective Effects of Vitamin E," *Photochem Photobiol,* 58(2), August 1993, p. 304-312.

This review article notes that numerous in vitro and in vivo studies in different animals species have shown that vitamins E and C offer protective effects against light-induced cataracts as well as sugar and steroid cataracts.

> —H. Gerster, "Antioxidant Vitamins in Cataract Prevention," *Z Ernahrungswiss,* 28(1), March 1989, p. 56-75.

Celiac Disease

This case study describes a woman suffering from adult onset celiac disease with a deficiency in vitamin E who experienced improvement in cerebellar symptoms as a result of vitamin E therapy.

> —A. Mauro, et al., "Cerebellar Syndrome in Adult Celiac Disease with Vitamin E Deficiency," *Acta Neurol Scand,* 84(2), August 1991, p. 167-170.

Cholestasis

This study found that the intravenous treatment of children with chronic cholestatic liver disease with doses of 50 to 100 mg of vitamin E every three to seven days, over a 32-month interval, resulted in the correction of abnormal blood cell peroxide hemolysis induced by vitamin E deficiency as well as the arrest of clinical progression of spinocerebellar degeneration. Additional studies have shown that vitamin E produced significant improvement in neurological disorders in patients under similar conditions.

> —D.H. Perlmutter, et al., "Intramuscular Vitamin E Repletion in Children with Chronic Cholestasis," *American Journal of Dis Child,* 141(2), February 1987, p. 170-174.

This study examined the relationship between vitamin E deficiency and children with prolonged neonatal cholestatic disorders. Results showed that 64% of the intrahepatic and 77% of the extrahepatic cholestasis patients suffered from vitamin E deficiencies. Results also found that prior to age 1, all children had normal neurological functions but neurological abnormalities became present in roughly 50% of vitamin E deficient children between the ages of 1-3. By age 3, all vitamin E deficient children had acquired neurologic abnormalities.

> —R.J. Sokol, et al., "Frequency and Clinical Progression of the Vitamin E Deficiency

Neurologic Disorder in Children with Prolonged Neonatal Cholestasis," *American Journal of Dis Child,* 139(12), December 1985, p. 1211-1215.

Results of this study showed that low intraluminal bile acid concentrations caused malabsorption and deficiency of vitamin E in children with prolonged severe cholestasis and that intramuscular vitamin E can be used in both the prevention and therapy of vitamin E deficiency caused neurologic abnormalities.
— R.J. Sokol, et al., "Mechanism Causing Vitamin E Deficiency During Chronic Childhood Cholestasis," *Gastroenterology,* 85(5), November 1983, p. 1172-1182.

Results of this study found that the water-soluble oral form of vitamin E, d-alpha-tocopheryl polyethylene glycol 1000 succinate (TPGS) given in doses of 15-25 IU/kg per day may be effective in both correcting and preventing deficiencies in vitamin E during severe childhood cholestasis.
— R.J. Sokol, et al., "Treatment of Vitamin E Deficiency During Chronic Childhood Cholestasis with Oral D-alpha-tocopheryl Polyethylene Glycol-1000 Succinate," *Gastroenterology,* 93(5), November 1987, p. 975-985.

This study examined the safety and efficacy of 25 IU kg per day of d-alpha-tocopheryl polyethylene glycol 1000 succinate (TPGS) in correcting vitamin E deficiency in children with chronic cholestasis unresponsive to oral treatment with vitamin E in other forms. Results showed that TPGS therapy produced a normalization of vitamin E status of all children in the study and that 25 experienced improvements in neurological functions, 27 experienced stabilization of neurological functions, and just 2 showed signs of worsening or neurological functions after an average therapy length of 2.5 years.
— R.J. Sokol, et al., "Multicenter Trial of D-alpha-tocopheryl Polyethylene Glycol 1000 Succinate for Treatment of Vitamin E Deficiency in Children with Chronic Cholestasis," *Gastroenterology,* 104(6), June 1993, p. 1727-1735.

Results of this study found that intramuscular injections of alpha-tocopherol were effective in improving neurologic disease in 3 of 4 children suffering from chronic cholestasis and serum deficiencies of vitamin E. Oral supplementation with high doses of vitamin E led to similar results in the fourth child.
— M.A. Guggenheim, et al., "Progressive Neuromuscular Disease in Children with Chronic Cholestasis and Vitamin E Deficiency: Diagnosis and Treatment with Alpha-tocopherol," *Journal of Pediatrics,* 100(1), p. 51-8

This study examined the effects of long-term correction of vitamin E deficiency on neurologic function in children suffering from chronic cholestasis. Results showed that all experienced vitamin E repletion either by intramuscular injection of 0.8 to 2.0 IU per kilogram per day or oral doses of up 120 IU per kilogram of body weight per day.
— R.J. Sokol, et al., "Improved Neurologic Function after Long-term Correction of Vitamin E Deficiency in Children with Chronic Cholestasis," *New England Journal of Medicine,* 313(25), December 19, 1985, p. 1580-1586.

Results of this study showed that high oral doses of vitamin E slowed the progression of neurological abnormalities in 2 of three patients with intrahepatic cholestasis.
— M. Nakagawa, et al., "Familial Intrahepatic Cholestasis Associated with Progressive Neuro-

muscular Disease and Vitamin E Deficiency,'' *Journal of Pediatric Gastroenterol Nutr,* 3(3), June 1984, p. 385-389.

Cystic Fibrosis

This study reports on two cases of adult patients with cystic fibrosis suffering from severe vitamin E deficiency and neurologic disease. Results found that neurologic deficits were partially corrected with intramuscular injections of vitamin E.

—M.D. Sitrin, et al., ''Vitamin E Deficiency and Neurologic Disease in Adults with Cystic Fibrosis,'' *Annals of Internal Medicine,* 107(1), July 1987, p. 51-54.

Results of this study showed that cystic fibrosis patients and patients with biliary atresia require supplementation with vitamin E to maintain a normal integrity of axons related to the gracile and possibly other sensory nuclei.

—J.H. Sung, et al., ''Axonal Dystrophy in the Gracile Nucleus in Congenital Biliary Atresia and Cystic Fibrosis (mucoviscidosis): Beneficial Effect of Vitamin E Therapy,'' *Journal Neuropathol Exp Neurol,* 39(5), September 1980, p. 584-597.

This study noted the prevalence and effects of vitamin E deficiency in patients with cystic fibrosis and recommends early supplementation in cystic fibrosis patients with pancreatic insufficiency in order to prevent neurologic dysfunction.

—H.A. Cynamon, et al., ''Effect of Vitamin E Deficiency on Neurologic Function in Patients with Cystic Fibrosis,'' *Journal of Pediatrics,* 113(4), October 1988, p. 637-640.

Results of this study found that the serum concentrations of vitamin E were all but undetectable in four patients with chronic steatorrhoe, two of whom had cystic fibrosis and two chronic cirrhosis of childhood. In one patient, substantial improvement was seen following the restoration of normal vitamin E levels by parenteral therapy.

—E. Elias, et al., ''Association of Spinocerebellar Disorders with Cystic Fibrosis or Chronic Childhood Cholestasis and Very Low Serum Vitamin E,'' *Lancet,* 2(8259), December 12, 1981, p. 1319-1321.

This study assessed the vitamin E status of 22 patients with cystic fibrosis. Results showed that for a given concentration of plasma or erythrocyte alpha-tocopherol, erythrocytes of patients with cystic fibrosis were more susceptible to peroxide-induced haemolysis relative to controls. The authors thus argue that such susceptibility should be countered by supplementation with vitamin E to maintain higher than normal concentrations of circulating alpha-tocopherol-greater than 4.8 mmol alpha-tocopherol/mol cholesterol.

—D.R. James, et al., ''Increased Susceptibility to Peroxide-Induced Haemolysis with Normal Vitamin E Concentrations in Cystic Fibrosis,'' *Clin Chim Acta,* 204(1-3), December 31, 1991, p. 279-290.

Diabetes

In this placebo-controlled, double-blind study, the effects of supplementation with 1 g of vitamin E per day for 35 days on type 1 diabetics were examined. Results showed that the vitamin E diminished

ADP-induced platelet aggregation and suggested that such effects were partly mediated through a diminution of the cyclooxygenase activity.

—C. Colette, et al., "Platelet Function in Type I Diabetes: Effects of Supplementation with Large Doses of Vitamin E," *American Journal of Clinical Nutrition,* 47(2), February 1988, p. 256-261.

In this study, 10 healthy and 15 non-insulin-dependent diabetics received an oral glucose tolerance test and a euglycemic hyperinsulinemic glucose clamp before and after supplementation with 900 mg/day for 4 months of vitamin E. Results showed the supplementation reduced oxidative stress as well as improved insulin action.

—G. Paolisso, et al., "Pharmacologic Doses of Vitamin E Improve Insulin Action in Healthy Subjects and Non-insulin-dependent Diabetic Patients," *American Journal of Clinical Nutrition,* 57(5), May 1993, p. 650-656.

Results of this study showed that treatment with d-alpha-tocopherol can prevent diabetes-induced abnormalities in rat retinal blood flow.

—M. Kunisaki, et al., "Vitamin E Prevents Diabetes-induced Abnormal Retinal Blood Flow via the Diacylglycerol-protein Kinase C Pathway," *American Journal of Physiology,* 269(2 Pt 1), August 1995, p. E239-46.

This four year follow-up study of Finnish middle-aged men examined whether or not vitamin E status is a risk factor for incident non-insulin dependent diabetes. Results showed that a low lipid standardized plasma vitamin E concentration was associated with a 3.9 fold risk of diabetes. For every decrement of 1 mumol/l of uncategorized unstandardized vitamin E concentration there was an increment of 22% in diabetes risk. According to the authors, such findings are consistent with the theory that free radical stress is a causative factor of non-insulin dependent diabetes mellitus.

—J.T. Salonen, et al., "Increased Risk of Non-insulin Dependent Diabetes Mellitus at Low Plasma Vitamin E Concentrations: A Four Year Follow up Study in Men," *British Medical Journal,* 311(7013), October 28, 1995, p. 1124-1127.

Results of this study showed that low platelet vitamin E levels might play a role in the increased thromboxane synthesis demonstrated by platelets in type I diabetics.

—C.W. Karpen, et al., "Interrelation of Platelet Vitamin E and Thromboxane Synthesis in Type I Diabetes Mellitus," *Diabetes,* 33(3), March 1984, p. 239-243.

This study found that the level of vitamin E in platelets was significantly reduced in diabetics relative to controls. Results also found that vitamin E content in platelets from both controls and diabetics showed inverse correlations with the rate of platelet aggregations as well as thromboxane B2 production during aggregation. Such findings, according to the authors, suggest that reduction in vitamin E in diabetic platelets can contribute to the mechanisms of the enhanced platelet thromboxane and aggregation which relate to the development of vascular complications.

—J. Watanabe, et al., "Effect of Vitamin E on Platelet Aggregation in Diabetes Mellitus," *Thromb Haemost,* 51(3), July 29, 1984, p. 313-316.

Results of this study on diabetic rats have shown that the activation of PKC activities in the vascular cells and tissues induced by hyperglycemia by lowering DAG levels can be prevented by D-alpha-tocopherol.

>—M. Kunisaki, "Normalization of Diacylglycerol-protein Kinase C Activation by Vitamin E in Aorta of Diabetic Rats and Cultured Rat Smooth Muscle Cells Exposed to Elevated Glucose Levels," *Diabetes,* 43(11), November 1994, p. 1372-1377.

Results of this study showed that dietary supplementation of large amounts of vitamin E in streptozocin-induced diabetic rats eliminated lipid peroxidation accumulation in the plasma and the liver, returned the plasma triglycerides toward normal levels, and increased the activity of lipoprotein lipase. Such findings, according to the authors, suggest vitamin E increases the total hepatic triglyceride lipase activity possibly by protecting the membrane-bound lipase against peroxidative damage.

>—K.A. Pritchard, Jr., et al., "Triglyceride-lowering Effect of Dietary Vitamin E in Streptozocin-Induced Diabetic Rats: Increased Lipoprotein Lipase Activity in Livers of Diabetic Rats Fed High Dietary Vitamin E," *Diabetes,* 35(3), March 1986, p. 278-281.

Results of this study suggest the existence of a relationship in type I diabetics between low vitamin E content and increased 12-HETE synthesis in platelets.

>—C.W. Karpen, et al., "Production of 12-hydroxyeicosatetraenoic Acid and Vitamin E Status in Platelets from Type I Human Diabetic Subjects," *Diabetes,* 34(6), June 1985, p. 526-531.

Results of this study showed that rats given vitamin E before being administered either streptozotocin or alloxan provided protection against the diabetogenic effects of each. It was also observed that rats with a depleted antioxidant state due to a vitamin E and selenium-deficient diet showed increased diabetogenic susceptibility to normally nondiabetogenic doses of streptozotocin.

>—A.E. Slonim, et al., "Modification of Chemically Induced Diabetes in Rats by Vitamin E: Supplementation Minimizes and Depletion Enhances Development of Diabetes," *Journal of Clinical Investigation,* 71(5), May 1983, p. 1282-1288.

Results of this study found that a diet containing 1000 IU/kg of vitamin E reduced the incidence of diabetes in non-obese diabetic mice.

>—A.R. Hayward, et al., "Vitamin E Supplementation Reduces the Incidence of Diabetes but Not Insulitis in NOD Mice," *Journal of Laboratory and Clinical Medicine,* 119(5), May 1992, p. 503-507.

In this study, four months worth of vitamin E supplementation resulted in a significant improvement in glucose utilization and hepatic response to insulin in both normal subjects as well as diabetics.

>—B. Caballero, "Vitamin E Improves the Action of Insulin," *Nutr Rev,* 51(11), November 1993, p. 339-340.

Results of this study found that vitamin E and taurine attenuated diabetic glomerulosclerosis by interfering with the bioactivation of transforming growth factor-6.

>—H. Trachtman, et al., "Antioxidants Reverse the Antiproliferative Effect of High Glucose and Advanced Glycosylation End Products in Cultured Rat Mesangial Cells," *Biochem Biophys Res Commun,* 199(1), February 28, 1994, p. 346-352.

Results of this study showed that protein glycation was inhibited by vitamin E and indicated the potential of using vitamin E to obtain the inhibition of nonenzymatic glycation.

> —A. Ceriello, et al., "A Preliminary Note on Inhibiting Effect of Alpha-tocopherol on Protein Glycation," *Diabete Metab*, 14(1), January-February 1988, p. 40-42.

Results of this study showed that daily doses of 600 mg of vitamin E may improve platelet function and prostaglandin metabolism and platelet function in diabetics as well as have positive effects on the development of vascular complications related to diabetes.

> —M. Kunisaki, et al., "Effects of Vitamin E Administration on Platelet Function in Diabetes Mellitus," *Diabetes Research*, 14(1), May 1990, p. 37-42.

This study examined the effects of vitamin E on glycosylated hemoglobin levels in streptozotocin-diabetic rats. Results showed that vitamin E treatment significantly suppressed the increase in glycosylated hemoglobin in rats receiving intraperitoneal injections of vitamin E on days 1, 4, 7, 11, 14, 18 and 21 at doses of 500 mg/kg and 1000 mg/kg respectively.

> —I. Ozden, et al., "The Effect of Vitamin E on Glycosylated Hemoglobin Levels in Diabetic Rats: A Preliminary Report," *Diabetes Res*, 12(3), November 1989, p. 123-124.

In this study, diabetic and nondiabetic rats were supplemented with vitamin E beginning 3 days following streptozotocin injection. Results showed the serum lipid peroxide levels expressed as thiobarbituric acid reactants were significantly higher in diabetic rats fed a control diet than in nondiabetic rats fed a control diet while diabetic rats receiving supplemental vitamin E showed levels that were reduced to normal. In the diabetic rats on both the control and supplemented diets, the fluorescence and thermal rupture time of collagen were increased significantly relative to nondiabetic rats.

> —Y. Aoki, et al. "Protective Effect of Vitamin E Supplementation on Increased Thermal Stability of Collagen in Diabetic Rats," *Diabetologia*, 35(10), October 1992, p. 913-916.

Results of this study found that high levels of vitamin E exerts an ameliorating influence of diabetic PG12/TXA2 imbalance.

> —V.A. Gilbert, et al., "Differential Effects of Megavitamin E on Prostacyclin and Thromboxane Synthesis in Streptozotocin-induced Diabetic Rats," *Horm Metab Res*, 15(7), July 1983, p. 320-325.

This study examined whether supplementation of non-obese diabetic mice with vitamin E could retard the selective destruction of pancreatic beta cells leading to type 1 diabetes. Results showed that vitamin E delayed the onset of the disease but did not reduce its incidence by 30 weeks of age.

> —P.E. Beales, et al., "Vitamin E Delays Diabetes Onset in the Non-obese Diabetic Mouse," *Horm Metab Res*, 26(10), October 1994, p. 450-452.

This double-blind, placebo-controlled, crossover study examined the antiplatelet effects of 200 mg of tocopherol given to NIDDM subjects for 6 weeks. Results showed that tocopherol suppressed platelet aggregation of whole blood ex vivo, suggesting tocopherol's platelet aggregation inhibitory effects may in part be achieved via interferences with fibrinogen binding towards its receptor.

> —H.P. Wu, et al., "Effect of Tocopherol on Platelet Aggregation in Non-insulin-dependent Diabetes Mellitus: Ex Vivo and in Vitro Studies," *Journal of Formos Med Assoc*, 91(3), March 1992, p. 270-275.

This study examined whether vitamin E could reverse the high glucose's promotion of lipid peroxidation and stimulation of the production of collagen by culture mesangial cells in vitro. Results showed that 100 microM of vitamin E achieved both. The authors argue that such findings suggest that vitamin E works as an endogenous antioxidant agent in the kidney to limit glomerulosclerosis in diabetic nephropathy.

>—H. Trachtman, "Vitamin E Prevents Glucose-induced Lipid Peroxidation and Increased Collagen Production in Cultured Rat Mesangial Cells," *Microvascular Research,* 47(2), March 1994, p. 232-239.

Results of this study showed that 1000 mg daily doses of vitamin E inhibited platelet activity in type 1 diabetics.

>—A. Dmoszynska-Giannopoulou, et al., [Effect of Vitamin E on the Function of Blood Platelets in Patients with Diabetes Mellitus], *Pol Tyg Lek,* 44(21-22), May 22-29, 1989, p. 496-498.

Results of this study showed that treatment with 8 micrograms/kg a day of vitamin E for 2 weeks improved pulmonary hemodynamics, lipid metabolism, and lipid peroxidation in patients with diabetic nephroangiopathy.

>—M.D. Dzhavad-zade, et al., [Disorders of Pulmonary Hemodynamics in Patients with Diabetic Nephroangiopathy and its Correction with Antioxidants], *Probl Endokrinol,* 38(2), March-April 1992, p. 20-22.

Results of this study showed that the use of alpha-tocopherol acetate significantly decreased lipid peroxidation activity in middle-aged patients with insulin independent diabetes.

>—R.M. Mamedgasanov and S.A. Rakhmani, [Dynamics of Lipid Peroxidation in Patients with Noninsulin-dependent Diabetes Mellitus], *Probl Endokrinol,* 35(1), January-February 1989, p. 19-21.

Results of this study found that, irrespective of therapy type, the administration of vitamin E in daily doses ranging between 600 and 1200 mg to type II diabetics stimulated pancreatic insulin-producing function and was conducive to normalization of lipid peroxidation.

>—M.I. Balabolkin, et al., [Effect of High Doses of Tocopherol on the Processes of Lipid Peroxidation and Insulin Secretion in Patients with Non-insulin-dependent Diabetes Mellitus], *Probl Endokrinol,* 40(3), May-June 1994, p. 10-12.

Results of this study showed that supplementation with doses of 300 mg per day of alpha-tocopherol acetate normalized processes of lipid peroxidation in red cell membranes and blood plasma lipid content, reduced the blood plasma level of lipid peroxidation products and the content of total lipids in red cell membranes in diabetics.

>—N.S. Kuznetsov, et al., [The Use of Antioxidants (Alpha-tocopherol Acetate) in the Treatment of Diabetes Mellitus], *Probl Endokrinol,* 39(2), March-April 1993, p. 9-11.

Results of this study showed that six-week injections of 100 mg/100 g per body weight of alpha-tocopherol with 48 hour intervals immediately after development of streptozotocin-induced diabetes prevented the development of diabetic angiopathy in rats.

>—G.F. Zadkova, et al., [Effect of Alpha-tocopherol on the Development of Diabetic Angiopa-

thy, Platelet Aggregation and Status of the Prostacyclin-thromboxane System in Rats with Streptozotocin Diabetes], *Probl Endokrinol,* 39(5), September-October 1993, p. 40-43.

Results of this study showed that vitamin E was significantly reduced in platelets obtained from diabetics relative to controls. Vitamin E content in platelets in diabetics as well as controls showed inverse correlations with both the rate of platelet aggregation and thromboxane B2 production during aggregation. Based on these findings, the authors suggest that reduced vitamin E levels in diabetic platelets may contribute to the mechanism of the enhanced platelet thromboxane A2 production and aggregation which results in vascular complications.

> —J. Watanabe, et al., "Effect of Vitamin E on Platelet Aggregation in Diabetes Mellitus," *Tohoku Journal Exp Med,* 143(2), June 1984, p. 161-169.

Results of this study showed that liver function in diabetics was positively effected by the administration of vitamin E.

> —O.I. Splavskii, [Effectiveness of Vitamin E in the Combined Therapy of the Hepatobiliary System Lesions in Diabetes Mellitus], *Vopr Pitan,* (6), November-December 1982, p. 36-39.

This review article makes the following observations with respect to vitamin E and diabetic atherosclerosis: Decreased platelet vitamin E levels have been associated with increased aggregation, and vitamin E appears to regulate arachidonic acid metabolism in platelets. Studies have shown that platelet vitamin E levels in diabetics have a tendency to be reduced with platelet aggregation increases. Supplementation with several hundred IU of vitamin E has been shown to significantly reduce lipid peroxidation and platelet aggregation in insulin and noninsulin dependent diabetics. In nondiabetics, low doses of vitamin E (200 IU) have bee seen to significantly decrease platelet adhesion and inhibit the formation of protruding pseudopods.

> —H. Gerster, et al., "Prevention of Platelet Dysfunction by Vitamin E in Diabetic Atherosclerosis," *Z Ernahrungswiss,* 32(4), December 1993, p. 243-261.

Disseminated Granuloma Anulare

This case study describes the successful treatment of a patient with disseminated granuloma anulare by local application of a vitamin E emulsion. Within 12 days, the patient showed noticeable improvement.

> —R.K. Goldstein, et al., [Local Treatment of Disseminated Granuloma Anulare with a Vitamin E Emulsion], *Hautarzt,* 42(3), March 1991, p. 176-178.

Endotoxemia

Results of this study showed that a combination of 250 mg/kg of Indomethacin and 100 mg/kg of alpha-tocopherol improved survival in endotoxic rats injected intravenously with lipopolysaccharide from Escherichia coli at 10, 20 and 30 mg/kg dose levels significantly.

> —R.B. Ashorobi and P.A. Williams, "Indomethacin and Alpha-tocopherol Enhanced Survival in Endotoxic Rats," *Central African Journal of Medicine,* 41(7), July 1995, p. 216-219.

Enteritis

Results of this study showed that vitamin E administered either as a chronic oral systemic pretreatment or as a brief topical application is a potential protectant against acute irradiation enteritis.

> —I. Felemovicius, et al., "Intestinal Radioprotection by Vitamin E (Alpha-tocopherol)," *Ann Surg,* 222(4), October 1995, p. 504-510.

Results of this study found that vitamin E treatment protected rat gastrointestinal mucosa against absorptive injury induced by radiation.

—L.R. Empey, et al., "Mucosal Protective Effects of Vitamin E and Misoprostol During Acute Radiation-induced Enteritis in Rats," *Dig Dis Sci,* 37(2), February 1992, p. 205-214.

Results of this study found that deficiencies in vitamin E and selenium may be a factor in eosinophilic enteritis and eosinophilia development in rats.

—C.B. Hong and C.K. Chow, "Induction of Eosinophilic Enteritis and Eosinophilia in Rats by Vitamin E and Selenium Deficiency," *Exp Mol Pathol,* 48(2), April 1988, p. 182-192.

Epilepsy

This placebo-controlled study found that in 24 epileptic children refractory to antiepileptic drugs (AEDs) with generalized tonic-clonic and other types of seizures, the administration of 400 IU per day of vitamin E to existing AEDs produced a significant reduction of seizures in 10 out of 12 cases compared to controls.

—A.O Ogunmekan and P.A. Hwang, "A Randomized, Double-blind, Placebo-controlled, Clinical Trial of D-alpha-tocopheryl Acetate (Vitamin E), as Add-on therapy, for Epilepsy in Children," *Epilepsia,* 30(1), January-February 1989, p. 84-89.

In this study, 600 mg of alpha-tocopherol were given to 17 epileptics once a day who had previously displayed resistance to standard anticonvulant and psychotropic therapy. Results showed that all patients benefited from the treatment after one month, with effects first being manifest in the appearance of adequate emotional-volitional activity and then in a reduced frequency of epileptic seizures. Generalized seizures were arrested completely in four patients and the prevalence and severity of affective phenomena were reduced in five.

—V.M. Kovalenko, et al., [Alpha-tocopherol in the Complex Treatment of Several Forms of Epilepsy], *Zh Nevropatol Psikhiatr,* 84(6), 1984, p. 892-897.

Results of this study showed that epileptics administered lithium and vitamin E experienced decreases in lipid peroxidation, elevated content of total and free cholesterol of red cell membranes and an increased superoxide dismutase activity in the blood as well as showing improvements in EEG parameters. Such effects resulted in a reduction in the frequency of epileptic attacks and an affective calming of patients.

—A.A. Megrabian, et al., [Use of Lithium Carbonate and Vitamin E in the Complex Treatment of Epileptics], *Zh Nevropatol Psikhiatr,* 86(9), 1986, p. 1407-1410.

Gastric Mucosal Injury

Results of this study found that alpha-tocopherol may be effective in the prevention of oxidative alteration in the gastric mucosa of rats.

—I. Kurose, et al., "Fluorographic Study on the Oxidative Stress in the Process of Gastric Mucosal Injury: Attenuating Effect of Vitamin E," *Journal of Gastroenterol Hepatol,* 8(3), May-June 1993, p. 254-258.

Gastritis

This study examined the activity of Cu/Zn superoxide dismutase (SOD) and catalase (CAT) in gastric mucosa of patients with various degree of chronic gastritis. Among other things, the results showed that the application of vitamin E significantly reduced activities of SOD and CAT.

> —I. Beno, et al., "The Activity of Cu/Zn-superoxide Dismutase and Catalase of Gastric Mucosa in Chronic Gastritis, and the Effect of Alpha-tocopherol," *Bratisl Lek Listy,* 95(1), January 1994, p. 9-14.

Gastrointestinal Disease

This review article notes that protective effects of vitamins A, C, and E have been demonstrated in the treatment of patients with gastroduodenal ulcer and gastric cancer.

> —J. Feher and L. Pronai, [The Role of Free Radical Scavengers in Gastrointestinal Diseases], *Orv Hetil,* 34(13), March 28, 1993, p. 693-696.

General

This general review article notes that vitamin E is considered nature's most effective lipid soluble, chain breaking antioxidant which protects cell membranes from peroxidative damage. The authors also point out that research indicates optimal vitamin E intake can protect against the high free radical concentration caused by lifestyle patterns and air pollutants.

> —L. Packer, "Protective Role of Vitamin E in Biological Systems," *American Journal of Clinical Nutrition,* 53(4 Suppl), April 1991, p. 1050S-1055S.

Results of this study showed that treatment with vitamin E prevented the decrement in hypothalamic beta-endorphin concentrations resulting from arcuate beta-endorphin cell loss. Results also showed that vitamin prevented the onset of persistent vaginal comification and polycystic ovarian condition which can be due to EV-induced hypothalamic pathology.

> —G.C. Desjardins, et al., "Vitamin E Protects Hypothalamic Beta-endorphin Neurons from Estradiol Neurotoxicity," *Endocrinology,* 131(5), November 1992, p. 2482-2484.

This review article makes the following observations about the importance of vitamin E: it is an essentail nutrient for animals and humans because of it not being synthesized in the body. Vitamin E and selenium's biochemical actions are concerned with prevention of peroxidative damage to cells and subcellular elements, thus helping the body maintain its normal defense mechanisms against environmental insult and disease.

> —M.L. Scott, "Advances in Our Understanding of Vitamin E," *Federal Proceedings,* 39(10), August 1980, p. 2736-2739.

Results of this group of studies showed that the turnover of ATP + ADP, cAMP, 5'-AMP and adenosine was greater in tocopherol-deficient rabbits relative to controls and that the administration of tocopherol to tocopherol-deficient rabbits restored the turnover of cAMP to values that were almost normal.

> —U.S. Srivastava, et al., "Turnover of Cyclic Adenosine-5'-monophosphate is Elevated in Skeletal Muscle of Vitamin E-Deficient Rabbits," *Journal of Nutrition,* 122(10), October 1992, p. 1935-1941.

Results of this study found that reductions of PGE2 synthesis in the brains of rats with fish oil feeding were relatively weak in relation to other tissues except when combined with the supplementation of vitamin E in high doses.

> —M. Meydani, et al., "Influence of Dietary Fat, Vitamin E, Ethoxyquin and Indomethacin on the Synthesis of Prostaglandin E2 in Brain Regions of Mice," *Journal of Nutrition,* 121(4), April 1991, p. 438-444.

This study examined the effects of dietary vitamin E-depletion and repletion on the cyclooxygenase activity in the semitendinosus muscle of rabbits. Results showed that vitamin E deficiency significantly reduced cyclooxygenase activity without changing the PGE2/PGF2 ratio. Cyclooxygenase activity was quickly returned to normal within 48 hours of oral tocopherol acetate supplementation.

> —A.C. Chan, et al., "The Effects of Vitamin E Depletion and Repletion on Prostaglandin Synthesis in Semitendinosus Muscle of Young Rabbits," *Journal of Nutrition,* 110(1), January 1980, p. 66-73.

Results of this study found that vitamin E's protective effects against fatty acid-mediated endothelial cell injury may be related to its ability to prevent the induction of peroximosal beta-oxidation enzymes and in turn the formation of excess hydrogen peroxide.

> —B. Hennig, et al., "Effect of Vitamin E on Linoleic Acid-mediated Induction of Peroxisomal Enzymes in Cultured Porcine Endothelial Cells," *Journal of Nutrition,* 120(4), April 1990, p. 331-337.

Results of this study showed that the activity of the lipoxygenase pathway of human neutrophils in vitro is bidirectionally modulated by vitamin E. Alpha-tocopherol concentrations at normal levels in plasma were seen to enhance the lipoxygenation of arachidonic acid, while higher concentrations produced a suppressive effect consistent with its role as a hyroperoxide scavenger.

> —E.J. Goetzl, "Vitamin E Modulates the Lipoxygenation of Arachidonic Acid in Leukocytes," *Nature,* 288(5787), November 13, 1980, p. 183-185.

Results of this study found that, under conditions of toxic insult, cellular vitamin E maintained cell viability in isolated rat hepatocytes.

> —M.W. Fariss, et al., "Vitamin E Reversal of the Effect of Extracellular Calcium on Chemically Induced Toxicity in Hepatocytes," *Science,* 227(4688), February 15, 1985, p. 751-754.

Results of this study found that alpha-tocopherol or CoQ10 functions cooperatively with endogenous antioxidants to prevent lipid peroxidation-induced tissue damage in endotoxemia.

> —K. Sugino, et al., "Changes in the Levels of Endogenous Antioxidants in the Liver of Mice with Experimental Endotoxemia and the Protective Effects of the Antioxidants," *Surgery,* 105(2 Pt 1), February 1989, p. 200-206.

This study examined the effects of vitamin E on the rate of lipid peroxidation and lipase activity in the discrete areas of the brain and spinal cord of rats. Results showed that the administration of alpha-tocopherol by itself significantly reduced lipid peroxidation and lipase activity, and when given with metasystox it showed similar effects.

> —K. Tayyaba and M. Hasan, "Vitamin E Protects Against Metasystox-induced Adverse

Effect on Lipid Metabolism in the Rat Brain and Spinal Cord," *Acta Pharmacol Toxicol,* 57(3), September 1985, p. 190-196.

This study examined the effects of combined supplementation with 20 mg/kg of vitamin E, 50 mg/kg of anthocyans, and 200 mg/kg of pyracetam on post lethal irradiation survival and post sublethal irradiation blood formation in mice. Results showed that pretreatment with mixture increased survival rate by·50%.
> —M. Minkova, et al., "Antiradiation Properties of Alpha-tocopherol, Anthocyans, and Pyracetam Administered Combined as a Pretreatment Course," *Acta Physiol Pharmacol Bulg,* 16(4), 1990, p. 31-36.

This review article notes that vitamin E inhibits the aggregatory responses of blood platelets to aggregating agents in vitro, following a period of preincubation necessary for the compound's uptake by the cells. It also noted, however, that alpha-tocopherol's antiaggregatory activity does not seem to be entirely dependent on the inhibition of thromboxane formation.
> —C. Galli and A. Socini, "Biological Actions and Possible Uses of Vitamin E," *Acta Vitaminol Enzymol,* 4(3), 1982, p. 245-251.

This lengthy review article makes the following observations with respect to the clinical uses of vitamin E: its early administration to low birth weight infants alleviates symptoms of retinopathy of prematurity as well as a reduce incidence of intraventricular hemorrhage. It prevents or reverses areflexia, ataxia, and sensory neuropathy when given to children with cholestatic liver disease before 3 years old. It helps prevent neuropathy and retinopathy related to cystic fibrosis and abetalipoproteinemia. Studies have shown that vitamin E given to G-6-P-D-deficient subjects increased levels of hemoglobin while reducing the number of irreversibly sickled cells in sickle-cell anemia patients. Platelet aggregation, platelet adhesion to collagen, and platelet thromboxane production have all been shown to be reduced by vitamin E while prostacyclin production has been increased. Lastly, it has been documented that high levels of vitamin E in the blood have been inversely correlated with death from breast cancer, ischemic heart disease and cancer, and a lower incidence of infections.
> —L.J. Machlin, "Clinical Uses of Vitamin E," *Acta Vitaminol Enzymol,* 7 Suppl, 1985, p. 33-43.

This review article notes research findings suggesting that vitamin E prevents or minimizes peroxidative damage in biological systems.
> —L. Packer and S. Landvik, "Vitamin E: Introduction to Biochemistry and Health Benefits," *Annals of the New York Academy of Sciences,* 570, 1989, p. 1-6.

Results of this study showed that the daily ingestion of 200 mg of vitamin E for 4 months decreased serum peroxide levels in the elderly by an average of 14%, and by 20% when combined with 400 mg of vitamin C. After a year of supplementation the rates of reduction were 26% and 25%, respectively.
> —M. Wartanowicz, et al., "The Effect of Alpha-tocopherol and Ascorbic Acid on the Serum Lipid Peroxide Level in Elderly People," *Anna Nutr Metab,* 28(3), 1984, p. 186-191.

Results of this study showed that the radical scavenger activity of erythrocyte membranes was stimulated in healthy subjects after 30 days by supplementation with vitamin E, C, and beta-carotene.
> —C. Regnault, et al., "Influence of Beta Carotene, Vitamin E, and Vitamin C on Endogenous

Antioxidant Defenses in Erythrocytes," *Ann Pharmacother,* 27(11), November 1993, p. 1349-1350.

This study examined the carbon centered and hydrogen radicals in the skeletal muscle of rats receiving supplemental vitamin E. Results showed that vitamin E quenched such free radicals directly.

    —M. Hiramatsu, et al., "Decreased Carbon Centered and Hydrogen Radicals in Skeletal Muscle of Vitamin E Supplemented Rats," *Biochem Biophys Res Commun,* 179(2), September 16, 1991, p. 859-864.

Results of this study found that pretreatment with vitamin E 24 hours prior to exposure to Na2CrO4 decreased DNA single strand breaks by carcinogenic chromate compounds.

    —M. Sugiyama, "Effects of Vitamin E and Vitamin B2 on Chromate-induced DNA Lesions," *Biological Trace Element Research,* 21, July-September, 1989, p. 399-404.

Results of this study showed that supplementation with vitamin E reversed vitamin E deficiency-induced impairment of endothelial cell function in rats.

    —A. Rubino and G. Burnstock, "Recovery After Dietary Vitamin E Supplementation of Impaired Endothelial Function in Vitamin E-Deficient Rats," *British Journal of Pharmacology,* 112(2), June 1994, p. 515-518.

Results of this study showed that vitamin E supplementation protected the scavenging systems of rats from the injurious effects of 6-OHDA.

    —A.S. Perumal, et al., "Vitamin E Attenuates the Toxic Effects of 6-hydroxydopamine on Free Radical Scavenging Systems in Rat Brain," *Brain Res Bull,* 29(5), November 1992, p. 699-701.

Results of this study showed that the pretreatment of rats with 50 mg/kg, im of vitamin E restored thioglycollate-induced monocyte migration levels to those of controls and partially reversed LPS-induced inhibition of monocyte phagocytosis in vivo.

    —N.P. Rocha, "Vitamin E Stimulates Endotoxin-inhibited Monocyte Migration and Phagocytosis in Vivo," *Braz Journal of Med Biol Res,* 22(11), 1989, p. 1401-1403.

This general review article on vitamin E notes that studies have found that supplementary vitamin E has been associated with a reduced risk of certain cancers or cardiovascular diseases with similar effects not being seen from dietary vitamin E.

    —L.J. Machlin, "Critical Assessment of the Epidemiological Data Concerning the Impact of Antioxidant Nutrients on Cancer and Cardiovascular Disease," *Crit Rev Food Sci Nutr,* 35(1-2), 1995, p. 41-50.

Results of this study showed that a single dose of 1 mg/kg of alpha-tocopherol administered to mice intravenously 3 and 24 hours prior to radiation as well as a 10 mg/kg intramuscular dose of oily alpha-tocopherol acetate increased their rates of 30-day survival.

    —A.V. Samoilov, et al., [The Radioprotective and Antioxidant Properties of Solubilized Alpha-tocopherol Acetate], *Eksp Klin Farmakol,* 55(4), July-August, 1992, p. 42-44.

This study found that the working capacity of rats was significantly increased for two weeks by a single intravenous injection of solubilized alpha-tocopherol acetate in doses ranging between 25-100 mg/kg.

—A.V. Samoilov, et al., [The Effect of Solubilized Alpha-tocopherol Acetate on Resistance to Experimental Physical Loading], *Eksp Klin Farmakol,* 55(2), March-April 1992, p. 39-40.

Results of this study found that the resistance of pancreatic islet cells to toxic doses of nitric oxide was improved significantly by their preincubation with alpha-tocopherol.

—V. Burkart, et al., "Suppression of Nitric Oxide Toxicity in Islet Cells by Alpha-tocopherol," *FEBS Lett,* 364(3), May 15, 1995, p. 259-263.

Results of this study showed that rats fed a vitamin E and selenium supplemented diet experienced strong protection against heme protein oxidation relative to rats fed a diet deficient in antioxidants.

—H. Chen and A.L. Tappel, "Protection by Vitamin E Selenium, Trolox C, Ascorbic Acid Palmitate, Acetylcysteine, Coenzyme Q, Beta-carotene, Canthaxanthin, and (+)- Catechin Against Oxidative Damage to Liver Slices Measured by Oxidized Heme Proteins," *Free Radic Biol Med,* 16(4), April 1994, p. 437-444.

Results of this study showed that rats fed a vitamin E and selenium supplemented diet experienced strong protection against oxidative tissue damage relative to rats fed a diet deficient in antioxidants. Rats fed diets with very high quantities of the fat soluble antioxidants vitamin E, coenzyme Q10, ascorbic acid 6-palmitate, beta-carotene; and the water soluble antioxidants selenium, acetylcysteine, trolox C, coenzyme Q0 and (+)- catechin, experienced ever greater protection.

—H. Chen and A.L. Tappel, "Vitamin E, Selenium, Trolox C, Ascorbic Acid Palmitate, Acetylcysteine, Coenzyme Q, Beta-carotene, Canthaxanthin, and (+)- Catechin Protect Against Oxidative Damage to Kidney, Heart, Lung and Spleen," *Free Radic Res,* 22(2), February 1995, p. 177-186.

Results of this study showed that vitamin E added to cultured A431 epidermoid cells exposed to UVB (120-2400 J/m2) inhibited surface blebbing and cell detachment from substrate and was most effective in stimulating the recovery of cells when added post UVB irradiation.

—E. Straface, et al., "Vitamin E Prevents UVB-induced Cell Blebbing and Cell Death in A431 Epidermoid Cells," *International Journal of Radiat Biol,* 68(5), November 1995, p. 579-587.

This general review article makes the following observations with respect to vitamin E: vitamin E deficiencies have been seen in patients with varieties of enteropathies, hemolytic anemias, acute respiratory distress syndrome, hepatitis, Gaucher's disease, and neurological dysfunction resulting from lipid malabsorption. Studies have shown that patients with G6PD deficiency, sickle-cell anemia, and beta-thalassemia have experienced improved hematological parameters from supplementation with 800 IU of vitamin E per day. Supplementation with 300 IU/day for 3-6 months has improved walking distances and blood flow in patients with intermittent claudication. Studies have also shown improvements in PMS, arthritis, and tardive dyskinesia in patients receiving 300-600 IU per day of vitamin E. Lastly, epidemiological data points to an inverse association between high levels of serum vitamin E and infections, cancer, and cardiovascular disease.

—L.J. Machlin, "Use and Safety of Elevated Dosages of Vitamin E in Adults," *International Journal of Vitamin Nut Res Suppl,* 30, 1989, p. 56-68.

Results of this study showed that vitamin E and selenium administered by injection in large doses into sponges subcutaneously implanted into rats reduced collagen breakdown and arrested the maturation of granulation tissue.

    —B. Asman, et al., "Reduction of Collagen Degradation in Experimental Granulation Tissue by Vitamin E and Selenium," *Journal of Clinical Periodontol,* 21(1), January 1994, p. 45-47.

In this study, healthy subjects received 1 week of supplementation with fish oil (containing 40 mg/kg body weight per day of eicosapentaenoic and docosahexaenoic acid), 800 IU of D-alpha-tocopherol per day, or both. Results showed that supplementation with either fish oil or vitamin E reduced endogenous leukotriene production and that increased leukotriene generation was associated with a depletion of vitamin E.

    —C. Denzlinger, et al., "Modulation of the Endogenous Leukotriene Production by Fish Oil and Vitamin E," *Journal of Lipid Mediat Cell Signal,* 11(2), March 1995, p. 119-132.

Results of this study found that a diet of vitamin E enriched egg yolk experienced a prevented hemolysis and lipid peroxidation in young and old rats as well as atrophy of testes in old rats.

    —Y. Yoshizawa, et al., "Effects of Vitamin E-enriched Egg Yolk on Lipid Peroxidation, Hemolysis and Serum Lipid Concentration in Young and Old Rats," *Journal of Nutr Sci Vitaminol,* 37(3), June 1991, p. 213-227.

This study examined vitamin E's effects on the differentiation of T cell differentiation in the rat thymus. Results showed that the ratio of CD4+CD8-/CD4-CD8+ T cells increased significantly in the high vitamin E fed rats and significantly decreased in rats fed diets that were vitamin E-free compared to that of the rats receiving a regular diet.

    —S. Moriguchi, et al., "Vitamin E is an Important Factor in T Cell Differentiation in Thymus of F344 Rats," *Journal of Nutr Sci Vitaminol,* 39(5), October 1993, p. 451-463.

This study examined the effects vitamin E on the modulation of keratinocytes in rats. Results showed that a 30% vitamin E ointment alleviated erythema and protected keratinocytes from cell damage induced by a 1% lauroylsarcosine ointment. Treatment with 100 mg/ml proved effective against lauroylsarcosine ointment-induced proliferative reduction of cultured keratinocytes as well.

    —T. Shimizu, et al., "Effect of Vitamin E on Keratinocyte-modulation Induced by Lauroylsarcosine," *Japanese Journal of Pharmacology,* 67(4), April 1995, p. 291-295.

This review article makes note of the well-documented findings in the literature that high doses of vitamin E, selenium, and vitamin C have significant immunostimulant, anti-inflammatory, and anticarcinogenic effects which may protect ischemic or hypoxic tissue structural integrity and have antithrombotic effects.

    —E.J. Crary and M.F. McCarty, "Potential Clinical Applications for High-dose Nutritional Antioxidants," *Medical Hypotheses,* 13(1), January 1984, p. 77-98.

This study examined the effects of vitamin E supplementation in uremic patients being treated with intermittent hemodialysis for positive effects on cell membrane-receptor response. Results showed that oxidative damage decreased following vitamin E treatment and peripheral mononucleur cell membranes contained greater amounts of some unsaturated fatty acids.

—R. Lubrano, et al., "Vitamin E Supplementation and Oxidative Status of Peripheral Blood Mononuclear Cells and Lymphocyte Subsets in Hemodialysis Patients," *Nutrition,* 8(2), March-April 1992, p. 94-97.

Results of this in vitro study found that alpha-tocopherol dramatically effected multiple endothelial cells functions involved in hemostasis.

—N. Huang, et al., "Alpha-tocopherol, A Potent Modulator of Endothelial Cell Function," *Thromb Research,* 50(4), May 15, 1988, p. 547-557.

This review article on the function of vitamin E in physical exercise makes the following observations: it is important for good skeletal muscle health. It is the major lipid-soluble chainbreaking antioxidant in lipid cell membranes and protects muscle tissue in aerobic exercise during which an acceleration is seen free radical creation. High doses of vitamin E reduced oxidative tissue damage in vitamin-E deficient animals is made worse from endurance training. Studies have shown that vitamin E supplemented individuals fared better during a Himalayan expedition than controls.

—H. Gerster, "Function of Vitamin E in Physical Exercise: A Review," *Z Ernahrungswiss,* 30(2), June 1991, p. 89-97.

Glomerulosclerosis

Results of this study found that d-alpha-tocopherol ameliorated glomerulosclerosis and improved hyperlipidemia in rats with adriamycin-induced progressive renal failure.

—M. Washio, et al., "Alpha Tocopherol Improves Focal Glomerulosclerosis in Rats with Adriamycin-induced Progressive Renal Failure," *Nephron,* 68(3), 1994, p. 347-352.

Glutathione Synthesis

In this placebo-controlled study, 1000 IU per day of oral vitamin E was given to normal volunteers. Results showed that significant subsequent increases in their red blood cell glutathione levels relative to controls.

—C. Costagliola, et al., "Vitamin E and Red Blood Cell Glutathione," *Metabolism,* 34(8), August 1985, p. 712-714.

Hearing Loss

This review article cites studies noting the efficacy of a vitamin E and A combination in decibel improvement of the pure-tone threshold in sensorineural hearing-loss patients. Effects are especially strong when hearing loss are the result of presbyaccusis.

—G. Romeo, "The Therapeutic Effect of Vitamins A and E in Neurosensory Hearing Loss," *Acta Vitaminol Enzymol,* 7 Suppl, 1985, p. 85-92.

Results of this study showed that patients with presbycusis experienced improvement in symptoms following treatment with vitamins A and E for 28-48 days.

—G. Romeo and M. Giorgetti, [Therapeutic Effects of Vitamin A Associated with Vitamin E in Perceptual Hearing Loss], *Acta Vitaminol Enzymol,* 7(1-2), 1985, p. 139-143.

Hemodialysis

Results of this study showed that uremic patients in chronic hemodialysis treated with vitamin E experienced a decrease of RBC MDA levels, an increase of RBC vitamin E concentrations, a decreased saturated fatty acid to unsaturated fatty acid ratio, and a significant increase of packed RBC volume.

> —O. Giardini, et al., "Effects of Alpha-tocopherol Administration on Red Blood Cell Membrane Lipid Peroxidation in Hemodialysis Patients," *Clin Nephrol,* 21(3), March 1984, p. 174-177.

Hemolysis

Results of this study showed that 4 weeks of supplementation with 800 units of vitamin E supplementation offered some protection against dapsone-induced hemolysis in dermatitis herpetiformis patients.

> —R. Prussick, et al., "The Protective Effect of Vitamin E on the Hemolysis Associated with Dapsone Treatment in Patients with Dermatitis Herpetiformis," *Arch Dermatol,* 128(2), February 1992, p. 210-213.

This study found that supplementation with doses of 800 IU of vitamin E per day alone and in combination with 25 mg of selenium for 2 months resulted a significant change towards normalization of hematologic status in children with mild chronic hemolysis.

> —M. Hafez, et al., "Improved Erythrocyte Survival with Combined Vitamin E and Selenium Therapy in Children with Glucose-6-phosphate Dehydrogenase Deficiency and Mild Chronic Hemolysis," *Journal of Pediatrics,* 108(4), April 1986, p. 558-561.

Results of this study showed that 3 months of supplementation with vitamin E in patients with Mediterranean glucose-6-phosphate dehydrogenase deficiency reduced chronic hemolysis as seen from an improvement of red-cell lifespan, improved red-cell half life, increased hemoglobin concentration, and reduced reticulocytosis.

> —L. Corash, et al., "Reduced Chronic Hemolysis During High-dose Vitamin E Administration in Mediterranean-type Glucose-6-phosphate Dehydrogenase Deficiency," *New England Journal of Medicine,* 303(8), August 21, 1980, p. 416-420.

This study reports on the single case of Coombs-negative, non-immune severe hemolytic anemia during cyclosporine therapy after allogenic bone marrow transplantation for severe aplastic anemia in which intravascular hemolysis was effectively treated using vitamin E.

> —E. Azuma, et al., "Acute Hemolysis During Cyclosporine Therapy Successfully Treated with Vitamin E," *Bone Marrow Transplant,* 16(2), August 1995, p. 321-322.

Results of this study found that 300 mg per day of vitamin E given to patients with chronic hemodialysis for one month significantly reduced plasma and erythrocyte lipid peroxidation.

> —A.S. Yalcin, et al., "The Effect of Vitamin E Therapy on Plasma and Erythrocyte Lipid Peroxidation in Chronic Hemodialysis Patients," *Clin Chim Acta,* 185(1), October 31, 1989, p. 109-112.

Hepatitis

Results of this study showed that endogenous vitamin E in the membranes and a water soluble vitamin E analogue added with a radical initiator suppressed hepatic damage induced by perfusion of radical generating azo compounds in rats.

—H. Yasuda, et al., "Hepatic Damage Induced by Perfusion of Radical Generating Azo Compound and its Inhibition by Vitamin E," *Chem Biol Interact,* 97(1), June 30, 1995, p. 11-23.

This study found that patients with acute hepatitis taking vitamin E in doses of 200 mg/d after 10 days experienced strong anti-lipid peroxidization.

—Y.C. Han, [Study of Anti-lipid Peroxidation of Vitamin E in Human Body], *Chung Hua Yu Fang I Hsueh Tsa Chih,* 27(3), May 1993, p. 132-134.

This article on hepatitis makes the following observations with respect to the use of tocopherol acetate and splenin in treating viral hepatitis B: it ensures a marked immunomodulating effect consisting in control of T-lymphopenia, normalization of helper-suppresser ratio, reduction of circulating immune complexes and a tendency to restoration of normal ratio between separate fractions of immune complexes, stimulation of phagocytic activity of monocytes of the peripheral blood.

—V.M. Frolov, et al., [The Tocopherol Acetate and Splenin Correction of the Immunological Disorders in Patients with Viral Hepatitis B], *Vrach Delo,* (4), April 1992, p. 90-91.

Hepatoxicity

Results of this study showed that cholesteryl hemisuccinate and alpha-tocopherol proved to be strong cytoprotective agents against CC14 hepatoxicity in vivo.

—M.W. Fariss, et al., "Protection Against Carbon Tetrachloride-induced Hepatoxicity by Pretreating Rats with the Hemisuccinate Esters of Tocopherol and Cholesterol," *Environ Health Perspect,* 101(6), November 1993, p. 528-536.

Homozygous Beta-Thalassemia

Results of this study showed that the administration of 300 mg per day of vitamin E for 15 days to patients with beta-thalassemic homozygotes between the ages of 2-14 reduced RBC oxidative damage. Effects were strongest in patients administered vitamin E parenterally.

—O. Giardini, et al., "Biochemical and Clinical Effects of Vitamin E Administration in Homozygous Beta-thalassemia," *Acta Vitaminol Enzymol,* 7(1-2), 1985, p. 55-60.

Hormone Production

This study examined the role of vitamin E in the endocrine system, in particular the pituitary-gonadal axis, in humans and rats. Results showed the following: pituitary content and basal plasma level of FSH and LH were significantly lower in vitamin E deficient rats than controls. Vitamin E supplemented rats had significantly higher FSH and LH content in pituitary tissue than controls. In normal males, Basal plasma testosterone and F.T.I were increased following oral vitamin E supplementation.

—F. Umeda, et al., "Effect of Vitamin E on Function of Pituitary-gonadal Axis in Male Rats and Human Subjects," *Endocrinol Jpn,* 29(3), June 1982, p. 287-292.

Hyperlipidemia

This study examined the effect of daily 8.56 mg/kg per body weight of vitamin E treatment for 9 days in experimental hyperlipidemia in rats. Results showed vitamin E increased the liver's natural scavenger capacity and decreased the level of thiobarbituric acid reactive products and dien conjugates.

> —E.M. Horvath, et al., [Antioxidant Effect of Vitamin E in Experimental Hyperlipidemia], *Orv Hetil,* 134(32), August 8, 1993, p. 1757-1760.

Immune Enhancement

This double-blind, placebo-controlled study examined the effects of supplementation with 800 mg of vitamin E for 30 days on immune response in older healthy adults. Results showed supplementation improved immune responsiveness through an apparent mediation by a decrease in PGE2 and/or other lipid-peroxidation products.

> —S.N. Meydani, et al., "Vitamin E Supplementation Enhances Cell-mediated Immunity in Healthy Elderly Subjects," *American Journal of Clinical Nutrition,* 52(3), September 1990, p. 557-563.

Results of this study on the effects of vitamin E on the immune system of chickens found that vitamin E may be ameliorating avian erythroblastosis virus-induced T-cell dysfunctions by decreasing PGE2 and increasing IL-1 produced by macrophages and by increasing IL-2 expression by T cells.

> —K. Kline, et al., "Vitamin E Modulation of Avian Retrovirus Induced Immune Dysfunctions: Possible Mechanisms," *FASEB Journal,* 4(4), 1990, p. A1051.

This study reports on a single case of severe vitamin E deficiency in a patient which developed secondary to an intestinal malabsorptive disorder. Impairment of T-cell function and polyneuropathy in vivo and in vitro were also observed. Results showed that repletion of the vitamin E deficiency dramatically improved T-cell function and modestly improved neuropathy.

> —K.V. Kowdley, et al., "Vitamin E Deficiency and Impaired Cellular Immunity Related to Intestinal Fat Malabsorption," *Gastroenterology,* 102(6), June 1992, p. 2139-2142.

Results of this study found that there may be macrophage-activating factor-like material in the lavage fluid of lungs of high vitamin E-fed rats (100-2500 mg/kg) and that such diet may activate splenic lymphocytes and alveolar macrophages.

> —S. Moriguchi, et al., "High Dietary Intakes of Vitamin E and Cellular Immune Functions in Rats," *Journal of Nutrition,* 120(9), September 1990, p. 1096-1102.

Results of this study showed that guinea pigs fed vitamin E-deficient diets had both T and B cell responses that were significantly depressed relative to diets adequate in vitamin E.

> —A. Bendich, et al., "Interaction of Dietary Vitamin C and Vitamin E on Guinea Pig Immune Responses to Mitogens," *Journal of Nutrition,* 114(9), September 1984, p. 1588-1593.

This study found that spontaneously hypertensive rats had depressed splenic mitogen responses as well as lower splenic vitamin E when compared to normotensive rats fed a stock diet. 17 weeks on a semipurifed, vitamin E deficient diet resulted in depressed T and B cell splenic mitogen responses in both groups of rats relative to rats fed stock diets or diets supplemented with vitamin E.

> —A. Bendich, et al., "Effect of Dietary Level of Vitamin E on the Immune System of the

Spontaneously Hypertensive (SHR) and Normotensive Wistar Kyoto (WKY) Rat,'' *Journal of Nutrition,* 113(10), October 1983, p. 1920-1926.

Results of this study found that the administration of 25 mg/kg daily of d-alpha-tocopheryl-polyethylene-glycol-1000 succinate to enhance absorption of cyclosporin could be an effective means of decreasing the high cost of immunosuppression in recipients of pediatric liver transplants.
— R.J. Sokol, et al., ''Improvement of Cyclosporin Absorption in Children after Liver Transplantation by Means of Water-soluble Vitamin E,'' *Lancet,* 338(8761), July 17, 1991, p. 212-214.

Results of this double-blind, placebo-controlled study found that healthy older adults taking 800 mg of vitamin E for 30 days experienced an improvement in some in vivo and in vitro parameters of the immune function relative to controls.
— ''Vitamin E Supplementation Enhances Immune Response in the Elderly,'' *Nutr Rev,* 50(3), March 1992, p. 85-87.

Results of this placebo-controlled study found that supplementation with vitamins A, C, and E in elderly long-stay patients improved the aspects of cell-mediated immune function.
— N.D. Penn, et al., ''The Effect of Dietary Supplementation with Vitamins A, C and E on Cell-mediated Immune Function in Elderly Long-stay Patients: A Randomized Controlled Trial,'' *Age Ageing,* 20(3), May 1991, p. 169-174.

This review article on the role of vitamin E in immune response makes the following observations: supplementation with vitamin E augments the efficiency of phagocytosis and enhances cell-mediated immunity. With respect to vitamin E's delivery system, a targeted delivery to localized immunocompetent cells in adjuvant formulations has proven far more effective that a general dispersed delivery in a diet. In sheep, studies have shown vitamin E to offer more protection than conventional vaccines against enterotoxemia and epididymitis.
— R.P. Tengerdy, ''The Role of Vitamin E in Immune Response and Disease Resistance,'' *Annals of the New York Academy of Sciences,* 587, 1990, p. 24-33.

The review article stressed the importance of vitamin E for optimal immune function and notes that animals fed diets deficient in vitamin E have been shown to suffer adverse effects to the immune system. Supplementation has been observed to reverse such effects and enhance the immune response. This article also makes the following observations: vitamin E can partially overcome the immunosuppressive effects of PUFA in high levels. Vitamin C protects vitamin E tissue levels and may play a role in vitamin E's immunoenhancing properties.
— A. Bendich, ''Vitamin E and Immune Functions,'' *Basic Life Sci,* 49, 1988, p. 615-620.

This study examined lipid peroxidation and vitamin E levels in the peripheral blood mononuclear cells of hemodialysis patients. Results showed lowered vitamin E levels and significant increases of PBMC malonyldialdehyde. PBMC MDA levels were returned to normal following vitamin E supplementation for 15 days.
— M. Taccone-Gallucci, et al., ''Vitamin E Supplementation in Hemodialysis Patients: Effects on Peripheral Blood Mononuclear Cells Lipid Peroxidation and Immune Response,'' *Clinical Nephrol,* 25(2), February 1986, p. 81-86.

This study examined the immunomodulating effects of 40 mg/kg of vitamin E give to patients 3.5 hours prior to open heart surgery. Results showed that patients given the vitamin E experienced a decreased rate of immunodepression in the postoperative period relative to controls.

> —O.S. Gaidova, et al., [The Immunomodulating Properties of Vitamin E in Surgery Involving Artificial Circulation], *Grud Serdechnososudistaia Khir,* (12), December 1990, p. 30-33.

This study examined the effects on calve immune responses of vitamin E injections from birth up through 12 weeks at doses of 0. 900, 1800, and 2700. Results demonstrated a trend in greater concentrations of IgG1 and IgG2 with increases in vitamin E. IgM was also observed to be significantly greater for calves receiving 2700 IU of vitamin E relative to controls.

> —M. Hidiroglou, et al., "Possible Roles of Vitamin E in Immune Response of Calves," *International Journal of Vitam Nutr Research,* 62(4), 1992, p. 308-311.

Results of this study showed that supplementation with 30 ppm or 500 ppm of vitamin E for 6 weeks enhanced the immune response of aged mice and that such effects were likely mediated by a decrease in prostaglandin synthesis.

> —S.N. Meydani, et al., "Vitamin E Supplementation Suppresses Prostaglandin E1(2) Synthesis and Enhances the Immune Response of Aged Mice," *Mech Ageing Dev,* 34(2), April 1986, p. 191-201.

This study examined the effects of vitamin E in high doses on blood and spleen leukocytes in mice. Results showed that 7 weeks of vitamin E supplementation in young mice produced a reduction in CD4+ and CD5+ SIgM+ (putative Fc-receptor positive) T cells and B1 cells in blood. Reductions were also observed in the splenic lymphocyte subsets.

> —D. Brohee and P. Neve, "Effect of Dietary High Doses of Vitamin E on Lymphocyte Subsets in Young and Old CBA Mice," *Mech Ageing Dev,* 76(2-3), October 20, 1994, p. 189-200.

Results of this study found that RRR-alpha-tocopheryl succinate was shown to be an effective in vitro modulator of retrovirus-induced immune dysfunction in erythroblastosis virus-infected chickens.

> —K. Kline and B.G. Sanders, "RRR-alpha-tocopheryl Succinate Enhances T Cell Mitogen-induced Proliferation and Reduces Suppresser Activity in Spleen Cells Derived from AEV-Infected Chickens," *Nutri Cancer,* 15(2), 1991, p. 73-85.

Results of this study found that mice exposed to chronic alcohol consumption with compromised immune responses experienced a complete restoration of immune status following 3 days of supplementation with 5 IU of vitamin E. Guinea pigs supplemented with 50 IU of vitamin E showed similar results.

> —K.D. Pletsityi, et al., [The Immunocorrecting Effect of Vitamin E During Ethanol Intoxication], *Vopr Med Khim,* 40(3), May-June 1994, p. 51-53.

This article notes that studies have shown that the administration of vitamin E to mice, rabbits, and guinea-pigs increases the T-lymphocyte content in the peripheral blood without any effects on B lymphocyte content and also stimulates natural killers of spleen lymphocytes.

> —K.D. Pletsityi, et al., [Effect of Vitamin E on T and B Lymphocyte Numbers in the Peripheral

Blood and Various Indicators of Nonspecific Immunity], *Vopr Pitan,* (4), July-August 1984, p. 42-44.

Infections

This study examined the antioxidative role of vitamin E and glutathione redox cycle (GSH) in normal human cultured skin fibroblasts infected by virulent Mycoplasma pneumoniae. Results found that host cell GSH redox cycle and vitamin supplementation limits the oxidative damage induced in M. pneumoniae-infected cells due to the increase in intracellular levels of H_2O_2 and O_2.

—M. Almagor, et al., ''Protective Effects of the Glutathione Redox Cycle and Vitamin E on Cultured Fibroblasts Infected by Mycoplasma Pneumoniae,'' *Infect Immun,* 52(1), April 1986, p. 240-244.

Infertility

Results of this double-blind, placebo-controlled study found that supplementation with 600 mg per day of vitamin E for 3 months significantly improved, as measured by the zona binding test, the in vitro function of human spermatozoa.

—E. Kessopoulou, et al., ''A Double-blind Randomized Placebo Cross-over Controlled Trial Using the Antioxidant Vitamin E to Treat Reactive Oxygen Species Associated Male Infertility,'' *Fertil Steril,* 64(4), October 1995, p. 825-831.

Influenza

Results of this study showed that the use of reaferon in combination with alpha-tocopherol in infected with influenza A virus-infected mice led to reduced mortality rate, boost in the reaferon's antiviral effects, and led to near total normalization of lipid peroxidation processes in the pulmonary tissues and blood plasma.

—N.G. Pertseva, et al., [The Effect of Reaferon and Alpha-tocopherol on Lipid Peroxidation in Experimental Influenza], *Vopr Virusol,* 40(2), March-April 1995, p. 59-62.

Keloids

Results of this study found that the combination of vitamin E and silicone gel sheets produced significant improvement in the treatment of hypertrophic scars or keloids in humans.

—B. Palmieri, et al., ''Vitamin E Added Silicone Gel Sheets for Treatment of Hypertrophic Scars and Keloids,'' *International Journal of Dermatology,* 34(7), July 1995, p. 506-509.

Keshan Disease

This study examined the effects of vitamin E (150 ppm) and selenium (0.1 ppm) supplemenation on myocardial mitochondria in rats fed grains from an endemic area of Keshan disease. Results showed that supplementation protected the myocardial mitochondria from lipid peroxidation induced damage.

—S.Y. Liu, [Protective Effects of Vitamin E and Selenium on Myocardial Mitochondria in Rats—a Study on the Pathogenic Factors and Pathogenesis of Keshan Disease], *Chung Hua Yu Fang I Hsueh Tsa Chih,* 24(4), July 1990, p. 214-216.

This study examined the effects of alpha-tocopherol and selenium supplementation on liver damage in rats induced by dietary grains from an endemic area of Keshan disease. Results showed that supplementation with either alpha-tocopherol or selenium reversed changes in serum enzymes and prevented increases in lipid peroxidation in the liver. Results also showed supplementation to reduce sensitivity to ischemic damages.

> —S.Y. Lui, et al., "Effects of Selenium and Alpha-tocopherol on Liver Damage Induced by Feeding Grains from an Endemic Area of Keshan Disease in Rats," *Mol Cell Biochem,* 132(2), March 30, 1994, p. 109-115.

Kidney Disease/Damage

Results of this study found that the injection of alpha-tocopherol as well as the synthetic antioxidants ional, diludin, and 6-mercurascan prevented the development of lesions during acute renal ischemia and subsequent reperfusion.

> —M.V. Bilenko, et al., [Use of Antioxidants to Prevent Damage During Acute Ischemia and Reperfusion of the Kidneys], *Biull Eksp Biol Med,* 96(9), September 1983, p. 8-11.

Results of this study showed that that the pretreatment of rats with alpha-tocopherol and lidocaine significantly reduced levels of ischemic cell necrosis in the liver as well as led to the retention of microsomal monooxygenase depression by phenobarbital in remote periods following acute hepatic ischemia.

> —O.R. Grek, et al., [Prevention, Using Alpha-tocopherol and Lidocaine, of Damage to the Monooxygenase System Activity and Ultrastructure of Hepatocytes Following Acute Ischemia of the Liver], *Biull Eksp Biol Med,* 104(12), December 1987, p. 669-671.

This study examined the effects of vitamin E supplementation (100 IU/KG) for 12 weeks on the severity of chronic puromycin aminonucleoside nephropathy (PAN) in rats. Results showed rats receiving the supplemented diet experienced an increased hematocrit as well as a 50% reduction in urinary total protein and albumin excretion and stabilization of the serum albumin, cholesterol, and triglyceride concentrations. Results also found a 69% higher rate of inulin clearance in supplemented animals and that phosphate reabsorption and beta 2-microglobulin excretion improved relative to controls. Glomerulosclerosis decreased in supplemented rats as was tubulointestinal scarring.

> —H. Trachtman, et al., "Dietary Vitamin E Supplementation Ameliorates Renal Injury in Chronic Puromycin Aminonucleoside Nephropathy," *Journal of the American Society of Nephrol* (1995 Apr) 5(10), April 1995, p. 1811-1819.

Results of this study found that vitamin E deficiency induced lipid peroxidation and glutathione depletion can cause injuries to the kidneys in rats.

> —K. Hagiwara, et al., "Kidney Injury Induced by Lipid Peroxide Produced by Vitamin E Deficiency and GSH Depletion in Rats," *Journal of Nutr Science Vitaminol,* 37(1), February 1991, p. 99-107

Results of this study found that a daily antioxidant combination of 0.2 mg/100 g of vitamin E, 5 mg/100 g of NAO, and 50 mg/100 g of DMTU along with endotoxin can be beneficial in the arrest of progressive renal damage associated with endotoxin plus entamicin in rats.

> —Y. Zurovsky and C. Haber, "Antioxidants Attenuate Endotoxin-gentamicin Induced Acute Renal Failure in Rats," *Scandinavian Journal of Urol Nephrol,* 29(2), June 1995, p. 147-154.

Lead Intoxication

This study examined the potential use of vitamin E in treating or preventing lead intoxication in rats. Results found that the simultaneous supplemenation of vitamin E with lead significantly reduced the inhibition of blood ALAD activity, brain DA and 5-HIAA levels, elevation of urinary ALA excretion, and blood and liver lead concentrations.

> —M. Dhawan, et al., "Preventive and Therapeutic Role of Vitamin E in Chronic Plumbism," *Biomed Environ Science,* 2(4), December 1989, p. 335-340.

Leg Cramps

This double-blind, placebo-controlled study compared the efficacy of vitamin E (400 IU per day) and quinine (325 mg per day) in treating leg cramps in dialysis patients. Results found the two treatments to be equally effective, prompting the authors to recommend vitamin E be the favored treatment due to its lack of side effects.

> —A.O. Roca, et al., "Dialysis Leg Cramps: Efficacy of Quinine Versus Vitamin E," *ASAIO Journal,* 38(3), July-September 1992, p. M481-485.

Liver Disease/Damage

Results of this study showed that intravenous therapy with liposomes containing vitamin E reduced mortality by close to 90% in rats given a lethal dose of CC14 relative to controls.

> —T. Yao, et al., "Inhibition of Carbon Tetrachloride-induced Liver Injury by Liposomes Containing Vitamin E," *American Journal of Physiology,* 267(3 Pt 1), September 1994, p. G476-G484.

Results of this study found that supplementation with 700 mg/kg per day of alpha-tocopherol prevented the hydrazine-induced formation of megamitochondria in the liver of rats.

> —J. Antosiewicz, et al., "Suppression of the Hydrazine-induced Formation of Megamitochondria in the Rat Liver by Alpha-tocopherol," *Exp Mol Pathol,* 60(3), June 1994, p. 173-187.

Results of this study found that the pretreatment of CC14 injected mice with alpha-tocopherol significantly inhibited acute hepatic injury caused by reactive oxygen intermediate production. Pretreatment was also observed to decrease NF-kappa B binding to levels approaching those found in normal mice.

> —S.L. Liu, et al., "Vitamin E Therapy of Acute CCl4-induced Hepatic Injury in Mice is Associated with Inhibition of Nuclear Factor Kappa B Binding," *Hepatology,* 22(5), November 1995, p. 1474-1481.

This study examined the effects of supplemental increases in the content of vitamin E in the liver on chronic liver damage and carbon-tetrachloride-induced cirrhosis in the rat. Results showed that supplementation significantly reduced oxidative liver damage and offered a significant level of protection against carbon tetrachloride-induced chronic liver damage and cirrhosis.

> —M. Parola, et al., "Vitamin E Dietary Supplementation Protects Against Carbon Tetrachloride-induced Chronic Liver Damage and Cirrhosis," *Hepatology,* 16(4), October 1992, p. 1014-1021.

Results of this study showed that mice fed normal levels of vitamin E and DPPD (30 mg/kg) for 9 months were not protected against the detrimental oxidative effects of selenite while mice fed 300 mg/kg of vitamin E demonstrated an ability to suppress such oxidative effects.

—A.S. Csallany, et al., "Effect of Selenite, Vitamin E and N,N'-diphenyl-p-phenylenediamine on Liver Organic Solvent-soluble Lipofuscin Pigments in Mice," *Journal of Nutrition,* 114(9), September 1984, p. 1582-1587.

Results of this study found a negative correlation between vitamin E in the liver and dietary iron concentration in mice. Subcutaneous supplementation with 20 mg/kg of vitamin E 24 hours before a lethal dose of iron prevented iron-induced liver damage without altering hepatic iron stores, offering 100% protection. Similar vitamin E doses administered intravenously following iron intoxication enhanced survival up to 90% as well.

—F.O. Omara and B.R. Blakley, "Vitamin E is Protective Against Iron Toxicity and Iron-induced Hepatic Vitamin E Depletion in Mice," *Journal of Nutrition,* 123(10), October 1993, p. 1649-1655.

This study examined the effects of pretreatment with alpha-tocopherol on cellular free radical metabolism during hepatic ischemia and subsequent reperfusion in rats. Results showed that alpha-tocopherol administered in doses of 10 mg/kg for 3 days enhanced the rate of survival to 45.5%.

—S. Marubayashi, et al., "Role of Free Radicals in Ischemic Rat Liver Cell Injury: Prevention of Damage by Alpha-tocopherol Administration," *Surgery,* 99(2), February 1986, p. 184-192.

Results of this study showed that liver damage is strongly associated to low plasma levels of alpha-tocopherol and that the antioxidant properties of vitamin E was able to reduce the frequency of liver dysfunction in PiMZ carriers at two but not at five months of age.

—K. Pittschieler, "Vitamin E and Liver Damage in MZ Heterozygous Infants with Alpha 1-antitrypsin Deficiency," *Acta Paediatr,* 82(3), March 1993, p. 228-232.

This study examined the effects of supplementation with vitamin E for 28 days on ethanol and cod liver oil induced lipid peroxidation in rats. Results found that in rats fed ethanol supplemented with vitamin E ethane expiration over a 3-hour period was reduced by 96%. An 89% reduction of ethane exhalation was observed in CLO-fed rats supplemented with vitamin E. Rats fed ethanol plus vitamin E showed a reduction of 96% of hepatic conjugated fatty acid dienes levels relative to rats fed ethanol diets without supplementation.

—O.E. Odeleye, et al., "Vitamin E Reduction of Lipid Peroxidation Products in Rats Fed Cod Liver Oil and Ethanol," *Alcohol,* 8(4), July-August, 1991, p. 273-277.

Results of this study showed that the administration of vitamin E, sodium selenite, infusion of Astragulus L., and vitamin E combinations with sodium selenite in particular arrested the occurrence of hepatotoxic properties of tetracycline in rats. Based on these findings, the authors suggest vitamin E be used in combination with selenium containing preparations in treatment and prophylaxis of tetracycline-induced damages of the liver.

—N.P. Skakun and Ilu Vysotskii, [Vitamin E and Selenium-containing Preparations in the Prevention Treatment of Tetracycline-induced Lesions of the Liver], *Antibiotiki,* 28(8), August 1983, p. 608-612.

Results of this study found that vitamin E had protective effect on liver disorders in rats by inhibiting lysosomal enzyme liberation and lipid peroxidation.

> —T. Yoshikawa, et al., "Effects of Vitamin E on D-galactosamine-induced or Carbon Tetra-chloride-induced Hepatotoxicity," *Digestion*, 25(4), 1982, p. 222-229.

Results of this study showed that preventive administration of alpha-tocopherol, lidocaine, contrykal and their combinations provided the most protection against thermal ischemia of the liver in rats as compared to their use separately.

> —V.I. Sharapov, et al., [Prevention of Damages to the Microsomal Monooxygenases in Thermal Ischemia of the Liver by the Separate and Combined use of Alpha-tocopherol, Lidocaine and Kontrikal], *Farmakol Toksikol,* 50(2), March-April 1987, p. 107-111.

This study examined the effects of vitamin E deficiency on fatty acid compositions of total lipids and phospholipids in the tissues of rats. Results showed that increased TAG in the liver of vitamin E deficient rats were restored to normal with supplementation of 20 mg of alpha-tocopheryl acetate/kg diet.

> —W.H. Saypil, et al., "Free Radical-induced Liver Injury. I. Effects of Dietary Vitamin E Deficiency on Triacylglycerol Level and its Fatty Acid Profile in Rat Liver," *Free Radic Res Commun,* 14(5-6), 1991, p. 315-322.

Results of this study showed that halothane-induced liver damage in guinea pigs was suppressed by inhibiting lipid peroxidation as a consequence of supplementation with vitamin E.

> —N. Sato, et al., "Suppressive Effect of Vitamin E on Lipid Peroxidation in Halothane-Administered Guinea Pig Liver," *In Vivo,* 6(5), September-October 1992, p. 503-505.

Results of this study showed that pretreatment with vitamin E protected rats from alterations induced by CC14 on liver membranes and that such effects were likely associated with the antioxidant activity of vitamin E.

> —I. Martinez-Calva, et al., "Vitamin E Improves Membrane Lipid Alterations Induced by CCl4 Intoxication," *Journal of Applied Toxicology,* 4(5), October 1984, p. 270-272.

This study assessed the vitamin E status of adults with chronic liver disease. Results found that low levels of vitamin E were most prevalent in patients with primary biliary cirrhosis (44%) and other chronic liver diseases (32%). Vitamin E supplementation restored serum vitamin E levels to normal in patients showing less severe biochemical deficiencies.

> —G.P. Jeffrey, et al., "Vitamin E Deficiency and its Clinical Significance in Adults with Primary Biliary Cirrhosis and Other Forms of Chronic Liver Disease," *Journal of Hepatology,* 4(3), June 1987, p. 307-317.

Results of this study found that supplementation with 300 mg of DL-alpha-tocopherol/kg improved early fat and collagen accumulation in the liver of rats, decreased SGPT level, and improved survival in the D-galactosamine experimental model of acute liver injury in both conventional and germ-free rats.

> —L. Sclafani, et al., "Protective Effect of Vitamin E in Rats with Acute Liver Injury," *JPEN Journal of Parenteral Enteral Nutrition,* 10(2), March-April 1986, p. 184-187.

This study examined the effect of single administration of alpha-tocopherol at a dose of 50 mg/kg on lipid peroxidation, content of alpha-tocopherol in liver tissue and on the activities of some enzymes in rat serum under conditions of acute blood loss. Results showed that alpha-tocopherol proved to be suitable for pathogenic correction of metabolic impairments in acute blood loss.

> —S.B. Matveev, et al., [Effect of Alpha-Tocopherol on Lipid Peroxidation in the Liver in Acute Blood Loss], *Vopr Med Khim,* 38(3), May-June 1992, p. 18-20.

Methylmercury Toxicity

This study examined whether or not vitamin E diminished the genotoxicity of MeHg in hamsters. Daily injections of 2.0 mg/kg of methylmercury chloride and/or vitamin E were given to hamsters for 3 weeks. Autopsy results showed a high incidence of chromosomal damage in hamsters given MeHg only as opposed to those given vitamin E in which such damage was totally eliminated.

> —M.M. Gilbert, et al., "Protective Effect of Vitamin E on Genotoxicity of Methylmercury," *Journal of Toxicol Environ Health,* 12(4-6), October-December 1983, p. 767-773.

Mucositis

This double-blind, placebo-controlled study examined the efficacy of vitamin E in the treatment of chemotherapy-induced mucositis in malignancy patients. Results showed total resolution of oral lesions in six of nine patients who took vitamin E. By contrast, eight of nine patients receiving a placebo showed no resolution of lesions.

> —R.G. Wadleigh, et al., "Vitamin E in the Treatment of Chemotherapy-induced Mucositis," *American Journal of Medicine,* 92(5), May 1992, p. 481-484.

Muscle Disease/Damage

This review article notes that vitamin E has been shown to decrease the amount of damage which occurs in isolated skeletal muscles following a given stress.

> —M.J. Jackson, et al., "Vitamin E and Muscle Diseases," *Journal of Inherit Metab Dis,* 8 Suppl 1, 1985, p. 84-87.

Results of this study found that the susceptibility to exercise-induced muscle damage is enhanced by a deficiency of vitamin E more in male rats than in female rats. The authors attribute such differences to oestradiol's protective effect that remains operative in female rats during a disturbance in vitamin E status.

> —G.J. Amelink, et al., "Exercise-induced Muscle Damage in the Rat: The Effect of Vitamin E Deficiency," *Pflugers Arch,* 419(3-4), October 1991, p. 304-309.

Myotonic Dystrophy

This study reports on the cases of five patients with myotonic dystrophy who experienced subjective benefits with respect to grip strength, normalized gait, and physical capacity following treatment with 4 mg per day of Na2SeO3 and 600 mg of vitamin E.

> —G. Orndahl, et al., "Myotonic Dystrophy Treated with Selenium and Vitamin E," *Acta Med Scand,* 219(4), 1986, p. 407-414.

Nephrotoxicity

Results of this study found that vitamin E offered protection against iron-induced toxicity in rats.
   —S. Okada, et al., ''Nephrotoxicity and its Prevention by Vitamin E in Ferric Nitrilotriacetate-promoted Lipid Peroxidation,'' *Biochim Biophys Acta,* 922(1), October 31, 1987, p. 28-33.

Neurological Function

This review article identifies three lines of evidence indicating vitamin E's importance for normal neurological function. The first concerns vitamin E's efficacy in delaying, preventing, and/or reversing neurological complications associated with abetalipoproteinaemia. The second concerns other chronic disorders of fat absorption with severe vitamin E deficiency that can be improved with vitamin E supplementation. The third line of evidence deals with the fact that the neuropathological changes observed in vitamin-E-deficient states in man are similar to those in monkeys and rats with vitamin E deficiencies.
   —D.P. Muller, et al., ''Vitamin E and Neurological Function,'' *Lancet,* 1(8318), January 29, 1983, p. 225-228.

This review article notes the findings of studies in patients with abetalipoproteinaemia, other chronic and severe fat malabsorptive states and a selective defect in vitamin E absorption, together with neuropathological studies in the vitamin E deficient human, monkey and rat which have found that vitamin E is important for normal neurological function.
   —D.P. Muller, ''Vitamin E—Its Role in Neurological Function,'' *Postgraduate Medical Journal,* 62(724), February 1986, p. 107-112.

This review article notes that due to chronic vitamin E malabsorption, children with cystic fibrosis, chronic cholestasis, abetalipoproteinemia, and short bowel syndrome are at risk for developing of neurologic deficits caused by vitamin E deficiency. Studies have shown that in susceptible individuals correction of such deficiencies can prevent, stabilize or reverse neurological dysfunction.
   —R.J. Sokol, ''Vitamin E and Neurologic Deficits,'' *Adv Pediatr,* 37, 1990, p. 119-148.

This review article cites studies supporting the view that vitamin E is necessary for optimal development and maintenance of the integrity and function of the skeletal muscle and human nervous system.
   —R.J. Sokol, ''Vitamin E Deficiency and Neurologic Disease,'' *Annu Rev Nutr,* 8, 1988, p. 351-373.

This study examined the effect of vitamin E on ischemic neuronal damage in the gerbil. Alpha-tocopherol was administered intravenously to gerbils at doses of either 50 or 100 mg/kg immediately after induced cerebral ischemia. Results showed alpha-tocopherol prevented ischemia-induced neuronal death.
   —H. Hara, et al., ''Protective Effect of Alpha-tocopherol on Ischemic Neuronal Damage in the Gerbil Hippocampus,'' *Brain Research,* 510(2), March 5, 1990, p. 335-338.

This review article discusses the increasing body of evidence linking the importance of vitamin E for normal neurological function. Some observations made include: development of the spinocerebellar syndrome associated with abetalipoproteinemia may be prevented by therapy with vitamin E. A neurological disorder similar to that seen in abetalipoproteinemia, comprising progressive ataxia, hyporeflexia, and proprioceptive loss, has been described in children and adults with chronic fat malabsorption and vitamin E deficiency. The neuropathological changes in such patients resemble those seen in vitamin E-deficient monkeys.

> —A.E. Harding, ''Vitamin E and the Nervous System,'' *Critical Reviews in Neurobiology,* 3(1), 1987, p. 89-103.

This study reports on a single case of a ten-year-old girl suffering from obstructive jaundice during the newborn period and lasting 4 years. Beginning at 6 she developed a progressive neurological syndrome which was arrested following supplementation with vitamin E over a 2.5 year period.

> —B.W. Lloyd and V. Dubowitz, ''Progressive Neurological Disorder Associated with Obstructive Jaundice and Vitamin E Deficiency,'' *Neuropediatrics,* 13(3), August 1992, p. 155-157.

This study examined the effects of alpha-tocopherol on fetal rat brain neurons in tissue culture. Results showed that alpha-tocopherol may play a role in regulating neuronal survival and neurite formation in the central nervous system.

> —M. Nakajima, et al., ''Alpha-tocopherol Supports the Survival and Neurite Extension of Neurons Cultured from Various Regions of Fetal Rat Brain,'' *Neuroscience Letters,* 133(1), November 25, 1991, p. 49-52.

Results of this study found that vitamin E and phenytoin had protective action against ischemic neuronal damage in the hippocampal slice of the guinea pig. The two drugs combined together proved more effective than either used alone.

> —M. Amagasa, et al., [Protective Effect of Various Agents Against Ischemic Neuronal Damage in Guinea Pig Hippocampal Neurons Studied in Vitro], *No Shinkei Geka,* 16(12), November 1988, p. 1363-1371.

Results of this study found that a deficiency in vitamin E can trigger results leading to the appearance of new neurons in rats.

> —T. Cecchini, et al., ''Increased Number of Dorsal Root Ganglion Neurons in Vitamin-E-Deficient Rats,'' *Somatosens Mot Research,* 10(4), 1993, p. 433-443.

This study reports on a single case of a 4-year-old girl deficient in vitamin E suffering from congenital nerve deafness, pancreatic insufficiency and incapacitating ataxia. Ataxia disappeared and electrphysiological variables were normalized following intramuscular injections of vitamin E.

> —G. Davidai, et al., ''Hypovitaminosis E Induced Neuropathy in Exocrine Pancreatic Failure,'' *Arch Dis Child,* 61(9), September 1986, p. 901-903.

This study reports on the case of a single patient who benefited from vitamin E supplementation as a means of treating motor sensory polyneuropathy with a recurrent remittent course, normal CSF and reduced motor and sensory conduction velocities.

> —L. Palmucci, et al., ''Neuropathy Secondary to Vitamin E Deficiency in Acquired Intestinal Malabsorption,'' *Italian Journal of Neurol Sci,* 9(6), December 1988, p. 599-602.

Results of this study showed that vitamin E supplementation could have neuroprotective effects in the septohippocampal cholinergic system of rats.

> —G. Wortwein, et al., ''Vitamin E Prevents the Place Learning Deficit and the Cholinergic Hypofunction Induced by AF64A,'' *Exp Neurol,* 125(1), January 1994, p. 15-21.

Neutrophil Function

Results of this study showed that vitamin E use protected neutrophil phagocytic function to a certain extent in severely burned patients.

> —J. Chai, et al., [Protective Effects of Vitamin E on Impaired Neutrophil Phagocytic Function in Patients with Severe Burn], *Chung Hua Cheng Hsing Shao Shang Wai Ko Tsa Chih,* 11(1), January 1995, p. 32-35.

Results of this study showed that four daily injections of 100 mg of vitamin E promoted neutrophils return to the circulation after chemotactic challenge in rabbits and did so by reducing their adherence to endothelium.

> —J.E. Lafuze, et al., "The Effect of Vitamin E on Rabbit Neutrophil Activation," *Ciba Found Symp,* 101, 1983, p. 130-146.

Newborns

Results of this study found that supplementation with 20 mg of vitamin E/kg im soon after birth protected preterm babies against intraventricular hemorrhage.

> —M. Chiswick, et al., "Vitamin E Supplementation and Periventricular Hemorrhage in the Newborn," *American Journal of Clinical Nutrition,* 53(1 Suppl), January 1991, p. 370S-372S.

Results of this study found that a deficiency in vitamin E is one feature associated with intra-uterine growth retardation and prematurity.

> —R.S. Shah, et al., "Vitamin E Status of the Newborn in Relation to Gestational Age, Birth Weight and Maternal Vitamin E Status," *British Journal of Nutrition,* 58(2), September 1987, p. 191-198.

In this study, babies of less than 32 weeks gestation received 25 mg/kg of vitamin E intramuscularly after birth. Results showed that the incidence of intraventricular hemorrhage was lower in these babies relative to controls. The authors argue that such findings suggest vitamin E protects endothelial cell membranes from disruption and oxidative damage and limits the magnitude of hemorrhage and its spread into the ventricles from subependyma in premature babies.

> —M.L. Chiswick, et al., "Protective Effect of Vitamin E (DL-alpha-tocopherol) Against Intraventricular Haemorrhage in Premature Babies," *British Medical Journal,* 287(6385), July 9, 1983, p. 81-84.

This placebo-controlled study examined the effects of vitamin E on severity of retinopathy of prematurity in low birth weight infants. Results showed some decrease in ROP among infants treated with vitamin E relative to controls.

> —L. Johnson, et al., "Effect of Sustained Pharmacologic Vitamin E Levels on Incidence and Severity of Retinopathy of Prematurity: A Controlled Clinical Trial," *Journal of Pediatrics,* 114(5), May 1989, p. 827-838.

This study examined the effects of vitamin E prophylaxis and treatment on the sequelae of severe retinopathy of prematurity in infants treated with cryotherapy. Results showed vitamin E combined with cryotherapy decreased the severity and sequale of threshold retinopathy of prematurity.

> —L. Johnson, et al., "Severe Retinopathy of Prematurity in Infants with Birth Weights Less

than 1250 Grams: Incidence and Outcome of Treatment with Pharmacologic Serum Levels of Vitamin E in Addition to Cryotherapy from 1985 to 1991,'' *Journal of Pediatrics,* 127(4), October 1995, p. 632-639.

This study examined the effects of daily intramuscular supplementation with 20 mg/kg of vitamin E on the prevention of periventricular haemorrhage in babies at or less than 32 weeks gestation. Results showed that supplemenation during the first 3 days of life was associated with a reduction in hydrogen peroxide haemolysis of red blood cells in vitro. Concerning babies without hemorrhage upon beginning the study, those supplemented with vitamin E showed a lower rate of intraventricular haemorrhage than controls as well as a lower combined frequency of intraventricular and parenchumal haemorrhage.

—S. Sinha, et al., ''Vitamin E Supplementation Reduces Frequency of Periventricular Haemor-rhage in Very Preterm Babies,'' *Lancet,* 1(8531), February 28, 1987, p. 466-471.

This double-blind, placebo-controlled study examined the effects of early intramuscular vitamin E supplementation (100 mg/kg per day) for 8 weeks on the incidence of intraventricular hemorrhage in low birth weight infants. Results showed that the incidence and the severity of intraventricular hemor-rhage were significantly reduced in supplemented infants relative to controls, findings which indicate vitamin E may be a key factor in protecting CNS microcirculation from the effects of hypoxic/ischemic injury.

—M.E. Speer, et al., ''Intraventricular Hemorrhage and Vitamin E in the Very Low-birth-weight Infant: Evidence for Efficacy of Early Intramuscular Vitamin E Administration,'' *Pediatrics,* 74(6), December 1984, p. 1107-1112.

In this study, 100 low birth weight infants treated with 100 mg/kg per day of dl-alpha-tocopheryl acetate were compared with 75 low birth weight infants receiving 5 mg/kg per day of dl-alpha-tocopherol in the same setting in order to test the efficacy of oral vitamin E in preventing severe retrolental fibroplasia. Results found that the severity of retrolental fibroplasia was reduced significantly in infants receiving the treatment dose of vitamin E relative to controls.

—H.M. Hittner, et al., ''Retrolental Fibroplasia: Further Clinical Evidence and Ultrastructural Support for Efficacy of Vitamin E in the Preterm Infant,'' *Pediatrics,* 71(3), March 1983, p. 423-432.

This placebo-controlled, double-blind study examined the effects of intramuscular vitamin E (100 mg/kg per day) on intracranial hemorrhage and mortality in low birth weight neonates. Results showed significantly lower levels of intracranial hemorrhage and mortality in neonates treated with vitamin E relative to controls.

—W.H. Fish, et al., ''Effect of Intramuscular Vitamin E on Mortality and Intracranial Hemor-rhage in Neonates of 1000 Grams or Less,'' *Pediatrics,* 85(4), April 1990, p. 578-584.

Results of this study found that oral supplementation with 100 mg/kg per day of vitamin E proved retinal protection against the development of severe retrolental fibroplasia in infants when started on day one of life and maintained until the completion of vascularization.

—H.M. Hittner, et al., ''Retrolental Fibroplasia and Vitamin E in the Preterm Infant—comparison of Oral Versus intramuscular:Oral Administration,'' *Pediatrics,* 73(2), February 1984, p. 238-249.

This study examined the effects of oral vitamin E pretreatment on the tolerance of hearts to ischemia in newborn piglets. Results found that treatment did improve ischemic tolerance of newborn myocardium.

> —D. Shum-Tim, et al., "Oral Vitamin E Prophylaxis in the Protection of Newborn Myocardium from Global Ischemia," *Surgery,* 112(2), August 1992, p. 441-450.

Results of this study found that vitamin E administered in doses of 120mg/kg during the first 13 days following birth may be used to accelerate the normalization of phagocytic function in the neonatal period in premature newborns.

> —G. Chirico, et al., "Deficiency of Neutrophil Phagocytosis in Premature Infants: Effect of Vitamin E Supplementation," *Acta Paediatr Scand,* 72(4), July 1983, p. 521-524.

In this study, vitamin E was shown to be a key protective factor against accumulation of lipoperoxides and abnormal synthesis in the liver tissues of rats during early stages following birth.

> —T. Yoshioka, et al., "Protective Effect of Vitamin E Against Lipoperoxides in Developing Rats," *Biol Neonate,* 51(3), 1987, p. 170-176.

Results of this study showed that vitamin E offered protection of neuronal development in X-irradiated rat fetuses.

> —H. Tanaka, et al., "The Protective Effects of Vitamin E Against Microcephaly in Rats X-Irradiated in Utero: Dendritic Branches," *Brain Development,* 8(3), 1986, p. 301-304.

This study examined the role, if any, of vitamin E deficiency in the hypercoagulability of neonatal blood. Results showed a significant correlation between plasma vitamin E and whole blood clotting time of cord blood and clotting time was prolonged with the addition of standard vitamin E to the cord blood in vitro. Based on these findings, the authors argue that a plasma vitamin E deficiency can shorten whole blood clotting time in newborns.

> —S.K. Jain, et al., "Vitamin E and the Hypercoagulability of Neonatal Blood," *Clin Chim Acta,* 225(2), March 1994, p. 97-103.

This study found evidence of retinal damage associated with the clinical observation of Retinopathy of Prematurity grade III in preterm infants receiving the minimum amount of vitamin E recommended by the American Academy of Pediatrics which is 5 mg/kg per day, and exposed to high concentration/ duration of oxygen at birth. By contrast, matched infants receiving 100 mg/kg per day of vitamin E showed no signs of retinopathy.

> —W.A. Monaco, "Ultrastructural Evaluation of the Retina in Retinopathy of Prematurity and Correlations with Vitamin E Therapy," *Current Eye Research,* 2(2), 1982-1983, p. 123-139.

This study reports on the results of three clinical trials involving low birth weight infants and an ultrastructural data base of whole eye donations which point to efficacy of vitamin E in suppressing the development of severe retrolent fibroplasia. It was shown that only continuous vitamin E supplementation to adult physiological levels from the first hours of life suppresses severe ROP development.

> —H.M. Hittner, et al., "Suppression of Severe Retinopathy of Prematurity with Vitamin E Supplementation: Ultrastructural Mechanism of Clinical Efficacy," *Ophthalmology,* 91(12), December 1984, p. 1512-1523.

This study examined the effects of vitamin E on the neonatal surfactant system in rabbits exposed to air or hyperoxia during the first 48 hours of life. Results found that 100 mg/kg of vitamin E administered at 1 and 24 hours of life abolished the negative effects of hyperoxia.

> —J.A. Ward and R.J. Roberts, ''Vitamin E Inhibition of the Effects of Hyperoxia on the Pulmonary Surfactant System of the Newborn Rabbit,'' *Pediatric Research,* 18(4), April 1984, p. 329-334.

Nutritional Pancreatic Atrophy

This study examined the relationship between dietary vitamin E and development of nutritional pancreatic atrophy in chicks with a deficiency in selenium. Results showed that supplementation with 500 or 1000 IU VE/kg prevented both nutritional pancreatic atrophy and the growth depression associated with it. At least 300 IU of vitamin E was needed to overcome the growth depression associated with severe selenium deficiency.

> —M.E. Whitacre, et al., ''Influence of Dietary Vitamin E on Nutritional Pancreatic Atrophy in Selenium-Deficient Chicks,'' *Journal of Nutrition,* 117(3), March 1987, p. 460-467.

Osteoarthritis

In this placebo-controlled, double-blind study, osteoarthritis patients were treated with 400 IE per day of d-alpha-tocopherylacetate for six weeks. Results showed that those taking the vitamin E experienced more pain relief and more improvement in mobility than controls.

> —G. Blankenhorn, [Clinical Effectiveness of Spondyvit (vitamin E) in Activated Arthroses: A Multicenter Placebo-controlled Double-blind Study], *Z Orthop,* 124(3), May-June 1986, p. 340-343.

This double-blind study examined the known antiphlogistic in vitro effects of 400 mg of vitamin E for 3 weeks in osteoarthritis patients relative to treatment with 50 mg of Diclofenac three times daily. Results found no significant differences between the two drugs, with each proving to be equally effective in pain reduction, increasing walking time, reducing the circumference of the knee joints, and increasing joint mobility.

> —O. Scherak, et al., [High Dosage Vitamin E Therapy in Patients with Activated Arthrosis], *Z Rheumatol,* 49(6), November-December 1990, p. 369-373.

This study examined the action of tocopherol administered in doses of 600 mg per day for 10 days in patients with osteoarthritis. Results showed positive effects in 52% of those receiving the supplementation compared to only 4% among patients given placebo.

> —I. Machtey and L. Ouaknine, ''Tocopherol in Osteoarthritis: A Controlled Pilot Study,'' *Journal of the American Geriatric Society* (1978 Jul) 26(7), July 1978, p. 328-330.

Parkinson's Disease

In this pilot study, a combination of alpha-tocopherol and ascorbate in high doses were given to early Parkinson's disease patients. Results found that Parkinson's progression may be slowed by the administration of such antioxidants.

> —S. Fahn, ''A Pilot Trial of High-dose Alpha-tocopherol and Ascorbate in Early Parkinson's Disease,'' *Ann Neurol,* 32(Suppl), 1992, p. S128-S132.

Results of this study indicated prolonged and severe vitamin E deficiency can produce a loss of nigrostriatal nerve terminals which suggests that oxidative stress may play a role in the etiology of Parkinson's disease.

—D.T. Dexter, et al., "Nigrostriatal Function in Vitamin E Deficiency: Clinical, Experimental, and Positron Emission Tomographic Studies," *Ann Neurol,* 35(3), March 1994, p. 298-303.

This study demonstrated the key role vitamin E plays in the prevention of membrane lipid peroxidation and the potential relationship between membrane lipid peroxidation and Parkinson's disease.

—M. Tanaka, et al., "Aging of the Brain and Vitamin E," *Journal of Nutr Sci Vitaminol,* Spec No, 1992, p. 240-243.

Periodontal Health

Results of this study showed that rats administered 100 mg of dl-alpha-tocopherol acetate twice a week for up to 4 weeks after they were subjected to pulp exposures that were capped with zinc oxide and eugenol experienced more healing than controls subjected to the same procedures.

—C. Niamonitos, et al., "Effects of Vitamin E Dietary Supplements on the Exposed Dental Pulp in Rats," *Oral Surg Oral Med Oral Pathol,* 59(6), June 1985, p. 627-636.

Results of this study suggest supplementation with vitamin E may play a role in maintaining periodontal health in rice rats.

—M.E. Cohen and D.M. Meyer, "Effect of Dietary Vitamin E Supplementation and Rotational Stress on Alveolar Bone Loss in Rice Rats," *Arch Oral Biol,* 38(7), July 1993, p. 601-606.

Peripheral Neuropathy

This study measured the alpha-tocopherol content in biopsy specimens of sural nerve and adipose tissue from symptomatic vitamin E deficient patients and control patients without vitamin E deficiency but with neurologic diseases. Results showed a significant reduction in tissue tocopherol content in vitamin E deficient patients relative to controls. Histologic degeneration in three of five vitamin E deficient patients was preceded by low tocopherol content of the nerves which indicates that low nerve tocopherol content may have been responsible for nerve injury.

—M.G. Traber, et al., "Lack of Tocopherol in Peripheral Nerves of Vitamin E-deficient Patients with Peripheral Neuropathy," *New England Journal of Medicine,* 317(5), July 30, 1987, p. 262-265.

Peritoneal Adhesions

This study examined whether or not there is a synergistic beneficial effect of vitamin E and sodium carboxymethyl cellulose solution (SCMC) in the reduction of postoperative adhesions in rats. Results found there to indeed be such a synergistic beneficial effect.

—O. Hemadeh, et al., "Prevention of Peritoneal Adhesions by Administration of Sodium Carboxymethyl Cellulose and Oral Vitamin E," *Surgery,* 114(5), November 1993, p. 907-910.

Pesticides

Results of this study found that vitamin E protected human lysomal membranes in vitro against the toxic effects of dichlorvus more effectively than did the nucleolar structure in these cells.

—M. Grabarczyk and J. Kopec-Szlezak, ''Protective Action of Vitamin E on the Subcellular Structures of Lymphocytes Intoxicated with Pesticides in Vitro,'' *Mater Med Pol,* 24(4), October-December 1992, p. 237-239.

Physical Performance

This study notes that vitamin E promotes an economical energy metabolism and acts as a stabilizing antioxidant in membranes, both of which are leading to its use to enhance physical performance. A group of high altitude mountain climbers was substituted with 2 x 200 mg dl-alpha-tocopheryl acetate for 10 weeks during an expedition. Results found vitamin E to have a beneficial effect on physical performance and cell protection in the climbers relative to a group of matched controls.

—I. Simon-Schnass and H. Pabst, ''Influence of Vitamin E on Physical Performance,'' *International Journal of Vitam Nutr Research,* 58(1), 1988, p. 49-54.

PMS

Results of this double-blind, placebo-controlled study found that two months of treatment with either 150, 300, or 600 IU of vitamin E per day in women with benign breast cancer improved severe PMS symptoms relative to controls.

—R.S. London, et al., ''The Effect of Alpha-tocopherol on Premenstrual Symptomatology: A Double-blind Study,'' *Journal of the American College of Nutrition,* 2(2), 1983, p. 115-122.

Results of this double-blind, placebo-controlled study showed that women treated daily with 400 IU of d-alpha-tocopherol for three cycles experienced significant improvements in certain affective and physical symptoms of PMS relative to controls.

—R.S. London, et al., ''Efficacy of Alpha-tocopherol in the Treatment of the Premenstrual Syndrome,'' *Journal of Reproductive Medicine,* 32(6), June 1987, p. 400-404.

Pregnancy

This study examined the relationship between abnormal pregnancy and reduced levels of vitamin E in healthy women. Results showed lower maternal levels of vitamin E in abnormal pregnancies.

—U. von Mandach, et al., ''Maternal and Cord Serum Vitamin E Levels in Normal and Abnormal Pregnancy,'' *International Journal of Vitam Nutr Research,* 64(1), 1994, p. 26-32.

Results of this study found that vitamin E is a key factor in platelet function regulation during pregnancy and may play a role, by inhibiting platelet aggregation, in maintaining placental microcirculation

—S. Akada, et al., [The Role of Vitamin E During Pregnancy—anti-platelet Aggregation Activity of Alpha-tocopherol], *Nippon Sanka Fujinka Gakkai Zasshi,* 43(5), May 1991, p. 523-528.

Results of this study found that vitamin E may have a protective effect on fetal ischemic distress caused by clamping the uterotubal vessels of pregnant rats by decreasing lipid peroxides.

—H. Iwasa, [Effect of Dietary Level of Vitamin E on Protection of Fetus Against Ischemic

Distress Induced by Clamping the Uterotubal Vessels of Pregnant Rats], *Nippon Sanka Fujinka Gakkai Zasshi,* 42(5), May 1990, p. 422-428.

Proliferative Vitreoretinopathy

Results of this study found that supplementation with 100 microM of alpha-tocopherol inhibited the proliferation of human retinal pigment epithelium (RPE) in culture without exerting cytotoxic effects. According to the authors, such findings could explain why vitamin E supplements have been seen to adversely effect light-damaged retinas as well as the course of retinitis pigmentosa. The authors suggest vitamin E could be a useful treatment for PVR since supplementation with vitamin E can raise the RPE concentration of alpha-tocopherol well above 100 microM.

—D. Mojon, et al., "Vitamin E Inhibits Retinal Pigment Epithelium Cell Proliferation in Vitro," *Ophthalmic Research,* 26(5), 1994, p. 304-309.

Pulmonary Health

Results of this study showed that rats given 50 mg/kg of vitamin E upon the start of progressing inflammatory injury protected against oxidant damage in the lung and attenuated the degree of lung injury.

—R. Demling, et al., "Alpha-tocopherol Attenuates Lung Edema and Lipid Peroxidation Caused by Acute Zymosan-induced Peritonitis," *Surgery,* 117(2), February 1995, p. 226-231.

Results of this study found that the supplementation of vitamin E and selenium reduced susceptibiliy to pulmonary oxygen poisoning in rats.

—L.N. North, et al., "Effect of Dietary Vitamin E or Selenium on Prostaglandin Dehydrogenase in Hyperoxic Rat Lung," *Aviat Space Environ Medicine,* 55(7), July 1984, p. 617-619.

This study showed that vitamin E delivered directly to the lung in a liposomal formulation 24 hours before the administration of paraquat, protected the lung against damage induced by paraquat.

—Z.E. Suntres, et al., "Protective Effect of Liposome-associated Alpha-tocopherol Against Paraquat-Induced Acute Lung Toxicity," *Biochem Pharmacol,* 44(9), November 3, 1992, p. 1811-1818.

Results of the series of studies reported in this paper found that vitamins E and C reduced lipid peroxidation and preserved the elastase inhibitory capacity of the lower respiratory tract fluid during oxidant stress in human subjects.

—V. Mohsenin, "Lipid Peroxidation and Antielastase Activity in the Lung Under Oxidant Stress: Role of Antioxidant Defenses," *Journal of Applied Physiology,* 70(4), April 1991, p. 1456-1462.

Results of this study showed that vitamin E and glutathione protected against peroxidation in the lung microsomal membranes of rats.

—D.P. Franco and S.G. Jenkinson, "Rat Lung Microsomal Lipid Peroxidation: Effects of Vitamin E and Reduced Glutathione," *Journal of Applied Physiology,* 61(2), August 1986, p. 785-790.

This study examined the effects of liposome-associated alpha-tocopherol on paraquat-induced pulmonary damage in rats. Results showed that rats treated with alpha-tocopherol liposomes 24 hours after paraquat administration increased significantly the concentrations of pulmonary alpha-tocopherol, reduced changes in lipid peroxidation induced by paraquat, concentration of GSH, and lung angiotensin converting enzyme and alkaline phosphatase activities.

> —Z.E. Suntres and P.N. Shek, "Liposomal Alpha-tocopherol Alleviates the Progression of Paraquat-Induced Lung Damage," *Journal of Drug Target,* 2(6), 1995, p. 493-500.

Respiration

This placebo-controlled study examined the effects of 900 IU of vitamin E for 6 weeks on the respiratory health of smokers. Results showed that the generation of oxidants by activated phagocytes seemed to be inhibited by the vitamin E supplementation.

> —G.A. Richards, et al., "Investigation of the Effects of Oral Administration of Vitamin E and Beta-Carotene on the Chemiluminescence Responses and the Frequency of Sister Chromatid Exchanges in Circulating Leukocytes from Cigarette Smokers," *American Review of Respiratory Disease,* 142(3), September 1990, p. 648-654.

This study found that 6 weeks of treatment with vitamin E improved the clinical status and normalized the proportion of OKT+4 T lymphocytes and the ratio of OKT+4 to OKT+8 cells in the peripheral blood of children suffering from respiratory tract infections.

> —E. Skopinska-Rozewska, et al., "The Effect of Vitamin E Treatment on the Incidence of OKT+4 Lymphocytes in the Peripheral Blood of Children with Chronic Respiratory Tract Infections," *Archives of Immunol Ther Exp,* 35(2), 1987, p. 207-210.

Retinal Degeneration/Light Damage

Results of this study showed that the mortality rate of new rats with inheritable retinal degeneration was reduced by 73% following supplementation with alpha-tocopherol. First week survival rates jumped from 72.3% to 92.5% when the dosage of supplemental vitamin E was increased from 50 to 100 IU/kg.

> —C.D. Eckhert, "Differential Effects of Riboflavin and RRR-alpha-tocopheryl Acetate on the Survival of Newborn RCS Rats with Inheritable Retinal Degeneration," *Journal of Nutrition,* 117(1), January 1987, p. 208-211.

Results of this study showed that the development of experimental retina degeneration is accompanied by lipid peroxidation intensification and that vitamin injections prior to and following monoidoacetic acid and oxygenous intoxication leads to lipid peroxdiation suppression.

> —N.M. Magomedov, et al., [Study of Lipid Peroxidation in Experimental Retinal Degeneration], *Biull Eksp Biol Med,* 95(3), March 1983, p. 37-39.

Results of this study showed that the administration of vitamin E or beta-carotene both prevented the increase of retinal lipid peroxide in rats caused by exposure to 18,175 lx with amelioration of the photic injury to the retinal structures.

> —W.H. Chen and H.R. Zhang, [Photogenic Retinal Damage and its Medicinal Prevention: Lipid Peroxide Studies], *Chung Hua Yen Ko Tsa Chih,* 30(2), March 1994, p. 125-127.

In this study, alpha-tocopherol was systemically administered before 60 minutes of xenon light exposure to the retinas of rabbits. Results found that light exposure increased the number of free radicals in the inner retina and that such free radicals were suppressed by alpha-tocopherol.

—J. Kozaki, et al., [Protective Effect of Alpha-tocopherol in Retinal Light Damage of Pigmented Rabbits—evaluation by Nitro Blue Tetrazolium Staining], *Nippon Ganka Gakkai Zasshi,* 99(2), February 1995, p. 161-165.

Results of this study found that the reperfusion-induced ionic imbalance was reduced and the recovery of retinal ion contents improved in the rat retina following chronic administration of vitamin E (50, 100, and 200 mg/kg, i.v.), superoxide dismutase (7500, 15,000, and 30,000 U/kg, i.v.), and EGB 761 (50, 100, and 200 mg/kg, orally) for 10 days.

—M.E. Szabo, et al., ''Modification of Reperfusion-induced Ionic Imbalance by Free Radical Scavengers in Spontaneously Hypertensive Rat Retina,'' *Free Radic Biol Medicine,* 13(6), December 1992, p. 609-620.

Retrolental Fibroplasia

This study examined the effects of intramuscular vitamin E on the severity and frequency of retrolental fibroplasia in low birth weight neonates. Results showed that the early use of vitamin E significantly reduced the severity of retrolental fibroplasia and eye damage that follows from it.

—N.N. Finer, et al., ''Effect of Intramuscular Vitamin E on Frequency and Severity of Retrolental Fibroplasia: A Controlled Trial,'' *Lancet,* 1(8281), May 15, 1982, p. 1087-1091.

This double-blind study examined the effects of oral vitamin E administration on retrolental fibroplasia in low weight, preterm infants with respiratory distress. Results found that infants given 100 mg of vitamin E per day experienced a significant reduction in the severity of retolental fibroplasia.

—H.M. Hittner, et al., ''Retrolental Fibroplasia: Efficacy of Vitamin E in a Double-blind Clinical Study of Preterm Infants,'' *New England Journal of Medicine,* 305(23), December 3, 1981, p. 1365-1371.

Sexual Function

Results of this study found that 8 weeks of supplementation with 300 mg per day of vitamin E lowered prolactin levels in uremic hemodialysis patients relative to controls. The authors suggest such effects could be due to the inhibition of central prolactin secretion.

—M. Yeksan, et al., ''Effect of Vitamin E Therapy on Sexual Functions of Uremic Patients in Hemodialysis,'' *International Journal of Artif Organs,* 15(11), November 1992, p. 648-652.

Short Bowel Syndrome

This study reports on a single case of a 64-year-old man suffering from severe vitamin E deficiency caused by chronic steatorrhea. Clinical improvement was seen a few months after vitamin E status was returned to normal following vitamin E supplementation.

—L. Howard, et al., ''Reversible Neurological Symptoms Caused by Vitamin E Deficiency in a Patient with Short Bowel Syndrome,'' *American Journal of Clinical Nutrition,* 36(6), December 1982, p. 1243-1249.

In this case study of a 71-year-old patient with severe vitamin E deficiency and fat malabsorption secondary to short bowel syndrome, results showed that supplementation with 400 IU per day of the water-soluble form of vitamin E, tocopheryl succinate polyethylene glycol 1000 (TPGS), had the following effects: normalized plasma alpha-tocopherol concentrations, raised adipose tissue alpha-tocopherol concentrations, and prevented the progression of vitamin E deficiency-related neurological abnormalities.

> —M.G. Traber, et al., ''Efficacy of Water-soluble Vitamin E in the Treatment of Vitamin E Malabsorption in Short-bowel Syndrome,'' *American Journal of Clinical Nutrition,* 59(6), June 1994, p. 1270-1274.

Sickle Cell Anemia

This review article argues that red cell susceptibility to peroxidation is enhanced by a deficiency in vitamin E and that such a deficiency promotes a troublesome cycle in patients with sickle cell anemia. The authors suggest vitamin E supplementation may be clinically beneficial for such patients.

> —D. Chiu, et al., ''Peroxidation, Vitamin E, and Sickle-cell Anemia,'' *Annals of the New York Academy of Sciences,* 393, 1982, p. 323-335.

Results of this study found significantly depressed levels of vitamins E and C in patients with sickle cell anemia. Such findings, the authors argue, may be responsible for such manifestations in sickle cell patients as an increased susceptibility to haemolysis and infection.

> —E.U. Essien, ''Plasma Levels of Retinol, Ascorbic Acid and Alpha-tocopherol in Sickle Cell Anemia,'' *Central African Journal of Medicine,* 41(2), February 1995, p. 48-50.

Results of this study found a significant deficiency of vitamin E in children with sickle cell anemia relative to age-matched controls.

> —I.O. Ndombi and S.N. Kinoti, ''Serum Vitamin E and the Sickling Status in Children with Sickle Cell Anaemia,'' *East African Medical Journal,* 67(10), October 1990, p. 720-725.

Results of this study found that low plasma vitamin E levels in sickle cell anemia patients might be related to reduced levels of lipoprotein carriers.

> —W.L. Stone, et al., ''Plasma-vitamin E and Low Plasma Lipoprotein Levels in Sickle Cell Anemia Patients,'' *Journal of the Association of the Academy of Minor Phys,* 1(2), 1990, p. 12-16.

Skin

This study examined the effects of vitamin E deficiency on lipid peroxide levels and the solubility of collagen in rats. After 3-6 months on a vitamin E deficient diet, results showed that the lipid peroxide content in the skin and subcutaneous was dramatically increased in deficient rats relative to controls. UV irradiation effects on the lipid peroxide content in skin of vitamin E deficient rats was also noticeably more damaging than in controls. In rats deficient in vitamin E for 6 months, the amount of insoluble collagen in the skin was increased more than those deficient for just 3 months.

> —A. Igarashi, et al., ''The Effects of Vitamin E Deficiency on Rat Skin,'' *British Journal of Dermatology,* 121(1), July 1989, p. 43-49.

Results of this study found that topical as well as dietary vitamin E were effective in protecting the epidermis of hairless mice against ultraviolet radiation-induced early damage.

—I.R. Record, et al., "The Influence of Topical and Systemic Vitamin E on Ultraviolet Light-induced Skin Damage in Hairless Mice," *Nutr Cancer,* 16(3-4), 1991, p. 219-225.

This study examined the effects of dl-alpha-tocopherol on ultraviolet light, 280-320 nm (UVB)-induced damage of human skin fibroblasts. Results showed that dl-alpha-tocopherol protected human skin fibroblasts against UVB's cytotoxic effects by its relation to the inhibition of UV-induced lipid peroxidation and/or its antioxidant effects.

—S. Kondo, et al., "Protective Effect of dl-alpha-tocopherol on the Cytotoxicity of Ultraviolet B Against Human Skin Fibroblasts in Vitro," *Photodermatol Photoimmunol Photomed,* 7(4), August 1990, p. 173-177.

This study examined whether or not tocopherol could minimize UV-induced damage to the epidermis in mice. Mice were treated topically with ethanol alone or a 1:1 mixture of tocopherol: ethanol in does of 0.1ml once a day for 1 week followed by irradiation with 0.30 mW/cm2 of UV-B. Results showed that Schiff base formation was reduced by 15% from control and 13% from vehicle as a result of tocopherol treatment. The same treatment increased epidermal thickness significantly by 52% over control and 63% over vehicle. Based on these findings, the authors conclude that topical tocopherol may decrease UV radiation-induced epidermal damage.

—M. Axelrod, et al., "Tocopherol Decreases Epidermal Damage from Ultraviolet Radiation," *FASEB Journal,* 4(4), 1990, p. A1139.

Smoking

Results of this study found that vitamin E may be a key antioxidant for the lower respiratory tract and that young smokers deficient in vitamin E may be predisposed to an enhanced oxidant attack on their lung parenchymal cells.

—E.R. Pacht, et al., "Deficiency of Vitamin E in the Alveolar Fluid of Cigarette Smokers: Influence on Alveolar Macrophage Cytotoxicity," *Journal of Clinical Investigations,* 77(3), March 1986, p. 789-796.

This study examined the effects of dietary vitamin E (100 or 200 ppm) for 4-8 weeks prior to cigarette smoking on cellular susceptibility to cigarette smoke in rats. Results showed more susceptibility to the harmful effects of cigarette smoke in rats deprived of dietary vitamin E than those receiving supplemenation.

—C.K. Chow, "Dietary Vitamin E and Cigaretted Smokings," *ACS Symp Ser,* (277), 1985, p. 229-239.

This study examined the effects of 100 ppm of dietary vitamin E supplemented for 4-5 weeks on cellular susceptibility to cigarette smoking in rats. Results showed higher mortality rates in vitamin E-deficient rats than those receiving supplementation and that there was greater alteration of biochemical parameters like reduced glutathione and related enzymes in the lungs of deficient rats.

—C.K. Chow, et al., "Dietary Vitamin E and Pulmonary Biochemical Responses of Rats to Cigarette Smoking," *Environ Research,* 34(1), June 1984, p. 8-17.

This study addressed changes induced by tobacco smoke in the lungs of vitamin E-depleted weanling rats. Results showed that when linked to tobacco exposure, vitamin E depletion may impair lung development.

—Y. Uejima, et al., "Influences of Tobacco Smoke and Vitamin E Depletion on the Distal Lung of Weanling Rats," *Experimental Lung Research,* 21(4), July-August 1995, p. 631-642.

This study examined the effects of vitamin E on lipid peroxidation in healthy smokers. Results found that supplemenation with 800 mg per day of vitamin E for two weeks decreased BPO in smokers.

—E. Hoshino, et al., "Vitamin E Suppresses Increased Lipid Peroxidation in Cigarette Smokers," *JPEN Journal of Parenter Enteral Nutr,* 14(3), May-June 1990, p. 300-305.

Spinal Cord Injury

Results of this study found that the combination of alpha-tocopherol and selenium or methylprednisolone sodium succinate (MPSS) by itself may protect damaged spinal cord tissue by limiting perturbation of membrane lipid metabolism which contributes to tissue necrosis and functional deficit of spinal cord injury.

—R.D. Saunders, et al., "Effects of Methylprednisolone and the Combination of Alpha-tocopherol and Selenium on Arachidonic Acid Metabolism and Lipid Peroxidation in Traumatized Spinal Cord Tissue," *Journal of Neurochemistry,* 49(1), July 1987, p. 24-31.

Results of this study showed that pretreatment with the vitamin E and selenium or methylprednisolone sodium succinate partially inhibited lipolysis and prostanoid production, prevented the loss of cholesterol, and that vitamin E and selenium protected the spinal cord from injury in cats.

—D.K. Anderson, et al., "Lipid Hydrolysis and Peroxidation in Injured Spinal Cord: Partial Protection with Methylprednisolone or Vitamin E and Selenium," *Central Nervous System Trauma,* 2(4), Winter 1985, p. 257-267.

This study examined the effects of vitamin E deficiency on compression injury of the spinal cord associated with ischemia in rats. Results found that vitamin E deficiency enhanced spinal cord injury-induced motor disturbances. Spinal cord blood flow also proved to be reduced in vitamin E deficient rats relative to controls as was the rate of recovery of injury.

—Y. Taoka, et al., "Influence of Dietary Vitamin E Deficiency on Compression Injury of Rat Spinal Cord," *Journal of Nutr Sci Vitaminol,* 36(3), June 1990, p. 217-226.

Spinocerebeller Dysfunction

This study reports on the single case of a 72-year-old vitamin E deficient male with severe malabsorption, progressive retinopathy and spinocerebellar degeneration 32 years after gastric surgery. Clinical improvements were seen following treatment with antibiotics and vitamin E supplementation.

—M.F. Brin, et al., "Blind Loop Syndrome, Vitamin E Malabsorption, and Spinocerebellar Degeneration," *Neurology,* 35(3), March 1985, p. 338-342.

Spondylosis

This double-blind study examined the effect of antioxidative roles of vitamins E and A on the degenerative process occurring in spondylosis in humans. Results showed that 100 mg of vitamin E given daily for three weeks significantly increased serum vitamin E levels and relieved pain completely. Such findings, according to the authors, point to vitamin E as an effective treatment for spondylosis.

    —Z. Mahmud and S.M. Ali, "Role of Vitamin A and E in Spondylosis," *Bangladesh Med Res Counc Bull,* 18(1), April 1992, p. 47-59.

Streatorrhoea

This study reports on the case of a 44-year-old woman with persistent severe steatorrhoea who experienced a surprise improvement in the slurring of speech and unsteadiness of gait following supplementation with vitamin E.

    —D.J. Evans, et al., "Symptomatic Vitamin E Deficiency Diagnosed after Histological Recognition of Myometrial Lipofuscinosis," *Lancet,* 346(8974), August 26, 1995, p. 545-546.

Stress

Results of this study showed supplementation with 300 mg/kg of alpha-tocopherol acetate for five days led a reduction in the stress enhancement of arachidonic acid level in the brain stem of rats.

    —Z. Chmela, et al., "Effect of Alpha-tocopherol, Pyridoxine and Dexpanthenol on the Stress Increase of Nonesterified Fatty Acids Levels in the Brain," *Acta Univ Palacki Olomuc Fac Med,* 136, 1993, p. 13-15.

Results of this study found 5 mg/kg of vitamin E and 50 mg/kg of dimethyl sulfoxide administered together prevented behavioral disturbances and disturbances of vegative functions created by chronic emotional stress in albino rats. Lipid peroxidation in blood serum and brain was also reduced as was cholesterol content in brain lipids, activated brain superoxide dismutase and nonenzymatic superoxide scavenging activity of the serum.

    —I.P. Levshina, et al., [Antistress Effects of Vitamin E and Dimethylsulfoxide During their Combined Administration in Low Doses], *Biull Eksp Biol Med,* 106(9), September 1988, p. 274-277.

This review article cites the results of one placebo-controlled study showing older men exposed to eccentric exercise-induced oxidative stress exhibited significantly lower levels of lipid peroxides in urine following 48 days of vitamin E supplementation relative to controls.

    —M. Meydani, et al., "Vitamin E Requirement in Relation to Dietary Fish Oil and Oxidative Stress in Elderly," *EXS,* 62, 1992, p. 411-418.

This study examined the ability of dietary vitamin E to increase global antioxidant capacity and decrease lipid peroxidation in guinea pigs. Results found that supplementation at levels 6 times higher than minimum daily requirements for guinea pigs increased protection against hepatic lipid peroxidation and did not lead endogenous antioxidant defences being depressed.

    —S. Cadenas, et al., "Vitamin E Protects Guinea Pig Liver from Lipid Peroxidation without Depressing Levels of Antioxidants," *International Journal of Biochemistry and Cell Biology,* 27(11), November 1995, p. 1175-1181.

This placebo-controlled study examined the effects of vitamin E supplementation for 5 months on the physical performance of top class cyclists. Results showed that while physical performance was not improved, supplementation did lead to a reduction in the CK in serum relative to controls as well as a reduction in malondialdehyde serum levels.

—L. Rokitzki, et al., "Alpha-Tocopherol Supplementation in Racing Cyclists During Extreme Endurance Training," *International Journal of Sport Nutrition,* 4(3), September 1994, p. 253-64.

Results of this study showed that supplementation with 1200 mg daily of vitamin E for 14 days prior to exhaustive running prevented exercise-induced DNA damage in humans resulting from oxidative stress.

—A. Hartmann, et al., "Vitamin E Prevents Exercise-induced DNA Damage," *Mutation Research,* 346(4), April 1995, p. 195-202.

This study examined the effects of alpha-tocopherol on lipid peroxidation and steroidogenesis in the adrenal cortices of rats and rabbits exposed to stress. Results found that vitamin E inhibited lipid peroxidation under chronic stress and reduced the release of steroids under acute stress while maintaining their levels when the stress became chronic.

—N.A. Doroshkevich, et al., [Effect of Alpha-tocopherol on Adrenal Cortex Functions Under Stress], *Ukr Biokhim Zh,* 63(5), September-October 1991, p. 79-83.

Results of this study showed that the preadministration of alpha-tocopherol into rats prior to stress prevented the corticosterone elevation as well as the catecholamine decrease in heart muscle and adrenal glands.

—V.A. Petrova, et al., [Limiting Stress Activation of the Adrenergic and Pituitary-adrenal Systems by Alpha-tocopherol], *Vopr Med Khim,* 31(6), November-December 1985, p. 115-118.

Stroke

Results of this study showed that the intravenous injection of 20 mg/kg of alpha-tocopherol in rats 30 minutes prior to ligation of the carotid arteries significantly suppressed the rise in brain and serum lipid peroxides, improved the severely expressed neurological signs, and promoted ATP resynthesis.

—M. Yamamoto, et al., "A Possible Role of Lipid Peroxidation in Cellular Damages Caused by Cerebral Ischemia and the Protective Effect of Alpha-tocopherol Administration," *Stroke,* 14(6), November-December 1983, p. 977-982.

Tardive Dyskinesia

In this double-blind, placebo-controlled study, tardive dyskinesia patients were given up to 1600 IU per day of vitamin E for 6 weeks. In nine patients with tardive dyskinesia for five years or less, results found AIMS scores to be significantly lower than controls.

—M.F. Egan, et al., "Treatment of Tardive Dyskinesia with Vitamin E," *American Journal of Psychiatry,* 149(6), June 1992, p. 773-777.

Results of this double-blind, placebo-controlled study found that AIMS scores were significantly reduced following vitamin E supplementation in 8 tardive dyskinesia patients relative to controls.

—A.M. Elkashef, et al., "Vitamin E in the Treatment of Tardive Dyskinesia," *American Journal of Psychiatry,* 147(4), April 1990, p. 505-506.

Results of this double-blind, placebo-controlled study showed a significant reduction of AIMS scores in eleven patients with tardive dyskinesia who received supplementation with vitamin E for 12 weeks relative to controls.

>—L.M. Dabiri, et al., "Effectiveness of Vitamin E for Treatment of Long-term Tardive Dyskinesia," *American Journal of Psychiatry,* 151(6), June 1994, p. 925-926.

In this double-blind, placebo-controlled study, tardive dyskinesia patients received 1600 IU per day of vitamin E for 8-12 weeks. Results showed a significant reduction in AIMS scores relative to controls.

>—L.A. Adler, et al., "Vitamin E Treatment of Tardive Dyskinesia," *American Journal of Psychiatry,* 150(9), September 1993, p. 1405-1407.

Results of this study found that vitamin E administration to chronic haloperidol treatment in rats prevented the development of behavioral supersensitivity to apomorphine, prompting the authors to argue that the concomitant administration of vitamin E to neuroleptics in humans may serve to prevent the development of tardive dyskinesia.

>—W.F. Gattaz, et al., "Vitamin E Attenuates the Development of Haloperidol-induced Dopaminergic Hypersensitivity in Rats: Possible Implications for Tardive Dyskinesia," *Journal of Neural Transm Gen Sect,* 92(2-3), 1993, p. 197-201.

This article reviewed the effects of vitamin E on tardive dyskinesia and Parkinson's disease. Double-blind, placebo-controlled studies have shown doses of up to 1600 IU per day improved symptoms in patients with tardive dyskinesia. With respect to Parkinson's disease, studies have found that 2000 IU per day of vitamin effectively slowed disease progression while not being able to entirely prevent it.

>—L. Bischot, et al., "Vitamin E in Extrapyramidal Disorders," *Pharm World Science,* 15(4), August 20, 1993, p. 146-150.

Results of this placebo-controlled study showed that vitamin E supplementation significantly improved the symptoms associated with tardive dyskinesia over a 36 week period.

>—L.A. Adler, et al., "Vitamin E in Tardive Dyskinesia: Time Course of Effect after Placebo Substitution," *Psychopharmacol Bulletin,* 29(3), 1993, p. 371-374.

Results of this placebo-controlled study found a significant reduction in AIMS scores in patients with persistent tardive dyskinesia receiving vitamin E supplementation relative to controls.

>—J.B. Lohr, et al., "Vitamin E in the Treatment of Tardive Dyskinesia: The Possible Involvement of Free Radical Mechanisms," *Schizophrenia Bulletin,* 14(2), 1988, p. 291-296.

This study examined the effects of selenium and vitamin E on experimentally-induced dyskinesia in rats. Results showed that treatment with both nutrients individually reduced IDPN induced dyskinesia and the combination of both together produce a near total absence of symptoms.

>—M. Tariq, et al., "Effect of Selenium and Vitamin E on Iminodipropionitrile Induced Dyskinesia in Rats," *International Journal of Neuroscience,* 78(3-4), October 1994, p. 185-192.

Thalassemia

Results of this study found that vitamin E deficiency in the serum of thalassaemic patients is easily corrected by oral supplementation of the vitamin.

—L. Bianco, et al., [The Role of Vitamin E in the Therapy of Thalassemia], *Pediatr Med Chir,* 8(1), January-February 1986, p. 23-26.

Thymus Damage

Results of this study found that supplementation with vitamin E in young chicks prior to exposure to a sublethal dose of gamma radiation improved recovery time in damage of the thymus.

—K. Rana, et al., "Radioprotection of Chick Thymus by Vitamin E," Indian *Journal of Experimental Biology,* 31(10), October 1993, p. 847-849.

Thyroid Dysfunction

This study measured serum lipoperoxides in malnourished children, adults with hyperthyroidism, adults with hypothyroidism, as well as normal adults. Results showed that lipid peroxide serum levels are related to concentrations of vitamin E.

—S. Krishnamurthy and D. Prasanna, "Serum Vitamin E and Lipid Peroxides in Malnutrition, Hyper and Hypothyroidism," *Acta Vitaminol Enzymol,* 6(1), 1984, p. 17-21.

This study examined the concentrations of vitamin E and malonic dialdehyde in the blood serum in patients with diffuse goiter of various degree of severity. Results found that patients with moderate and severe types of thyrotoxicosis had decreased vitamin E concentrations relative to controls.

—IuK Danis, et al., [Vitamin E and Malondialdehyde in the Blood Serum of Thyrotoxicosis Patients], *Probl Endokrinol,* 36(5), September-October 1990, p. 21-24.

Tuberculosis

Results of this study found that alpha-tocopherol administration prevented the occurrence of noticeable respiratory insufficiency contributing to its elimination in fibrocavernous tuberculosis patients.

—I.G. Gur'eva, et al., [Antioxidants—Effective Pathogenetic Agents in the Combined Therapy of Pulmonary Tuberculosis], *Ter Arkh,* 59(7), 1987, p. 72-74.

Ulcerative Colitis

This study reports on the case of a patient with chronic continuous ulcerative colitis whose condition was dramatically improved following treatment with 3 g per day of alpha-tocopherylquinone coupled with a low-fat diet.

—J.D. Bennet, "Use of Alpha-tocopherylquinone in the Treatment of Ulcerative Colitis," *Gut* (1986 Jun) 27(6), June 1986, p. 695-697.

Ulcers

Results of this study found that alpha-tocopherol administration prevented duodenal ulcer development in rats in 75% of cases treated.

—S.A. Morenkova, et al., [Effect of Vagotomy, Alpha-tocopherol and Arachidene on Lipid

Peroxidation in Various Areas of the Gastroduodenal Zone in Rats with Experimental Peptic Ulcer], *Biull Eksp Biol Med*, 103(5), May 1987, p. 532-534.

Results of this study showed that rats pretreated with vitamin E experienced a significant inhibition of gastric lesions induced by hypothermic restraint stress, indomethacin, reserpine, hydrochloric acid, sodium chloride and ethanol.
— M. Tariq, "Gastric Anti-ulcer and Cytoprotective Effect of Vitamin E in Rats," *Res Commun Chem Pathol Pharmacol*, 60(1), April 1988, p. 87-96.

Uveitis

Results of this study found that rats supplemented with vitamin E experienced less intraocular inflammation when sensitized to S antigen at 9 weeks relative to controls.
— G. Pararajasegaram, et al., "Suppression of S antigen-induced Uveitis by Vitamin E Supplementation," *Ophthalmic Research*, 23(3), 1991, p. 121-127.

Veno-Occlusive Disease

This study reports on the case of a 44-year-old woman treated with vitamin E and glutamine following her developing severe veno-occlusive disease after a bone marrow transplant. Results showed the clinical and biochemical signs of severe hepatic dysfunction were reversed by the therapy.
— T.V. Nattakom, et al., "Use of Vitamin E and Glutamine in the Successful Treatment of Severe Veno-occlusive Disease Following Bone Marrow Transplantation," *Nutr Clinical Practice*, 10(1), February 1995, p. 16-18.

Vision

This study examined the effects of vitamin E and taurine on the fluidity of membranes from frog retinal rod outer segments and of liposomes prepared with lecithin or with lipids from outer segment membranes. With respect to alpha-tocopherol, results showed that it increased the DPH anisotropy parameter in each preparation and modified the breakpoint temperature of Arrhenius plots of DPH anisotropy, and reduced the activation energy.
— J. Moran, et al., "Effect of Tocopherol and Taurine on Membrane Fluidity of Retinal Rod Outer Segments," *Exp Eye Research*, 45(6), December 1987, p. 769-776.

Results of this study showed that concentrations of 10(-3) M of vitamin E protected rat lenses from the damaging effects of lysophosphatidylcholine in vitro.
— T. Libondi, et al., "In Vitro Effect of Alpha-tocopherol on Lysophosphatidylcholine-induced Lens Damage," *Exp Eye Research*, 40(5), May 1985, p. 661-666.

Results of this study showed vitamin E administration doubled the survival time of isolated perfused rabbit corneal endothelium.
— O. Neuwirth-Lux and F. Billson, "Vitamin E and Rabbit Corneal Endothelial Cell Survival," *Aust N Z Journal of Ophthalmology*, 15(4), November 1987, p. 309-314.

Results of this study found that intramuscular injections of vitamin E proved to be effective in the reduction of thiobarbituric-acid-reactive substances and leukocyte-derived myeloperoxidase activity in the vitreous body of the eye.
— A.J. Augustin, et al., "Evidence for the Prevention of Oxidative Tissue Damage in the

Inner Eye by Vitamins E and C," *German Journal of Ophthalmology,* 1(6), 1992, p. 394-398.

Vitiligo

In this study, vitamin E and photochemotherapy were combined in the attempt to shorten treatment time in vitiligo patients. Results found treatment time was subsequently reduced twofold relative to normal treatment time.

—IuN Koshevenko, [alpha-Tocopherol in the Combined Treatment of Vitiligo], *Vestn Dermatol Venerol,* (10), 1989, p. 70-72.

Wound Healing

Results of this study found that mice supplemented with 300 IU/kg of vitamin E experienced a significant reduction in the incidence and degree of adhesions relative to controls.

—P. Kagoma, et al., "The Effect of Vitamin E on Experimentally Induced Peritoneal Adhesions in Mice," *Arch Surg,* 120(8), August 1985, p. 949-951.

In this study, vitamin E was administered to burned mice every other day over a 2 week period. Results showed that treatment with either parenteral vitamin E in corn oil or topical vitamin E in dimethyl sulphoxide improved cell-mediated immunity to a major degree relative to controls.

—C. Rundus, et al., "Vitamin E Improves Cell-mediated Immunity in the Burned Mouse: A Preliminary Study," *Burns Incl Therm Inj,* 11(1), October 1984, p. 11-15.

Results of this series of clinical and experimental studies indicated that cellular and humoral immunity were stimulate by supplementation with vitamin E in rats and humans suffering burns.

—M. Haberal, et al., "The Effects of Vitamin E on Immune Regulation after Thermal Injury," *Burns Incl Therm Injuries,* 14(5), October 1988, p. 388-393.

In this study, burn patients were pretreated with vitamin E, zinc, and selenium alone and in combination for 30 minutes. Results found that treatment with each and all three together significantly prevented an increase in the release of acid phosphates in the burn patients.

—M. Haberal, et al., "The Stabilizing Effect of Vitamin E, Selenium and Zinc on Leucocyte Membrane Permeability: A Study in Vitro," *Burns Incl Therm Inj,* 13(2), April 1987, p. 118-122.

This study examined the effects of vitamin E on the healing of wounds exposed to preoperative ionizing radiation in rats. Results showed that as levels of supplemental vitamin E were increased so was the breaking strength of wounds.

—D.L. Taren, et al., "Increasing the Breaking Strength of Wounds Exposed to Preoperative Irradiation Using Vitamin E Supplementation," *International Journal of Vitam Nutr Research,* 57(2), 1987, p. 133-137.

Results of this study showed that rats receiving 60 IU per day of d-alpha-tocopherol acetate experienced more rapid healing of gingival wounds than controls after 7 days.

—J.E. Kim and G. Shklar, "The Effect of Vitamin E on the Healing of Gingival Wounds in Rats," *Journal of Periodontology,* 54(5), May 1983, p. 305-308.

Results of this study showed that healing time in pigs with irradiated skin wounds was significantly reduced following pretreatment with vitamin E or vitamin E treatment of the wound dressing relative to controls.

—G.A. Simon, et al., "Wound Healing after Laser Injury to Skin—the Effect of Occlusion and Vitamin E," *Journal of Pharm Science,* 83(8), August 1994, p. 1101-1106.

Results of this study found that burned guinea pigs supplemented with vitamin E experienced beneficial effects on the maintenance of intestinal mucosa and erythrocyte counts over a wide range.

—K. Kuroiwa, et al., "Metabolic and Immune Effect of Vitamin E Supplementation After Burn," *JPEN Journal of Parenter Enteral Nutrition,* 15(1), January-February 1991, p. 22-26.

Yellow Nail Syndrome

This double-blind study on a single patient with yellow nail syndrome examined the effects of topical vitamin E solution for 6 months on this condition. Results found that nails treated with an active solution containing DL-alpha-tocopherol in dimethly sulfoxide showed major improvement and increases in nail growth.

—H.C. Williams, et al., "Successful Use of Topical Vitamin E Solution in the Treatment of Nail Changes in Yellow Nail Syndrome," *Arch Dermatol,* 127(7), July 1991, p. 1023-1028.

■ VITAMIN K

AIDS/HIV

This study examined the effects of napthoquinone (Vitamin K series) compounds on HIV-1 induced syncytia formation and replication in vitro. Results showed that the bacterially produced vitamin K, MK-7, inhibited syncytia formation in MT-2 infected cells at concentration between 5 and 1 ug per ml similar to AZT.

—L.F. Qualtiere, et al., "Menaquinone (bacterial vitamin K) Inhibits HIV-1 Induced Syncytia Formation but Not HIV-1 Replication," *International Conference on AIDS,* 5, June 4-9, 1989, p. 566.

Cancer

This study examined the effects of vitamin K on the growth and morphology of mouse neuroblastoma (P2), mouse melanoma (B-16) and rat glioma (C-6) cells in vitro. Results showed that vitamin K3 inhibited the growth each cell type and did not produce any morphological differentiation.

—K.N. Prasad, et al., "Vitamin K3 (Menadione) Inhibits the Growth of Mammalian Tumor Cells in Culture," *Life Science,* 29(13), 1981, p. 1387-1392.

This study notes the inhibitory effects of vitamin K on carboxylation, growth and gene expression in the human hepatoma cell line Hep 3B and argues they may be direct due to a free radical process or be mediated via vitamin K dependent carboxylated proteins.

—B.I. Carr, et al., "The Vitamins K: A Novel Family of Naturally-occurring Cell Growth

Inhibitors," *Procceedings of the Annual Meeting of the American Associations of Cancer Researchers,* 35, 1994, p. A230.

Cardiovascular/Coronary Heart Disease

This study examined the effects of vitamin K analogues on human platelet aggregation. Results showed them to be strong inhibitors of aggregation due to arachidonate, collagen, ADP, and thrombin.

—G.J. Blackwell, et al., "Inhibition of Human Platelet Aggregation by Vitamin K," *Thromb Research,* 37(1), January 1, 1985, p. 103-114.

Results of this study showed that the antenatal use of 10 mg of intramuscular every 5 days prior to delivery of vitamin K by mothers destined to deliver infants less than 32 weeks gestation led to a significant reduction in the prothrombin time and partial thromboplastin time. Based on these findings, the authors concluded that vitamin K can reduce intraventricular hemorrhage severity in neonates under 1500 gm.

—W.J. Morales, et al., "The Use of Antenatal Vitamin K in the Prevention of Early Neonatal Intraventricular Hemorrhage," *American Journal of Obstet Gynecol,* 159(3), September 1988, p. 774-779.

■ ZINC

Acne

This double-blind, placebo-controlled study examined the effects of 135 mg of oral zinc sulfate per day by itself and coupled with 300,000 IU of vitamin A per day on acne lesions. Results showed significant reductions in the number of papules, pustules, and infiltrates in the zinc-treated subjects after 4 weeks.

—G. Michaelsson, et al., "Effects of Oral Zinc and Vitamin A in Acne," *Arch Dermatol,* 113(1), January 1977, p. 31-36.

Results of this, double-blind, placebo-controlled study showed that acne vulgaris patients receiving 0.4 g per day of oral zinc sulphate experienced significantly better results than controls following 12 weeks of treatment.

—L. Hillstrom, et al., "Comparison of Oral Treatment with Zinc Sulphate and Placebo in Acne Vulgaris," *British Journal of Dermatology,* 97(6), December 1977, p. 679-684.

Results of this double-blind study found that both oral zinc and tetracycline were equally effective in reducing acne over a period of 12 weeks, reducing severity by upwards of 70%.

—G. Michaelsson, et al., "A Double-blind Study of the Effect of Zinc and Oxytetracycline in Acne Vulgaris," *British Journal of Dermatology,* 97(5), November 1977, p. 561-566.

Results of this double-blind, placebo-controlled study found that acne vulgaris patients receiving 600 mg per day of zinc sulphate for 12 weeks experienced significant improvement with respect to the number of papules, infiltrates and cysts relative to controls.

—K.C. Verma, et al., "Oral Zinc Sulphate Therapy in Acne Vulgaris: A Double-blind Trial," *Acta Derm Venereol,* 60(4), 1980, p. 337-340.

This double-blind, placebo-controlled study examined the effects of 0.6 grams of zinc sulphate per day on acne vulgaris patients. Results showed significant improvements after 6 weeks.
— K. Goransson, et al., "Oral Zinc in Acne Vulgaris: A Clinical and Methodological Study," *Acta Derm Venereol,* 58(5), 1978, p. 443-448.

Acrodermatitis Enteropathica

This article reports on the case of a 7-year-old boy with acrodermatitis enteropathica who experienced complete recovery with respect to skin lesions, diarrhea, and hair loss following oral zinc sulfate therapy.
— V.M. Der Kaloustian, et al., "Oral Treatment of Acrodermatitis Enteropathica with Zinc Sulfate," *American Journal of Dis Child,* 130(4), April 1976, p. 421-423.

This article reports on the case of a 21-year-old woman with acrodermatitis enteropathica since the age of 3 months who experienced significant improvement following oral zinc therapy.
— W.S. Lynch & H.H. Roenigk, Jr. "Acrodermatitis Enteropathica. Successful Zinc Therapy," *Arch Dermatol,* 112(9), September 1976, p. 1304-1307.

This article reports on a single case of a patient with acrodermatitis enteropathic who experienced initial benefits from diiodohydroxyquin therapy, but such benefits were not maintained when treatment was discontinued after three months. The administration of zinc sulfate in its place produced a complete recovery in 48 hours.
— A.G. Campo, Jr. & C.J. McDonald, "Treatment of Acrodermatitis Enteropathica with Zinc Sulfate," *Arch Dermatol,* 112(5), May 1976, p. 687-689.

This article reports on the case of a woman with acrodermatitis enteropathica who experienced a total remission of disease following 220 mg of oral zinc sulfate three times a day.
— K.H. Neldner, et al., "Zinc Therapy of Acrodermatitis Enteropathica," *New England Journal of Medicine,* 292(17), April 24, 1975, p. 879-882.

This article reports on the case of a 22-month-old child with acrodermatitis enteropathica suffering from generalized oral and cutaneous candidiasis. Following the failure of drug treatment including nystatin, iodochlorhydroxyquin-hydrocortisone, topical clotrimazole, procaine penicillin G, then methicillin sodium and gentamicin sulfate; the child was given 50 mg t.i.d. of zinc sulfate. Results showed a 99% recovery of skin lesions following the zinc treatment.
— G.A. Steiner, "Successful Treatment of Acrodermatitis Enteropathica with Zinc Sulfate," *American Journal of Hosp Pharm,* 35(12), December 1978, p. 1535-1538.

This article reports on the case of a 6-month-old with acrodermatitis enteropathica who was successfully treated with 100 mg per day of oral zinc sulphate up to the age of 2.5 years.
— M.H. Marandian, et al., [Enteropathic Acrodermatitis Treated with Zinc Sulfate], *Arch Fr Pediatr,* 35(8), October 1978, p. 870-874.

This article reports on the case of an infant with acrodermatitis enteropathica suffering from severe diarrhea. Results showed that 100 mg per day of oral zinc for 11 days led to a complete recovery of skin lesions.

—D. Leupold, et al., "Zinc Therapy in a Acrodermatitis Enteropathica," *Helv Paediatr Acta,* 31(2), August 1976, p. 109-115.

AIDS/HIV

Results of this study showed that normalization of deficient zinc status was associated with significant increases in CD4 count and improved functional immune parameters among homosexual male patients with HIV.

—R.S. Beach, et al., "Effect of Zinc Normalization on Immunological Function in Early HIV-1 Infection," *International Conference on AIDS,* 7(1), June 16-21, 1991, p. 330.

Results of this study showed that administration of 200 mg per day of oral zinc sulphate had immunostimulant T-cell effects in asymptomatic patients with HIV infection.

—F. Ancarani, et al., "Zinc Therapy in HIV Infected Subjects," *International Conference on AIDS,* 9(1), June 6-11, 1993, p. 493.

Results of this study demonstrated zinc can inhibit renin and protease from HIV-1. Such inhibition, the authors suggest, may explain some of the benefits seen in AIDS patients following zinc therapy.

—Z.Y. Zhang, et al., "Zinc Inhibition of Renin and the Protease from Human Immunodeficiency Virus Type 1," *Biochemistry,* 30(36), September 10, 1991, p. 8717-8721.

Alcoholic Cirrhosis

Results of this study indicated that the administration of 200 mg per day in zinc sulfate improved responsiveness to delayed hypersensitivity skin tests in patients suffering from alcoholic cirrhosis.

—H. Labadie, et al., "Does Oral Zinc Improve the Cellular Immunity of Patients with Alcoholic Cirrhosis?" *Gastroenterol Clin Biol,* 10(12), December 1986, p. 799-803.

Anorexia

Results of this study showed that 45-90 mg per day of zinc sulfate had positive effects with respect to weight gain in anorexic females between the ages of 14-26.

—S. Safai-Kutti, "Oral Zinc Supplementation in Anorexia Nervosa," *Acta Psychiatr Scand Suppl,* 361, 1990p. 14-17.

This article reports on the case of a 16-year-old girl hospitalized for anorexia who experienced significant benefits following initial treatment with 40 mumol per day of intravenous zinc for 7 days which was then reduced to oral intake of 15 mg of elemental zinc per day for 60 days.

—H. Yamaguchi, et al., "Anorexia Nervosa Responding to Zinc Supplementation: A Case Report," *Gastroenterol Jpn,* 27(4), August 1992, p. 554-558.

Results of this study found that zinc deficiency is common among adolescent anorexics and that supplementation with 50 mg per day of elemental zinc improved symptoms of anxiety and depression among such patients.

> —R.L. Katz, et al., "Zinc Deficiency in Anorexia Nervosa," *Journal of Adolescent Health Care,* 8(5), September 1987, p. 400-406.

Arthritis

Results of this double-blind, placebo-controlled study showed that peroral zinc sulphate administered to psoriatic arthritis patients over a 24 week period led to a reduction in joint pains and swelling, and increased mobility.

> —O.J. Clemmensen, et al., "Psoriatic Arthritis Treated with Oral Zinc Sulphate," *British Journal of Dermatology,* 103(4), October 1980, p. 411-415.

In this double-blind, placebo-controlled study, 220 mg of zinc sulphate was administered thrice daily over a period of 12 weeks to patients suffering from chronic, refractory rheumatoid arthritis. Results showed significant improvements in patients taking the zinc with respect to joint swelling, morning stiffness, walking time, and subjective patient reports of own conditions.

> —P.A. Simkin, "Oral Zinc Sulphate in Rheumatoid Arthritis," *Lancet,* 2(7985), September 11, 1976, 539-542.

In this study, psoriatic arthritis patients received 600 mg per day of oral zinc sulphate for 6 months. Results showed significant reductions in the number of swollen and tender joints, the need for nosteroidal anti-inflammatory drugs, and erythrocyte sedimentation rate relative to controls.

> —A. Frigo, et al., [Zinc Sulfate in the Treatment of Psoriatic Arthritis], *Recenti Prog Med,* 80(11), November 1989, p. 577-581.

Birth Weight

Results of this double-blind, placebo-controlled study showed that 25 mg of zinc per day in pregnant African American women was associated with increased infant birth weights and head circumferences relative to controls.

> —R.L. Goldenberg, et al., "The Effect of Zinc Supplementation on Pregnancy Outcome," *JAMA,* 274(6), August 9, 1995, p. 463-468.

Cancer

In this study, 250 mg per day of oral zinc gluconate were given to patients with ARC or with malignancy in remission and with severe and stable CD4 lymphoid cells cytopenia over a period of three weeks. Results showed that the therapy increased CD8 lymphoid cell subsets in patients where they were low and reduced them in patients where they were high.

> —G. Mathe, et al., "A Phase II Trial of Immunorestoration with Zinc Gluconate in Immunode-pressed Cancer Patients," *Biomed Pharmacother,* 40(10). 1986, p. 383-385.

Cardiovascular/Coronary Heart Disease

This double-blind, placebo-controlled study examined the effects of oral zinc at doses of either 50 mg per day or 75 mg per day over a 12 week period on serum total cholesterol, lipoprotein-cholesterol fractions, and serum triglycerides in white males. Results indicated that serum high-density-lipoprotein cholesterol levels of those receiving the 50 mg and the 75 mg dose showed significant reductions after 12 weeks.

> —M.R. Black, et al., "Zinc Supplements and Serum Lipids in Young Adult White Males," *American Journal of Clinical Nutrition,* 47(6), June 1988, p. 970-975.

Results of this double-blind, placebo-controlled study showed that the oral administration of 200 mg three times per day of zinc sulphate significantly reduced serum cholesterol and beta-lipoproteins and significantly increased alpha-lipoproteins in stablized ischemic heart disease patients.

> —D.R. Shah, et al., "Effect of Oral Zinc Sulphate on Serum Lipids and Lipoproteins in Human Subjects," *Indian Journal of Physiol Pharmocol,* 32(1), January-March 1988, p. 47-50.

Cerebral Palsy

Results of this study showed that children with cerebral paralysis between the ages of 3-14 years experienced improved metabolic processes, clinical health status, and enhanced body defense properties following supplemental zinc sulfate relative to controls.

> —E.D. Zhukovskaia, et al., [Zinc Sulfate in the Complex Treatment of Children with Cerebral Palsy], *Zh Nevropatol Psikhiatr Im S S Korsakova,* 91(8), 1991, p. 15-17.

Childhood Growth

This double-blind, placebo-controlled study examined the effects of 10 mg per day of zinc over a 5 month period on the growth, incidence of infections and circulating insulin-like growth factor concentrations in undernourished Vietnamese children. Results showed significant increases in height and weight relative to controls. Relative risk of infection was decreased 3-fold for diarrhea and 2.5-fold for respiratory infections.

> —N.X. Ninh, et al., "Zinc Supplementation Increases Growth and Circulating Insulin-like Growth Factor I (IGF-I) in Growth-retarded Vietnamese Children," *American Journal of Clinical Nutrition,* 63(4), April 1996, p. 514-519.

This double-blind, placebo-controlled study examined the effects of 2 mg/kg per day of zinc on the growth and immune function of marasmic infants. After 60 days, results showed that weight-for-length gain in infants receiving zinc measured 9% of standard compared to 3% for controls. Rate of infections was significantly lower in the zinc group relative to controls

> —C. Castillo-Duran, et al., "Controlled Trial of Zinc Supplementation During Recovery from Malnutrition: Effects on Growth and Immune Function," *American Journal of Clinical Nutrition,* 45(3), March 1987, p. 602-608.

This double-blind, placebo-controlled study examined the effects of 3 mg per day of zinc on postnatal growth of Chilean infants born small for gestational age. Results showed those infants receiving zinc over a 6 month period exhibited greater weight gain and linear growth relative to controls.

> —C. Castillo-Duran, et al., "Zinc Supplementation and Growth of Infants Born Small for Gestational Age," *Journal of Pediatrics,* 127(2), August 1995, p. 206-211.

Results of this double-blind, placebo-controlled study showed that low birth weight toddlers receiving supplemental zinc exhibited significant improvements in weight gain relative to controls over a period of 6 months.

—P.A. Walravens, et al., "Zinc Supplementation in Infants with a Nutritional Pattern of Failure to Thrive: A Double-blind, Controlled Study," *Pediatrics,* 83(4), April 1989, p. 532-538.

Common Cold

This article reviewed data from 10 studies on the use of zinc in treating the common cold. Results showed consistent beneficial effects when zinc was administered in the form of zinc gluconate lozenges.

—J.C. Godfrey, et al., "Zinc for Treating the Common Cold: Review of all Clinical Trials Since 1984," *Altern Ther Health Med,* 2(6), November 1996, p. 63-72.

Results of this double-blind, placebo-controlled study found that that zinc gluconate taken in the form of a lozenge every two hours containing 13.3 mg significantly reduced the duration of symptoms of the common cold.

—S.B. Mossad, et al., Zinc Gluconate Lozenges for Treating the Common Cold. A Randomized, Double-blind, Placebo-controlled Study," *Annals of Internal Medicine,* 125(2), July 15, 1996, p. 81-88.

Diaper Rash

Results of this double-blind, placebo-controlled study showed that 10 mg per day of oral zinc over a period of 4 months significantly reduced the incidence of diaper rash in newborns.

—P.J. Collipp, "Effect of Oral Zinc Supplements on Diaper Rash in Normal Infants," *Journal of Medical Association Ga,* 78(9), September 1989, p. 621-623.

Diarrhea

This double-blind, placebo-controlled study examined the effects of 20 mg per day of elemental zinc on diarrhea in children in India between the ages of 6-35 months. Results showed significant reductions in both the severity and duration of diarrhea relative to controls.

—S. Sazawal, et al., "Zinc Supplementation in Young Children with Acute Diarrhea in India," *New England Journal of Medicine,* 333(13), September 28, 1995, p. 839-844.

Results of this study indicated that oral zinc supplementation significantly reduced the incidence of persistent diarrhea in poor children between 13-35 months of age in India.

—S. Sazawal, et al., "Zinc Supplementation Reduces the Incidence of Persistent Diarrhea and Dysentery among Low Socioeconomic Children in India," *Journal of Nutrition,* 126(2), February 1996, p. 443-450.

Eczema

This article reports on the case of an elderly female with nonulcerating severe stasis eczema who experienced significant benefits following 220 mg per day of oral zinc therapy.

—C.W. Owens, et al., "A Severe 'Stasis Eczema', Associated with Low Plasma Zinc, Treated Successfully with Oral Zinc," *British Journal of Dermatology,* 105(4), October 1981, p. 461-464.

Gonadal Function

In this double-blind, placebo-controlled study, stable patients undergoing hemodialysis three times a week received 50 mg of elemental zinc over a period of 6 months. Results showed significant increases in plasma zinc, serum testosterone, and sperm count relative to controls. Patients administered showed improvements in potency, libido, and frequency of intercourse.

—S.K. Mahajan, et al., "Effect of Oral Zinc Therapy on Gonadal Function in Hemodialysis Patients. A Double-blind Study," *Annals of Internal Medicine,* 97(3), September 1982, p. 357-361.

Head Injury

Results of this double-blind study found that supplemental zinc administered immediately after injury was associated with more rapid neurologic recovery and visceral protein concentrations in severe closed head injury patients relative to controls.

—B. Young, et al., "Zinc Supplementation is Associated with Improved Neurologic Recovery Rate and Visceral Protein Levels of Patients with Severe Closed Head Injury," *Journal of Neurotrauma,* 13(1), January 1996, p. 25-34.

Herpes

Results of this study showed that zinc sulphate solution had preventive effects on recurrent herpes simplex of the skin (0.025-0.05% concentrations) and oral mucous membrane (0.01-0.025%).

—I. Brody, "Topical Treatment of Recurrent Herpes Simplex and Post-herpetic Erythema Multiforme with Low Concentrations of Zinc Sulphate Solution," *British Journal of Dermatology,* 104(2), February 1981, p. 191-194.

In this study, patients experiencing recurrent herpes simplex skin infections were treated with a 4% topical zinc solution. Results showed a total remission in pain, tingling and burning stopped completely within 24 hours of treatment in all patients.

—A. Wahba, "Topical Application of Zinc-solutions: A New Treatment for Herpes Simplex Infections of the Skin?" *Acta Derm Venereol,* 60(2), 1980, p. 175-177.

Results of this double-blind, placebo-controlled study showed that zinc sulfate added to gel was significantly more effective in alleviating symptoms associated with herpes labialis recidivans than the use of gel only.

—W. Kneist, et al., [Clinical Double-blind Trial of Topical Zinc Sulfate for Herpes Labialis Recidivans], *Arzneimittelforschung,* 45(5), May 1995, p. 624-626.

Immune Enhancement

This study examined the effects of 440 mg per day for a month in subjects over the age of 70 on age-associated immune dysfunction. Results showed significant improvements with respect to the number of circulating T lymphocytes, delayed cutaneous hypersensitivity reactions to purified protein derivative, Candidin and streptokinase-streptodornase, and immunoglobulin G (IgG) antibody response to tetanus vaccine relative to controls.

—J. Duchateau, et al., "Beneficial Effects of Oral Zinc Supplementation on the Immune Response of Old People," *American Journal of Medicine,* 70(5), May 1981, p. 1001-1004.

Infertility

Results of this study showed that treatment of male infertility patients with oral zinc sulfate improved sperm motility.

—A.A. Caldamone, et al., "Seminal Zinc and Male Infertility," *Urology,* 13(3), March 1979, p. 280-281.

Results of this study indicated that the administration of 440 mg per day of zinc sulfate over a period of between 60 days to 2 years had beneficial effects on male patients experiencing infertility, particularly following variocelectomy.

—H. Takihara, et al., "Zinc Sulfate Therapy for Infertile Male with or without Varicocelectomy," *Urology,* 29(6), June 1987, p. 638-641.

Inflammatory Bowel Disease

This double-blind study examined the effects of in vivo treatment with zinc in natural killer cell activity in patients with inflammatory bowel disease. Results showed the zinc exhibited long-lasting effects, leading to a reduction in peripheral blood natural killer cell activity.

—Y. Van de Wal, et al., "Effect of Zinc Therapy on Natural Killer Cell Activity in Inflammatory Bowel Disease," *Aliment Pharmacol Ther,* 7(3), June 1993, p. 281-286.

Lead Intoxication

Results of this study indicated that the combination of supplemental zinc and thiamine was effective in countering the ill effects of lead-intoxication in rats.

—S.J. Flora, et al., "Thiamine and Zinc in Prevention or Therapy of Lead Intoxication," *Journal of Int Med Res,* 17(1), Jan-Feb 1989, p. 68-75.

Leprosy

This study examined the effects of oral zinc supplementation in erthema nodosum leprosy patients over a period of four months. Results showed the zinc treatment led to improved frequency, duration, and severity of reactions to prednisolone therapy as well as a reduced dependency on the steroid itself.

—P.M. Mahajan, et al., "Oral Zinc Therapy in Recurrent Erythema Nodosum Leprosum: A Clinical Study," *Indian Journal of Leprosy,* 66(1), January-March 1994, p. 51-57.

In this study, oral zinc was administered to patients with multibacillary leprosy as an immunostimulant in addition to conventional antileprosy drugs and compared to patients treated with the drugs alone. Results showed quicker improvement in patients receiving the zinc.

—N.K. Mathur, et al., "Oral Zinc as an Adjunct to Dapsone in Lepromatous Leprosy," *International Journal of Leprosy and Other Mycobacterial Disease,* 52(3), September 1984, p. 331-338.

Lung Damage

This study examined the effects of 114 mg/L per day of orally administered zinc on experimental-induced lung collagen in rats. Results showed the zinc inhibited lung prolyl hydroxylase activity and prevented the increases in lung collagen content.

—H. Anttinen, et al., "Prevention by Zinc of Rat Lung Collagen Accumulation in Carbon Tetrachloride Injury," *Am Rev Respir Disease,* 132(3), September 1985, p. 536-540.

Macular Degeneration

Results of this double-blind, placebo-controlled study showed that the oral administration of zinc led to significantly less visual loss among patients with drusen or macular degeneration relative to controls over a period of 12 to 24 months.

—D.A. Newsome, et al., "Oral Zinc in Macular Degeneration," *Arch Ophthalmol,* 106(2), February 1988, p. 192-198.

Obesity

Results of this study showed that the administration of 600 mg of zinc sulfate and/or 0.1 mg thyroxine per day had significant weight reduction effects in obese subjects over an eight week period.

—M.D. Chen, et al., [Zinc Sulfate and Thyroxine Treatment on the Obese Patients], *Chung Hua I Hsueh Tsa Chih,* 48(3), September 1991, p. 210-216.

Sickle Cell Anemia

Results of this study showed zinc therapy corrected hyperammonemia in sickle cell anemia patients.

—A.S. Prasad, et al., "Effect of Zinc on Hyperammonemia in Sickle Cell Anemia Subjects," *American Journal of Hematology,* 7(4), 1979, p. 323-327.

This study examined the effects of zinc on the 51Cr survival of red blood cells taken from homozygous sickle cell anemia patients and transfused into rats. Results showed that administered to rats at plasma levels just above those presently obtained in patients increased sickle cell anemia red blood cell survival.

—E.B. Schoomaker, et al., "Zinc in the Treatment of Homozygous Sickle Cell Anemia: Studies in an Animal Model," *American Journal of Hematology,* 1(1), 1976, p. 45-57.

Results of this controlled study found that supplemental zinc significantly improved body weight and growth in 14-19 year old sickle cell anemia patients.

—A.S. Prasad, "Zinc Deficiency in Sickle Cell Disease," *Prog Clin Biol Res,* 165, 1984, p. 49-58.

Results of this study showed that zinc supplementation led to improvements in sickle cell anemia patients with respect to weight gain, serum testosterone level, plasma ammonia level, and abnormal dark adaptation.

—A.S. Prasad, "Zinc Deficiency and Effects of Zinc Supplementation on Sickle Cell Anemia Subjects," *Prog Clin Biol Res,* 55, 1981, p. 99-122.

Stress

Results of this study found that the administration of zinc ameliorated the effects of chronic stress in mice with respect to immunocompetence, growth, and corporal weight.

—F. Garcia Tamayo, et al., "Zinc Administration Prevents Wasting in Stressed Mice," *Arch Med Res,* 27(3), Autumn 1996, p. 319-325.

Stroke

Results of this study showed that the oral administration of zinc, zinc protoporphyrin, and protoporphyrin exhibited protective effects on the rat brain when given early in a temporary focal ischemia model.

—Y.J. Zhao, et al., ''Zinc Protoporphyrin, Zinc Ion, and Protoporphyrin Reduce Focal Cerebral Ischemia,'' *Stroke,* 27(12), December 1996, p. 2299-3303.

Taste Disorder

Results of this double-blind, placebo-controlled study showed that patients suffering from taste disorder experienced significant improvements following 4 months of supplementation with oral zinc gluconate.

—S. Yoshida, et al., ''A Double-blind Study of the Therapeutic Efficacy of Zinc Gluconate on Taste Disorder,'' *Auris Nasus Larynx,* 18(2), 1991, p. 153-161.

Results of this double-blind, placebo-controlled study showed that patients suffering from idiopathic taste disorder experienced significant improvements following supplementation with oral zinc picolinate.

—F. Sakai, et al., [Therapeutic Efficacy of Zinc Picolinate in Patients with Taste Disorders], *Nippon Jibiinkoka Gakkai Kaiho,* 98(7), July 1995, p. 1135-1139.

Ulcerative Stomatitis

This article reports on the case of a 15-year-old boy suffering from ulcerative stomatitis that did not respond to conventional treatment. The administration of 3 X 50 mg of zinc sulphate given per os per day over a period of 3 months led to normalization of the lymphoblast transformation rate and the permanent elimination of symptoms.

—L. Endre, ''Successful Treatment of Recurrent Ulcerative Stomatitis, Associated with Cellular Immune Defect and Hypozincaemia, by Oral Administration of Zinc Sulfate,'' *Orv Heitl,* 131(9), March 4, 1990, p. 475-477.

Ulcers

In this double-blind, placebo-controlled study, benign gastric ulcer patients received thrice daily doses of 220 mg of zinc sulphate over a period of three weeks. Results showed that patients taking zinc sulphate had an ulcer healing rate three times higher than controls.

—D.J. Frommer, ''The Healing of Gastric Ulcers by Zinc Sulphate,'' *Medical Journal of Aust,* 2(21), November 22, 1975, p. 793-796.

In this randomized, double-blind, placebo-controlled study, geriatric patients with either arterial and/ or venous leg ulcers were treated with a gauze compress medicated with 400 mcg of zinc oxide. Results showed zinc-treated patients responded significantly better than controls, exhibiting a 83% improvement rate.

—H.E. Stromberg & M.S. Agren, ''Topical Zinc Oxide Treatment Improves Arterial and Venous Leg Ulcers,'' *British Journal of Dermatology,* 111(4), October 1984, p. 461-468.

Wilson's Disease

Results of this study showed that the administration of 50 mg of zinc three times per day was effective in controlling copper balance in patients suffering from Wilson's disease.

>   —G.M. Hill, et al., "Treatment of Wilson's Disease with Zinc. I. Oral Zinc Therapy Regimens," *Hepatology,* 7(3), May-June 1987, p. 522-528.

Results of this study showed that 220 mg of oral zinc per day reduced symptoms associated with Wilson's disease and led to normal urinary copper excretions in 5 of 5 patients examined.

>   —L. Rossaro, et al., "Zinc Therapy in Wilson's Disease: Observations in Five Patients," *American Journal of Gastroenterology,* 85(6), June 1990, p. 665-668.

Results of this study found that supplemental zinc normalized serum uric acid metabolism in patients suffering from Wilson's disease by improving dysfunctions of the liver.

>   —S. Umeki, et al., "Oral Zinc Therapy Normalizes Serum Uric Acid Level in Wilson's Disease Patients," *American Journal of Medical Science,* 292(5), November 1986, p. 289-292.

HERBAL SUPERSTARS

■ ALOE

Anti-inflammatory Effects

Results of this study showed that the topical administration of small amounts of aloe vera inhibited inflammation in a croton oil-induced edema assay, with decolorized aloe proving more effective than colorized.

> —R.H. Davis, et al., "Processed Aloe Vera Administered Topically Inhibits Inflammation," *Journal of the American Podiatry Medical Association,* 79(8), August 1989, p. 395-397.

Results of this study showed the oral administration of aloe vera exhibited anti-inflammatory effects in rats across a variety of inflammation models.

> —R.H. Davis, et al., "Anti-inflammatory Activity of Aloe Vera Against a Spectrum of Irritants," *Journal of American Podiatry Medical Association,* 79(6), June 1989, p. 263-276.

This study reported the isolation of a new anti-inflammatory agent identified as 8-[C-beta-D-]2-O-(E)- cinnamoyl]glucopyranosyl]-2- [(R)-2-hydroxypropyl]-7-methoxy-5-methylchromone (1) from Aloe barbadensis Miller using a murine ear model.

> —J.A. Hutter, et al., "Antiinflammatory C-glucosyl Chromone from Aloe Barbadensis," *Journal of Natural Products,* 59(5), May 1996, p. 541-543.

Arthritis

Results of this study showed that Aloctin A, a glycoprotein isolated from Aloe arborescens Mill, inhibited adjuvant arthritis in rats and carrageenin-induced edema in rats.

> —H. Saito, et al., "Pharmacological Studies on a Plant Lectin Aloctin A. II. Inhibitory Effect of Aloctin A on Experimental Models of Inflammation in Rats," *Japanese Journal of Pharmacology,* 32(1), February 1982, p. 139-142.

Cancer

Results of this study showed that the intravenous and intracutaneous administration of the immuno-modulator fraction, Alva, extracted from Aloe vahombe exhibited anticancer effects in mice.

> —L. Ralamboranto, et al., [Immunomodulating Properties of an Extract Isolated and Partially Purified from Aloe Vahombe. 3. Study of Antitumoral Properties and Contribution to the

Chemical Nature and Active Principle], *Arch Inst Pasteur Madagascar,* 50(1), 1982, p. 227-256.

In this study, both enriched and highly purified forms of acemannan was intraperitoneally administered to female rats which had received implanted sarcoma cells. Sarcoma grew in 100% of control rats leading to death in 20-46 days. By contrast, 40% of the acemannan-treated rats survived, and tumors in these rats showed vascular congestion, edema, polymorphonuclear leukocyte infiltration, and central necrosing foci with hemorrhage and peripheral fibrosis.

—S.Y. Peng, et al., ''Decreased Mortality of Norman Murine Sarcoma in Mice Treated with the Immunomodulator, Acemannan,'' *Mol Biother,* 3(2), June 1991, p. 79-87.

Results of this study showed that succus aloes reduced tumor mass, metastatic foci and metastasis frequency at different stages of tumor progress in mice and rats.

—N.V. Gribel' & V.G. Pashinskii, [Antimetastatic Properties of Aloe Juice], *Vopr Onkol,* 32(12), 1986, p. 38-40.

Results of this study found that aloe (2500 mg/kg per day for 6 days) significantly inhibited BPDE-I-DNA adduct formation and DNA repair in ICR mice and suggest it may play a chemopreventive role in cancer of humans.

—H.S. Kim, et al., ''Chemopreventive Effect of Aloe in Male ICR Mice Treated with Benzo(a)pyrene,'' *Proceedings of the Annual Meeting of the American Association of Cancer Research,* 35, 1994, p. A1937.

Cardiovascular/Coronary Heart Disease

In this 5 year study of 5,000 atheromatous heart disease patients, results showed that dietary intake of Husk of Isabgol and aloe vera to the diet led to a marked reduction in total serum cholesterol, serum trigylcerides, fasting and post prandial blood sugar level in diabetic patients. Clinical profiles showed decreased frequency of anginal attacks and gradually, the drugs, like verapamil, nifedipine, beta-blockers and nitrates, were tapered.

—O.P. Agarwal, ''Prevention of Atheromatous Heart Disease,'' *Angiology,* 36(8), August 1985, p. 485-492.

Constipation

In this double-blind, placebo-controlled study, 35 men and women suffering from constipation received capsules containing celandin-aloevera-psyllium for a period of 28 days. Results found that subjects in the celandin, aloevera and psyllium group, experienced more frequent bowel movements, the stools were softer and laxative dependence was reduced. All such parameters were unchanged in those receiving placebo.

—H.S. Odes and Z. Madar, ''A Double-blind Tiral of a Celandin, Aloevera and Psyllium Laxative Preparation in Adult Patients with Constipation,'' *Digestion,* 49(2), 1991, p. 65-71.

Contraception

Results of this study showed that 7.5% and 10% concentrations of lyophilized aloe barbadensis exhibited spermicidal activity, suggesting such concentrations may be a useful vaginal contraceptive.

—M.S. Fahim & M. Wang, ''Zinc Acetate and Lyophilized Aloe Barbadensis as Vaginal Contraceptive,'' *Contraception,* 53(4), April 1996, p. 231-236.

Diabetes

Noting that the dried sap of the aloe plant to be a traditional diabetic remedy in the Arabian peninusla, this study examined its ability to reduce blood glucose levels in 5 non-insulin-dependent diabetics and in Swiss albino mice made diabetic with alloxan. Results showed that the intake of 1/2 teaspoon of aloes daily for 4-14 weeks signficantly reduced the fasting serum glucose level fell in all patients. Fasting plasma glucose was significantly reduced in diabetic mice by glibenclamide and aloes after 3 days.

—N. Ghannam, et al., "The Antidiabetic Activity of Aloes: Preliminary Clinical and Experimental Observations," *Hormone Research,* 24(4), 1986, p. 288-294.

In this study, the anti-inflammatory activity of aloe vera and gibberellin was measured in streptozotocin-induced diabetic mice by measuring the inhibition of polymorphonuclear leukocyte infiltration into a site of gelatin-induced inflammation over a dose range of 2 to 100 mg/kg. Results found that Aloe and gibberellin both inhibited inflammation in a dose-response manner. Based on these findings, the authors suggest that gibberellin or a gibberellin-like substance is an active anti-inflammatory component in aloe vera.

—R.H. Davis & N.P. Maro, "Aloe Vera and Gibberellin. Anti-inflammatory Activity in Diabetes," *Journal of the American Podiatry Medical Association,* 79(1), January 1989, p. 24-26.

This study examined the effects of exudate of Aloe barbadensis leaves (oral administration of 500 mg/kg) and its bitter principle (ip administration of 5 mg/kg) on plasma glucose levels of alloxan-diabetic mice. Results showed that the hypoglycemic effect of a single oral dose of aloes on serum glucose level was insignificant in while that of the bitter principle was highly significant and extended over a period of 24 hours.

—M.A. Ajabnoor, "Effect of Aloes on Blood Glucose Levels in Normal and Alloxan Diabetic Mice," *Journal of Ethnopharmacology,* 28(2), February 1990, p. 215-220.

This study found that five non-insulin-dependent diabetics experienced a mean reduction in fasting blood sugar of 273 to 151 mg/dl following 14 weeks of taking a half teaspoon 4 times daily of aloes.

—Nadia Gnhannam, et al., "The Antidiabetic Activity of Aloes," *Hormone Research,* 24, 1986, p. 288-294.

Frostbite

Results of this study found aloe vera cream to be an effective therapy for improving tissue survival in rabbits following frostbite injury.

—M.B. Miller & P.J. Koltai, "Treatment of Experimental Frostbite with Pentoxifylline and Aloe Vera Cream," *Arch Otolaryngol Head Neck Surg,* 121(6), June 1995, p. 678-680.

Gastric Lesions

This study examined the effects of aloctin A, a glycoprotein isolated from leaves of Aloe arborescens MILL, on the gastric secretion and acute gastric lesions in rats. Results showed that the intravenous administration of aloctin A inhibited the volume of gastric juice, acid and pepsin output in pylorus-ligated rats, development of Shay ulcers, indomethacin-induced gastric lesions, and water-immersion stress-induced lesions in rats.

—H. Saito, et al., [Effects of Aloe Extracts, Aloctin A, on Gastric Secretion and on Experimental Gastric Lesions in Rats], *Yakugaku Zasshi,* 109(5), May 1989, p. 335-339.

General

Results of this study found that the intravenous administration of a partially purified extract of Aloe vahombe leaves protected mice against infection of bacteria, parasites, and fungus, (Candida albicans).

—J.Y. Brossat, et al., [Immunostimulating Properties of an Extract Isolated from Aloe Vahombe. 2. Protection in Mice by Fraction F1 against Infections by Listeria Monocytogenes, Yersinia pestis, Candida Albicans and Plasmodium Berghei], *Arch Inst Pasteur Madagascar,* 48(1), 1981, p. 11-34.

This review article on the aloe vera plant and its products notes that the plant contains numerous pharmacologically active ingredients, including a carboxypeptidase that inactivates bradykinin in vitro, salicylates, and a substance(s) that inhibits thromboxane formation in vivo. The scientific literature supports the antibacterial and antifungal effects for these and other substance in aloe vera as well the plants use in the treatment of human radiation ulcers and stasis ulcers and burn and frostbite injuries in animals.

—A.D. Klein & N.S. Penneys, "Aloe Vera," *Journal of the American Academy of Dermatology,* 18(4 Pt 1), April 1988, p. 714-720.

Skin Damage

This double-blind, placebo-controlled study examined the effects of a 0.5% Aloe vera extract in a hydrophilic cream on psoriasis patients. Results showed that the topical administration of the cream three times per day for five straight days over a period of 16 weeks led to a cure in 85% of patients compared to a 6.6% cure rate among controls.

—T.A. Syed, et al., "Management of Psoriasis with Aloe Vera Extract in a Hydrophilic Cream: A Placebo-controlled, Double-blind Study," *Trop Med Int Health,* 1(4), August 1996, p. 505-509.

Results of this set of studies found that Aloe barbadensis gel extract topically applied to the skin of UV-irradiated mice ameliorated immune suppression without causing DNA damage.

—F.M. Strickland, et al., "Prevention of Ultraviolet Radiation-induced Suppression of Contact and Delayed Hypersensitivity by Aloe Barbadensis Gel Extract," *Journal of Invest. Dermatology,* 102(2), February 1994, p. 197-204.

This study examined the protective effects of Aloe arborescens on soft X-irradiated induced skin injury in mice. Results found Aloe to have significant protective effects.

—Y. Sato, et al., "Studies on Chemical Protectors Against Radiation. XXXI Protection Effects of Aloe Arborescens on Skin Injury Induced by X-irradiation," *Yakugaku Zasshi,* 110(11), November 1990, p. 876-884.

Wound Healing

Results of this study showed that 300 mg/kg of mannose-6-phosphate, the primary sugar in Aloe gel, improved wound healing relative to saline controls.

—R.H. Davis, et al., "Anti-inflammatory and Wound Healing Activity of a Growth Substance in Aloe Vera," *Journal of the American Podiatry Medical Association,* 84(2), February 1994, p. 77-81.

Results of this study found that guinea pigs suffering from burns experienced a significantly faster healing rate when treated with aloe gel extract compared to those treated with either aspirin or Silvadine.

—M. Rodriguez-Bigas, N.I. Cruz, and A. Suarez, "Comparative Evaluation of AloeVera in the Management of Burn Wounds in Guinea Pigs," *Plast Reconst Surg,* 81(3), March 1988, p. 386-389.

Results of this study found that both the oral and topical administration of aloe vera proved to be an effective means of wound healing in mice suffering from biopsy punched induced verterbal column injury.

—R.H. Davis, et al., "Wound Healing: Oral and Topical Activity of Aloe Vera," *Journal of American Podiatry Medical Association,* 79(11), November 1989, p. 559-562.

Results of this study found that daily intake of 100 and 300 mg/kg of aloe vera for 4 days blocked the wound healing suppression of hydrocortisone acetate in mice up to 100% using the wound tensile strength assay.

—R.H. Davies, et al., "Aloe Vera, Hydrocortisone, and Sterol Influences on Wound Tensile Strength and Anti-inflammation," *Journal of the American Podiatry Medical Association,* 84(12), December 1994, p. 614-621.

Results of this study on full-face dermabrasion found that overall wound healing was approximately 72 hours faster on those sites treated with a polyethylene oxide gel dressing saturated with stabilized aloe vera compared to that without the aloe vera.

—J.E. Fulton, Jr., "The Stimulation of Postdermabrasion Wound Healing with Stabilized Aloe Vera Gel-polyethylene Oxide Dressing," *Journal of Dermatol Surg Oncology,* 16(5), May 1990, p. 460-467.

In this study, 27 patients with partial thickness burn wounds were treated with aloe vera gel compared with vaseline gauze. Results found that aloe vera gel treated lesions healed more rapidly than the vaseline gauze area, with the average time of healing in the aloe gel area being 11.89 days and 18.19 days for the vaseline gauze treated wound. A significant difference.

—V. Visuthiokosol, et al., "Effect of Aloe Vera Gel to Healing of Burn Wound a Clinical and Histologic Study," *Journal of the Medical Association of Thailand,* 78(8), August 1995, p. 403-409.

■ ASTRAGALUS

Antimicrobial Activity

Results of this study reported the isolation of two new antimicrobial isoflavans from the roots of Astragalus alexandrinus and A. trigonus—1-[(3R)-7,8-dimethoxybenzopyranyl]-4- hydroxybenzoquinone (astragaluquinone) and (3S)-7,1'-dihydroxy-8,3'-dimethoxyisoflavan (8-methoxyvestitol).

>   —N.A. el-Sebakhy, et al., "Antimicrobial Isoflavans from Astragalus Species," *Phytochemistry,* 36(6), August 1994, p. 1387-1389.

Cancer

Results of this study found that the Astragalus membraneceus fraction, F3, exhibited significant immunorestorative effects on mononucleur cells taken from cancer patients. Similar results were seen in vivo using a rat model.

>   —D.T. Chu, et al., [Immune Restoration of Local Xenogeneic Graft-versus-host Reaction in Cancer Patients in Vitro and Reversal of Cyclophosphamide-induced Immune Suppression in the Rat in Vivo by Fractionated Astragalus Membranaceus], *Chung Hsi I Chieh Ho Tsa Chih,* 9(6), June 1989, p. 351-354.

Results of this study showed that the antitumor activity of LAK cells was greatly enhanced by the action of Shengmaisan with Astragalus membranaceus at concentrations of 100 micrograms/ml.

>   —T.H. Zhao, [Positive Modulating Action of Shengmaisan with Astragalus Membranaceus on Anti-tumor Activity of LAK Cells], *Chung Kuo Chung Hsi I Chieh Ho Tsa Chih,* 13(8), August 1993, p. 471-472.

Results of this study found Astragalus polysaccharide and Radis hedysair polysaccharide exhibited immunopotentiating effects in mice.

>   —J. Wang, et al., "Enhancing Effect of Antitumor Polysaccharide from Astragalus or Radix Hedysarum on C3 Cleavage Production of Macrophages in Mice," *Japanese Journal of Pharmacology,* 51(3), November 1989, p. 432-434.

Cardiovascular/Coronary Heart Disease

Results of this study showed that Astragalus membranaceus inhibited lipid peroxidation in rat heart mitochondria when administered at concentrations of 2 mg dried herb/ml mitochondrial suspension.

>   —C.Y. Hong, et al., "Astragalus Membranaceus and Polygonum Multiflorum Protect Rat Heart Mitochondria Against Lipid Peroxidation," *American Journal of Chinese Medicine,* 22(1), 1994, p. 63-70.

Results of this study found that the Astragalus compound, 3-Nitropropionic acid (NPA), elicited a dose-dependent relaxation of precontracted rabbit aortic rings and had vasodilator and antihypertensive properties that were independent of animal species.

>   —C. Castillo, et al., [An Analysis of the Antihypertensive Properties of 3-nitropropionic Acid, a Compound from Plants in the Genus Astragalus], *Arch Inst Cardiol Mex,* 63(1), January-February 1993, p. 11-16.

Results of this study showed that Astragalus membranaceus had significant protective effects against Coxsackie B virus-induced acute myocarditis in rats when administered early on during the infection period.

—W.L. Yuan, et al., "Effect of Astragalus Membranaceus on Electric Activities of Cultured Rat Beating Heart Cells Infected with Coxsackie B-2 Virus," *Chinese Medical Journal,* 103(3), March 1990, p. 177-182.

Results of this study showed that Astragalus membranaceus exhibited inhibitory effects on Coxsackie B virus propagation and protected the myocardium in mouse myocarditis.

—Y.Z. Yang, et al., "Treatment of Experimental Coxsackie B-3 Viral Myocarditis with Astragalus Membranaceus in Mice," *Chinese Medical Journal,* 103(1), January 1990, p. 14-18.

Results of this study indicated that Astragalus membranaceus exhibited beneficial effects with respect to the prevention and treatment of coxsackie B virus-induced acute myocarditis in mice.

—T. Rui, et al., "Effect of Astragalus Membranaceus on Electrophysiological Activities of Acute Experimental Coxsackie B-3 Viral Myocarditis in Mice," *Chinese Med Sci Journal,* 8(4), December 1993, p. 203-206.

Results of this study found that Astragalus membranaceus exhibited useful effects with respect to prevention and treatment of acute myocarditis induced by coxsackie B-2 virus in vitro.

—W.L. Yuan, et al., [Effect of Astragalus Membranaceus on Electrical Activities of Coxsackie B-2 virus-infected Rat Myocardial Cells in Culture], *Chung Hsi I Chieh Ho Tsa Chih,* 9(6), June 1989, p. 355-357.

In this study, 19 congestive heart failure patients received treatment with Astragalus membranceus ingredient, the astragaloside IV (XGA). Results showed relief in chest distress and dispnea in 15 patients after 2 weeks of treatment. Improvements were also seen with respect to left ventricular modeling, left ventricular end-diastolic volume, and left ventricular end-systolic volume, and heart rate.

—H.M. Luo, et., [Nuclear Cardiology Study on Effective Ingredients of Astragalus Membranaceus in Treating Heart Failure], *Chung Kuo Chung Hsi I Chieh Ho Tsa Chih,* 15(12), December 1995, p. 707-709.

Results of this study found that the administration of Astragalus membranaceus decreased the ratio of pre-ejection period/left ventricular ejection time, increased superoxide dismutase activity of red blood cells, and reduced the lipid peroxidation content of plasma in acute myocardial infarction patients.

—L.X. Chen, et al., [Effects of Astragalus Membranaceus on Left Ventricular Function and Oxygen Free Radical in Acute Myocardial Infarction Patients and Mechanism of its Cardiotonic Action], *Chung Kuo Chung Hsi I Chieh Ho Tsa Chih,* 15(3), March 1995, p. 141-143.

Results of this study found that treatment with Astragalus membranaceus was a successful therapy for ischemic heart disease patients, proving more effective than Nifedipine and Tab.

—S.Q. Li, et al., [Clinical Observation on the Treatment of Ischemic Heart Disease with Astragalus Membranaceus], *Chung Kuo Chung Hsi I Chieh Ho Tsa Chih,* 15(2), February 1995, p. 77-80.

Results of this study indicated that Astragalus membranaceus exhibited beneficial effects with respect to the prevention and treatment of coxsackie B3 virus-induced acute myocarditis in mice.

> —T. Rui, et al., [Effect of Astragalus Membranaceus on Electrophysiological Activities of Acute Experimental Coxsackie B3 Viral myocarditis in Mice], *Chung Kuo Chung Hsi I Chieh Ho Tsa Chih,* 14(5), May 1994, p. 292-294.

Results of this study found that Astragalus membranaceus reduced secondary Ca2+ damages, improved abnormal myocardial electric activity, and inhibited the replication of Coxsackie virus B3 in myocardium of cultured neonatal rat heart cells.

> —Q. Guo, et al., [Effect of Astragalus Membranaceus on Ca2+ influx al and Coxsackie Virus B3 RNA Replication in Cultured Neonatal Rat Heart Cells], *Chung Kuo Chung Hsi I Chieh Ho Tsa Chih,* 15(8), August 1995, p. 483-485.

Results of this study found that Radix Astragalus lowered collagen content in the aorta and lung of old rats to levels comparable to those found in young rats.

> —P. Xu, et al., [Effect of Radix Astragalus on the Contents of Collagen in the Aorta and Lung of Old Rats], *Chung Kuo Chung Yao Tsa Chih,* 16(1), January 1991, p. 49-50.

Results of this study found that Atenolol, dibunol, Astragalus dasyanthus pall. reduced the myocardial damage area at permanent and transient ischemia following coronary arterial ligation in rats.

> —A.N. Kudrin, et al., [Effect of Atenolol, Dibunol, Peroxidase and Astragalus Dasynthus on the Morphometric Parameters of Myocardial Infarction], *Farmakol Toksikol,* 50(6), November-December 1987, p. 47-51.

Digestion

Results of this study found that Astragalus membranaceus strengthened muscle tonus and enhanced movement in the dog small intestine.

> —D.Z. Yang, [Effect of Astragalus Membranaceus on Myoelectric Activity of Small Intestine], *Chung Kuo Chung Hsi I Chieh Ho Tsa Chih,* 13(10), October 1993, p. 616-617.

Results of this study showed that Astragalus membraceus root led to the recovery of ozone-induced intestinal flora imbalance in senile mice.

> —M. Yan, et al., [Changes of Intestinal Flora in Senile Mouse Models and the Antagonistic Activity of the Root of Astragalus Membraceus], *Chung Kuo Chung Yao Tsa Chih,* 20(10), October 1995, p. 624-626.

General

Results of this study showed that administration of 250 mg/kg ip per day of Astragalus polysaccharide and 50 mg/kg sc of ginsenosides of ginseng stems and leaves from 0-3 days posttrauma significantly elevated the lymphocytes membrane fluidity of plasmalemma, mitochondria and microsome from spleen, thymus and mesenteric lymph nodes in traumatized mice. Results also showed the treatment reduced lipid peroxide levels, and increased superoxide dismutase activities in serum and lymphocytes from such animals.

> —H. Liang, et al., [Effects of Astragalus Polysaccharides and Ginsenosides of Ginseng Stems

and Leaves on Lymphocytes Membrane Fluidity and Lipid Peroxidation in Traumatized Mice], *Chung Kuo Chung Yao Tsa Chih,* 20(9), September 1995, p. 558-560.

Immune Function

Results of this study showed that the injection of Astragalus membranaceus extract into normal mice or immunodepressed mice enhanced the antibody response to a T-dependent antigen.

—K.S. Zhao, et al., "Enhancement of the Immune Response in Mice by Astragalus Membranaceus Extracts," *Immunopharmacology,* 20(3), November-December 1990, p. 225-233.

Results of this study found that the Astragalus membranaceus fraction, F3, exhibited a marked immune potentiating activity in rats.

—D.T. Chu, et al., "Immunotherapy with Chinese Medicinal Herbs. II. Reversal of Cyclophosphamide-Induced Immune Suppression by Administration of Fractionated Astragalus Membranaceus in Vivo," *Journal of Clinical Lab Immunol,* 25(3), March 1988, p. 125-129.

Results of this study showed that forced running exercises and the administration of Astragalus enhanced immune function in mice

—H. Sugiura, et al., [Effects of Exercise in the Growing Stage in Mice and of Astragalus Membranaceus on Immune Functions], *Nippon Eiseigaku Zasshi,* 47(6), February 1993, p. 1021-1031.

Leucopenia

This study examined the effects of pure Astragalus in patients suffering from leucopenia. Results showed that patients receiving 10 ml equaled to 15 g of Astragalus twice per day for 8 weeks experienced an 82.76% rate of effectiveness. Patients receiving 10 ml equaled to 5 g of Astragalus over the same schedule experienced a 47.3% rate of effectiveness.

—X.S. Weng, et al., [Treatment of Leucopenia with Pure Astragalus Preparation—an Analysis of 115 Leucopenic Cases], *Chung Kuo Chung Hsi I Chieh Ho Tsa Chih,* 15(8), August 1995, p. 462-464.

Liver Damage

Results of this study showed that the saponins ASI, SK extracted from the root of Astragalus membranaceous Bge and Astragalus sieversianus Pull provided protection against chemical-induced liver injury in mice.

—Y.D. Zhang, et al., [Effects of Astragalus (ASI, SK) on Experimental Liver Injury], *Yao Hsueh Hsueh Pao,* 27(6), 1992, p. 401-406.

Lupus

Results of this study showed that pre-incubation of peripheral blood mononuclear cells with Astragalus membranaceus and Tripterygium hypoglaucum or a combination of both stimulated NK cytotoxicity in lupus patients as well as healthy control donors in a dose dependent manner.

—X.Z. Zhao, [Effects of Astragalus Membranaceus and Tripterygium Hypoglancum on Natural Killer Cell Activity of Peripheral Blood Mononuclear in Systemic Lupus Erythematosus], *Chung Kuo Chung Hsi I Chieh Ho Tsa Chih,* 12(11), November 1992, p. 669-671.

Memory

Results of this study found that an aqueous Astragalus membranaceus extract improved anisodine-induced impairment on memory acquisition and alcohol-induced memory retrieval deficit in step down behavior of mice.

—G.X. Hong, et al.,[Memory-improving Effect of Aqueous Extract of Astragalus Membranaceus (Fisch.) Bge.], *Chung Kuo Chung Yao Tsa Chih,* 19(11), November 1994, p. 687-688.

Reproduction

Results of this study showed that Astragalus membranaceus increased semen sperm motility relative to controls when administered at 10 mg/ml in vitro.

—C.Y. Hong, et al., "Astragalus Membranaceus Stimulates Human Sperm Motility in Vitro," *American Journal of Chinese Medicine,* 20(3-4), 1992, p. 289-294.

Wound Healing

Results of this study found that Astragalus polysaccharides exhibited restorative effects on damaged cell mediated immunity in rats following burn injury.

—H. Liang, et al., [The Effect of Astragalus Polysaccharides (APS) on Cell Mediated Immunity (CMI) in Burned Mice], *Chung Hua Cheng Hsing Shao Shang Wai Ko Tsa Chih,* 10(2), March 1994, p. 138-141.

■ BEE PROPOLIS

Antibacterial Effects

Results of this study indicated that propolis exhibited antibacterial activity against various commonly encountered cocci and Gram-positive rods such as human tubercle bacillus.

—J.M. Grange & R.W. Davey "Antibacterial Properties of Propolis (Bee Glue)," *Journal of the Royal Society of Medicine,* 83(3), March 1990, p. 159-160.

Results of this study showed there to be synergy between the antibiotic effects of propolis and antibiotics to antibiotic resistant strains of Staphylococcus aureus.

—T.A. Shub, et al., [Effect of Propolis on Staphylococcus Aureus Strains Resistant to Antibiotics], *Antibiotiki,* 26(4), April 1981, p. 268-271.

Results of this study showed the ethanol extract of propolis to have lethal effects on Trichomonas vaginalis in vitro and also on Toxoplasma gondii, the latter after 24 hours of contact.

—J. Starzyk, et al., "Biological Properties and Clinical Application of Propolis. II. Studies on the Antiprotozoan Activity of Ethanol Extract of Propolis," *Arzneimittelforschung,* 27(6), 1977, p. 1198-1199.

Results of this study showed propolis exhibited antimicrobial effects against strains isolated from the respiratory tracts of human patients suffering from infections.

—F. Focht, et al., "Bactericidal Effect of Propolis in Vitro Against Agents Causing Upper Respiratory Tract Infections," *Arzneimittelforschung,* 43(8), August 1993, p. 921-923.

Results of this study identified antibacterial activity in some Brazilian propolis fractions.
> —V. Bankova, et al., "Chemical Composition and Antibacterial Activity of Brazilian Propolis," *Z Naturforsch*, 50(3-4), March-April 1995, p. 167-172.

Results of this study identified antibacterial activity in some Brazilian propolis fractions.
> —V. Bankova, et al., "Antibacterial Diterpenic Acids from Brazilian Propolis," *Z Naturforsch*, 51(5-6), May-June 1996, p. 277-280.

Anti-inflammatory Effects

Results of this study showed that a 13% aqueous extract administered orally exhibited anti-inflammatory effects on a carrageenan rat paw oedema model and on adjuvant-induced arthritis in rats.
> —M.T. Khayyal, et al., "Mechanisms Involved in the Antiinflammatory Effect of Propolis Extract," *Drugs Exp Clin Res*, 19(5), 1993, p. 197-203.

Bone Loss

Results of this study found an increased rate of ossification in cases of artificially induced bone tissue loss following treatment with ethanol extract of propolis.
> —A. Stojko, et al., "Biological Properties and Clinical Application of Propolis. VIII. Experimental Observation on the Influence of Ethanol Extract of Propolis (EEP) on the Regeneration of Bone Tissue," *Arzneimittelforschung*, 28(1), 1978, p. 35-37.

Cancer

Results of this study showed that PMS-1, a tumoricidal substance isolated from Brazilian propolis, decreased DMBA-induced skin tumor incidence and growth in mice.
> —T. Mitamura, et al., "Effects of a New Clerodane Diterpenoid Isolated from Propolis on Chemically Induced Skin Tumors in Mice," *Anticancer Research*, 16(5A), September-October 1996, p. 2669-2672.

Results of this study showed that propolis exhibited BRM-like antitumor activities in vitro.
> —T. Hanaya, et al., "Biological Effects of Propolis on Macrophage Function and Tumor Growth," *Proceedings of the Annual Meeting of the American Association of Cancer Researchers*, 35, 1994, p. A2938.

Results of this study showed that an ethanolic extract of propolis exhibited antitumoral effects in mice-bearing Ehrlich carcinoma.
> —S. Scheller, et al., "Antitumoral Property of Ethanolic Extract of Propolis in Mice-bearing Ehrlich Carcinoma, As Compared to Bleomycin," *Z Naturforsch*, 44(11-12), November-December 1981, p. 1063-1065.

Cardiovascular/Coronary Heart Disease

Results of this study examined the effects of 50 and 100 mg/kg of propolis on doxurubicin-induced cardiomyopathy in rats. Results showed that propolis pretreatment produced significant cardioprotective effects.
> —S. Chopra, et al., "Propolis Protects Against Doxorubicin-induced Myocardiopathy in Rats," *Exp Mol Pathol*, 62(3), June 1995, p. 190-198.

Cervicitis

Results of this double-blind study showed that 5% propolis dressings applied to vaginal dressings for 10 days had significant positive effects on women suffering from acute cervicitis relative to controls.

—E. Santana Perez, et al., [Vaginal Parasites and Acute Cervicitis: Local Treatment with Propolis. Preliminary Report], *Rev Cubana Enferm,* 11(1), June-January 1995, p. 51-56.

Dental Health

Results of this study showed that an ethanol extract of propolis stimulated the regenerative process on damaged dental pulp and led to a decrease in circulatory system disorders and degenerative processes.

—S. Scheller, et al. "Biological Properties and Clinical Application of Propolis. IX. Experimental Observation on the Influence of Ethanol Extract of Propolis (EEP) on Dental Pulp Regeneration," *Arzneimittelforschung,* 28(2), 1978, p. 289-291.

This study examined the effects of propolis on the growth and glucosyltransferase activity of Streptococcus sobrinus 6715, Streptococcus mutans PS14 and Streptococcus cricetus OMZ61 in vitro. The effects of propolis on the dental caries of S. sobrinus 6715-infected rats were examined as well. Results showed antimicrobial activity against S. sobrinus, S. mutans and S. cricetus, with inhibitions seen for both water-insoluble glucan synthesis and glucosyltransferase activity. Dental caries were also reduced by propolis.

—K. Ikeno, et al., "Effects of Propolis on Dental Caries in Rats," *Caries Research,* 25(5), 1991, p. 347-351.

Results of this study found that the topical administration of propolis hydro-alcoholic solution increased the rate of epithelial repair following tooth removal in rats.

—O. Magro Filho & A.C. de Carvalho, "Application of Propolis to Dental Sockets and Skin Wounds," *J Nihon Univ Sch Dent,* 32(1), March 1990, p. 4-13.

This article notes that clinical and X-ray exams point to the efficacy of a 4% alcohol solution of bee glue added to root-canal fillings in severe cases of periodontitis.

—S.V. Kosenko & TIu Kosovich, [The Treatment of Periodontitis with Prolonged-action Propolis Preparations (clinical x-ray research)], *Stomatologiia,* 69(2), March-April 1990, p. 27-29.

Flu

Results of this study showed that the administration of an aqueous propolis extract 3 hours following the inoculation of mice with an influenza virus led to a reduction in HA titer and reduction in mortality and increased mean survival time.

—V. Esanu, et al., "The Effect of an Aqueous Propolis Extract, of Rutin and of a Rutin-quercetin Mixture on Experimental Influenza Virus Infection in Mice," *Virologie,* 32(3), July-September 1981, p. 213-215.

General

This studies reviews the medicinal properties of ethanolic extract of propolis and demonstrated the extract's ability to inhibit luminol-H2O2 chemiluminescence in vitro.

—W. Krol, et al., "Anti-oxidant Property of Ethanolic Extract of Propolis (EEP) as Evaluated by Inhibiting the Chemiluminescence Oxidation of Luminol,'' *Biochem Int,* 21(4), 1990, p. 593-597.

This review article notes that numerous pharmaceutical properties have been attributed to propolis, including anti-inflammatory, antiviral, immunostimulatory and carcinostatic activities.
—D. Grunberger, et al., ''Preferential Cytotoxicity on Tumor Cells by Caffeic Acid Phenethyl Ester Stomatologiia Isolated from Propolis,'' *Experientia,* 44(3), March 15, 1988, p. 230-232.

This study examined the effects of various propolis extracts on the parasite T. cruzi. Results showed that ethanolic extracts and dimethylsulphoxide extracts both proved effective against T. cruzi. In addition to these findings, the treatment of infected peritoneal macrophages and heart muscle cells with ethanol extracts inhibited infection levels.
—K.O. Higashi & S.L. de Castro, ''Propolis Extracts are Effective Against Trypanosoma Cruzi and have an Impact on its Interaction with Host Cells,'' *Journal of Ethnopharmacol,* 43(2), July 8, 1994, p. 149-155.

Results of this study found the ethanolic extracts of two forms of Cuban propolis exhibited strong scavenging activity against oxygen radicals.
—C Pascual, et al., ''Scavenging Action of Propolis Extract Against Oxygen Radicals,'' *Journal of Ethnopharmacology,* 41(1-2), January 1994, p. 9-13.

Results of this study showed that continuous administration of propolis stabilized free radical lipid peroxidation in salmonellosis.
—L.B. Okonenko, [Propolis as an Inhibitor of Free Radical Lipid Oxidation in Salmonellosis], *Vopr Med Khim,* 32(3), May-June 1986, p. 45-48.

Results of this study showed the intraperitoneally administration of an ethanoic extract of propolis provided protection against gamma irradiation in mice.
—S. Scheller, et al., ''The Ability of Ethanolic Extract of Propolis (EEP) to Protect Mice Against Gamma Irradiation,'' *Z Naturforsch,* 44(11-12), November-December 1989, p. 1049-1052.

Giardiasis

Results of this study found propolis ranging in concentration strength from 10%-30% to be an effective treatment for patients suffering from giardiasis.
—C. Miyares, et al., [Clinical Trial with a Preparation Based on Propolis ''propolisina'' in Human Giardiasis], *Acta Gastroenterol Latinoam,* 18(3), 1988, p. 195-201.

Herpes

Results of this showed that the propolis constituent, 3-methyl-but-2-enyl caffeate, reduced the viral titer of herpes simplex virus 1 by 3 log110 and reduced viral DNA synthesis 32-fold.
—M. Amoros, et al., ''Comparison of the Anti-herpes Simplex Virus Activities of Propolis and 3-methyl-but-2-enyl Caffeate,'' *Journal of Natural Products,* 57(5), May 1994, p. 644-647.

Results of this study found that ocular medical propolis films applied behind the lower eyelids before bed over a period of 10-15 days cut recovery time in half in patients with postherpetic trophic keratitis and/or postherpetic nebula.

> —IuF Maichuk, et al., [The Use of Ocular Drug Films of Propolis in the Sequelae of Ophthalmic Herpes], *Voen Med Zh*, (12), December 1995, p. 36-39.

Liver Damage

Results of this study found that rats treated with 100 mg/kg of Cuban red propolis extract experienced hepatoprotective effects against CC14-induced liver damage.

> —N. Merino, et al., "Histopathological Evaluation on the Effect of Red Propolis on Liver Damage Induced by CCl4 in Rats," *Arch Med Res,* 27(3), Autumn 1996, p. 285-289.

Results of this study indicated that propolis exhibited beneficial antioxidative properties in rats suffering from toxic liver damage and acute hepatic ischemia.

> —S.M. Drogovoz, et al., [The Liver-protective Properties of the Pediatric Drug Form of Propolis in Animals of Different Age Groups], *Eksp Klin Farmakol,* 57(4), July-August 1994, p. 39-42.

Stroke

Results of this study indicated that apitherapy proved to be an effective treatment in patients suffering from ischemic insults.

> —V.A. Samoliuk, [The Indices of the Antioxidant System and the Status of the Cerebral Blood Supply in Patients with an Ischemic Stroke on Apitherapy], *Vrach Delo,* (1-2), January-February 1995, p. 68-70.

Tuberculosis

Results of this study showed that apitherapy had positive effects on pulmonary tuberculosis in-patients.

> —G.D. Masterov, [Apitherapy in the Combined Treatment of Patients with Pulmonary Tuberculosis Taking into Account the Hpophyseal-adrenal System Indices], *Vrach Delo,* (1-2), January-February 1995, p. 120-122.

Wound Healing

Results of this study showed that a propolis mouth rinse exhibited pain-killing and anti-inflammatory effects and proved beneficial in the repair of intra-buccal surgical wounds in patients following sulcoplasty by modified Kazanjian techniques.

> —O. Magro-Filho & A.C. de Carvalho, "Topical Effect of Propolis in the Repair of Sulcoplasties by the Modified Kazanjian Technique. Cytological and Clinical Evaluation," *J Nihon Univ Sch Dent,* 36(2), June 1994, p. 102-111.

Results of this study showed propolis to be an effective treatment in patients suffering from panaritium, abscesses, phlegmons, and infectious wounds.

> —N.I. Tsarev, et al., [Use of Propolis in the Treatment of Local Supportive Infection], *Vestn Khir,* 134(5), May 1985, p. 119-122.

■ GARLIC/ONION

Aging

This study utilized the Hayflick system of cellular aging in culture in order to test garlic for its anti-ageing effects on long-term growth characteristics, morphology and acromolecular synthesis of human skin fibroblasts. Results found that adding garlic extract into the normal cell culture medium can support serial subculturing for over more than 55 population doublings in 475 days, and that this treatment has some youth-preserving, anti-aging and beneficial effects on human fibroblasts in terms of maximum proliferative capacity and morphological characteristics. Similar or lesser doses of garlic extracts are growth inhibitory for cancerous cells that could not be grown over longer periods in the presence of garlic.

> —L. Svendsen, et al., "Testing Garlic for Possible Anti-ageing Effects on Long-term Growth Characteristics, Morphology and Macromolecular Synthesis of Human Fibroblasts in Culture," *Journal of Ethnopharmacology,* 43(2), July 8, 1994, p. 125-133.

AIDS/HIV

Results of this study showed that 7 of 10 HIV positive patients receiving 5 g per day of aged garlic extract over a period of 6 weeks followed by 6 weeks of 10 g per day experienced significant improvements in immune parameters and opportunistic infections.

> —T. Abdullah, et al., "Garlic as an Antimicrobial and Immune Modulator in AIDS," *International Conference on AIDS,* 5, June 4-9, 1989, p. 466.

Asthma

Noting previous research studies supporting the use of onions as treatment for bee stings, to inhibit platelet aggreation; this study found that a crude ethanolic onion extract produced clear protective effects against allergen-induced bronchial obstruction in guinea pigs.

> —Dorsch, et al., "Antiasthmatic Effects of Onion Extracts—Detection of Benzyl - and other Isothiocyanates (Mustard Oils) as Antiasthmatic Compounds of Plant Origin," *European Journal of Pharmacology,* 107, 1985, p. 17-24.

Cancer

This study examined the antimutagenic/anticarcinogenic, immune enhancing, antitumor and antifungal effects of a crude extract and organosulfur compound of garlic. Results showed that rat liver mutagenesis was inhibited by the administration of diallyl sulfide and ajeone, each at 100 ug/ml, and garlic extract at 12.5 mg/ml. Garlic extract was also shown to inhibit binding of [3H]AFB1 to calf thymus DNA and the formation of specific AFB1-DNA adducts while also controlling candida albicans.

> —P.P. Tadi, "Anticarcinogenic, Antitumor, and Antifungal Properties of Allium Sativum," *Dissertion Abstracts International,* 52(8), 1992, p. 4144.

This study examined the effects of 6 organosulfur compounds present in garlic for their ability to alter the growth of canine mammary tumor cells in culture. Results showed that diallysulfide and diallyldisulfide inhibited growth by 30% and 37%, respectively, at a final concentration of 0.05 after a 24 hour incubation. Treatment with diallytrisulfide (0.05 mM) inhibited growth by 50% after 24 hour incubation. Increasing diallytrisulfide to 0.5 mM decreased growth by 81%.

—S.G. Sundaram & J.A. Milner, "Antitumor Effects of Organosulfur Compounds Present in Garlic Against Canine Mammary Tumor Cells," *FASEB Journal,* 6(4), 1992, p. A1391.

Results of this study involving 120,852 subjects between the ages of 55-69 showed a strong inverse association between the consumption of onions and incidence of stomach cancer.

—E. Dorant, et al., "Consumption of Onions and a Reduced Risk of Stomach Carcinoma," *Gastroenterology,* 110(1), January 1996, p. 12-20.

Results of this case-control study involving interviews with 564 Chinese stomach cancer patients showed a significant decrease in gastric cancer risk with increasing consumption of allium vegetables. Subjects scoring in the highest quartile of intake experienced only 40% of the risk of those in the bottom quartile.

—W.C. You, et al., "Allium Vegetables and Reduced Risk of Stomach Cancer," *Journal of the National Cancer Institute,* 81(2), January 18, 1989, p. 162-164.

This study examined the chemopreventive action of garlic extract on DMBA-induced complete skin carcinogenesis in mice. Results showed that garlic extract topically applied twice daily for 3 days every week prior to DMBA significantly reduced incidences of tumors.

—A.R. Rao, et al., "Inhibition of Skin Tumors in DMBA-induced Complete Carciogenesis System in Mice by Garlic," *Indian Journal of Experimental Biology,* 28(5), May 1990, p. 405-408.

In this series of studies, onion extracts were added to cell cultures of an epidermoid carcinoma cell line derived from hamster buccal pouch carcinoma. Results showed an inhibition of tumor growth at a concentration level of 25% beginning 24 hours after incubation with a clear decrease in tumor proliferation after birth both 4 and 10 days of incubation.

—K. Niukian, et al., "In Vitro Inhibitory Effect of Onion Extract on Hamster Buccal Pouch Carcinomas," *Nutrit Cancer,* 10(3), 1987, p. 137-144.

Results of this study showed that onion extract was found to significantly delay DMBA-induced tumor formation in hamsters receiving onion extracts via their drinking water.

—K. Niukan, et al., "Effects of Onion Extract on the Development of Hamster Buccal Pouch Carcinomas as Expressed in Tumor Burden," *Nutr Cancer,* 9(2-3), 1987, p. 171-176.

This study examined the anticarcinogenic activities of regular garlic and selenium-enriched garlic DMBA exposed rats. With respect to regular garlic, results showed that a continuous treatment stating prior to DMBA and persisting through the life of the study proved most effective in tumor suppression. Rats fed the selenium enriched garlic experienced the lowest overall rate of mammary tumors.

—C. Ip, et al., "Mammary Cancer Prevention by Regular Garlic and Selenium-enriched Garlic," *Nutr Cancer,* 17(3), 1992, p. 279-286.

Results of this study found that garlic extract inhibited one of the earliest phenomena caused by 12-0-tetradecanoyl-phorbol-13 acetate, a tumor promoter, in vitro, ie, the enhancement of phospholipid metabolism. Results also showed garlic suppressed the first stage of tumor promotion in two-stage mouse skin carcnogenesis in vivo.

> —H. Nishino, et al., ''Antitumor-promoting Activity of Garlic Extracts,'' *Oncology,* 46(4), 1989, p. 277-280.

In this study, the effects of diallyl sulfide and dially disulfide, oil-soluble constituents of garlic and onion, on DMBA-induced and 12,0-tetradecanoylphorbol-13-acetate-promoted skin tumor formation were examined in mice. Results found that Topical application of diallyl sulfide or diallyl disulfide significantly inhibited skin papilloma formation from the ninth week of promotion and significantly increased the rate of survival.

> —C. Dwivedi, et al., ''Chemoprevention of Chemcially Induced Skin Tumor Development by Diallyl Sulfide,'' *Pharm Research,* 9(12), December 1992, p. 1668-1770.

This study investigated the optimal dose of garlic during long-term feeding and its preventive and therapeutic effects on DMH-induced colon cancer in rats. Results showed the incidence of colon tumor was significantly decreased in rats fed with 2.5%, 5% and 10% garlic diets thus the minimal optimal dose of garlic to inhibit colon cancer was 2.5% with the equivalent dose of this concentration in humans being 4.76 g/m2 body surface/day.

> —J.Y. Cheng, et al., ''Opitmal Dose of Garlic to Inhibit Dimethylhydrazine-induced Colon Cancer,'' *World Journal of Surgery,* 19(4), July-August 1995, p. 621-625.

Results of this study suggest garlic possesses anticancer effects by 10 direct actions on tumor cell metabolism, by inhibiting the initiating and promotion phases of cancer and by modulating immune response in the host.

> —B. Lau, et al., ''Allium Sativum (Garlic) and Cancer Prevention,'' *Nutrition Research,* 10, 1990, p. 937-948.

Results of this set of two studies found that garlic and its constituents S-allylcysteine and diallyldisulfide inhibited MNU-induced mammary cancer in female rats.

> —J.Z. Liu, et al., ''Dietary Garlic Inhibits Mammary Carcinogenesis Induced by N-methylni-trosourea,'' *FASEB Journal,* 9(4), 1995, p. A991.

Results of this study showed that diallyl disulfide, an oil soluble organosulfur compound of processed garlic, inhibited human colon tumor cell growth both in vivo and in vitro.

> —S.G. Sundaram & J.A. Milner, ''Diallyl Disulfide Present in Garlic Oil Inhibits Both in Vitro and in Vivo Growth of Human Colon Tumor Cells,'' *FASEB Journal,* 9(4), 1995, p. A869.

Results of this study found garlic powder inhibited the binding of N-nitroso compounds to liver and mammary DNA in female rats.

> —X.Y. Lin, et al., ''Dietary Garlic Powder Suppresses the in Vivo Formation of DNA Adducts Induced by N-nitroso Compounds in Liver and Mammary Tissues,'' *FASEB Journal,* 6(4), 1992, p. A1392.

Results of this study showed that Ehrlich carcinoma cells exposed to a freshly ground garlic extract and then transplanted into mice did not produce ascites tumors and all mice survived over a test period of ten weeks. Mice treated with freshly prepared tumor cells exposed to fresh GE over 1-week intervals acquired resistance against Ehrlich ascites carcinoma cells and none of the mice developed tumors. By contrast, all controls developed ascites tumors and died within a month.

—M. Fujiwara & T. Natata, "Induction of Tumour Immunity with Tumour Cells Treated Extract of Garlic (Allium Sativum)," *Nature,* 216(5110), 1967, p. 83-84.

Results of this study found that diallyl sufide exhibited protective effects against DMBA-induced forestomach tumors in the hamster buccal pouch.

—M. Nagabhushan, et al., "Anticarcinogenic Action of Diallyl Sulfide in Hamster Pouch and Forestomach," *Third International Congress on Engineered Oral Cancer, January 22-25, 1994, Madras, India,* 1994, p. 67.

Results of this study showed that garlic and amino acids significantly inhibited Ehrlich ascites tumor cell growth in tumor-bearing mice and extended survival time by as much as 50%.

—Y.M. Choy, et al., "Effect of Garlic, Chinese Medicinal Drugs and Amino Acids on Growth of Ehrlich Ascites Tumor Cells in Mice," *American Journal of Chinese Medicine,* 11(1-4), 1983, p. 69-73.

Results of this study showed that treatment with diallyl disulfide, an organosulfur garlic compound, significantly inhibited the growth of H-ras oncogene transformed tumors in nude mice. Diallyl disulfide significantly inhibited hepatic and tumoral 3-hydroxy-3-methylglutaryl coenzyme A reductase activity as well.

—S.V. Singh, et al., "Novel Anti-carcinogenic Activity of an Organosulfide from Garlic: Inhibition of H-RAS Oncogene Transformed Tumor Growth in Vivo by Diallyl Disulfide is Associated with Inhibition of p21H-ras Processing," *Biochem Biophys Res Commun,* 225(2), August 14, 1996, p. 660-665.

Results of this study showed that diallyl disulfide, an oil-soluble organosulfur compound in garlic, inhibited the growth of human neoplastic cells in vitro.

—S.G. ndaram & J.A. Milner, "Diallyl Disulfide Inhibits the Proliferation of Human Tumor Cells in Culture," *Biochim Biophys Acta,* 1315(1), January 17, 1996, p. 15-20.

Results of this study showed that ajeone, an organosulfur compound derived from garlic, inhibited mutagenesis induced by both benzo[a]pyrene (B[a]P) and 4-nitro-1,2-phenylenediamine (NPD) in a dose-dependent manner.

—K. Ishikawa, et al., "Antimutagenic Effects of Ajoene, an Organosulfur Compound Derived from Garlic," *Biosci Biotechnol Biochem,* 60(12), December 1996, p. 2086-2088.

Results of this study showed that the topical administration of garlic oil applied at the start of benzo[a]pyrene (B(a)P)-induced skin carcinogenesis in female albino mice reduced the number of tumor-bearing animals as well as the number of tumors per animal.

—A.S. Sadhana, et al., "Inhibitory Action of Garlic Oil on the Initiation of Benzo[a]pyrene-induced Skin Carcinogenesis in Mice," *Cancer Letters,* 40(2), June 15, 1988, p. 193-197.

Results of this study showed that garlic exhibited significant inhibitory effects on MCA-induced cancer of the uterine cervix in young albino mice.

    —S.P. Hussain, et al., "Chemopreventive Action of Garlic on Methylcholanthrene-induced Carcinogenesis in the Uterine Cervix of Mice," *Cancer Letters,* 49(2), February 1990, p. 175-180.

Results of this study showed that garlic powder and its components S-allyl cysteine diallyl disulfide significantly inhibited MNU-induced mammary carcinogenesis in female rats.

    —E.M. Schaffer, et al., "Garlic and Associated Allyl Sulfur Components Inhibit N-methyl-N-nitrosourea Induced Rat Mammary Carcinogenesis," *Cancer Letters,* 102(1-2), April 19, 1996, p. 199-204.

Results of this study showed that diallyl sulfide, a component of garlic, exhibited anticarcinogenic effects on squamous mucosa of the hamster.

    —M. Nagabhushan, et al., "Anticarcinogenic Action of Diallyl Sulfide in Hamster Buccal Pouch and Forestomach," *Cancer Letters,* 66(3), October 21, 1992, p. 207-216.

Results of this study showed that diallyl sulfide pretreatment significantly reduced the incidence of NNK-induced lung tumors and tumor multiplicity in mice.

    —J.Y. Hong, et al., "Inhibitory Effects of Diallyl Sulfide on the Metabolism and Tumorigenicity of the Tobacco-specific Carcinogen 4-(methylnitrosamino)-1-(3-pyridyl)-1-butanone (NNK) in A/J mouse Lung," *Carcinogenesis,* 13(5), May 1992, p. 901-904.

Results of this study found the garlic component diallyl sulfide significantly inhibited the incidence and frequency of dimthylhydrazine-induced colorectal adenocarcinomas in mice.

    —M.J. Wargovich, et al., "Diallyl Sulfide, a Flavor Component of Garlic (Allium Sativum), Inhibits Dimethylhydrazine-induced Colon Cancer," *Carcinogenesis,* 8(3), March 1987, p. 487-489.

This study examined the effects of garlic powder on DMBA-induced mammary tumors and mammary DMBA-DNA adducts in rats. Results showed that garlic significantly delayed first tumor onset and decreased total incidence of mammary tumors. Additionally, garlic inhibited in vivo binding of DMBA to mammary cell DNA.

    —J. Liu, et al., "Inhibition of 7,12-dimethylbenz[a]anthracene-induced Mammary Tumors and DNA Adducts by Garlic Powder," *Carcinogenesis,* 13(10), October 1992, p. 1847-1851.

Results of this study showed that diallyl sulfide, a natural extract of garlic, inhibited MNNG-induced gastric cancer in rats.

    —P.J. Hu, [Protective Effect of Diallyl Sulfide, a Natural Extract of Garlic, on MNNG-induced Damage of Rat Glandular Stomach Mucosa], *Chung Hua Chung Liu Tsa Chih,* 12(6), November 1990, p. 429-431.

Results of this study found that a topically applied garlic extract inhibited DMBA-induced oral carcinogenesis in hamsters.

    —C.L. Meng & K.W. Shyu, "Inhibition of Experimental Carcinogenesis by Painting with Garlic Extract," *Nutr Cancer,* 14(3-4), 1990, p. 207-217.

Results of this study showed that both onion oil and garlic inhibited DMBA-induced skin papilloma production in mice.

—J.P. Perchellet, et al., "Inhibition of DMBA-induced Mouse Skin Tumorigenesis by Garlic Oil and Inhibition of Two Tumor-promotion Stages by Garlic and Onion Oils," *Nutr Cancer,* 14(3-4), 1990, p. 183-193.

Results of this study showed that an extract of onion exhibited inhibitory activity against an oral carcinoma cell line in vitro.

—K. Niukian, et al., "In Vitro Inhibitory Effect of Onion Extract on Hamster Buccal Pouch Carcinogenesis," *Nutr Cancer,* 10(3), 1987, p. 137-144.

Results of this study showed that the topical administration of an onion extract delayed the formation of DMBA-induced tumors in hamsters.

—K. Niukian, et al., "Effects of Onion Extract on the Development of Hamster Buccal Pouch Carcinomas as Expressed in Tumor Burden," *Nutr Cancer,* 9(2-3), 1987, p. 171-176.

Results of this study showed diallyl sulfide inhibited the incidence of MNU-induced tracheal carcinoma in rats.

—C.J. Detrisac, et al., "Garlic Oil Constituents in the Prevention of Mammary and Respiratory Cancer," *Proceedings of the Annual Meeting of the American Association of Cancer Researchers,* 32, 1991, p. A791.

Results of this study showed that sulfur-containing garlic compounds prevented the development of AOM-induced colonic aberrant crypts in rats.

—S. Hatono, et al., "Chemopreventive Activity of Sulfur-containing Compounds Derived from Garlic," *Proceedings of the Annual Meeting of the American Association of Cancer Researchers,* 34, 1993, p. A744.

Results of this study showed that the natural garlic compound diallyl sulfide significantly inhibited AOM-induced aberrant colonic crypts in rats.

—M.J. Wargovich, et al., "New Agents for Colon Cancer Prevention Efficacy Studies Using Carcinogen-Induced Aberrant Crypt Foci in the Rat," *Proceedings of the Annual Meeting of the American Association of Cancer Researchers,* 33, 1992, p. A1010.

Results of this study showed that diallyl sulfide pretreatment significantly reduced the incidence of NNK-induced lung tumors and tumor multiplicity in mice.

—J.Y. Hong, et al., "Inhibitory Effects of Diallyl Sulfide on the Metabolism and Tumorigenicity of the Tobacco-specific Carcinogen 4-(methylnitrosamino)-1-(3-pyridyl)-1-butanone (NNK) in A/J mouse Lung," *Carcinogenesis,* 13(5), May 1992, p. 901-904.

Results of this study found that garlic exhibited significant inhibitory effects on DMBA-induced carcinogenesis in hamsters.

—K.W. Shyu & C.L. Meng, "The Inhibitory Effect of Oral Administration of Garlic on Experimental Carcinogenesis in Hamster Buccal Pouches by DMBA Painting," *Proc Natl Sci Counc Repub China,* 11(2), April 1987, p. 137-147.

Candida

Results of this study showed that the garlic fraction, ajoene, inhibited the growth of aspergillus niger and candida albicans in vitro.

> —S. Yoshida, et al., "Antifungal Activity of Ajoene Derived from Garlic," *Appl Environ Microbiol,* 53(3), March 1987, p. 615-617.

Results of this study showed that an aqueous garlic extract inhibited the growth of candida albicans in vitro.

> —M. Adetumbi, et al., "Allium Sativum (garlic) Inhibits Lipid Synthesis by Candida Albicans," *Antimicrob Agents Chemother,* 30(3), September 1986, p. 499-501.

Cardiovascular/Coronary Heart Disease

This study examined the effect of raw garlic on serum cholesterol, fibrinolytic activity and clotting time in 50 medical students. Subjects were given 10 g of raw garlic per day following breakfast for two months. Results showed a significant decrease in serum cholesterol and an increase in clotting time and fibrinolytic activity relative to controls.

> —J.V. Gadkari & V.D. Joshi, "Effect of Ingestion of Raw Garlic on Serum Cholesterol Level, Clotting Time and Fibrinolytic Activity in Normal Subjects," *Journal of Postgraduate Medicine,* 37(3), July 1991, p. 128-131.

Results of this study found that a group of 20 healthy volunteers fed garlic for 6 months followed by 2 months without garlic experienced significantly lower serum cholesterol and triglyceride levels. A group of 62 coronary heart disease patients with high serum cholesterol fed garlic for 10 months experienced a significant decrease in serum cholesterol levels relative to controls.

> —A. Bordia, "Effect of Garlic on Blood Lipids in Patients with Coronary Heart Disease," *American Journal of Clinical Nutrition,* 34(10), October 1981, p. 2100-2103.

In this double-blind, placebo-controlled study, 42 healthy middle-age adults with a serum total cholesterol level of greater than or equal to 220 mg/dl received 300 mg three times a day of standardized garlic powder in tablet form. Results found that the garlic treatment significantly reduced serum total cholesterol levels relative to controls.

> —A.K. Jain, et al., "Can Garlic Reduce Levels of Serum Lipids? A Controlled Clinical Study," *American Journal of Medicine,* 94(6), June 1993, p. 632-635.

The meta-analysis of 5 placebo-controlled studies examined the effects of garlic on total serum cholesterol levels in subjects with cholesterol levels greater than 5.17 mmol/L (200 mg/dL). Results showed that garlic was effective in reducing total cholesterol levels and is best used at doses ranging from one half to one clove per day.

> —S. Warhafsky, et al., "Effect of Garlic on Total Serum Cholesterol. A Meta-analysis," *Annals of Internal Medicine,* 119(7 Pt 1), October 1, 1993, p. 599-605.

Results of this series of studies showed that garlic increased the excretion of neutral and acidic steroids and exerts hypocholesterolemic effects into rats fed high-cholesterol diets.

> —M.S. Chi, et al., "Effects of Garlic on Lipid Metabolism in Rats Fed Cholesterol or Lard," *Journal of Nutrition,* 112(2), February 1982, p. 241-248.

Results of this study found both garlic and onion significantly inhibited the rise in serum cholesterol, serum triglycerides, and serum beta lipoproteins, serum phospholipids and significantly enhanced the fibrinolytic activity in healthy rabbits.

> —G.S. Sainani, et al., "Onion, Garlic, and Experimental Atherosclerosis," *Japanese Heart Journal,* 20(3), May 1979, p. 351-357.

In this study, a garlic powder extract was added to smooth muscle cells cultured from atherosclerotic plaques of human aorta. Results showed that over a 24 hour incubation period, the extract significantly decreased the level of cholesterol esters and free cholesterol in the cultured cells and inhibited their proliferative activity. Results also showed the extract significantly reduced cholesterol accumulation and inhibited cell proliferation stimulated by blood serum taken from patients with angiographically assessed coronary atherosclerosis. This study examined garlic s effects on blood atherogenicity of coronary atherosclerosis patients ex vivo as well. Results found that blood serum taken 2 hours following an oral administration of 300 mg garlic powder tablet caused substantially less cholesterol accumulation in cultured cells.

> —A.N. Orekhov, et al., "Direct Anti-atherosclerosis-related Effects of Garlic," *Annals of Medince,* 27(1), February 1995, p. 63-65.

This study examined the effects of essential oils extracted from 2 g of raw onion per kg of body weight and 1 g of raw garlic per kg body weight on experimental induced atherosclerosis in rabbits. Results showed the extracts to be effective in significantly reducing the rise in serum cholesterol levels over a 4 month experimental period. Results also showed that fibrinolytic activity significantly increased with onion and garlic while feeding only cholesterol actually decreased it, and onion and garlic cut aortic atheroma in half.

> —A. Bordia, et al., "Effect of Essential Oil of Onion and Garlic on Experimental Atherosclerosis in Rabbits," *Atherosclerosis,* 26(3), March 1977, p. 379-386.

In this double blind, placebo controlled study of 40 hypercholesterolaemic outpatients, results showed that patients taking 900 mg of garlic powder per day for 4 months demonstrated significantly lower total cholesterol, triglycerides and blood pressure levels than controls.

> —G. Vorberg & B. Schneider, "Therapy with Garlic: Results of a Placebo-controlled, Double-blind Study," *British Journal of Clinical Pract Symp Suppl,* 69, August 1990, p. 7-11.

In this double-blind, placebo-controlled study, 47 mild hypertension patients received either a garlic powder preparation or placebo for 12 weeks. Results showed a significant decrease in supine diastolic blood pressure in the garlic group relative to controls as well as significant reductions in serum cholesterol and triglyceride levels.

> —W. Auer, et al., "Hypertension and Hyperlipdaemia: Garlic Helps in Mild Cases," *British Journal of Clinical Pract Symp Suppl,* 69, August 1990, p. 3-6.

This study examined the effects of garlic juice on smooth and cardiac muscles of rabbits and guinea pigs. Results showed that garlic juice inhibited the contractions of rabbit and guinea pig aortic rings induced by norepinephrine in Ca(2+)-containing Krebs-Henseleit solutions; and it inhibited the contraction of rabbit and guinea pig tracheal smooth muscles induced by acetylcholine and histamine, respectively, in both Ca(2+)-free and Ca(2+)-containing Krebs- Henseleit solutions. Results also showed garlic juice inhibited the spontaneous movements of rabbit jejunum and guinea pig ileum and inhibited the force of contraction of isolated rabbit hearts in a concentration-dependent manner. All inhibitions were reversible.

> —M.B. Aqel, et al., "Direct Relaxant Effects of Garlic Juice on Smooth and Cardiac Muscles," *Journal of Ethnopharmacology,* 33(1-2), May-June 1991, p. 13-19.

This study evaluated a popular garlic preparation containing 1.3% allicin at a 2400 mg dose in 9 severe hypertension patients. Results showed that sitting blood pressure fell 7/16 (+/-3/2 SD) mm Hg at peak effect approximately 5 hours after the dose, with a significant decrease in diastolic blood pressure from 5-14 hours following the dose.

> —F.G. McMahon & R. Vargas, "Can Garlic Lower Blood Pressure? A Pilot Study," *Pharmacotherapy,* 13(4), July-August 1993, p. 406-407.

This study examined the effects of eating one fresh clove of garlic per day for 16 weeks on platelet thromboxane production in a group of middle-aged men. Results showed there to be an approximately 20% reduction of serum cholesterol and 80% reduction in serum thromboxane following garlic consumption.

> —M. Ali & M. Thomson, "Consumption of a Garlic Clove a Day Could be Beneficial in Preventing Thrombosis," *Prostaglandins Leukot Essent Fatty Acids,* 53(3), September 1995, p. 211-212.

Results of this double-blind, placebo-controlled study on subjects with cerebrovascular risk factors showed that daily ingestion of 800 mg of powdered garlic over 4 weeks led to a significant inhibition of the pathologicaly increased ratio of cirulating platelet aggregates and of spontaneous platelet aggregation.

> —H. Kieswetter, et al., "Effect of Garlic on Platelet Aggregation in Patients with Increased Risk of Juvenille Ischaemic Attack," *European Journal of Pharmacology,* 45, 1993, p. 333-336.

This meta-analysis of eight trials on the effects of 600-900 mg per day of dried garlic powder administered for 12 weeks on blood pressure found that it was of benefit in some patients with hypertension.

> —C.A. Silagy & A.W. Neil, "A Meta-Analysis of the Effect of Garlic on Blood Pressure," *Journal of Hypertension,* 12, 1994, p. 463-468.

This study examined the effects of a 2400 mg dose of garlic preparation containing 1.3% allicin on 9 patients with severe hypertension. Results showed drops in sitting blood pressure of 7/16 (+/- 3/2 SD) mm Hg at peak effect approximately 5 hours after the dose. Significant drops in diastolic blood pressure occurred 5-14 hours following the dose.

> —F.G. McMahon & R. Vargas, "Can Garlic Lower Blood Pressure? A Pilot Study," *Pharmacotherapy,* 13(4), July-August 1993, p. 406-407.

Results of this in vitro study indicate that ajoene, isolated from the extracts of garlic, prevents thrombus formation both at low and high shear rate in circulated whole blood. Such effects appear to be dependent on ajoene's inhibition of fibrinogen binding. The authors conclude that ajoene might be useful in the acute prevention of thrombus formation induced by vascular damage.

> —R. Apitz-Castro, et al., "Effect of Ajoene, the Major Antiplatelet Compound from Garlic, on Platelet Thrombus Formation," *Thrombosis Research,* 68, 1992, p. 145-155.

Cognitive Function

Results of this study showed that the chronic dietary administration of aged garlic extract improved spatial learning in senescence-accelerated mice.

> —T. Moriguchi, et al., "Aged Garlic Extract Prolongs Longevity and Improves Spatial Memory Deficit in Senescence-accelerated Mouse," *Biol Pharm Bull,* 19(2), February 1996, p. 305-307.

Results of this study showed that the chronic dietary administration of aged garlic extract improved memory retention in senescence-accelerated mice.

> —T. Moriguchi, et al., "Prolongation of Life Span and Improved Learning in the Senescence Accelerated Mouse Produced by Aged Garlic Extract," *Biol Pharm Bull,* 17(12), December 1994, p. 1589-1594.

Cytomegalovirus

This study examined the in vitro antiviral activity of garlic extract on human cytomegalovirus by tissue culture, plaque reduction and early antigen assay. Results found a dose dependent inhibitory effect when garlic was applied simultaneously with cytomegalovirus.

> —N.L. Guo, et al., "Demonstration of the Anti-viral Activity of Garlic Extract Against Human Cytomegalovirus in Vitro," *Chinese Medical Journal,* 106(2), February 1993, p. 93-96.

Diabetes

Results of this study showed that S-methyl cysteine sulphoxide, a sulphur containing amino acid isolated from onion exhibited antidiabetic and antihyperlipidemic effects in rats.

> —K. Kumari, et al., "Antidiabetic and Hypolipidemic Effects of S-methyl Cysteine Sulfoxide Isolated from Allium Cepa Linn," *Indian J Biochem Biophys,* 32(1), February 1995, p. 49-54.

Results of this study showed that S-allyl cysteine sulphoxide, a sulphur containing amino acid of garlic which is the precursor of allicin and garlic oil, exhibited significant antidiabetic effects in rats.

> —C.G. Sheela & K.T. Augusti, "Antidiabetic Effects of S-allyl Cysteine Sulphoxide Isolated from Garlic Allium Sativum Linn," *Indian Journal of Exp Biol,* 30(6), June 1992, p. 523-526.

In this study, the administration of S-allyl cysteine sulphoxide (SACS), a sulphur containing amino acid of garlic which is the precursor of allicin and garlic oil, to rats at doses of 200 mg/kg per body weight significantly reduced the concentration of serum lipids, blood glucose and activities of serum enzymes like alkaline phosphatase, acid phosphatase and lactate dehydrogenase and liver glucose-6-

phosphatase. Results also showed that it significantly increased liver and intestinal HMG CoA reducatase activity liver hexokinase activity.

> —C.G. Sheela & K.T. Augusti, "Antidiabetic Effects of S-Allyl Cysteine Sulphoxide Isolated from Garlic Allium Sativum Linn," *Indian Journal of Experimental Biology,* 30(6), June 1992, p. 523-526.

This study found that rats intravenously administered 50 mg per day of garlic oil showed a 64% reduction in blood and urine glucose levels after 29 days compared to controls. Reduction in the elevated serum total esterified fatty acids and serum cholesterol levels were also seen in the diabetic rats on garlic oil.

> —G.I. Adoga & M.B. Ibrahim, "Effect of Garlic Oil on Some Biochemical Parameters in Streptozotoicn-Induced Diabetic Rats," *Medical Sciences Research,* 18, 1990, p. 859-860.

This study examined the blood sugar lowering effects of an ether-soluble and steam-volatile hypoglycemic principle from common onions in alloxan-induced diabetic rabbits. Results showed the principle to have significant blood sugar lowering effects relative to controls.

> —K.T. Augusti, "Studies on the Effects of Hypoglycemic Principle from Allium Cepa Linn.," *Indian Journal of Medical Research,* 61, July 1973, p. 1066-1071.

General

Results of this study showed that the garlic compound ajoene exhibited broad-spectrum antimicrobial activity in vitro, inhibiting the growth of such bacteria as Bacillus cereus, Bacillus subtilis, Mycobacterium smegmatis, Streptomyces griseus, Staphylococcus aureus, Lactobacillus plantarum, Escherichia coli, Klebsiella pneumoniae, and Xanthomonas maltophilia.

> —R. Naganawa, et al., "Inhibition of Microbial Growth by Ajoene, a Sulfur-containing Compound Derived from Garlic," *Appl Environ Microbiol,* 62(11), November 1996, p. 4238-4242.

Results of this study showed that aqueous extracts of both garlic and onion exhibited inhibitory effects on various Gram-positive organisms, Gram-negative organisms, and fungi. Garlic exhibited the strongest such effects of the two.

> —E.I. Elnima, et al., "The Antimicrobial Activity of Garlic and Onion Extracts," *Pharmazie,* 38(11), November 1983, p. 747-748.

This study examined the in vitro effects of garlic on H202-induced oxidant injury in bovine pulmonary artery endothelial cells. Results suggest that aged garlic extract contains certain radical scavengers that could be beneficial for prevention of cancer, atherosclerosis, and for retardation of the aging process.

> —T. Yamasaki, et al., "Garlic Extract Protects Vascular Endothelial Cells from Oxidant Injury," *Proceedings of the Annual Meeting of the American Association of Cancer Researchers,* 34, 1993, p. A3299.

The effects of aged garlic extract (AGE) on longetivity and learning and memory performances were studied in the senescence accelerated mouse (SAM). A solid diet containing 2% (w/w) AGE was given to SAM from 2 months of age. The survival ratio of SAM P8, senescence accelerated animals, treated with AGE was significantly higher than that of untreated controls. AGE, however, did not affect the life span of SAM R1, a remescence-resistant strain. AGE had no effect on body weight and motor activity. In the passive and conditioned avoidance tests, AGE markedly improved a memory acquisition process in the step-down test and in an acquisition stage in lever-press test in SAM R1. These results suggest the possibility that AGE might be useful for treating physiological aging and age-related memory deficits in humans.

> —T. Moriguchi, et al., ''Prolongation of Life Span and Improved Learning in the Senescence Accelerated Mouse Produced by Aged Garlic Extract,'' *Biol Pharm Bull,* 17(12), December 1994, p. 1589-1594.

In an in vitro study, the effects of garlic extract and one of its components S-allyl cysteine (SAC) was evaluated for its effect on hydrogen peroxide-induced injury using bovine pulmonary artery endothelial cells. Pretreatment with the age garlic extract (AGE) at 2 to 4 mg/ml and 4 mg/ml significantly reveresed the loss of cell viability induced by 50 and 100 um of H202 AGE or SAC also exhibited a dose-dependent inhibition of both LDL release and lipid peroxidation induced by 50 um of H202 . These results showed that both AGE and SAC can protect vascular endeothelial cells from oxidant injury. The data suggest that these compound may be useful for the retardation of aging process and for the prevention of cancer in atherosclerosis.

> —T. Yamasaki, ''Garlic Compounds Protect Vascular Endothelial Cells from Hydrogen Peroxide-Induced Oxidant Injury,'' *Phytotherapy Research,* 8, 1994, p. 408-412.

Results of this study found that alloxan diabetic rats orally administered a combination of onion, garlic, sulfoxide amino acids, S-methylycsteine sulfoxide, and S-allycysteine sulfoxide experienced an amelioration of symptoms relative to rats treated with glibebclamide and insulin.

> —C.G. Sheela, et al., ''Anti-diabetic Effects of Onion and Garlic Sulfoxide Amino Acids in Rats,'' *Planta Med,* 61, 1995, p. 356-357.

Hepatopulmonary Syndrome

This study reports on the case of a patient with severe hepatopulmonary syndrome who failed somatostatin therapy and declined liver transplantation, but took large daily doses of powdered garlic. Following the garlic consumption, she has experienced partial palliation of her symptoms and some objective signs of improvement over 18 months.

> —S.H. Caldwell, et al., ''Ancient Remedies Revisted: Does Allium Sativum Palliate the Hepatopulmonary Syndrome?'' *Journal of Clnical Gastroenterology,* 15(3), October 1992, p. 248-250.

Liver Damage

In this study, 10 organosulfur compound from garlic and onions were studied for their modifying effects on dietthlnitrosamine-induced neoplasia of liver in rats. Results showed that high doses of diallyl sulfide, diallyl trisulfide, allyl methyl sulfide, allyl methyl trisulfide, and dipropyl sulfide had enhancing effects on focus formation while high doses of methyl propyl disulfide and propylene sulfide significantly decreased the number of glutathione S-transferase placental form-positive foci.

> —N. Takada, et al., ''Enhancement by Organosulfur Compounds from Garlic and Onions of Diethylnitrosamine-induced Gluthathione S-transferase Positive Foci in the Rat Liver,'' *Cancer Research,* 54(11), June 1, 1994, p. 2895-2899.

Meningitis

Results of this study showed that the intravenous administration of a garlic extract in two cryptococcal meningitis patients and three additional patients with other forms of meningitis increased plasma titers of anti-Cryptococcus neoformans activity twofold over preinfusion titers.

> —L.E. Davis, et al., ''Antifungal Activity in Human Cerebrospinal Fluid and Plasma after Intravenous Administration of Allium Sativum,'' *Antimicrob Agents Chemother,* 34(4), April 1990, p. 651-653.

■ GINKGO BILOBA

Aging

Results of this study indicated that Ginkgo biloba extract had a restorative effect on the neuronal membrane of in aging rats.

> —F. Huguet, et al., ''Decreased cerebral 5-HT1A Receptors During Ageing: Reversal by Ginkgo Biloba Extract (EGb 761),'' *Journal of Pharm Pharmacol,* 46(4), April 1994, p. 316-318.

Results of this double-blind, placebo-controlled, found that Ginkgo biloba extract proved effective against aging-induced cerebral disorders in humans.

> —J. Taillandier, et al., [Treatment of Cerebral Aging Disorders with Ginkgo Biloba Extract. A Longitudinal Multicenter Double-blind Drug vs. Placebo Study], *Presse Med,* 15(31), September 25, 1986, p. 1583-1587.

This review article cites numerous studies supporting the use of Ginkgo biloba in the treatment of various conditions associated with cerebral aging.

> —M. Allard, [Treatment of the Disorders of Aging with Ginkgo Biloba Extract. From Pharmacology to Clinical Medicine], *Presse Med,* 15(31), September 25, 1986, p. 1540-1545.

Anti-Clastogenic Effects

Results of this study showed that the administration of Ginkgo biloba leaves at doses of 120 mg per day for 2 months reduced plasma clastogenic activity to control levels when measured on the first day following treatment in workers exposed to high levels of radiation from the Chernobyl accident. Such positive effects lasted for a minimum of 7 months.

> —I. Emerit, et al., ''Clastogenic Factors in the Plasma of Chernobyl Accident Recovery Workers: Anticlastogenic Effect of Ginkgo Biloba Extract,'' *Radiat Res,* 144(2), November 1995, p. 198-205.

Results of this study of a small number of Chernobyl workers exposed to radiation showed either regression or total disappearance of plasma clastogenic factors following two months of Gingko biloba extract administered in doses of 120 per day.

> —I. Emerit, et al., ''Radiation-induced Clastogenic Factors: Anticlastogenic Effect of Ginkgo Biloba Extract,'' *Free Radic Biol Med,* 18(6), June 1995, p. 985-991.

Brain Function/Injury

Results of this study found that rats suffering from brain lesions which received treatment with 100 mg/kg Ginkgo biloba extract (GBE) intraperitoneally for 30 days experienced less impairment and a reduction in brain swellings induced by lesions than rats treated with saline or sham controls.

> —M.J. Attella, et al., "Ginkgo Biloba Extract Facilitates Recovery from Penetrating Brain Injury in Adult Male Rats," *Exp Neurol*, 105(1), July 1989, p. 62-71.

This study examined the effects of 100 mg/kg per os of Ginkgo biloba extract for 14 days on electroconvulsive shock induced accumulation of free fatty acids and diacylglycerols in the cerebral cortex and hippocampus of rats. Results found that Ginkgo biloba extract reduced the FFA pool size by 33% and increased the DAG pool by 36% in the hippocampus. A delay of 10 s to 1 min was seen in the rise of DAG content triggered in the cortex and hippocampus by ECS following Gingko biloba treatment, while DAG content showed a more rapid decrease following tonic seizure in rats treated with Gingko biloba relative to sham controls in the hippocampus and cortex.

> —E.B. Rodriguez de Turco, et al., "Decreased Electroconvulsive Shock-induced Diacylglycerols and Free Fatty Acid Accumulation in the Rat Brain by Ginkgo Biloba Extract (EGb 761): Selective Effect in Hippocampus as Compared with Cerebral Cortex," *Journal of Neurochemistry,* 61(4), October 1993, p. 1438-1444.

This study examined the effects of Ginkgo biloba on cerebral edema in rats intoxicated with triethyltin chloride. Results showed severe edema with extensive vacuolization in the cerebral and cerebellar white matter, while significant decrease in these manifestations were seen of the cytotoxic edema when rats received the Ginkgo bilobo extract. Such findings prompted the authors to conclude that Ginkgo biloba extract has a protective effect on cytotoxic edema development in the brain's white matter.

> —M. Otani, et al., "Effect of an Extract of Ginkgo Biloba on Triethyltin-induced Cerebral Edema," *Acta Neuropathol,* 69(1-2), 1986, p. 54-65.

Results of this study found that rats pretreated with a Ginkgo Biloba extract prior to unilateral embolization of the brain experienced suppressed effects of the embolization relative to controls which was due to an apparent increase in the blood flow associated with normalization of cellular energy.

> —L.M. Le Poncin, et al., "Effects of Ginkgo Biloba on Changes Induced by Quantitative Cerebral Microembolization in Rats," *Arch Int Pharmacodyn Ther,* 243(2), February 1980, p. 236-244.

In this double-blind, placebo-controlled study, patients with classical symptoms of organic syndrome were tested for the therapeutic effects of Ginkgo biloba extract administered in doses of 120 mg per day for 8 weeks. Results showed a significant improvement after 4 and 8 weeks of therapy with respect to both saccadic test and the psychometric tests relative to controls.

> —B. Hofferberth, [The Effect of Ginkgo Biloba Extract on Neurophysiological and Psychometric Measurement Results in Patients with Psychotic Organic Brain Syndrome. A Double-blind Study Against Placebo], *Arzneimittelforschung,* 39(8), August 1989, p. 918-922.

Results of this meta-analysis involving 7 double-blind, placebo-controlled clinical trials found Ginkgo biloba extract (mean dose of 150 mg per day) significantly effective in reducing clinical symptoms associated with cerebrovascular insufficiency in old age.

> —W. Hopfenmuller, [Evidence for a Therapeutic Effect of Ginkgo Biloba Special Extract.

Meta-analysis of 11 Clinical Studies in Patients with Cerebrovascular Insufficiency in Old Age], *Arzneimittelforschung,* 44(9), September 1994, p. 1005-1013.

This double-blind, placebo-controlled study examined the effects of 120 mg per day of Ginkgo biloba extract on the central nervous system in geriatric patients with cerebral insufficiency. Results found that chronic Ginkgo biloba extract supplementation led to clear improvement in vigilance as measured in the resting EEG among a subclassification of the subjects.
—B. Gessner, et al., "Study of the Long-term Action of a Ginkgo Biloba Extract on Vigilance and Mental Performance as Determined by Means of Quantitative Pharmaco-EEG and Psycho-metric Measurements," *Arzneimittelforschung,* 35(9), 1985, p. 1459-1465.

This review article cites numerous studies supporting the effectiveness of Ginkgo biloba extract (mean dose being 120 mg per day for 4-6 weeks) in the treatment of cerebral insufficiency.
—J. Kleijnen & P. Knipschild, "Ginkgo Biloba for Cerebral Insufficiency," *British Journal of Clinical Pharmacology,* 34(4), October 1992, p. 352-358.

Results of this study showed the Ginkgo biloba extract significantly improved the NaNO and memory impaired by scopolamine in mice.
—C. Chen, et al., [Improvement of Memory in Mice by Extracts from Leaves of Ginkgo Biloba L.], *Chung Kuo Chung Yao Tsa Chih,* 16(11), November 1991, p. 681-683.

Results of this double-blind, placebo-controlled study found that elderly subjects with age-related memory impairment experienced significant improvement in the speed of information processing following treatment with either 320 or 600 mg of Ginkgo biloba extract 1 hour prior to performing a dual-code test.
—H. Allain, et al., "Effect of Two Doses of Ginkgo Biloba Extract (EGb 761) on the Dual-coding Test in Elderly Subjects," *Clin Ther,* 15(3), May-June 1993, p. 549-558.

In this double-blind, placebo-controlled study, patients over 50 with some level of memory impairment received treatment with oral doses of 120 mg of Ginkgo biloba per day. Results found that Ginkgo biloba had significant beneficial effects on cognitive function at both 12 and 24 weeks.
—G.S. Rai, et al., "A Double-blind, Placebo Controlled Study of Ginkgo Biloba Extract ('tanakan') in Elderly Outpatients with Mild to Moderate Memory Impairment," *Curr Med Res Opin,* 12(6), 1991, p. 350-355.

Results of this double-blind, placebo-controlled study showed that Ginkgo biloba extract significantly improved memory after 6 weeks of treatment and learning rate after 24 weeks in cerebral insufficiency outpatients.
—E. Grassel, [Effect of Ginkgo-biloba Extract on Mental Performance: Double-blind Study Using Computerized Measurement Conditions in Patients with Cerebral Insufficiency], *Fortschr Med,* 110(5), February 20, 1992, p. 73-76.

Results of this double-blind, placebo-controlled study of cerebral insufficiency inpatients with depressive mood noted as a leading symptom found that those treated with 160 mg per day of Ginkgo biloba extract experienced a significantly greater degree of clinical improvement than controls.
—F. Eckmann, [Cerebral Insufficiency—Treatment with Ginkgo-biloba Extract. Time of

Onset of Effect in a Double-blind Study with 60 Inpatients], *Fortschr Med,* 108(29), October 10, 1990, p. 557-560.

Results of this randomized, 6-week study of 80 elderly, cererbrovascular disorder patients found that both Ginkgo biloba extract and dihydroergotoxine treatment led to improvements with no significant difference seen between them.

    —G. Gerhardt, et al., [Drug Therapy of Disorders of Cerebral Performance: Randomized Comparative Study of Dihydroergotoxine and Ginkgo Biloba Extract], *Fortschr Med,* 108(19), June 30, 1990, p. 384-388.

In this double-blind, placebo-controlled study, healthy female subjects were given Ginkgo biloba extract in doses of either 120, 240, or 600 mg per day. Results showed significant improvements in memory as measured by the Sternberg technique following treatment with 600 mg of Ginkgo biloba relative to controls.

    —Z. Subhan & I. Hindmarch, ''The Psychopharmacological Effects of Ginkgo Biloba Extract in Normal Healthy Volunteers,'' *International Journal of Clinical Pharmacology Research,* 4(2), 1984, p. 89-93.

Results of this study indicated that Ginkgo biloba extract was effective in aiding recovery of brain function in cats following unilateral vestibular neurectomy.

    —B. Tighilet & M. Lacour, ''Pharmacological Activity of the Ginkgo Biloba Extract (EGb 761) on Equilibrium Function Recovery in the Unilateral Vestibular Neurectomized Cat,'' *Journal of Vestib Research,* 5(3), May-June 1995, p. 187-200.

Results of this study indicated that Ginkgo biloba leaves can decreased increases in oxidative metabolism of rat brain neurons induced by Ca(2+).

    —Y. Oyama, et al., ''Ca(2+)-induced Increase in Oxidative Metabolism of Dissociated Brain Neurons: Effect of Extract of Ginkgo Biloba Leaves,'' *Japanese Journal of Pharmacology,* 61(4), April 1993, p. 367-370.

Results of this study found that visual field damage caused by a chronic lack of blood flow could be reversed by treatment with Ginkgo biloba extract at doses of 160 mg per day for 4 weeks.

    —A. Raabe, et al., [Therapeutic Follow-up Using Automatic Perimetry in Chronic Cerebroretinal Ischemia in Elderly Patients. Prospective Double-blind Study with Graduated Dose Ginkgo Biloba Treatment (EGb 761)], *Klin Monatsbl Augenheilkd,* 199(6), December 1991, p. 432-438.

Results of this study showed that Ginkgo biloba leaf extract produced reversible inhibition of brain monoamine in rats which the authors argue may be a factor responsible for Ginkgo biloba's reported anxiolytic and antistress activities.

    —H.L. White, et al., ''Extracts of Ginkgo Biloba Leaves Inhibit Monoamine Oxidase,'' *Life Sci,* 58(16), 1996, p. 1315-1321.

This study examined the effects of Ginkgo biloba extract on the levels of blood glucose, local cerebral blood flow, and cerebral glucose concentration and consumption. Results found the extract reduced the concentration of cortical glucose and did not change other substrate levels, indicating Ginkgo biloba can inhibit glucose and may play a role in its capacity to protect brain tissue from hypoxic or ischemic damage.

> —J. Krieglstein, et al., "Influence of an Extract of Ginkgo Biloba on Cerebral Blood Flow and Metabolism," *Life Sci,* 39(24), December 15, 1986, p. 2327-2334.

This study examined the effects of Ginkgo biloba extract on the acquisition, performance and retention of mice in an appetite operant condition exercise designed to enhance memory. Results showed that the extract administered at 100 mg/kg per day for a total of 18 weeks enhanced memory processes.

> —E. Winter, "Effects of an Extract of Ginkgo Biloba on Learning and Memory in Mice," *Pharmacol Biochem Behavior,* 38(1), January 1991, p. 109-114.

Results of this series of studies involving rats and mice indicated that the antihypoxidotic activity of Ginkgo biloba extract is carried in its non-flavone fraction.

> —H. Oberpichler, et al., "Effects of Ginkgo Biloba Constituents Related to Protection Against Brain Damage Caused by Hypoxia," *Pharmacol Res Commun,* 20(5), May 1988, p. 349-368.

Results of this study showed that chronic treatment with Ginkgo biloba extract reduced 3H-dihyroalpren-olol binding density as well as in adenulate cyclase activity stimulate by isoproterenol in the cerebral cortex of rats.

> —N. Brunello, et al., "Effects of an Extract of Ginkgo Biloba on Noradrenergic Systems of Rat Cerebral Cortex," *Pharmacol Res Commun,* 17(11), November 1985, p. 1063-1072.

Results of this study showed that Panax ginseng and Ginkgo biloba administered in combination improved the retention of learned behavior in rats in a dose-dependent manner.

> —V.D. Petkov, et al., "Memory Effects of Standardized Extracts of Panax Ginseng (G115), Ginkgo Biloba (GK 501) and their Combination Gincosan (PHL-00701)," *Planta Med,* 59(2), April 1993, p. 106-114.

The authors of this extensive review article on the clinical psychopharmacology of Gingko biloba extract concluded that the extract appears to be effective in treating vascular disorders, dementia, and cognitive disorders secondary to depression. The authors also suggest that there are no risks associated with taking the drug in doses well above its recommended levels.

> —D.M. Warburton, [Clinical Psychopharmacology of Ginkgo Biloba Extract], *Presse Med,* 15(31), September 25, 1986, p. 1595-1604.

Results of this double-blind, placebo-controlled study found that Ginkgo biloba extract administered to patients suffering from senile macular degeneration showed significant improvements in lost distance visual acuity relative to controls.

> —D.A. Lebuisson, et al., [Treatment of Senile Macular Degeneration with Ginkgo Biloba Extract. A Preliminary Double-blind Drug vs. Placebo Study], *Presse Med,* 15(31), September 25, 1986, p. 1556-1558.

Results of this study found the administration of Ginkgo biloba to gerbils with experimentally-induced cerebral ischameia led to significant degrees of normalization of mitochondrial respiration, diminution of cerebral oedema, correlation of the accompanying ionic perturbation, and near complete functional restoration as seen by a normal neurological index.

 —B. Spinnewyn, et al., [Effects of Ginkgo Biloba Extract on a Cerebral Ischemia Model in Gerbils], *Presse Med,* 15(31), September 25, 1986, p. 1511-1555.

This review article notes that Ginkgo biloba extract limits cerebral oedema formation (be if of cytotoxic or vasogenic origin) and suppresses its neurological consequences.

 —A. Etienne, et al., [Mechanism of Action of Ginkgo Biloba Extract in Experimental Cerebral Edema] *Presse Med,* 15(31), September 25, 1986, p. 1506-1510.

Results of this study showed Ginkgo biloba extract given to rats partly reestablished glucose consumption in rats subject to either normobaric hypoxia or catotid clamping.

 —J.R. Rapin, et al., [Cerebral Glucose Consumption. The Effect of Ginkgo Biloba Extract], *Presse Med,* 15(31), September 25, 1986, p. 1494-1497.

Results of this study showed that the chronic administration of Ginkgo biloba extract to aged rats increased the muscarinic receptor population in the hippocampus.

 —J.E. Taylor, [Neuromediator Binding to Receptors in the Rat Brain. The Effect of Chronic Administration of Ginkgo Biloba Extract], *Presse Med,* 15(31), September 25, 1986, p. 149-1493.

Results of this study showed that Ginkgo biloba extract exerts a specific effect on the noradrenergic system and on beta-receptors which suggest central effects of a drug acting on cerebral aging, connected specifically to reactivation of the noradrenergic system in the cerebral cortex.

 —G. Racagni, et al., [Neuromediator Changes During Cerebral Aging. The Effect of Ginkgo Biloba Extract] *Presse Med,* 15(31), September 25, 1986, p. 1488-1490.

Results of this study indicated Ginkgo biloba extract proved beneficial in Parkinsonian patients with additional signs of SDAT.

 —E.W. Funfgeld, ''A Natural and Broad Spectrum Nootropic Substance for Treatment of SDAT—the Ginkgo Biloba Extract,'' *Prog Clin Biol Res,* 317, 1989, p. 1247-1260.

This study notes that rats undergoing simultaneous ligature of both carotid arteries results in certain death and about a 50% fatality rate when ligatures are separated by a four day time period. However, when rats receive extracts of Ginkgo biloba leaves prior to the procedure, dopamine synthesis is increased and survival rate is improved.

 —M. Le Poncin-Lafitte, et al., [Cerebral Ischemia after Ligature of Both Carotid Arteries in Rats: Effect of Ginkgo Biloba Extracts], *Sem Hop,* 58(7), February 18, 1982, p. 403-406.

Results of this study showed that pretreatment with Ginkgo biloba leaves partially suppressed the effects of unilateral embolization in the brain of rats.

 —J.R. Rapin, et al., [Experimental Model of Cerebral Ischemia Preventive Activity of Ginkgo Biloba Extract], *Sem Hop,* 55(43-44), December 18-25, 1979, p. 2047-2050.

This review article cites clinical studies supporting efficacy of Ginkgo biloba extracts in the treatment of cerebral insufficiency and atherosclerotic disease of the peripheral arteries.

—A. Z'Brun, [Ginkgo— Myth and Reality], *Schweiz Rundsch Med Prax,* 84(1), January 3, 1995, p. 1-6.

Cardiovascular/Coronary Heart Disease

Results of this study showed that Ginkgo biloba extract improved contractile function following global ischemia in the isolated working heart of rats due its ability to inhibit the formation of oxygen radicals.

—A. Tosaki, et al., "Ginkgo Biloba Extract (EGb 761) Improves Postischemic Function in Isolated Preconditioned Working Rat Hearts," *Coronary Artery Disease,* 5(5), May 1994, p. 443-450.

Results of this showed that the administration of Ginkgo biloba extract over a period of 3 months provided protective effects on the hypoxic myocardium in rats.

—K. Punkt, et al., "Changes of Enzyme Activities in the Rat Myocardium Caused by Experimental Hypoxia With and Without Ginkgo Biloba Extract EGb 761 Pretreatment. A Cytophotometrical Study," *Acta Histochem,* 97(1), January 1995, p. 67-79.

Results of this meta-analysis demonstrated significant therapeutic effects of Ginkgo biloba extract administered to patients suffering from peripheral arterial disease.

—B. Schneider, [Ginkgo biloba extract in peripheral arterial diseases. Meta-analysis of Controlled Clinical Studies], *Arzneimittelforschung,* 42(4), April 1992, p. 428-436.

Results of this single-blind, placebo-controlled study found Ginkgo biloba extract significantly decreased erythrocyte aggregation and increased blood flow in the nail fold capillaries of healthy subjects.

—F. Jung, et al., "Effect of Ginkgo Biloba on Fluidity of Blood and Peripheral Microcirculation in Volunteers," *Arzneimittelforschung,* 40(5), May 1990, p. 589-593.

In this double-blind, placebo-controlled study, patients suffering from peripheral arteriopathy experienced significant improvements in degree of pain free walking distance, maximum walking distance and plethylsmography recordings relative to controls.

—U. Bauer, "6-Month Double-blind Randomised Clinical Trial of Ginkgo Biloba Extract Versus Placebo in Two Parallel Groups in Patients Suffering from Peripheral Arterial Insufficiency," *Arzneimittelforschung,* 34(6), 1984, p. 716-720.

Results of this double-blind, placebo-controlled study showed that the administration of Ginkgo biloba extract for 14 days led to significant improvements in hypoxic hypoxia fixation time of saccadic eye movements and complex choice reaction time in healthy male subjects. The authors argue such findings may be taken as a hypoxia-protective phenomenon.

—K. Schaffler & P.W. Reeh, [Double Blind Study of the Hypoxia Protective effect of a Standardized Ginkgo Biloba Preparation after Repeated Administration in Healthy Subjects] *Arzneimittelforschung,* 35(8), 1985, p. 1283-1286.

This study examined Ginkgo biloba's cardioprotective effects on myocardial ischemia-reperfusion injury in rabbits. Results showed that 10 mg/kg of Ginkgo biloba injected in the coronary artery significantly inhibited increases in lipid peroxidation relative to rabbits receiving saline perfusion. Treatment with Ginkgo biloba also significantly suppressed decreases in tissue type plasminogen activator and the increase in plasminogen activator inhibitor-1 caused by ischemia-reperfusion.

> —J.G. Shen & D.Y. Zhou, "Efficiency of Ginkgo Biloba Extract in Antioxidant Protection Against Myocardial Ischemia and Reperfusion Injury," *Biochem Mol Biol Int,* 35(1), January 1995, p. 125-134.

Results of this study showed that Ginkgo biloba extract inhibited hypoxia-induced reductions in ATP content in endothelial cells in vitro.

> —D. Janssens, et al., "Protection of Hypoxia-induced ATP Decrease in Endothelial Cells by Ginkgo Biloba Extract and Bilobalide," *Biochem Pharmacol,* 50(7), September 28, 1995, p. 991-995.

Results of this study showed that the water-soluble constituents of Ginkgo biloba episperm 100 or 200 mg/kg po inhibited passive cutaneous allergic response in mice. The same doses administered to rats ip inhibited mast cell degranulation. In guinea pigs, it antagonized the antigen-induced contractile effect of isolated ileum smooth muscles and inhibited the deliverance of SRS-A from anaphylactic lung.

> —H. Zhang, et al., [Anti-anaphylactic Pharmacological Action of Water-soluble Constituents of Ginkgo Biloba L. Episperm], *Chung Kuo Chung Yao Tsa Chih,* 15(8), August 1990, p. 496-497.

Results of this study found that the administration of 240 mg per day of Ginkgo biloba for 12 weeks to patients with a history of elevated fibrinogen levels and plasma viscosity as well as a host of different underlying diseases led to significant improvement in fibrinogen levels and hemorrheological properties.

> —S. Witte, et al., [Improvement of Hemorheology with Ginkgo Biloba Extract. Decreasing a Cardiovascular Risk Factor], *Fortschr Med,* 110(13), May 10, 1992, p. 247-250.

Results of this study showed that a single injection of Ginkgo biloba extract at doses of either 50, 100, 150, or 200 mg had positive effects on whole blood visco-eslasticity and microcirculation in patients with pathological visco-elasticity values.

> —P. Koltringer, et al., [Hemorheologic Effects of Ginkgo Biloba Extract EGb 761. Dose-dependent Effect of EGb 761 on Microcirculation and Viscoelasticity of Blood], *Fortschr Med,* 111(10), April 10, 1993, p. 170-172.

Results of this study found that Ginkgo biloba extract provided protection against cardiac ischemia reperfusion injury in isolated rat hearts.

> —N. Haramaki, et al., "Effects of Natural Antioxidant Ginkgo Biloba Extract (EGB 761) on Myocardial Ischemia-reperfusion Injury," *Free Radic Biol Med,* 16(6), June 1994, p. 789-794.

Results of this study showed that Ginkgo biloba extract prevented early ventricular tachycardia by coronary reperfusion in dogs.

> —H.M. Lo, et al., "Effect of EGb 761, a Ginkgo Biloba Extract, on Early Arrhythmia Induced

by Coronary Occlusion and Reperfusion in Dogs,'' *Journal of Formos Medical Association,* 93(7), July 1994, p. 592-597.

In this double-blind, placebo-controlled study, arthritis patients received treatment with Ginkgo biloba extract for sixty-five weeks. Results showed that Ginkgo biloba extract provided significantly more pain relief and walking tolerance after 6 months of taking it than placebo.

> —U. Bauer, [Ginkgo Biloba Extract in the Treatment of Arteriopathy of the Lower Extremities. A 65-week Trial], *Presse Med,* 15(31), September 25, 1986, p. 1546-1549.

This review article makes the following observations with respect to the vascular impact of Ginkgo biloba extract: Its preferential tissue effect in ischaemic areas is primarily explained its direct impact on both arteries and veins, with the drenergic vasoregulatory system and the vascular endothelium being the preferential targets for arterial impact. The extract reinforces the physiological vasoregulation of the sympathetic nervous system directly, by acting on neuromediator release, and indirectly, by inhibiting their extraneuronal degradation by catechol-orthomethyltransferase. It stimulates the release of endogenous relaxing factors like endothelium-derived relaxing factors and prostacyclin. Its action on the venous system has a venoconstrictor component that maintains the degree of parietal tonus essential to the dynamic clearing of toxic metabolites accumulated during tissue ischaemia.

> —M. Auguet, et al., [Pharmacological Bases of the Vascular Impact of Ginkgo Biloba Extract], *Presse Med,* 15(31), September 25, 1986, p. 1524-1528.

Results of this study found that Ginkgo biloba extract injected into rabbits suppressed the vasospasm induced by the topic application of autologous serum on the surface of the brain in a dose-dependent manner.

> —S. Reuse-Blom & K. Drieu, [Effect of Ginkgo Biloba Extract on Arteriolar Spasm in Rabbits], *Presse Med,* 15(31), September 25, 1986, p. 1520-1523.

Results of this study showed that Ginkgo biloba extract induced a significant reduction in the intensity of ventricular fibrillation during reperfusion stage in an in vitro model of ischaemia-reperfusion. The extract also provided protection action against the ischaemia-induced electrocardiographic disorders on normal or hypertrophied hearts in vivo.

> —J.M. Guillon, et al.., [Effects of Ginkgo Biloba Extract on 2 Models of Experimental Myocardial Ischemia], *Presse Med,* 15(31), September 25, 1986, p. 1516-1519.

This article comments on the fact that Ginkgo biloba extract appears to uniformly improve the ultrastructural qualities of vestibular sensorial epithelia when fixed by vascular perfusions. The author suggests that such improvements may be consequential to the effects of the extract on capillary permeability and general microcirculation.

> —J. Raymond, [Effects of Ginkgo Biloba Extract on the Morphological Preservation of Vestibular Sensory Epithelia in Mice], *Presse Med,* 15(31), September 25, 1986, p. 1484-1487.

This study notes that Ginkgo biloba extract has been found to be capable of partially antagonizing the ability of sodium lactate applied on the pia-mater of rabbits to induce the appearance of venous platelets thrombi.

> —M.G. Borzeix, et al., [Researches on the Antiaggregative Activity of Ginkgo Biloba Extract], *Sem Hop,* 56(7-8), February 18-25, 1980, p. 393-398.

In this study, 15 patients with arteriosclerotic lesions in the extracranial brain received an infusion of 250 ml physiological NaCl and 25 ml Ginkgo biloba extract while 15 other patients received 250 ml NaCl only. Results showed that significant increases in perfusion in response to Ginkgo biloba extract relative to controls.

> —P. Koltringer, et al., [Microcirculation in Parenteral Ginkgo Biloba Extract Therapy], Wien *Klin Wochenschr,* 101(6), March 17, 1989, p. 198-200.

Claudication

This review of ten controlled trials on the effects of Ginkgo biloba in the treatment of intermittent claudication concluded the therapy to be effective, but noted the studies reviewed were not of high methodological quality.

> —E. Erns, [Ginkgo Biloba in Treatment of Intermittent Claudication. A Systematic Research Based on Controlled Studies in the Literature], *Fortschr Med,* 114(8), March 20, 1996, p. 85-87.

Results of this double-blind, placebo-controlled study found 120 mg per day of Gingko biloba extract administered for 3 months led to improvements in some cognitive functions in elderly patients with moderate arterial insufficiency.

> —H. Drabaek, et al., [The Effect of Ginkgo Biloba Extract in Patients with Intermittent Claudication], *Ugeskr Laeger,* 158(27), July 1, 1986, p. 3928-3931.

Diabetes

This double-blind, placebo-controlled study examined the effects of Ginkgo biloba on early diabetic retinopathy associated with a blue-yellow dyschromatopsia. Results showed statistical improvement among patients receiving the Ginkgo biloba relative to controls.

> —P. Lanthony & J.P. Cosson, [The Course of Color Vision in Early Diabetic Retinopathy Treated with Ginkgo Biloba Extract. A Preliminary Double-blind Versus Placebo Study], *J Fr Ophtalmol,* 11(10), 1988, 671-674.

Results of this study showed that alloxan-induced diabetic rats treated with Gingko biloba experienced a significantly greater amplitude in electoretinograms than controls.

> —M. Doly, et al., [Effect of Ginkgo Biloba Extract on the Electrophysiology of the Isolated Retina from a Diabetic Rat], *Presse Med,* 15(31), September 25, 1986, p. 1480-1483.

Edema

Results of this study showed that treatment of women suffering from idiopathic cyclic oedema with Ginkgo biloba extract led to complete correction of the biological anomaly in 10 cases receiving oral and 5 receiving intravenous administration.

> —G. Lagrue, et al., [Idiopathic Cyclic Edema. The Role of Capillary Hyperpermeability and its Correction by Ginkgo Biloba Extract], *Presse Med,* 15(31), September 25, 1986, p. 1550-1553.

General

Results of this study found Ginkgo biloba extract to be a scavenger of nitric oxide in vitro acellular systems.

> —L. Marcocci, et al., "The Nitric Oxide-scavenging Properties of Ginkgo Biloba Extract EGb 761," *Biochem Biophys Res Commun,* 201(2), June 15, 1994, p. 748-755.

Results of this study found that Ginkgo biloba extract can prevent radical mediated damage to human membranes caused by cyclosporin A.

> —S.A. Barth, et al., "Influences of Ginkgo Biloba on Cyclosporin A Induced Lipid Peroxidation in Human Liver Microsomes in Comparison to Vitamin E, Glutathione and N-acetylcysteine," *Biochem Pharmacol,* 41(10), May 15, 1991, p. 1521-1526.

Results of this study found that Ginkgo Biloba extract is an effective peroxyl radical scavenger.

> —I. Maitra, et al., "Peroxyl Radical Scavenging Activity of Ginkgo Biloba Extract EGb 761," *Biochem Pharmacol,* 49(11), May 26, 1995, p. 1649-1655.

Results of this study showed that Ginkgo biloba extract's antioxidant activities provided protection against lipoperoxidation of the retina in rats.

> —M.T. Droy-Lefaix, et al., "Protective Effect of Ginkgo Biloba Extract (EGB 761) on Free Radical-Induced Changes in the Electroretinogram of Isolated Rat Retina," *Drugs Exp Clin Res,* 17(12), 1991, p. 571-574.

This study examined the action of Ginkgo biloba extract against superoxide anion under in vitro conditions. Results showed the extract to have an O2- scavenging effect as well as superoxide dismutase activity.

> —J. Pincemail, et al., "Superoxide Anion Scavenging Effect and Superoxide Dismutase Activity of Ginkgo Biloba Extract," *Experientia,* 45(8), August 15, 1989, p. 708-712.

This study examined Ginkgo biloba extract for the release of activated oxygen species during human neutrophils stimulation by a soluble agonist. Results showed that Ginkgo biloba slowed O2 consumption by its inhibitory action on NADPH-oxidase. Results also found that, because of this action, superoxide anion (O-.2) and hydrogen peroxide production was significantly decreased when the PMNs stimulation was done in the presence of the extract at concentrations of 500, 250 and 125 micrograms/ml, while hydroxyl regeneration was decreased at concentrations as low as 15.6 micrograms Gbe/ml, which indicates that the extract also had activity of myeloperoxidase contained in neutrophils.

> —J. Pincemail, et al., "Ginkgo Biloba Extract Inhibits Oxygen Species Production Generated by Phorbol Myristate Acetate Stimulated Human Leukocytes," *Experientia,* 43(2), February 15, 1987, p. 181-184.

Results of this study showed that Ginkgo biloba extract provided protection against free radical attack in vitro following the exposure of rat liver microsomes to UV-C irradiation.

> —E. Dumont, et al., "UV-C Irradiation-induced Peroxidative Degradation of Microsomal Fatty Acids and Proteins: Protection by an Extract of Ginkgo Biloba (EGb 761)," *Free Radic Biol Med,* 13(3), September 1992, p. 197-203.

This review article cites studies supporting the use of Ginkgo biloba in the treatment of hypoxia/ischemia, seizure activity, and peripheral nerve damage.

> —P.F. Smith, et al., ''The Neuroprotective Properties of the Ginkgo Biloba Leaf: A Review of the Possible Relationship to Platelet-activating Factor (PAF),'' *Journal of Ethnopharmacology,* 50(3), March 1996, p. 131-139.

This study examined an extract of Ginkgo biloba's antioxidant activity on healthy human erythrocyte membranes. Results showed that the extract administered at doses of 0, 25, 50, 125, 250 and 500 micrograms/ml indicated its antioxidant potential increased in a dose-dependent manner.

> —K. Kose & P. Dogan, ''Lipoperoxidation Induced by Hydrogen Peroxide in Human Erythrocyte Membranes. 1. Protective Effect of Ginkgo Biloba Extract (EGb 761),'' *Journal of International Medical Research,* 23(1), January-February 1995, p. 1-8.

Results of this case control study showed that Ginkgo biloba extract had a significant protective effect against experimental retinal damage in rabbits.

> —S. Pritz-Hohmeier, et al., ''Effect of In Vivo Application of the Ginkgo Biloba Extract EGb 761 (Rokan) on the Susceptibility of Mammalian Retinal Cells to Proteolytic Enzymes,'' *Ophthalmic Research,* 26(2), 1994, p. 80-86.

Results of this study indicated that Ginkgo biloba extract had excitatory effects on the lateral vestibular nuclei neurons in guinea pigs.

> —T. Yabe, et al., ''Effects of Ginkgo Biloba Extract (EGb 761) on the Guinea Pig Vestibular System,'' *Pharmacol Biochem Behav,* 42(4), August 1992, p. 595-604.

This study examined the effects of 50 mg/kg ip per day of Ginkgo biloba extract on vestibular compensation in unilateral vestibular neurectomized cats. Results found cats treated with the extract recovered faster than controls and that treatment significantly accelerated postural and locomotor balance recovery.

> —M. Lacour, et al., ''Plasticity Mechanisms in Vestibular Compensation in the Cat are Improved by an Extract of Ginkgo Biloba (EGb 761),'' *Pharmacol Biochem Behav,* 40(2), October 1991, p. 367-379.

This article notes that a flavanol glycosides containing Ginkgo bilob L. extract induces a concentration-dependent relaxation of guinea-pig trachea in vitro and antagonizes in vivo bronchoconstriction induced by various agonists.

> —L. Puglisi, et al., ''Pharmacology of Natural Compounds. I. Smooth Muscle Relaxant Activity Induced by a Ginkgo Biloba L. Extract on Guinea-pig Trachea,'' *Pharmacol Res Commun,* 20(7), July 1988, p. 573-589.

Results of this double-blind, placebo-controlled study showed that vertiginous patients treated with Ginkgo biloba extract over 3 months experienced a significant improvement in the intensity, frequency and duration of their condition relative to controls.

> —J.P. Haguenauer, et al., [Treatment of Equilibrium Disorders with Ginkgo Biloba Extract. A Multicenter Double-blind Drug vs. Placebo Study], *Presse Med,* 15(31), September 25, 1986, p. 1569-1572.

This article notes that intravenous administration of Ginkgo biloba extract resulted in dramatic recovery in severe cases of hypovolaemic shock related to monoclonal.

> —G. Lagrue, et al., [Recurrent Shock with Monoclonal Gammopathy. Treatment in the Acute and Chronic Phases with Oral and Parenteral Ginkgo Biloba Extract], *Presse Med,* 15(31), September 25, 1986, p. 1554-1555.

This review article notes that experimental models of ischaemia, oedema and hypoxia, have shown that Ginkgo biloba extract reduced vascular, tissular and metabolic disturbances along with neurological and behavioral consequences associated with them.

> —F. Clostre, [From the Body to the Cell Membrane: The Different Levels of Pharmacological Action of Ginkgo Biloba Extract], *Presse Med,* 15(31), September 25, 1986, p. 1529-1538.

This review article notes that studies have shown Ginkgo biloba to have significant positive effects on the central nervous systems as well as in the treatment of dementia.

> —T. Itil & D. Martorano, ''Natural Substances in Psychiatry (Ginkgo Biloba in Dementia),'' *Psychopharmacol Bull,* 31(1), 1995, p. 147-158.

Hair Growth

Results of this study showed that Ginkgo biloba extract promoted hair regrowth in rats.

> —N. Kobayashi, et al., [Effect of Leaves of Ginkgo Biloba on Hair Regrowth in C3H Strain Mice], *Yakugaku Zasshi,* 113(10), October 1993, p. 718-724.

Hearing Loss

In this study, patients with idiopathic sudden hearing loss existing no longer than 10 days were given treatment with either Ginkgo EGb 761 (Tebonin) + HAES or Naftidrofuryl (Dusodril)+HAES. Results showed that, after one week of observation, 40% of the patients in both treatment groups experienced a complete remission of hearing loss.

> —F. Hoffmann, et al., [Ginkgo Extract EGb 761 (tenobin)/HAES versus Naftidrofuryl (Dusodril)/HAES. A Randomized Study of Therapy of Sudden Deafness], *Laryngorhinootologie,* 73(3), March 1994, p. 149-152.

Results of this double-blind study showed treatment with both Ginkgo biloba extract of nicegoline led to significant recovery in patients with acute cochlear deafness caused by ischemia, with the effects of Ginkgo biloba being markedly stronger.

> —C. Dubreuil, [Therapeutic Trial in Acute Cochlear Deafness. A Comparative Study of Ginkgo Biloba Extract and Nicergoline], *Presse Med,* 15(31), September 25, 1986, p. 1559-1561.

Hepatitis

Results of this study showed that Ginkgo biloba Composita arrested the development of liver fibrosis of chronic hepatitis.

> —W. Li, et al., [Preliminary Study on Early Fibrosis of Chronic Hepatitis B Treated with Ginkgo Biloba Composita], *Chung Kuo Chung Hsi I Chieh Ho Tsa Chih,* 15(10), October 1995, p. 593-595.

Intestinal Disorders

Results of this study showed that Ginkgo biloba extract protected the intestinal mucosa of rats against ischaemic damage through the reduction of lipid peroxidation and neutrophil infiltration.

—T. Otamiri & C. Tagesson, "Ginkgo Biloba Extract Prevents Mucosal Damage Associated with Small-Intestinal Ischaemia," *Scandinavian Journal of Gastroenterology,* 24(6), August 1989, p. 666-670.

Neuropathy

In this study, 10 neuropathy patients with an autonomic disregulation of skin were intravenously administered a combination of 87.5 mg of Ginkgo biloba extract standardized to 21.0 mg Flavonglycosids and 3 mg folic acid over a period of 4 days. Results showed significant improvements in nerve function following treatment.

—P. Koltringer, et al., [Ginkgo Biloba Extract and Folic Acid in the Therapy of Changes Caused by Autonomic Neuropathy], *Acta Med Austriaca,* 16(2), 1989, p. 35-37.

PMS

This double-blind, placebo-controlled study examined the effects of Ginkgo biloba extract on congestive symptoms of PMS in a group of 165 women. Results showed the extract proved to be effective in relieving symptoms, particularly those associated with the breasts.

—A. Tamborini & R. Taurelle, [Value of Standardized Ginkgo Biloba Extract (EGb 761) in the Management of Congestive Symptoms of Premenstrual Syndrome], *Rev Fr Gynecol Obstet,* 88(7-9), July-September 1993, p. 447-457.

Pneumocystis Carinii

Results of these in vitro and in vivo studies showed that sesquiterpene bilobalide, extracted from Ginkgo biloba leaves, might be useful for therapy of and prophylaxis against P. carinii infections in humans.

—C. Atzori, et al., "Activity of Bilobalide, A Sesquiterpene from Ginkgo Biloba, on Pneumocystis Carinii," *Antimicrob Agents Chemothe,* 37(7), July 1993, p. 1492-1496.

Spinal Cord Injury

Results of this double-blind study found that Ginkgo biloba had protective effects against ischaemic spinal cord injury in rats due to its antioxidant activities.

—R.K. Koc, et al., "Lipid Peroxidation in Experimental Spinal Cord Injury. Comparison of Treatment with Ginkgo Biloba, TRH and Methylprednisolone," *Res Exp Med,* 195(2), 1995, p. 117-123.

Stress

This study examined the effects of sub-chronic cold stress on hippocampal 5-HT1A receptors functioning and potential protective effects of Ginkgo biloba extract in old isolated rats. Results showed that the extract prevented the stress-induced desensitization of 5-HT1A.

—F. Bolanos-Jimenez, et al., "Stress-induced 5-HT1A Receptor Desensitization: Protective

Effects of Ginkgo Biloba Extract (EGb 761)," *Fundam Clin Pharmacol,* 9(2), 1995, p. 169-174.

Results of this study found that Ginkgo biloba extract enhanced behavioral adaptation in the face of adverse environmental influences in rats. Such findings suggest it may be useful in the treatment of cognitive impairment in humans.
    —J.R. Rapin, et al., "Demonstration of the "Anti-stress" Activity of an Extract of Ginkgo Biloba (EGb 761) Using a Discrimination Learning Task," *Gen Pharmacol,* 25(5), September 1994, p. 1009-1016.

Results of this study found that mice administered 50 and 100 mg/kg per day of Ginkgo biloba extract prior to unavoidable shock exposure experienced a reduction in subsequent avoidance deficits in learned helplessness.
    —R.D. Porsolt, et al., "Effects of an Extract of Ginkgo Biloba (EGB 761) on "Learned Helplessness" and Other Models of Stress in Rodents," *Pharmacol Biochem Behav,* 36(4), August 1990, p. 963-971.

Tinnitus

Results of this double-blind, placebo-controlled study found that Ginkgo biloba extract treatment led to improvements among patients suffering from tinnitus.
    —B. Meyer, [Multicenter Randomized Double-blind Drug vs. Placebo Study of the Treatment of Tinnitus with Ginkgo Biloba Extract], *Presse Med,* 15(31), September 25, 1986, p. 1562-1564.

■ GINSENG

Adrenal Function

In this study, results of two experiments found that ginseng therapy restored the thyroid and adrenal functions inhibited by dexamethasone treatment in rats.
    —J.H. Lin, et al., "Effects of Ginseng on the Blood Chemistry Profile of Dexamethasone Treatment in Male Rats," *American Journal of Chinese Medicine,* 23(2), 1995, p. 167-172.

Aging

This single-blind study examined the antiaging activities of American ginseng, compound liquor in subjects over 60 years old. Results showed that symptoms of Kidney-Yang deficiency in the treated group were improved much better than controls, with the treated group experiencing a decrease in functional months of age from 751.77 +/- 5.215 to 743.53 +/- 5.144, the effective rate being 68.57%.
    —J. Chui & K.J. Chen, [American Ginseng Compound Liquor on Retard-aging Process], *Chung Hsi I Chih,* 11(8), August 1991, p. 457-460.

Results of this study indicated that 50 mg tablets of Ginseng-Rhizome taken three times a day for two months exhibited antisenility effects and led to the relief of age-related symptoms in a group of middle age and elderly subjects. In addition to these findings, the treatment had significant benefits with respect to coronary heart disease.

—X.Z. Zhao, [Antisenility Effect of Ginseng-rhizome Saponin], *Chung Hsi I Chieh Ho Tsa Chih,* 10(10), October 1990, p. 586-589.

Results of this study showed that Rg1 enhanced the proliferation of lymphocytes and the production of IL-2 in aged rats.

—M. Liu & J.T. Zhang, [Immunoregulatory Effects of Ginsenoside Rg1 in Aged Rats], *Yao Hsueh Hsueh Pao,* 30(11), November 1995, p. 818-823.

Results of this study showed that Rg1 significantly increased intracellular cAMP and cGMP levels in aged rats.

—M. Liu & J.T. Zhang, [Studies on the Mechanisms of Immunoregulatory Effects of Ginsenoside Rg1 in Aged Rats], *Yao Hsueh Hsueh Pao,* 31(2), 1996, p. 95-100.

AIDS/HIV

Results of this study showed that Korean red ginseng exhibited positive effects on immune markers in subjects infected with HIV.

—Y.K. Cho, et al., "The Effect of Red Ginseng and Zidovudine on HIV Patients," *International Conference on AIDS,* 10(1), August 7-12, 1994, p. 215.

Anti-inflammatory Effects

Results of this study showed that the administration of ginsenoside Ro at doses of 10, 50, and 200 mg/kg p.o. reduced chemically-induced acute paw edema in rats and chemically-induced vascular permeability in mice.

—H. Matsuda, et al., "Anti-inflammatory Activity of Ginsenoside Ro," *Planta Medicine,* 56(1), February 1990, p. 19-23.

Antinarcotic Effects

Results of this study found that the Panax ginseng extract G115 significantly inhibited the development of morphine-induced tolerance and physical dependence.

—H.S. Kim, et al., "Antinarcotic Effects of the Standardized Ginseng Extract G115 on Morphine," *Planta Medicine,* 56(2), April 1990, p. 158-163.

Blood Alcohol Clearance

Results of this study showed that the administration of an extract of Panax ginseng at doses of 3 g/ 65 kg body weight 40 minutes after last drink enhanced the rate of blood alcohol clearance in healthy male volunteers.

—F.C. Lee, et al., "Effects of Panax Ginseng on Blood Alcohol Clearance in Man," *Clin Exp Pharmacol Physiol,* 14(6), June 1987, p. 543-546.

Brain Damage

Results of this study showed that ginsenosides exhibited protective effect on cerebral ischemia-reperfusion injury in rats.

—G.X. Chu & X. Chen, "Anti-lipid Peroxidation and Protection of Ginsenosides Against

Cerebral Ischemia-reperfusion Injuries in Rats," *Chung Kuo Yao Li Hsueh Pao,* 11(2), March 1990, p. 119-123.

Results of this study showed that the ginsenoside Rb1 protected the rat brain from experimentally-induced ischemic and reperfusion injuries.

    —Y.G. Zhang & T.P. Liu, "Influences of Ginsenosides Rb1 and Rg1 on Reversible Focal Brain Ischemia in Rats," *Chung Kuo Yao Li Hsueh Pao,* 17(1), January 1996, p. 44-48.

Cancer

This study examined the effects of ginsenoside-Rb2 extracted from Panax ginseng on angiogenesis and metastasis produced by B16-BL6 melanoma cells in mice. Results showed that the intravenous administration of ginsenoside-Rb2 between 1 and 7 days following inoculation with tumor significantly reduced number of vessels oriented toward tumor mass. Oral ginsenoside-Rb 2 administration led to inhibition of tumor growth and neovascularization. Results also found that administration of ginsenoside-Rb2 following B16-BL6 melanoma cell inoculation produced a significant inhibition of lung metastasis relative to controls.

    —K. Sato, et al., "Inhibition of Tumor Angiogenesis and Metastasis by a Saponin of Panax Ginseng, Ginsenoside-Rb2," *Biol Pharm Bull,* 17(5), May 1994, p. 635-639.

Results of this study found that the ginseng saponins, 20(R)- and 20(S)-ginsenoside-Rg3 inhibited lung metastasis of tumor cells both in in vitro and in vivo studies involving mice.

    —M. Mochizuki, et al., "Inhibitory Effect of Tumor Metastasis in Mice by Saponins, Ginsenoside-Rb2, 20(R)- and 20(S)-ginsenoside-Rg3, of Red Ginseng," *Biol Pharm Bull,* 18(9), September 1995, p. 1197-1202.

Results of this study showed that the local use of bioginseng and germanium-selective drugs produced by cultivating ginseng radix cell in a medium containing organogermanium or a conventional medium were effective in inhibiting DMBA-induced squamous-cell carcinomas of the uterus cervix and vagina.

    —V.G. Bespalov, et al., [The Inhibition of the Development of Experimental Tumors of the Cervix Uteri and Vagina by Using Tinctures of the Cultured-cell Biomass of the Ginseng Root and its Germanium-Selective Stocks], *Biull Eksp Biol Med,* 116(11), November 1993, p. 534-536.

Results of this study found that bio-ginseng reduced the rate of spontaneous SCE, mitomycin C-induced chromosome aberrations in Chinese hamster cells, and also protected ascitic tumor cells against the mutagen action of urea nitrosomethyl.

    —N.V. Umnova, et al., [Study of Antimutagenic Properties of Bio-ginseng in Mammalian Cells in Vitro and in Vivo], *Biull Eksp Biol Med,* 111(5), May 1991,. 507-509.

This study examined the effects of oral Korean red ginseng on chemical-induced carcingogenesis in newborn mice. Results showed that long-term use of the ginseng inhibited both the incidence and proliferation of tumors.

    —T.K. Yun, et al., "Anticarcinogenic Effect of Long-term Oral Administration of Red Ginseng on Newborn Mice Exposed to Various Chemical Carcinogens," *Cancer Detect Prev,* 6(6), 1983, p. 515-525.

Results of this Korean case-control study showed an inverse association between oral intake of different types of ginseng and the risk of various cancers in humans including lip, oral cavity, pharynx, esophageal, stomach, colorectal, liver, pancreatic, laryngeal, lung, and ovarian.

—T.K. Yun & S.Y. Choi, "Preventive Effect of Ginseng Intake Against Various Human Cancers: A Case-control Study on 1987 Pairs," *Cancer Epidemiol Biomarkers Prev,* 4(4), June 1995, p. 401-408.

Results of this study reported the isolation of a new type of cell growth inhibitory substance from the root of Panax ginseng. Findings showed that the extract administered intramuscularly produced significant inhibition of melanoma tumor growth in mice.

—M. Katano, et al., [Cell Growth Inhibitory Substance Isolated from Panax Ginseng Root: Panaxytriol], *Gan To Kagaku Ryoho,* 17(5), May 1990, p. 1045-1049.

Results of this Korean case-control study found an inverse association between a history of ginseng intake and the risk of cancer in human subjects. Ginseng extract and powder proved more effective than fresh sliced ginseng, the juice, or tea in reducing cancer risk.

—T.K. Yun & S.Y. Choi, "A Case-control Study of Ginseng Intake and Cancer," *International Journal of Epidemiology,* 19(4), December 1990, p. 871-876.

Results of this study showed that the Panax ginseng ginsenoside Rh2 inhibited tumor incidence and growth in nude mice bearing HRA cells.

—T. Tode, et al., "Inhibitory Effects by Oral Administration of Ginsenoside Rh2 on the Growth of Human Ovarian Cancer Cells in Nude Mice," *Journal of Cancer Research and Clinical Oncology,* 120(1-2), 1993, p. 24-26.

Results of this study showed that Panax ginseng significantly inhibited DEN-induced hepatocellular carcinoma and extended time of survival in rats.

—X. Li, et al., [Effects of Ginseng on Hepatocellular Carcinoma in Rats Induced by Diethylnitrosamine—A Further study], *Journal of Tongji Med Univ,* 11(2), 1991, p. 73-80.

Results of this study showed that the administration of ether extracts of Korean Panax ginseng at doses of 500 mg/d x 7->11 ip started at 1 day following tumor inoculation led to significant tumor inhibition in mice with solid Sarcoma 180 or adenocarcinoma 755. Ethanol extracts also exhibited significant effects against S-180.

—K.D. Lee & R.P. Huemer, "Antitumoral Activity of Panax Ginseng Extracts," *Japanese Journal of Pharmacol,* 21(3), 1971, p. 299-302.

Results of this study showed that treatment with the ethanol-insoluble fraction of ginseng, Fr. 3, significantly inhibited the incidence of lung tumors in young male mice.

—Y.S. Lee, et al., "Inhibition of Autochthonous Tumor by Ethanol Insoluble Fraction from Panax Ginseng as an Immunomodulator," *Planta Med,* 59(6), December 1993, p. 521-524.

Results of this large-scale study found a significant inverse association between the consumption of ginseng and risk of gastric and lung cancer in adults over the age of 40.

—T.K. Yun & S.Y Choi, "A Prospective Study on Ginseng Intake and Cancer in a Ginseng

Cultivation Area,'' *Proceedings of the Annual Meeting of American Association of Cancer Researchers,* 37, 1996, p. A1906.

Cardiovascular/Coronary Heart Disease

Results of this study showed that injections of ginseng principles fraction 4 reduced elevated plasma levels of cholesterol and triglyceride.

—M. Yamamoto, et al., ''Plasma Lipid-lowering Action of Ginseng Saponins and Mechanism of the Action,'' *American Journal of Chinese Medicine,* 11(1-4), 1983, p. 84-87.

Results of this study showed that Panax ginseng delayed experimentally-induced impairment of rat heart mitochondria and muscle contraction deterioration.

—H.T. Toh, ''Improved Isolated Heart Contractility and Mitochondrial Oxidation after Chronic Treatment with Panax Ginseng in Rats,'' *American Journal of Chinese Medicine,* 22(3-4), 1994, p. 275-284.

Results of this study showed that total ginsenoside and ginsenoside Rb protected against myocardiac ischemic and reperfusion injuries in open heart surgery patients.

—Y. Zhan, et al., [Protective Effects of Ginsenoside on Myocardiac Ischemic and Reperfusion Injuries], *Chung Hua I Hsueh Tsa Chih,* 74(10), October 1994, p. 626-628.

Results of this study found that ginsenosides attenuated ischemic myocardium and protected against reperfusion injury of myocardium in dogs.

—J. Zhang, et al., [Protective Effects of Ginsenosides in Myocardial Ischemia and Reperfusion Injury], *Chung Hua Nei Ko Tsa Chih,* 29(11), November 1990, p. 653-655.

Results of this study found that red ginseng was a safe and effective treatment in patients suffering from congestive heart failure and proved to be synergistic with digoxin in exhibiting even stronger improvement of hemodynamical and biological indexes.

—D.Z. Ding, et al., [Effects of Red Ginseng on the Congestive Heart Failure and its Mechanism], *Chung Kuo Chung Hsi I Chieh Ho Tsa Chih,* 15(6), June 1995, p. 325-327.

Results of this study found that Wisconsion ginseng root powder added to the diet was effective in lowering total serum cholesterol levels of white leghorn chickens.

—A.A. Qureshi, et al., ''Suppression of Cholesterogenesis and Reduction of LDL Cholesterol by Dietary Ginseng and its Fractions in Chicken Liver,'' *Atherosclerosis,* 48, 1983, p. 81-94.

Cognitive Function

This study examined the neuroprotective effects of ginseng roots in 5-minute ischemic gerbils. Red ginseng powder, crude ginseng saponin, crude ginseng non-saponin, and pure ginsenosides Rb1, Rg1 and Ro were administered 7 days prior to ischemia. Results showed that red ginseng and crude ginseng saponin prevented delayed neuronal death.

—T.C Wen, et al., ''Ginseng Root Prevents Learning Disability and Neuronal Loss in Gerbils with 5-minute Forebrain Ischemia,'' *Acta Neuropathol,* 91(1), 1996, p. 15-22.

Results of this study showed that the ginseng containing herbal prescription improved memory retention disorder in the senescence accelerated mouse on a passive avoidance test, increased conditioned avoidance rate in lever press test.

—N. Nishiyama, et al., ''An Herbal Prescription, S-113m, Consisting of Biota, Ginseng and Schizandra, Improves Learning Performance in Senescence Accelerated Mouse,'' *Biol Pharm Bull,* 19(3), March 1996, p. 388-393.

Results of this study showed that the administration of 8 g/kg per day of a Panax ginseng extract over a period of 12-33 days reduced impairment of learning performance on a radial maze task in aged rats.

—H. Nitta, et al., ''Panax Ginseng Extract Improves the Performance of Aged Fischer 344 Rats in Radial Maze Task but not in Operant Brightness Discrimination Task,'' *Biol Pharm Bull,* 18(9), September 1995, p. 1286-1288.

Results of this study found that 50 mg/kg x 7d of ginseng root saponins enhanced the memory and learning of male rats. The same dosage of ginseng stem-leaf saponins had even stronger effects on antielectroconvulsive shock-induced memory impairment.

—A. Wang, et al., [Effects of Chinese Ginseng Root and Stem-leaf Saponins on Learning, Memory and Biogenic Monoamines of Brain in Rats], *Chung Kuo Chung Yao Tsa Chih,* 20(8), August 1995, p. 493-495.

Results of this study showed that repeated administrations of ginseng stem-leaves saponins to rats facilitated learning and memory acquisition in rats.

—T.C. Ma, et al., ''Effects of Ginseng Stem-leaves Saponins on One-way Avoidance Behavior in Rats,'' *Chung Kuo Yao Li Hsueh Pao,* 12(5), September 1991, p. 403-406.

Results of this study showed that the oral administration standardized extracts of Panax ginseng, Ginkgo biloba, and their combination Gincosan exhibited positive effects on learning and memory in young and old rats.

—V.D. Petkov, et al., ''Memory Effects of Standardized Extracts of Panax Ginseng (G115), Ginkgo Biloba (GK 501) and their Combination Gincosan (PHL-00701),'' *Planta Med,* 59(2), April 1993, p. 106-114.

Diabetes

This study examined the effects of a 0.2/200 g ginseng solution on antiperoxidation in myocardium and erythrocytes of streptozocin-induced diabetic rats over a period in 15-16 days. Results showed a significant reduction in the levels of fasting blood-glucose and lipid peroxide in myocardium and erythrocytes relative to controls.

—Z.C. Xie, et al., [Effect of Ginseng on Antiperoxidate Injury in Myocardium and Erythrocytes in Streptozocin-induced Diabetic Rats], *Chung Kuo Chung Hsi I Chieh Ho Tsa Chih,* 13(5), May 1993, p. 289-290.

Results of this study showed that the administration of 50-200 mg/kg ip or sc of ginseng polysaccharides led to a decrease in blood glucose and liver glycogen in mice.

—M. Yang, et al., [Effects of Ginseng Polysaccharides on Reducing Blood Glucose and Liver Glycogen], *Chung Kuo Yao Li Hsueh Pao,* 11(6), November 1990, p. 520-524.

Results of this study identified five substances in ginseng with hypoglycemic and insulin-mimetic principles as evidenced by their effects on both normal and diabetic mice.

> —T.B. Ng & H.W. Yeung, "Hypoglycemic Constituents of Panax Ginseng," *Gen Pharmacol*, 16(6), 1985, p. 549-552.

Results of this study found that an H20 extract of American ginseng roots produced significant hypoglycemic effects on mice.

> —Y. Oshima, et al., "Isolation and Hypoglycemic Activity of Quinquefolans A, B, and C, Glycans of Panax Quinquefolium Roots," *Journal of National Products*, 50(2), March-April 1987, p. 188-190.

Results of this study showed that the intraperitoneal injection of a Siberian ginseng aqueous extract significantly reduced plasma-sugar levels in mice.

> —H. Hikino, et al., "Isolation and Hypoglycemic Activity of Eleutherans A, B, C, D, E, F, and G: Glycans of Eleutherococcus Senticosus Roots," *Journal of Natural Products*, 49(2), March-April 1986, p. 293-297.

Results of this study showed that drugs extracted from ginseng leaves and roots exhibited marked antidiabetic and hepatoprotective effects in rats and mice.

> —V.V. Davydov, et al., [Efficacy of Ginseng Drugs in Experimental Insulin-dependent Diabetes and Toxic Hepatitis], *Patol Fiziol Eksp Ter*, (5), September-October 1990, p. 49-52.

Results of this study showed that 50-200 mg/kg of intravenous ginseng polypeptide isolated from Panax ginseng root reduced blood sugar levels and liver glycogen in rats.

> —B.X. Wang, et al., [Studies on the Hypoglycemic Effect of Ginseng Polypeptide], *Yao Hsueh Hsueh Pao*, 25(6), 1990, p. 401-405.

This review article notes that five substances have been identified as being hypoglycemic and insulino-mimetic principles in ginseng. These are: adenosine, a carboxylic acid, a peptide with a molecular weight of 1400 and lacking in basic amino acid residues, and a fraction designated DPG-3-2 prepared from the water extract of ginseng. The structuree of panaxan A has been partially elucidated and the glycans have been demonstrated to elicit hypoglycemia in both normal and diabetic mice. DPG-3-2 exerted its hypoglycemic action or provoked insulin secretion in diabetic and glucose-loaded normal mice while having no effect on normal mice. Adenosine, the carboxylic acid and the molecular weight 1400 peptide inhibited catecholamine-induced lipolysis in rat epididymal fat pads. EPG-3-2, a fraction related to DPG-3-2, also exhibited antilipolytic activity.

> —T.B. Ng & H.W. Yeung, "Hypoglycemic Consituents of Panax Ginseng," *General Pharmacology*, 16(6), 1985, p. 549-552.

This placebo-controlled study examined the effects of 100 or 200 mg per day of ginseng taken for 8 weeks by newly diagnosed non-insulin-dependent diabetics. Results showed that ginseng elevated mood, improved psychophysical performance, and reduced fasting glucose and body weight. The 200 mg dose improved glycated hemoglobin, serum PIIINP, and physical activity.

> —E.A. Sotaniemi, et al., "Ginseng Therapy in Non-Insulin-Dependent Diabetic Patients," *Diabetic Care*, 18(10), October 1995, p. 1373-1375.

In this study, an acetic acid extract of ginseng root powder enhanced glucose-induced insulin release from an isolated pancreas in the rat.

—Tao Zhang, et al., "Ginseng Root: Evidence for Numerous Regulatory Peptides in Insulino-tropic Activity," *Biomedical Research,* 11(1), 1990, p. 49-54.

Results of this study found that a water extract of American ginseng roots administered to mice produced significant hypoglycemic acitivty.

—Y. Oshima, et al., "Isolation and Hypoglycemic Activity of Quinquefolans A, B, and C, Glycans of Panax Quinquefolium Roots," *Journal of Natural Products,* 50(2), March-April 1987, p. 198-190.

General

Results of this study found that the administration of ginseng extract for 10 days improved learning, memory and physical performance in rats.

—V.D. Petkov, et al., "Effects of Standardized Ginseng Extract on Learning, Memory and Capabilities," *American Journal of Chinese Medicine,* 15(1-2), 1987, p. 19-29.

Results of this double-blind, placebo-controlled study found that the consumption of two capsules containing a preparation of ginseng extract, dimethylaminoethanol bitartrate, vitamins, minerals, and trace elements per day for six weeks increased work capacity due to improved muscular oxygen utilization in healthy male sports teachers.

—G. Pieralisi, et al., "Effects of a Standardized Ginseng Extract Combined with Dimethylami-noethanol Bitartrate, Vitamins, Minerals, and Trace Elements on Physical Performance During Exercise," *Clin Ther* 13(3), May-June 1991, p. 373-382.

This article reviews over 300 studies on ginseng published in China since 1982. Results of such studies have found ginseng to possess a large variety of therapeutic effects on the body including benefits to the central nervous system, cardiovascular system and endocrine secretion, immune function, stress, aging, etc.

—C.X. Liu, et al., "Recent Advances on Ginseng Research in China," *Journal of Ethnophar-macology,* 36(1), February 1992, p. 27-38.

This article notes that experiments have shown that PQS (0.03-3 mg/ml) inhibits the contractility of papillary muscle of guinea pigs, and on depolarized sample of papillary muscle with high potassium, PQS (0.03-o.3 mg/ml) can increase this contractility. Monomer saponin-Re (10 mg/kg), -Rb3 (30 mg/kg) can inhibit the hemodynamic indication of rats, but psuedogisenoside-F11 (10 mg/kg) acts the other way around. These results prove that PQS contains two components of opposite actions.

—X. Chen, et al., [The Effects of Panax Quinquefolium Saponin (PQS) and its Monomer Ginsenoside on Hart], *Chung Kuo Chung Yao Tsa Chih,* 19(10), October 1994, p. 7-20.

Immune Function

Results of this study showed that Panax ginseng exhibited steroid-like activity in vitro and that it may have potentiating effects on T-cell immunity when combined with hydrocortisone.

—S.K. Chong, et al., "In Vitro Effect of Panax Ginseng on Phytohaemagglutinin-induced

Lymphocyte Transformation,'' *International Arch Allergy Appl Immunol,* 73(3), 1984, p. 216-220.

This double-blind, placebo-controlled study examined the effects of Panax ginseng extracts on cell-mediated immune functions in healthy volunteers. Results showed that the consumption of one capsule every 12 hours for 8 weeks of either 100 mg of aqueous ginseng extract or 100 mg of standardized extract led to significant enhancements in chemotaxis, phagocytosis index, phagocytosis fraction, and intracellular killing.

—F. Scaglione, et al., ''Immunomodulatory Effects of Two Extracts of Panax Ginseng,'' *Drugs Exp Clin Research,* 16(10), 1990, p. 537-542.

Results of this study indicated that Panax ginseng possessed immunomodulatory properties in mice. The strongest effects were seen with respect to natural killer cell activity.

—J.Y. Kim, et al., ''Panax Ginseng as a Potential Immunomodulator: Studies in Mice,'' *Immunopharmacol Immunotoxicol,* 12(2), 1990, p. 257-276.

Results of this study showed that the administration of 10 mg/kg of ginsenoside Rg1 over three straight days prior to sheep red cell exposure in mice produced an increase in the number of spleen plaque-forming cells, the titers of sera hemagglutinins and the number of antigen-reactive T-cells. Results also showed that ginsenoside Rg1 increased the number of T-helper cells relative to the total T-cell number and the splenocyte natural killer activity. An augmentation of the production of IL-1 by macrophages was induced by ginsenoside Rg1 as well, and it exhibited direct mitogenic effect on microcultured thymus cells.

—B. Kenarova, et al., ''Immunomodulating Activity of Ginsenoside Rg1 from Panax Ginseng,'' *Japanese Journal of Pharmacology,* 54(4), December 1990, p. 447-454.

This study makes the following observations with respect to the traditional Chinese drugs Ginsenoside. Ginsenoside promotes phagocytic activity of plaque-forming cells, enhances the mitogenesis of T and B lymphocytes primed by mitogens, is involved in the NKC-IFN-IL-2 regulatory system, inhibits tumor cell growth, and antagonizes the suppression of ADCC and NK cytotoxicities in mice with surgical stress.

—G. Yang & Y. Yu, ''Immunopotentiating Effect of Traditional Chinese Drugs—Ginsenoside and Glycyrrhiza Polysaccharide,'' *Proceedings of the Chin Acad Med Sci Peking Union Med Coll,* 5(4), 1990, p. 188-193.

Kidney Damage

Results of this study showed that pretreatment with ginsenosides at intravenous doses of 30 mg/kg body weight 10 minutes prior to warm ischemia had protective effects on the renal function of rabbits.

—Y. Zhang, [Protective Effects of Ginsenosides on Warm Ischemic Damages of the Rabbit Kidney], *Chung Hua I Hsueh Tsa Chih,* 72(2), February 1992, p. 84-85, 127-128.

Sexual Function

Results of this double-blind, placebo-controlled study found that the administration of Korean red ginseng had significant positive effects with respect to penile rigidity and girth, libido and subjective reports of satisfaction relative to controls in patients suffering from erectile dysfunction.

—H.K. Choi, et al., "Clinical Efficacy of Korean Red Ginseng for Erectile Dysfunction," *International Journal of Impotence Research*, 7(3), September 1995, p. 181-186.

Sleep

Results of this study showed that chronic treatment with Panax ginseng extract significantly stabilized sleep-waking disturbances in male rats relative to controls.

—S.P. Lee, et al., "Chronic Intake of Panax Ginseng Extract Stabilizes Sleep and Wakefulness in Food-Deprived Rats," *Neurosci Letters*, 111(1-2), March 26, 1990, p. 217-221.

Stress

This study examined the effects of a Chinese ginseng preparation administered over a period 16-18 days in the drinking water and injection 30-60 minutes prior to experiments in mice exposed to experimentally-induced stress. Results showed that the ginseng exhibited protective effects against shock induced by electroshock, heat, and fatigue.

—U. Banerjee & J.A. Izquierdo, "Antistress and Antifatigue Properties of Panax Ginseng: Comparison with Piracetam," *Acta Physiol Lat Am*, 32(4), 1982, p. 277-285.

Results of this study showed that Vietnamese ginseng crude saponin suppressed the effects of psychological stress in mice.

—T.T. Nguyen, et al., "Crude Saponin Extracted from Vietnamese Ginseng and its Major Constituent Majonoside-R2 attenuate the Psychological Stress- and Foot-shock Stress-induced Antinociception in Mice," *Pharmacol Biochem Behav*, 52(2), October 1995, p. 427-432.

Ulcers

Results of this study showed that a methanol extract of Panax japonicus rhizome exhibited antiulcer effects in rats.

—J. Yamahara, et al., "Anti-ulcer Action of Panax Japonicus Rhizome," *Journal of Ethnopharmacology*, 19(1), January-February 1987, p. 95-101.

Results of this study showed that the Panax ginseng leaf polysaccharide fraction, GL-4, inhibited chemically-induced gastric lesion formation in mice and rats at oral doses of 50 to 200 mg/kg and subcutaneous doses of 50-100 mg/kg.

—X.B. Sun, et al., "Anti-ulcer Activity and Mode of Action of the Polysaccharide Fraction from the Leaves of Panax Ginseng," *Planta Med*, 58(5), October 1992, p. 432-435.

■ GREEN TEA

Cancer

In this case-control study, smoking, alcohol, and green tea were examined as potential stomach cancer risk factors in patients already diagnosed with the disease. Results showed smoking of cigarettes and the consumption of alcohol were associated with an increased risk of stomach cancer while an inverse association was found between the consumption of green tea and stomach cancer.

> —B.T. Ji, et al., "The Influence of Cigarette Smoking, Alcohol, and Green Tea Consumption on the Risk of Carcinoma of the Cardia and Distal Stomach in Shanghai, China," *Cancer,* 77(12), June 15, 1996, p. 2449-2457.

This study examined the inhibitory effects of EGCG and green tea extract chemical-induced duodenal carcinogenesis in mice and glandular stomach and colon cancer in rats. Results found rodent gastrointestinal tract cancer was inhibited by both EGCG and green tea extract.

> —T. Yamane, et al., "Inhibitory Effects and Toxicity of Green Tea Polyphenols for Gastrointestinal Carcinogenesis," *Cancer,* 77(8 Suppl), April 15, 1996, p. 1662-1667.

Results of this study showed that the oral intake of a polyphenolic fraction isolated from green tea in drinking water produced an increase in the activities of antioxidant and phase II enzymes in skin, small bowel, liver, and the lungs of mice. In addition, mice fed the green tea extract for one month experienced a significant increase in glutathione peroxidase, catalase, and quinone reductase activities in small bowel, liver, and lungs, and glutathione S-transferase in small bowel and liver. Based on these findings, the authors suggest green tea may contain chemopreventive properties.

> —S.G. Khan, et al., "Enhancement of Antioxidant and Phase II Enzymes by Oral Feeding of Green Tea Polyphenols in Drinking Water to SKH-1 Hairless Mice: Possible Role in Cancer Chemoprevention," *Cancer Research,* 52(14), July 15, 1992, p. 4050-4052.

This study examined green tea's effects on the tobacco-specific nitrosamine 4-(methylnitrosamino)-1-(3-pyridyl)-1-butanone (NNK)-induced lung tumorigenesis in mice. Over a period of 13 weeks, mice were either administered 2% tea, 560 ppm EGCG, or 1120 ppm caffeine in drinking water. Results showed that NNK-exposed mice developed 22.5 lung adenomas per mouse compared to NNK-treated mice that drank green tea or EGCG as drinking water which developed an average of only 12.2 and 16.1 tumors per mouse, respectively — a significant difference.

> —Y. Xu, et al., "Inhibition of Tobacco-specific Nitrosamine-induced Lung Tumorigenesis in A/J Mice by Green Tea and its Major Polyphenol as Antioxidants," *Cancer Research,* 52(14), July 15, 1992, p. 3875-3879.

This study examined the effects of topically applied green tea extract on experimental-induced skin tumors in mice. Results found the extract inhibited tumor activity in a dose-dependent fashion. Researchers also showed that green tea's major constituent, (-)epigallocatechin-3-gallate (EGCG), produced the strongest inhibition of all specific green tea constituents tested.

> —R. Agarwal, et al., "Inhibition of Skin Tumor Promoter-caused Induction of Epidermal Ornithine Decarboxylase in SENCAR Mice by Polyphenolic Fraction Isolated from Green

Tea and its Individual Epicatechin Derivatives,'' *Cancer Research,* 52(13), July 1, 1992, p. 3582-3588.

This study examined the effects of green and black tea on chemical-induced cancer in mice. Results showed that mice had an average of 8.3 forestomach and 2.5 lung tumors per mice after chemical exposure. For those exposed mice also given green tea as their sole drinking water source, pulmonary tumor rates decreased 44% and tumor multiplicity by 60%. Forestomach tumors dropped by 26% with a 63% drop in tumor multiplicity. Similar results were seen with respect to black tea as well.

—Z.Y. Wang, et al., ''Inhibition of N-nitrosodiethylamine- and 4-(methylnitrosamino)-1-(3-pyridyl)-1-butanone-induced Tumorigenesis in A/J Mice by Green Tea and Black Tea,'' *Cancer Research,* 52(7), April 1, 1992, p. 1943-1947.

Results of this study found that mice given 1.25 or 2.5% green tea extract as the sole source of drinking water prior to exposure to ultraviolet B light experienced a dose-dependent inhibition of skin lesions relative to controls. Similar results were seen in DMBA exposed mice administered green tea as well.

—Z.Y., Wang, et al., ''Inhibitory Effect of Green Tea in the Drinking Water on Tumorigenesis by Ultraviolet Light and 12-O-tetradecanoylphorbol-13-acetate in the Skin of SKH-1 Mice,'' *Cancer Research,* 52(5), March 1, 1992, p. 1162-1170.

This study examined the in vitro and in vivo effects of decaffeinated black and green teas, and the components of tea on mice exposed to experimental carcinogens. Results showed that extracts from both green and black tea as well as their fractions inhibited NNK oxidation and NNK-induced DNA methylation when added to mixtures that included lung microsomes from mice. (-)-Epigallocatechin-3-gallate was the most potent inhibitor of the tea components examined,

—S.T. Shi, et al., ''Effects of Green Tea and Black Tea on 4-(methylnitrosamino)-1-(3-pyridyl)-1-butanone Bioactivation, DNA Methylation, and Lung Tumorigenesis in A/J Mice,'' *Cancer Research,* 54(17), September 1, 1994, p. 4641-4647.

This study compared the effects of black, green, decaffeinated black and decaffeinated green tea on UVB-induced skin carcinogenesis in DMBA-initiated mice. Results showed that UVB-induced skin tumor formation was significantly inhibited by oral administration of 0.63 or 1.25% black tea, green tea, decaffeinated black tea, or decaffeinated green tea as the sole source of drinking fluid 2 weeks prior to and during 31 weeks of UVB treatment. In addition to tumor formation, tumor size was significantly inhibited by the different tea preparations as well.

—Z.Y. Wang, et al., ''Inhibitory Effects of Black Tea, Green Tea, Decaffeinated Black Tea, and Decaffeinated Green Tea on Ultraviolet B Light-induced Skin Carcinogenesis in 7,12-dimethylbenz[a]anthracene-initiated SKH-1 Mice,'' *Cancer Research,* 54(13), July 1, 1994, p. 3428-3435.

This study examined the effects of a topical green tea extract on chemical-induced skin papillomas in mice. Results showed that the extract had both chemopreventive effects against tumor initiation and contains significant protective effects against the progression of tumors as well.

—S.K. Katiyar, et al., ''Protection Against Malignant Conversion of Chemically Induced Benign Skin Papillomas to Squamous Cell Carcinomas in SENCAR Mice by a Polyphenolic

Fraction Isolated from Green Tea,'' *Cancer Research,* 53(22), November 15, 1993, p. 5409-5412.

This study examined the effects of green tea extract on chemical-induced skin tumor promotion in mice. Results showed that topical application of extract doses between 1-24 mg 30 minutes prior to carcinogen exposure led to significant, dose-dependent protection against tumor promotion.

> —S.K. Katiyar, et al., ''Inhibition of 12-O-tetradecanoylphorbol-13-acetate-caused Tumor Promotion in 7,12-dimethylbenz[a]anthracene-initiated SENCAR Mouse Skin by a Polyphenolic Fraction Isolated from Green Tea,'' *Cancer Research,* 52(24), December 15, 1992, p. 6890-6897.

This article reports on the results of ten separate studies which, when taken together, indicated that the oral administration of green tea, i.p. administration of a green tea polyphenol fraction, or i.p. administration of (-)-epigallocatechin gallate either inhibited skin papilloma growth and/or led to their regression in micee exposed to chemical carcinogens.

> —Z.Y. Wang, et al., ''Inhibitory Effect of Green Tea on the Growth of Established Skin Papillomas in Mice,'' *Cancer Research,* 52(23), December 1, 1992, p. 6657-6665.

This study examined the effects of a polyphenolic fraction taken from green tea topically administered to chemical-induced skin tumors in mice 30 minutes prior to carcinogen exposure. Results found the extract inhibited tumor formation and growth.

> —S.K. Katiyar, et al., ''Inhibition of 12-O-tetradecanoylphorbol-13-acetate and Other Skin tumor-promoter-caused Induction of Epidermal Interleukin-1 Alpha mRNA and Protein Expression in SENCAR Mice by Green Tea Polyphenols,'' *Journal of Invest Dermatol,* 105(3), September 1995, p. 394-398.

This review article cites numerous animal studies supporting the anti-skin cancer activities of green tea.

> —H. Mukhtar, et al., ''Green Tea and Skin—anticarcinogenic Effects,'' *Journal of Invest Dermatol,* 102(1), January 1994, p. 3-7.

This population based, case-control study examined the effects of green tea consumption on the risk of esophageal cancer in a group of 902 esophageal cancer patients between the ages of 30-74. Results showed green tea consumption had a significant, dose-dependent protective effect against esophageal cancer in women and significant protective effects in male and female smokers.

> —Y.T. Gao, et al., ''Reduced Risk of Esophageal Cancer Associated with Green Tea Consumption,'' *Journal of the National Cancer Institute,* 86(11), June 1, 1994, p. 855-858.

Results of this study found that green tea polyphenols and EGCg inhibited chemical-induced gastrointestinal tract cancer in rats.

> —Y. Yamane, et al., ''Inhibition of Gastrointestinal Carcinogenesis by EGCg and Green Tea Polyphenols,'' *Current Strategies of Cancer Chemoprevention, 13th International Symposium on Cancer,* July 6-9, 1993, Sapporo, Japan, 1993, p. 22.

Results of this in vitro study showed the polyphenol EGCG, extracted from green tea, differentially downregulated aberrant hyperprolieration in myc oncogene and MTV-initiated cells.

—R. Araki, et al., "Chemoprevention of Mammary Preneoplasia. In Vitro Effects of a Green Tea Polyphenol," *Annals of the New York Academy of Science,* 768, September 30, 1995, p. 215-222.

Results of this series of studies found that the polyphenol EGCG, extracted from green tea, successfully inhibited chemical-induced lung tumorigenesis in rats.

—F.L. Chung, et al., "Inhibition of Tobacco-specific Nitrosamine-induced Lung Tumorigenesis by Compounds Derived from Cruciferous Vegetables and Green Tea," *Annals of the New York Academy of Sciences,* 686, May 28, 1993, p. 186-201.

Results of this study found that the incidence of chemical-induced lung carcinoma was reduced and mean survival time of carcinmoa survival increased in rats administered 2% green tea extract for life than in those (controls) not consuming green tea.

—S.Q. Luo, et al., "Inhibitory Effect of Green Tea Extract on the Carcinogenesis Induced by Asbestos Plus Benzo(a)pyrene in Rat," *Biomed Environ Sci,* 8(1), March 1995, p. 54-58.

This population-based, case-controlled study examined the effects of drinking green tea on the risk of stomach cancer in subjects under the age of 80. Results showed an inverse association between the two variables.

—G.P. Yu, et al., "Green-tea Consumption and Risk of Stomach Cancer: A Population-based Case-control Study in Shanghai, China," *Cancer Causes Control,* 6(6), November 1995, p. 532-538.

This study examined the chemopreventive effects of green tea and coffee among cigarette smokers in healthy males between the ages of 20 and 52. Results showed that the frequencies of sisterchromatid exchange (SCE) in mitogen-stimulated peripheral lymphocytes were elevated significantly in smokers compared to nonsmokers while the frequency of SCE in smokers who consumed green tea was comparable to that of nonsmokers, suggesting green tea can block the cigarette-induced increase in the frequency of SCE.

—J.S. Shim, et al., "Chemopreventive Effect of Green Tea (Camellia sinensis) among Cigarette Smokers," *Cancer Epidemiol Biomarkers Prev,* 4(4), June 1995, p. 387-391.

Results of this study showed that (-)-Epigallocatechin gallate (EGCG), the main polyphenolic constituent of green tea, inhibited metastasis of mouse B16 melanoma cell lines,

—S. Taniguchi, et al., "Effect of (-)-epigallocatechin Gallate, the Main Constituent of Green Tea, on Lung Metastasis with Mouse B16 Melanoma Cell Lines," *Cancer Letters,* 65(1), July 31, 1992, p. 51-54.

Results of this study showed that tannic acid and green tea polyphenols provided significant protective effects against chemical-induced skin tumorigenesis in mice.

—W.A. Khan, et al., "Inhibition of the Skin Tumorigenicity of (+/-)-7 beta,8 Alpha- Dihydroxy-9 alpha,10 alpha-epoxy-7,8,9,10-tetrahydrobenzo[a]pyrene by Tannic Acid, Green Tea Polyphenols and Quercetin in Sencar Mice," *Cancer Letters,* 42(1-2), September-October 1988, p. 7-12.

This study examined the effects of natural antioxidants on chemical-induced mammary gland carcinogenesis in rats. Results showed significantly higher survival rates in the rats treated with antioxidants relative to those on a basal diet only. Those administered green tea experienced a survival rate of 93.8%. which contrasted strongly with a 33% survival rate of the basal diet only rats.

> —M. Hirose, et al., "Inhibition of Mammary Gland Carcinogenesis by Green Tea Catechins and other Naturally Occurring Antioxidants in Female Sprague-Dawley Rats Pretreated with 7,12-dimethylbenz[alpha]anthracene," *Cancer Letters,* 83(1-2), August 15, 1984, p. 149-156.

Results of this study showed that the administration of green tea infusion led to a decrease in the number of lung colonies of mouse Lewis lung carcinoma cells in a spontaneous metastasis system.

> —M. Sazuka, et al., "Inhibitory Effects of Green Tea Infusion on In Vitro Invasion and In Vivo Metastasis of Mouse Lung Carcinoma Cells," *Cancer Letters,* 98(1), November 27, 1995, p. 27-31.

Results of this study showed that epicatechin derivatives of green tea possess antioxidant activity which may contribute to green tea's well-documented anticarcinogenic effects.

> —S.K. Katiyar, et al., "Inhibition of Spontaneous and Photo-enhanced Lipid Peroxidation in Mouse Epidermal Microsomes by Epicatechin Derivatives from Green Tea," *Cancer Letters,* 79(1), April 29, 1994, p. 61-66.

Results of this study indicated that green tea has preventive effects on chemical-induced cancer of the large intestine in mice.

> —P. Yin, et al., "Experimental Studies of the Inhibitory effects of Green Tea Catechin on Mice Large Intestinal Cancers Induced by 1,2-dimethylhydrazine," *Cancer Letters,* 79(1), April 29, 1994, p. 33-38.

Results of this study found that small doses of green tea polyphenol fraction isolates administered 30 minutes prior to carcinogen exposure provided protection against internal organ tumorigenesis in mice.

> —S.K. Katiyar, et al., "Protective Effects of Green Tea Polyphenols Administered by Oral Incubation Against Chemical Carcinogen-induced Forestomach and Pulmonary Neoplasia in A/J Mice," *Cancer Letters,* 73(2-3), September 30, 1993, p. 167-172.

Results of this study showed that green tea extract inhibited tumor promotion by enhancing gap junctional intercellular communication in promoter-treated, rat liver epithelial cells.

> —K. Sigler and R.J. Ruch, "Enhancement of Gap Junctional Intercellular Communication in Tumor Promoter-treated Cells by Components of Green Tea," *Cancer Letters,* 69(1), April 15, 1993, p. 15-19.

Results of this study found that the topical application of a polyphenol fraction of green tea inhibited chemical-induced skin tumor initiation and promotion in mice. The topical application inhibited chemical-induced inflammation, ornithine decarboxylase activity, hyperplasia and hydrogen peroxide formation as well. The individual polyphenolic compounds in green tea (-)-epigallocatechin gallate, (-)-epigallocatechin and (-)-epicatechin gallate were also shown to inhibited mouse epidermis inflammation.

> —M.T. Huang, et al., "Inhibitory Effect of Topical Application of a Green Tea Polyphenol

Fraction on Tumor Initiation and Promotion in Mouse Skin,'' *Carcinogenesis,* 13(6), June 1992, p. 947-954.

Results of this study found that antioxidant catechins from green tea showed antioxidant activity toward hydrogen peroxide and superoxid oxide radical O2-, and prevented hydrogen peroxide and oxygen radical-induced cytotoxicity in mouse hepatocytes and human kertinocytes.

—R.J. Ruch, et al., ''Prevention of Cytotoxicity and Inhibition of Intercellular Communication by Antioxidant Catechins Isolated from Chinese Green Tea,'' *Carcinogenesis,* 10(6), June 1989, p. 1003-1008.

Results of this study showed that green tea polyphenols possess significant skin tumor inhibiting activity in mice exposed to chemical carcinogens.

—Z.Y. Wang, et al., ''Protection Against Polycyclic Aromatic Hydrocarbon-induced Skin Tumor Initiation in Mice by Green Tea Polyphenols,'' *Carcinogenesis,* 10(2), February 1989, p. 411-415.

This study administered green tea extracts as the sole source of drinking water to rats for 4 weeks. Results showed green tea increased the O-demethylation of methoxyresorufin and the dealkylations of ethoxyresorufin and pentoxyresorufin. Increases found in lauric acid and apoprotein levels of CYP1A2 and CYP4A1, and CN(-)-insensitive palmitoyl CoA oxidation as well.

—A. Bu-Abbas, et al., ''Selective Induction of Rat Hepatic CYP1 and CYP4 Proteins and of Peroxisomal Proliferation by Green Tea,'' *Carcinogenesis,* 15(11), November 1994, p. 2575-2579.

Results of this study found that various antioxidants, including green tea catechins, produced chemo-preventive effects against chemical-induced hepatocarcinogenesis in rats.

—M. Hirose, et al., ''Inhibitory Effects of 1-O-hexyl-2,3,5-trimethylhydroquinone (HTHQ), Green Tea Catechins and other Antioxidants on 2-amino-6-methyldipyrido[1,2-a:3',2'-d]imidazole (Glu-P-1)-induced Rat Hepatocarcinogenesis and Dose-dependent Inhibition by HTHQ of Lesion Induction by Glu-P-1 or 2-Amino-3,8-dimethylimidazo[4,5-f]quinoxaline (MeIQx),'' *Carcinogenesis,* 16(12), December 1995, p. 3049-3055.

This study examined the effects of green and black tea on esophageal cancer in rats. Results found that consumption of both teas inhibited chemical-induced tumorigenesis.

—Z.Y. Wang, et al., ''Inhibition of N-nitrosomethylbenzylamine-induced Esophageal Tumorigenesis in Rats by Green and Black Tea,'' *Carcinogenesis,* 16(9), September 1995, p. 2143-2148.

This study examined the effects of green tea polyphenols on stage I and II skin tumors promotion in mice. Results showed that topical application of green tea extract provided significant protection against the formation of skin papilloomas with respect to tumor growth and multiplicity.

—S.K. Katiyar, et al., ''Inhibition of Both Stage I and Stage II Skin Tumor Promotion in SENCAR Mice by a Polyphenolic Fraction Isolated from Green Tea: Inhibition Depends on the Duration of Polyphenol Treatment,'' *Carcinogenesis,* 14(12), December 1993, p. 2641-2643.

This study examined the chemopreventive effects of a green tea water extract against chemical-induced lung tumorigenesis in mice. Results showed clear protective effects against lung and forestomach tumors.

> —S.K. Katiyar, et al., "Protection Against N-nitrosodiethylamine and Benzo[a]pyrene-induced Forestomach and Lung Tumorigenesis in A/J Mice by Green Tea," *Carcinogenesis,* 14(5), May 1993, p. 849-855.

Results of this study showed that green tea polyphenols may act as cancer chemopreventive agents against stage I tumor promotion in mice.

> —S.K. Katiyar, et al., "Protection Against 12-O-tetradecanoylphorbol-13-acetate-caused Inflammation in SENCAR Mouse Ear Skin by Polyphenolic Fraction Isolated from Green Tea," *Carcinogenesis,* 14(3), March 1993, p. 361-365.

This study examined the effects of both oral and topical administration of green tea polyphenols ultraviolet radiation-induced skin cancer in mice. Results showed that both means of application significantly inhibited carcinogenesis, with oral administration providing the strongest level of protection.

> —Z.Y. Wang, et al., "Protection Against Ultraviolet B Radiation-induced Photocarcinogenesis in Hairless Mice by Green tea Polyphenols," *Carcinogenesis,* 12(8), August 1991, p. 1527-1530.

Results of this study showed that green tea extracts had stronger scavenging effects on active oxygen radicals that either vitamin C or vitamin E.

> —B.L. Zhao, et al., "Scavenging Effect of Extracts of Green Tea and Natural Antioxidants on Active Oxygen Radicals," *Cell Biophysics,* 14(2), April 1989, p. 175-185.

Results of this study showed that green tea epicatechin compounds inhibited the mutagenicity and/or chromosomal damage caused by different experimental carcinogens in both bacterial and rat cells.

> —S. Cheng, et al., "Progress in Studies on the Antimutagenicity and Anticarcinogenicity of Green Tea Epicatechins," *Chin Med Sci Journal,* 6(4), December 1991, p. 233-238.

Results of this study showed that green tea extract significantly inhibited radiolabeled thymidine and uridine transport in mouse leukemia cells and potentiated the inhibitory effect of AraC on mouse leukemia as well.

> —Y. Zhen, et al., "Green Tea Extract Inhibits Nucleoside Transport and Potentiates the Antitumor Effect of Antimetabolites," *Chin Med Sci Journal,* 6(1), March 1991, p. 1-5.

This study examined the effects of green tea, coffee, and levamisole on chemical-induced hepatocarcinogenesis in rats. Results showed that all three exhibited such effects, with green tea demonstrating the strongest protection against hepatocarcinogenesis.

> —Y. Li, [Comparative Study on the Inhibitory Effect of Green tea, Coffee and Levamisole on the Hepatocarcinogenic Action of Diethylnitrosamine], *Chung Hua Chung Liu Tsa Chih,* 13(3), May 1991, p. 193-195.

Results of this study showed that regular consumption of green tea may counteract the ill effects of mutagens and/or carcinogens produced in meat cooked under high temperature.

—X.L. Liu, [Genotoxicity of Fried Fish Extract, MeIQ and Inhibition by Green Tea Antioxidant], *Chung Hua Chung Liu Tsa Chih,* 12(3), May 1990, p. 170-173.

Results of this study showed that green tea extracts exhibited strong inhibitory effects against hepatocarcinogenesis in rats.

—G.Z. Qin, [Effects of Green Tea Extract on the Development of Aflatoxin B1-induced Precancerous enzyme-altered Hepatocellular Foci in Rats], *Chung Hua Yu Fang I Hsueh Tsa Chih,* 25(6), November 1991, p. 332-334.

Results of this study showed green tea extract exhibited significant antitumor effects against stomach cancer in rats.

—Y.S. Yan, [Effect of Chinese Green Tea Extracts on the Human Gastric Carcinoma Cell in Vitro], *Chung Hua Yu Fang I Hsueh Tsa Chih,* 24(2), March 1990, p. 80-82.

Results of this study showed that green tea extract inhibits gastrointestinal malignant tumors in rats as well as humans.

—Y.S. Yan, [The Experiment of Tumor-Inhibiting Effect of Green Tea Extract in Animal and Human Body], *Chung Hua Yu Fang I Hsueh Tsa Chih,* 27(3), May 1993, p. 129-131.

Results of this study found that green tea polyphenols exhibited strong antioxidant activity, significantly inhibiting chemical-induced edema in the skin of mice.

—S.J. Cheng, [Inhibitory Effect of Green Tea Extract on Promotion and Related Action of TPA], *Chung Kuo I Hsueh Ko Hsueh Yuan Hsueh Pao,* 11(4), August 1989, p. 259-264.

Results of this study showed that various flavonoid components of green tea, including (-)-epicatechin (EC), (-)-epigallocatechin (EGC), (-)-epicatechin-3-gallate (ECG), and (-)-epigallocatechin-3- gallate (EGCG) exhibited anticarcinogenetic effects in rats.

—Z.Y. Wang, et al., "Interaction of Epicatechins Derived from Green Tea with Rat Hepatic Cytochrome P-450," *Drug Metab Dispos,* 16(1), January-February 1988, p. 98-103.

This study examined the effects of various fruit juices, orange peel, green tea, and low dose vitamin C on endogenous N-nitrosation in Chinese subjects at high risk for gastric cancer. Results showed that endogenous nitrosation was strongly affected by the food compounds studied, pointing to their potential anticancer activities.

—G.P. Xu, et al., "Effects of Fruit Juices, Processed Vegetable Juice, Orange Peel and Green Tea on Endogenous Formation of N-nitrosoproline in Subjects from a High-risk Area for Gastric Cancer in Moping County, China," *European Journal of Cancer Prevention,* 2(4), July 1993, p. 327-335.

In this study, rats were given 2% green tea as their drinking water for 2 weeks prior to carcinogen exposure. Results showed that the green tea was effective in blocking hepatoxicity and DNA oxidative to the liver.

—"Preventive Effects of Green Tea Against Liver Oxidative DNA Damage and Hepatotoxicity in Rats Treated with 2-nitropropane,'' *Food Chem Toxicol,* 33(11), November 1995, p. 961-970.

Results of this study showed that green tea inhibited chemical-induced lung cancers in mice.
—D. Luo and Y. Li, [Preventive Effect of Green Tea on MNNG-induced Lung Cancers and Precancerous Lesions in LACA mice], *Hua Hsi I Ko Ta Hsueh Hsueh Pao,* 23(4), September 1992, p. 433-437.

This study examined the effects of green tea polyphenols on chemical-induced colon cancer in rats. Results showed that mean number of tumors and tumor incidence were significantly reduced in rats administered the green tea than controls.
—T. Yamane, et al., ''Inhibition of Azoxymethane-induced Colon Carcinogenesis in Rat by Green Tea Polyphenol Fraction,'' *Japanese Journal of Cancer Research,* 82(12), December 1991, p. 1336-1369.

Results of this study showed that the consumption of green tea for 10 days prior to carcinogen exposure led to the significant inhibition of pre-cancerous activity in the colon of rats.
—M. Inagake, et al., ''Inhibition of 1,2-dimethylhydrazine-induced Oxidative DNA Damage by Green Tea Extract in Rat,'' *Japanese Journal of Cancer Research,* 86(11), November 1995, p. 1106-1111.

This study examined the effects of green tea polyphenols on colon cancer in rats. Autopsy results showed rats consuming green tea extracts had significantly lower levels of colon cancer than did controls.
—T. Narisawa and Y. Fukaura, ''A Very Low Dose of Green Tea Polyphenols in Drinking Water Prevents N-methyl-N-nitrosourea-induced Colon Carcinogenesis in F344 Rats,'' *Japanese Journal of Cancer Research,* 84(10), October 1993, p. 1007-1009.

This review article notes that studies have clearly demonstrated green tea extract exhibits strong chemopreventive activity in humans in addition to experimental animals.
—A. Komor, et al., ''Anticarcinogenic Activity of Green Tea Polyphenols,'' *Japanese Journal of Clinical Oncology,* 23(3), June 1993, p. 186-190.

The results of this study showed that the administration of the green tea fraction, (-)-epigallocatechin 3-O-gallate (EGCG), to mice via drinking water prevented radiation-induced increase of lipid peroxides in the liver while also prolonging lifespan significantly following lethel levels of whole-body X-irradiation.
—S. Uchida, et al., ''Radioprotective Effects of (-)-epigallocatechin 3-O-gallate (Green-tea Tannin) in Mice,'' *Life Sci,* 50(2), 1992, p. 147-152.

Results of this study found that green tea extracts produced significant inhibition against occupational and dietary carcinogens in mice.
—A. Bu-Abbas, et al., ''Marked Antimutagenic Potential of Aqueous Green Tea Extracts: Mechanism of Action,'' *Mutagenesis,* 9(4), July 1994, p. 325-331.

Results of this study demonstrated the significant antimutation effects of green tea polyphenols in rats exposed to chemical carcinogens.

—Z.Y. Wang, et al., ''Antimutagenic Activity of Green Tea Polyphenols,'' *Mutation Research,* 223(3), July 1989, p. 273-285.

Results of this study showed that hot water extracts from green tea administered to rats 24 hours prior to carcinogen exposure significantly suppressed chromosome aberrations in rat bone marrow cells. Hot water extracts of either black tea or coffee did not produce inhibitory effects, nor did administration of tannic acid or ascorbic acid.

—Y. Ito, et al., ''Chromosome Aberrations Induced by Aflatoxin B1 in Rat Bone Marrow Cells in Vivo and their Suppression by Green Tea,'' *Mutation Research,* 222(3), March 1989, p. 253-261.

Results of this study showed that polyphenol extracts from both green and black tea inhibited chemical-induced mutagenicity in rats.

—Z. Apostolides, et al., ''Inhibition of 2-amino-1-methyl-6-phenylimidazo[4,5-b]pyridine (PhIP) Mutagenicity by Black and Green Tea Extracts and Polyphenols,'' *Mutation Research,* 359(3), April 4, 1996, p. 159-163.

Results of this study found that epigallo-catechin-gallate (EGCg) extracted from Japanese green tea decreased high spontaneous mutations due to altered DNA-polymerase III in a mutator strain of Bacillus subtilis.

—T. Kada, et al., ''Detection and Chemical Identification of Natural Bio-antimutagens. A Case of the Green Tea Factor,'' *Mutation Research,* 150(1-2), June-July 1985, p, 127-132.

Results of this study found that catechins extracted from tea significantly inhibited chemical-induced chromosome aberrations in mice and in CHO cells.

—Y.F. Sasaki, et al., ''The Clastogen-suppressing Effects of Green Tea, Po-lei tea and Rooibos tea in CHO Cells and Mice,'' *Mutation Research,* 286(2), April 1993, p. 221-232.

Results of this study found that (-)-epigallocatechin 3-O-gallate, a primary component of green tea, had an inhibitory effect on the proliferation of mesangial cells.

—T. Yokozawa, et al., ''Inhibitory Effect of Tannin in Green Tea on the Proliferation of Mesangial Cells,'' *Nephron,* 65(4), 1993, p. 596-600.

In this study, the effects of green tea consumption and topical application of tea extracts on chemical-induced mouse skin and lung cancer were examined. Results showed that daily tea consumption for 4-8 weeks significantly inhibited expression of NNK-induced c-myc, c-raf, and c-H-ras oncogenes. Results also found that topical application of EGCG an hour before topical exposure to TPA completely inhibited TPA-induced gene expression.

—G. Hu, et al., ''Inhibition of Oncogene Expression by Green tea and (-)- Epigallocatechin gallate in Mice,'' *Nutr Cancer,* 24(2), 1995, p. 203-209.

Results of this study showed that oral and topical administration of polyphenols taken from green tea had anticarcinogenic effects in mice exposed to ultraviolet B radiation.

—S.K. Katiyar, et al., ''Protection Against Ultraviolet-B Radiation-induced Local and Systemic Suppression of Contact Hypersensitivity and Edema Responses in C3H/HeN Mice by Green Tea Polyphenols," *Photochem Photobiol,* 62(5), November 1995, p. 855-361.

This study examined the protective effects of green tea polyphenols on UVB radiation-induced skin damage in mice. Results showed that mice fed green tea as their sole source of drinking water for 30 days and then exposed to UVB radiation experienced significant protection against cutaneous edema as well as induction of epidermal and cyclooxygenase activities.

—R. Agarwal, et al., "Protection Against Ultraviolet B Radiation-induced Effects in the Skin of SKH-1 Hairless Mice by a Polyphenolic Fraction Isolated from Green Tea," *Photochem Photobiol,* 58(5), November 1993, p. 695-700.

Results of this study showed that the topical application of a green tea polyphenol fraction inhibited chemical-induced tumor promotion in mice. Oral intake of a green tea as the sole source of drinking water inhibited UVB light-induced sunburn lesions, skin tumors, and nitrosodiethylamine-induced forestomach and lung tumors as well.

—A.H. Conney, et al., "Inhibitory Effect of Green Tea on Tumorigenesis by Chemicals and Ultraviolet Light," *Prev Med,* 21(3), May 1992, p. 361-369.

This study examined the effects of a catechin containing green tea extract on liver tumor promoters, induction of cytolethality, inhibition of gap junctional intercellular communication, and induction of cell proliferation. Results showed that the extract prevented the induction of hepatocyte cytolethality, the inhibition of gap junctional-mediated intercellular communication, and significantly decreased the labeling index in hepatic preneoplastic foci from animals treated with phenobarbital for 7 days.

—J.E. Klaunig, "Chemopreventive Effects of Green Tea Components on Hepatic Carcinogenesis," *Prev Med,* 21(4), July 1992, p. 510-519.

Results of this study found that the administration of green tea extract as the sole source of drinking water 1-2 weeks prior to UVB exposure significantly inhibited the formation of skin tumors in mice. The extract also inhibited the formation of DMBA induced skin tumors in a related experiment part of the same study. Size of tumors showed reductions as well as a result of the green tea extract.

—Z.Y., Wang, et al., "Inhibitory Effect OF Orally Administered Green Tea on Ultraviolet B Light (UV-B)-induced Carcingogenesis in the Skin of SKH-1 Mice," *Proceedings of the Annual Meeting of the American Association of Cancer Researchers,* 32, 1991, p. A773.

Results of this study found that the pretreatment of prostate carcinoma cell cultures with green tea polyphenols for one hour significantly inhibited testosterone-induced ODC activity and mRNA expression, suggesting green tea may be an effective means for the prevention of prostate cancer.

—R.R. Mohan, et al., "Testosterone Induces Ornithine Decarboxylase (ODC) Activity and mRNA Expression in Human Prostate Carcinoma Cell Line LNCaP: Inhibition by Green Tea," *Proceedings of the Annual Meeting of American Association Cancer Researchers,* 36, 1995, p. A1633.

Results of this study showed that the administration of green tea polypheonols 30 minutes prior to carcinogen exposure provided significant protection against chemical-induced forestomach and pulmonary tumorigenesis in mice relative to controls.

—S.K. Katiyar, et al., "Protection Against Diethylnitrosamine (DEN)- and benzo(a)pyrene

(BP)-Induced Forestomach and Pulmonary Neoplasia in A/J Mice by Limited Oral Intubation of Green Tea Polyphenols,'' *Proceedings of the Annual Meeting of the American Association of Cancer Researchers,* 35, 1994, p. A3731.

This study examined the effects of decaffeinated green tea and DASO2, a garlic-related chemical on chemical-induced lung tumorigenesis in mice. Results showed that a single dose of DASO2 administered 2 hours before carcinogen exposure significantly decreased tumor incidence and multiplicity. Green tea administration produced, similar significant effects.

> —Z.Y. Wang, et al., ''Inhibitory Effects of Diallyl Sulfone (DASO2) and Green Tea on Lung Tumorigenesis Induced by 4-(methylnitrosamino)-1-(3-pyridyl)-1-butanone(NNK) in A/J Mice,'' *Proceedings of the Annual Meeting of the American Association of Cancer Researchers,* 35, 1994, p. A3728.

This study examined the effects of the green tea polyphenol (-)-epigallocatechin gallate (EGCG) on c-myc oncogene-induced preneoplastic transformation in the mammary epithelial cells of mice. Results showed that EGCG may inhibit the post-initiational events of mammary cell transformation by altering the cellular metabolism of E2 in favor of 2-hydroxy estrone formation.

> —N.T. Telang, et al., ''Antipromotional Effect of a Green Tea Polyphenol on C-myc-transfected Mammary Epithelial Cells,'' *Proceedings of the Annual Meeting of the American Association of Cancer Researchers,* 35, 1994, p. A3692.

This study examined the effects of four different polyphenols found in green and black tea on canine mammary tumor cell growth in culture. Results showed that (-)-epigallocatechin gallate (EGCG) and (-)-epigallocatechin gallate sulfide (green tea) and theaflavins (TFs) and thearubigins (black tea) inhibited the growth of CMT-13 cells when added at 25 ppm or more for 24 hours or more. TFs proved to be the most effective, and the addition of glutathione prior to including EGCG or Tfs reduced severity of growth inhibition significantly.

> —K. Sakamotol, et al., ''Impact of Green or Black Tea Polyphenol on Canine Mammary Tumor cells in Culture,'' *Proceedings of the Annual Meeting of the American Association of Cancer Researchers,* 36, 1995, p. A3542.

This extensive review article cites numerous studies supporting the chemoprotective effects of green tea on stomach and esophageal cancer.

> —A.H. Conney, et al., ''Inhibitory Effects of Green and Black Tea on Carcinogenesis,'' *Proceedings of the Annual Meeting of the American Association of Cancer Researchers,* 36, 1995, p. 704-705.

This study examined the effects of green tea, black tea, and tea components NNK metabolic activation. Results showed polyphenol fractions from both kinds of tea inhibited NNK metabolism by more than 50%.

> —S.T. Shi, et al., ''Inhibitory Effects of Green Tea and Black Tea components on 4-(methyl-nitrosamino)-1-(3-pyridyl)-1-butanone (NNK) Metabolism and NNK-induced DNA Methyla-tion,'' *Proceedings of the Annual Meeting of the American Association of Cancer Researchers,* 34, 1993, p. A935.

This study examined the effects of decaffeinated green and black tea on esophageal tumorigenesis in rats. Results showed that the administration of both kind of tea significantly inhibited chemical-induced papilloma incidence and tumor size.

—Z.Y. Wang, et al., "Inhibition of N-nitrosomethylbenzylamine (NMBzA)-induced Esophageal Tumorigenesis in Rats by Decaffeinated Green Tea and Back Tea," *Proceedings of the Annual Meeting of the American Association of Cancer Researchers,* 34, 1993, p. A746.

Results of this study found that the topical application of green tea polyphenols 30 minutes before carcinogen exposure produced significant protection against enhanced malignant conversions in mice.

—S.K. Katiyar, et al., "Protection Against Malignant Conversion of Mouse Skin Papillomas to Carcinomas by Green Tea Polyphenols," *Proceedings of the Annual Meeting of the American Association of Cancer Researchers,* 34, 1993, p. A3308.

Results of this study showed that oral intake of green tea extract or polyphenolic fraction isolated from green tea significantly protected mice against chemical-induced forestomach and lung tumorigenesis.

—H. Mukhtar, et al., "Protection Against Diethylnitrosamine (DEN) and Benzo(alpha)pyrene (BP)-induced Forestomach and Lung Tumorigenesis in A/J Mice by Green Tea," *Proceedings of the Annual Meeting of the American Association of Cancer Researchers,* 34, 1993, p. A3307.

Cardiovascular/Coronary Heart Disease

In this study of 1371 Japanese men over 40, results showed an inverse association between the daily consumption of green tea and serum cholesterol levels. Consumption of more than 10 cups per day was correlated to a reduced concentration of hepatological markers in serum, aspartate aminotransferase, alanine transferase, and ferritin.

—K. Imai and K. Nakachi, "Cross Sectional Study of Effects of Drinking Green Tea on Cardiovascular and Liver Diseases," *British Medical Journal,* 310(6981), March 18, 1995, p. 693-696.

This study examined the antihypertensive effects of green tea, which is rich in GABA, in rats sensitive to salt. Results showed that rats consuming the green tea experienced a significant decrease in blood pressure relative to controls.

—Y. Abe, et al., "Effect of Green Tea Rich in Gamma-aminobutyric Acid on Blood Pressure of Dahl Salt-Sensitive Rats," *American Journal of Hypertension,* 8(1), January 1995, p. 74-79.

Results of this study found that green tea tannin mixture added to a medium of cultured smooth muscle cells suppressed the proliferation of the cells in a dose-dependent manner, as did green tea's main ingredient, (-)-epigallocatechin 3-O-gallate.

—T. Yokozawa, et al., "Effects of a Component of Green Tea on the Proliferation of Vascular Smooth Muscle Cells," *Biosci Biotechnol Biochem,* 59(11), November 1995, p. 2134-2136.

This study examined the effects of green tea extract on the collagen-induced aggregation of washed rabbit platelets. Results showed that the extract prolonged lag time and lowered submaximal aggregation dose dependently.

—Y. Sagesaka-Mitane, et al., "Platelet Aggregation Inhibitors in Hot Water Extract of Green Tea," *Chem Pharm Bull,* 38(3), March 1990, p. 790-793.

This study examined the effects of green tea catechins on lipid metabolism in rats fed a high-cholesterol diet. Results showed that catechins decreased plasma total cholesterol, cholesterol ester, total cholesterol—HDL- cholesterol, and atherogenic index (VLDL-+LDL-cholesterol/HDL-cholesterol).

> —K. Muramatsu, et al., "Effect of Green Tea Catechins on Plasma Cholesterol Level in Cholesterol-fed Rats," *Journal of Nutr Sci Vitaminol,* 32(6), December 1986, p. 613-622.

Results of this study found that mice treated with green tea extract experienced protection against an atherogenic-induced increase in serum cholesterol. The extract prevented increases in serum phospholipid and a decline of lecithin.

> —Y. Yamaguchi, et al., [Preventive Effects of Green Tea Extract on Lipid Abnormalities in Serum, Liver and Aorta of Mice Fed a Atherogenic Diet], *Nippon Yakurigaku Zasshi,* 97(6), June 1991, p. 329-337.

In this study of 1306 Japanese males, results found serum total cholesterol levels to be inversely related to the consumption of green tea.

> —S. Kono, et al., "Green Tea Consumption and Serum Lipid Profiles: A Cross-sectional Study in Northern Kyushu, Japan," *Prev Med,* 21(4), July 1992, p. 526-531.

Results of this study showed that rats administered unprocessed tea leaf extracts for 8 weeks experienced a significant reduction in thromboxane and cholesterol levels.

> —M. Ali, et al., "A Potent Thromboxane Formation Inhibitor in Green Tea Leaves," *Prostaglandins Leukot Essent Fatty Acids,* 40(4), August 1990, p. 281-283.

Dental Health

This study examined the effects of Japanese green tea on dental carries in vitro and in vivo. Results showed that green tea polyphenolic compounds inhibited the attachment of Streptococcus mutans strain JC-2 to saliva-coated hydroxyapatide discs. Results also found that rats infected with S mutans JC-2 (c) and fed a cariogenic diet and/or drinking water containing green tea polyphenols exhibited fewer caries than did controls.

> —S. Otake, et al., "Anticaries Effects of Polyphenolic Compounds from Japanese Green Tea," *Caries Research,* 25(6), 1991, p. 438-443.

Results of this study found Chinese green tea polyphenols are effective preventive agents against dental caries.

> —S.Q. You, [Study on Feasibility of Chinese Green tea Polyphenols (CTP) for Preventing Dental Caries], *Chung Hua Kou Chiang Hsueh Tsa Chih,* 28(4), July 1993, p. 197-199, p. 254.

This study examined the effects of green tea extract on the inhibition of dental caries in hamsters. Results showed that the fluoride in green tea may increase the cariostatic action in combination with other properties in the tea.

> —H. Yu, et al., "Anticariogenic Effects of Green Tea," *Fukuoka Igaku Zasshi,* 83(4), April 1992, p. 174-180.

General

Results of this study showed that both green and black tea exhibited antioxidant effects on tissue lipid peroxidation in rats.

> —M. Sano, et al., "Effect of Tea (Camellia sinensis L.) on Lipid Peroxidation in Rat Liver and Kidney: A Comparison of Green and Black Tea Feeding," *Biol Pharm Bull,* 18(7), July 1995, p. 1006-1008.

In this case-control study, five healthy adults ingested 300 ml of either green or black tea following an overnight fast. Results showed that both types of tea inhibited the in vitro peroxidation in a dose-dependent manner, with green tea showing a six times greater potency than black. Ingestion of both teas produced a significant increase of TRAP in vivo as well.

> —M. Serafini, et al., "In Vivo Antioxidant Effect of Green and Black Tea in Man," *European Journal of Clinical Nutrition,* 50(1), January 1996, p. 28-32.

Results of this study found that consumption of green and black tea as the sole liquid ingested led to significant reductions in the activity of transketolase in whole blood of rats. Liver transketolase activity was decreased only by green tea.

> —M. Ali, et al., "Effect of Consumption of Green and Black Tea on the Level of Various Enzymes in Rats," *Experientia,* 45(1), January 15, 1989, p. 112-114.

In this study, antibacterial and bactericidal actions of extracts of green tea were tested against 24 bacterial strains isolated from root canal infections. Results showed the extracts had antibacterial and bactericidal actions against many of the bacteria.

> —N. Horiba, et al., "A Pilot Study of Japanese Green Tea as a Medicament: Antibacterial and Bactericidal Effects," *Journal of Endod,* 17(3), March 1991, p. 122-124.

Results of this study showed that green tea extracts inhibited the growth of bacteria causing diarrheal diseases, including Staphylococcus aureus, S. epidermidis, Vibrio cholerae O1, V. cholerae non O1. V. parahaemolyticus, V. mimicus, Campylobacter jejuni and Plesiomonas shigelloides. Green tea exhibited antibacterial activity over S. aureus, V. parahaemolyticus and enteropathogenic E. coli as well.

> —M. Toda, et al., [Antibacterial and Bactericidal Activities of Japanese Green Tea], *Nippon Saikingaku Zasshi,* 44(4), July 1989, p. 669-672.

Liver Damage

This study examined the preventive effects of green tea extract on D-galactosamine (GalN)-induced hepatic injury in rats. Results showed the oral administration of green tea extract in doses of 50, 100, or 200 mg/kg 5 times each prior to GAIN injection significantly prevented the increase in GOT, GPT, and ALP activities. Extract administration also significantly prevented decreases in serum albumnin and total cholesterol. The authors concluded that such findings suggest that green tea could have ameliorating effects on hepatic dysfunction.

> —M. Hayashi, et al., [Effects of Green Tea Extract on Galactosamine-induced Hepatic Injury in Rats], *Nippon Yakurigaku Zasshi,* 100(5), November 1992, p. 391-399.

Pancreatitis

Results of this study found that green tea catechins exhibited protective effects on chemical-induced pancreatitis in rats.

—F. Takabayashi, et al., "The Effects of Green Tea Catechins (Polyphenon) on DL-ethionine-induced Acute Pancreatitis," *Pancreas,* 11(2), August 1995, p. 127-131.

Stroke

Results of this four year, follow-up study of 5,910 Japanese women who neither smoked nor drank alcohol showed that the rate of stroke and cerebral was at least twice as high as those consuming less than 5 cups or green tea daily compared to those consuming 5 or more cups per day.

—Y. Sato, et al., "Possible Contribution of Green Tea Drinking Habits to the Prevention of Stroke," *Tohoku Journal of Exp Med,* 157(4), April 1989, p. 337-343.

■ MISTLETOE

AIDS/HIV

Results of this study found that semi-purified aqueous extact of Viscum album had anti-HIV, immuno-modulating and anticancer activities in 12 symptomatic HIV disease patients followed for 6 years.

—R. Gorter, et al., "Anti-HIV and Immunomodulating Activities of Viscum Album," *International Conference on AIDS,* 8(3), July 19-24, 1992, p. 84.

Cancer

In this study, 3 groups of patients with advanced tumors received intravenously (in 250 ml saline infusion) 0.2 biological unit (BU)/kg, 1.0 BU/kg and 5.0 BU/kg of lectins, respectively. Results showed that significant differences were found between the three groups and that 1.0 BU/kg dose of lectins induced the greatest immunomodulation.

—K. Hostanska, et al., "Immunomodulatory Potency of Mistletoe Lectins in Cancer Patients: Results of a Dose Finding Study," *Molecular Biology of Hematopoiesis, 8th Sympsosium,* July 9-13, 1993, Basel Switzerland, 27, 1993.

This study examined the ability of immunomodulating mistletoe extract standardized for the galacto-sidespecific lectin (ML-1) to affect immunological parameters and neuroendocrinological parameters in 36 women with breast cancer. Results showed that regular subcutaneous injections of the optimal immunomodulating ML-1 dosage (1ng/kg body weight, twice a week) for 12 weeks induced a significant increase of beta-endorphin plasma levels, a reduced decrease of defined peripheral blood lymphatic subsets after standard chemotherapy, and an evidently increased in vitro cytokine release by mononuclear immune cells after adequate stimulation.

—B.M. Heiny, et al., "Mistletoe Extract Standardized for the Galactoside-specific Lectin (ML-1) Induces Beta-endorphin Release and Immunopotentiation in Breast Cancer Patients," *Anticancer Research,* 14(3B), May-June 1994, p. 1339-1342.

In this review article, the author notes that studies from their lab have demonstrated that mistletoe extact exhibits significant anticancer activity against a variety of experimental tumor systems, in vitro and in vivo, particularly those modeling for lung, breast and colon carcinomas.

—T.A. Khwaga, "Biopharmacological Studies of Different Components of Viscum Album (Mistletoe)," *Anticancer Research,* 10(5B), 1990, p. 1374-1375.

This study examined the antiproliferative effects of Viscum album C, Viscum album Qu and Viscum album M on melanoma cell lines. Results showed that mistletoe extacts can have some antiproliferative effect on melanoma cell lines.

—C. Gawlik, et al., "Antiproliferative Effect of Mistletoe-Extracts in Melanoma Cell Lines," *Anticancer Research,* 12(6A), 1992, p. 1882.

This study examined the cellular aspects of the immunomodulating activity of propriety mistletoe extract (Eurixor) standardized for mistletoe lectin-1 (ML-1) in 20 mammary cancer patients. Results showed that subcutaneous injections of the different dosages (0.5 and 1.0 ng ML-1/kg body weight, twice a week, for 5 weeks) led to statistically significant increases of defined peripheral blood lymphocyte subsets (helper T cells, natural killer cells) which are gerneally beleived to be involved in antitumor activity. The administration of either ML-1 concentration also enhanced the expression of activation markers such as interleukin-2 receptors and HLA/DR-antigens on peripheral blood T-lymphocytes.

—J. Beuth, et al., [Immunoactive Effects of Various Mistletoe Lectin-1 Dosages in Mammary Carcinoma Patients], *Arzeimittelforschung,* 45(4), April 1995, p. 505-507.

This study examined the effects of mistletoe preparations of the suspension cell cultures of human leukemia cells and of human myeloma cells. Results found a dose dependent reduction of their growth and a dose-dependent decrease of the percentage of viable cells after treatment for 72 hours.

—H. Haulesen & F. Mechelke, "The Influence of a Mistletoe Preparation on Suspension Cell Cultures of Human Leukemia and Human Myeloma Cells," *Arzmeimittelforshung,* 32(9), 1982, p. 1126-1127.

This study isolated a tumor reducing component from mistletoe extract (Iscador) and identified to be a peptide of approximate molecular weight 5000. The isolated peptide reduced the solid tumour induced by Dalton's lymphoma ascites tumour cells in mice and was highly cytotoxic to the DLA cells but was not cytotoxic to normal lymphocytes, indicating a cell dependent specificity.

—G. Kuttan, et al., "Isolation and Identification of a Tumour Reducing Component from Mistletoe Extract (Iscador)," *Cancer Letters,* 41(3), August 30, 1988, p. 307-314.

Results of this study found that an extact of Korean mistletoe inhibited tumour metastasis caused by haematogenous as well as non-haematogenous tumour cells, and that its antimetastic effect results from the suppression of tumour growth and the inhibition of tumour-induced agniogenesis by inducing TNF-alpha.

—T.J. Yoon, et al., "Inhibitory Effect of Korean Mistletoe (Viscum Album Coloratum) Extract on Tumour Angiogesis and Metastais of Heamatogenous and Non-haematogenous Tumour Cells in Mice," *Cancer Letters,* 97(1), October 20, 1995, p. 83-91.

Results of this study found that subcutaneous injections of low doses of mistletoe extact led to significant enhancement of peritoneal macrophage activity and significant weight gain of the thymus in mice. When enhancement of peritoneal macrophages activity and significant weight gain of the thymus in mice. When sarcoma L-1 and fibrosarcoma RAW 117 - H 10 cells were intravenously inoculated with the same extract, results showed significant reduction in the number of lung and liver tumor colonies relative to controls.

> —J. Beuth, et al., "Influence of Treatment with the Immunomodulatory Effective Dose of the Beta-Galactoside-specific Lectin from Mistletoe on Tumor Colonization in BALB/c-mice for Two Experimental Model Systems," *In Vivo,* 5(1), January-February 1991, p. 29-32.

This review article notes that mistletoe extracts have been found to possess significant antitumor activity, in vivo, against murine tumors, Lewis lung carcinoma, colon adenocarcinoma 38 and C3H mammary adenocarcinoma 16/C.

> —T.A. Khwaja, et al., "Recent Studies on the Anticancer Activities of Mistletoe and its Alkaloids," *Oncolocy,* 43(Suppl. 1), 1986, p. 42-50.

Results of this study of 40 oral cancer patients found T mali to be the most effective mistletoe preparation with a success rate of 76% and a reduction of clonal growth in vitro ranging from 51 to 94% following coincubation of cells and variable doses of drugs.

> —E. Wartenberg, et al., "Direct Antineoplastic Activity of Different Mistletoe Preparations Against Oral Cancer Cell in Vitro CPI-Based Matched-Pair Analyis," *Proceedings of the Annual Meeting of the American Association of Cancer Researchers,* 33, 1992, p. A1339.

This study compared the results of the postoperative treatment of 319 breast cancer patients treated with Iscador (Viscum album) are to 228 controls. Results showed that the survival of patients in the Iscador groups significantly better than controls.

> —R. Leroi, [Postoperative Treatment of Breast Cancer Patients with a Mistletoe Preparation], *Helv Chir Acta,* 44(3), 1977, p. 403-414.

This study examined the effects of galactoside-specific lectin from mistletoe (ML-1) on breast cancer patients. Subcutaneous injections of 1 mg/kg per body weight of the substance twice a week for 4 weeks significantly increased helper T-lymphocytes and natural killer cells and enhanced the expression of interleukin (II)-2 receptors on lymphatic cells. Similar effects were seen in vitro.

> —J. Beuth, et al., [Comparative Studies on the Immunoactive Action ofGalactoside-Specific Mistletoe Lectin: Pure Substance Compared to the Standardized Extract], *Arzneimittelforschung,* 43(2), February 1993, p. 166-169.

This study examined the effects of Isacador (a mistletoe, Viscum album extact) on the immunological parameters in the peripheral blood of patients with breast cancer. Results showed that phagocytic activity of granulocytes was significantly enhanced as were natural killer cell and antibody-dependent cell-mediated cytoxicity activities.

> —T. Hajto, "Immunomodulatory Effects of Iscador: A Viscum Album Preparation," *Oncology,* 43(Suppl 1), 1986, p. 51-65.

Breast cancer patients in this study were administered a single infusion of Iscador intravenously. Results showed that natural killer cell and antibody-dependent cell-mediated decreased significantly after 6 hours, but then significantly increased 24 hours later.

> —T. Hajto & C. Lanzrein, ''Natural Killer and Antibody-Dependent Cell-Mediated Cytotoxicity Activities and Large Granular Lymphocyte Frequencies in Viscum Album-Treated Breast Cancer Patients,'' *Oncology,* 43(2), 1986, p. 93-97.

In this placebo-controlled study, the effects of a mistletoe preparation were examined in advanced breast cancer patients. Those receiving the treatment showed significantly higher white blood cell counts and leukocyte levels compared to controls following the fourth cycle of chemotherapy.

> —B.M. Heiny, [Adjuvant Treatment with Standardized Misletoe Extract Reduces Leukopenia and Improves the Quality of Life of Patients with Advanced Carcinomas of the Breast Getting Palliative Chemotherapy], *Krebsmedizin,* 12, 1991, p. 3-14.

■ TURMERIC

AIDS/HIV

This study examined curcumin's effects on purified HIV-1 integrase. Results showed that curcumin had an inhibitory concentration 50 (IC50) for strand transfer of 40 microM and suggest that HIV-1 integrase inhibition might be involved in curcumin's antiviral effects study .

> —A. Mazumder, et al., ''Inhibition of Human Immunodeficiency Virus type-1 integrase by Curcumin,'' *Biochem Pharmacol,* 49(8), April 18, 1995, p. 1165-1170.

This article notes that curcumin is a modest inhibitor of HIV-1 (IC50 = 100 microM) and HIV-2 (IC50 = 250 microM) proteases.

> —Z. Sui, et al., ''Inhibition of the HIV-1 and HIV-2 proteases by Curcumin and Curcumin Boron Complexes,'' *Bioorg Med Chem,* 1(6), December 1993, p. 415-422.

Antifungal Activity

Results of this study found that turmeric oil exhibited antifungal activity against tichophyton-induced dermatophytosis in guinea pigs.

> —A. Apisariyakul, et al., ''Antifungal Activity of Turmeric Oil Extracted from Curcuma Longa (Zingiberaceae),'' *Journal of Ethnopharmacology,* 49(3), December 15, 1995, p. 163-169.

Anti-inflammatory Effects

Results of this placebo-controlled study showed that phenylbutazone and curcumin exhibited anti-inflammatory effects in patients with postoperative inflammation.

> —R.R. Satoskar, et al., ''Evaluation of Anti-inflammatory Property of Curcumin (Diferuloyl Methane) in Patients with Postoperative Inflammation,'' *International Journal of Clinical Pharmacology Ther Toxicol,* 24(12), December 1986, p. 651-654.

Cancer

Results of this study showed that curcumin exhibited inhibitory effects on TPA-induced tumor promotion in the epidermis of mice.

—M.T. Huang, et al., "Inhibitory Effects of Curcumin on in Vitro Lipoxygenase and Cyclooxygenase Activities in Mouse Epidermis," *Cancer Research,* 51(3), February 1, 1991, p. 813-819.

Results of this study indicated that the topical application of curcumin inhibited TPA-induced epidermal ornithine decarboxylase activity in female mice. In addition to these findings, the topical application of curcumin coupled with TPA twice a week over a period of 20 weeks to mice previously exposed to DMBA significantly inhibited the number of TPA-induced tumors.

—M.T. Huang, et al., "Inhibitory Effect of Curcumin, Chlorogenic Acid, Caffeic Acid, and Ferulic Acid on Tumor Promotion in Mouse Skin by 12-O-tetradecanoylphorbol-13-acetate," *Cancer Research,* 48(21), November 1, 1988, p. 5941-5946.

This study examined the chemopreventive effects of curcumin on azoxymethane-induced colon cancer in rats. Results showed that the curcumin significantly reduced the incidence of colon adenocarcinomas, the multiplicity of both invasive and noninvasive adenocarcinomas, and suppressed colon tumor volume relative to controls.

—C.V. Rao, et al., "Chemoprevention of Colon Carcinogenesis by Dietary Curcumin, a Naturally Occurring Plant Phenolic Compound," *Cancer Research,* January 15, 1995, p. 55(2), p. 259-266.

This study examined the effects of curcumin on experimentally-induced tumorigenesis in the forestomach, duodenum, and colon of mice. Results found that curcumin inhibited the number of tumors per mouse, tumor size, and the percentage of mice with tumors.

—M.T. Huang, et al., "Inhibitory Effects of Dietary Curcumin on Forestomach, Duodenal, and Colon Carcinogenesis in Mice," *Cancer Research,* 54(22), November 15, 1994, p. 5841-5847.

Results of this study showed that an aqueous extract of turmeric suppressed the mutagenicity of both direct- and indirect-acting mutagen, benzo(a)pyrene (B(a)P) in Salmonella typhimurium strains TA98 and TA100. In addition to these findings, aqueous turmeric extracts reduced incidence and multiplicity of B(a)P-induced forestomach tumors in mice, and curcumin was shown to inhibit B(a)P- DNA-adduct formation and B(a)P-induced strand breaks.

—M.A. Azuine, et al., "Mechanisms of Chemoprevention of Cancer by Turmeric," *Third International Conference on Mechanisms of Antimutagenesis and Anticarcinogenesis, May 5-10, 1991, Lucca, Italy,* 1991, p. 59.

Results of this study found that the topical administration of curcumin exhibited inhibitory effects on TPA-induced tumorigenesis in the skin of mice.

—A.H. Conney, et al., "Inhibitory Effect of Curcumin and Some Related Dietary Compounds on Tumor Promotion and Arachidonic Acid Metabolism in Mouse Skin," *Adv Enzyme Regul,* 31, 1991, p. 385-396.

Results of this study showed that curcumin induced apoptotic cell death in promyelocytic leukemia HL-60 cells at concentrations as low as 3.5 micrograms/ml.

—M.L. Kuo, et al., "Curcumin, An Antioxidant and Anti-tumor Promoter, Induces Apoptosis in Human Leukemia Cells," *Biochim Biophys Acta,* 1317(2), November 15, 1996, p. 95-100.

Results of this study found that the administration of curcumin in mice inhibited AOM-induced colonic neoplasia in mice.

—M.T. Huang, et al., "Effect of Dietary Curcumin and Ascorbyl Palmitate on Azoxymethanol-induced Colonic Epithelial Cell Proliferation and Focal Areas of Dysplasia," *Cancer Letters,* 64(2), June 15, 1992, p. 117-121.

Results of this study inhibited the DNA synthesis of human umbilical vein endothelial cells in vitro, pointing to its potential as a useful new therapy for cancer.

—A.K. Singh, et al., "Curcumin Inhibits the Proliferation and Cell Cycle Progression of Human Umbilical Vein Endothelial Cell," *Cancer Letters,* 107(1), October 1, 1996, p. 109-115.

Results of this study showed that curcumin exhibited inhibitory effects on TPA-induced skin cancer in mice.

—S.S. Kakar & D. Roy, "Curcumin Inhibits TPA Induced Expression of C-fos, C-jun and C-myc Proto-Oncogenes Messenger RNAs in Mouse Skin," *Cancer Letters,* 87(1), November 24, 1995, p. 85-89.

Results of this showed that the i.p. administration of 100 mg/kg and 200 mg/kg of curcumin significantly reduced the number of palpable DMBA-induced mammary tumors and mammary adenocarcinomas in rats.

—K. Singletary, et al., "Inhibition of 7,12-dimethylbenz[a]anthracene (DMBA)-induced Mammary Tumorigenesis and DMBA-DNA Adduct Formation by Curcumin," *Cancer Letters,* 103(2), June 5, 1996, p. 137-141.

Results of this study showed that a tumeric extract inhibited cell growth in Chinese Hamster Ovary cells and was cytotoxic to lymphocytes and Dalton's lymphoma cells.

—R. Kuttan, et al., "Potential Anticancer Activity of Turmeric," *Cancer Letters,* 29(2), November 1985, p. 197-202.

Results of this study showed the curcumin inhibited xanthine oxidase in vitro, xanthine oxidase being one a causative factor in PMA-mediated tumor promotion.

—J.K. Lin & C.A. Shih, "Inhibitory Effect of Curcumin on Xanthine Dehydrogenase/oxidase Induced by Phorbol-12-myristate-13-acetate in NIH3T3 Cells," *Carcinogenesis,* 15(8), August 1994, p. 1717-1721.

Results of this study found that the administration of curcumin mediated a dose-dependent inhibition of the incidence and multiplicity of AOM-induced colon adenomas in rats relative to controls.

—M.A. Pereira, et al., "Effects of the Phytochemicals, Curcumin and Quercetin, Upon Azoxymethane Induced Colon Cancer and 7,12-dimethylbenz[a]anthracene-induced Mammary Cancer in Rats," *Carcinogenesis,* 17(6), June 1996, p. 1305-1311.

Results of this study showed that curcumin had inhibitory effects on TPA-induced tumor promotion in DMBA-initiated mouse skin.

> —M.T. Huang, et al., "Effects of Curcumin, Demethoxycurcumin, Bisdemethoxycurcumin and Tetrahydrocurcumin on 12-O-tetradecanoylphorbol-13- Acetate-induced Tumor Promotion," *Carcinogenesis,* 16(10), October 1995, p. 2493-2497.

Results of this study showed that the topical application of 3 or 10 mumol of curcumin 5 min prior to the application of 20 nmol [3H]B[a]P inhibited the formation of [3H]B[a]P-DNA adducts in the epidermis of mice and inhibited the incidence and number of DMBA-induced skin tumors.

> —M.T. Huang, et al., "Inhibitory Effects of Curcumin on Tumor Initiation by Benzo[a]pyrene and 7,12-dimethylbenz[a]anthracene," *Carcinogenesis,* 13(11), November 1992, p. 2183-2186.

Results of this study showed that the oral administration of betel-leaf extract combined with turmeric had inhibitory effects on chemical-induced carcinogenesis in hamsters.

> —M.A. Azuine & S.V. Bhide, "Protective Single/combined Treatment with Betel Leaf and Turmeric Against Methyl (acetoxymethyl) Nitrosamine-induced Hamster Oral Carcinogenesis," *International Journal of Cancer,* 51(3), May 28, 1992, p. 412-415.

Results of this study showed that curcumin I inhibited benzopyrene- (BP) induced forestomach tumors and DMBA-induced TPA-promoted skin tumors in female mice, while curcumin III inhibited DMBA—induced skin tumors in bald mice.

> —M. Nagabhushan & S.V. Bhide, "Curcumin as an Inhibitor of Cancer," *Journal of the American College of Nutrition,* 11(2), April 1992, p. 192-198.

Results of this study showed that an aqueous turmeric extract and its constituents, curcumin-free aqueous turmeric extract and curcumin exhibited chemopreventive effects in female mice.

> —M.A. Azuine, et al., "Protective Role of Aqueous Turmeric Extract Against Mutagenicity of Direct-Acting Carcinogens as Well as Benzo [alpha] pyrene-induced Genotoxicity and Carcinogenicity," *Journal of Cancer Research and Clinical Oncology,* 118(6), 1992, p. 447-452.

Results of this study found that turmeric and catechin exhibited chemopreventive effects in golden hamsters and in mice.

> —M.A. Azuine & S.V. Bhide, "Adjuvant Chemoprevention of Experimental Cancer: Catechin and Dietary Turmeric in Forestomach and Oral Cancer Models," *Journal of Ethnopharmacology,* 44(3), December 1994, p. 211-217.

Results of this study showed turmeric to be an effective antimutagen in smokers, pointing to its potential as a chemopreventive agent.

> —K. Polasa, et al., "Effect of Turmeric on Urinary Mutagens in Smokers," *Mutagenesis,* 7(2), March 1992, p. p. 107-109.

Results of this study showed that curcumin I, II, and III inhibited mutagenesis and croton oil-induced tumor promotion in mice.

> —R.J. Anto, et al., "Antimutagenic and Anticarcinogenic Activity of Natural and Synthetic Curcuminoids," *Mutation Research* (1996 Sep 13) 370(2), September 13, 1996, p. 127-131.

Results of this study showed that curcumin suppressed UV irradiation-induced mutagenesis in Salmonella typhimurium and Eschericia coli strains in vitro.

> —Y. Oda, "Inhibitory Effect of Curcumin on SOS Functions Induced by UV Irradiation." *Mutation Research,* 348(2), October 1995, p. 67-73.

Results of this study showed that turmeric inhibited DMBA-induced skin tumors and BP-induced forestomach tumors in mice.

> —M.A. Azuine & S.V. Bhide, "Chemopreventive Effect of Turmeric Against Stomach and Skin Tumors Induced by Chemical Carcinogens in Swiss Mice," *Nutr Cancer,* 17(1), 1992, p. 77-83.

Results of this study showed that curcumin induced cell shrinkage, chromatin condensation, and DNA fragmentation, characteristics of apoptosis, in immortalized mouse embryo fibroblast NIH 3T3 erb B2 oncogene-transformed NIH 3T3, mouse sarcoma S180, human colon cancer cell HT-29, human kidney cancer cell 293, and human hepatocellular carcinoma Hep G2 cells.

> —M.C. Jiang, et al., "Curcumin Induces Apoptosis in Immortalized NIH 3T3 and Malignant Cancer Cell Lines," *Nutr Cancer,* 26(1), 1996, p. 111-120.

Results of this study found that the oral administration of curcumin inhibited benzo[a]pyrene (B[a]P)-induced forestomach tumorigenesis, ENNG-induced duodenal tumorigenesis, and AOM-induced colon tumorigenesis in mice.

> —M.T. Huang, et al., "Inhibitory Effect of Dietary Curcumin on Gastrointestinal Tumorigenesis in Mice," *Proceedings of the Annual Meeting of the American Association of Cancer Researchers,* 34, 1993, p. A3305.

Results of this study indicated that commercial, purified, and demethoxy—curcumin exhibited inhibited TPA-induced skin tumors in mice previously exposed to DMBA.

> —M.T. Huang, et al., "Effects of Derivatives of Curcumin on 12-O-Tetradecanolyphorbol-13-Acetate (TPA)-Induced Tumor Promotion in Mouse Epidermis and-Independent Growth of Cultured JB6 Cells," *Proceedings of the Annual Meeting of the American Association of Cancer Researchers,* 33, 1992, p. A994.

Results of this study found that patients with external cancerous lesions experienced significant relief following treatment with an ethanol turmeric extract and a curcumin ointment.

> —R. Kuttan, et al., "Turmeric and Curcumin as Topical Agents in Cancer Therapy," *Tumori,* 73(1), February 28, 1987, p. 29-31.

Cardiovascular/Coronary Heart Disease

Results of this study showed that ischaemia-induced changes in cat hearts were prevented by both curcumin and quinidine.

> —M. Dikshit, et al., "Prevention of Ischaemia-induced Biochemical Changes by Curcumin & Quinidine in the Cat Heart," *Indian Journal of Medical Research,* January 1995, p. 101.

Results of this study showed that the administration of 500 mg per day of curcumin for 7 days significantly reduced the level of serum lipid peroxides, increased HDL cholesterol, and decreased total serum cholesterol in healthy human subjects.

> —K.B. Soni & R. Kuttan, "Effect of Oral Curcumin Administration on Serum Peroxides and

Cholesterol Levels in Human Volunteers," *Indian J Physiol Pharmacol,* 36(4), October 1992, p. 273-275.

Results of this study showed that oral curcumin significantly reduced increased lipid peroxidation in different mouse organs including the brain, liver, lung, and kidney. Curcumin significantly reduced serum and tissue cholesterol levels in mice as well.

—K.K. Soudamini, et al., "Inhibition of Lipid Peroxidation and Cholesterol Levels in Mice by Curcumin," *Indian Journal of Physiol Pharmacol,* 36(4), October 1992, p. 239-243.

Results of this study showed that curcumin inhibited arachidonate, adrenaline, and collagen-induced platelet aggregation in human blood.

—K.C. Srivastava, et al., "Curcumin, A Major Component of Food Spice Turmeric (Curcuma longa) Inhibits Aggregation and Alters Eicosanoid Metabolism in Human Blood Platelets," *Prostaglandins Leukot Essent Fatty Acids,* 52(4), April 1995, p. 223-227.

Cataracts

Results of this in vitro study found that curcumin provided protection against lipid peroxidation-induced cataractogenesis in rat lenses.

—S. Awasthi, et al., "Curcumin Protects Against 4-hydroxy-2-trans-nonenal-induced Cataract Formation in Rat Lenses," *American Journal of Clinical Nutrition,* 64(5), November 1996, p. 761-766.

Diabetes

Results of this study indicated that dietary curcumin over an 8 week period led to an enhanced metabolic status across numerous diabetic conditions in albino rats relative to controls.

—P.S. Babu & K. Srinivasan, "Influence of Dietary Curcumin and Cholesterol on the Progression of Experimentally Induced Diabetes in Albino Rat," *Mol Cell Biochem,* 152(1), November 8, 1995, p. 13-21.

Gallstones

Results of this study found that mice fed a lithogenic diet supplemented with 0.5 per cent curcumin over a period of 10 weeks experienced a significantly decreased incidence of gallstone formation relative to controls as well as a significant reduction in biliary cholesterol concentration.

—M.S. Hussain & N. Chandrasekhara, "Effect on Curcumin on Cholesterol Gall-stone Induction in Mice," *Indian Journal Medical Research,* 96, October 1992, p. 288-291.

General

This study compared the ability of the natural curcuminoids (curcumin (CAS 458-37-7), demethoxycurcumin, bisdemethoxycurcumin) and acetylcurcumin to scavenge superoxide radicals and to interact with 1,1-diphenyl-2-picryl-hydrazyl (DPPH) stable free radicals. The results found curcumin to be the most potent scavenger of superoxide radicals.

—N. Sreejayan & M.N. Rao, "Free Radical Scavenging Activity of Curcuminoids," *Arzneimittelforschung,* 46(2), February 1996, p. 169-171.

Results of this study showed that turmeric reduced lipid peroxidation in male rats by enhancing antioxidant enzyme activities.

> —A.C. Reddy & B.R. Lokesh, "Effect of Dietary Turmeric (Curcuma longa) on Iron-induced Lipid Peroxidation in the Rat Liver," *Food Chem Toxicol,* 32(3), March 1994, p. 279-283.

Results of this study showed that demethoxycurcumin, bisdemethoxycurcumin and acetylcurcumin were equally effective in their ability to inhibit iron-stimulated lipid peroxidation in rat brain homogenate and rat liver microsomes.

> —Sreejayan & M.N Rao, "Curcuminoids as Potent Inhibitors of Lipid Peroxidation," *Journal of Pharm Pharmacol,* 46(12), December 1994, p. 1013-1016.

Results of this study showed that curcumin and an aqueous extract of turmeric were effective inhibitors of lipid peroxidation.

> —V.K. Shalini & L. Srinivas, "Lipid Peroxide Induced DNA Damage: Protection by Turmeric (Curcuma longa)," *Mol Cell Biochem,* 77(1), September 1987, p. 3-10.

Liver Damage

Results of this study showed that 30 mg/kg body weight of curcumin administered over a period of 10 days reduced the iron-induced liver damage in male rats by lowering lipid peroxidation.

> —A.C. Reddy & B.R. Lokesh, "Effect of Curcumin and Eugenol on Iron-induced Hepatic Toxicity in Rats," *Toxicology,* 107(1), January 22, 1996, p. 39-45.

■ YOHIMBINE

Anticonvulsant Effects

Results of this study showed that 10 mg/kg i.p. of yohimbine or desipramine exhibited anticonvulsant effects in genetically epilepsy-prone rats.

> —Q.S. Yan, et al., "Noradrenergic Mechanisms for the Anticonvulsant Effects of Desipramine and Yohimbine in Genetically Epilepsy-prone Rats: Studies with Microdialysis," *Brain Research,* 610(1), April 30, 1993, p. 24-31.

Results of this study showed that doses of 10 mg/kg of yohimbine exhibited significant anticonvulsant effects against clonidine-induced audiogenic seizure in rats.

> —U. Tacke & S. Kolonen, "The Effect of Clonidine and Yohimbine on Audiogenic Seizures (AGS) in Rats," *Pharmacol Res Commun,* 16(10), October 1984, p. 1019-1030.

Cardiovascular/Coronary Heart Disease

This study examined the effects of orally administered yohimbine on platelet aggregation in healthy subjects. Results showed that that a minimum dose of 8 mg of yohimbine significantly inhibited epinephrine-induced platelet aggregation. Such inhibitory effects were maintained for 10 hours following a 12 mg dose.

> —I. Berlin, et al., "The Alpha 2-adrenergic Receptor Antagonist Yohimbine Inhibits Epineph-

rine-induced Platelet Aggregation in Healthy Subjects,'' *Clinical Pharmacol Ther,* 49(4), April 1991, p. 362-369.

Results of this study showed that hypoxic rabbit hearts treated with 3 to 30 microM yohimbine experienced an enhancement of posthypoxic recovery of contractile function and suppression of the hypoxia- and reoxygenation-induced rise in resting tension. In addition to these findings, yohimbine inhibited hypoxia/reoxygenation-induced release of ATP metabolites, restored myocardial high-energy phosphates, and inhibited the reoxygenation-induced rise in tissue calcium.

—S. Takeo, et al., ''Beneficial Effects of Yohimbine on Posthypoxic Recovery of Cardiac Function and Myocardial Metabolism in Isolated Perfused Rabbit Hearts,'' *Journal Pharmacol Exp Ther,* 258(1), July 1, 1991, p. 94-102.

This study examined yohimbine's ability to increase sympathoadrenal discharge and blood pressure in patients with autonomic failure characterized by orthostatic hypotension. Results showed that 5 mg of oral yohimbine produced significant increases in mean systolic and diastolic blood pressure as well as mean heart rate.

—J. Onrot, et al., ''Oral Yohimbine in Human Autonomic Failure,'' *Neurology,* 37(2), February 1987, p. 215-220.

Results of this study showed that 1.6 mg/kg of yohimbine exhibited antiarrhymic effects in rats hypertenesive rats subjected to acute coronary artery ligation.

—J.C. Roegel, et al., ''Comparative Effects of Idazoxan, Prazosin, and Yohimbine on Coronary Ligation-induced Arrhythmias in Spontaneously Hypertensive Rats,'' *Journal of Cardiovascular Pharmacology,* 27(2), February 1996, p. 226-234.

Depression

Results of this double-blind, placebo-controlled study found that 4 mg/t.i.d. of yohimbine significantly increased in blood pressure in depression patients suffering from clomipramine-induced orthostatic hypotension.

—L. Lacomblez, et al., ''Effect of Yohimbine on Blood Pressure in Patients with Depression and Orthostatic Hypotension Induced by Clomipramine,'' *Clinical Pharmacol Ther,* 45(3), March 1989, p. 241-251.

Diabetes

Results of this study showed that intravenous administration of 0.1 and 0.3 mg/kg of yohimbine increased plasma insulin and reduced plasma glucose concentrations in dogs. Such findings point to yohimbine's potential as a treatment for non-insulin-dependent diabetics.

—W.H. Hsu, et al., ''Yohimbine Increases Plasma Insulin Concentrations of Dogs,'' *Proceedings of Soc Exp Biol Med,* 184(3), March 1987, p. 345-389.

Narcolepsy

Results of this study showed that an average dose of 8 mg/kg per day of yohimbine proved effective in maintaining subjective wakefulness for 8 consecutive working hours in narcolepsy patients.

—V. Wooten, ''Effectiveness of Yohimbine in Treating Narcolepsy,'' *South Med Journal,* 87(11), November 1994, p. 1065-1066.

Obesity

Results of this study showed that yohimbine exhibited significant anorectic effects in both obese and lean mice.

—M.F. Callahan, et al., "Yohimbine and Rauwolscine Reduce Food Intake of Genetically Obese and Lean Mice," *Pharmacol Biochem Behav,* 20(4), April 1984, p. 591-599.

Sexual Function

Results of this study showed yohimbine to be a potentially beneficial therapy for sexual side effects brought on by serotonin reuptake blockers in humans, with 5 of 6 psychiatric patients experiencing improvements in sexual function following yohimbine treatment.

—E. Hollander & A. McCarley, "Yohimbine Treatment of Sexual Side Effects Induced by Serotonin Reuptake Blockers," *Journal of Clinical Psychiatry,* 53(6), June 1992, p. 207-209.

This article reports on the case of a patient with obsessive compulsive disorder and depression who was experiencing clomipramine-induced anorgasmia. Treatment with yohimbine proved effective.

—J. Price & L.J. Grunhaus, "Treatment of Clomipramine-induced Anorgasmia with Yohimbine: A Case Report," *Journal of Clinical Psychiatry,* 51(1), January 1990, p. 32-33.

This double-blind, placebo-controlled study examined the effects of yohimbine hydrochloride on erectile dysfunction in patients suffering from impotence. Results showed that 14% of patients experienced full and sustained erections following 1 month of treatment with a maximum dose of 42.0 mg or yohimbine hydrochloride per day. Partial improvements were seen in 20% of the patients, and 65% experienced no improvements.

—J.G. Susset, et al., "Effect of Yohimbine Hydrochloride on Erectile Impotence: A Double-blind Study," *Journal of Urology,* 141(6), June 1989, p. 1360-1363.

This double-blind, placebo-controlled, partially crossover study examined the effects of 18 mg per day of yohimbine over a 10 week period in patients with psychogenic impotence. Results showed a 46% overall improvement rate in patients who received yohimbine.

—K. Reid, et al., "Double-blind Trial of Yohimbine in Treatment of Psychogenic Impotence," *Lancet* 2(8556), August 22, 1987, p. 421-423.

Results of this study showed that the administration of yohimbine hydrochloride enhanced sexual motivation in male rats. Rats exhibited increases in mounting performance in mating tests conducted after genital anesthetization, percentage of male rats ejaculating in their first heterosexual encounter, and induction of copulatory behavior in sexually inactive male rats.

—J.T. Clark, et al., "Enhancement of Sexual Motivation in Male Rats by Yohimbine," *Science,* 225(4664), August 24, 1984, p. 847-849.

This study reports on the results of 4 independent meta-analyses concerning the efficacy of yohimbine on erectile disorder. Results found yohimbine showed a consistent pattern of improving erectile function when compared to controls.

—M.P. Carey & B.T. Johnson, "Effectiveness of Yohimbine in the Treatment of Erectile Disorder: Four Meta-analytic Integrations," *Archives of Sexual Behavior,* 25(4), August 1996, p. 341-360.

This articles reviews the history of yohimbine's use as a treatment for sexual disorders of both sexes and notes studies have shown it to have some benefits relative to placebo.

—A.J. Riley, ''Yohimbine in the Treatment of Erectile Disorder,'' *British Journal of Clinical Practice,* 48(3), May-June 1994, p. 133-136.

Results of this study showed that male rats receiving intracerebroventricular injections with yohimbine hydrochloride experienced significant reductions in latency to initial mounting and significant increases in the number of mountings when presented with a receptive female for 30 minutes following administration.

—T.R. Saito, et al., ''Central Effects of Yohimbine on Copulatory Behavior in Aged Male Rats,'' *Jikken Dobutsu,* 40(3), July 1991, p. 337-341.

Results of this study showed that low doses of yohimbine enhanced the ejaculatory response in male dogs.

—A. Yonezawa, et al., ''Biphasic Effects of Yohimbine on the Ejaculatory Response in the Dog,'' *Life Sci,* 48(20), 1991, p. PL103-109.

Results of this study showed that the administration of 1-4 mg/kg of yohimbine improved age-induced sexual dysfunction in male rats.

—E.R. Smith & J.M. Davidson, ''Yohimbine Attenuates Aging-induced Sexual Deficiencies in Male Rats,'' *Physiol Behavior,* 47(4), April 1990, p. 631-634.

Results of this study showed that 2 mg/kg of yohimbine enhanced sexual motivation in male rats independent of testosterone levels.

—J.T. Clark, et al., ''Testosterone is Not Required for the Enhancement of Sexual Motivation by Yohimbine,'' *Physiol Behav,* 35(4), October 1985, p. 517-521.

In this double-blind, placebo-controlled, partial crossover study, patients with psychogenic impotence received 15 mg per day or oral yohimbine coupled with 50 mg per day of trazodone over two 8-week periods. Results showed that 71% of the patients experienced clinical improvements relative to controls and that such benefits were maintained by 58% of such patients after 3 months and 56% after 6 months.

—J.T. Clark, et al., ''Testosterone is Not Required for the Enhancement of Sexual Motivation by Yohimbine,'' *Physiol Behav,* 35(4), October 1985, p. 517-521.

ADDITIONAL HERBS

■ AMERICAN CREOSOTE BUSH

Antimicrobial Activity

Results of this study showed Larrea tridentata exhibited strong antimicrobial activity against numerous organisms, including L. monocytogenes, C. perfiringens, S. dysenteriae, Y. enterocoliticia, P. vulgaris, etc.

> —M. Angeles, Verastegui, et al., "Antimicrobial Activity of Extracts of Three Major Plants from the Chihuahan Desert," *Journal of Ethnopharmacology,* 52, 1996, p. 175-177.

Cancer

This study documents the case of an 85-year-old male who refused all medical treatment for a malignant melanoma in his right cheek with a larger cervical metastasis. Following 1 year of self-medication with an aqueous extract of creosote bush, the patients exhibited a dramatic regression of the tumor. A literature review by the authors revealed norhihydroguaiaretic acid (NDGA), a nontoxic food antioxidant, to be a key ingredient of the extract which has been shown to contain antitumor activity when combined with ascorbic acid in vivo.

> —C.R. Smart, et al., "An Interesting Observation on Nordihydroguaiaretic Acid (NSC-4291; NDGA) and a Patient with Malignant Melanoma — A Prelimary Report," *Cancer Chemotherpay Reports,* 53(2), April 1969, p. 147-151.

General

This extensive review article on Larrea tridenta notes that its active constituent, NDGA, has been the subject of numerous studies on its efficacy as an antioxidant, anti-inflammatory, anticarcinogen, antimicrobial agent, etc.; many of which have produced findings supporting its use and calling for the need for additional research into the overall health benefits of the plant in general.

> —F. Brinker, "Larrea Tridentata (D.C.) Colville (Chaparral or Creosote Bush)," *British Journal of Phytotherapy,* 3(1), 1993-1994, p. 10-30.

■ ANGELICA

Antibacterial Activity

Results of this study found xanthoangelol and 4-hydroxyderricin, two chalcone isolated from the root of Angelcia keiskei KOIDZUMI, showed antibacterial activities against gram-positive pathogenic bacteria.

> —Y. Inamori, et al., "Antibacterial Activity of Two Chalcones, Xanthoangelol and 4-Hydroxyderricin, Isolated from the Root of Angelica Keiskie KOIDZUMI," *Chem. Pharm.* Bull., 39(6), 1991, p. 1604-1605.

Cancer

This review article reports that potent antitumor promoter has been documented in the nonpolar extracts of the root of Ashita-Ba, Angelica Keiskei Koidz (Umbelliferae), which is a commonly eaten vegetable among the Japanese.

> —T. Okuyama, et al., "Anti-tumor-promotion by Principles Obtained from Angelica Keiskei," *Planta Medicine,* 57(3), June 1991, p. 242-246.

In this study, the antimutagenic activity of Angelica archangelica L. aqueous and alcohol extracts of thioTEPA against mutagencicity was examined by the micronucleus test in murine bone marrow cells. Results showed that the reduction of Thio-TEPA s mutagenic activity was more profound when the extracts were injected 2 hours before thio-TEPA treatment, as seen during simultaneous treatment. The observed reduction of micronuclear frequencies was reached levels as high as 77%.

> —R.A. Salikhova & G.G. Poroshenko, [Antimutagenic Properties of Angelica Archangelica L], *Vestn Ross Akad Med Nauk,* (1), 1995, p. 58-61.

This study examined the biological activities of immunostimulating polysacharide (AIP) from Angelica. Results found the antitumour activity of AIP was observed in terms of prolongation of the survival period of mice bearing Ehrlich ascites cells. The uptake of triated thymidine into murine and human spleen cells could be stimulated by AIP in a dose-dependent manner. Murine B cells were activated polycolonally by AIP and differentiated to antibody forming cells even in the absence of either helper T cells or macrophages.

> —Y. Kumazawa, et al., "Immunostimulating Polysaccharide Separated from Hot Water Extract of Angelica Acutiloba Kitagawa (Yamato Tohki)," *Immunology,* 47, 1982, p. 75-83.

Cardiovascular/Coronary Heart Disease

Results of this study found that 0.6 gm crude drug/kg of Angelica administration to rats vita peritoneal injection significantly reduced the incidence of ventricular premature beat and the total incidence of arrhythmia. Based on these findings, the authors suggest that angelica injection effectively protects against arrhythmia in rats during myocardial inschemia.

> —X.X. Zhuang, [Protectuve Effect of Angelica Injection on Arrhythmia During Myocardial Ischemia Reperfusion in Rat], *Chung Hsi I Chieh Ho Tsa Chih,* 11(6), June 1991, p. 360-361, 326.

In this study, the injection of aqueous extract of Angelica sinensis (AS), 50 mg/kg, 30 ml, were administered intravenously at rate of 0.4 ml/min by an infusion pump 10 min before the left anterior descending coronary artery of rabbit was ligated. Results found that Angelica provided clear protection against myocardial dysfunction and injury.

> —S.G. Chen, et al., [Protective Effects of Angelica Sinensis Injection on Myocardial Ischemia/ Reperfusion Injury in Rabbits], *Chung Kuo Chung Hsi I Chieh Ho Tsa Chih,* 15(8), August 1995, p. 486-488.

General

This study notes the isolation of a low molecular weight polysaccharide from the rhizome of Angelica sinensis (Oliv.). Diels (Umbelliferaer) which carries a molecular weight of approximately 3,000 and consists of protein (4.63%) and carbohydrate (85.85%) of which 5.2% is uronic acid. It's been shown to possess strong antitumor activity of Ehrlich Ascites tumor-bearing mice and to exhibit immunostimulating activities in vitro as well as in vivo.

> —Y.M. Choy, et al., "Immunopharmacological Studies of Low Molecular Weight Polysaccharide from Angelica Sinesis," *American Journal of Chinese Medicine,* 22(2), 1994, p.137-145.

Results of this study showed that Angelica pubescens roots anti-inflammatory and analgesic constituents were related to peripheral inhibition of inflammatory substances and to the influence on the central nervous system in humans.

> —Y.F. Chen, et al., "Anti-inflammatory and Analgesic Activities from Roots of Angelica pubescens," *Planta Med,* 61(1), February 1995, p. 2-8.

This review article cites numerous studies supporting the use of Angelica sinensis as an effective treatment for a variety of conditions including: PMS, dysmenorrhea, amenorrhea, cardiac arrhythmia, high blood pressure, anemia, and acute icteric hepatitis.

> —R. Belford/Courtney, "Comparison of Chinese and Western Uses of Angelica Sinensis," *Aust Journal of Med Herbalism,* 5(4), 1993, p. 87-91.

Results of this study showed that XT isolated from the dried roots of Angelica archangelica L., produced dose-dependent sedative activity in dogs, cats, rats, mice, and hamsters.

> —O.P. Sethi, et al., "Evaluation of Xanthotoxol for Central Nervous System Activity," *Journal of Ethnopharmacology,* 36(1992), p. 239-247.

Psoriasis

Results of this study found Angelica dahurica posesses photochemically active constiuents that proved to be a safe and effective treatment for adult patients suffering from psoriasis.

> —E.M. Farber, et al., (eds.), "The Treatment of Psoriasis with Extracts of Angelica Dahurica and UVA Irradiation," *Psoriasis: Proceedings of the Third International Symposium,* 1981, p. 401-402.

■ BILBERRY

Anti-inflammatory Effects

Results of this study showed that an oral preparation of vaccinium myrtillus exhibited significant vasoprotective and antioedema effects in rabbits and rats.

—A. Lietti, et al., "Studies on Vaccinium Myrtillus Anthocyanosides. I. Vasoprotective and Antiinflammatory Activity," *Arzneimittelforschung,* 26(), 1976, p. 829-832.

Cardiovascular/Coronary Heart Disease

Results of this study showed vaccinium myrtillus anthocyanosides to be effective promoters and enhancers of arteriolar rhythmic diameter changes in the hamster cheek pouch.

—A. Colantuoni, et al., "Effects of Vaccinium Myrtillus Anthocyanosides on Arterial Vasomotion," *Arzneimittelforschung,* 41(9), September 1991, p. 905-909.

Results of this study showed vaccinum myrtillus anthocyanosides reduced ischaemia reperfusion injury-induced microvascular impairments and improved capillary perfusion in the hamster cheek pouch.

—S. Bertuglia, et al., "Effect of Vaccinium Myrtillus Anthocyanosides on Ischaemia Reperfusion Injury in Hamster Cheek Pouch Microcirculation," *Pharmacol Research,* 31(3-4), March-April 1995, p. 183-187.

■ BLACK COHOSH

Depression

This article reports on the succesful use of black cohosh in tincture form as a treatment for depression in 3 different case studies.

—D. Frances, "Cimicifuga for Depression," *Medical Herbalism,* 7(1-2), Spring/Summer 1995, p. 1-2.

Measles

Cimicifuga-Pueraria decoction has been shown to effective in the early stages of measles. When used according to traditional Chinese Methods, additional studies have found it to be effective in influenza, mumps, measles complicated with pneumonia, congenital syphilis and tonsilitis as well.

—H.M. Chang & P.P. But (eds.), *Pharmacology and Applications of Chinese Materia Medica,* Hong Kong, World Scientific, 1986, p. 235-239.

Menopause

This study examined the effects of remifemin, an extract of Cimicifua racemosa, on LH and FSH secretion of menopausal women. Levels of LH, but not FSH were found to be reduced significantly in patients who received the extract. Subsequent animal experiments within the same study supported these results.

—E.M. Duker, et al., "Effects of Extracts from Cimicifuga Racemosa on Gonadotropin

Release in Menopausal Women and Ovariectomized Rats,'' *Planta Med,* 57(5), October 1991, p. 420-424.

This review article cites studies supporting the use of black cohosh as an estrogenic agent in the treatment of women suffering from menopausal symptoms.
—J.M. Snow, ''Cimicifuga Racemosa (L) Nutt. (Ranunculaceae),'' *The Protocol Journal of Botanical Medicine,* Spring 1996, p. 17-19.

Pregnancy

Clinical evidence suggests black cohosh relives the pain and distress of pregnancy, contributes to easy and quick uncomplicated deliveries, and promotes uterine involution and recovery.
—D.B. Mowrey, *The Scientific Validation of Herbal Medicine,* New Canaan, CT, Keats Publishing, 1986, p. 108.

■ BLACK WALNUT

Cancer

This study examined antitumor activities of compounds present in Juglans nigra (black walnut) in mice with spontaneous and/or transplanted tumors. Swiss-Wesbster mice with mammary adenocarcinomas were treated for 9 days (ip) with ellagic acid (50 mg/kg/d), juglone (10 mg/kg/d), a strong acids fraction (100 mg/kg/d) or a weak acids fraction (100 mg/kg/d); C57BL/65 mice with sc transplanted BW-10232 mammary adenocarcinoma were treated ip with total alkaloids (50 mg/kg/d x 12) or EA (10 mg/kg bid x 10 d). Results found that juglone decreased the tumor growth rate and body weight in mice with spontaneous tumors. Strong acids slightly decreased the growth rate of spontaneous tumors. Strong acids slightly decreased the growth rate of spontaneous tumors and ellagic acids depressed the growth of both tumors, especially the spontaneous tumors.
—U.C. Bhargava & B.A. Westfall, ''Antitumor Activity of Julans Nigra (Black Walnut) Extractives,'' *Journal of Pharm Science,* 57(10), 1968, p. 1674-1677.

In this study, ellagic acid, juglone, and isolated fractions of Juglans nigra were injected intraperitonally into mice bearing transplanted tumors for 9-12 days. Results showed such injections significantly inhibited the growth rate of tumors.
—U.C. Bhargava & B.A. Westfall, ''Antitumor Activity of Juglans Nigra (Black Walnut) Extract,'' *Journal of Pharmaceutical Sciences,* 57(10), October 1968, p. 1674-1677.

Cardiovascular/Coronary Heart Disease

This letter to The Lancet reports on the results of a single-blind study involving men consuming a diet high in walnuts (84 g per day). Results showed that the diet significantly lowered serum total cholesterol levels and low and high density cholesterol. The study also reported a 12% reduction in the ratio of low to high density lipoprotein cholesterol in those consuming the walnuts.
—1. D. McNamee, The Lancet, 341, March 13, 1993, p. 687; 2. J. Sabate, et al., ''Effects of Walnuts on Serum Lipid Levels and Blood Pressure in Normal Men,'' *New England Journal of Medicine,* 328, 1993, p. 603-607

General

Studies have shown black walnut bark to kill ringworm and tapeworm, lower blood pressure, and possess anticancer properties.

—D.B. Mowrey, *The Scientific Validation of Herbal Medicine,* New Canaan, CT, Keats Publishing, 1986, p. 230.

■ CARROT

Cancer

Results of this study showed cancer and death by diethlynitrosamine (DNEA)-induced hepatomas in rats were significantly delayed by the consumption of only carrots for several days a week.

—A. Reider, et al., "Delay of Diethylnitrosamine-Induced Hepatoma in Rats by Carrot Feeding," *Oncology,* 40, 1983, p. 120-123.

General

This study identified 6-Methoxymellein to be a common phytoalexin produced by carrot roots irrespective of the species challenging fungi and showed the compound to possess a broad antimicrobial spectrum and inhibit the growth of numerous bacteria, fungi, and yeasts.

—F. Kurosaki & A. Nishi, "Isolated and Antimicrobial Activity of the Phytoalexin 6-Methoxymellein from Culture Carrot Cells," *Phytochemistry,* 22(3), 1983, p. 669-672.

Liver Damage

This study examined the effects of carrot extract on carbon tetrachloride (CC14)-induced acute liver damage in mice. Results found that increased serum enzyme levels (viz. glutamate oxaloacetate transaminase, glutamate pyruvate transaminase, lactate dehydrogenase, alkaline phosphatase, sorbitol and glutamate, dehydrogenase) by CC14-induction to be significantly lowered due to pretreatment with the extract. Results also showed that the extract decreased the elevated serum bilirubin andurea content due to CC14 administration and increased activities of hepatic 5 -nucleotidase, acid phosphatase, acid ribouclease and decreased levels of succint dehydrogenase, glucose-6-phosphatase and cytochrome P-450 produced by CC14 were reversed by the extract in a dose-responsive way. The overall findings of this study revealed demonstrated that carrot could afford a significant protective action in the alleviation of CC14-induced hepatocellular injury.

—A. Bishayee, et al., "Hepatoprotective Activity of Carrot (Daucus carota L.) Against Carbon Tetrachloride Intoxication in Mouse Liver," *Journal of Ethnopharmacology,* 47(2), July 7, 1995, p. 69-74.

Uterine Contractions

Results of this study found that the methanolic fraction of the petrol extract of Daucus carota seeds produced inhibitory effects on spontaneous, oxytocin-induced contractions of the uterus in rats and histamine-induced responses of isolated guinea pig ileum.

—V.J. Dhar, "Studies on Daucus Caroto Seeds," *Fitoterapia,* LXI(3), 1990, p. 255-258.

■ COMMON PLANTAIN

Bronchitis

In this study, 25 chronic bronchitis patients received treated with Plantago major for a period of between 25-30 days. Results found a quick effect on subjective complaints and objective benefits in as many as 80% of the patients with no toxic effects.

> —M. Mateve, et al., [Clinical Trial of a Plantago Major Preparation in the Treatment of Chronic Bronchitis], *Vutr Boles,* 21(2), 1982, p. 133-137.

Cancer

Results of this study found that adding the polyphenolic complex from Plantago major plantastine to the diet of rats inhibited the carcinogenic activity of long-term liver exposure to amidopyrine and sodium nitrate.

> —E.D. Karpilovksaia, et al, [Inhibiting Effect of the Polyphenolic Complex from Plantago Major (Plantastine) on the Carcinogenic Effect of Endogenously Synthesized Nitrosodimethylamine], *Farmakol Toksikol,* 52(4), July-August 1989, p. 64-67.

In this case-controlled study a number of female mice were given subcutaneous injections of intracellular fluid of way-bread. Results showed there to be a significant difference between the frequency of tumor formation between the two groups, with the control rate of formation being 93.3% compared to 18.2% in the treated animals.

> —A. Lithander, "Intracellular Fluid of Waybread (Plantago major) as a Prophylactic for Mammary Cancer in Mice," *Tumour Biology,* 13(3), 1992, p.138-141.

General

This study examined the laxative properties of seeds from Plantago ovata, Plantago psyllium L, and Plantago major L. Results showed Plantago seeds to be a stronger purgative than linseed, with Plantago major being the most effective of those studied.

> —V.R. Wasicky, "Untersuchungen Der Samen Von Plantago Ovat A Forsk (P. Ispaghula Roxb.), P. Psyllium L. Und P. Major l. Var Cruent A Holuby Unter Dem Gesichtspunkt Ihrer Abfuhrwifkung," *Planta Med,* 9, 1961, p. 232-244.

This study examined the pharmacological properties of Passiflora incarnata in a variety of experimental animals. Results found the active substances of the plant produced a lowering of blood pressure and contraction of smooth muscle of the uterus and gut.

> —G.H. Ruggy & C.S. Smith, "A Pharmacological Study of the Active Principal of Passiflora Incarnata," *Journal of the American Pharmaceutical Association,* 29, 1947, p. 245-249.

This study examined the neuropharmalogical properties of a fluid extract of passiflora incarnata L. in rats. Results showed intraperitoneal injection significantly increased sleeping time and provided protection against the convulsive effects of pentylenetetrazole.

> —E. Speroni & A. Mingehti, "Neuropharmacological Activity of Extracts from Passiflora Incarnata," *Planta Medica,* 1988, p. 488-491.

Results of this study of the large Plantain leaf showed it exhibited anti-inflammatory action and affects epithelialization and destruction of the elements of impetigo and ecthyma of the skin when administered in ointment form.

—R.K. Aliev, ''A Wound Healing Preparation from the Leaves of the Large Plantain (Plantago Major L.),'' *American Journal of Pharmacology,* 122,1950, p. 24-26.

■ CRANBERRY

Cardiovascular/Coronary Heart Disease

Results of this found that a component of Viburnum opulus led to bradycardia, hypotension, and a reduction on myocardial contractility in dogs, cats, and rats.

—J.A. Nicholson, et al., ''Viopudial, a Hypotensive and Smooth Muscle Antispasmodic from Viburnum Opulus,'' *Proc. Soc. Exp. Biol. Med.,* 140(2), June 1972, p. 457-461.

This study showed components of the bark of Viburnum Opulus exhibited hypotensive action in cats and spasmolytic acitivity in rabbit intestines.

—W. Raszejowa & K. Szpunarowna, ''Consituents of the Bark of Viburnum Opulus and Some Pharmacodynamic Properties Thereof,'' *Acta Polon Pharm,* 16, 1959, p. 131-139.

General

This study isolated scopoletin from Viburnum opulus and Viburnum prunifolium and found it to have antispasmodic properties in an in an in vitro estrone-primed and BaCl2 stimulated rat uterus preparation.

—C.H. Jarboe, et al., ''Scopoletin, as Antispasmodic Component of Viburnum Opulus and Viburnum Prunifolium,'' *Journal of Med. Chem.,* 10(3), 1967, p. 488-489.

Urinary Tract Infection

Results of this study on 77 clinical isolates of Eschericihia coli found cranberry juice to be an effective inhibitor of bacterial adherence b 75% or more in over 60% of the clinical isolates. Mice given cranberry cocktail for 14 days also possessed urine which inhibited adherence of E. coli to uroepithelial cells by 80%. Results showed significant antiadherence activity could be in the urine of 15 of 22 human subjects 1 to 3 hours after drinking 15 ounces of cranberry cocktail as well.

—A.E. Sobota, ''Inhibition of Bacterial Adherence by Cranberry Juice: Potential use for the Treatment of Urinary Tract Infections,'' *Journal of Urology,* 131(5), May 1984, p. 1013-1016.

This study examined the effects of cranberry juice on the adherence of Escherichia coli expressing surface lectins of defined sugar specifically to yeasts, tissue culture cells, erythroyctes, and mouse peritoneal macrophages. Results showed that it inhibited the adherence of urinary isolates expressing type 1 fimbriae (mannose specific) and P fimbriae ecific for alpha-D-Gal(1—-4)-beta-D-Gal] and also inhibited yeast agglutination by purified type 1 fimbriae. In addition to cranberry juice; results found that orange juice, and pineapple juice inhibited adherence of type 1 fimbriated E. coli, as well, most likely because of their fructose content.

—D. Zafriri, et al., ''Inhibitory Activity of Cranberry Juice on Adherence of Type 1 and

Type P Fimbriated Escherichia Col to Eucaryotic Cells,'' *Antimicrobials Agents Chemotherapy,* 33(1), January 1989, p. 92-98.

Drinking 4 to 6 ounces of cranberry juice almost daily for 7 weeks was shown to prevent urinary tract infections in 19 of 28 nursing home patients. The remaining nine had trace or greater leukocytes and or nitrates in all their urine and significant colony counts of Gram negative bacilli even though they drank 4 to 6 ounces of cranberry juice. The authors suggest that cranberry juice is thus preventative rather than curative of urinary tract infections.

—L. Gibson, et al., ''Effectiveness of Cranberry Juice in Preventing Urinary Tract Infections in Long-Term Care Facility Patients,'' *The Journal of Naturopathic Medicine,* 2(1), 1991, p. 45-47.

In this placebo-controlled study, elderly women who consumed 300 ml per day of cranberry juice had an odds ration of bacteriuria with pyuria of 42% of the odds in controls. Odds of remaining bacteriuricpy-uric were 27% of control odds. based on the results, the authors suggest that cranberry juice may be effective in the treatment of urinary tract infections.

—Jerry Avorn, et al., ''Reduction of Bacteriuria and Pyruia after Ingestion of Cranberrry Juice,'' *JAMA,* 271(10), March 9, 1994, p. 751-754.

Results from this study found that 73% of subjects suffering from urinary tract infections who consumed 16 ounces of cranberry juice per day experience relief. Recurrence rate was 61% when the treatment was withdrawn.

—P.N. Prodromos, et al., ''Cranberry Juice in the Treatment of Urinary Tract Infections,'' *Southwest Medicine,* 47, 1968, p. 17.

This study of 7 juices including cranberry, blueberry, grapefruit, guava, mango, orange, and pineapple found that only two (cranberry and blueberry) possessed anti-Escherichia coli ahesis activity. The authors recommend both as treatments for bladder infection.

—Ofek, et al., ''Anti-Escheriica Adhesi Activity of Cranberry and Blueberry Juices,'' *New England Journal of Medicine,* 324(1599), 1991.

Results of this study found extracts of Viburnum opulus and Viburnum prunifolium acted as uterine relaxants in rats.

—C.H. Jarboe, et al., ''Uterine Relaxant Properties of Viburnum,'' *Nature,* 212(5064), November 19, 1966, p. 837.

■ DANDELION

Cancer

This study examined the antitumor effects of a non-dialyzable hot water extract, tof-CFr, isolated from dandelions in mice. Results showed that the Tof-CFr had antitumor effects on the allogenic ddY-Ehrlich tumor system and on the syngenieic C3H/Hef-MM46 tumor system when administered days 11-20 or 2-20 but not if administered days 1-10.

—K. Baba, et al., [Antitumor Activity of Hot Water Extract Dandelion,Taraxacum Officinale -

Correlation Between Antitumor Activity and Timing of Administration], *Yakugaku Zasshi,* 101(6), 1981, p. 538-543.

Diabetes

Dandelion root has been shown to cause hypoglycemic effects in animal studies. A likely explanation for this is that the dandelion root improves kidney function, particularly with respect to the kidney's ability to cleanse blood and resorb nutrients.

—D.B. Mowrey, *The Scientific Validation of Herbal Medicine,* New Canaan, CT, Keats Publishing, 1986, p. 67.

This study examined the blood glucose levels of rabbits following oral intake of whole, dried and powdered plants of the Portulaca olecarae, Linn and Taraxaxum offinale. Results found both plants taken as a powder had significant hypoglycemic effects in rabbits other than those treated with alloxan.

—M.S. Akhtar, et al., ''Effects of Portulaca Oleracae (Kulfa) and Taraxacum Offinale (Dhud-hal) in Normoglycaemic and Alloxan-Treated Hyperglycaemic Rabbits,'' *J.P.M.A.,* 35, July 1985.

General

This extensive review articlenotes numerous clinical studies supporting the use of Dandelion in treating conditions including liver problems, hepatitis, gallstones, kidney trouble, and weight loss. Animals studies have found Dandelion to increase bile excretion in rats and dogs, promote weight loss in mice, inhibit the growth of inoculated Ehrlich ascites cancer cells in mice, and posess hypotensive properties.

—E. Cordatos, ''Taraxacum Officinale,'' *Aust. Journal of Med. Herbalism,* 3(4), 1991, p. 64-73.

■ DWARF/SAW PALMETTO

Benign Prostatic Hyperplasia

This review article cites numerous studies supporting the use of saw palmetto berries and stinging nettle roots in the treatment of benign postatic hyperplasia.

—E. Koch & A. Biber, ''Pharmacological Effects of Sabal and Urtica Extracts as Basis for a Rational Medication of Benign Prostatic Hyperplasia,'' *Urologe,* 34(2), 1994, p. 90-95.

This study examined the effects of a 160 mg dose of Serona repens extract taken twice a day over 3 months by 505 benign prostatic hyperplasia patients. Results showed significant improvement after only 45 days. 88% of patients and physicians deemed the therapy to be effective after 90 days.

—J. Braeckman, ''The Extract of Seronoa Repens in the Treatment of Benign Prostatic Hyperplasia: A Multicenter Open Study,'' *Current Therapeutic Research,* 55(7), July 1994, p. 776-785.

Results of this study found that Serona repens lipid extract inhibited 5 beta-reducatase, 3- ketosteroid reductase and receptor binding and androgens in cultured human foreskin fibroblasts, suggesting it may be considered a new antiandrogenic compound as therapeutic for treating hirsutism, benign prostatic hypertrophy, and related conditions.

> —C. Sultan, et al., "Inhibition of Androgen Metabolism and Binding By A Liposterolic Extract of Serona Repens B in Human Foreskin Firboblasts," *Journal of Steroid Biochem,* 20(1), 1984, p. 515-519.

Results of this double-blind, placebo-controlled study found Serenoa repens extract to be significantly effective in improving the micturitional symptoms and the uroflowmetric records of patients suffering from stage I and stage II prostatic adenomoa relative to controls.

> —A. Tasca, et al., "Treatment of Obstructive Symptomatolgy in Prostatic Adenoma with an Extract of Serenoa Repens," 1988, (German translation, source not available).

General

Results of this study showed an acidic polysaccharide from Saw Palmetto at low dosages inhibited carrageenin-produced paw edema and pellet tests in rats.

> —H. Wagner, et al., "A New Anti-phlogistic Principle from Sabal Serrulata," *Planta Med.,* 41, 1981, p. 252-258.

■ ECHINACEA

Anti-inflammatory Effects

Results of this study found that a topically administered polysaccharide fraction obtained from Echinacea angustifolia roots exhibited anti-inflammatory effects on paw and ear oedema in mice.

> —A. Tubaro, et al., "Anti-inflammatory Activity of a Polysaccharidic Fraction of Echinacea Angustifolia," *Journal of Pharm Pharmacol,* 39(7), July 1987, p. 567-569.

Results of this study showed that fractions taken from an aqueous extract of echinacea angustifolia roots exhibited anti-inflammatory effects on ear oedema in mice.

> —E. Tragni, et al., "Anti-inflammatory Activity of Echinacea Angustifolia Fractions Separated on the Basis of Molecular Weight," *Pharmacol Res Commun,* 20 (Suppl 5), December 1988, p. 87-90.

Cancer

Results of this study showed that the Echinacea purpurea polysaccharide, acidic arabinogalactan, proved effective in activating macrophages to cytotoxicity against tumor cells and micro-organisms and induced macrophages to produce tumor necrosis factor, interleukin-1, and interferon-beta 2.

> —B. Luettig, et al., "Macrophage Activation by the Polysaccharide Arabinogalactan Isolated from Plant Cell Cultures of Echinacea Purpurea.," *Journal of National Cancer Institute,* 81(9), May 3, 1989, p. 669-675.

Immune Function

Results of this study showed that ethanolic extracts of Echinacea purpurea, E. pallida and E. angustifolia roots exhibited immunoglocial activity and significantly enhanced phagocytosis in vitro.

> —V.R. Bauer, et al., [Immunologic in Vivo and in Vitro Studies on Echinacea Extracts], *Arzneimittelforschung,* 38(2), February 1988, p. 276-281.

Results of this study showed that ethanolic extract from the roots Echinacea gloriosa L. (Moench), Echinacea angustifolia DC. and Rudbeckia speciosa Wenderoth exhibited immunomodulating activity in mice treated with the extracts over a period of five days.

> —M. Bukovsky, et al., [Immunomodulating Activity of Ethanol-water Extracts of the Roots of Echinacea Gloriosa L., Echinacea angustifolia DC. and Rudbeckia speciosa Wenderoth Tested on the Immune System in C57BL6 Inbred Mice], *Cesk Farm,* 42(4), August 1993, p. 184-187.

Results of this study indicated that polysaccharide isolates from Echinacea purpurea enhanced nonspecific immunity in immunodeficient mice.

> —C. Steinmuller, et al., "Polysaccharides Isolated from Plant Cell Cultures of Echinacea Purpurea Enhance the Resistance of Immunosuppressed Mice Against Systemic Infections with Candida Albicans and Listeria Monocytogenes," *International Journal of Immunopharmacol,* 15(5), July 1993, p. 605-614.

Skin Damage

Results of this study found that polyphenols of Echinacea species protected collagen against free radical damage, pointing to Echinacea's potential as a topical agent of prevention or treatment for UV radiation-induced skin damage.

> —R.M. Facino, et al., "Echinacoside and Caffeoyl Conjugates Protect Collagen from Free Radical-induced Degradation: A Potential Use of Echinacea Extracts in the Prevention of Skin Photodamage," *Planta Medicine,* 61(6), December 1995, p. 510-514.

■ EVENING PRIMROSE OIL

Arthritis

This study examined the serum concentration of lipids and composition of fatty acids in 18 patients following overnight fasting with rheumatoid arthritis treated for 12 weeks with either 20 ml of evening primrose oil containing 9% of gamma-linolenic acid or olive oil. Results showed decreases in the serum concentrations of oleic acid, eicosapentaenoic acid, andapolipoprotein B during treatment with evening primrose oil with increases seen in serum levels of linoleic acid, gamma-linolenic acid, dihomo-gamma-linolenic acid, and arachidonic acid.

> —J. Jantti, et al., "Evening Primrose Oil in Rheumatoid Arthritis: Changes in Serum Lipids and Fatty Acids," *Ann Rheum Disease,* 48(2), February 1989, p. 124-127.

In this double-blind, placebo-controlled study of rheumatoid arthritis patients with drug induced upper gastrointestinal lesions, results found that those receiving 6 g per day of evening oil experienced significant reductions in morning stiffness relative to controls.

—M. Brzeski, et al., ''Evening Primrose Oil in patients with Rheumatoid Arthritis and Side-effects of Non-steroidal Anti-inflammatory Drugs,'' *British Journal of Rheumatology,* 30(5), October 1991, p. 370-372.

Eczema

This double-blind, placebo-controlled study examined the effects of oral evening primrose oil on patients with atopic eczema. Results showed that those in the treatment group experienced a significant overall improvement in inflammation levels and percentage of body surface effected by the eczema relative to controls.

—M. Schlin-Karrila, et al., ''Evening Primrose Oil in the Treatment of Atopic Eczema: Effect on Clinical Status, Plasma Phospholipid Fatty Acids and Circulating Blood Prostaglandins,'' *British Journal of Dermatology,* 117(1), July 1987, p. 11-19.

Results of this study showed that children with atopic eczema who were treated with long-term oral evening primrose oil supplementation experienced improvements in their clinical conditions after 4 weeks and lasting up to 20 weeks.

—P.L. Biagi, et al., ''A Long-term Stud on the Use of Evening Primrose Oil (Efamol) in Atopic Children,'' *Drugs Exp Clinical Research,* 14(4), 1988, p. 285-290.

Diabetes

This study examined the effects of evening primrose oil (10 g/kg per day) on sciatic nerve pefusion and oxygenation in streptozotocin-diabetic rats. Results showed the treatment to be effective in preventing impairment of blood flow and endoneurial oxygenation.

—N.E. Cameron & M.A. Cotter, ''Effects of Evening Primrose Oil Treatment on Sciatic Nerve Blood Flow and Endoneurial Oxygen Tension in Streptozotocin-diabetic Rats,'' *Acta Diabetol,* 31(4), December 1994, p. 220-225.

Results of this case-control study of insulin dependent diabetics found that those given 3 g daily of linoleic-gamma-linilenic acid mixture experienced positive changes with respect to HDL-cholesterol and platelet adhesiveness relative to controls.

—R. Uccella, et al., [Action of Evening Primrose Oil on Cardiovascular Risk Factors in Insulin-dependent Diabetics], *Clin Ter,* 129(5), June 15, 1989, p. 381-388.

This study examined the effects of evening primrose oil and fish oil on glucose and lipid metabolism, prostaglandin levels and body composition in patients with non-insulin-dependent diabetes. Seven patients were administered 4 g of evening primrose oil, 2.4 g sardine oil and 200 mg of vitamin E for 4 weeks. Results showed significant differences in fasting plasma glucose, hemoglobin A1 c, total cholesterol, body weight and % body fat mass following treatment. In the treatment group, concentrations of (e) icosapentaenoic acid (EPA) increased significantly in all the lipoprotein fractions. Results also showed the ratio of 6-keto- PGF1 alpha and PGE1 to 11-dehydro-thromboxane B2 increased signficantly after the treatment.

> —R. Takahashi, et al., ''Evening Primrose Oil and Fish Oil in non-insulin-dependent-diabetes,'' *Prostaglandins Leukot Essent Fatty Acids,* 49(2), August 1993, p. 569-571.

Cardiovascular/Coronary Heart Disease

In this study, 4 week old spontaneously hypertensive rats were fed a diet supplemented with sunflowerseed oil, evening primrose oil, fish oil, or both fish oil and evening primrose oil for 22 weeks. Results found significant decreases in systolic blood pressure during and after supplementation with fish oil, evening primrose oil, or both given together. Results also indicated that serum triglycerides and total cholesterol levels were lowest after evening primrose oil followed by fish oil.

> —P. Singer, et al., ''Blood Pressure and Serum Lipids from SHR after Diets Supplemented with Evening Primrose, Sunflowered or Fish Oil,'' *Prostaglandings Leukot Essent Fatty Acids,* 40(1), May 1990, p. 17-20.

Dermatitis

In this study, cats suffering from papulocrusous dermatitis received either evening primrose oil or sunflower oil for 12 weeks. Results showed both treatment groups experienced improvements with those in the evening primrose group showing increased concentration of linoleic acid in erythrocyte phospholipid.

> —R.G. Harvey, ''A Comparison of Evening Primrose Oil and Sunflower Oil for the Management of Papulocrustous Dermatitis in Cats,'' *Vet Rec,* 133(23), December 4, 1993, p. 571-573.

In this study, 14 cats with crusting dermatoses received supplements with combinations of evening primrose oil and fish oil. Results showed improvements in cutaneous signs irregardless of treatment combination.

> —R.G. Harvey, ''Effects of Varying Proportions of Evening Primrose Oil and Fish Oil on Cats with Crusting Dermatosis,'' *Vet Rec,* 133(9), August 28, 1993, p. 208-211.

■ FEVERFEW

Candida

Results of this study showed that a feverfew extract inhibited phagocytosis of Candida guilliermondii and its overall killing in vitro.

> —L.M. Williamson, et al., ''Effect of Feverfew on Phagocytosis and Killing of Candida by Neutrophils,'' *Inflammation,* 12(1), February 1988, p. 11-16.

Cardiovascular/Coronary Heart Disease

This study examined the effects of a feverfew extract on the interaction of platelets with surfaces coated with human collagens of type III and IV (CIII, CIV), and on the integrity of the endothelial cell (EC) monolayer in perfused rabbit aorta. Results suggested feverfew may possess antithrombotic potential.

> —W. Loesche, et al., "Feverfew—An Antithrombotic Drug?" *Folia Haematol Int Mag Klin Morphol Blutforsch,* 115(1-2), 1988, p. 181-184.

General

Results of this study indicated that feverfew extracts inhibit platelet aggregation of and the platelet release reaction.

> —S. Heptinstall, et al., Guilliermondii "Inhibition of Platelet Behaviour Folia by Feverfew: A Mechanism of Action Involving Sulphydryl Groups," *Haematol Int Mag Klin Morphol Blutforsch,* 115(4), 1988, p. 447-479.

Migraine

Results this double-blind, placebo-controlled study showed that the consumption of fresh feverfew leaves daily by patients prevented migraines relative to controls.

> —E.S. Johnson, et al., "Efficacy of Feverfew as Prophylactic Treatment of Migraine," *British Medical Journal,* 291(6495), August 31, 1985, p. 569-573.

This double-blind, placebo-controlled, crossover study examined the effects of feverfew on migraines over a period of 4 months among a group of 59 volunteers. Results showed an association between feverfew intake and a reduced severity of migraine attacks and degree of vomiting.

> —J.J. Murphy, et al., "Randomised Double-blind Placebo-controlled Trial of Feverfew in Migraine Prevention," *Lancet,* 2(8604), July 23, 1988, p. 189-192.

■ FLAX

Cancer

Results of this study showed that 4 weeks of flaxseed flour feeding or defatted flaxseed meal (5% or 10%) in a high-fat diet to male rats led to a significant decrease in the formation of aberrant crypts and foci, and epithelial cell proliferation in the colon. A flaxseed diet significantly reduced the epithelial cell proliferation and nuclear aberration in female rat mammary glands as well.

> —M. Serraino, "Studies on the Effect of Flaxseed on Colon and Mammary Carcinogenesis," *Dissertation Abstracts International,* 53(8), 1993, p. 4041.

In this study, 3-week-old female rats received a high-fat diet with or without supplementation with 5% flaxseed. Results showed that the flaxseed provided protection against DMBA-induced tumors.

> —M.R. Serraino and L.U. Thompson, "The Effect of Flaxseed on the Initiation and Promotional Stages of Mammary Tumorigenesis," *FASEB Journal,* 5(5), 1991, p. A928.

Results of this study indicated that supplemental flaxseed reduced the risk of chemical-induced colon cancer in rats fed a high-fat diet.

> —M. Serraino & L.U. Thompson, "Flaxseed Supplementation and Early Markers of Colon Carcinogenesis," *Cancer Letters,* 63(2), April 15, 1992, p. 159-165.

Results of this study showed that supplemental flaxseed flour or defatted flaxseed meal (5% or 10%) significantly decreased the epithelial cell proliferation and nuclear aberrations in mammary glands of female rats fed a high-fat diet.

 —M. Serraino & L.U. Thompson, ''The Effect of Flaxseed Supplementation on Early Risk Markers for Mammary Carcinogenesis,'' *Cancer Letters,* 60(2), November 1991, p. 135-142.

This study examined the effects of flaxseed on chemical-induced mammary tumorigenesis in rats when administered beginning 13 weeks after carcinogenin exposure. Results showed a 50% reduction in tumor volume among those receiving flaxseed 7 weeks into the treatment.

 —L.U. Thompson, et al., ''Flaxseed and Its Lignan and Oil Components Reduce Mammary Tumor Growth at a Late Stage of Carcinogenesis,'' *Carcinogenesis,* 17(6), June 1996, p. 1373-1376.

Results of this study indicated that supplemental flaxseed exhibited protective effects against colon cancer in rats fed a high-fat diet.

 —M. Jenab & L.U. Thompson, ''The Influence of Flaxseed and Lignans on Colon Carcinogenesis and Beta-glucuronidase Activity,'' *Carcinogenesis,* 17(6), June 1996, p. 1343-1348.

Results of this study showed that rats fed 5% flaxseed flour in a high-fat diet at the promotional stage of DMBA-induced tumorigenesis experienced a significant decrease in tumor size.

 —M. Serraino & L.U. Thompson, ''The Effect of Flaxseed Supplementation on the Initiation and Promotional Stages of Mammary Tumorigenesis,'' *Nutrition Cancer,* 17(2), 1992, p. 153-159.

Cardiovascular/Coronary Heart Disease

In this study, healthy young males consumed either 40 g of flaxseed oil or sunflowerseed oil per day over a 23 day period. Results showed that platelet eicosapentaenoic acid doubled in subjects consuming flaxseed oil relative to no change in those taking sunflower seed oil.

 —M.A. Allman, et al., ''Supplementation with Flaxseed Oil Versus Sunflowerseed Oil in Healthy Young Men Consuming a Low Fat Diet: Effects on Platelet Composition and Function,'' *European Journal of Clinical Nutrition,* 49(3), March 1995, p. 169-178.

General

Results of this study found that the consumption of 50 g per day of flaxseed for 4 weeks increased bowel movements by 30% and reduced LDL cholesterol by as much as 8% in healthy young adults.

 —S.C. Cunnane, et al., ''Nutritional Attributes of Traditional Flaxseed in Healthy Young Adults,'' *American Journal of Clinical Nutrition,* 61(1), January 1995, p. 62-68.

Kidney Damage

Results of this study found that dietary flaxseed and flax oil attenuated renal function decline and reduced glomerular injury with favorable effects on blood pressure, plasma lipids, and urinary prostaglandins in rats subjected to 5/6 nephrectomy.

 —A.J. Ingram, et al., ''Effects of Flaxseed and Flax Oil Diets in a Rat-5/6 Renal Ablation Model,'' *American Journal of Kidney Disease,* 25(2), February 1995, p. 320-329.

Lupus

Results of this study showed that the consumption of 30 g of flaxseed per day had beneficial effects on kidney function, inflammatory, mechanisms and atherogenic mechanisms in patients suffering from lupus nephritis.

> —W.F. Clark, et al., "Flaxseed: A Potential Treatment for Lupus Nephritis," *Kidney Int,* 48(2), August 1995, p. 475-480.

■ GOLDENSEAL

Antimicrobial Activity

This study reports berberine sulfate to be a bacteriostatic for streptocpcco and that sub-MICs or berberine blocked the adherence of sterptococci to host cells, immobilized fibronectin, and hexadecane. Results showed that concentrations of berberine below its MIC caused an eightfold increase in release of lipoteichoic acid from the streptococci. Higher concentrations of berberine directly interfered with the adherence of streptococci to host cells either by preventing the complexing of lipoteichoci acid with fibronectin or byh dissolution of such complexes once they were formed.

> —D. Sun, et al., "Berberine Sulfate Blocks Adherence of Streptococcus pyogenes to Epithelial Cells, Fibronectin, and Hexadeceane," *Antimicrobial Agents and Chemotherapy,* 32(9), September 1988, p. 1370-1374.

Cancer

Results of this study found that berberine sulfate, an isoquinoline alkaloid from Hydrastis canadensis L., posessed antitumor-promoting activity in the two-stage carcinogenesis experiment on mouse skin.

> —H. Nishino, et al., "Berberine Sulfate Inhibits Tumor-Promoting Activity of Teleocidin in Two-Stage Carcinogenesis on Mouse Skin," *Oncology,* 43, 1986, P. 131-134.

Cardiovascular/Coronary Heart Disease

Results of this study showed that the administration of berberine in an intravenous bolus injection (1 mg/kg, within 3 minutes) followed by a constant infusion (0.2 mg/kg/min, 30 minutes) significantly increased the cardiac output and decreased LVEDP, diastolic blood pressure, and sytemic vascular resistance in dogs suffering from ischemic left ventricular failure.

> —H. Wei-min, et al., "Beneficial Effects of Berberine on Hemodynamics During Acute Ischemic Left Ventricular Failure in Dogs," *Chinese Medical Journal,* 105(12), 1992, p. 1014-1019.

Diarrhea

Results of this randomized, case-control study of 165 adult diarrhea patients due to enterotoxigenic Escherichia coli (ETEC) and Vibrio cholerae showed that those taking a single dose 400 mg of berberine sulfate, an isoquinoline alkaloid from Hydrastis canadensis L., experienced a signficant decrease in stool volume 8 hours following intake and a significant elimination of diarrhea 24 hours following intake compared to controls.

> —G.H. Rabbani, et al., "Randomized Controlled Trial of Berberine Sulfate Therapy for

Diarrhea due to Enterotoxigenic Escherichia coli and Vibrio cholerae,'' *The Journal of Infectious Diseases,* 155(5), May 1987, p. 979-984.

■ HAWTHORN

Acne

Results of this study found a flavonoid-containing, topical extract of Crataegus oxyacantha to be effective in the treatment of acne vulgaris or rosacea in humans.

    —M.G. Longhi, et al., ''Activity of Crataegus Oxyacantha Derivatives in Functional Dermo-cosmesis,'' *Fitoterapia,* L(2), 1984, p. 87-99.

Cardiovascular/Coronary Heart Disease

This study examined the influence of flavonoids from crataegus species (hawthorn, Rosaceae) on coronary flow, heart rate and left ventricular pressure as well as on the velocity of contraction and relaxation guinea pig hearts. Results found an increase of coronary flow caused by the O-glycosides luteolin-7-glucoside (186%), hypersoide (66%) and rutin (66%) as well as an increase of the relaxation velocity (positive lusitropsim) by luteolin-7-glucoside (104%), hyperoside (62%) and rutin (73%) were the major effects observed at a maxium concentration of 0.5 mmol/l.

    —M. Schussler, et a al., ''Myocardial Effects of Flavonoids from Crataegus Species,'' *Arzneimittelforschung,* 45(8), August 1995, p. 842-845.

Results of this placebo-controlled study showed that patients with stage II heart failure who received treatment with 600 mg per day of Hawthorn Extract LI 132 for 8 weeks experienced significant decreases in systolic pressure, heart rate, and the pressure-rate product relative to controls.

    —U. Schmidt, et al., ''Wirksamkeit des Extrak-tes LI 132 (600 mg/Tag) bei achitowchiger Therapie,'' *Munch. med. Wschr,* 136 (Suppl 1), 1994, p. S13-S19.

Results of this study found that a 0.05% Crataegus extract had a cardioprotective effect on the ischemic-reperfused heart in rats, and that the cardioprotective effect was not accompanied by an increase in coronary flow.

    —Y. Nasa, et al., ''Protective Effect of Crataegus Extract on the Cardiac Mechanical Dysfunction in Isolated Perfused Working Heart,'' *Arzneim Forsch/Drug Res,* 43(9), 1993, p. 945-949.

This placebo-controlled study gave 100 mg of Crataegus pinnatifida leaves to angina patients for 4 weeks. Results showed the treatment had an efficacy rate of 84.8% compared to 37% for controls, with 46.4% of the treatment group showing improvements in ECG readings relative to 3.3% improvement in controls.

    —W.L. Weng, et al., ''Therapeutic Effect of Crataegus Pinnatifida on 46 Cases of Angina Pectoris—A Double Blind Study,'' *Journal of Traditional Chinese Medicine,* 4(4), 1984, p. 293-294.

This study examined the hypotensive effects in rats of an aqueos extract of Crataegus oxyacantha leaves. Results showed the herb given at a median effective dose of of 31 mg/kg significantly decreased the rates of systolic, diastolic, and mean blood pressure while having no effect on heart rate.

> —A.S. Abdulghani, et al., "Hypotensive Effect of Crataegus Oxyacantha," *International Journal of Crude Drug Research,* 25(4), 1987, p. 216-220.

In this double-blind, placebo-controlled study, middle-age chronic heart failure patients received a daily dose of 600 mg of Crataegus extract for 8 weeks. Results showed significant reductions in systolic blood pressure and heart rate relative to controls.

> —U. Schmidt, et al., "Efficacy of Hawthorn (Crataegus) Preparation of LI 132 in 78 Patients with Chronic Congesitive Heart Failure Defined as NYHA Functional Class II," *Phytomedicine,* 1, 1994, p. 17-24.

■ HIBISCUS

Cardiovascular/Coronary Heart Disease

Results of this study found that a crude hydroalcoholic extract from Hibiscus sabdariffa L. calyces exhibited an appreciable enzyme-inhibiting activity towards the Angiotensin I Converting Enzyme (ACE) in vitro, attributable to flavones.

> —M. Jonadet, et al., [In Vitro Enzyme Inhibitory and In Vivo Cardioprotective Activities of Hibiscus (Hibiscus sabdariffa L.)], *Journal of Pharm Belg,* 45(2), March-April 1990, p.120-124.

Results of this study showed that the administration of Karkade had marked cholesterol lowering effects in male rats fed a high-cholesterol diet over a period of 12 weeks.

> —S.S. el-Saadany, et al., "Biochemical Dynamics and Hypocholesterolemic Action of Hibiscus Sabdariffa (Karkade)," *Nahrung,* 35(6), 1991, p. 567-576.

Contraception

In this study, 250-1000 mg/kg body weight per day of a benzene extract of Hibiscus rosa-senensis was given to mice from day 1 through 4 of postcoitus. Results showed a dose-dependent increase in the rate of implantation failure.

> —S.N. Kabir, et al., "Flowers of Hibiscus Rosa-sinensis, A Potential Source of Contragestative Agent: I. Effect of Benzene Extract on Implantation of Mouse," *Contraception,* 29(4), April 1984, p. 385-397.

In this study, 1 gm/kg body weight per day of a benzene extract of Hibiscus rosa-senensis was given to mice from day 5 through 8 of gestation. Results showed a the extract led to termination of pregnancy in approximately 92% of the mice.

> —A. Pakrashi A, et al., "Flowers of Hibiscus Rosa-sinensis, a Potential Source of Contragestative Agent. III: Interceptive Effect of Benzene Extract in Mouse," *Contraception,* 34(5), November 1986, p. 523-536.

General

This study examined the protective effects of hibiscus protocatechuic acid, a simple phenolic compound isolated from Hibiscus sabdariffa L., against tert-butylhydroperoxide-induced oxidative damage in a primary culture of rat hepatocytes. Results showed that it provided protection against cytotoxicity and genotoxicity of hepatocytes induced by t-BHP.

> —T.H. Tseng, et al., "Hibiscus Protocatechuic Acid Protects Against Oxidative Damage Induced by tert-butylhydroperoxide in Rat Primary Hepatocytes," *Chem Biol Interact*, 101(2), August 14, 1996, p. 137-148.

■ LICORICE

Antiviral Effects

This article notes that investigations in antiviral action of plant extracts have found that a component of Glycyrrhiza glabra roots, found to be glycyrrhizie acid, is active against viruses. The articel reports the drugs inhibits growth and cytopathology of several unrelated DNA and RNA viruses, while not affecting cell activity and ability to replicate. In addition, glycyrrhizic acid inactivates herpes simplex virus particles irreversibly.

> —R. Pompei, et al., "Glycyrrhizic Acid Inhibits Virus Growth and Inactivates Virus Particles," *Nature*, 281(5733), October 25, 1979, p. 689-690.

Diabetes

In this study, 10 steptozotocine induced diabetic rats were treated with baicalin 150 mg/kg per day and liquid extract of licorice (LEL) 7.5 ml/kg per day for one week. Results showed that oral baicalin and licorice significantly reduced sorbitol levels in RBC without affecting blood glucose levels and that the sorbitol levels were restored to original values one week after discontinuing the treatment.

> —Y.P. Zhou & J.Q. Zhang, "Oral Baicalin and Liquid Extract of Licorice Reduce Sorbitol Levels in Red Blood Cell of Diabetic Rats," *Chinese Medical Journal*, 102(3), March 1989, p. 203-206.

This study examined the effects of glycyrrhizine in low doses on hyperkalemia in 8 NIDDM patients. Results showed the mean serum potassium concentration decreased from 5.3+/-0.3 (SD) mEq/1 to 4.9 +/- 0.2 mEq/1 shen 15 g of calcium polysterene sulfonate, a potassium-binding resin, was given per day, and it decreased significantly to 4.4 +/- 0.4 mEq/1 with 150 mg/day of glycyrrhizine therapy.

> —T. Murakami & T. Uchikawa, "Effect of Glycrrhizine on Hyperkalemia Due to Hyporeninemic Hypoaldosteronism in Diabetes Mellitus," *Life Sciences*, 53(5), 1993, p. 63-68.

Herpes

This study found that, at high concentrations in vitro, glycyrrhizic acid, a compound of liquorice root, inhibits the growth and effects of the herpes simplex virus.

> —R. Pompeii, et al., "Antiviral Activity of Glycyrrhizic Acid," *Experientia*, 36, 1980, p. 304.

This study examined the effects of glycyrrhizin on the resistance of thermally injured mice to opportunistic herpes simplex virus type 1. Results found that glycyrrhizin may reverse the increased susceptibility to herpes simplex virus type 1 infection through the induction of CD4+ contrasuppressor T cells.

—T. Utsunomiya, et al., "Glycyrrhizin Improves the Resistance of Thermally Injured Mice to Opportunistic Infection of Herpes Simplex Virus Type I," *Immunology Letters,* 44, 1995, p. 59-66.

■ LOVAGE

Anti-inflammatory Effects

Results of this study found that tetramethylpyrazine (TMP) and ferulic acid (FA) (an alkaloid and phenolic compound contained in Ligusticum wallichii, respectively) significantly inhibited carrageenin-induced edema in rats. Both compounds also inhibted the number of writhes induced by acetic acid, suggesting they each have anti-inflammatory and analgesic effects.

—Y. Ozaki, "Antiinflammatory Effect of Tetramethylpyrazine and Ferulic Acid," *Chem. Pharm. Bull.,* 40(4), 1992, p. 954-956.

Cardiovascular/Coronary Heart Disease

Clincial research has found Lingusticum chuanxiong in tablet form to be a significantly effective treatment in patients suffering from anginia pectoris and high blood pressure, as well as those suffering from ischemic cerebrovascular disease. When taken at doses of 3-9 g daily as an oral decoction, extract, or tincture, studies have shown it to be an effective treatment for headache, vertigo, and prolonged postpartum lochia.

—H.M. Chang & P.P. But, *Pharmacology and Applications of Chinese Materia Medica,* Vol 1, Hong Kong, World Scientific, 1986.

General

Pharmalogical and clinical research has found that Lovage root has a sedative effect on rats when given in oral doses of 25-50 g/kg. Intramuscular injections of the root has been shown to significantly decrease blood pressure in anesthetized animals. Small doses of a 10% solution have been shown to stimulate pregnant rabbit uterus specimans with large amounts stopping contractile effects entirely. The herb also possesses known antibacterial properties, as research has demonstrated in vitro inhibitory effects against bacteria including Shigella sonnei, Pseudomonas aeruginosa, Salmonella typhi, and Virbrio cholerae.

—D. Bensky & A. Gamble (eds.), *Chinese Herbal Medicine Materia Medica,* Seattle, Eastland Press, 1986, p. 382-384.

Uterine Contractions

Results of this study found that tetramethylpyrazine (TMP) and ferulic acid (FA) (an alkaloid and phenolic compound contained in Ligusticum wallichii, respectively) significantly inhibited uterine movement in rats when administered perorally and intravenously, respectively. When combined in doses insufficient to individually inhibit, the two compounds inhibited uterine contractions synergistically as well.

> —Y. Ozaki & J.P. Ma, "Inhibitory Effects of Tetramethylpyrazine and Ferulic Acid on Spontaneous Movement of Rat Uterus in Situ," *Chem. Pharm. Bull.,* 38(6), 1990, p. 1620-1623.

■ MOTHERWORT

Cancer

Results of this study found that absorbed and unabsorbed motherwort fractions separated by ion exchange resins suppressed the incidence and growth of palpable mammary tumors in mice.

> —H. Nagasawa, et al., "Further Study on the Effects of Motherwort (Leonurus sibiricus L) on Preneoplastic and Neoplastic Mammary Gland respect Growth in Multiparous GR/A Mice," *Anticancer Research,* 12(1), p January-February 1992, p. 141-143.

Results of this study showed that intake of a .5% motherwort methanol extract via drinking water suppressed the development of mammary cancers originating from hyperplastic alveolar nodules in mice while also reducing the incidence uterine adenomyosis. The same treatment, however, enhanced development of pregnancy-dependent mammary tumors.

> —H. Nagasawa, et al., "Effects of Motherwort (Leonurus sibiricus L) on Preneoplastic and Neoplastic Mammary Gland Growth in Multiparous GR/A Mice," *Anticancer Research,* 10(4), July-August 1990, p. 1019-1023.

Cardiovascular/Coronary Heart Disease

This study examined motherwort's effects on blood hyperviscosity in 105 patients. Results showed the herb administered intravenously in doses of 10 ml in 250 mil of 5% glucose over a period of 15 days produced clinical benefits with respect to reduced blood mammary viscosity and in fibrinogen volume as well as an increase in the deformability of Rbc, decreased time of Rbc electrophoresis, and enhanced antiplatelet aggregation.

> —Q.Z. Zou, et al., "Effect of Motherwort on Blood Hyperviscosity," American *Journal of Chinese Medicine,* 17(1-2), 1989, 65-70.

General

This article notes that searches of both modern phytochemical references and ancient Chinese medical references point to the efficacy of motherwort leaves as a uterotonic.

> —Y.C. Kong, et al., "Isolation of the Uterotonic Principle from Leonurus Artemisia, the Chinese Motherwort," *American Journal of Chinese Medicine,* 4(4), Winter 1976, p. 373-382.

Results of this study showed that the decoction of Carthamus tinctorius, Angelica sinensis and Leonurus sibiricus (motherwort) has stimulating action on the mouse uterus in vitro.

> —M. Shi, et al., [Stimulating Action of Carthamus Tinctorius L., Angelica Sinensis (Oliv.)

Diels and Leonurus sibiricus L. on the Uterus], *Chung Kuo Chung Yao Tsa Chih,* 20(3), March 1995, p. 173-175.

■ PEPPERMINT

General

This double-blind, placebo-controlled study examined the effects of peppermint oil and eucalyptus oil preparations on neurophysiological, psychological and experimental algesimetric parameters 32 healthy subjects. Results showed that combination preparations increased cognitive performance, had a muscle-relaxing and mentally relaxing effect, and had a significant analgesic effect with a reduction in sensitivity to headache.

> —H. Gobel, et al., "Effect of Peppermint and Eucalyptus Oil Preparations on Neurophysiological and Experimental Algesimetric Headache Parameters," *Cephalalgia,* 14(3), June 1994, p. 228-234.

Results of this study found that peppermint extract had clear sedative effects when administered to mice in a saline solution.

> —R. Della Loggia, et al., "Evaluation of Some Pharmacological Activities of a Peppermint Extract," *Fitoterapia,* LXI(3), 1990, p. 215-221.

Herpes

Peppermint has been shown to inhibit and kill the herpes simplex virus, among many other microorganisms.

> —D.B. Mowrey, *The Scientific Validation of Herbal Medicine,* New Canaan, CT, Keats Publishing, 1986, p. 73.

Irritable Bowel Syndrome

This double-blind, crossover study found peppermint oil in enteric-coated capsules to be effective in reducing abdominal symptoms associated with irritable bowel syndrome.

> —"Treating Irritable Bowel Syndrome with Peppermint Oil," *British Medical Journal,* October 6, 1979, p. 835-836.

Ulcers

This case-control study demonstrated that peppermint oil dramatically inhibited basal secretions in peptic ulcer patients.

> —J. Meyer, et al., "Action of Oil of Peppermint on the Secretion and Motility of the Stomach in Man" *Archives of Internal Medicine,* 56, 1945, p. 88-97.

■ PUMPKIN

Acute Schistosomiasis

This study reports on the efficacy of pumpkin seed treatment in 89 acute schistomiasis cases. Symptoms common to the condition include fever, chills, sweating, anorexia, cough, abdominal pain, urticaria, enlarged and tender liver and splenomegaly. When administered in 80 g doses three times daily for one month, pumpkin seed proved to be highly effective, particularly with respect to fever, anorexia, liver tenderness.

> —C. Hsueh-Chang & H. Ming, ''Pumpkin Seed (Cucurbita Moschata) in the Treatment of Acute Schistosomiasis,'' *Chinese Medical Journal,* 80, February 1960, p. 115-120.

Benign Prostatic Hyperplasia

Results of this double-blind, placebo-controlled study of 53 prostatic hyperplasia patients found that a Curbicin preparation, taken from pumpkin seeds and dwarf palm plants, significantly improved urinary flow, micturition time, residual urine, and frequency of micturition relative to controls.

> —B.E. Carbin, et al., ''Treatment of Benign Prostatic Hyperplasia with Phytosterols,'' *British Journal of Urology,* 66, 1990, p. 639-641.

General

This study evaluating the nutrive value of pumpkin seeds concluded that pumpkin seed products are an excellent source of high digestibility proteins; are rich in Ca, K, P, Mg, Fe, Zn, and contain high amounts of niacin and thiamine; and posess a well-balanced essential amino acid composition.

> —E.H. Mansour, et al., ''Nutrive Value of Pumpkin (Cucurbita pepo Kakai 35) Seed Products,'' *Journal of Sci. Food Agriculture,* 61, 1993, p. 73-78.

■ RED CLOVER

Cancer

In this study, an assay was done on the effects on the metabolism of [3H]benzo(a)pyrene [B(a)P] in hamster embryo cell cultures. Results showed that the 95% ethyl alcohol extract of Trifolium pratense L Leguminose, red clover, significantly inhibited the metabolism of B(a)P and decreased the level of binding of B(a)P to DNA by 30 to 40%. Such findings suggest red clover may possess chemopreventive properties.

> —J.M. Cassady, et al., ''Use of a Mammalian Cell Culture Benzo(a)pyrene Metabolism Assay for the Detection of Potential Anticarcinogens from Natural Products: Inhibition of Metabolism by Biochanin A, an Isoflavone from Trifolium pratense L,'' *Cancer Research,* 48, November 15, 1988, p. 6257-6261.

This study examined the effects of coumarin in various prostate tumour models and evaluate its endocrine properties. Results showed that coumarin administered three times a week at doses of 40 mg/kg inhibited the growth of Noble Nb-R prostate tumours of the rat. Results found coumarin possessed antimetastic activity in a Dunning R3327-MatLu tumour model as well.

> —A. Maucher, et al., ''Evaluation of the Antitumour Activity of Coumarin in Prostate Cancer Models,'' *Journal of Cancer Research and Clinical Oncology,* 119, 1993, p. 150-154.

In this study, 45 metastatic renal cell cancer patients were given 100 mg per day of coumarin and 300 mg of cimetide 4 times per day. Results found both to be safe and effective agents for the treatment of the disease.

> —M.E. Marshal, et al., "Treatment of Metastatic Renal Cell Carcinoma with Coumarin (1,2-Benzopyrone) and Cimetide: A Pilot Study," *Journal of Clinical Oncology,* 5f(6), June 1987, p. 862-866.

■ RHUBARB

Antibacterial Effects

In this study, extracts of 178 Chinese herbs were screened for their antibacterial activity against Bacteroides fragilis a major anaerobic microorganism in the intestinal flora of humans. Results showed that rhubarb root (Rheum officinale) was the only one found to have signficant activity and the purified substances was identified as rhein.

> —J. Cyong, et al., "Anti-Bacteriodes Fragilis Substance from Rhubarb," *Journal of Ethnopharmacology,* 19(3), May 1987, p. 279-283.

Cancer

Results of this study found three aglycone fractions isolated from Indonesian rhubarb inhibited the growth of human breast carcinoma cells and exhibited cytotoxic activity against HeLa epitholid carcinoma cells.

> —I. Kubo, et al., "Cytotoxic Anthraquinones from Rheum Palmatum," *Phytochemistry,* 31, 1992, p. 1063-1065.

Cardiovascular/Coronary Heart Disease

This double-blind, placebo-controlled study gave 0.75 mg or processed rhubarb to pregnant women at risk for preganancy induced hypertension from the 28th week of gestation up through delivery. Results found that only 5.7% of the women taking rhubarb developed hypternsion compared to 20.8% of controls. Plasma fibronectin and levels of plasminogen activator inhibitor were significantly decreased relative to controls after 9-10 weeks of treatment as well. Significant decreases in antithrombin levels were also seen in those taking rhubarb compared to controls.

> —Z.J. Zhang, et al., [Low-Dose of Processed Rhubarb in Preventing Pregnancy Induced Hypertension], *Chung Hua Fu Chan Ko Tsa Chih,* 29(8), August 1994, p. 463-464, 509.

Results of this study demonstrated a positive correlation between the sennoside A content of various rhubarbs and their cathartic effects in rats.

> —S. Harima, et al., "Study of Various Rhubarbs Regarding the Cathartic Effect and Endotoxin-Induced Disseminated Intravascular Coagulation," *Biol. Pharm. Bull.,* 17(11), 1994, p. 1522-1525.

General

Clinical studies have supported the use of the traditional Chinese drug, Dahuang, derived from Rheum palmatum L., Rheum tanguticum, or Rheum officinale Baill, in the treatment of acute inflammations and fever, abdominal distension, constipation, mental confusion, delirium, acute biliary infection, acute pancreatitis, acute appendicitis, hepaptitis, typhoid fever, dystentry, internal and external bleeding, burns, boils, cellulitis, dermatitis, herpes zoster, and numerous other conditions.

—H.M. Chang & P.P. But, (eds.), *Pharmacology and Applications of Chinese Materia Medica,* vol 1., World Scientific, 1986, p. 72-83.

Hemorrhagic Pancreatitis

Results of this study showed that rhubarb was an effective means of treating experimentally-induced hemorrhagic pancreatitis in rabbits.

—S. Ren, [Role of a Virus in Hemorrhagic Pancreatitis and the Therapeutic Effect of Rhubarb], *Chung Hsi I Chieh Ho Tsa Chih,* 10(3), March 1990, p.162-163.

Immune Enhancement

Results of this study showed that the oral administration of rhubarb increased the delayed hypersensitivity response induced by bovine serum albumin and proliferation response of murine spleen cell to Con A and lipoplysaccharide, suggesting rhubarb may enhance immune response.

—L. Ma, [Experimental Study on the Immunomodulatory Effects of Rhubarb], *Chung Hsi I Chieh Ho Tsa Chih,* 11(7), July 1991, p. 418-419.

Kidney Damage

This article argues that treatment of chronic renal failure with rhubarb and adjuvant drugs combined with other appropriate measures alleviates the suffering of the patients and improves the quality of their survival.

—Z. Kang, et al., ''Observation of Therapeutic Effect in 50 Cases of Chronic Renal Failure Treated with Rhubarb and Adjuvant Drugs,'' *Journal of Traditional Chinese Medicine,* 13(4), December 1993, p. 249-252.

This case-controlled study examined the effects of the Chinese herbal drug, Rheum E. compared to Captopril on patients suffering from chronic renal failure. Results found that long-term oral ingestion of Rheum E at low doses was beneficial compared to controls and that Rheum E in combination with Captopril is the best choice for treating chronic renal failure.

—J.H. Zang, et al., ''Clinical Effects of Rheum and Captopril on Preventing Progression of Chronic Renal Failure,'' *Chinese Medical Journal,* 103(10), 1990, p. 788-793.

■ ROSEMARY

Cancer

Results of this study showed that the topical application of a rosemary leaf extract significantly inhibited chemical-induced tumor initiation and tumor promotion in the of mice.

—M.T. Huang, et al., ''Inhibition of Skin Tumorigenesis by Rosemary and its Constituents Carnosol and Ursolic Acid,'' *Cancer Research,* 54(3), February 1, 1994, p. 701-708.

Results of this study showed that rosemary reduced DMBA metabolite binding to mammary cell DNA in 55 day old rats.

—H. Amagase, et al., "Dietary Rosemary Suppresses 7,12-dimethylbenz(a)anthracene Binding to Rat Mammary Cell DNA," *Journal of Nutrition Carnosol,* 126(5), May 1996, p. 1475-1480.

Results of this study showed that supplemental rosemary extract significantly reduced the incidence of DMBA-induced mammary tumors in vivo. Supplemental 0.5% and 1.0% extracts significantly inhibited total in vivo binding of skin DMBA to epithelial cells as well.

—K.W. Singletary & J.M. Nelshoppen, "Inhibition of 7,12-dimethylbenz[a]anthracene (DMBA)-induced Mammary Tumorigenesis and of in Vivo Formation of Mammary DMBA-DNA Adducts by Rosemary Extract," *Cancer Letters,* 60(2), November 1991, p. 169-175.

Results of this study showed that the rosemary constituent, carnosol, significantly inhibited DMBA-induced mammary carcinogeneis in rats.

—K. Singletary, et al., "Inhibition by Rosemary and of 7,12-dimethylbenz[a]anthracene (DMBA)-induced Rat Mammary Tumorigenesis and in Vivo DMBA-DNA Adduct Formation," *Cancer Letters,* 104(1), 1996, p. 43-48.

This study examined the means by which constituents of rosemary inhibit the initiation of carcinogenesis by the procarcinogen benzo[a]pyrene (B[a]P) in human bronchial epithelial cells. Results showed that 6 micrograms/ml of whole rosemary extract or an equivalent concentration of its constituents, carnosol or carnosic acid, inhibited DNA adduct formation by 80% after 6 h co-incubation with 1.5 muM B[a]P.

—E.A. Offord, et al., "Rosemary Components Inhibit Benzo[a]pyrene-induced Genotoxicity in Human Bronchial Cells," *Carcinogenesis,* 16(9), September 1995, p. 2057-2062.

Results of this study showed that dietary rosemary inhibited DMBA-induced mammary carcinogenesis and azoxymethane-induced colon carcinogenesis in mice.

—M.T. Huang, et al., "Inhibitory Effect of Dietary Rosemary on Mammary and Colon Carcinogenesis in Mice," *Proceedings of the Annual Meeting of the American Association Cancer Researchers,* 36, 1995, p. A3514.

■ ST. JOHN'S WORT

Alcoholism

In this study, hypericum herbal infusion was used in combination with rational psychotherapy of depressive manifestations in 57 outpatients with alcoholism and concomitant diseases of digestive organs. Results found that 2 months of daily intake proved to be effective.

—A.A. Krylov & A.N. Ibatov, [The Use of an Infusion of St. John's Wort in the Combined Treatment of Alcoholics with Peptic Ulcer and Chronic Gastritis], *Vrach Delo,* (2-3), February-March 1993, p. 146-148.

Depression

Results of this meta-analysis involving 23 randomized studies, 15 of which were placebo-controlled, found that hypericum extacts proved significantly effective in the treatment of patients suffering from moderate to mildly severe depression.

—K. Linde, et al., "St John's Wort for Depression—an Overview and Meta-analysis of Randomised Clinical Trials," *British Medical Journal,* 313(7052), August 3, 1996, p. 253-258.

Results of this study showed that the administration of a hypericum extract to middle-aged women suffering from depression led to improvements in anxiety, dysphoric mood, anorexia, hypersomnia, insomnia, loss of interest and feelings of worthlessness.

—H. Muldner & M. Zoller, [Antidepressive Effect of a Hypericum Extract Standardized to an Active Hypericine Complex. Biochemical and Clinical Studies], *Arzneimittelforschung,* 34(8), 1984, p. 918-920.

Results of this study showed that extracts of hypericum perforatum exhibited positive effects on numerous measures of depressive activity in mice.

—S.N. Okpanyi & M.L. Weischer, [Animal Experiments on the Psychotropic Action of a Hypericum Extract], *Arzneimittelforschung,* 37(1), January 1987, p. 10-13.

Results of this double-blind, placebo-controlled study involving 97 depression outpatients showed that 100 to 120 mg of hypericum extract led to noticeable improvement in 70% of the patients.

—B. Witte, et al., [Treatment of Depressive Symptoms with a High Concentration Hypericum Preparation. A Multicenter Placebo-controlled Double-blind Study], *Fortschr Med,* 113(28), October 10, 1995, p. 404-408.

Results of this double-blind, placebo-controlled study showed that 3 x 300 mg of hypericum extract over a period of 4 weeks led to significant improvements in depression outpatients relative to controls.

—H. Sommer & G. Harrer, "Placebo-controlled Double-blind Study Examining the Effectiveness of an Hypericum Preparation in 105 Mildly Depressed Patients," *Journal of Geriatr Psychiatry Neurol,* 7 (Suppl 1), October 1994, p. S9-11.

This study evaluated the effects of a 4-week treatment program with hypericum extract in 3,250 patients suffering from various levels of depression. Results showed that 30% of the patients experienced improvement while receiving the therapy.

—H. Woelk, et al., "Benefits and Risks of the Hypericum Extract LI 160: Drug Monitoring Study with 3250 Patients," *Journal of Geriatr Psychiatry Neuro,* 7 (Suppl 1), October 1994, p. S34-S38.

Results of this study showed that treatment with 900 mg per day of hypericum coupled with two hours of daily light therapy significantly reduced symptoms of depression in patients suffering from seasonal affective disorder.

—B. Martinez, et al., "Hypericum in the Treatment of Seasonal Affective Disorders," *Journal of Geriatr Psychiatry Neurol,* 7 (Suppl 1), October 1994, p. S29-S33.

Results of this double-blind, placebo-controlled study showed that treatment with hypericum extract over a period of 4 weeks led to significant improvements in patients suffering from depression.
—K.D. Hansgen, et al., "Multicenter Double-blind Study Examining the Antidepressant Effectiveness of the Hypericum Extract LI 160," *Journal of Geriatr Psychiatry Neurol,* 7 (Suppl 1), October 1994, p. S15-18.

This review article notes that recent studies have shown that St. John's wort is a clinically effective depression treatment equal to standard medication and without its negative side effects.
—E. Ernst, [St. John's Wort as Antidepressive Therapy], *Fortschr Med,* 113(25), September 10, 1995, p. 354-355.

This placebo-controlled, randomized, double-blind study examined the effects of a St. John's wort extract, LI 160, on patients suffering from moderateley severe depression. 66% of those receiving treatment responded positively versus only 26.7% of the controls.
—U. Schmidt & H. Sommer, [St. John's Wort Extract in the Ambulatory Therapy of Depression: Attention and Reaction Ability are Preserved], *Fortschr Med,* 111(19), July 10, 1993, p. 339-342.

This study compared the antidepressive-anxiolytic effects of a Valerian root and St. John's wort extract to amitriptyline. Results showed the herbal extract to be equally as effective as the amitriptyline, prompting the authors to argue for the use of phytomedicines in treating the depression and mood disorders.
—K.O. Hiller & V. Rahlfs, "Therapeutische Aquivalenz Eines Hochdosierten Phytoharmakons mit Amitriptylin bei Angstlich-Depressiven Verstimmugen - Reanalyse einer Randomisierten Studie unter Besonderer Beachtung Biometrischer und Klinischer Aspekte," *Forsch-Komplementarmed,* 2(3), 1995, p. 123-132.

In this randomized, double-blind study, placebo-controlled study, 300 mg of the hyperium extract LI 160 was administered to depression patients 3 times daily for 4 weeks. The treatment group showed significant improvement compared to controls, with 70% showing no symptoms after 4 weeks.
—W.D. Hubner, et al., "Hypericum Treatment of Mild Depression with Somatic Symptoms," *Journal of Geriatr Psychiatry Neurol,* 7(Suppl), October 1994, p. 1: S12-4.

General

Results of this study found that hypericum perforatum L. reduced the intesity level of enzymatic and non-enzymatic processes of lipid peroxidation of rat liver microsomes in vitro and in vivo.
—A.V. Smysthliaeva, et al., [The Modification of a Radiation Lesion in Animals with an Aqueous Extract of Hypericum Perforatum L. 2.,], *Biol Nauki,* (4), 1992, p. 9-13.

Herpes

In this study, an SHS-174 preparation, a lyophized infusion from flowers of Sambucus nigra L., aerial parts of Hypericum performatum L., and roots of Saponaria officinalis (100 g; 70 g; 40 g) exhibited an antiherpes simplex virus type1 effect in vitro. The preparation contains flavonoids, triterpene saponins, phenolic acids, tannins and polysaccharide which could be responsible for its antiviral properties.

—J. Serkedjieva, et al., "Antiviral Activity of the Infusion (SHS-174) from Flowers of Sambucus Nigra L., Aerial Parts of Hypericum Perforatum, L, and Roots of Saponaria Offinalis L against Influenza and Herpes Simplex Viruses," *Phytotherapy Research*, 4(3), 1990, p. 97-100.

■ STINGING NETTLE

Benign Prostatic Hyperplasia

This study examined the effects of organic-solvent extracts of Urtica dioica (Urticaceae) on the Na+, K(+)- ATPase of the tissue of benign prostatic hyperplasia (BPH) were investigated. Results indicated that some hydrophobic consituents such as steroids in the stinging nettle roots inhibited the membrane Na+, K(+)- ATPase activity of the prostate, which may suppress prostate-cell metabolism and growth.

—T. Hirano, et al., "Effects of Stinging Nettle Root Extracts and their Steroidal Components on the Na+,K(+)-ATPase of the Benign Prostatic Hyperplasia," *Planta Med*, 60(1), February 1994, p. 30-33.

Noting that extracts from stinging nettle roots have been used to treat benign prostatic hyperplasia, this study examined what if any specific extracts from the plant are capable of modulating the binding of sex hormone-binding globulin to its receptor on the prostate membranes of humans. Results found that of four substances studied, only an aqueos extract was active, with inhibition beginning at approximately 0.6 mg/ml and total inhibition binding occuring at 10 mg/ml.

—D.J. Hyrb, et al., "The Effect of Extracts of the Roots of the Stinging Nettle (Urtica dioica) on the Interaction of SHBG with its Receptor on Human Prostatic Membranes," *Planta Med.*, 61, 1995, p. 31-32.

Results of this study showed that benign prostatic hyperplasia patients who received capsules containing either 300 mg of Urtica dioica root extract combined with 25 mg of Pygeum africanum bark extract or two capsules with half this dose twice a day over a period of 8 weeks experienced significant reductions in symptoms related to the condition.

—T. Krzeski, et al., "Combined Extracts of Urtica diocia and Pygeum Africanum in the Treatment of Benign Prostatic Hyperplasia: Double-Blind Comparison of Two Doses," *Clinical Therapeutics*, 15(6), 1993, p. 1011-1020.

Results of this study found the fluid of Urtica dioca and Urtica urens roots were effective in significantly alleviating symptoms of prostatic adenoma in men over 60 years of age, particularly nocturnia. Results were strongest in those with less severe conditions.

—P. Belaiche & O. Lievoux, "Clinical Studies on the Palliative Treatment of Prostatic Adenoma with Extract of Urtica Root," *Phytotherapy Research*, 5, 1991, p. 267-269.

This double-blind, placebo-controlled study examined the effects of a freeze-dried stinging nettle extract on patients suffering from allergic rhinitis. Results found that the extract was rated more effective by patients as well as by a global assessment than placebo.

—P. Belaiche & O. Lievoux, "Clinical Studies on the Palliative Treatment of Prostatic Adenoma with Extract of Urtica Root," *Phytotherapy Research*, 5, 1991, p. 267-269.

■ SUNFLOWER

Cardiovascular/Coronary Heart Disease

Results of this study found that intake of a linoleic acid-rich diet, applying 12% sunflower seed oil in rat food pellet for 4 weeks, decreased the occurrence of life-threatening arrhythmias both during the acute phase of myocardial ischemia and during reperfusion in anesthetized rats.

> —I. Lepran & L. Szekeres, ''Effect of Dietary Sunflower Seed Oil on the Severity of Reperfu-sion-induced Arrthymias in Anesthetized Rats,'' *Journal of Cardiovascular Pharmacology,* 19(1), January 1992, p. 40-44.

Dermatitis

This study reports on the cases of three patients deficient in essential fatty acids due to chronic malabsorption, two suffering from scaly dermatitis. Results showed that the cutaneous application of sunflower-seed oil to their right arms for 2 weeks led to a major increase in the level of linoleic acid in their epidermal lecithin, significant lowering in the rate of transepidermal water loss, and the disappearance of scaly lesions.

> —C. Prottey, et al., ''Correction of the Cutaneous Manifestations of Essential Fatty Acid Deficiency in Man by Application of Sunflower-Seed Oil to the Skin,'' *The Journal of Investigative Dermatology,* 64, 1975, p. 228-234.

■ TEA TREE OIL

Acne

Results of this single-blind, randomized study found that 5% tea-tree oil and 5% benzoyl peroxide significantly ameliorated acne in patients by decreasing the number of inflamed and non-inflamed lesions.

> —I.B. Bassett, et al., ''A Comparative Study of Tea-tree Benzoylperoxide Oil Versus in the Treatment of Acne,'' *Medical Journal of Australia,* 153(8), October 15, 1990, p. 455-458.

Results of this study found tea tree oil to be effective in removing transient skin flora in vitro.

> —K.A. Hammer, et al., ''Susceptibility of Transient and Commensal Skin Flora to the Essential Oil of Melaleuca Alternifolia,'' *American Journal of Infect Control,* 24(3), June 1996, p. 186-189.

In this study, the tea-tree oils, terpinen-4-ol, alpha- terpineol and alpha-pinene were shown to be active against Staphylococcus aureus, Staph. epidermis and Propionibacterium acnes.

> —A. Raman, et al., ''Antimicrobial Effects of Tea-tree Oil and its Major Components on Staphylococcus Aureus, Staph. Epidermidis and Propionibacterium Acnes,'' *Lett Appl Microbiol,* 21(4), October 1995, p. 242-245.

■ VALERIAN

Antidepressant Effects

In this study, the psychotropic effects of "Hokkai-Kisso", i.e. roots of Japanese valerian, were compared with those of diazepam and imipramine. Results showed that valerian extract may be considered an antidepressant due to its action on the central nervous system of mice.
> —T. Sakamoto, et al., "Psychotropic Effects of Japanese Valerian Root Extract," *Chemical Pharmacology Bulletin,* 40(3), March 1992, p. 758-761.

Results of this study showed that a methanol extract of the roots of Valerian fauriei exhibited antidepressant activity in mice.
> —Y. Oshima, et al., "Antidepressant Principles of Valerian Fauriei Roots," *Chemical Pharm Bulletin,* 43(1), January 1995, p. 169-170.

Sleep

This double-blind, placebo-controlled study examined the effects of valerian root on sleep measures in 128 subjects. Results showed that valerian led to significant reduction in subjectively evaluated sleep latency scores and significantly enhanced the quality of sleep.
> —P.D. Leatherwood, et al., "AAqueous Extract of Valerian Root Improves Sleep Quality in Man," *Pharmacol Biochem Behavior,* 17(1), July 1982, p. 65-71.

Results of this double-blind, placebo-controlled study found a significant positive effect of a valerian preparation and improved sleep.
> —O. Lindahl & L. Lindwall, "Double Blind Study of a Valerian Preparation," *Pharmacol Biochem Behavior,* 32(4), April 1989, p. 1065-1066.

This study examined the effect of an aqueous extract of valerain root on sleep in healthy, young subjects. Results showed that doses of both 450 mg and 900 mg of valerian extract reduced perceived sleep latency and wake time after sleep onset under home conditions.
> —G. Balderer & A.A. Borbely, "Effect of Valerian on Human Sleep," *Psychopharmacology,* 87(4), 1985, p. 406-409.

THERAPEUTIC AMINO ACIDS

■ ALANINE

Diabetes

Results of this placebo-controlled study found that supplemental alanine and terbutaline led to sustained glucose recovery from hypoglycemia in IDDM patients.

> —B.V. Wiethop & C.E. Cryer, "Alanine and Terbutaline in Treatment of Hypoglycemia in IDDM," *Diabetes Care,* 16(8), August 1993, p. 1131-1136.

Diarrhea

Results of this study found that an oral rehydration solution containing L-alanine proved more effective than standard solution without L-alanine in alleviating diarrhea symptoms associated with enterotoxigenic E coli and V cholerae in male patients.

> —F.C. Patra, et al., "Oral Rehydration Formula Containing Alanine and Glucose for Treatment of Diarrhoea: A Controlled Trial," *BMJ,* 298(6684), May 20, 1989, p. 1353-1356.

Liver Damage

Results of this study showed that alanine exhibited beneficial effects in the treatment of experimentally-induced liver failure in rats.

> —K. Maezono, et al., "Effect of Alanine on D-galactosamine-induced Acute Liver Failure in Rats," *Hepatology,* 24(5), November 1996, p. 1211-1216.

■ ARGININE

Brain Injury

Results of this study showed that intravenous nitro-l-arginine delayed onset of ischemic injury in rats by retarding cytotoxic brain edema.

> —E. Kozniewska, et al., "NG-nitro-L-arginine Delays the Development of Brain Injury During Focal Ischemia in Rats," *Stroke,* 26(2), February 1995, p. 282-288.

Cancer

This study examined the effects of dietary L-arginine on the growth and development of Ehrlich Ascites tumor cells in mice. Results showed that significant inhibitions in the growth of tumor-bearing mice fed a purified casein diet supplemented with 5% arginine as well as in the number of free tumor cells growing in the mice.

> —J.A. Milner & L.V. Stepanovich, "Inhibitory Effect of Dietary Arginine on Growth of Ehrlich Ascites Tumor Cells in Mice," *Journal of Nutrition,* 109(3), March 1979, p. 489-494.

Results of this study found that the administration of 30 g per day of L-arginine for 3 days significantly enhanced host defenses in breast cancer patients.

> —J. Brittenden, et al., "L-arginine Stimulates Host Defenses in Patients with Breast Cancer," *Surgery* 115(2), February 1994, p. 205-212.

Results of this study showed that arginine supplementation exhibited antitumor activity in mice inoculated with murine sarcoma virus.

> —G. Rettura, et al., "Supplemental Arginine Increases Thymic Cellularity in Normal and Murine Sarcoma Virus-inoculated Mice and Increases the Resistance to Murine Sarcoma Virus Tumor," *JPEN J Parenter Enteral Nutr,* 3(6), November-December 1979, p. 409-416.

Results of this study found that supplementation with an arginine-enriched solution suppressed tumor growth and metastasis in rats.

> —K. Tachibana, et al., "Evaluation of the Effect of Arginine-enriched Amino Acid Solution on Tumor Growth," *JPEN J Parenter Enteral Nutr,* 9(4), July-August 1985, p. 428-434.

Cardiovascular/Coronary Heart Disease

Results of this study showed that arginine significantly reduced the size of myocardial infarct following ischemia and reperfusion in rats exposed to environmental tobacco smoke.

> —B. Zhu, et al., "L-arginine Decreases Infarct Size in Rats Exposed to Environmental Tobacco Smoke," *American Heart Journal,* 132(1 Pt 1), July 1996, p. 91-100.

Results of this study showed that the administration of L-arginine reduced infarct size in rats subjected to distal middle cerebral arterial and ipsilateral common carotid arterial occlusion by 31%.

> —E. Morikawa, et al., "L-arginine Decreases Infarct Size Caused by Middle Cerebral Arterial Occlusion in SHR," *American Journal of Physiol,* 263(5 Pt 2), November 1992, p. H1632-1635.

Results of this study showed that L-arginine decreased lipid peroxidation, plasma levels of soluble adhesion molecules, myocardial stunning, and arrhythmias in pig heart during ischemia/reperfusion.

> —D.T. Engelman, et al., "L-arginine Reduces Endothelial Inflammation and Myocardial Stunning During Ischemia/reperfusion," *Ann Thorac Surg,* 60(5), November 1995, p. 1275-1281.

Results of this double-blind, placebo-controlled study found that the oral administration of oral L-arginine hydrochloride at doses of 5.6 to 12.6 g per day over a period of 6 weeks had positive effects in heart failure patients.

> —T.S. Rector, et al., "Randomized, Double-blind, Placebo-controlled Study of Supplemental Oral L-arginine in Patients with Heart Failure," *Circulation,* 93(12), June 15, 1996, p. 2135-2141.

Results of this study showed that the administration of L-arginine prevented hypertension in Dahl salt-sensitive rats.

> —A. Patel, et al., "L-arginine Administration Normalizes Pressure Natriuresis in Hypertensive Dahl Rats," *Hypertension,* 22(6), December 1993, p. 863-869.

In this study, 12 congestive heart failure patients brought on by coronary artery disease received 20 g of intravenous L-arginine. Results showed a significant increase in stroke volume and cardiac output with no change in heart rate. Significant reducts were seen in mean arterial blood pressure and systemic vascular resistance as well.

> —B. Koifman, et al., "Improvement of Cardiac Performance by Intravenous Infusion of L-arginine in Patients with Moderate Congestive Heart Failure," *Journal of Am Coll Cardiol,* 26(5), November 1, 1995, p. 1251-1256.

Results of this placebo-controlled study showed that the administration of 7 g of L-arginine 3 times per day over a period of 4 weeks led to significantly improvements in endothelium-dependent dilation in hypercholesterolemic young adults.

> —P. Clarkson, et al., "Oral L-arginine Improves Endothelium-dependent Dilation in Hyper-cholesterolemic Young Adults," *Journal of Clinical Investigation,* 97(8), April 15, 1996, p. 1989-1994.

In this study, 5 infants with PPHN were infused with a 500 mg/kg dose of L-arginine over a period of 30 minutes. Results suggested L-arginine may be an effective treatment for infants with this condition.

> —M.J. McCaffrey, et al., "Effect of L-arginine Infusion on Infants with Persistent Pulmonary Hypertension of the Newborn," *Biol Neonate,* 67(4), 1995, p. 240-243.

Results of this study indicated that exogenous L-arginine had vasodilatory effects in patients suffering from various forms of hypertension.

> —K. Hishikawa, et al., "L-arginine as an Antihypertensive Agent," *Journal of Cardiovascular Pharmacol,* 20(Suppl 12), 1992, p. S196-S197.

Results of this study showed L-arginine attenuated transplant arteriosclerosis in rabbits.

> —H. Lou, et al., "L-arginine Prevents Heart Transplant Arteriosclerosis by Modulating the Vascular Cell Proliferative Response to Insulin-like Growth Factor-I and Interleukin-6," *Journal of Heart Lung Transplant,* 15(12), December 1996, p. 1248-1257.

Results of this study found that L-arginine had positive effects on cerebral metabolic recovery following deep hypothermic circulatory arrest in a piglet model.

> —T. Hiramatsu, et al., "Cerebral Metabolic Recovery from a Deep Hypothermic Circulatory

Arrest after Treatment with Arginine and Nitro-arginine Methyl Ester,'' *Journal of Thorac Cardiovascular Surgery,* 112(3), September 1996, p. 698-707.

Results of this study showed that the administration of 12 mg/kg of NG-methyl-L-arginine followed by 4 mg/kg every 4 hours reversed IL-2-induced hypotensive effects in three patients with metastatic renal cell carcinoma.

—R.G. Kilbourn, et al., ''NG-methyl-L-arginine, an Inhibitor of Nitric Oxide Synthase, Reverses Interleukin-2-Induced Hypotension,'' *Crit Care Med,* 23(6), June 1995, p. 1018-1024.

General

Results of this study found that L-arginine and its derivative reduced intraoccular pressure in rabbits.

—G.C. Chiou, et al., ''Ocular Hypotensive Effects of L-arginine and its Derivatives and their Actions on Ocular Blood Flow,'' *Ocul Pharmacol Ther,* 11(1), Spring 1995, p. 1-10.

This review article notes that both animal and human studies point to the beneficial effects of L-arginine on nitrogen metabolism, wound healing, and host defenses.

—J. Brittenden, et al., ''L-arginine and Malignant Disease: A Potential Therapeutic Role?'' *European Journal of Surg Oncology,* 20(2), April 1994, p. 189-192.

Results of this study showed that the administrated of 4 g per day of chlorhydrate arginine for six months had beneficial effects on children suffering from short constitutional stature.

—A.M. Pittari, et al., ''Therapy with Arginine Chlorohydrate in Children with Short Constitutional Stature,'' *Minerva Pediatr,* 45(1-2), January-February 1993, p. 61-65.

Hepatitis

Results of this double-blind, placebo-controlled study found that the administration of three 400 mg tablets of arginine tidiacicate over a period of 30 days had positive effects on symptoms associated with chronic persistent hepatitis in human subjects.

—S. Rizzo, ''Clinical Trial with Arginine Tidiacicate in Symptomatic Chronic Persistent Hepatitis,'' *International Journal of Clin Pharmacol Res,* 6(3), 1986, p. 225-230.

Infertility

Results of this study found that the administration of 80 ml of 10% L-arginine HCL daily per os over a 6 month period improved sperm motility in infertile men.

—M. Scibona, et al., ''L-arginine and Male Infertility,'' *Minerva Urol Nefrol,* 46(4), December 1994, p. 251-253.

Intestinal Damage

Results of this study found that arginine-derived nitrous oxide mediated the restitution of intestinal mucosa by minimizing cell injury during reperfusion in rats.

—F. Raul, et al., ''Beneficial Effects of L-arginine on Intestinal Epithelial Restitution after Ischemic Damage in Rats,'' *Digestion,* 56(5), 1995, p. 400-405.

Results of this study found that the intragastric administration of 32.5-300 mg/kg per day of L-arginine accelerated the healing of acetic acid-induced gastric ulcers.

> —T. Brzozowski, et al., "Healing of Chronic Gastric Ulcerations by L-arginine. Role of Nitric Oxide, Prostaglandins, Gastrin and Polyamines," *Digestion,* 56(6), 1995, p. 463-471.

Results of this study showed that the administration of L-arginine had protective effects against endothelin-1-induced gastric mucosal ulcers in rats.

> —S. Lazaratos, et al., "L-arginine and Endogenous Nitric Oxide Protect the Gastric Mucosa from Endothelin-1-induced Gastric Ulcers in Rats," *Journal of Gastroenterol,* 30(5), October 1995, p. 578-584.

Results of this study showed that pretreatment with L-arginine ameliorated survival and led to improvements in mucosal barrier function in rats following intestinal ischemia/reperfusion.

> —R. Schleiffer & F. Raul, "Prophylactic Administration of L-arginine Improves the Intestinal Barrier Function after Mesentric Ischaemia," *Gut,* 39(2), August 1996, p. 194-198.

Kidney Damage

Results of this study showed that supplemental L-arginine administered over a period of 6 weeks ameliorated the progression of kidney disease in female rats.

> —A.A. Reyes, et al., "Dietary Supplementation with L-arginine Ameliorates the Progression of Renal Disease in Rats with Subtotal Nephrectomy," *American Journal of Kidney Dis,* 20(2), August 1992, p. 168-176.

Liver Damage

Results of this study found that oral arginine administration led to significant improvements in experimentally-induced acute liver injury in rats.

> —D. Adawi, et al., "Oral Arginine Supplementation in Acute Liver Injury," *Nutrition,* 12(7-8), July-August 1996, p. 529-533.

Pain

Results of this study found that the intravenous administration of a 10% solution, 300 ml (30 g)/patient L-arginine over a 60-70 minute period produced significant analgesiac effects in patients suffering from different types of pain.

> —A. Harima, et al., "Analgesic Effect of L-arginine in Patients with Persistent Pain," *European Neuropsychopharmacol,* 1(4), December 1991, p. 529-533.

Stress

Results of this study found that the administration of arginine within 3 days of cold exposure in rats exhibited protective effects against numerous physiologic measures of stress associated with the exposure.

> —A.A. Krichevskaia, et al., "Evaluation of the Effectiveness of the Protective Effect of Arginine in Cold Stress," *Vopr Med Khim,* 31(6), November-December 1985, p. 50-53.

Uterine Contractions

Results of this study found that supplemental L-arginine significantly reduced the number of contractions in women suffering from preterm onset of uterine contractions relative to controls.

—F. Facchinetti, et al., "L-arginine Infusion Reduces Preterm Uterine Contractions," *Journal of Perinat Med,* 24(3), 1996, p. 283-285.

Vein Graft Intimal Hyperplasia

Results of this study showed that the administration of oral L-arginine significantly decreased intimal hyperplasia and preserved nitric oxide mediated relaxation in experimental vein grafts in rabbits.

—M.G. Davies, et al., "Reduction of Experimental Vein Graft Intimal Hyperplasia and Preservation of Nitric Oxide-Mediated Relaxation by the Nitric Oxide Precursor L-arginine," *Surgery,* 116(3), 1994, p. 557-568.

Wound Healing

Results of this study indicated that supplemental arginine had beneficial effects on guinea pigs suffering from burn injury.

—H. Saito, et al., "Metabolic and Immune Effects of Dietary Arginine Supplementation after Burn," *Arch Surg,* 122(7), July 1987, p. 784-789.

Results of this study showed that supplemental arginine at levels totaling 2% of nutritional energy significantly enhanced the T lymphocyte response to PHA, CD4 phenotype expression, CD4/CD8 ratio, IL-2 production and IL-2 receptor expression in burn patients relative to controls.

—S.L. Lu, "Effect of Arginine Supplementation on T-lymphocyte Function in Burn Patients," *Chung Hua Cheng Hsing Shao Shang Wai Ko Tsa Chih,* 9(5), September 1993, p. 368-371.

■ ASPARTIC ACID

Cardiovascular/Coronary Heart Disease

Results of this study showed that supplementation with aspartate and glutamate reduced infarct size and enhanced regional function in pig hearts during reperfusion.

—R.M. Engelman, et al., "Reduction of Infarct Size by Systemic Amino Acid Supplementation During Reperfusion," *Journal of Thorac Cardiovasc Surg,* 101(5), May 1991, p. 855-859.

Results of this study showed that aspartate enrichment of glutamate-blood cardioplegia improved recovery after severe ischemic/reperfusion in canine hearts.

—E.R. Rosenkranz, et al., "Safety of Prolonged Aortic Clamping with Blood Cardioplegia. III. Aspartate Enrichment of Glutamate-blood Cardioplegia in Energy-depleted Hearts after Ischemic and Reperfusion Injury," *Journal of Thorac Cardiovasc Surg,* 91(3), March 1986, p. 428-435.

Results of this study showed that the administration of aspartate and glutamate had protective effects on isolated cat hearts during myocardial ischemia.

—L.R. Bush, et al., "Comparative Effects of Aspartate and Glutamate During Myocardial Ischemia," *Pharmacology,* 23(6), 1981, p. 297-304.

Cancer

Results of this study indicated that PALA exhibited antitumor effects against sarcoma, colon cancer, melanoma, and ovarian cancer in mice..
> —M. Rozencweig, et al., "N-(Phosphonacetyl)-L-Aspartate (PALA): Current Status, Recent Results," *Cancer Research,* 74, 1980, p. 72-77.

Hypoxia

Results of this study found that the intradermal administration of L-Aspartate in mice 2-3 minutes prior to placement to a hypoxic chamber was extended mean lifespan by 38% and delayed hypoxic convulsions by 38-40%.
> —I.I. Abu-Asali, et al., [The Possible Participation of the GABA Metabolic System in the Mechanisms of the Protective Action of L-aspartate in Hypoxia in an Enclosed Space], *Eksp Klin Farmakol,* 55(4), July-August 1992, p. 36-38.

Liver Damage

This article reports on the case of a seven-year-old girl with slowly progressive motor neurological impairment severe hepatic pyruvate carboxylase deficiency. Seven years of therapy with aspartic acid and thiamine led to biochemical improvement and a stable neurological condition.
> —M.G. Baal, et al., "A Patient with Pyruvate Carboxylase Deficiency in the Liver: Treatment with Aspartic Acid and Thiamine," *Dev Med Child Neurol,* 23(4), August 1981, p. 521-530.

Results of this study showed that aspartate and glutamate significantly reduced carbon tetrachloride induced liver necrosis in rats.
> —J. Singh, et al., "Effect of Aspartate and Glutamate on Carbon Tetrachloride Induced Liver Damage in Rats," *Indian Journal of Exp Biol,* 28(12), December 1990, p. 1180-1183.

Opiate Addiction

This study examined the effects of aspartic acid on the development of morphine dependence and withdrawal in rats. Results showed that the treatment prevented the alterations induced by morphine during the development of physical dependence and tolerance.
> —H. Koyuncuoglu, et al., "Antagonizing Effect of Aspartic Acid on the Development of Physical Dependence on and Tolerance to Morphine in the Rat," *Arzneimittelforschung,* 27(9), 1977, p. 1676-1679.

Results of this study found that 8 g of L-aspartic acid taken for 7 days following the appearance of opiate withdrawal proved significantly better in alleviating such symptoms in addicts than did the more conventional treatment of daily chlorpromazine and diazepam.
> —A.I. Sener, et al., "Comparison of the Suppressive Effects of L-aspartic Acid and Chlorpromazine + Diazepam Treatments on Opiate Abstinence Syndrome Signs in Men," *Arzneimittelforschung,* 36(11), November 1986, p. 1684-1686.

This study reports on the case of two patients addicted to codeine, two to heroin, and four to opium tincture who received 2 g of oral L-aspartic acid 4 times per day for up to 5 days. Results showed that none of the patients exhibited signs of abstinence syndrome or feelings of need for the drug they had previously been addicted to.

—H. Koyuncuoglu, "The Treatment with L-aspartic Acid of Persons Addicted to Opiates," *Bull Narc,* 35(1), January-March 1983, p. 11-15.

■ CYSTEINE

Cancer

Results of this double-blind, placebo-controlled study found that L-cysteine exhibited preventive effects against leukopenic complications associated with radiotherapy in cancer patients.

—K. Jingum et al., "Protective Effect of L-cysteine Upon Leukopenic Syndrome due to Radiotherapy," *Nippon Gan Chiryo Gakkai Shi,* 16(4), 1981, p. 681-693.

Dermatitis

Results of this study showed that cysteine was an effective treatment against allergic contact dermatitis caused by parthenin in guinea pigs.

—J. Picman & A.K. Picman, "Treatment of Dermatitis from Parthenin," *Contact Dermatitis,* 13(1), July 1985, p. 9-13.

Leg Ulcer

Results of this double-blind, placebo-controlled study showed that hypostatic leg ulceration patients treated with a topical cream containing l-cysteine, glycine, and dl-threonin 3 times per week over a period of 12 weeks experienced a significantly increased rate of healing relative to patients being treated with cream base alone.

—S.G. Harvey, et al., "L-cysteine, Glycine and Dl-threonine in the Treatment of Hypostatic Leg Ulceration: A Placebo-controlled Study," *Pharmatherapeutica,* 4(4), 1985, p. 227-230.

■ GLUTAMIC ACID

Adrenal Function

In this study, a dose of 1/100 of the LD50 of glutamic acid was injected in the form of sodium salt into rats for 7 days 8-12-days following injections of dexazone. Results found that the glutamic acid coupled with dexazone reduced the inhibitory effect of dexazone without averting its inhibitory effect on the central nervous system. Results also indicated that prolonged injections of glutamic acid following dexazone treatment promoted more rapid and overall adrenal function.

—L.S. Mitianina, et al., [Effect of Glutamic Acid on the Course of Recovery Processes in the Adrenal Cortex], *Farmakol Toksikol,* 47(6), November-December, 1984, p. 63-67.

Asthma

Results of this study showed that bronchial asthma patients treated with aevit and glutamic acid experienced clinical improvements relative to those receiving conventional therapy alone or couple with glucocorticoids.

> —I.G. Daniliak, et al., [Aevit and Glutamic Acid in the Treatment of Patients with Bronchial Asthma], *Klin Med,* 73(5), 1995, p. 50-53.

Cancer

This review article cites results from numerous studies indicating supplemental glutamine decreases tumor growth in vivo due to its stimulatory effects on the immune system.

> —V.S. Klimberg & J.L. McClellan, "Glutamine, Cancer, and its Therapy," *American Journal of Surgery,* 172(5), November 1996, p. 418-424.

Results of this study found that patients undergoing chemotherapy who also received a suspension of L-glutamine in the form of a 4 g swish and swallow twice a day beginning with the first day of chemotherapy and lasting 28 days or 4 days past the resolution of any post-chemotherapy mucositis experienced a significant reduction in the severity of stomatitis induced by the chemotherapy.

> —K.M. Skubitz & P.M. Anderson, "Oral Glutamine to Prevent Chemotherapy Induced Stomatitis: A Pilot Study," *Journal of Lab Clin Medicine,* 127(2), February 1996, p. 223-228.

Results of this study showed that diets supplemented with glutamine before, during, and after radiotherapy protected rats from radiation injury.

> —F.G. Campos, "Protective Effects of Glutamine Enriched Diets on Acute Enteritis," *Nutr Hosp,* 11(3), May-June 1996, p. 167-177.

Results of this study showed that glutamine supplementation boosted the selectivity of antitumor drugs in rats by protecting normal tissues from and sensitizing tumor cells to injury caused from chemotherapy.

> —T.V. Nattakom, et al., "Use of Vitamin E and Glutamine in the Successful Treatment of Severe Veno-Occlusive Disease Following Bone Marrow Transplantation," *Nutr Clin Pract,* 10(1), Feb 1995, p. 16-18.

Results of this study found that L-glutamic acid exhibited strong anti-tumoral activity in vivo against L1210 leukemia and B16 melanoma and total cytoxicity against L1210 cells in culture. L-glutamic acid caused concentration-dependent inhibition of L1210 cell growth in vitro. Additional results found that L-glutamic acid prolonged survival time of mice with L1210 leukemia or a solid tumor, the B16 melanoma in vivo.

> —J. Vila, et al., "In Vitro and in Vivo Anti-tumor Activity of L-glutamic Acid Gamma-monohydroxamate Against L1210 Leukemia and B16 Melanoma," *International Journal of Cancer,* 45(4), April 15, 1990, p. 737-743.

Cardiovascular/Coronary Heart Disease

Results of this study found that the administration of 2 mM glutamate led to an association between enhanced postischemic cardiac performance and improved production of alpha-ketoglutarate and succinate in rabbits.

> —J.A. Bittl & K.I. Shine, "Protection of Ischemic Rabbit Myocardium by Glutamic Acid," *American Journal of Physiol,* 245(3), September 1983, p. H406-412.

Results of this study found that the administration of glutamate coupled with high dose glucose-insulin-potassium is an effective and safe treatment in patients with reversible cardiac failure.

> —R. Svedjeholm, et al., "Glutamate and High-dose Glucose-insulin-potassium (GIK) in the Treatment of Severe Cardiac Failure after Cardiac Operations," *Ann Thorac Surg,* 59(2 Suppl), February 1995, p. S23-S30.

This study examined the effects on cardiac function and metabolism in the working rat heart of adding glutamic acid to a cardioplegic solution containing 20 mM K+ . Results showed the treatment led to improved ATP and creatine phosphate content, prompting the authors to argue that the addition of glutamic acid may be beneficial with respect to open heart surgery.

> —O.I. Pisarenko, et al., "Protective Effect of Glutamic Acid on Cardiac Function and Metabolism During Cardioplegia and Reperfusion," *Basic Research in Cardiology,* 78(5), September-October 1983, p. 534-543.

This study examined the effects of intravenous glutamic acid (3 mg/kg/min) on cardiac contractile function during short-term ischemia and subsequent reperfusion in dogs. Results found the treatment had beneficial effects on the ischemic, but not normal heart.

> —O.I. Pisarenko, et al., "Function and Metabolism of Dog Heart in Ischemia and in Subsequent Reperfusion: Effect of Exogenous Glutamic Acid," *Pflugers Arch,* 405(4), December 1985, p. 377-383.

Colonic Mucosa Injury

Results of this study showed that L-glutamine stimulated repair mechanisms of colonic mucosa in rats following acid injury.

> —W. Scheppach, et al., "Effect of L-glutamine and N-butyrate on the Restitution of Rat Colonic Mucosa after Acid Induced Injury," *Gut,* 38(6), June 1996, p. 878-885.

Diabetes

This study examined the in vivo effects of glutamate on glycemia and insulinemia in both fasted rats and those on a normal diet. Results showed that intravenous glutamate at doses of 9 and 30 mg/kg increased insulinemia in anesthetized fed rats. The intragastric administration of glutamate at 200 mg/kg elicited a transient insulin response in conscious fed rats while having no effect in conscious fasted rats.

> —G. Bertrand, et al., "Glutamate Stimulates Insulin Secretion and Improves Glucose Tolerance in Rats," *American Journal of Physiology,* 269(3 Pt 1), September 1995, p. E551-E556.

Results of this study showed glutamic acid decarboxylase to be an autoantigen in insulin dependent diabetes melitus and that it can prevent onset of the disease in prediabetic mice when administered as an immunization.

> —J.F. Elliott, et al., "Immunization with the Larger Isoform of Mouse Glutamic Acid Decarboxylase (GAD67) Prevents Autoimmune Diabetes in NOD Mice," *Diabetes,* 43(12), December 1994, p. 1494-1499.

Results of this study found that 100 micrograms of glutamic acid decarboxylase significantly delayed the onset of diabetes in NOD female mice relative to controls.

> —J.S. Petersen, et al., "Neonatal Tolerization with Glutamic Acid Decarboxylase but Not

with Bovine Serum Albumin Delays the Onset of Diabetes in NOD Mice,'' *Diabetes*, 43(12), December 1994, p. 1478-1484.

General

This study examined the effects of glutamic acid in rats with experimental silicosis and asbestosis. Results showed the treatment significantly reduced fibrinogenic changes in lung tissue of rats exposed to asbestos and quartz dust.

—G.V. Aronova, et al., [Antifibrotic Effect of Inifibrotic Effect of Glutamic Acid in Experimental Acid in Experimental Silicosis and Asbestosis] *Gig Tr Prof Zabol*, (1), 1980, p. 12-15.

Results of this study indicated that glutamic acid can modulate rat hepatocyte response sensitivity to mitogens in primary culture.

—K. Hasegawa, et al., ''Glutamic Acid Potentiates Hepatocyte Response to Mitogens in Primary Culture,'' *Journal of Cellular Physiology*, 158(2), February 1994, p. 365-373.

Results of this double-blind, placebo-controlled study found that athletes consuming drinks containing glutamine immediately and 2 hours after exercise experienced a lower incidence of infections 7 days following exercise than controls.

—L.M. Castell, et al., ''Does Glutamine Have a Role in Reducing Infections in Athletes?'' *European Journal of Applied of Physiology*, 73(5), 1996, p. 488-490.

Results of this study showed that supplemental glutamine exhibited preventive effects against gut-origin sepsis in mice following burn injury.

—L. Gianotti, et al., ''Oral Glutamine Decreases Bacterial Translocation and Improves Survival in Experimental Gut-Origin Sepsis,'' *Japanese Journal of Parenter Enter Nutrition*, 19(1), January-February 1995, p. 69-74.

Liver Damage

Results of this study found that the administration of large doses of gamma-ethylester of glutamic acid to patients suffering from liver failure produced significantly positive effects with respect to such symptoms as tremors, confusion, restlessness, and reductions in blood ammonia levels.

—G. Santagati, et al., [Glutamic Acid Gamma-ethyl Ester in High Doses in the Treatment of High Blood Ammonia Levels in Severe Hepatic Failure], *Minerva Med*, 69(20), April 28, 1978, p. 1367-1374.

Neurotoxicity

Results of this double-blind, placebo-controlled study found that 1500 mg per day of glutamic acid administered orally reduced vincristine-induced neurotoxicity in cancer patients.

—D.V. Jackson, et al., ''Amelioration of Vincristine Neurotoxicity by Glutamic Acid,'' *American Journal of Medicine*, 84(6), June 1988, p. 1016-1022.

Results of this study showed glutamate to be an effective neuroprotectant against vincristine-induced toxicity in rats.

—F.M. Boyle, et al., ''Prevention of Vincristine Neuropathy with Glutamate: An in Vivo

Model,'' *Procceedings of the Annual Meeting of the American Association of Cancer Researchers,* 35, 1994, p. A1476.

Occupational Fluorosis

This study examined the effects of glutamic acid on occupational fluorosis in cryolite production workers. Results showed the treatment effective in preventing progression of metabolic disorders.

—T.D. Grekhova, et al., [Effectiveness of Glutamate in the Treatment of Early Manifestations of Occupational Fluorosis], *Med Tr Prom Ekol,* (8), 1994, p. 20-23.

Rhinitis

This study examined the effects of Mg salt of N-acetyl-aspartyl- glutamic acid taken for 15 days in patients with allergic rhinitis. Results showed the drug to be effective and well tolerated.

—A. Miadonna, et al., [Evaluation of the Efficacy of the Magnesium Salt of N-acetyl-aspartyl-glutamic Acid in the Treatment of Acute Rhinitis], *Clin Ter,* 131(3), November 15, 1989, p. 173-176.

Short Bowel Syndrome

Results of this study found that a protocol involving growth hormone, glutamine and a high-carbohydrate, low-fat diet proved effective in treating surgical patients suffering from short-bowel syndrome or related problems of the GI tract.

—T.A. Byrne, et al., ''A New Treatment for Patients with Short-Bowel Syndrome. Growth Hormone, Glutamine, and a Modified Diet,'' *Annals Surg,* 222(3), September 1995, p. 243-254.

Tinnitus

Results of this study indicated that the intravenous administration of glutamic acid and glutamic acid diethylester worked to suppress certain forms of tinnitus in human patients relative to controls.

—K. Ehrenberger & R. Brix, ''Glutamic Acid and Glutamic Acid Diethylester in Tinnitus Treatment,'' *Acta Otolaryngol,* 95(5-6), May-June 1983, p. 599-605.

Virchowan Leprosy

This study compared the effects of short-term activities of the Brazilian made imidphtalic glutamic acid and of the triancinolone in the therapy of the hansenic reaction of the Virchowian hanseniasis in Brazilian patients. Results showed that both drugs were equally effective, each reducing hospital time per patient from 8 to 3 days.

—E. de Almeida Neto, [Comparative Study of the Therapeutic Activity of Glutamic Acid Phthalimide and the Therapeutic Activity of Triamcinolone in the Treatment of Hansen's Reaction of Virchowian Leprosy], *Hansenol Int,* 6(2), December 1981, p. 114-121.

Wound Injury

Results of this study showed that early glutamine supplementation can prevent stress ulcer problems associated with severe thermal injury in major burn patients.

—R. Yan, et al., ''Early Enteral Feeding and Supplement of Glutamine Prevent Occurrence of Stress Ulcer Following Severe Thermal Injury,'' *Chung Hua Cheng Hsing Shao Shang Wai Ko Tsa Chih,* 11(3), May 1995, p. 189-192.

■ GLYCINE

Leg Ulcer

Results of this double-blind, placebo-controlled study showed that hypostatic leg ulceration patients treated with a topical cream containing l-cysteine, glycine, and dl-threonin 3 times per week over a period of 12 weeks experienced a significantly increased rate of healing relative to patients being treated with cream base alone.

—S.G. Harvey, et al., ''L-cysteine, Glycine and Dl-threonine in the Treatment of Hypostatic Leg Ulceration: A Placebo-controlled Study,'' *Pharmatherapeutica,* 4(4), 1985, p. 227-230.

Schizophrenia

Results of this double-blind, placebo-controlled study involving 14 chronic schizophrenics on medication found that the administration of glycine led to significant improvements in symptoms associated with the disease.

—D.C. Javitt, et al., ''Amelioration of Negative Symptoms in Schizophrenia by Glycine,'' *American Journal of Psychiatry,* 151(8), August 1994, p. 1234-1236.

This article notes that three previous studies have found that 0.4-0.8 g/kg/day doses of glycine coupled with neuroleptics lead to improvements in symptoms associated with schizophrenia.

—U. Heresco-Levy, et al., ''Glycinergic Augmentation of NMDA Receptor-mediated Neurotransmission in the Treatment of Schizophrenia,'' *Psychopharmacol Bull,* 32(4), 1996, p. 731-740.

Stress

Results of this study showed that derivatives of glycine reduced the activation of lipid peroxidation in stress, the duration of the alarm stage of the stress reaction, and stress damage to the heart.

—V.V. Malyshev, et al., ''The Limitation of Lipid Hyperperoxidation and the Prevention of Stressor Damages to the Heart by Glycine Derivatives,'' *Eksp Klin Farmakol,* 59(5), September-October 1996, p. 23-25.

■ HISTIDINE

Cardiovascular/Coronary Heart Disease

Results of this study showed that the intravenous administration of histidine exhibited protective effects on cardiac and brain function during cerebral thrombosis in rats.

—S.Q. Li, et al., ''Histidine Ameliorated Brain Edema and Cardiac Dysfunction During Local Thrombotic Cerebral Ischemia in Rats,'' *Chung Kuo Yao Li Hsueh Pao,* 16(2), March 1995, p. 156-159.

Results of this study found that histidine exhibited antioxidative activity both in vitro and in vivo in rat hearts under conditions of myocardial injury due to ischemia and reperfusion.

—Q. Cai, et al., "Antioxidative Properties of Histidine and its Effects on Myocardial Injury During Ischemia/Reperfusion in Isolated Rat Heart," *Journal Cardiovasc Pharmacol*, 25(1), January 1995, p. 147-155.

Menkes' Kinky-Hair Disease

This article reports on the case of a Menkes' kinky-hair disease patient who received copper histidine treatment from a young age and subsequently didn't suffer from the progressive mental deterioration and early death common to such patients.

—T.A. Waslen, et al., "Menkes' Kinky-hair Disease: Radiologic Findings in a Patient Treated with Copper Histidinate," *Can Assoc Radiol Journal*, 46(2), April 1995, p. 114-117.

This article reports on the case of an 8.5-year-old male Menkes' disease patient treated alternately with intramuscular copper-histidine and oral D-penicillamine. The boy exhibited a surprisingly mild form of the disease which the authors attribute to the treatment.

—D. Nadal & K. Baerlocher, "Menkes' Disease: Long-term Treatment with Copper and D-penicillamine," *European Journal of Pediatrics*, 147(6), August 1988, p. 621-625.

■ ORNITHINE

Aging

Results of this double-blind, placebo-controlled study found that 10 g per day of ornithine oxoglutarate administered for 2 months to ambulatory elderly patients recovering from acute illnesses led to significant improvements in appetite, body weight, quality of life, medical cost, and measures of independence.

—P. Brocker, et al., "A Two-centre, Randomized, Double-blind Trial of Ornithine Oxoglutarate in 194 Elderly, Ambulatory, Convalescent Subjects," *Age Ageing*, 23(4), July 1994, p. 303-306.

Cancer

Results of this study showed that the p.o. administration of DL-alpha-difluoromethylornithine significantly inhibited cultured human small cell lung carcinoma growth in mice.

—G.D. Luk, et al., "Successful Treatment with DL-alpha-difluoromethylornithine in Established Human Small Cell Variant Lung Carcinoma Implants in Athymic Mice," *Cancer Res*, 43(9), September 1983, p. 4239-4243.

Results of this single-blind, placebo-controlled study showed that the oral administration of 18 g per day of alpha-difluoromethylornithine over a period of one month had positive effects on patients suffering from chronic non-suppurative, culture-negative prostatitis.

—U. Dunzendorfer, "alpha-Difluoromethylornithine (alpha DFMO) and Phenoxybenzamine Hydrochloride in the Treatment of Chronic Non-suppurative Prostatitis," *Arzneimittelforschung*, 31(2), 1981, p. 382-385.

Results of this study indicated alpha-difluoromethylornithine exhibited chemopreventive effects against human colonic cancer cell in vitro.

> —A.N. Kingsnorth, et al., ''Effects of Alpha-difluoromethylornithine and 5-fluorouracil on the Proliferation of a Human Colon Adenocarcinoma Cell Line,'' *Cancer Research,* 43(9), September 19983, p. 4035-4058.

Results of this study found that alpha-difluoromethylornithine reduced TPA-induced hyperplasia and TPA-induced increases in DNA synthesis in mice, suggesting it may have potential as an effective new cancer therapy in humans.

> —M. Takigawa, et al., ''Inhibition of Mouse Skin Tumor Promotion and of Promoter-stimulated Epidermal Polyamine Biosynthesis by Alpha-difluoromethylornithine,'' *Cancer Research,* 43(8), August 1983, p. 3732-3738.

Results of this study showed that the administration of D,L-2-difluoromethylornithine via drinking water inhibited experimentally-induced mammary gland carcinomas in rats during the stage of tumor promotion.

> —H.J. Thompson, et al., ''Effect of Concentration of D,L-2-difluoromethylornithine on Murine Mammary Carcinogenesis,'' *Cancer Research,* 45(3), March 1985, p. 1170-1173.

Results of this study showed that alpha-difluoromethylornithine exhibited inhibitory effects on urinary bladder carcinogenesis in male rats.

> —Y. Homma, et al., ''Inhibition of Carcinogenesis by Alpha-difluoromethylornithine in Heterotopically Transplanted Rat Urinary Bladders,'' *Cancer Research,* 45(2), February 1995, p. 648-652.

Results of this study showed that ornithine alpha-ketoglutarate improved muscle protein balance in tumor bearing rats by decreasing breakdown and total amino acid release of incubated EPI.

> —T. Le Bricon, et al., ''Ornithine Alpha-ketoglutarate Limits Muscle Protein Breakdown without Stimulating Tumor Growth in Rats Bearing Yoshida Ascites Hepatoma,'' *Metabolism,* 43(7), July 1994, p. 899-905.

Results of this study showed that a 1% solution of D,L-alpha-difluoromethylornithine significantly suppressed the development of chemically-induced mammary gland carcinomas in rats.

> —H.J. Thompson, et al., ''Effect of D,L-alpha-difluoromethylornithine on Murine Mammary Carcinogenesis,'' *Carcinogenesis,* 5(12), December 1984, p. 1649-1651.

Results of this study found that the administration of DL-alpha-difluoromethylornithine had dramatic inhibitory effects against lung metastases and tumor growth in mice.

> —J. Bartholeyns, et al., ''Treatment of Metastatic Lewis Lung Carcinoma with DL-alpha-difluoromethylornithine,'' *European Journal of Cancer Clin Oncol,* 19(4), April 1983, p. 567-572.

Results of this placebo-controlled study found that a 10% w/w topical solution of DFMO applied for 6 months decreased incidence of severe actinic keratosis in patients experiencing the disease on the forearms.

> —D.S. Alberts, et al., ''Positive Randomized, Double Blinded, Placebo Controlled Study

of Topical Difluoromethyl Ornithine (DFMO) in the Chemoprevention of Skin Cancer,'' *Proceedings of the Annual Meeting of the American Society of Clinical Oncology,* 15, 1996, p. A342.

Contraception

Results of this study showed that intraperitoneal doses of 200 mg/kg twice per day of alpha-difluoromethylornithine (DFMO) during days 4-7 of pregnancy caused inhibition of embryogenesis in rats and a failure to deliver any pups.

—P.R. Reddy & V. Rukmini, ''Alpha-difluoromethylornithine as a Postcoitally Effective Antifertility Agent in Female Rats,'' *Contraception,* 24(2), August 1981, p. 215-221.

Encephalopathy

Results of this study showed that the oral administration of 34 mmol per day of ornithine salts of branched-chain ketoacids over a period of 7-10 days significantly improved electroencephalographic abnormalities and clinical grade of encephalopathy in patients suffering from chronic portal-systemic encephalopathy.

—H.F. Herlong, et al., ''The Use of Ornithine Salts of Branched-chain Ketoacids in Portal-systemic Encephalopathy,'' *Ann Intern Med,* 93(4), October 1980, p. 545-550.

Small Intestine Damage

Results of this study showed that ornithine decarboxylase is a key factor in the repair process and restoration of small intestine mucosal function in rats following ischemia-reperfusion.

—K. Fujimoto, et al., ''Ornithine Decarboxylase is Involved in Repair of Small Intestine after Ischemia-Reperfusion in Rats,'' *American Journal of Physiol,* 261(3 Pt 1), September 1991, p. G523-G529.

Surgical Trauma

Results of this study showed that the administration of glutamine and ornithine-alpha-ketoglutarate as part of the amino acid supply reduced the loss of muscle glutamine from 40% to 25% in skeletal muscle of human patients following elective surgery.

—J. Wernerman, et al., ''Glutamine and Ornithine-alpha-ketoglutarate but Not Branched-chain Amino Acids Reduce the Loss of Muscle Glutamine after Surgical Trauma,'' *Metabolism,* 38(8 Suppl 1), August 1989, p. 63-66.

Wound Healing

Results of this study found that ornithine alpha-ketoglutarate exhibited immunomodulatory effects in rats with severe burn injuries.

—M. Roch-Arveiller, et al., ''Immunomodulatory Effects of Ornithine Alpha-ketoglutarate in Rats with Burn Injuries,'' *Arch Surg,* 131(7), July 1996, p. 718-723.

■ TYROSINE

Anaphylactic Shock

Results of this study found that oral tyrosine prevented anaphylaxis in guinea pigs.
>—M.A. Mchedlishvili, et al., "Tyrosine Inhibition of Anaphylactic Shock in Guinea Pigs," *Biull Eksp Biol Med,* 102(10), October 1986, p. 410-412.

Cardiovascular/Coronary Heart Disease

Results of this study showed that the administration of tyrosine increased blood pressure in hypotensive rats.
>—L.A. Conlay, et al., "Tyrosine Increases Blood Pressure in Hypotensive Rats," *Science,* 212(4494), May 1, 1981, p. 559-560.

Results of this study found that intravenous tyrosine exhibited protective effects against ventricular arrhythmias in canine hearts.
>—N.A. Scott, et al., "Tyrosine Administration Decreases Vulnerability to Ventricular Fibrillation in the Normal Canine Heart," *Science,* 211(4483), February 13, 1981, p. 727-729.

Depression

Results of this study showed that 3200 mg of oral tyrosine per day proved effective in the treatment of dopamine-dependent depression.
>—J. Mouret, et al., "L-tyrosine Cures, Immediate and Long Term, Dopamine-dependent Depressions. Clinical and Polygraphic Studies," *C R Acad Sci III,* 306(3), 1988, p. 93-98.

Narcolepsy

Results of this study showed that the administration of oral tyrosine over a period of six months led to the elimination of 8 out 8 subjects receiving the treatment.
>—J. Mouret, et al., "Treatment of Narcolepsy with L-tyrosine," *Lancet,* 2(8626-8627), December 24-31, 1988, p. 1458-1459.

Stress

Results of this study showed that 100 mg/kg of tyrosine significantly reduced stress symptoms associated with 4.5 hours of exposure to cold and hypoxia in human subjects.
>—L.E. Banderet & H.R. Lieberman, "Treatment with Tyrosine, a Neurotransmitter Precursor, Reduces Environmental Stress in Humans," *Brain Res Bull,* 22(4), April 1989, p. 759-762.

ESSENTIAL AMINO ACIDS

■ ISOLEUCINE

Amyotrophic Lateral Sclerosis

Results of this double-blind, placebo-controlled study found that amyotrophic lateral sclerosis patients who received daily oral administration of a mix of 12 g of L-leucine, 8 g of L-isoleucine, and 6.4 g of L-valine experienced significant improvements in muscle strength and walking ability.

>—A. Plaitakis, et al., "Pilot Trial of Branched-chain Aminoacids in Amyotrophic Lateral Sclerosis," *Lancet,* 1(8593), May 7, 1988, p. 1015-1058.

Brain Damage

Results of this double-blind study showed that the administration of a mixture of valine, isoleucine, and leucine to phenylketonuria patients over a 3 month period can inhibit phenylalanine from entering the brain and reduce its toxic effects on the central nervous system.

>—H.K. Berry, et al., "Valine, Isoleucine, and Leucine. A New Treatment for Phenylketonuria," *American Journal of Dis Child,* 144(5), May 1990, p. 539-543.

■ LEUCINE

Phenylketonuria

Results of this double-blind study showed that the administration of valine, isoleucine, and leucine to adolescents and young adults with phenylketonuria had positive effects.

>—H.K. Berry, et al., "Valine, Isoleucine, and Leucine. A New Treatment for Phenylketonuria," *American Journal of Dis Child,* 144(5), May 1990, p. 539-543.

■ LYSINE

Biliary Colic

Results of this double-blind, placebo-controlled study showed that biliary colic patients experienced significant reductions in pain following 1.8 g of supplemental lysine acetylsalicylate and 200 mg of ketoprofen via intravenous bolus.

>—M. Magrini, et al., "Successful Treatment of Biliary Colic with Intravenous Ketoprofen or Lysine Acetylsalicylate," *Curr Med Res Opin,* 9(7), 1985, p. 454-460.

Herpes

Results of this double-blind, placebo-controlled study found that 1000 mg of oral 1-lysine per day administered over a period of 12 months led to significant reductions in lesion frequency in patients suffering from recurrent herpes simplex labialis.

> —D.J. Thein & W.C. Hurt, "Lysine as a Prophylactic Agent in the Treatment of Recurrent Herpes Simplex Labialis," *Oral Surg Oral Med Oral Pathol,* 58(6), December 1994, p. 659-666.

Results of this double-blind, placebo-controlled study found that 1248 mg of oral 1-lysine monohydrochloride per day decreased the recurrence rate of herpes simplex attacks in nonimmunocompromised hosts.

> —M.A. McCune, et al., "Treatment of Recurrent Herpes Simplex Infections with L-lysine Monohydrochloride," *Cutis,* 34(4), October 1984, p. 366-373.

Results of this double-blind, placebo-controlled study found that 1000 mg tablets of oral 1-lysine monohydrochloride taken three times per day over a period of six months decreased the recurrence rate of herpes simplex attacks in human subjects.

> —R.S. Griffith, et al., "Success of L-lysine Therapy in Frequently Recurrent Herpes Simplex Infection. Treatment and Prophylaxis," *Dermatologica,* 175(4), 1987, p. 183-190.

Results of this study showed that an average dose of 936 mg of lysine per day administered over a 6 month period prevented recurrence or reduced the frequency of herpes infection in subjects suffering from cold sores, canker sores, and genital herpes.

> —D.E. Walsh, et al., "Subjective Response to Lysine in the Therapy of Herpes Simplex," *Journal of Antimicrob Chemother,* 12(5), November 1983, p. 489-496.

Migraines

Results of this double-blind, placebo-controlled study found oral lysine acetylsalicylate combined with metroclopramide to be an effective treatment for migraines in human patients.

> —H. Chabriat, et al., "Combined Oral Lysine Acetylsalicylate and Metoclopramide in the Acute Treatment of Migraine: A Multicentre Double-blind Placebo-controlled Study," *Cephalalgia,* 14(4), August 1994, p. 297-300.

Postoperative Pain

Results of this study found that the intravenous administration of acetylsalicylate of lysine to obstetrical and gynecological surgery patients exhibited beneficial effects with respect to postoperative pain in 77.4% of the patients examined.

> —G. Ramella, et al., "Lysine Acetylsalicylate in the Treatment of Postoperative Pain in Obstetric and Gynecological Surgery," *Minerva Anestesiol,* 47(1-2), January-February 1981, p. 33-36.

Rheumatic Disorders

Results of this study showed that 320 mg per day of ketoprofen lysine had beneficial effects on patients suffering from various rheumatic disorders.

—M. Chevallard, et al., "Effectiveness and Tolerability of Ketoprofen Lysine, Once a Day, in Patients with Rheumatic Disorders," *Drugs Exp Clin Res,* 13(5), 1987, p. 293-296.

■ METHIONINE

Cancer

Results of this study showed that supplemental methionine prevented the induction of hepatocarcinogenesis in rats.

—T. Tsujiuchi, et al., "Prevention by Methionine of Enhancement of Hepatocarcinogenesis by Coadministration of a Choline-deficient L-amino Acid-defined Diet and Ethionine in Rats," *Japanese Journal of Cancer Research,* 86(12), December 1995, p. 1136-1142.

Hepatitis

This article reports on the case of a middle-aged woman with halothane induced hepatitis resulting from gastric surgery to remedy obesity. Treatment with methionine quickly cured her jaundice.

—J.A. Windsor & G. Wynne-Jones, "Halothane Hepatitis and Prompt Resolution with Methionine Therapy: Case Report," *New Zealand Medical Journal,* 101(851), August 10, 1988, p. 502-503.

Lead Poisoning

Results of this study found methionine to be an effective supportive therapy against lead poisoning in rats.

—D.N. Kachru, et al., "Influence of Methionine Supplementation in Chelation of Lead in Rats," *Biomed Environ Sci,* 2(3), September 1989, p. 265-270.

Neuropathy

This article reports on the case of a patient with severe myeloneuropathy and macrocytic anemia associated with a low vitamin B12 serum levels resulting from nitrous exposure who benefited from methionine treatment.

—C.B. Stacy, et al., "Methionine in the Treatment of Nitrous-oxide-induced Neuropathy and Myeloneuropathy," *Journal of Neurol,* 239(7), August 1992, p. 401-403.

Paracetamol Poisoning

Results of this study found the oral administration of methionine to be as effective as acetylcysteine in the prevention of severe liver damage and death following overdose of acetaminophen when administered within ten hours of acetiminophen ingestion.

—J.A.Vale, et al., "Treatment of Acetaminophen Poisoning. The Use of Oral Methionine," *Arch Intern Med,* 141(3 Spec No), February 23, 1981, p. 394-396.

Results of this study indicated that methionine administered at doses of 2-5 g every 4 hours up to 10 total g beginning within ten hours of paracetamol overdose was effective in limiting the frequency and severity of hepatic damage associated with such patients.

> —P. Crome, et al., "Oral Methionine in the Treatment of Severe Paracetamol (Acetaminophen) Overdose," *Lancet,* 2(7990), October 6, 1976, p. 829-830.

Results of this 4-year study found early methionine administration to be effective in reducing liver damage associated with paracetamol overdose in young patients.

> —K.J. Breen, et al., "Paracetamol Self-poisoning: Diagnosis, Management, and Outcome," *Medical Journal of Aust,* 1(2), January 23, 1982, p. 77-79.

■ PHENYLALANINE

Cancer

Results of this study showed that the oral administration of 6% phenylalanine following 25 weeks of carcinogen exposure significantly reduced the incidence and number of glandular stomach adenocarcinomas in rats.

> —H. Iishi, et al., "Protection by Oral Phenylalanine Against Gastric Carcinogenesis Induced by N-methyl-N'-nitro-N-nitrosoguanidine in Wistar Rats," *British Journal of Cancer,* 62(2), August 1990, p. 173-176.

Results of this study showed that the administration of 250 mg of D-phenylalanine 3 times per day over a period of 15 days prevented acute or incident pain in cancer patients.

> —G. Donzelle, et al., "Curing Trial of Complicated Oncologic Pain by D-phenylalanine," *Anesth Analg,* 38(11-12), 1981, p. 655-658.

Depression

Results of this double-blind, placebo-controlled study showed that the administration of 150-200 mg/ 24 hours of DL-phenylalanine over a period of 30 days exhibited antidepressive effects in depressed patients.

> —H. Beckmann, et al., "DL-phenylalanine Versus Imipramine: A Double-blind Controlled Study," *Arch Psychiatr Nervenkr,* 227(1), July 4, 1979, p. 49-58.

Results of this study showed that the administration of 75-200 mg per day of DL-phenylalanine over a period of 20 days exhibited antidepressive effects in patients suffering from depression.

> —H. Beckmann & E. Ludolph, "DL-phenylalanine as an Antidepressant. Open Study," *Arzneimittelforschung,* 28(8), 1978, p. 1283-1284.

Results of this study found that the intravenous and oral administration of 5-10 mg per day of L-deprenyl coupled with 250 mg per day of phenylalanine had positive effects on patients suffering from unipolar depression.

> —W. Birkmayer, et al., "L-deprenyl Plus L-phenylalanine in the Treatment of Depression," *Journal of Neural Transm,* 59(1), 1984, p. 81-87.

Ulcer

Results of this study showed that the administration of phenylalaninol prevented stress and indomethacin induced gastric ulcers in rats.
>—H. Hashizume, et al., "Effects of Phenylalaninol on Centrally Induced Gastric Acid Secretion," *Chem Pharm Bull,* 40(11), November 1992, p. 3113-3114.

Vitiligo

Results of this study showed that 50 mg/kg of phenylalanine coupled with UVA exposure proved to be an effective therapy for vitiligo.
>—R.H. Cormane, et al., "Phenylalanine and UVA Light for the Treatment of Vitiligo," *Arch Dermatol Res,* 277(2), 1985, p. 126-130.

Results of this study showed that oral L-phenylalanine coupled with UVA exposure proved to be a safe and effective therapy for vitiligo in children.
>—C.H. Schulpis, et al., "Phenylalanine Plus Ultraviolet Light: Preliminary Report of a Promising Treatment for Childhood Vitiligo," *Pediatr Dermatol,* 6(4), December 1989, p. 332-335.

Results of this study showed that 50 mg/kg of phenylalanine coupled with UVA exposure proved to be an effective therapy for vitiligo.
>—B. Thiele, et al., "Repigmentation Treatment of Vitiligo with L-phenylalanine and UVA Irradiation," *Z Hautkr,* 62(7), April 1, 1987, p. 519-523.

■ TRYPTOPHAN

Cancer

Results of this study showed that DL-tryptophan counteracted benzidine's carcinogenic effects in mice and significantly inhibited the onset of hepatomas.
>—M. Miyakawa & O. Yoshida, "Protective Effects of DL-Tryptophan on Benzidine-induced Hepatic Tumor in Mice," *Gan,* 71(2), 1980, p. 265-268.

This article reports on the case of a 56-year-old woman hospitalized due to carcinoid crisis. Treatment with 3.4 g per day of tryptophan improved her consciousness level which had been comatose prior to administration.
>—A.L. Harris & I.E. Smith, "Tryptophan in the Treatment of Carcinoid Crisis," *Cancer Chemother Pharmacol,* 10(2), 1983, p. 137-139.

Cardiovascular/Coronary Heart Disease

Results of this study indicated that tryptophan significantly protected against the development of DOCA-induced hypertension, polydipsia, and cardiac hypertrophy in rats.
>—M.J. Fregly & D.C. Fater, "Prevention of DOCA-induced Hypertension in Rats by Chronic Treatment with Tryptophan," *Clin Exp Pharmacol Physiol,* 13(11-12), November-December 1986, p. 767-776.

Results of this study showed that the administration of L-tryptophan significantly protected rats from the onset of hypertension caused by bilateral encapsulation of the kidneys.

—M.J. Fregly, et al., "Effect of Chronic Dietary Treatment with L-tryptophan on the Development of Renal Hypertension in Rats," *Pharmacology,* 36(2), 1988, p. 91-100.

Depression

This review article notes studies have shown that L-tryptophan may be useful in mild cases of depression and improve the depressed mood of Parkinsonian patients.

—B. Boman, "L-tryptophan: A Rational Anti-depressant and a Natural Hypnotic?," *Aust N Z J Psychiatry,* 22(1), March 1988, p. 83-97.

Results of this study indicated that L-tryptophan coupled with lithium had beneficial effects on patients suffering from endogenous depression.

—P. Honore, et al., "Lithium + L-tryptophan Compared with Amitriptyline in Endogenous Depression," *Journal of Affect Disord,* 4(1), March 1982, p. 79-82.

Results of this study showed that the administration of 8 g per day of tryptophan over a period of 4 weeks had antidepressive effects in patients suffering from moderate depression.

—R.N. Herrington, et al., "Comparative Trial of L-tryptophan and Amitriptyline in Depressive Illness," *Psychol Med,* 6(4), November 1976, p. 673-678.

Mania

Results of this double-blind, placebo-controlled study showed that 12 g per day of L-tryptophan administered over a period of 1 week led to a significant reduction in manic symptoms in newly admitted manic patients.

—G. Chouinard, et al., "A Controlled Clinical Trial of L-tryptophan in Acute Mania," *Biol Psychiatry,* 20(5), May 1985, p. 546-557.

Menstruation

Results of this study showed that the administration of 6 g per day of L-tryptophan led to a significant amelioration of symptoms associated with luteal phase dysphoric disorder.

—S. Steinberg, et al., "Tryptophan in the Treatment of Late Luteal Phase Dysphoric Disorder: A Pilot Study," *Journal of Psychiatry Neurosci,* 19(2), March 1994, p. 114-119.

Obsessive Compulsive Disorder

Results of this study showed that patients suffering from symptoms associated with obsessive-compulsive disorder that were resistant to clomipramine experienced improvement following treatment with lithium or L-tryptophan.

—S.A. Rasmussen, "Lithium and Tryptophan Augmentation in Clomipramine-resistant Obsessive-compulsive Disorder," *American Journal of Psychiatry,* 141(10), October 1984, p. 1283-1285.

Pain

Results of this study showed that tryptophan relieved pain in patients suffering from recurrent and diminished sensory deficits stemming from rhizotomy and cordotomy.
> —R.B. King, ''Pain and Tryptophan,'' *Journal of Neurosurg,* 53(1), July 1980, p. 44-52.

Results of this study showed that the administration of 3 g of tryptophan over a period of 24 hours led to significant pain reduction pain in patients requiring nonsurgical endodonitc therapy.
> —S.E. Shpeen, et al., ''The Effect of Tryptophan on Postoperative Endodontic Pain,'' *Oral Surg Oral Med Oral Pathol,* 58(4), October 1984, p. 446-449.

Results of this study showed that L-tryptophan supplementation significantly reduced experimentally-induced ischemic pain in 3 out of 11 subjects examined.
> —T. Nurmikko, et al., ''Effect of L-tryptophan Supplementation on Ischemic Pain,'' *Acupunct Electrother Res,* 9(1), 1984, p. 45-55.

This article reports on the case of a patient with chronic pain and unipolar and cyclothymic disorders or showed marked improvement following the administration of 1000 mg of tryptophan every 4 hours and high carbohydrate, low protein meal diet.
> —R.J. Hedaya, ''Pharmacokinetic Factors in the Clinical Use of Tryptophan,'' *Journal of Clin Psychopharmacol,* 4(6), December 1984, p. 347-348.

Parkinson's Disease

Results of this study showed that the administration of L-tryptophan at doses of 150-450 mg per day ameloriated paranoid hallucinations associated with L-Dopa treatment in Parkinson's disease patients.
> —J.M. Rabey, et al., ''L-tryptophan Administration in L-dopa-induced Hallucinations in Elderly Parkinsonian Patients,'' *Gerontology,* 23(6), 1977, p. 438-444.

Results of this study showed that supplementation with L-tryptophan at the start levodopa therapy may help preventing levodopa-induced motor complications common to Parkinson's disease patients.
> —R. Sandyk & H. Fisher, ''L-tryptophan Supplementation in Parkinson's Disease,'' *Int Journal of Neurosci,* 45(3-4), April 1989, p. 215-219.

Schizophrenia

This article reviews clinical findings concerning the role of L-tryptophan in potentiating the effects of lithium carbonate on schizoaffective patients. One double-blind, placebo-controlled study in particular found the combined treatment with lithium and L-tryptophan resulted in significant improvements in such patients.
> —T.D. Brewerton & V.I. Reus, ''Lithium Carbonate and L-tryptophan in the Treatment of Bipolar and Schizoaffective Disorders,'' *American Journal of Psychiatry,* 140(6), June 1983, p. 757-760.

Sleep

This article reports on the case of three patients with isolated sleep paralysis which was able to be controlled by L-tryptophan alone or in combination with amitriptyline.
> —S. Snyder & G. Hams, ''Serotoninergic Agents in the Treatment of Isolated Sleep Paralysis,'' *American Journal of Psychiatry,* 139(9), September 1982, p. 1202-1203.

This review article notes that both animal and human studies have showed L-tryptophan can reduce sleep latency.

—E. Hartmann, "L-tryptophan: A Rational Hypnotic with Clinical Potential," *American Journal of Psychiatry,* 134(4), April 1977, p. 366-370.

Results of this study showed that the administration of 1 g of L-tryptophan significantly reduced sleep latency in mild insomniacs.

—E. Hartmann & C.L. Spinweber, "Sleep Induced by L-tryptophan. Effect of Dosages within the Normal Dietary Intake," *Journal of Nerv Ment Dis,* 167(8), August 1979, p. 497-499.

Results of this double-blind, placebo-controlled study found the repetitive administration of 3 X 2 g of L-tryptophan led to significant improvements in severe chronic insomniacs.

—D. Schneider-Helmert, "Interval Therapy with L-tryptophan in Severe Chronic Insomniacs. A Predictive Laboratory Study," *Pharmacopsychiatry,* 16(3), 1981, p. 162-173.

Results of this study showed that the administration of 2 g of L-tryptophan over a period of 4 weeks significantly improved sleeping patterns and mood in patients suffering from chronic insomnia.

—K. Demisch, et al., "Treatment of Severe Chronic Insomnia with L-tryptophan and Varying Sleeping Times," *Pharmacopsychiatry,* 20(6), November 1987, p. 245-248.

Results of this double-blind, placebo-controlled study found that the administration of l-tryptophane at doses of either 1 g or 3 g per night significantly reduced sleep latency in patients suffering from insomnia to unfamiliar sleeping location.

—E. Hartmann & R. Elion, "The Insomnia of 'Sleeping in a Strange Place': Effects of l-tryptophane," *Psychopharmacology,* 53(2), July 18, 1977, p. 131-133.

This review article notes that studies have shown doses of L-tryptophan ranging from 1 to 15 g to be effective in reducing sleep onset time in patients suffering from insomnia.

—D. Schneider-Helmert & C.L. Spinweber, "Evaluation of L-tryptophan for Treatment of Insomnia: A Review," *Psychopharmacology,* 89(1), 1986, p. 1-7.

Smoking Cessation

Results of this study indicated that the administration of tryptophan to patients trying to quit smoking led to a reduction in total number of daily cigarettes and in symptoms of withdrawal and anxiety relative to controls.

—D.J. Bowen, et al., "Tryptophan and High-carbohydrate Diets as Adjuncts to Smoking Cessation Therapy," *Journal of Behav Med,* 14(2), April 1991, p. 97-110.

Tardive Dyskinesia

This article reports on the case of a patients with neuroleptic-induced tardive dyskinesia who experienced a major improvement following supplemental L-tryptophan.

—R. Sandyk, et al., "L-tryptophan in Neuroleptic-induced Tardive Dyskinesia," *Int Journal Neurosci,* 42(1-2), September 1988, p. 127-130.

■ VALINE

Phenylketonuria

Results of this double-blind study showed that the administration of valine, isoleucine, and leucine to adolescents and young adults with phenylketonuria had positive effects.

—H.K. Berry, et al., "Valine, Isoleucine, and Leucine. A New Treatment for Phenylketonuria," *American Journal of Dis Child,* 144(5), May 1990, p. 539-543.

INTRODUCTION/ PHYTOCHEMICALS

Phytochemicals are substances found in edible plants that exhibit potential benefits in the prevention and treatment of disease. There are thousands of phytochemicals in the foods we eat and scientists are just beginning to discover their healing properties. According to the *Journal of the American Dietetic Association* (April 1995):

> *It is the position of the American Dietetic Association (ADA) that specific substances in foods (e.g. phytochemicals as naturally occurring components and functional food components) may have a beneficial role in health as part of a varied diet. The Association supports research regarding the health benefits and risks of these substances. Dietetics professionals will continue to work with the food industry and government to ensure that the public has accurate scientific information in this emerging field.*

The report goes on to say that phytochemicals are present in many frequently consumed foods, especially fruits, vegetables, grains, legumes, and seeds, as well as in such less common foods as licorice, soy, and green tea. In addition to naturally occurring phytochemicals, scientists are developing what they call *functional foods* which consist of any food or food ingredient providing health benefits beyond the traditional nutrients it contains.

Phytochemicals and functional food components have been associated with the prevention and/or treatment of at least four of the leading causes of death in the country — cancer, diabetes, cardiovascular disease, and hypertension — and with the prevention and/or treatment of other medical ailments including neural tube defects, osteoporosis, abnormal bowel function, and arthritis (*Journal of the American Dietetic Association,* April 1995). Dr. Potter, professor of epidemiology and director of the University of Minnesota Cancer Prevention Research unit, has been studying the relationship between diet and cancer for more than 15 years. Like scientists worldwide, he has found that people whose diets are heavy in fruits and vegetables have lower rates of most cancers. Limonene in citrus fruits, for example, is known to increase the production of enzymes that help the body dispose of potentially carcinogenic substances. Even the National Cancer Institute estimates that one in three cancer deaths are diet related and that 8 of 10 cancers have a nutrition/diet component.

Phytochemicals have been actively used by pharmaceutical companies in making many of their products. According to a report in *Business Week* (February 15, 1993), 25% of modern pharmaceuticals are derived in some way from plants. The heart medicine digitalis and the cancer drugs vinicistine and taxol are just some examples. Pharmaceutical companies may soon be motivated to isolate components in foods into pills or supplement form to market the individual elements for their health benefits. However, due to regulatory problems, such companies will have to market naturally occurring components as drugs.

What makes phytochemicals new in the public ranks is their potential health benefits before people get sick, and the saving of both lives and health-care dollars as a direct result of their use. Unfortunately, according to Dr. Stephen L. DeFelic, head of the Foundation for Innovation in Medicine, the field is still in its infancy because of too few large-scale clinical trials focusing on the health benefits of foods. Since phytochemicals aren't patentable, companies are reluctant to finance something that could cost as much as $200 million for each test.

Nevertheless, epidemiological evidence and small human trials point to benefits which may well be sleeping giants in the nutrition arena. Such is the case with licorice root. In one USDA study, licorice root, an extract, proved to be 50 times sweeter than sugar without promoting tooth decay. It contains prostaglandin inhibitors that may guard against cancer and ulcers, and it is being pursued by many companies that want to use it as a food additive. In another study, Michael Gould, professor of human oncology at the University of Wisconsin Medical School, has found that d-limonene, the major component of orange peel oil, protects rats against breast cancer. In addition to findings such as these, the ADA report notes that well-designed clinical trials indicate the beneficial effects associated with high fruit and vegetable diets cannot be duplicated by nutritional supplementation alone. Clearly, there is more benefits to be had in the healthy foods we eat than is obtained from the most common nutrients often associated with them such as vitamins C, E, A, Beta-Carotene, etc.

The material on phytochemicals that follows has been obtained from the extensive electronic database assembled by Stephen M. Beckstrom and James A. Duke at the *National Germplasm Resources Laboratory, Agriculture Research Service, United States Department of Agriculture*. This database is accessible on the World Wide Web at:

(http://www.ars-grin.gov/ngrlsb/)

FRUIT/PHYTOCHEMICALS

Phytochemicals are as important, if not more important, than vitamins, minerals, and enzymes. Each fruit and vegetable has from several dozen to nearly 200 different phytochemicals. Each of these phytochemicals has the capacity to prevent cancer, kill viruses and bacteria, stimulate the immune system, and cleanse and rebuild our bodies. Some plants, such as broccoli, soy beans, cabbage, cauliflower, kale, and mustard greens have multiple anticancer phytochemicals. The way to use them would be to first determine what condition you want helped, then look it up in the index. You will see a list of the different recommended foods and their individual phytochemicals. Therefore you can construct a meal plan or juice therapy that would contain the most beneficial anticancer phytochemicals in dosages that have therapeutic benefit.

■ ACEROLA

Chemical Constituents of Malphigia glabra L. (Malpighiaceae)

ASCORBIC ACID Fruit 16,228—172,231 ppm
ASH Fruit 2,000—42,000 ppm
BETA-CAROTENE Fruit 3—69 ppm
CALCIUM Fruit 120—1,400 ppm
CARBOHYDRATES Fruit—778,000 ppm
FAT Fruit 3,000—34,924 ppm
FIBER Fruit 4,000—46,566 ppm
IRON Fruit 2—28 ppm
KILOCALORIES Fruit 320—3,725/kg
MAGNESIUM Fruit 180—2,095 ppm
NIACIN Fruit 4—47 ppm
PANTOTHENIC-ACID Fruit 3—36 ppm
PHOSPHORUS Fruit 110—1,280 ppm
POTASSIUM Fruit 828—24,345 ppm
PROTEIN Fruit 4,000—46,566 ppm
RIBOFLAVIN Fruit 0.6—7 ppm
SODIUM Fruit 0.2—2.3 ppm

THIAMIN Fruit 0.2—2.3 ppm
VITAMIN B6 Fruit 0.09—1.04 ppm
WATER Fruit 914,000—923,000 ppm

■ APPLE

Chemical Constituents of Malus domestica BORKH (Rosaceae)

1,3,3,-TRIMETHYL-DIOXA-2,7-
    BICYCLO(2,2,1)HEPTANE Fruit
1-MONO-LINOLEIN Seed
2-METHYL-2-3-EPOXY-PENTANE Fruit
2-METHYL-BUT-2-EN-1-AL Fruit
2-METHYL-BUT-3-EN-1-OL Fruit
2-METHYL-PROPEN-1-AL Fruit
3,4-BENZOPYRENE Fruit
3-HYDROXY-OCTYL-BETA-D-
    GLUCOSIDE Fruit
6-METHYL-HEPTEN-5-EN-2-ONE Fruit

ABSCISIC-ACID Fruit
ALANINE Fruit 70—435 ppm
ALPHA-ALANINE Fruit
ALPHA-LINOLENIC-ACID Fruit 180—1,120
    ppm
ALPHA-TOCOPHEROL Fruit 2—37 ppm
ALUMINUM Fruit 0.4—129 ppm
AMMONIA(NH3) Fruit Epidermis 235—1,029
    ppm
AMYGDALIN Seed 6,000—13,800 ppm
ANILINE Fruit 1.5 ppm
ANILINE Fruit Epidermis 1.7 ppm
ARGININE Fruit 60—373 ppm
ARSENIC Fruit 0.001—0.43 ppm
ASCORBIC-ACID Fruit 20—402 ppm
ASCORBIDASE Plant
ASH Fruit 2,300—43,000 ppm
ASPARAGINE Fruit 171 ppm
ASPARTIC-ACID Fruit 210—2,115 ppm
AVICULARIN Fruit
BARIUM Fruit 0.22—8.6 ppm
BENZL-AMINE Fruit Epidermis 0.6 ppm
BENZLAMINE Fruit 0.3—3 ppm
BETA-ALANINE Fruit
BETA-CAROTENE Fruit 0—76 ppm
BORON Fruit 1—110 ppm
BROMINE Fruit
CADMIUM Fruit 0.002—0.026 ppm
CAFFEIC-ACID Fruit 85—1,270 ppm
CALCIUM Fruit 43—570 ppm
CARBOHYDRATES Fruit 152,250—948,550
CHLOROGENIC-ACID Fruit
CHLOROPHYLL Fruit 0—1 ppm
CHROMIUM Fruit 0.005—0.3 ppm
COBALT Fruit 0.24—4 ppm
COPPER Fruit 0.24—4 ppm
COUMARIC-ACID Plant
CUTIN Fruit Epidermis
CYANIDIN-3,5-DIGLUCOSIDE Cotyledon
D-CATECHIN Fruit
DIETHYLAMINE Fruit 3 ppm
DIGALACTOSYL-DIGLYCERIDE Fruit 49—
    107 ppm
DIHYDROXYTRICARBALLYCLIC-ACID
    Fruit 1 ppm

DIPHOSPHATIDYL-GLYCEROL Fruit 4—6
    ppm
EO Fruit 25—35 ppm
ESTRAGOLE Essential Oil
ESTRONE Seed 0.1—0.13 ppm
ETHYLAMINE Fruit 3 ppm
FARNESENE Fruit Epidermis
FAT Fruit 3,210—34,200 ppm
FAT Seed 180,000—230,000 ppm
FERULIC-ACID Fruit 4—95 ppm
FIBER Fruit 5,200—49,636 ppm
FIBER Fruit 131,000 ppm
FLUORINE Fruit 0.1—2.1 ppm
FOLACIN Fruit 0.02—0.2 ppm
FRUCTOSE Fruit 50,100—60,800 ppm
GLUCOSE Fruit 17,200—18,200 ppm
GLUTAMIC-ACID Fruit 156—1,244 ppm
HISTIDINE Fruit 30—187 ppm
HYDROXYCINNAMIC-ACID Fruit 1,340 ppm
HYPEROSIDE Fruit
IRON Fruit 1.1—123 ppm
ISOLEUCINE Fruit 50—497 ppm
ISOQUERCITRIN Fruit
JASMONIC-ACID Fruit
KILOCALORIES Fruit 3,419/kg
L-EPICATECHIN Fruit
LAURIC-ACID Fruit 10—63 ppm
LEAD Fruit 0.002—64 ppm
LEUCINE Fruit 120—746 ppm
LINOLENIC-ACID Fruit 870—5,411 ppm
LITHIUM Fruit 0.044—0.172 ppm
LUTEIN Fruit 0.4—5 ppm
LUTEOXANTHIN Fruit
LYSINE Fruit 20—746 ppm
MAGNESIUM Fruit 48—478 ppm
MALVIDIN-MONOGLYCOSIDE Plant
MANGANESE Fruit 0—29 ppm
MERCURY Fruit 0—0.02 ppm
METHYL-2-XI-ACETOXY-20-BETA-
    HYDROXY-URSONATE Fruit Epidermis
METHYL-VINYL-KETONE Fruit
METHYLAMINE Fruit Epidermis 4.5 ppm
MEVALONIC-ACID Fruit 30—36 ppm
MOLYBDENUM Fruit—0.077—0.43 ppm

MUFA Fruit 150—935 ppm
MYRISTIC-ACID Fruit 20—124 ppm
N-METHYL-BETA-PHENETHYLAMINE Fruit 1.2 ppm
N-METHYL-PHENETHYLAMINE Exocarp 1.3 ppm
N-METHYL-PHENETHYLAMINE Fruit 1.2 ppm
N-PENTYL-AMINE Fruit 0.3 ppm
NEOXANTHIN Fruit Epidermis
NIACIN Fruit 1—7 ppm
NICKEL Fruit 0.004—0.645 ppm
NITROGEN Fruit 280—4,000 ppm
OLEIC-ACID Fruit 140—871 ppm
P-COUMARIC-ACID Fruit 15—460 ppm
P-COUMARYL-QUINIC-ACID Fruit
P-HYDROXYBENZOIC-ACID Fruit
PALMITIC-ACID Fruit 480—2,986 ppm
PALMITOLEIC-ACID Fruit 10—62 ppm
PANTOTHENIC-ACID Fruit 1—4 ppm
PECTIN Fruit 1,400—66,585 ppm
PHENYLALANINE Fruit 50—311 ppm
PHLORETAMIDE Fruit
PHLORETIN-4'-0-BETA-D-GLUCOPYRANOSIDE Fruit 6,486 ppm
PHLORETIN-XYLOGLUCOSIDE Fruit
PHOSPHATIDYL-CHOLINE Fruit 189—214 ppm
PHOSPHATIDYL-ETHONALOAMINE Fruit 101—124 ppm
PHOSPHATIDYL-GLYCEROL Fruit 8—27 ppm
PHOSPHATIDYL-INOSITOL Fruit 53—59 ppm
PHOSPHATIDYLSERINE Fruit 4 ppm
PHOSPHATIDYLIC-ACID Fruit 3—6 ppm
PHOSPHORUS Fruit 68—925 ppm
PHYTOSTEROLS Fruit 120—745 ppm
POTASSIUM Fruit 1,110—12,140 ppm
PROTEIN Fruit 1,870—12,140 ppm
PROTOCATECHUIC-ACID Fruit
PUFA Fruit 1,050—6,535 ppm
PYRROLIDINE Fruit Epidermis 1.5 ppm
QUERCETIN Pericarp 58—263 ppm

QUERCETIN-3-O-ALPHA-GALACTOSIDE Fruit Epidermis
QUERCETIN-3-O-XYLOSIDE Fruit Epidermis
QUERCITRIN Fruit
REYNOUTRIN Fruit
RIBOFLAVIN Fruit 1 ppm
RUBIDIUM Fruit 0.27—10 ppm
RUTIN Fruit Epidermis
SELENIUM Fruit
SERINE Fruit 80—497 ppm
SFA Fruit 580—3,610 ppm
SILICON Fruit 1—70 ppm
SILVER Fruit 0.011—0.086 ppm
SINAPIC-ACID Fruit
SODIUM Fruit 0—133 ppm
SORBITOL Leaf
STEARIC-ACID Fruit 70—435 ppm
STRONTIUM Fruit 0.165—8.6 ppm
SUCCINIC-ACID Plant
SUCROSE Fruit 24,000—36,200 ppm
SUGAR Fruit 60,100—166,000 ppm
SULFUR Fruit 1.65—23 ppm
THIAMIN Fruit 1—2 ppm
THREONINE Fruit 30—435 ppm
TITANIUM Fruit 0.055—3 ppm
TRANS-ABSCISIC-ACID Fruit
TRYPTOPHAN Fruit 20—124 ppm
TYROSINE Fruit 40—249 ppm
URONIC-ACID Fruit 7—1,440 ppm
URSOLIC-ACID Fruit Epidermis
VALINE Fruit 40—560 ppm
VITAMIN B6 Fruit 1—3 ppm
VOMIFOLIOL-L-O-BETA-D-XYLOPYRANOSYL-6-O-BETA-D-GLUCOPYRANOSIDE B WATER Fruit 809,000 ppm
ZINC Fruit 0—35 ppm
ZIRCONIUM Fruit 0.22—0.86 ppm

■ APRICOT

Chemical Constituents of Prunus armeniaca L. (Rosaceae)

ACETIC-ACID Essential Oil
ALANINE Fruit 680—4,980 ppm
ALPHA-TERPINEOL Essential Oil
AMYLASE Fruit
ARGININE Fruit 450—3,300 ppm
ASCORBIC-ACID Fruit 100—745 ppm
ASH Fruit 7,000—105,000 ppm
ASPARTIC-ACID Fruit 3,140—23,000 ppm
BENZYL-ALCOHOL Fruit
BETA-CAROTENE Fruit 13—189 ppm
BORON Fruit 1—70 ppm
CAFFEIC-ACID Plant
CALCIUM Fruit 134—1,899 ppm
CALCIUM-PECTATE Fruit 10,000 ppm
CAPRONIC-ACID Fruit
CARBOHYDRATES Fruit 111,200—873,000 ppm
CHLOROGENIC-ACID Fruit
CIS-EPOXYDIHYDROLINALOOL Plant
CITRIC-ACID Fruit
CYANIDIN Plant
CYSTINE Fruit 30—220 ppm
DELTA-OCTALACTONE Fruit
EMULSIN Fruit
FAT Fruit 2,200—41,000 ppm
FIBER Fruit 6,000—132,000 ppm
FOLACIN Fruit 0.07—0.7 ppm
FRUCTOSE Fruit 14,000—42,000 ppm
GAMMA-CAPRALACTONE Fruit
GAMMA-CAPRALACTONE Fruit
GAMMA-CAROTENE Fruit
GAMMA-DECALACTONE Plant
GERANIAL Essential Oil
GERANIOL Essential Oil
GLUCOSE Fruit 32,000—48,000 ppm
GLUTAMIC-ACID Fruit 1,570—11,500 ppm
GLYCINE Fruit 400—2,930 ppm
HISTIDINE Fruit 270—1,980 ppm
INVERTASE Fruit
IODINE Fruit 0.05 ppm
IRON Fruit 5—79 ppm
ISOBUTYRIC-ACID Fruit
ISOLEUCINE Fruit 410—3,000 ppm
ISOQUERCITRIN Fruit

KILOCALORIES Fruit 480—3,515/kg
LEUCINE Fruit 770—5,640 ppm
LIMONENE Essential Oil
LINALOOL Fruit
LINOLEIC-ACID Fruit 770—5,640 ppm
LYCOPENE Fruit
LYSINE Fruit 970—7,105 ppm
M-INOSITOL Plant
MAGNESIUM Fruit 76—615 ppm
MALIC-ACID Fruit 7,000—22,000 ppm
METHIONINE Fruit 60—440 ppm
MUFA Fruit 170—1,245 ppm
MYRCENE Essential Oil
NEOCHLOROGENIC-ACID Fruit
NIACIN Fruit 6-61 ppm
OLEIC-ACID Fruit 170—1,245 ppm
PALMITIC-ACID Fruit 240—1,760 ppm
PANTOTHENIC-ACID Fruit 2.4—17.6 ppm
PHENYLALANINE Fruit 520—3,810 ppm
PHOSPHORUS Fruit 180—2,982 ppm
PHYTOSTEROLS Fruit 180—1320 ppm
POTASSIUM Fruit 2,824—22,565 ppm
PROLINE Fruit 1,010—7,400 ppm
PROTEIN Fruit 10,000—127,000 ppm
PUFA Fruit 770—5,640 ppm
QUERCITIN Fruit
QUERCITIN-3-DIGLUCOSIDE Fruit
QUINIC-ACID Fruit
RIBOFLAVIN Fruit 0.4—4.4 ppm
SERINE Fruit 830—6,080 ppm
SFA Fruit 270—1,980 ppm
SODIUM Fruit 10—88 ppm
STEARIC-ACID Fruit 30—220 ppm
SUCCINIC-ACID Fruit
SUCROSE Fruit 14,000—54,000 ppm
TANNIN Fruit 600—1,000 ppm
TARTARIC-ACID Fruit
TERPINOLENE Essential Oil
THIAMIN Fruit 0.3—2.5 ppm
THREONINE Fruit 470—3,445 ppm
TRANS-2-HEXENAL Essential Oil
TRANS-EPOXYDIHYDROLINALOOL Fruit
TRYPTOPHAN Fruit 150—1,100 ppm
TYROSINE Fruit 290—2,125 ppm

VALINE Fruit 470—3,445 ppm
VITAMIN B6 Fruit 0.5—4 ppm
WATER Fruit 963,500 ppm
XYLOSE Plant

■ BANANA

Chemical Constituents of Musa x paradisiaca
(Musaceae)

(24S-24-METHYL-25-
  DEHYDROCHOLESTEROL Fruit
24-METHYLCHOLESTEROL Fruit
24-METHYLENE-31-NOR-5ALPHA-
  CYCLOARTAN-3-ONE Fruit
24-METHYLENE-31-NOR-5ALPHA-
  LANOST-9(11)-3BETA-OL Fruit
24-METHYLENECHOLESTEROL Fruit
24-METHYLENECYCLOARTENOL Fruit
24-METHYLENEPOLLINASTANOL Fruit
31-NORCYCLOLAUDENOL Fruit
31-NORCYCLOLAUDENONE Fruit
6G-BETA-D-
  FRUCTOFURANOSYLSUCROSE Fruit
ACETIC-ACID Fruit
ALANINE Fruit 390—1,515 ppm
ALPHA-LINOLENIC-ACID Fruit 330—1,282
  ppm
ALUMINUM Fruit 1—35 ppm
ANHYDROGALACTURONIC-ACID Fruit
ARABINOSE Fruit
ARGININE Fruit 470—1,826 ppm
ARSENIC Fruit 0.04—0.35 ppm
ASCORBIC-ACID Fruit 88—367 ppm
ASH Fruit 7,100—31,900 ppm
ASH Shoot 11,710—158,300 ppm
ASPARTIC-ACID Fruit 1,130—4,390 ppm
BETA-CAROTENE Fruit 0.4—2.1 ppm
BORIC-ACID Fruit
BORON Fruit 1—17.7 ppm
BROMINE Fruit 0.3—27 ppm
CADMIUM Fruit
CALCIUM Fruit 40—460 ppm
CAPRIC-ACID Fruit 10—39 ppm

CARBOYDRATES Fruit 234,300—910,256
  ppm
CHOLESTEROL Fruit
CHROMIUM Fruit 0.02—0.15 ppm
CITRIC-ACID Fruit
COBALT Fruit
COPPER Fruit 1—7 ppm
CYANIDIN Inflorescence
CYCLOARTENOL Fruit
CYCLOEUCALENONE Fruit
CYCLOLAUDENOL Fruit
CYSTINE Fruit 170—660 ppm
DELPHINIDIN Inflorescence
DOPA Fruit
DOPAMINE Fruit
FAT Fruit 3,450—23,693 ppm
FIBER Fruit 5,000—19,425 ppm
FLUORINE Fruit 0.1—0.4 ppm
FOLACIN Fruit 0.2—0.9 ppm
FORMIC-ACID Fruit
FRUCTOSE Fruit 35,000 ppm
GADOLEIC-ACID Plant
GALACTOSE Fruit
GAMMA-GUANIDINOBUTYRIC-ACID Fruit
GLUCOSE Fruit 45,000 ppm
GLUTAMIC-ACID Fruit 1,110—4,312 ppm
GLYCINE Fruit 370—1,437 ppm
HISTIDINE Fruit 810—3,147 ppm
INDOLE-3-ACETIC-ACID Fruit
IRON Fruit 3—25 ppm
ISOFUCISTEROL Fruit
ISOLEUCINE Fruit 330—1,282 ppm
ISOVALERIANIC-ACID Plant
KAEMPFEROL Fruit
KILOCALORIES Fruit 920—3,574/kg
LAURIC-ACID Fruit 20—78 ppm
LEAD Fruit 20—0.2 ppm
LEUCINE Fruit 710—2,758 ppm
LINOLEIC-ACID Fruit 560—2,176 ppm
LYSINE Fruit 480—1,865 ppm
MAGNESIUM Fruit 277—1,465 ppm
MALIC-ACID Fruit 530—3,730 ppm
MALVIDIN Inflorescence
MANGANESE Fruit 1.4—18 ppm
MERCURY Fruit 0.001—0.007 ppm
METHIONINE Fruit 110—427 ppm

MOLYBDENUM Fruit
MUFA Fruit 410—1,593 ppm
MYRISTIC-ACID Fruit 30—117 ppm
NIACIN Fruit 5—23 ppm
NICKEL Fruit 0.01—0.1 ppm
NITROGEN Fruit 1,600—15,000 ppm
NOREPINEPHRINE Fruit
OBTUSIFOLIOL Fruit
OLEIC-ACID Fruit 270—1,049 ppm
PALMITIC-ACID Fruit 1,250—4,856 ppm
PALMITOLEIC-ACID Fruit 120—466 ppm
PANTOTHENIC-ACID Fruit 2.6—10.1 ppm
PELARGONIDIN Inflorescence
PETUNIDIN Inflorescence
PHENYLALANINE Fruit 200—1,190 ppm
PHYTOSTEROLS Fruit 160—622 ppm
POTASSIUM Fruit 3,100—16,150 ppm
PROLINE Fruit 400—1,554 ppm
PROTEIN Fruit 10,040—41,026 ppm
PUFA Fruit 890—3,458 ppm
QUERCETIN Fruit
RHAMNOSE Fruit
RIBOFLAVIN Fruit 1—3.9 ppm
RUBIDIUM Fruit 2.5—20 ppm
RUTIN Fruit
SELENIUM Fruit 0.001—0.04 ppm
SERINE Fruit 470—1,826 ppm
SEROTONIN Fruit
SFA Fruit 1,850—7,187 ppm
SILICON Fruit 70—350 ppm
SITOSATEROL Fruit
SODIUM Fruit 6—44 ppm
STEARIC-ACID Fruit 60—233 ppm
STIGMASTEROL Fruit
SUCROSE Fruit 119,000 ppm
SULFUR Fruit 78—500 ppm
TARTARIC-ACID Fruit
THIAMIN Fruit 0.45—1.7 ppm
THREONINE Fruit 340—1,321 ppm
TRYPTOPHAN Fruit 120—466 ppm
TYROSINE Fruit 240—932 ppm
VALINE Fruit 470—1,826 ppm
VITAMIN B6 Fruit 6—22.5 ppm
WATER Fruit 738,790—746,410 ppm
XYLOSE Fruit
ZINC Fruit 1.5—10 ppm

■ BITTER MELON

Chemical Constituents of Momordica charantia
L. (Cucurbitaceae)

5-HYDROXYTRYPTAMINE Fruit
ALKALOIDS Fruit 380 ppm
ASCORBIC-ACID Fruit 570—36,447 ppm
ASCORBIGEN Fruit
ASH Fruit 4,000—142,000 ppm
BETA-CAROTENE Fruit 18 ppm
BETA-SITOSTEROL Fruit
BETA-SITOSTEROL-D-GLUCOSIDE Fruit
CALCIUM Fruit 130—4,333 ppm
CARBOHYDRATES Fruit 47,000—763,000 ppm
CHARANTIN Fruit 1,500 ppm
CHOLESTEROL Fruit
CITRULLINE Fruit
COPPER Fruit 30 ppm
CRYPTOXANTHIN Fruit
DIOSGENIN Tissue Culture
ELASTEROL Plant
FIBER Fruit 10,000—257,800 ppm
FLAVOCHROME Fruit
FLUORIDE Fruit 0.2—0.5 ppm
FLUORINE Fruit 4.8 ppm
GABA Fruit
GALACTURONIC-ACID Fruit
IODINE Fruit 0.41 ppm
IRON Fruit 2—560 ppm
KILOCALORIES Fruit 190—3,290/kg
KILOCALORIES Fruit 440—3,020/kg
LANOSTEROL Fruit
LEAD Fruit 5 ppm
LUTEIN Fruit
LYCOPENE Fruit
MAGNESIUM Fruit 195—3,800 ppm
MANGANESE Fruit 10 ppm
MOMORDICIN Fruit
MOMORDICOSIDE-F-1 Fruit
MOMORDICOSIDE-F-2 Fruit
MOMORDICOSIDE-G Fruit
MOMORDICOSIDE-I Fruit
MUTACHROME Fruit
NIACIN Fruit 3—50 ppm

NICKEL Fruit 10 ppm
NITROGEN Fruit 33,800 ppm
OXALATE Fruit 185—1,444 ppm
OXALIC-ACID Fruit 5 ppm
PECTIN Fruit
PEROXIDASE Fruit
PHOSPHORUS Fruit 320—8,333 ppm
PIPECOLIC-ACID Fruit
POLYPEPTIDE-P Fruit
POTASSIUM Fruit 2,700—45,000 ppm
PROTEIN Fruit 9,000—181,000 ppm
RIBOFLAVIN Fruit 0.4—9 ppm
RUBIXANTHIN Fruit
SODIUM Fruit 20—333 ppm
STIGMASTA-5,25-DIEN-3-BETA-OL Plant
STIGMASTEROL Fruit
SUGARS Fruit 35,000—45,000 ppm
THIAMIN Fruit 0.2—12 ppm
TITANIUM Fruit 100 ppm
WATER Fruit 795,000—934,000 ppm
ZEAXANTHIN Fruit
ZEINOXANTHIN Fruit

■ BITTER ORANGE

Chemical Constituents of Citrus aurantium L.
(Rutaceae)

4-TERPINENOL Pericarp
6,7-DIMETHOXYCOUMARIN Fruit
AURANETIN Fruit
AURANTIAMARIN Fruit
BERGAPTEN Fruit
CALCIUM Fruit 3,710—4,230 ppm
CITRANTIN Fruit
CITRIC-ACID Fruit
COPPER Fruit 4—10 ppm
COUMARIN Fruit
DELTA-LIMONENE Fruit
DUODECYLALDEYDE Pericarp
EO Fruit 7,000—25,000 ppm
FORMIC-ACID Pericarp
GAMMA-TERPINENE Pericarp
HESPERIDIN Fruit 700—2,500 ppm
IRON Fruit 60—260 ppm

ISOHESPERIDIN Fruit
MANGANESE Fruit 8 ppm
NARINGIN Fruit
NEOHESPERIDIN Fruit
NOBILETIN Fruit
NONANOL Pericarp
NONYLALDEHYDE Pericarp
OCTALDEHYDE Pericarp
OCTANOL Pericarp
PELARGONALDEHYDE Pericarp
PELARGONIC-ACID Pericarp
PENTANOL Pericarp
PHELLANDRENE Pericarp
POTASSIUM Fruit 7,020—13,800 ppm
SABINENE Pericarp
SINENSETINE Pericarp
SODIUM Fruit 54—116 ppm
TANGERETIN Pericarp
TANNIN Fruit
TERPENYLACETATE Pericarp
TERPINOLENE Pericarp
VIOLAXANTHIN Pericarp
ZEAXANTHIN Fruit
ZINC Fruit 16 ppm

■ BLACKBERRY

Chemical Constituents of Rubus fruticosus
(Rasaceae)

BORON Fruit 0.1—21 ppm
CHLOROGENIC-ACID Fruit
FERULIC-ACID Fruit
NEOCHLOROGENIC-ACID Fruit

■ BLACK CHERRY

Chemical Constituents of Prunus serotina EHRH
(Rosaceae)

ACETYLCHOLINE Plant
CAFFEIC-ACID Plant
CYANIDIN Plant

■ BLACK CURRANT

Chemical Constituents of Ribes nigrum L. (Grossulariaceae)

(+)-CATECHIN Fruit 5,500—13,800 ppm
(+)-GALLOCATECHIN Fruit
1,8-CINEOLE Fruit
1-METHYL-4-ISOPROPYLBENZOL Plant
1-PENTEN-3-OL Fruit
2-BUTANOL Fruit
2-BUTANONE Fruit
2-HEXENAL Fruit
2-METHYL-3-BUTEN-2-OL Fruit
2-METHYL-PROPANOL
2-PENTANOL Fruit
3-METHYL-2-BUTEN-1-OL Fruit
3-METHYL-BUTANOL Fruit
ACETALDEHYDE Fruit
ACETIC-ACID Fruit
ACETONE Fruit
ALPHA-ALANINE Fruit Juice 210 ppm
ALPHA-LINOLENIC-ACID Fruit 720—3,988 ppm
ALPHA-PINENE Fruit
ALPHA-TERPINENE Fruit
ALPHA-TERPINEOL Fruit
ALPHA-TOCOPHEROL Fruit 22—120 ppm
ALUMINUM Fruit 3—65 ppm
ANTHOCYANINS Fruit 10,000—40,000 ppm
ANTHOCYANOSIDES Fruit 3,000 ppm
ARGININE Fruit Juice 35 ppm
ARSENIC Fruit 0.01—0.06 ppm
ASCORBIC-ACID Fruit 1,200—10,030 ppm
ASH Fruit 8,050—61,100 ppm
ASPARAGINE Fruit Juice 87 ppm
ASPARTIC-ACID Fruit Juice 23 ppm
BENZALDEHYDE Fruit
BETA-ALANINE Fruit Juice 12 ppm
BETA-CAROTENE Fruit 1—8 ppm
BETA-PHELLANDRENE Fruit
BETA-PINENE Fruit
BORON Fruit 1—64 ppm
BROMINE Fruit
BUTANOL Fruit
BUTYL-ACETATE Fruit

BUTYL-FORMIATE Fruit
BUTYRALDEHYDE Fruit
CADMIUM Fruit 0.001—0.01 ppm
CAFFEIC-ACID Fruit
CALCIUM Fruit 502—4,720 ppm
CALCIUM-PECTATE Fruit 9,000—17,000 ppm
CAMPHENE Fruit
CARBOHYDRATES Fruit 153,800—852,050 ppm
CARYOPHYLLENE Fruit
CHLOROGENIC-ACID Fruit
CHROMIUM Fruit 0.01—0.27 ppm
CINNAMIC-ACID Fruit
CIS-BETA-OCIMENE Fruit
CIS-HEX-3-EN-1-OL Plant
CITRIC-ACID Fruit 35,000 ppm
CITRONELLOL Fruit
CITRONELLYL-ACETATE Fruit
COBALT Fruit 0.002—0.027 ppm
COPPER Fruit 0.6—7 ppm
CYANIDIN Plant
CYANIDIN-3-DIGLUCOSIDE Fruit
CYANIDIN-3-GLUCOSIDE Fruit
CYANIDIN-3-RUTINOSIDE Fruit
CYANIDIN-MONOGLUCOSIDE Fruit
DACTYLIFRIC-ACID Fruit
DELPHINIDIN Plant
DELPHINIDIN-3-DIGLUCOSIDE Fruit
DELPHINIDIN-3-GLUCOSIDE Fruit
DELPHINIDIN-3-RUTINOSIDE Fruit
DELTA-3-CARENE Fruit
ETHANOL Fruit
ETHYL-ACETATE Fruit
ETHYL-BENZOATE Fruit
ETHYL-BUTYRATE Fruit
FAT Fruit 3,150—27,977 ppm
FERULIC-ACID Fruit
FIBER Fruit 24,000—133,000 ppm
FLUORINE Fruit 0.1—2.8 ppm
FORMALDEHYDE Fruit
FORMIC-ACID Fruit
FRUCTOSE Fruit 36,700 ppm
GAMMA-LINOLENIC-ACID Seed 47,500—57,950 ppm
GENTISIC-ACID Fruit

GERANIOL Fruit
GLUCOSE Fruit 23,500 ppm
GLUTAMIC-ACID Fruit Juice 210 ppm
GLYCOLLIC-ACID Fruit
HARDWICKIC-ACID Fruit
HEXANOL Fruit
HUMULENE Fruit
HUMULENE Leaf 4 ppm
INDOLEACETIC-ACID Seed
INVERT-SUGARS Fruit 60,000—80,000 ppm
IRON Fruit 11—108 ppm
ISO-AMYBUTYRATE Fruit
ISOLEUCINE Fruit Juice 28 ppm
ISOQUERCITRIN Fruit
KAEMPFEROL Fruit
LEAD Fruit 0.04—0.6 ppm
LEUCINE Fruit Juice 28 ppm
LIMONENE Fruit
LINOLEIC-ACID Fruit 1,070—5,928 ppm
LUTEIN Fruit 4.4—22 ppm
MAGNESIUM Fruit 220—1,720 ppm
MANGANESE Fruit 0.5—27 ppm
MERCURY Fruit 0—0.01 ppm
METHANOL Fruit
METHYL-BENZOATE Fruit
METHYL-BUTYRATE Fruit
METHYL-N-HEXENOATE Fruit
METHYL-SALICYLATE Fruit
METHYL-SALICYLATE Leaf
MOLYBDENUM Fruit 0.01—0.6 ppm
MYRCENE Fruit
MYRICETIN Fruit
NEOCHLOROGENIC-ACID Fruit
NIACIN Fruit 3—17 ppm
NICKEL Fruit 0.101 ppm
NITROGEN Fruit 1,800—12,775 ppm
NORVALINE Fruit Juice 17 ppm
O-COUMARIC-ACID Fruit
OCT-1-EN-3-OL Fruit
OLEIC-ACID Fruit 560—3,102 ppm
P-COUMARIC-ACID Fruit
P-CYMENE Fruit
P-CYMENOL-(4) Fruit
P-METHYLISOPROPENYLBENZOL Fruit
PALMITIC-ACID Fruit 200—1,108 ppm
PALMITOLEIC-ACID Fruit 70—388 ppm

PANTOTHENIC ACID Fruit 4—22 ppm
PECTIN Fruit
PECTINESTERASE Fruit
PENTANAL Fruit
PENTANOL Fruit
PHOSPHORUS Fruit
POTASSIUM Fruit 3,100—21,110 ppm
PROLINE Fruit Juice 98 ppm
PROPANOL Fruit
PROTEIN Fruit 12,000—88,640 ppm
PROTOCATECHUIC-ACID Fruit
QUERCETIN Fruit
QUERCETIN-3-GLUCOSDIE Fruit
QUERCETRIN Fruit
RIBOFLAVIN Fruit 1—3 ppm
RUBIDIUM Fruit 1—2 ppm
RUTIN Fruit
SELENIUM Fruit
SERINE Fruit Juice 60 ppm
SILICON Fruit 10—220 ppm
SODIUM Fruit 20—111 ppm
STEARIC-ACID Fruit 70—388 ppm
STYROL Fruit
SUCROSE Fruit 6,200 ppm
SUGARS Fruit 15,800—106,400 ppm
SULFUR Fruit 200—1,385 ppm
SYRINGIC-ACID Fruit
TERPINENE Fruit
TERPINENOL-(4) Fruit
TERPINOLENE Fruit
THIAMIN Fruit 1—3 ppm
THREONINE Fruit Juice 17 ppm
TRANS-BETA-OCIMENE Fruit
TRANS-CHLOROGENIC-ACID Fruit
TRANS-HEX-2-EN-1-OL Fruit
VALINE Fruit 170 ppm
VITAMIN B6 Fruit 1—4 ppm
WATER Fruit 815,220—824,000 ppm
ZINC Fruit 2—21 ppm

■ CANTALOUPE

Chemical Constituents of Cucumis melo L.
(Cucurbitaceae)

3,4-DIMETHOXY-ACETOPHENONE-ISOMER Petiole

3-PHENYL-PROPYL-ACETATE Petiole

ACETALDEHYDE Petiole

ADENOSINE Fruit

ALPHA-CAROTENE Fruit

ALPHA-TOCOPHEROL Fruit 1.4—14 ppm

ALUMINUM Fruit 26—77 ppm

ARACHIDIC-ACID Cotyledon 10,200—55,300 ppm

ARSENIC Fruit 0.004—0.006 ppm

ASCORBIC-ACID Fruit 397—4,370 ppm

ASH Fruit 6,950—110,000 ppm

BARIUM Fruit 1.3—7.7 ppm

BENZALDEHYDE Petiole

BENZYL-ACETATE Petiole

BENZYL-PROPIONATE Petiole

BETA-CAROTENE Fruit 0.2—201 ppm

BETA-CRYPTOXANTHIN Fruit

BETA-IONONE Petiole

BETA-PYRAZOL-1-YL-ALANINE Fruit

BORON Fruit 1—16.5 ppm

BUTYL-ACETATE Petiole

CADMIUM Fruit 0.017—0.044 ppm

CALCIUM Fruit 96—3,080 ppm

CARBOHYDRATES Fruit 83,600—818,026 ppm

CHROMIUM Fruit 0.13—0.165 ppm

CINNAMIC-ACETATE Petiole

CIS,CIS-3,6-NONADIEN-1-OL Fruit

CIS-3-NONEN-1-OL Fruit

CIS-6-NONEN-1-OL Fruit

CIS-6-NONENAL Fruit

CIS-CIS-NONA-3,6-DIENYL-ACETATE Petiole

CITRULLINE Fruit 142—241 ppm

COBALT Fruit 0.087—0.11 ppm

COPPER Fruit 0.4—7.7 ppm

CUCURBITACIN-B Fruit

CUCURBITACIN-E Fruit

EPSILON-CAROTENE Fruit

ETHANOL Petiole

ETHYL-(METHYLTHIO)-ACETATE Petiole

ETHYL-2-METHYL-BUTYRATER Petiole

ETHYL-ACETATE Petiole

ETHYL-DECANOATE Petiole

FAT Fruit 2,600—29,355 ppm

FIBER Fruit 3,180—39,357 ppm

FOLACIN Fruit 0.1—1.9 ppm

GAMMA-GLUTAMYL-BETA-PYRAZOL-1-YL-ALANINE Fruit

GLOBULIN Fruit 26,000 ppm

HEPTYL-ACETATE Petiole

HEXYL-ACETATE Petiole

HISTAMINE Juice

IRON Fruit 2—55 ppm

ISOBUTYL-ACETATE Petiole

ISOFRAXIDIN Plant

KILOCALORIES Fruit 350—3,425/kg

LEAD Fruit 1.74—2.2 ppm

LINOLEIC-ACID Cotyledon 56,100—726,700 ppm

LINOLENIC-ACID Cotyledon 200,500—219,000 ppm

LITHIUM Fruit 0.348—0.44 ppm

MAGNESIUM Fruit 92—3,300 ppm

MANGANESE Fruit 0.4—7.7 ppm

MERCURY Fruit 0.001—0.001 ppm

MOLYBDENUM Fruit 0.609—0.77 ppm

MYRISTIC-ACID Fruit 1,500—8,920 ppm

NIACIN Fruit 4.6—68 ppm

NICKEL Fruit 0.87—1.1 ppm

NONAN-1-OL Fruit

NONANAL Fruit

NONYL-ACETATE Petiole

OCTYL-ACETATE Petiole

OLEIC-ACID Cotyledon 40,500—195,300 ppm

PALMITIC-ACID Cotyledon 122,000—532,300 ppm

PANTOTHENIC-ACID Fruit 1.2—14 ppm

PHOSPHORUS Fruit 121—2,640 ppm

PHYSETOLIC-ACID Cotyledon

PHYTOSTEROLS Fruit 100—978 ppm

POTASSIUM Fruit 3,018—44,000 ppm

PROPYL-ACETATE Petiole

PROTEIN Fruit 8,410—89,924 ppm

RIBOFLAVIN Fruit 0.2—2.4 ppm

RUTIN Plant

SELENIUM Fruit 0.003—0.004 ppm

SILVER Fruit 0.087—0.11 ppm

SODIUM Fruit 66—1,115 ppm

STEARIC-ACID Cotyledon 10,100—61,400 ppm
STRONTIUM Fruit 2.6—16.5 ppm
SUGAR Fruit 20,000—30,000 ppm
SULFUR Fruit 139—198 ppm
THIAMIN Fruit 0.3—4.4 ppm
TITANIUM Fruit 0.435—2.2 ppm
TRANS,CIS-2,6-NONADIEN-1-OL Fruit
TRANS,CIS-2,6-NONADIENAL Fruit
TRANS-2-NONEN-1-OL Fruit
TRANS-2-NONENAL Fruit
VITAMIN B6 Fruit 1—13 ppm
WATER Fruit 896,000—938,000 ppm
ZINC Fruit 1.5—31 ppm
ZIRCONIUM Fruit 1.7—2.2 ppm

■ CAMU-CAMU OR RUMBERRY

Chemical Constituents of Myrciaria dubia (Myrtaceae)

ASCORBIC-ACID Fruit 20,890—499,000 ppm
ASH Fruit 2,000—33,335 ppm
BETA-CAROTENE Fruit
CALCIUM Fruit 270—4,500 ppm
CARBOHYDRATES Fruit 45,000—933,335 ppm
FIBER Fruit 5,000—100,000 ppm
IRON Fruit 5—85 ppm
KILOCALORIES Fruit 160—2,665/kg
NIACIN Fruit 6—100 ppm
PHOSPHORUS Fruit 150—2,835 ppm
PROTEIN Fruit 5,000—83,330 ppm
RIBOFLAVIN Fruit 0.4—6.7 ppm
THIAMIN Fruit 0.1—1.7 ppm
WATER Fruit 930,000—940,000 ppm

■ COCONUT

Chemical Constituents of Cocus nucifera L (Arecaceae)

1,3-DIPHENYLUREA Seed
ALPHA-TOCOPHEROL Oil 18 ppm

ALUMINUM Seed 7.2 ppm
ANTIMONY Seed 0.1 ppm
ARSENIC Seed 0.02 ppm
ASCORBIC-ACID Seed 20—88 ppm
ASH Seed 9,000—22,000 ppm
BARIUM Seed 0.1 ppm
BORON Seed 3—5.2 ppm
BROMINE Seed 4 ppm
CADMIUM Seed 0.03 ppm
CALCIUM Seed 71—476 ppm
CALCIUM-OXIDE Leaf 2,700 ppm
CAPRIC-ACID Seed 2,628—69,473
CAPROIC-ACID Seed 117—3,595 ppm
CAPRYLIC-ACID Seed 3,154—68,305
CARBOHYDRATES Seed 94,000—331,000 ppm
CESIUM Seed 0.1 ppm
CHLORINE Seed 1,007 ppm
CITRIC-ACID Seed
COBALT Seed 0.2 ppm
COPPER Seed 3.2—33 ppm
D-GALACTOSE Seed
D-GALACTURONIC-ACID Seed
EUROPIUM Seed 0.1 ppm
FAT Seed 58,400—719,000
FERULIC-ACID Leaf
FIBER Seed 30,000—115,000 ppm
FLUORINE Seed 2.7 ppm
FRUCTOSE Resin Exudate Sap 21,000 ppm
GABA Seed
GALACTOMANNAN Seed 16,000 ppm
GAMMA-TOCOPHEROL Oil
GLUCOSE Resin Exudate Sap 2,400 ppm
GOLD Plant
INOSITOL Resin Exudate Sap 690 ppm
IODINE Seed 0.3 ppm
IRON Seed 23—33 ppm
KILOCALORIES Seed 2,960—7,050/kg
L-RHAMNOSE Seed
LANTHANUM Seed 0.03 ppm
LAURIC-ACID Seed
LEAD Seed 0.7 ppm
LIGNIN Hull Husk 294,000 ppm
LINOLEIC-ACID Seed 584—18,694 ppm
LUTETIUM Seed 0.01 ppm
MAGNESIUM Seed 770 ppm

MALIC-ACID Seed
MANGANESE Seed 9—21 ppm
MANNAN Seed
MERCURY Seed 0.1 ppm
MESOINOSITOL Endosperm 100 ppm
MOLYBDENUM Seed 0.03 ppm
MYRISTIC-ACID Seed 7,650—133,015 ppm
NIACIN Seed 5—10 ppm
NICKEL Seed 2.1 ppm
OLEIC-ACID Seed 2,920—58,958 ppm
PALMITIC-ACID Seed 4,380—75,495 ppm
PECTIN Seed
PHOSPHORUS Seed 830—2,400 ppm
PHOSPHORUS-OXIDE (P205) Leaf 1,700 ppm
PHYTOSTEROLS Seed
POTASSIUM Seed 2,650—11,491 ppm
POTASSIUM-OXIDE (K20) Leaf 52,300 ppm
PROTEIN Seed 32,000—77,000 ppm
QUINIC-ACID Seed
RAFFINOSE Resin Exudate Sap 900 ppm
RIBOFLAVIN Seed 0.2—0.7 ppm
RUBIDIUM Seed 16 ppm
SAMARIUM Seed 0.04 ppm
SCANDIUM Seed 0.002 ppm
SCYLLITOL Endosperm 500 ppm
SELENIUM Seed 0.02 ppm
SHIKIMIC-ACID Seed
SILICON Seed 370 ppm
SODIUM Seed 145—626 ppm
SORBITOL Endosperm 15,000 ppm
SQUALENE Seed
STEARIC-ACID Seed 584—23,008 ppm
STRONTIUM Seed 2.8 ppm
SUCCINIC-ACID Seed
SUCROSE Resin Exudate Sap 134,000 ppm
SULFUR Seed 440—1,370 ppm
TANTALUM Plant
THIAMIN Seed 0.3—1 ppm
THRORIUM Plant
TIN Seed 1.5 ppm
TITANIUM Seed 5.6 ppm
TRIDECANOIC-ACID Seed
TUNGSTEN Seed 0.3 ppm
UNDECANOIC-ACID Seed
VANADIUM Seed 0.004 ppm
VITAMIN E Seed 2 ppm

WATER Seed 363,000—546,000 ppm
YTTERBIUM Seed 0.1 ppm
ZINC Seed 13—17 ppm

■ CRANBERRY

Chemical Constituents of Vaccinium macrocarpon (Ericaceae)

2-METHYL-BUTYRIC-ACID Fruit
ALPHA-TERPINEOL Fruit
ALPHA-TOCOPHEROL Fruit 9—81 ppm
ALUMINUM Fruit 2 —15 ppm
ANISALDEHYDE Fruit
ANTHOCYANODISES Fruit
ASCORBIC-ACID Fruit 75—1,003 ppm
ASH Fruit 1,800—17,000 ppm
BENZALDEHYDE Fruit
BENZOIC-ACID Fruit
BENZYL-ALCOHOL Fruit
BENZYL-BENZOATE Fruit
BETA-CAROTENE Fruit 0.2—2.6 ppm
BORON Fruit 1—8 ppm
CADMIUM Fruit 0.03—0.23 ppm
CALCIUM Fruit 70—1,157 ppm
CARBOHYDRATES Fruit 108,000—942,050 ppm
CATECHINS Fruit
CHLOROGENIC-ACID Fruit
CHROMIUM Fruit 0.01—0.08 ppm
COBALT Fruit
COPPER Fruit 0.5—4.7 ppm
CYANIDIN-3-ARABINOSIDE Fruit
CYANIDIN-3-GALACTOSIDE Fruit
CYANIDIN-3-GLUCOSIDE Fruit
EUGENOL Fruit
FAT Fruit 2,000—58,000 ppm
FIBER Fruit 12,000—116,000 ppm
FOLACIN Fruit 0.1—0.2 ppm
IRON Fruit 2—41 ppm
KILOCALORIES Fruit 490—3,800 ppm
LEAD Fruit 0.2—2 ppm
LUTEIN Fruit 0.28—2 ppm
MAGNESIUM Fruit 50—690 ppm
MALIC-ACID Fruit

MANGANESE Fruit 1.4—200 ppm
MERCURY Fruit 0.001—0.007 ppm
MOLYBDENUM Fruit 0.1—0.7 ppm
NIACIN Fruit 1—8.3 ppm
NICKEL Fruit 0.05—0.38 ppm
NITROGEN Fruit 650—5,000 ppm
OXALIC-ACID Fruit
OXYCOCCRIYANINE Fruit
PANTOTHENIC-ACID Fruit 2.2—16 ppm
PEONIDIN-3-ARABINOSIDE Fruit
PEONIDIN-3-GALACTOSIDE Fruit
PEONIDIN-3-GLUCOSIDE Fruit
PHOSPHORUS Fruit 90—1,075 ppm
POTASSIUM Fruit 250—6,777 ppm
PROTEIN Fruit 3,900—33,000 ppm
QUERCETIN Fruit 100—250 ppm
QUINIC-ACID Fruit
RIBOFLAVIN Fruit 0.2—1.7 ppm
RUBIDIUM Fruit 0.5—3.5 ppm
SELENIUM Fruit
SODIUM Fruit 10—165 ppm
SULFUR Fruit 65—500 ppm
THIAMIN Fruit 0.3—2.5 ppm
VITAMIN B6 Fruit 0.6—5.4 ppm
WATER Fruit 865,400—879,000 ppm
ZINC Fruit 1—19 ppm

■ FIG

Chemical Constituents of Ficus carica L. (Moraceae)

ACIDS Fruit 1,000—4,400 ppm
ALANINE Fruit 450—2,154 ppm
ALKALOIDS Fruit 500 ppm
APIGENIN-GLYCOSIDES Fruit
ARABINOSE Fruit
ARACHIDIC-ACID Seed 2,520—3,150 ppm
ARGININE Fruit 170—814 ppm
ABSCORBIC-ACID Fruit 20—2,013 ppm
ASH Fruit 5,000—57,000 ppm
ASPARTIC-ACID Fruit 1,760—3,447 ppm
BETA-CAROTENE Fruit 0.3—16 ppm
BORIC-ACID Fruit
BORON Fruit 1—100 ppm

CAFFEIC-ACID Plant
CALCIUM Fruit 350—4,228 ppm
CARBOHYDRATES Fruit 98,000—918,143 ppm
CEROTINIC-ACID Latex Exudate
CHLOROPHYLL-A Fruit
CHLOROPHYLL-B Fruit
CITRIC-ACID Fruit 1,000—4,400 ppm
COPPER Fruit 0.6—3.6 ppm
CYSTINE Fruit 120—574 ppm
FAT Fruit 2,000—24,000 ppm
FAT Seed 240,000—300,000 ppm
FERULIC-ACID Plant
FIBER Fruit 12,000—154,000 ppm
FRUCTOSE Fruit 22,950 ppm
FUMARIC-ACID Fruit
GLUCOSE Fruit 31,050 ppm
GLUTAMIC-ACID Fruit 720—3,447 ppm
GLYCINE Fruit 250—1,197 ppm
GLYCOSIDES Fruit 500 ppm
GUAIAZULENE Root
HEMICEULLOLOSE Fruit 11,200 ppm
HISTIDINE Fruit 110—527 ppm
INVERT-SUGAR Fruit 500,000—700,000 ppm
IRON Fruit 3—57 ppm
ISOLEUCINE Fruit 230—1,101 ppm
ISOSCHAFTOSIDE Fruit
KAEMPFEROL Plant
KILOCALORIES Fruit 420—3,600/kg
LEUCINE Fruit 330—1,580 ppm
LINOLEIC-ACID Fruit 1,440—6,893 ppm
LINOLEIC-ACID Seed 84,000—105,000 ppm
LINOLENIC-ACID Seed 115,200—144,000 ppm
LIPASE Latex Exudate
LUPEOL Leaf
LUTEIN Fruit
LYSINE Fruit 300—1,436 ppm
MAGNESIUM Fruit 158—872 ppm
MALIC-ACID Fruit 30,200 ppm
MALONIC-ACID Fruit
MANGANESE Fruit 1—7 ppm
METHIONINE Fruit 60—287 ppm
MUCILAGE Fruit 8,000 ppm
MUFA Fruit 660—3,159 ppm
MYRISTIC-ACID Fruit 20—96 ppm

NIACIN Fruit 3—32 ppm
OLEIC-ACID Fruit 660—3,159 ppm
OLEIC-ACID Seed 47,520—59,400 ppm
OXALIC-ACID Fruit
PALMITIC-ACID Fruit 460—2,202 ppm
PALMITIC-ACID Seed 12,552—15,690 ppm
PANTOTHENIC-ACID Fruit 3—14 ppm
PECTIN Fruit 18,000—50,000 ppm
PENTOSANS Fruit 8,300 ppm
PHENYLALANINE Fruit 180—862 ppm
PHOSPHORUS Fruit 129—2,764 ppm
PHYTOSTEROLS Fruit 310—1,484 ppm
POTASSIUM Fruit 1,770—11,662 ppm
PROLINE Fruit 490—2,346 ppm
PROTEASE Latex Exudate
PROTEIN Fruit 7,220—130,000 ppm
PUFA Fruit 1,440—6,893 ppm
PYRROLIDINE-CARBOXYLIC-ACID Fruit
QUERCETIN Plant
QUINIC-ACID Fruit
RIBOFLAVIN Fruit 0—5.7 ppm
SCHAFTOSIDE Fruit
SERINE Fruit 370—1,771 ppm
SFA Fruit 600—2,872 ppm
SODIUM Fruit 10—366 ppm
STEARIC-ACID Fruit 120—574 ppm
STEARIC-ACID Seed 5,232—6,540 ppm
SUCCINC-ACID Fruit
SUCROSE Fruit 2,250 ppm
THIAMIN Fruit 0—3.3 ppm
THREONINE Fruit 240—1,149 ppm
TRYPTOPHAN Fruit 60—287 ppm
TYROSINE Fruit 320—1,532 ppm
VALINE Fruit 280—1,340 ppm
VIOLAXANTHIN Fruit
VITAMIN B6 Fruit 1—5.4 ppm
WATER Fruit 775,000—877,000 ppm
ZINC Fruit 1—7 ppm

■ GRAPE

Chemical Constituents of Vitis vinifera L. (Vitaceae)

(-)-EPICATECHIN Fruit
(-)-EPICATECHIN-3-GALLATE Seed
(-)-GALLOCATECHIN Leaf
(DL)-GALLOCATECHIN Leaf
2,2,6-TRIMETHYL-8-(1-HYDRFOXY-
    ETHYL)-7-OXA-BICYCLO-(4,3,0)-NONA-
    4,9-DIENE Fruit
2,6-DIMETHYL-TRANS,TRANS-OCTA-2,6-
    DIEN-1,8-DIOL Fruit
2,6-DIMETHYL-TRANS-OCTA-2,7-DIEN-
    1,6-DIOL-6-O-ALPHA-D-
    ARABINOFURANOYL-BETA-D
    -BETA-D-GLUCOPYRANOSIDE Fruit
2,6-DIMETHYL-TRANS-OCTA-2,7-DIEN-
    1,6-DIOL-BETA-D-
    GLUCOPYRANDOSIDE Plant
2-METHOXY-3-ISOBUTYL-PYRAZINE Stem
2-PHENYLETHAN-1-OL Leaf
2-PHENYLETHAN-2-OL-6-BETA-D-
    APIOFURANOSYL-BETA-D-
    GLUCOSIDE Fruit
2-PHENYLETHYL-AMINE Fruit Juice
24-METHYL-CYCLOARTENOL Stem
3,7-DIMETHYL-OCT-1-ENE-3,6,7-TRIOL
    Fruit
3,7-DIMETHYL-OCT-1-ENE-3,7-DIOL Fruit
3,7-DIMETHYL-OCTA-1,5,7-TRIEN-3-OL
    Fruit
3,7-DIMETHYL-OCTA-1,5-DIEN-3,7-DIOL
    Fruit
3,7-DIMETHYL-OCTA-1,6-DIEN-3,5-DIOL
    Fruit
3,7-DIMETHYL-OCTA-1,7-DIEN-3,6-DIOL
    Fruit
3-HYDROXY-BETA-DAMASCONE   Fruit
    Juice
30-NOR-LUPAN-3-BETA-OL-20-ONE Root
9-HYDROXY-MEGASTIGM-4,6,7-TRIEN-3-
    ONE Fruit Juice
A-HEMICELLULOSE Fruit
ABSCISSIC-ACID Fruit

ACETIC-ACID Fruit 1,500—2,000 ppm
ACETIC-ACID Leaf
ACUMINOSIDE Fruit Juice
ALANINE Fruit 280—1,440 ppm
ALPHA-3-OXO-DAMASCONE Fruit Juice
ALPHA-3-OXO-IONONE Fruit Juice
ALPHA-AMYL-AMINE Fruit Juice
ALPHA-AMYRIN Stem
ALPHA-CAROTENE Fruit
ALPHA-HYDROXY-CAROTENE Fruit
ALPHA-LINOLENIC-ACID Fruit 390—2,006 ppm
ALPHA-TERPINEOL Leaf Essential Oil 108,000 ppm
ALPHA-TOCOPHEROL Fruit 6—31 ppm
ALPHA-VINIFERIN Leaf 23,400 ppm
ALUMINUM Fruit 1—154 ppm
ALUMINUM Stem 1,030 ppm
ANTHERAXANTHIN Fruit
ANTHOCYANINS Fruit
ARGININE Fruit 490—2,520 ppm
ARSENIC Fruit 0.001—0.889 ppm
ASCORBIC-ACID Fruit 99—600 ppm
ASCORBIC-ACID Leaf 3,490—3,870 ppm
ASCORBIC-ACID Stem 310 ppm
ASCORBIC-ACID-OXIDASE Fruit
ASH Fruit 4,290—77,000 ppm
ASH Stem 88,000 ppm
ASPARTIC-ACID Fruit 810—4,167 ppm
B-HEMICELLULOSE Fruit
BARIUM Fruit 0.66—15.4 ppm
BENZOIC-ACID Fruit
BENZYL-6-0-BETA-D-APIOFURANOSYL-BETA-D-GLUCOSIDE Fruit Juice
BENZYL-ALCOHOL Leaf
BEYZYL-ALCOHOL-6-O-L-ARABINOFURANOSYL-BETA-D-GLUCOPYRANOSIDE Leaf
BENZYL-ALCOHOL-BETA-D-GLUCOSIDE Leaf
BENZYL-ALCOHOL-BETA-D-RUTINOSIDE Leaf
BETA-AMYRIN Stem
BETA-CAROTENE Fruit 0.5—2.1 ppm
BETA-CAROTENE Stem 43 ppm
BETA-IONONE Fruit

BETA-PHENYLETHATNOL-6-BETA-D-ARABINOFURANOSYL-BETA-D-GLUCOPYRANOSIDE Fruit Juice
BETA-PHENYLETHANOL-BETA-D-GLUCOSIDE Fruit Juice
BETA-PHENYLETHANOL-BETA-D-RUTINOSIDE Fruit Juice
BETA-SITOSTEROL Fruit
BETAIN Fruit Juice
BETULINIC-ACID Fruit
BIOTIN Fruit
BORON Fruit 1—50 ppm
BREVILAGIN-I Leaf 533 ppm
BROMINE Fruit
CADMIUM Fruit 0.001—0.231 ppm
CAFFEIC-ACID Fruit
CAFFEOYL-TARTRATE Fruit
CAFFEYLTARTARIC-ACID Fruit
CALCIUM Fruit 92—4,774 ppm
CALCIUM Stem 17,700 ppm
CALCIUM-PECTATE Leaf 69,000 ppm
CARBOHYDRATES Fruit 177,700—914,095 ppm
CATALASE Fruit
CATECHOL-OXIDASE Fruit
CHLOROGENIC-ACID Fruit
CHOLESTEROL Fruit
CHROMIUM Fruit 0.005—0.385 ppm
CHROMIUM Stem 9 ppm
CINNAMIC-ACID Fruit
CIS-CAFFEIC-ACID Fruit
CITRIC-ACID Fruit
CITRIC-ACID Leaf
CITRONELLOL Leaf
CITROSTADIENOL Stem
COBALT Fruit 0.005—0.22 ppm
COBALT Stem 33 ppm
COPPER Fruit 0.7—11.6 ppm
COUMARIN Fruit
CRYPTOCHLOROGENIC-ACID Fruit
CRYPTOXANTHIN Fruit
CYANIDIN Fruit
CYANIDIN-3-GALACTOSIDE Fruit
CYANIDIN-3-GLUCOSIDE Fruit
CYCLOARTENOL Stem
CYSTINE Fruit 110—566 ppm

D-CATECHIN Fruit
D-CATECHIN Leaf
DAMASCENONE Fruit Juice
DELPHINIDIN Plant
DELPHINIDIN-3,5-DIGLUCOSIDE Fruit
DELPHINIDIN-3-(6-P-COUMAROGYLGLUCOSIDE) Fruit
DELPHINIDIN-3-(P-COUMAROYLGLUCOSIDE)-5-GLUCOSIDE Fruit
DELPHINIDIN-3-BETA-D-GLUCOSIDE Fruit
DELPHINIDIN-3-CAFFEOYLGLUCOSIDE Fruit
DIETHYL-AMINE Fruit Juice
DIHYDROFURAN-I Fruit Juice
DIHYDROPHASEIC-ACID-4'-BETA-D-GLUCOSIDE Fruit
DIMETHYL-AMINE Fruit Juice
ELEMOL-ACETATE Leaf Essential Oil 130.2 ppm
ELLAGIC-ACID Fruit
ENOMELANIN Fruit
ENOTANNIN Seed
EPICATECHIN-3-GALLATE Fruit
EPSIOLON-VINIFERIN Leaf 30,900 ppm
ERGOSTEROL Fruit
ETHYL-AMINE Fruit Juice
FAT Fruit 5,010—33,898 ppm
FAT Seed 60,000—200,000 ppm
FERULIC-ACID Fruit
FIBER Fruit 4,210—24,640 ppm
FLAVONOIDS Leaf 40,000—50,000 ppm
FLUORINE Fruit 0.1—0.6 ppm
FOLACIN Fruit 0.03—0.23 ppm
FORMIC-ACID Fruit
FR Fruit
FRUCTOSE Fruit
FUMARIC-ACID Leaf
GABA Fruit
GALACTOSE Fruit
GALACTURONIC-ACID Fruit
GALLIC-ACID Fruit
GAMMA-CAROTENE Fruit
GENTISIC-ACID Hull Husk
GERANIOL Fruit
GERANIOL Leaf Essential Oil 145,200 ppm

GERANIAL-6-O-ALPHA-L-ARABINOFURANOSYL-BETA-D-GLUCOPYRANOSIDE Fruit
GERANIOL-6-O-ALPHA-L-RHAMNOPYRANOSYL-BETA-D-GLUCOPYRANODISE Fruit
GERANIOL-BETA-D-GLUCOSIDE Fruit Juice
GERMANICOL Stem
GLUCOSE Fruit
GLUCOSE-6-PHOSPHATE-DEHYDROGENASE Fruit
GLUTAMIC-ACID Fruit 1,380—7,099 ppm
GLYCERIC-ACID Leaf
GLYCINE Fruit 200—1,029 ppm
HENTRIACONTAINE Fruit
HEPTACOSAN-1-OL Root
HEXOKINASE Fruit
HIRSUTRIN Leaf
HISTIDINE Fruit 240—1,235 ppm
HYDROXY-CITRONELLOL Essential Oil
INOSITOL Leaf
IRON Fruit 1.5—154 ppm
IRON Stem 900 ppm
ISOAMYL-AMINE Fruit Juice
ISOBUTYL-AMINE Fruit Juice
ISOCHLOROGENIC-ACID Fruit
ISOLEUCINE Fruit 50—257 ppm
ISOQUERCETRIN Leaf
ISOVITILAGIN Leaf 163 ppm
JU Plant
KAEMPFEROL Leaf
KAEMPFEROL-3-MONOGLUCOSIDE Fruit
LACTIC-ACID Fruit
LEAD Fruit 0.02—9 ppm
LEUCINE Fruit 140—720 ppm
LEUCOANTHOCYANIDOLE Fruit
LEUCOYANIDIN Plant
LIMONENE Plant
LINALOOL Fruit
LINALOOL Leaf Essential Oil 273,000 ppm
LINALOOL-6-0-ALPHA-L-ARABINOFURANOSYL-BETA-D-GLUCOPYRANOSIDE Fruit
LINALOOL-6-0-ALPHA-L-RHAMNOPYRANOSYL-BETA-D-GLUCOPYRANOSIDE Fruit

LINALOOL-6-0-BETA-D-APIOFURANOSYL-BETA-D-GLUCOSIDE Fruit Juice
LINALOOL-BETA-D-GLUCOSIDE Fruit Juice
LINOLEIC-ACID Fruit 1,300—6,687 ppm
LINOLEIC-ACID Seed 33,000—110,000 ppm
LITHIUM Fruit 0.088—0.308 ppm
LUPEOL Leaf
LUTEIN Fruit 0.7—7 ppm
LUTEIN-5-6-EPOXIDE Fruit
LUTEIN-5-8-EPOXIDE Fruit
LUTEOLIN Leaf
LUTEOXANTHIN Fruit
LYCOPENE Fruit
LYSINE Fruit 150—772 ppm
MAGNESIUM Fruit 58—2,310 ppm
MAGNESIUM Stem 4,360 ppm
MALIC-ACID Fruit 1,500—2,000 ppm
MALIC-ACID Plant
MALVIDIN Fruit
MALVIDIN-3-(6-P-COUMARYOYLGLUCOSIDE)-5-GLUCOSIDE Fruit
MALVIDIN-3-(P-COUMAROYLGLUCOSIDE) Fruit
MALVIDIN-3-CAFFEYLGLUCOSIDE Fruit
MALVIDIN-3-CHLOROGENIC-ACID-GLUCOSIDE Fruit
MALVIDIN-3-GLUCOSIDE Fruit
MALVIDIN-3-O-BETA-D-GLUCOSIDE Fruit
MANGANESE Fruit 0.5—54 ppm
MANGANESE Stem 986 ppm
MEGASTIGM-5-EN-7-YNE-3,9-DIOL Fruit Juice
MELIBIOSE Fruit
MERCURY Fruit 0—0.011 ppm
METHIONINE Fruit 220—1,132 ppm
MOLYBDENUM Fruit 0.1—0.539 ppm
MONO-P-COUMARYL-ACID Fruit
MONO-P-COUMARYL-ACID Leaf
MONOCAFFEIC-ACID Fruit
MONOCAFFEIC-ACID Leaf
MONOFERULYLSUCCINIC-ACID Leaf
MUFA Fruit 230—1,183 ppm
MUTATOXANTHIN Fruit
MYRICETIN Fruit

MYRICETIN-3-MONOGLUCOSIDE Fruit
MYRISTIC-ACID Fruit 50—257 ppm
N-PROPYL-AMINE Fruit Juice
NEOCHLOROGENIC-ACID Fruit
NEOXANTHIN Fruit
NEROL Leaf
NEROL-6-0-ALPHA-L-ARABINOFURANOSYL-BETA-D-GLUCOPYRANOSIDE Fruit
NEROL-6-0-ALPHA-L-RHAMNOPYRANOSYL-BETA-D-GLUCOPYRANOSIDE Fruit
NEROL-6-0-BETA-D-APIOFURANOSYL-BETA-D-GLUCOSIDE Fruit Juice
NEROL-BETA-D-GLUCOSIDE Fruit Juice
NIACIN Fruit 3—15.4 ppm
NIACIN Stem
NICKEL Fruit 0.01—0.77 ppm
NITROGEN Fruit 1,100—7,220 ppm
NONACOSANE Fruit
O-HYDROXYBENZOIC-ACID Hull Husk
OBTUSIFOLIOL Stem
OCTAN-1-OL Stem
OENIN Petiole
OLEANOLIC-ACID Leaf Wax
OLEANOLIC-ACID-METHYL-ESTER Leaf
OLEANOLIC-ALDEHYDE Stem
OLEIC-ACID Plant 230—1,183 ppm
OLEIC-ACID Seed 22,200—74,000 ppm
OXALIC-ACID Fruit 34 ppm
P-COUMARIC-ACID Fruit
P-COUMAROYL-CIS-TARTRATE Fruit
P-COUMAROYL-TRANS-TARTRATE Fruit
P-HYDROXYBENZOIC-ACID Hull Husk
PAEONIDIN Fruit
PAEONIDIN-3-(6-P-COUMAROYLGLUCOSIDE) Fruit
PAEONIDIN-3-5,-DIGLUCOSIDE Fruit
PAEONIDIN-3-CAFFEOYLGLUCOSIDE Fruit
PAEONIDIN-3-O-BETA-D-GLUCOSIDE Fruit
PALMITIC-ACID Fruit 1,620—8,333 ppm
PALMITIC-ACID Seed 3,300—11,000 ppm
PANTOTHENIC-ACID Fruit 0.2—1.3 ppm
PECTIN Fruit 300—3,900 ppm

PECTIN-METHYL-ESTERASE Fruit
PELARGONIDIN Fruit
PEROXIDASE Fruit
PETUNIDIN-3,5-DIGLUCOSIDE Fruit
PETUNIDIN-3-(6-P-
  COUMAROYLGLUCOSIDE) Fruit
PETUNIDIN-3-CAFFEOYLGLUCOSIDE
  Plant
PETUNIDIN-3-GLUCOSIDE Fruit
PETUNIDIN-3-O-BETA-D-GLUCOSIDE Fruit
PHENYLALANINE Fruit 140—720 ppm
PHOSPHORUS Fruit 117—1,848 ppm
PHOSPHORUS Stem 1,710 ppm
PHYTOENE Fruit
PHYTOFLUENE Fruit
PHYTOSTEROLS Fruit 40—206 ppm
POLYPHENOL-OXIDE Fruit
POTASSIUM Fruit 1,784—24,640 ppm
POTASSIUM Stem 20,100 ppm
PROCYANIDIN-B-2-3'-O-GALLATE Fruit
PROCYANIDINS Fruit
PROLINE Fruit 220—1,132 ppm
PROTEIN Fruit 6,350—35,236 ppm
PROTEIN Seed 70,000—100,000 ppm
PROTEIN Stem 89,000 ppm
PROTOPECTINASE Fruit
PTEROSTILBENE Leaf
PUFA Fruit 1,690—8,693 ppm
PYROPHOSPHATASE-NUCLEOTIDE Root
PYRROLIDINE Fruit Juice
QUERCETIN Fruit
QUERCETIN-GLUCURONOSIDE Fruit
QUERCITRIN Leaf
QUINIC-ACID Fruit
QUINIC-ACID Leaf
RAFFINOSE Fruit
RESVERATROL Leaf 90,400 ppm
RIBOFLAVIN Plant 0.5—3.2 ppm
RIBOFLAVIN Stem 6.9 ppm
ROSEOSIDE Fruit
RUBIDIUM Fruit 0.4—5.5 ppm
RUTIN Leaf
SALICYLIC-ACID Root
SELENIUM Fruit 0—0.012 ppm
SELENIUM Stem
SERINE Fruit 320—1,646 ppm

SFA Fruit 1,890—9,722 ppm
SHIKIMIC-ACID Leaf
SILICON Fruit 1—28 ppm
SILICON Stem 365 ppm
SILVER Fruit 0.022—0.077 ppm
SINAPIC-ACID Root
SODIUM Fruit 2—454 ppm
SODIUM Stem 156 ppm
SQUALENE Seed
STACHYOSE Fruit
STEARIC-ACID Seed 1,440—4,800 ppm
STIGMASTEROL Plant
STRONTIUM Fruit 1.54—38.5 ppm
SUCCINDEHYDROGENASE Fruit
SUCCINIC-ACID Fruit
SUGAR Fruit 30,000—189,000 ppm
SULFUR Fruit 7—888 ppm
SYRINGIC-ACID Hull Husk
TANNIN Seed
TARAXASTEROL Leaf
TARAXEROL Leaf
TARTARIC-ACID Fruit 15—20 ppm
TARTARIC-ACID-CAFFEOYL-ESTER Fruit
  15—20 ppm
THIAMIN Fruit 0.8—4.9 ppm
THIAMIN Stem 11 ppm
THREONINE Fruit 180—926 ppm
TIN Stem 12 ppm
TITANIUM Fruit 0.11—7.7 ppm
TRANS-CAFFEIC-ACID Fruit
TRIACONTAN-1-OL Root
TRIACONTAN-1-OL-TRIDECANOATE Root
TRYPTOPHAN Fruit 30—154 ppm
TYROSINE Fruit 120—617 ppm
URSOLIC-ALDEHYDE Stem
VALINE Fruit 180—926 ppm
VANILLIC-ACID Hull Husk
VIOLAXANTHIN Fruit
VITAMIN B6 Fruit 1—6 ppm
VITILAGIN Leaf 89 ppm
VITISPIRANE Plant
VOMIFOLIOL Fruit
WATER Fruit 761,000—897,000 ppm
WATER Stem 792,000 ppm
XYLOSE Fruit
ZEAXANTHIN Fruit

ZINC Fruit 0.4—27 ppm
ZINC Stem 75 ppm
ZIRCONIUM Fruit 0.44—1.54 ppm

■ GRAPEFRUIT

Chemical Constituents of Citrus paradisi (Rutaceae)

(+)-6-ISO-PROPENYL-4,8-ALPHA-DIMETHYL-4-ALPHA-(R)-5,6-(R)-7,8,8-ALPHA(R)-HEXAHYDRO-2-(1H)NAPTHALENONE Fruit
(+)-8,9-DIDEHYDRO-ALPHA-VETIVONE Fruit
(+)-8,9-DIDEHYDRO-NOOTKATONE Fruit
(+)-ALPHA-CYPERONE Fruit
(+)-ALPHA-VETIVONE Fruit
(-)-10-EPI-ALPHA-CYPERONE Fruit
1,10-DIHYDRO-ALPHA-VETIVONE Fruit
24-METHYLENE-CYCLOARTENOL Pericarp
24-METHYLENE-LOPHENOL Pericarp
3',4',5,6,7,8-HEXAMETHOXYFLAVONE Pericarp
3-HYDROXY-ETHYL-HEXANOATE Fruit
4',5,6,7,8-PENTAMETHOXY-FLAVONE Pericarp
4',5,6,7-TETRAHYDROXY-FLAVONE-8-O-BETA-D-GLUCOSIDE Fruit
4',5,7-TRIHYDROXY-FLAVONE-6-C-GLUCOSIDE Fruit
4',5-DIHYDROXY-FLAVONE-7-O-BETA-D-RHAMNOSYL-GLUCOSIDE Fruit
5-(3,7-DIMETHYL-6-EPOXY-2-OCTENYL)-OXYPSORALEN Pericarp
5-(6,7-DIHYDROXY-3,7-DIMETHYL-2-OCTENYL)-OXYPSORALEN Pericarp
5-HYDROXY-4'-METHOXY-FLAVANONE-7-O-BETA-D-RHAMNOSYL-GLUCOSIDE Fruit
7-(3,7-DIMETHYL-6-EPOXY-OCT-TRANS-2-ENYL)-OXYCOUMARIN Pericarp
7-GERANYL-OXYCOUMARIN Pericarp
7-METHOXY-8(2,3-DIHYDROXY-ISOPENTYL)-COUMARIN Pericarp
7-METHOXY-8(2,3-EPOXY-ISOPENTENYL)-COUMARIN Pericarp
7-OBACUNOL Seed 8—9 ppm
ACETIC-ACID Fruit
AESCULETIN Fruit
ALANINE Fruit 90 ppm
ALPHA-AMINO-BUTYRIC-ACID Fruit 190 ppm
ALPHA-CAROTENE Fruit
ALPHA-CYTOXANTHIN Fruit
ALPHA-LINOLENIC-ACID Fruit 50—550 ppm
ALPHA-PINENE Fruit
ALPHA-TOCOPHEROL Fruit 3—29 ppm
ALUMINUM Fruit 1—330 ppm
APIGENIN-7-O-BETA-D-RUTINOSIDE Leaf 5 ppm
ARABAN Fruit
ARGININE Fruit 470—760 ppm
ARSENIC Fruit 0.001—4.4 ppm
ASCORBIC-ACID Fruit 337—3,862 ppm
ASH Fruit 3,050—53,000 ppm
ASPARAGINE Fruit 420 ppm
ASPARTIC-ACID Fruit 810—4,700 ppm
BARIUM Fruit 0.44—22 ppm
BERGAMOTTIN Pericarp
BERGAPTOL Fruit
BETA-CAROTENE Fruit 0—5 ppm
BETA-SITOSTEROL Fruit
BORON Fruit 1—33 ppm
BROMINE Fruit
CADMIUM Fruit 0.002—0.066 ppm
CAFFEIC-ACID Fruit 40—51 ppm
CAFFEINE Flower 29 ppm
CALCIUM Fruit 117—4,270 ppm
CAMPESTEROL Fruit
CARBOHYDRATES Fruit 80,800—948,000 ppm
CARYOPHYLLENE Fruit
CATECHOL Plant
CHALCONASE Fruit
CHLORINE Plant 6 ppm
CHOLESTEROL Fruit
CHROMIUM Fruit 0.002—0.55 ppm
CIS-LINALOOL-OXIDE Fruit
CITRAL Fruit

CITRIC-ACID Fruit 11,900—21,000 ppm
CITROSTADIENOL Pericarp
COBALT Fruit 0.005—0.22 ppm
CONIFERIN Pericarp
COPPER Fruit 0—7.7 ppm
CRYPTOXANTHIN Fruit 0.03—0.3 ppm
CYCLOARTENOL Pericarp
CYSTINE Fruit 2 ppm
D-LIMONENE Plant 9,000 ppm
DEACETYL-NOMILIN Seed
DEACETYL-NOMILINIC-ACID-17-O-BETA-
    D-GLUCOSIDE Seed
DECYL-ALDEHYDE Fruit
DECYLIC-ACID Fruit
DEOXY-LIMONOL Seed 8 ppm
DIHYDROKAEMPFEROL Fruit
EO Fruit 6,000—10,000 ppm
EPI-ISO-OBACUNOIC-ACID-17-O-BETA-D-
    GLUCOSIDE Seed
ERIODICTYOL Fruit
FAT Fruit 1,000—19,000 ppm
FERULIC-ACID Fruit 30—34 ppm
FIBER Fruit 2,000—44,000 ppm
FLUORINE Fruit 0.03—0.9 ppm
FRIEDELIN Pericarp
GALACTURONIC-ACID Fruit
GAMMA-CAROTENE Fruit
GERANIAL Fruit 420—700 ppm
GERANYL-ACETATE Fruit
GLUCOSE Fruit 19,500 ppm
GLUTAMIC-ACID Fruit 220—2,800 ppm
GLYCINE Fruit
HEPTULOSE Pericarp
HESPERETIN Fruit
HESPEREDIN Fruit
HISTIDINE Fruit 140 ppm
HORDENENE Fruit
HUMULENE Fruit
IRON Fruit 1—88 ppm
ISO-OBACUNOIC-ACID-17-O-BETA-D-
    GLUCOSIDE Seed
ISOMERANZIN Pericarp
ISORHAMNETIN Fruit
ISOSAKURANETIN Fruit
KAEMPFEROL Fruit
KILOCALORIES Fruit 1,724/kg

LEAD Fruit 0.02—7.7 ppm
LEUCINES Fruit 240 ppm
LIMONIN Fruit
LIMONOATE-A-RING-LACTONE Fruit
LIMONOL Seed 23 ppm
LINALOOL Fruit
LINALYL-ACETATE Fruit
LINOLEIC-ACID Fruit 190—2,090 ppm
LITHIUM Fruit 0.088—2.31 ppm
LUTEIN Fruit 0.095—0.95 ppm
LYCOPENE Fruit
LYSINE Fruit 160—1,760 ppm
MAGNESIUM Fruit 15—1,360 ppm
MALIC-ACID Fruit 400—600 ppm
MALONIC-ACID Fruit
MANGANESE Fruit 0—5 ppm
MANNOSE Fruit
MERANZIN Pericarp
MERANZIN-HYDRATE Pericarp
MERCURY Fruit 0—0.001 ppm
METHIONINE Fruit 3—222 ppm
METHYL-ANTHRALINATE Fruit
MOLYBDENUM Fruit 0.1—0.77 ppm
MYRCENE Fruit 72—190 ppm
N-DODECASANE Fruit
N-DORIACONTANE Fruit
N-EICOSANE Fruit
N-HENEICOSANE Fruit
N-HENTRIACONTANE Fruit
N-HEPTACOSANE Fruit
N-HEXACOSANE Fruit
N-METHYL-TYRAMINE Fruit
N-NONACOSANE Fruit
N-NONYL-ALCOHOL Fruit
N-OCTACOSANE Fruit
N-OCTYL-ACETATE Fruit
N-OCTYL-ALCOHOL Fruit
N-PENTACOSANE Fruit
N-PENTATRIACONTANE Pericarp
N-TETRACOSANE Fruit
N-TETRATRIANCONTANE Pericarp
N-TRIACONTANE Fruit
NARINGENIN Fruit
NARINGENIN-7-BETA-(4-BETA-D-
    GLUCOSYL)-NEOHESPERIDOSIDE Fruit

NARINGENIN-7-BETA-(4-BETA-D-
GLUCOSYL)-RUTINOSIDE Fruit
NARINGENIN-7-O-BETA-D-RUTINOSIDE
Fruit
NARINGENIN-RUTINOSIDE Fruit
NARINGIN Fruit 245 ppm
NARINGIN Pericarp 4,500—14,000 ppm
NARINGIN Seed 200 ppm
NARINGIN-4-BETA-D-GLUCOSIDE Plant
NARIRUTIN Fruit
NEOHESPERIDIN Fruit
NERAL Fruit 136—210 ppm
NEUROSPORENE Fruit
NIACIN Fruit 2—44 ppm
NICKEL Fruit 0.04—7.7 ppm
NITROGEN Fruit 990—16,360 ppm
NOMILIN Seed
NOMILINIC-ACID Plant
NOMILINIC-ACID-17-O-BETA-D-
GLUCOSIDE Seed
OBACUNONE Seed
OCTYL-ALDEHYDE Fruit
OCTYLIC-ACID Fruit
OLEIC-ACID Fruit 120—1,320 ppm
OXALIC-ACID Plant
P-COUMARIC-ACID Fruit 0—53 ppm
P-MENTH-1-ENE-8-THIOL Fruit
PALMITIC-ACID Fruit 120—1,320 ppm
PALMITOLEIC-ACID Fruit 10—110 ppm
PANTOTHENIC-ACID Plant 3—31 ppm
PARADISOL Fruit
PECTIN Fruit
PENTAN-1-OL Fruit
PHENYLALANINE Fruit
PHLORIN Plant
PHLOROGLUCINOL Fruit
PHOSPHORUS Fruit 76—2,545 ppm
PHYTOENE Fruit
POLYGALACTURONIC-ACID Fruit
PONCIRIN Fruit
POTASSIUM Fruit 1,300—16,360 ppm
PROLINE Fruit 590 ppm
PROTEIN Fruit 6,000—70,290 ppm
PSI-CAROTENE Plant
QUERCETIN Fruit
QUINIC-ACID Fruit

RHOIFOLIN Leaf
RIBOFLAVIN Fruit 0—5 ppm
RUBIDIUM Fruit 0.26 ppm—22 ppm
SALICYLATES Fruit 0—70 ppm
SCOPOLETIN Fruit
SELENIUM Fruit 0—0.027 ppm
SERINE Fruit 150—3,100 ppm
SILICON Fruit
SILVER Fruit 0.022—0.11 ppm
SINAPIC-ACID Fruit 4—5 ppm
SODIUM Fruit 0—175 ppm
STEARIC-ACID Fruit 10—110 ppm
STIGMASTEROL Fruit
STRONTIUM Fruit 3.3—220 ppm
SUBAPHYLLIN Fruit
SUCROSE Fruit 21,400 ppm
SUGARS Fruit 33,000—99,600 ppm
SULFUR Fruit 7—2,090 ppm
SYNEPHERINE Fruit
THIAMIN Fruit 0—6 ppm
THREONINE Fruit 100 ppm
TIN Fruit 0.66—3.3 ppm
TITANIUM Fruit 0.11—7.7 ppm
TRANS-OBACUNOIC-ACID-17-O-BETA-D-
GLUCOSIDE Seed
TRYPTOPHAN Fruit 20—220 ppm
TYRAMINE Fruit
TYROSINE Fruit 61 ppm
UMBELLIFERONE Fruit
URONIC-ACID Fruit
VALINE Fruit 240 ppm
WATER Fruit 847,000—930,000 ppm
XANTHYLETINE Fruit
XYLAN Fruit
XYLOSE Fruit
ZETA-CAROTENE Fruit
ZINC Fruit 0—9 ppm
ZIRCONIUM Fruit 0.44—2.2 ppm

■ GUAVA

Chemical Constituents of Psidium guajava L. (Myrtaceae)

ACETONE Fruit
ALANINE Fruit 410—2,952 ppm
ALPHA-HUMULENE Fruit
ALPHA-LINOLENIC-ACID Fruit 710—5,112 ppm
ALPHA-SELINENE Fruit
ARABAN Fruit
ARABINOSE Fruit
ARABINOSE-HEXAHYDROXYDIPHENYL-ACID-ESTER Fruit 1,000 ppm
ARGININE Fruit 210—1,512 ppm
ASCORBIC-ACID Fruit 200—14,300 ppm
ASCORBIGEN Fruit 253—2,145 ppm
ASH Fruit 6,000—43,200 ppm
ASH Seed 30,000 ppm
ASPARTICA-ACID Fruit 520—3,744 ppm
BENZALDEHYDE Fruit
BENZENE Fruit
BETA-BISABOLENE Fruit
BETA-CAROTENE Fruit 3—46 ppm
BETA-CARYOPHYLLENE Fruit
BETA-COPAENE Fruit
BETA-FARNESENE Fruit
BETA-HYMULENE Fruit
BETA-IONONE Fruit
BETA-PINENE Fruit
BETA-SELINENE Fruit
BUTANOL Fruit
CALCIUM Fruit 180—1,582 ppm
CARBOHYDRATES Fruit 118,800—855,360 ppm
CHLORINE Fruit 40 ppm
CINNAMYLACETATE Fruit
CITRAL Fruit
CITRIC-ACID Fruit
COPPER Fruit 1—9 ppm
D-GALACTOSE Fruit
D-GALACTURONIC-ACID Fruit
DELTA-CADINENE Fruit
ELLAGIC-ACID Fruit
FAT Fruit 6,000—43,200 ppm

FAT Seed 100,000—143,000 ppm
FIBER Fruit 56,000—403,200 ppm
FIBER Seed 424,000 ppm
FRUCTOSE Fruit
GALLIC-ACID Fruit
GLUCOSE Seed 1,000 ppm
GLUTAMIC-ACID Fruit 1,070—7,704 ppm
GLYCINE Fruit 410—2,952 ppm
HISTIDINE Fruit 70—504 ppm
IRON Fruit 3—24 ppm
ISOLEUCINE Fruit 300—2,160 ppm
KILOCALORIES Fruit 510—3,670/kg
L-MALIC-ACID Fruit
LACTIC-ACID Fruit
LEUCINE Fruit 550—3,960 ppm
LEUCOCYANIDINS Fruit 1,000 ppm
LIMONENE Fruit
LINOLEIC-ACID Fruit 1,820—13,104 ppm
LINOLEIC-ACID Seed 13,900 ppm
LINOLENIC-ACID Seed 200 ppm
LYSINE Fruit 230—1,656 ppm
MAGNESIUM Fruit 98—735 ppm
MANGANESE Fruit 1—12 ppm
MECOCYANIN Fruit
METHIONINE Plant 50—360 ppm
METHYLCINNAMATE Fruit
METHYLISOPROPYLKETONE Fruit
MUFA Fruit 55—3,955 ppm
MYRISTIC-ACID Fruit 120—864 ppm
NIACIN Fruit 12—86 ppm
OLEIC-ACID Fruit 520—3,744 ppm
OLEIC-SEED 27,900 ppm
OXALIC-ACID Fruit 140 ppm
PALMITIC-ACID Fruit 1,440—10,368 ppm
PALMITOLEIC-ACID Fruit 30—216 ppm
PANTOTHENIC-ACID Fruit 2—11 ppm
PECTIN Fruit 3,000—16,000 ppm
PHENYLALANINE Fruit 20—144 ppm
PHOSPHORUS Fruit 235—1,905 ppm
PHYTIN-PHOSPHORUS Fruit 127—1,029 ppm
POTASSIUM Fruit 2,672—21,658 ppm
PROLINE Fruit 250—1,800 ppm
PROTEIN Fruit 8,200—59,000 ppm
PROTEIN Seed 152,000 ppm
PUFA Fruit 2,530—18,200 ppm

RHAMNOSE Fruit
RIBOFLAVIN Fruit 1—4 ppm
SERINE Fruit 240—1,728 ppm
SEQUIGUAVENE Plant
SFA Fruit 1,720—12,375 ppm
SODIUM Fruit 26—246 ppm
STARCH Seed 132,000 ppm
STEARIC-ACID Fruit 160—1,152 ppm
SUCROSE Fruit
SULFUR Fruit 140 ppm
TANNINS Seed 14,000 ppm
THIAMIN Fruit 1—4 ppm
THREONINE Fruit 310—2,232 ppm
TRYPTOPHAN Fruit 70—504 ppm
TYROSINE Fruit 100—720 ppm
VALINE Fruit 280—2,016 ppm
VITAMIN B6 Fruit 1—10 ppm
WATER Fruit 854,000—868,000 ppm
WATER Seed 103,000 ppm
XYLOSE Fruit
ZINC Fruit 2—200 ppm

■ KIWI

Chemical Constituents of Actinidia Chinensis
(Actinidiaceae)

ACTINIDIN Fruit
ACTINDINE Fruit
AFZELICHIN Plant
ASCORBIC-ACID Fruit 750—6,370 ppm
ASH Fruit 4,500—41,600 ppm
BETA-CAROTENE Fruit 0.4—6 ppm
BETA-SITOSTEROL Plant
CALCIUM Fruit 160—1,910 ppm
CARBOHYDRATES Fruit 148,800—877,900 ppm
CAROTENOIDS Fruit 5—42 ppm
CHROMIUM Fruit
CRYPTOXANTHIN Fruit 0.037—0.185 ppm
CYANIDIN Plant
DELPHINDIN Plant
FAT Fruit 700—38,400 ppm
FIBER Fruit 11,000—64,900 ppm
FOLACIN Fruit

GLUCOSE Fruit
IRON Fruit 3—30 ppm
KILOCALORIES Fruit 620—3,600/kg
LEVULOSE Fruit
LUTEIN Fruit
MAGNESIUM Fruit 300—1,770 ppm
NEOCHROME Fruit
NEOXANTHIN Fruit
NIACIN Fruit 5—30 ppm
P-COUMARIC-ACID Plant
PECTIN Fruit 4,200—24,800 ppm
PHOSPHOROUS Fruit 300—3,060 ppm
POTASSIUM Fruit 3,320—19,600 ppm
PROTEIN Fruit 7,900—62,830 ppm
QUERCETIN Plant
QUINIC-ACID Fruit
RIBOFLAVIN Fruit 0.5—3 ppm
SODIUM Fruit 50—295 ppm
SUCCINIC-ACID Plant
TANNIN Fruit 9,500 ppm
THIAMIN Fruit 0.2—1 ppm
TOCOPHEROL Fruit
VIOLAXANTHIN Fruit
WATER Fruit 812,000—837,000 ppm
ZEAXANTHIN Fruit

■ LEMON

Chemical Consituents of Citrus limon L. (Rutaceae)

2',4',5-TRIHYDROXY-FLAVONONE-7-O-BETA-D-GLUCOSYL-RHAMNOSIDE Pericarp
3-(4-HYDROXY-3-METHOXY-PHENYL)-1-GLUCOSYL-PROP-2-ENE Pericarp
3-HEXEN-1-OL Essential Oil
4',5,7-TRIHYDROXY-3',8-DIMETHOXY-FLAVONE-3-O-BETA-D-GLUCOSIDE Pericarp
4',5,7-TRIHYDROXY-3',8-DIMETHOXY-FLAVONE-3-O-BETA-D-GLUCOSYL-RHAMNOSIDE
4',7-DIHYDROXY-3'-METHOXY-

FLAVONE-8-O-BETA-D-GLUCOSYL-
RHAMNOSIDE Pericarp

5,7-DIMETHYOXYOXYCOUMARIN Essential Oil

5-GERANOXY-7-METHOXYCOUMARIN Essential Oil 630 ppm

5-GERANOXY-7-METHOXYPSORALEN Essential Oil

5-GERANYL-OXYPSORALEN Pericarp

5-ISOPENTENOXY-7-METHOXYCOUMARIN Essential Oil

6,7-DIMETHYOXYCOUMARIN Bark 162 ppm

6-8-DI-C-GLUCOSYL-DIOSMETIN Pericarp

6-C-GLUCOSYL-DIOSMETIN Pericarp

7-PENTAHYDROXY-2',3',5',5'-PENTAHYDROXY-FLAVANONE-7-(6-O-ALPHA-L-RHAMNOSYL-BETA-D-GLUCOSIDE Pericarp

ALPHA-L-RHAMNOSYL-BETA-D-GLUCOSE Pericarp

8-C-GLUCOSYL-DIOSMETIN Pericarp

8-GERAN-OXYPSORALEN Pericarp

ACETIC-ACID Essential Oil

ADENOSINE Pericarp

ALPHA-BERGAMOTENE Essential Oil 250 ppm

ALPHA-COPAENE Essential Oil

ALPHA-CUBEBENE Essential Oil

ALPHA-HUMULENE Essential Oil 10 ppm

ALPHA-PHELLANDRENE Essential Oil 20 ppm

ALPHA-PINENE Essential Oil 40—500 ppm

ALPHA-PINENE Leaf Oil 500—2,000 ppm

ALPHA-PINENE Pericarp Essential Oil 5,000—14,000 ppm

ALPHA-TERPINENE Essential Oil 70 ppm

ALPHA-TERPINENE Pericarp

ALPHA-TERPINEOL Essential Oil 6—50 ppm

ALPHA-TERPINEOL Leaf Essential Oil 11,000—125,000 ppm

ALPHA-TERPINEOL Pericarp Essential Oil 4,000—73,000 ppm

ALPHA-TERPINYL-PROPIONATE Essential Oil

ALPHA-THUJENE Essential Oil 16—40 ppm

BERGAMOTENE Essential Oil 16—40 ppm

BERGAMOTTIN Essential Oil 649 ppm

BERGAPTEN Essential Oil 10 ppm

BETA-BISABOLENE Essential Oil 23—400 ppm

BETA-CAROTENE Fruit 0—2 ppm

BETA-ELEMENE Essential Oil

BETA-HUMULENE Essential Oil 10 ppm

BETA-PHELLANDRENE Essential Oil 80 ppm

BETA-PINENE Essential Oil 40—1,270 ppm

BYAKANGELICIN Essential Oil 29 ppm

BYAKANGELICOL Essential Oil

CADINENE Essential Oil

CAFFEIC-ACID Fruit 21—35 ppm

CAFFEINE Flower 50 ppm

CAMPHENE Essential Oil 2—50 ppm

CARBOHYDRATES Fruit 111,000—863,000 ppm

CARVEOL Essential Oil

CARVONE Essential Oil

CARYOPHYLLENE Essential Oil 11—28 ppm

CIS-LIMONENE-1,2,-OXIDE Essential Oil

CITRAL Essential Oil 250—300 ppm

CITRIC-ACID Fruit 59,500 ppm

CITROPTEN Fruit

CITRUSIN-A Pericarp

CITRUSIN-B Pericarp

CITRUSIN-C Pericarp

CONFERIN Pericarp

D-GALACTURONIC-ACID Fruit

DEACETYL-NOMILIN-17-O-BETA-D-GLUCOPYRANOSIDE Seed

DECAN1-AL Pericarp

DECANAL Essential Oil

DECANOIC-ACID Essential Oil

DECANOL Essential Oil

DELTA-CARENE Essential Oil

DICONIFERYL-ALCOHOL-4-BETA-D-GLUCOSIDE Pericarp

DIOSMIN Fruit 5 ppm

DODECANAL Essential Oil 10 ppm

DODECANOIC-ACID Essential Oil

EPIJASMONIC-ACID-METHYL-ESTER Pericarp

ERIOCITRIN Fruit 1 ppm

ERIODICTYOSIDE Fruit

FARNESENE Essential Oil
FAT Fruit 28,000 ppm
FAT Seed 300,000—400,000 ppm
FERULIC-ACID Fruit 14—40 ppm
FIBER Fruit 17,000—47,000 ppm
GAMMA-TERPINENE Essential Oil 290—1,400 ppm
GAMMA-TERPINENE Pericarp Essential Oil 12,000—58,000 ppm
GERANIAL Essential 42—236 ppm
GERANIOL Essential oil
GERANYL-ACETATE Essential Oil 12—310 ppm
GERANYL-BUTYRATE Essential Oil
GERANYL-FORMATE Essential Oil
HEPTADECANAL Essential Oil
HEPTANAL Essential Oil 4 ppm
HESPERIDIN Fruit 44 ppm
HEPSERIDIN Pericarp 68,800 ppm
HESPERIDOSIDE Fruit
HEXADECANAL Essential Oil
HEXANAL Essential Oil
HEXANOL Essential Oil
IMPERATORIN Fruit
IRON Fruit 23—72 ppm
ISOIMPERATORIN Essential Oil
ISOLIMOCITROL Pericarp
ISOVITEXIN Pericarp
JASMONIC-ACID-METHYL-ESTER Pericarp
KILOCALORIES Fruit 2,640/kg
LAURALDEHYDE Fruit
LIMETTIN Essential Oil 295 ppm
LIMOCITRIN Pericarp
LIMOCITRIN-3-(6-0-ALPHA-L-RHAMNOSYL-BETA-D-GLUCOSIDE) Pericarp
LIMOCITROL Pericarp
LIMONENE Essential Oil 2,796—8,000 ppm
LIMONENE Pericarp Essential Oil 512,000—774,000 ppm
LIMONIN Fruit
LIMONIN Seed
LIMONIN-17-O-BETA-D-GLUCOPYRANOSIDE Seed
LIMONOATE-A-RING-LACTONE Fruit
LINALOOL Essential Oil 8—30 ppm

LINALOOL Pericarp Essential Oil 7,000—110,000 ppm
LINALYL-ACETATE Essential Oil
LUTEIN Fruit 0.12—1.2 ppm
MENTH-1-EN-9-OL Essential Oil
METHYL-HEPTANONE Essential Oil
METHYL-HEPTENONE Leaf Essential Oil 6,000 ppm
MUCILAGE Fruit
MYRCENE Essential Oil 65—1,270 ppm
NARINGIN Pericarp
NARINGOSIDE Fruit
NARIRUTIN Pericarp
NEOHESPERIDIN Pericarp
NERAL Essential Oil 27—130 ppm
NEROL-ACETATE Essential Oil 16—310 ppm
NERYL-FORMATE Essential Oil 20 ppm
NIACIN Fruit
NOMILIN Seed
NOMILIN-17-O-BETA-D-GLUCOPYRANOSIDE Seed
NONAN-1-AL Essential Oil 3—7 ppm
NONANAL Essential Oil 9—30 ppm
NONYL-ALDEHYDE Essential Oil
O-PHENYLPHENOL Essential Oil
OBACUNONE Seed
OBACUNONE-17-O-BETA-D-GLUCOPYRANOSIDE Seed
OCIMENE Leaf Essential Oil 10,000 ppm
OCTAN-1-AL Pericarp
OCTANOIC-ACID Essential Oil
OCTANOL Essential Oil 10—15 ppm
OCTYL-ACETATE Essential Oil
OCTYLALDEHYDE Essential Oil
OXYPEUCEDANIN Essential Oil 207 ppm
OXYPEUCEDANIN-HYDRATE Essential Oil 64 ppm
P-COUMARIC-ACID Fruit 6—102 ppm
P-CYMENE Essential Oil 12—31 ppm
P-CYMOL Essential Oil
P-MENTHA-1,8-DIEN-9-YL-ACETATE Essential Oil
P-MENTHA-2,8-DIEN-1-OL Essential Oil
PECTIN Pericarp
PENTADECANAL Essential Oil
PERILLALDEHYDE Fruit

PHELLOPTERIN Essential Oil
PHOSPHORUS Fruit 100—1,979 ppm
POTASSIUM Fruit 14,700 ppm
PROTEIN Fruit 10,000—111,000 ppm
QUERCETIN-3,5-DIGLUCOSIDE Plant
RIBOFLAVIN Fruit 2—3 ppm
RUTIN Fruit 1—2 ppm
SABINENE Essential Oil 50—175 ppm
SALICYLATES Fruit
SELINENE Essential Oil
SINAPIC-ACID Fruit 14 —18 ppm
SODIUM Fruit 470 ppm
SYRINGEN Pericarp
TERPINEN-4-OL Essential Oil 1—40 ppm
TERPINEN-4-OL Leaf Essential Oil 10,000 ppm
TERPINEN-4-OL Pericarp Essential Oil
    1,000—11,000 ppm
TERPINOLENE Essential Oil 14—120 ppm
TETRADECANAL Essential Oil
TETRADECANE Essential Oil
TETRAHYDROGERANIOL Essential Oil 10 ppm
THIAMIN Fruit 4—6 ppm
THYMOL Pericarp Essential Oil 53,000—
    111,000 ppm
TRANS-LIMONENE-1,2-OXIDE Essential Oil
TRIDECANAL Essential Oil
UNDECANAL Essential Oil
VICENIN-2 Pericarp
WATER Fruit 850,000—894,000 ppm

■ LIME

Chemical Constituents of Tilia sp. (Tiliaceae)

ASH Fruit 21,000—66,000 ppm
ASH Fruit 114,000—130,000 ppm
ASPARAGINE Fruit
FAT Fruit 30,000—580,000 ppm
FIBER Fruit 135,000—423,000 ppm
GLUTAMIC-ACID Fruit
GLYCINE Fruit
PROTEIN Fruit 36,000—113,000 ppm
WATER Fruit 681,000 ppm

■ LOQUAT

Chemical Constituents of Eriobotrya japonica
(Rosaceae)

ASCORBIC-ACID Fruit 10—840 ppm
ASH Fruit 4,000—44,000 ppm
BETA-CAROTENE Fruit 2.6—68 ppm
CALCIUM Fruit 180—2,381 ppm
CARBOYDRATES Fruit 102,000—919,000
    ppm
CRYPTOXANTHIN Fruit
D-(+)-TARTARIC-ACID Fruit
D-SORBITOL Leaf 2,000 ppm
DL-LACTIC-ACID Fruit
FAT Fruit 2,000—50,000 ppm
FIBER Fruit 5,000—71,000 ppm
IRON Fruit 20—67 ppm
KAEMPFEROL Plant
KILOCALORIES Fruit 400—3,700/kg
LEVULOSE Fruit
NEO-BETA-CAROTENE Fruit
NEO-BETA-CAROTENE-B Fruit
NEO-BETA-CAROTENE-U Fruit
NIACIN Fruit 2—25 ppm
PHOSPHORUS Fruit 140 2,667 ppm
POTASSIUM Fruit 2,600—27,632 ppm
PROTEIN Fruit 2,000—56,000 ppm
RIBOFLAVIN Fruit 0.4—4.2 ppm
SODIUM Fruit 40—351 ppm
SUCCINIC-ACID Fruit
SUCROSE Fruit
THIAMIN Fruit 0.2—1.8 ppm
WATER Fruit 865,000—886,000 ppm

■ MANDARIN/TANGARINE

Chemical Constituents of Citrus reticulata (Rutaceae)

1,8-CINEOLE Fruit 0—76 ppm
3,5,5-TRIMETHYLBENZYL-ALCOHOL Fruit
    3 ppm
ACETALDEHYDE Fruit 0—2 ppm
ALANINE Fruit 70—2,740 ppm

ALPHA-CAROTENE Fruit 0.2—2 ppm
ALPHA-COPAENE Fruit—2 ppm
ALPHA-LINOLENIC-ACID Fruit 100—806 ppm
ALPHA-PHELLANDRENE Fruit 3—32 ppm
ALPHA-PINENE Fruit 30—393 ppm
ALPHA-SELINENE Fruit 2 ppm
ALPHA-SINESAL Fruit 1—32 ppm
ALPHA-TERPINENE Fruit 4—42 ppm
ALPHA-TERPINEOL Fruit 2—110 ppm
ALPHA-TERPINYL-ACETATE Fruit 1—5 ppm
ALPHA-THUJENE Fruit 46—58 ppm
ALPHA-TOCOPHEROL Fruit 3—31 ppm
ALPHA-YLANGENE Fruit 1 ppm
ALUMINUM Fruit 1—15 ppm
ARGININE Fruit 440—3,546 ppm
ARSENIC Fruit 0.04—0.3 ppm
ASORBIC-ACID Fruit 280—3,684 ppm
ASH Fruit 3,900—31,525 ppm
ASPARAGINE Fruit 180—850 ppm
ASPARTIC-ACID Fruit 240—6,206 ppm
BENZYL-ALCOHOL Fruit 1—2 ppm
BETA-APOCAROTENOL Fruit 1—44 ppm
BETA-CITRAURIN Fruit
BETA-ELEMENE Fruit 1—80 ppm
BETA-PINENE Fruit 90—210 ppm
BETA-SESQUIPHELLANDRENE Fruit 20 ppm
BETA-TERPINEOL Fruit 40 ppm
BORON Fruit 1 —14 ppm
BROMINE Fruit 1 ppm
CADMIUM Fruit
CALAMIN Plant
CALCIUM Fruit 140—3,077 ppm
CAMPHENE Fruit 1—40 ppm
CARBOHYDRATES Fruit 102,000—901,914 ppm
CARVONE Fruit 0—3 ppm
CARYOPHYLLENE Fruit—9 ppm
CHLORINE Fruit 24 ppm
CHROMIUM Fruit 0.01—0.08 ppm
CIS-30-HEXENOL Fruit 1 ppm
CIS-CARVEOL Fruit 1—4 ppm
CITRIC-ACID Fruit 8,600—12,200 ppm
CITRONELLAL Fruit 1—20 ppm

CITRONELLIC-ACID Fruit
CITRONELLOL Fruit 1—50 ppm
CITRONELLYL-ACETATE Fruit 4—10 ppm
COBALT Fruit
COPPER Fruit 0—4.8 ppm
CYSTINE Fruit 70—564 ppm
DECANAL Fruit 3—90 ppm
DECANOIC-ACID Fruit 3 ppm
DECANOL Fruit 4 ppm
DECYL-ACETATE Fruit 1—5 ppm
DELTA-3-CARENE Fruit 1—6 ppm
DELTA-CADINENE Fruit 20 ppm
DELTA-ELEMENE Fruit 6—10 ppm
DIMETHYL-ANTHRALINATE Fruit 90 ppm
DODECANAL Fruit 1—15 ppm
DODECANOIC-ACID Fruit 1 ppm
DODECANOL Fruit 1 ppm
EO Fruit 10,000 ppm
ETHANOL Fruit 0—183 ppm
EUPATILIN Fruit
FAT Fruit 1,900—22,000 ppm
FERULOYL-PUTRESCINE Fruit
FIBER Fruit 1,890—43,000 ppm
FLUORINE Fruit 0.1—0.76 ppm
FOLACIN Fruit 0—2 ppm
GAMMA-AMINOBUTRYIC-ACID Fruit 180 ppm
GAMMA-CADANINE Fruit 2 ppm
GAMMA-ELEMENE Fruit 15—20 ppm
GAMMA-SELINE Fruit 1 ppm
GAMMA-TERPINENE Fruit 210—2,014 ppm
GERANIAL Fruit 6—30 ppm
GERANIOL Fruit 1—4 ppm
GERANYL-ACETATE Fruit 1 —18 ppm
GLUTAMIC-ACID Fruit 160—5,158 ppm
GLYCINE Fruit 20—5,158 ppm
HEPTANOIC-ACID Fruit 1 ppm
HEPTANOL Fruit 1—2 ppm
HISTIDINE Fruit 440—3,546 ppm
HUMULENE Fruit 5 ppm
IRON Fruit 1—79 ppm
ISOLEUCINE Fruit 170—1,370 ppm
ISOPYLEGOL Fruit 50—1,290 ppm
LIMONENE Fruit 6,500—9,400 ppm
LINALOOL Fruit 3—610 ppm
LINOLEIC-ACID Fruit 270—2,176 ppm

LONGIFOLENE Fruit 1 ppm
LUTEIN Fruit 0.2—2 ppm
LYSINE Fruit 40—2,579 ppm
MAGNESIUM Fruit 111—1,416 ppm
MALIC-ACID Fruit 1,800—2,100 ppm
MALONIC-ACID Fruit
MANGANESE Fruit 0—4.6 ppm
MERCURY Fruit
METHIONINE Fruit 130—1,048 ppm
METHYL-HEPTENONE Fruit 1 ppm
METHYL-N-METHYLANTHRALINATE
    Fruit 1—33 ppm
METHYL-THYMOL Fruit 10 ppm
MOLYBDENUM Fruit
MYRCENE Fruit 46—760 ppm
MYRISTIC-ACID Fruit 10—80 ppm
N-METHYL-TYRAMINE Fruit 0—58 ppm
NERAL Fruit 2—6 ppm
NEROL Fruit 1—5 ppm
NERYL-ACETATE Fruit 1 —10 ppm
NIACIN Fruit 1—35 ppm
NICKEL Fruit 0.01—0.3 ppm
NITROGEN Fruit 1,600—13,075 ppm
NOBELITIN Fruit
NONANAL Fruit 1—8 ppm
NONANOIC-ACID Fruit 1 ppm
NONANOL Fruit 2—10 ppm
NOOTKATONE Fruit 1 ppm
OCIMENE Fruit 8 ppm
OCTANAL Fruit 4—30 ppm
OCTANOIC-ACID Fruit 4 ppm
OCTANOL Fruit 9 ppm
OCTOPAMINE Fruit 1—2 ppm
OCTYL-ACETATE Fruit 2—4 ppm
OLEIC-ACID Fruit 300—2,418 ppm
OXALIC-ACID Fruit
P-CYMENE Fruit 14—820 ppm
P-MENTHA-1-EN-9-YL-ACETATE Fruit
PALMITIC-ACID Fruit 40—320 ppm
PANTOTHENIC-ACID Fruit 2—16 ppm
PERILLALSEHYDE Fruit 0—10 ppm
PHENYLALANINE Fruit 50—1,693 ppm
PHOSPHORUS Fruit 90—1,385 ppm
POTASSIUM Fruit 1,200—13,127 ppm
PROLINE Fruit 310—2,499 ppm
PROTEIN Fruit 6,130—80,228 ppm

QUINIC-ACID Fruit
RETICULAXANATHIN Fruit
RETROCULAMIN Plant
RIBOFLAVIN Fruit 0—4 ppm
RUBIDIUM Fruit 0.25—2.4 ppm
SABINENE Fruit 40—210 ppm
SABINENE-HYDRATE Fruit 1—20 ppm
SALICYLATES Fruit 5—50 ppm
SELENIUM Fruit
SERINE Fruit 120—1,773 ppm
SILICON Fruit 3—23 ppm
SODIUM Fruit 8—154 ppm
STEARIC-ACID Fruit 10—80 ppm
SUGARS Fruit 69,400—113,600 ppm
SULFUR Fruit 130—1,000 ppm
SYNEPHERINE Fruit 50—280 ppm
TANGERAXANTHIN Fruit
TANGERITIN Fruit
TERPINEN-4-OL Fruit 2—110 ppm
TERPINEOLINE Fruit 4—110 ppm
TETRADECANAL Fruit 5 ppm
THIAMIN Fruit 1—8 ppm
THREONINE Fruit 100—806 ppm
THYMOL Fruit 1—20 ppm
THYMYL-METHYL-ETHER Fruit 10 ppm
TRANS-CARVEOL Fruit 0—4 ppm
TRYPTOPHAN Fruit 60—484 ppm
TYRAMINE Fruit 1 ppm
TYROSINE Fruit 110—887 ppm
UNDECANOIC-ACID Fruit 1 ppm
UNDECANOL Fruit 1 ppm
VALINE Fruit 20—2,176 ppm
VITAMIN B6
WATER Fruit 879,720—886,000 ppm
ZEAXANTHIN Fruit
ZINC Fruit 0.8—8 ppm

■ MANGO

Chemical Constituents of Mangifera indica L.
(Anacardiaceae)

ALANINE Fruit 510—5,650 ppm
ARGININE Fruit 190—3,400 ppm
ASCORBIC-ACID Fruit 30—1,760 ppm

ASH Fruit 4,700—29,140 ppm
ASPARTIC-ACID Fruit 420—4,100 ppm
BETA-CAROTENE Fruit 11—96 ppm
BORON Fruit 0.5—17.5 ppm
CALCIUM Fruit 92—1,400 ppm
CARBOYDRATES Fruit 170,000—929,390 ppm
CAROTENOIDS Fruit 10—165 ppm
CATALASE Fruit
CHLORINE Fruit 205 ppm
CITRIC-ACID Fruit
COPPER Fruit 1.1—16.6 ppm
CYSTINE Fruit 70—350 ppm
FAT Fruit 1,000—16,890 ppm
FIBER Fruit 8,000—49,000 ppm
FRUCTOSE Fruit 25,700—48,300 ppm
FURFUROL Resin Exudate Sap 18,000 ppm
GABA Fruit
GLUCOSE Fruit 10,000—43,300 ppm
GLUTAMIC-ACID Fruit 600—6,800 ppm
GLYCINE Fruit 210—1,900 ppm
HISTIDINE Fruit 120—1,200 ppm
IODINE Fruit 0.016 ppm
IRON Fruit 1—243 ppm
ISOLEUCINE Fruit 180—2,000 ppm
KILOCALORIES Fruit 590—3,554/kg
LAURIC-ACID Fruit 10—55 ppm
LEUCINE Fruit 310—2,950 ppm
LINOLEIC-ACID Fruit 140—765 ppm
LINOLENIC-ACID Fruit 370—2.023 ppm
LYSINE Fruit 410—3,200 ppm
MAGNESIUM Fruit 84—875 ppm
MALIC-ACID Fruit 6,700—36,600 ppm
MANGANESE Fruit 0.2—12.2 ppm
MANGIFERIC-ACID Fruit
MANGIFERINE Fruit
METHIONINE Fruit 50—550 ppm
MUFA Fruit 1,010—5,522 ppm
MYRISTIC-ACID Fruit 90—492 ppm
NEO-BETA-CAROTENE-B Fruit 19.2 ppm
NEO-BETA-CAROTENE-U Fruit 7.3 ppm
NEOXANTHOPHYLL Fruit
NIACIN Fruit 6.5—63 ppm
OLEIC-ACID Fruit 540—2,950 ppm
OXALIC-ACID Fruit 300 ppm
PALMITIC-ACID Fruit 520—2,843 ppm

PALMITOLEIC-ACID Fruit 1.6—8.8 ppm
PEROXIDASE Fruit
PHENYLALANINE Fruit 170—3,700 ppm
PHOSPHORUS Fruit 103—1,050 ppm
PHYTIN Fruit
POTASSIUM Fruit 1,080—9,475 ppm
PROLINE Fruit 180—2,000 ppm
PROTEIN Fruit 5,000—60,000 ppm
PUFA Fruit 510—2,788 ppm
RIBOFLAVIN Fruit 0.5—3.3. ppm
SERINE Fruit 220—3,150 ppm
SFA Fruit 660—3,608 ppm
SODIUM Fruit 13—143 ppm
STEARIC-ACID Fruit 30—164 ppm
SUCCINIC-ACID Fruit
SUCROSE Fruit 66,700—125,800 ppm
SUGARS Fruit 112,000—205,000 ppm
SULFUR Fruit 70—615 ppm
THIAMIN Fruit 0.4—3.4 ppm
THREONINE Fruit 190—2,250 ppm
TRYPTOPHAN Fruit 80—700 ppm
TYROSINE Fruit 100—1,600 ppm
VALINE Fruit 260—2,700 ppm
VITAMIN B6 Fruit 1.3—7.3 ppm
WATER Fruit 754,300—900,000 ppm
XANTHYOPHYLL Fruit 42 ppm
ZINC Fruit 0.4—11.4 ppm

■ ORANGE

Chemical Constituents of Citrus sinensis L. (Rutaceae)

2'-TRANS-O-FERULOYL-GALACTARIC-ACID Pericarp
2'-TRANS-O-P-COUMAROYL-GALACTARIC-ACID Pericarp
2'-TRANS-O-P-COUMAROYL-GLUCARIC-ACID Pericarp
2-METHYL-1-PROPANOL Fruit Juice 0—0.07 ppm
2-TRANS-O-FERULOYL-GLUCARIC-ACID Pericarp
3,3',4,5,6,7,8-HEPTAMETHOXY-FLAVONE Fruit

3-HYDROXY-ETHYL-HEXANOATE Fruit
3-METHYL-BUT-1-ENE Essential Oil
3-METHYL-BUTAN-1-OL Fruit
4-(3-METHYL-2-BUTENOXY)-ISO-NITROSO-ACETOPHENONE Pericarp 48 ppm
5,6-DIHYDRO-BETA-BETA-CAROTEN-3,3',5,6-TETROL Fruit Juice
5,8-EPOXY-5,5',8-TETRAHYDRO-BETA,BETA-CAROTEN-3,3',5',6'-TETROL Plant
5,8-EPOXY-5,8-DIHYDRO-8'-APO-BETA-ACOTEN-3,10-DIOL Fruit Juice
ACETALDEHYDE Fruit Juice 3—15 ppm
ALANINE Fruit 30—3,775 ppm
ALPHA-BERGAMOTENE Fruit 6 ppm
ALPHA-CAROTENE Fruit 0.19—1.9 ppm
ALPHA-COPAENE Pericarp
ALPHA-HYDROXY-CAROTENE Pericarp
ALPHA-LINOLENIC-ACID Fruit 70—528 ppm
ALPHA-PINENE Fruit 10—60 ppm
ALPHA-SINESAL Fruit 3 ppm
ALPHA-SINESAL Pericarp
ALPHA-TERPINEOL Fruit 10—50 ppm
ALPHA-TERPINEOL Fruit Juice 0.09—1.1 ppm
ALPHA-TOCOPHEROL Fruit 4—29 ppm
ALUMINUM Fruit 1—165 ppm
ANTHERAXANTHIN Fruit
APOVIOLAXANTH-10'-AL Pericarp
ARABAN Fruit
ARGININE Fruit 230—4,908 ppm
ARSENIC Fruit 0.001—0.154 ppm
ASCORBIC-ACID Fruit 500—4,071 ppm
ASH Fruit 4,100—36,920 ppm
ASPARAGINE Fruit 200—1,800 ppm
ASPARTIC-ACID Fruit 70—8,607 ppm
AURAPTENE Fruit
AURAXANTHIN Fruit 0—4 ppm
BARIUM Fruit 0.54—16.5 ppm
BERGAPTOL Fruit
BETA-APO-8'-CAROTINAL Pericarp
BETA-APO-CAROTEN-8-AL Pericarp
BETA-CAROTENE Fruit 1—28 ppm
BETA-CITRAURIN Pericarp
BETA-CRYTOXANTHIN Fruit

BETA-CUBEBENE Fruit 10 ppm
BETA-ELEMENE Fruit 6 ppm
BETA-SINESAL Pericarp
BETA-SITOSTEROL Fruit
BETA-ZEACAROTENE Pericarp
BETAINE Fruit 390—630 ppm
BORON Fruit 1.89—27.5 ppm
BROMINE Fruit
BUTYRIC-ACID Fruit
CADMIUM Fruit 0.001—0.138 ppm
CAFFEIC-ACID Fruit 36—50 ppm
CALCIUM Fruit 210—5,615 ppm
CAMPESTEROL Fruit
CAPRIC-ACID Fruit
CAPROIC-ACID Fruit
CAPRYLIC-ACID Fruit
CARBOHYDRATES Fruit 99,000—887,125 ppm
CAROTENOIDS Fruit 12—35 ppm
CARVONE Fruit 2—10 ppm
CARYOPHYLLENE Pericarp
CHLORINE Fruit 12—32 ppm
CHOLESTEROL Fruit
CHOLINE Fruit 70—160 ppm
CHROMIUM Fruit 0.005—0.385 ppm
CITRIC-ACID Fruit 5,600—9,800 ppm
CITRONELLAL Fruit 0—55 ppm
CITRUSINS Plant
COBALT Fruit 0.001—0.005 ppm
CONIFERIN Pericarp
COPPER Fruit 0.44—5.5 ppm
CRYPTOFLAVIN Pericarp
CRYPTOXANTHIN Fruit
CRYPTOXANTHIN-5,5',6,6'-DIEPOXIDE Pericarp
CYANIDIN-3-GLUCOSIDE Fruit
CYSTINE Fruit 100—755 ppm
DEACETYL-NOMILIN Seed
DECANAL Fruit 10—60 ppm
DECANAL Fruit Juice 0—0.15 ppm
DELPHINIDIN-3-GLUCOSIDE Fruit
DELTA-CADINENE Pericarp
DIHUDROXKAEMPFEROL-4'-METHYL-ETHER-7-O-RHAMNOSIDE Fruit
DIOSMIN Pericarp
DODECANAL Fruit 5—20 ppm

EO Fruit 10,000 ppm
EPOXY-NOOTKATONE Pericarp
EPOXY-VALENCENE Fruit
ETA-CAROTENE Pericarp
ETHANOL Fruit Juice 64—900 ppm
ETHYL-ACETATE Fruit Juice 0.01—0.58 ppm
ETHYL-BUTYRATE Fruit Juice 0.08—1.02 ppm
FARNESENE Fruit Juice 0.08—1.02 ppm
FARNESENE Fruit 2—7 ppm
FAT Fruit 1,100—16,000 ppm
FERULIC-ACID Fruit 10—19 ppm
FERULOYL-PUTRESCINE Fruit 0—5 ppm
FIBER Fruit 3,740—47,000 ppm
FLAVOXANTHIN Pericarp
FLUORINE Fruit 0.04—0.76 ppm
FOLACIN Fruit 0—2 ppm
FR Juice
FRUCTOSE Fruit 23,800 ppm
GALACTAN Fruit
GALACTOSE Fruit
GALACTURONIC-ACID Fruit
GAMMA-AMINOBUTYRIC-ACID Fruit 40—730 ppm
GAMMA-TERPINENE Fruit 10 ppm
GAMMA-TERPINENE Fruit Juice 0.04—0.46 ppm
GERANIAL Fruit 6—350 ppm
GERANIOL Fruit 0—50 ppm
GLUCOSAN Fruit
GLUCOSE Fruit 23,600 ppm
GLUTAMIC-ACID Fruit 60—7,097 ppm
GLUTAMINE Fruit 30—630 ppm
GLYCINE Fruit 50—7,097 ppm
HEPTANAL Fruit 3—5 ppm
HEPTULOSE Fruit
HESPERIDIN Pericarp 40,600—63,500 ppm
HESPERIDIN-7-O-ALPHA-L-RHAMNO-GLUCOSIDE Fruit
HEXANAL Fruit 1—2 ppm
HEXANAL Fruit Juice 0.02—0.65 ppm
HEXANOL Fruit Juice 0.02—0.22 ppm
HISTIDINE Fruit 180—1,359 ppm
HORDENINE Fruit
IRON Fruit 1—8 ppm
ISOCAPROIC-ACID Fruit

ISOLEUCINE Fruit 250—1,888 ppm
ISOLUTEIN Pericarp
ISOPENTENYL-PSORALENS Fruit
ISOPRENE Essential Oil
ISORHOIFOLIN Pericarp
ISOSAKURANETIN Fruit
JASMONIC-ACID Fruit
LEAD Fruit 0.02—1.1 ppm
LEUCINE Fruit 230—1,136 ppm
LIMONENE Fruit 8,300—9,700 ppm
LIMONENE Fruit Juice 1—278 ppm
LIMONEXIC-ACID Fruit
LIMONIN Fruit
LIMONOATE-A-RING-LACTIONS Fruit
LINALOOL Fruit 30—530 ppm
LINALOOL Fruit Juice 0.15—4.69 ppm
LINOLEIC-ACID Fruit 180—1,359 ppm
LITHIUM Fruit 0.108—1.54 ppm
LOCHNOCARPOL-A Root
LUTEIN Fruit 0—3 ppm
LUTEOLIN-7-O-ALPHA-L-RHAMNO-GLUCOSIDE Fruit
LUTEOXANTHINS Fruit 0—6 ppm
LYSINE Fruit 470—3,548 ppm
MAGNESIUM Fruit 98—1,075 ppm
MALIC-ACID Fruit 600—2,000 ppm
MALONIC-ACID Plant
MANGANESE Fruit 0—8 ppm
MANNOSE Fruit
MERANZINE Fruit
MERCURY Fruit 0—0.001 ppm
METHANOL Fruit Juice 0.8—80 ppm
METHIONINE Fruit 200—1,510 ppm
METHYL-BUTYRATE Fruit Juice 0.01—0.1 ppm
MEVALONIC-ACID Fruit 0.5 ppm
MEVALONIC-ACID Pericarp 6 ppm
MOLYBDENUM Fruit 0.1—0.385 ppm
MUTATOCHROME Fruit
MUTATOXANTHIN Fruit 2 ppm
MYRCENE Fruit 69—210 ppm
N-METHYL-TYRAMINE Fruit 0—2 ppm
NARINGENIN Pericarp 35,000—45,800 ppm
NARINGENIN-4-BETA-D-GLUCOSIDE Plant
NARINGENIN-RUTINOSIDE

NARINGENIN-RUTINOSIDE-4-BETA-D-
  GLUCOSIDE Fruit
NARINGIN Fruit
NARINGIN-7-O-ALPHA-L-RHAMNO-
  GLUCOSIDE Fruit
NARIRUTIN Pericarp
NEO-BETA-CAROTENE Pericarp
NEOCHROME-A Pericarp
NEOCRHOME-B Pericarp
NEOHESPERIDIN-DIHYDROCHALCONE
  Pericarp
NEOPONCIRIN Pericarp
NEOXANTHIN-A Pericarp
NEOXANTHIN-B Pericarp
NERAL Fruit 1—20 ppm
NERYL-ACETATE Fruit 10 ppm
NERYL-FORMATE Fruit 10 ppm
NEUROSPORIN Pericarp
NIACIN Fruit
NICKEL Fruit 0.01—0.55 ppm
NITROGEN Fruit 500—13,845 ppm
NOBELITIN Fruit
NOMILIN Seed
NONANAL Fruit 6—20 ppm
NONANOL Fruit 10 ppm
NOOTKATOL Fruit
NOOTKATONE Fruit 1 ppm
OBACUNONE Seed
OCTAN-1-AL Fruit
OCTANAL Fruit 20—280 ppm
OCTANAL Fruit Juice 0—0.28 ppm
OCTOPAMINE Fruit 0—1 ppm
OCTYL-ACETATE Fruit 10 ppm
OLEIC-ACID Fruit 20—1,510 ppm
OXALIC-ACID Fruit 87 ppm
P-COUMARIC-ACID Fruit—17 ppm
P-CYMENE Fruit 20 ppm
PALMITIC-ACID Fruit 130—982 ppm
PALMITOLEIC ACID Fruit 30—226 ppm
PANTOTHENIC-ACID Fruit 2—19 ppm
PECTIN Fruit 1,300—5,900 ppm
PECTINESTERASE Fruit
PERILLALDEHYDE Fruit 2 ppm
PHENYLALANINE Fruit 310—2,340 ppm
PHOSPHORUS Fruit 136—1,980 ppm
PHYTOENE Fruit 0—2 ppm

PHYTOFLUENCE Fruit 0—4 ppm
POLYGALACTURONIC-ACID Fruit
POTASSIUM Fruit 1,400—13,772 ppm
PROLINE Fruit 60—3,473 ppm
PROTEIN Fruit 9,260—78,000 ppm
QUINIC-ACID Fruit
RIBOFLAVIN Fruit 0—3 ppm
RUBIDIUM Fruit 0.1—7.7 ppm
RUTIN Pericarp 6,100 ppm
SABINENE Fruit 10—60 ppm
SABINENE Fruit Juice 0—0.15 ppm
SCUTELLAREIN Fruit
SELENIUM 0—0.002 ppm
SERINE Fruit 40—2,410 ppm
SILICON Fruit
SILVER 0.027—0.055 ppm
SINAPIC-ACID Fruit 7—19 ppm
SINENSETIN Plant
SODIUM Fruit 0—29 ppm
STACHYDRINE Fruit
STIGMASTEROL Fruit
STRONTIUM Fruit 0.054—110 ppm
SUBAPHYLLIN Fruit
SUCCINIC-ACID Fruit
SUCROSE Fruit 47,000 ppm
SUGARS Fruit 39,600—119,800 ppm
SULFUR Fruit 46—1,000 ppm
SYNEPHRINE Fruit 15—43 ppm
TANGERETIN Fruit
TAU-CAROTENE Pericarp
TERPINEN-4-OL Fruit 6—550 ppm
TERPINOLENE Fruit 10 ppm
TETRA-O-METHYL-SCUTELLAREIN Fruit
TETRADECANAL Fruit 5—9 ppm
THIAMIN Fruit 1—7 ppm
THREONINE Fruit 150—1,132 ppm
TITANIUM Fruit 0.135—3.85 ppm
TRANS-2-HEXENOL Fruit Juice 0—0.1 ppm
TRYPTOPHAN Fruit 90—680 ppm
TYRAMINE Fruit 0—1 ppm
TYROSINE Fruit 160—1,208 ppm
URONIC-ACID Fruit
VALENCENE Fruit 10—20 ppm
VALENCENE Fruit Juice 0.04—15.3 ppm
VALENCIAXANTHIN Fruit 3 ppm
VALINE Fruit 100—3,020 ppm

VIOLAXANTHIN Fruit
VITAMIN B6 Fruit 1—5 ppm
VITEXIN-XYLOSIDE Fruit
WATER Fruit 839,000—898,000 ppm
XYLAN Fruit
XYLOSE Fruit
ZEAXANTHIN Fruit 2 ppm
ZETA-CAROTENE Fruit 0—2 ppm
ZINC Fruit 0.9—13 ppm
ZIRCONIUM Fruit 0.5—1.1 ppm

■ PAPAYA

Chemical Constituents of Carica papaya (Caricaceae)

(E)-BETA-OCIMENE Fruit
(Z)-BETA-OCIMENE Fruit
3-METHYL-BUTYL-BENZOATE Fruit
4-HYDROXY-4-METHYL-PENTAN-2-ONE Fruit
4-TERPINEOL Fruit
5,6-MONOEPOXI-BETA-CAROTENE Fruit
6-METHYLKEPT-5-EN-2-ONE Fruit
ALANINE Fruit 140—1,253 ppm
ALPHA-LINOLENIC-ACID Fruit 250—2,238 ppm
ALPHA-PHELLANDRENE Fruit
ALPHA-TERPINENE Fruit
AMYL-ACETATE Fruit
ARGININE Fruit 100—895 ppm
ASCORBIC-ACID Fruit 330—5,732 ppm
ASH Fruit 5,800—57,280 ppm
ASPARTIC-ACID Fruit 490—4,387 ppm
BENZALDEHYDE Fruit
BENZYL-ISOTHIOCYANATE Fruit
BETA-CAROTENE Fruit 10 -123 ppm
BETA-PHELLANDRENE Fruit
BORON Fruit 5—15 ppm
BUTYL-ALCOHOL Fruit
BUTYL-BENZOATE Fruit
BUTYL-HEXANOATE Fruit
CALCIUM Fruit 100—2,792 ppm
CALLOSE Latex Exudate
CAOUTCHOUC Latex Exudate 45,000 ppm

CARBOHYDRATES Fruit 95,000—991,000 ppm
CARYOPHYLLEN Fruit
CHRYSANTHEMEXANTHIN Fruit
CHYMOPAPAIN-A Latex Exudate
CHYMOPAPAIN-B Latex Exudate
CITRIC-ACID Fruit
COPPER Fruit 0.1—5 ppm
COTININE Plant
D-GALACTOSE Fruit
D-GALACTURONIC-ACID Fruit
DECANAL Fruit
DEHYDROCARPAMINES Plant
EO Seed 900 ppm
EPSILON-CAROTENE
ETHYL-ACETATE Fruit
ETHYL-ALCOHOL Fruit
ETHYL-BENZOATE Fruit
ETHYL-BUTYRATE Fruit
ETHYL-OCTOATE Fruit
FAT Fruit 980—22,000 ppm
FAT Latex Exudate 24,000 ppm
FIBER Fruit 6,960 ppm
GAMMA-CAROTENE Fruit
GAMMA-OCTALACTONE Fruit
GAMMA-TERPINENE Fruit
GERANYL-ACETONE Fruit
GERMACRENE-D Fruit
GLUCOTROPAEOLIN Plant
GLUTAMIC-ACID Fruit
GLYCINE Fruit 180—1,611 ppm
HEPTAN-2-ONE Fruit
HEPTANAL Fruit
HEXANAL Fruit
HISTIDINE Fruit 50—448 ppm
IRON Fruit 0.8—38 ppm
ISOAMYL-ACETATE Fruit
ISOLUECINE Fruit 80—716 ppm
KILOCALORIES Fruit 390—3,491/kg
KRYPTOFLAVIN Fruit
KRYPTOXANTHIN Fruit
LAURIC-ACID Fruit 10—90 ppm
LEUCINE Fruit 160—1,432 ppm
LINALOOL Fruit
LINALOOL-OXIDE-A Fruit
LINALOOL-OXIDE-B Fruit

LINOLEIC-ACID Fruit 60—537 ppm
LYCOPENE Fruit
LYSINE Fruit 250—2,238 ppm
MAGNESIUM Fruit 82—1,058 ppm
MALIC-ACID Fruit
MALIC-ACID Latex Exudate 4,400 ppm
MANGANESE Fruit 0.1—1.1 ppm
METHIONINE Fruit 20—179 ppm
METHYL-ACETATE Fruit
METHYL-ALCOHOL Fruit
METHYL-GERANATE Fruit
METHYL-HEXANOATE Fruit
METHYL-OCTANOATE Fruit
METHYL-SALICYLATE Fruit
METHYL-THIOCYANATE Fruit
MUFA Fruit 380—3,402 ppm
MUTATOCHROM Fruit
MYOSMINE Plant
MYRCENE Fruit
MYRISTIC-ACID Fruit 70—627 ppm
N-ACETYL-HEXOSAMIDASE Latex Exudate
NEOXANTHIN Fruit
NIACIN Fruit 3—33 ppm
NICOTINE Plant
NONANAL Fruit
OCTANAL Fruit
OLEIC-ACID Fruit 180—1,611 ppm
PALMITIC-ACID Fruit 320—2,865 ppm
PALMITOLEIC-ACID Fruit 200—1,790 ppm
PANTOTHENIC-ACID Fruit 2—19 ppm
PAPAIN Fruit
PAPAIN Latex Exudate 53,000 ppm
PENTADECANE Fruit
PENTAN-2,4-DIONE Fruit
PHENYLACETONITRILE Fruit
PHENYLALANINE Fruit 90—806 ppm
PHOSPHORUS Fruit 45—1,260 ppm
PHYTOENE Fruit
PHYTOFLUENE Fruit
POTASSIUM Fruit 2,294—25,469 ppm
PROLINE Fruit 100—895 ppm
PROP-2-YL-BUTYRATE Fruit
PROPYL-ALCOHOL Fruit
PROTEIN Fruit 5,000—57,370 ppm
PUFA Fruit 310—2,775 ppm
RESIN Latex Exudate 28,000 ppm

RIBOFLAVIN Fruit 0.3—3 ppm
SERINE Fruit 150—1,343 ppm
SFA Fruit 430—3,850 ppm
SODIUM Fruit 26—554 ppm
SODIUM Leaf 160—711 ppm
STEARIC-ACID Fruit 20—179 ppm
SUCROSE Fruit
SULFUR Fruit 300—900 ppm
TARTARIC-ACID Fruit
TERPINOLENE Fruit
THIAMIN Fruit 0.2—2.6 ppm
THREONINE Fruit 110—985 ppm
TRIACETIN Fruit
TRYPTOPHAN Fruit 80—716 ppm
TYROSINE Fruit 50—448 ppm
VALINE Fruit 100—895 ppm
VIOLAXANTHIN Fruit
VITAMIN B6 Fruit 0.2—1.7 ppm
WATER Fruit 865,000—918,300 ppm
WATER Latex Exudate 750,000 ppm
ZEAXANTHIN Fruit
ZINC Fruit 1.8—5.4 ppm

■ PASSIONFRUIT

Chemical Constituents of Passiflora edulis (Passifloraceae)

ALKALOIDS Fruit 120—7,000 ppm
ARACHIDIC-ACID Seed 780 ppm
ASCORBIC-ACID Fruit 300—1,205 ppm
ASH Fruit 8,000—32,000 ppm
ASH Seed 18,400 ppm
BETA-CAROTENE Fruit 4—17 ppm
CALCIUM Fruit 130—1,190 ppm
CALCIUM Seed 800 ppm
CARBOHYDRATES Fruit 212,000—851,000
CAROTENOIDS Fruit 580—11,600 ppm
CATALASE Fruit
CITRIC-ACID Fruit 20,000—45,600 ppm
EO Fruit Juice 23—43 ppm
ETHYL-BUTYRATE Fruit
ETHYL-CAPROATE Fruit Juice 14—30 ppm
FAT Fruit 7,000—28,000 ppm
FAT Seed 230,000—238,000 ppm

FIBER Fruit Juice 500—12,000 ppm
FIBER Seed 537,000 ppm
FLAVONOIDS Fruit 10,000—10,600 ppm
HARMAN Fruit 7,001 ppm
IRON Fruit 16—64 ppm
IRON Seed 180 ppm
KILOCALORIES Fruit 900—3,610/kg
LINOLEIC-ACID Seed 137,770 ppm
LINOLENIC-ACID Seed 12,420 ppm
MALIC-ACID Fruit 1,200—3,800 ppm
N-HEXYL-BUTYRATE Fruit Juice 3—6 ppm
N-HEXYL-CAPROATE Fruit Juice 14—30 ppm
NIACIN Fruit 15—60 ppm
NITROGEN Plant 960—1,920 ppm
OLEIC-ACID Seed 43,700 ppm
PALMITIC-ACID Seed 15,595 ppm
PECTIN Petiole 24,000—140,000 ppm
PECTIN-METHYLESTERASE Fruit
PELARGONIDIN-3-DIGLUCOSIDE Petiole 14 ppm
PHENOLASE Fruit
PHOSPHORUS Fruit 480—2,570 ppm
PHOSPHORUS Seed 6,400 ppm
POTASSIUM Fruit 3,480—13,975 ppm
PROTEIN Fruit 22,000—88,000 ppm
PROTEIN Fruit 111,000 ppm
RIBOFLAVIN Fruit 1—5 ppm
SFA Seed 20,470 ppm
SODIUM Fruit 280—1,124 ppm
STEARIC-ACID Seed 4,050 ppm
THIAMIN Fruit 0—1.4 ppm
WATER Fruit 751,000—790,000 ppm
WATER Seed 54,000 ppm
XANTHOPHYLLIS Fruit 60—2,495 ppm

■ PAWPAW

Chemical Constituents of Asimina triloba L. (Annonaceae)

(E)(E)-FARNESOL Fruit 0—0.058 ppm
(E)(E)-FARNESYL-ACETATE Fruit 0—0.001 ppm
(E)(E)-FARNESYL-BUTANOATE Fruit 0—0.001 ppm
(E)(E)-FARNESYL-HEXANOATE Fruit 0—0.06 ppm
(E)(E)-FARNESYL-OCTANOATE Fruit 0—0.041 ppm
(Z)-HEX-3-EN-1-OL Fruit 0—0.041 ppm
2-THEYL-HEX-AN-1-OL Fruit 0—0.004 ppm
3-({HEPTYLCARBONYL}OXY)BUTAN-2-ONE Fruit 0—0.74 ppm
3-({PENTYLCARBONYL}OXY)BUTAN-2-ONE Fruit 0—1.305 ppm
3-({PROPYLCARBONYL}OXY)BUTAN-2-ONE Fruit 0—2.407 ppm
3-ACETOXYBUTAN-2-ONE Fruit 0—0.108 ppm
3-HYDROXYBUTAN-2-ONE Fruit 0.001—3.123 ppm
4-HEXANOLIDE Fruit 0—0.453 ppm
4-OCTANOLIDE Fruit 0—0.024 ppm
ALANINE Fruit 523—5,331 ppm
ARGININE Fruit 240—2,336 ppm
ASCORBIC-ACID Fruit 76—893 ppm
ASH Fruit 6,000—22,000 ppm
ASIMICIN Seed
ASIMILOBINE Plant
ASIMINE Seed
ASPARTIC-ACID Fruit 424—5,167 ppm
BETA-CAROTENE Fruit 0.4—2.5 ppm
BUTANE-2,3-DIOL-MONOBUTANOATE-1 Fruit 0—0.473 ppm
BUTANE-2,3-DIOL-MONOBUTANOATE-2 Fruit 0—0.588 ppm
BUTANE-2,3-DIOL-MONOHEXANOATE-1 Fruit 0—0.489 ppm
BUTANE-2,3-DIOL-MONOHEXANOATE-2 Fruit 0—1.121 ppm
BUTANE-2,3-DIOL-MONOOCTANOATE-1 Fruit 0—0.23 ppm
BUTANE-2,3-DIOL-MONOOCTANOATE-2 Fruit 0—0.239 ppm
BUTYL-(E)-BUT-2-ENOATE Fruit 0—0.845 ppm
BUTYL-OCTANOATE Fruit 0—0.048 ppm
BUTYRIC-ACID Fruit 0—0.001 ppm
CALCIUM Fruit 530—3,248 ppm

CARBOHYDRATES Fruit 168,000—854,000 ppm
CITRONELLOL Fruit 0—0.024 ppm
COREXIMINE Plant
CYANIDIN Plant
DECANOIC-ACID Fruit 0.01—0.662 ppm
DIBUTYL-PHTHALATE Fruit 0.02—0.036 ppm
DODECANOIC-ACID Fruit 0.012—0.135 ppm
ETHYL-(E)(E)-HEXA-2,4-DIENOATE Fruit 0—0.047 ppm
ETHYL-(E)-BUT-2-ENOATE Fruit 0—0.291 ppm
EHTYL-(Z)-HEX-4-ENOATE Fruit 0—0.352 ppm
ETHYL-(Z)-OCT-4-ENOATE Fruit 0—0.716 ppm
ETHYL-3-HYDROXYHEXANOATE Fruit 0—0.676 ppm
ETHYL-ACETATE Fruit 0.008—0.143 ppm
ETHYL-BUTANOATE Fruit 0.002—7.109 ppm
ETHYL-DECANOATE Fruit 0.003—1.92 ppm
ETHYL-HEXA-2,4-DIENOATE Fruit 0—0.155 ppm
ETHYL-HEXADECANOATE Fruit 0.001—0.06 ppm
ETHYL-HEXANOATE Fruit 0.006—62.864 ppm
ETHYL-NICOTINATE Fruit 0—0.036 ppm
ETHYL-OCTANOATE Fruit 0.02—24.609 ppm
ETHYL-TETRADECANOATE Fruit 0—0.215 ppm
FAT Fruit 6,000—59,000 ppm
FIBER Fruit 14,000—150,000 ppm
FRUCTOSE Fruit 13,000—119,658 ppm
GERANIOL Fruit 0—1.305 ppm
GERANYL-HEXANOATE Fruit 0—0.047 ppm
GERANYL-OCTANOATE Fruit 0—0.012 ppm
GLUCOSE Fruit 18,000—170,940 ppm
GLUTAMIC-ACID Fruit 622—7,332 ppm
GLYCINE Fruit 389—3,501 ppm
HALF-CYSTINE Fruit 14—336 ppm
HEXADECANOIC-ACID Fruit 0—0.23 ppm
HEXANOIC-ACID Fruit 0—0.001 ppm

HEXYL-OCTANOATE Fruit 0—0.027 ppm
HISTIDINE Fruit 124—1,336 ppm
HYDROXYPROLINE Fruit 70—836 ppm
IRON Fruit 68—308 ppm
ISOCORYDINE Plant
ISOLEUCINE Fruit 373—4,166 ppm
KCALS Fruit 770—3,400 ppm
LEUCINE Fruit 466—5,002 ppm
LIMONENE Fruit 0.027—0.548 ppm
LINOLEIC-ACID Fruit 480—6,018 ppm
LINOLENIC-ACID Fruit 840—14,396 ppm
LYSINE Fruit 339—3,831 ppm
MAGNESIUM Fruit 1,090—5,128 ppm
MANGANESE Fruit 25—111 ppm
METHIONINE Fruit 70—836 ppm
METHYL-(E)(E)-FARNESATE Fruit 0.048—0.304 ppm
METHYL-(E)-OCTANOATE Fruit 0.031—6.179 ppm
METHYL-(Z)-OCT-2-ENOATE Fruit 0—0.036 ppm
METHYL-BUTANOATE Fruit 0.047—0.119 ppm
METHYL-CYCLOHEXANE Fruit 0.063—0.196 ppm
METHYL-DECANOATE Fruit 0—0.107 ppm
METHYL-DODECANOATE Fruit 0—0.06 ppm
METHYL-GERANATE Fruit 0—0.453 ppm
METHYL-HEXANOATE Fruit 0—5.344 ppm
METHYL-OCTANOATE Fruit 0.031—6.179 ppm
METHYL-TETRADECANOATE Fruit 0—0.058 ppm
MYRISTIC-ACID Fruit 306—4,956 ppm
OCTANOIC-ACID Fruit 0—0.001 ppm
OLEIC-ACID Fruit 1,392—24,780 ppm
PALMITIC-ACID Fruit 1,080—14,396 ppm
PALMITOLEIC Fruit 348—6,018 ppm
PHENYLALANINE Fruit 294—3,001 ppm
PHOSPHORUS Fruit 420—2,265 ppm
POTASSIUM Fruit 3,140—15,726 ppm
PROLINE Fruit 282—3,648 ppm
PROPYL-BUTANOATE Fruit 0—0.068 ppm
PROPYL-HEXANOATE Fruit 0—0.167 ppm
PROTEIN Fruit 8,000—61,000 ppm

QUERCETIN-3-GLUCOSIDE Plant
SERINE Fruit 354—3,666 ppm
STEARIC-ACID Fruit 102—2,124 ppm
SUCROSE Fruit 60,000—545,000 ppm
SULFUR Fruit 620—3,333 ppm
TETRADECANOIC-ACID Fruit 0.059—0.162 ppm
TETRADECEN-1-OL Fruit 0—0.147 ppm
THREONINE Fruit 254—2,812 ppm
TOULENE Fruit 0.001—0.024 ppm
TRYPTOPHAN Fruit 35—536 ppm
TYROSINE Fruit 140—1,501 ppm
VALINE Fruit 334—3,661 ppm
WATER Fruit 695,000—766,000 ppm
ZINC Fruit 9—38 ppm

■ PEACH

Chemical Constituents of Prunus persica L. (Rosaceae)

A-DECALACTONE Fruit
ACETIC-ACID Fruit
ALANINE Fruit 420—3,402 ppm
ALPHA-TOCOPHEROL Fruit 10—86 ppm
ALUMINUM Fruit 2.25—1,050 ppm
ANTHOCYANIDIN Fruit
ARGININE Fruit 180—1,458 ppm
ARSENIC Fruit 0.001—0.053 ppm
ASCORBIC-ACID Fruit 14—1,127 ppm
ASH Bark 63,000 ppm
ASH Fruit 4,000—150,000 ppm
ASPARTIC-ACID Fruit 1,170—8,586 ppm
BARIUM Fruit 0.045—30 ppm
BENZALDEHYDE Fruit
BENZYL-ACETATE Fruit
BENZYL-ALCOHOL Fruit
BETA-CAROTENE Fruit 0—30 ppm
BORON Fruit 1—150 ppm
BROMINE Fruit
CADMIUM Fruit 0—0.45 ppm
CALCIUM Fruit 18—8,850 ppm
CARBOHYDRATES Fruit 111,000—910,000 ppm
CHROMIUM Fruit 0.01—2.25 ppm

CITRIC-ACID Fruit
COBALT Fruit 0.005—0.45 ppm
COPPER Fruit 0.3—30 ppm
CYANIDIN-3-MONOGLUCOSIDE Fruit
CYSTINE Fruit 60—486 ppm
ETHANOL Fruit
ETHYL-ACETATE Fruit
ETHYL-BENZOATE Fruit
FAT Fruit 860—18,000 ppm
FIBER Fruit 6,210—162,000 ppm
FLAVONOL-GLYCOSIDE Fruit 10 ppm
FLUORINE Fruit 0.1—0.8 ppm
FOLACIN Fruit 0.031—0.303 ppm
FORMIC-ACID Fruit
GAMMA-HEPTALACTONE Fruit
GAMMA-HEXALACTONE Fruit
GAMMA-OCTALACTONE Plant
GLUTAMIC-ACID Fruit 1,060—8,586 ppm
GLYCINE Fruit 240—1,944 ppm
HEXANOIC-ACID Fruit
HEXYL-ACID Fruit
HEXYL-ACETATE Fruit
HEXYL-FORMATE Fruit
HISTIDINE Fruit 130—1,053 ppm
IRON Fruit 1—99 ppm
ISOLEUCINE Fruit 200—1,620 ppm
ISOVALERIANIC-ACID Fruit
L-ARABINOSE Gum
L-MALIC-ACID Fruit
L-RHAMNOSE Gum
LEAD Fruit 0.3—3 ppm
LEUCINE Fruit 400—3,240 ppm
LINOLEIC-ACID Fruit 440—3,565 ppm
LINOLENIC-ACID Fruit 10—80 ppm
LITHIUM Fruit 0.06—0.6 ppm
LUTEIN Fruit 0.14—2.8 ppm
LYCOPENE Fruit
LYSINE Fruit 230—1,863 ppm
MAGNESIUM Fruit 68—850 ppm
MALONIC-ACID Fruit
MANGANESE Fruit 0—22.5 ppm
MERCURY Fruit 0—0.007 ppm
METHIONINE Fruit 170—1,377 ppm
METHYL-ACETATE Fruit
MOLYBDENUM Fruit 0.1—1.05 ppm
MUFA Fruit 340—2,755 ppm

NIACIN Fruit 10—82 ppm
NICKEL Fruit 0.15—4.5 ppm
NITROGEN Fruit 1,400—13,075 ppm
OLEIC-ACID Fruit 340—2,755 ppm
PALMITIC-ACID Fruit 90—730 ppm
PANTOTHENIC-ACID Fruit 2—14 ppm
PECTINS Fruit 8,600 ppm
PENTANOIC-ACID Fruit
PENTYL-ACETATE Fruit
PHOSPHORUS Fruit 90—2,000 ppm
PHYTIN-PHOSPHORUS Fruit 10 ppm
PHYTOSTEROLS Fruit 100—810 ppm
POTASSIUM Fruit 1,275—22,072 ppm
PROLINE Fruit 290—2,349 ppm
PROTEIN Fruit 290—2,349 ppm
PUFA Fruit 450—3,645 ppm
QUERCETIN-3-DIGLUCOSIDE Fruit
QUERCETIN-3-GALACTOSIDE Fruit
QUERCETIN-3-GLUCOSIDE Fruit
QUERCETIN-3-RHAMNOSIDE Fruit
QUERCETIN-3-RUTINOSIDE Fruit
RIBOFLAVIN Fruit 1—4 ppm
SELENIUM Fruit 0—0.003 ppm
SERINE Fruit 320—2,592 ppm
SFA Fruit 100—810 ppm
SILICON Fruit 4—30 ppm
SILVER Fruit 0.015 ppm—0.3 ppm
SODIUM Fruit 0—366 ppm
STEARIC-ACID Fruit 10—80 ppm
STRONTIUM Fruit 0.225—45 ppm
SUCROSE Fruit 20,000—100,000 ppm
SULFUR Fruit 3—700 ppm
TANNIN Fruit 8,000 ppm
THIAMIN Fruit 1—2 ppm
THREONINE Fruit 270—2,187 ppm
TITANIUM Fruit 0.075—30 ppm
TRANS-2-HEXENYL-ACETATE Fruit
TRYPTOPHAN Fruit 20—162 ppm
TYROSINE Fruit 180—1,458 ppm
VALINE Fruit 380—3,078 ppm
VITAMIN B6 Fruit 0.2—1.6 ppm
WATER Fruit 835,000—964,000 ppm
ZEAXANTHIN Fruit
ZINC Fruit 0.45—37.5 ppm
ZIRCONIUM Fruit 0.3—4.5 ppm

■PEAR

Chemical Constituents of Pyrus communis L.
(Rosaceae)

4-HYDROXYMETHYLPROLINE Fruit
ALANINE Fruit 130—803 ppm
ALPHA-LINOLENIC-ACID Fruit 10—62 ppm
ALPHA-PYRUFURAN Plant
ALPHA-TOCOPHEROL Fruit 0.6—31 ppm
ALUMINUM Fruit 1—105 ppm
ARGININE Fruit 70—432 ppm
ARSENIC Fruit 0.001—0.06 ppm
ASCORBIC-ACID Fruit 40—250 ppm
ASH Fruit 2,720—40,000 ppm
ASPARTIC-ACID Fruit 770—4,756 ppm
BARIUM Fruit 0.045—11 ppm
BETA-CAROTENE Fruit 0.17—1.7 ppm
BETA-PHENYLETHYLAMINE Fruit
BORON Fruit 1—82 ppm
BROMINE Fruit 1—82 ppm
CADMIUM Fruit 0—0.125 ppm
CAFFEIC-ACID Fruit 43—19,700 ppm
CALCIUM Fruit 68—1,776 ppm
CARBOHYDRATES Fruit 151,000—933,292
  ppm
CHROMIUM Fruit 0.002—0.555 ppm
CITRIC-ACID Fruit
COBALT Fruit 0.015—0.111 ppm
COPPER Fruit 0.45—11.1 ppm
CYANIDIN-3-GALACTOSIDE Epidermis
CYTSINE Fruit 40—247 ppm
EPIFRIEDELIN Fruit
FAT Fruit 2,790—32,198 ppm
FIBER Fruit 14,000—86,473 ppm
FLUORINE Fruit
FOLACIN Fruit 0.06—0.5 ppm
FRIEDELIN Fruit
GADOLEIC-ACID Fruit 10—62 ppm
GLUTAMIC-ACID Fruit 280—1,729 ppm
GLYCINE Fruit 110—679 ppm
HISTIDINE Fruit 40—247 ppm
IRON Fruit 0.9—37 ppm
LEAD Fruit 0.02—1.11 ppm
LEUCINE Fruit 200—1,235 ppm
LINOLEIC-ACID Fruit 930—5,744 ppm

LITHIUM Fruit 0.06—0.185 ppm
LUTEIN Fruit 1—11 ppm
LYSINE Fruit 140—865 ppm
MAGNESIUM Fruit 54—1,110 ppm
MALIC-ACID Fruit
MANGANESE Fruit 0.3—5.55 ppm
MERCURY Fruit 0—0.019 ppm
METHIONINE Fruit 50—309 ppm
MOLYBDENUM Fruit 0.1—0.26 ppm
MUFA Fruit 840—5,188 ppm
NIACIN Fruit 1—6 ppm
NICKEL Fruit 0.1—1.11 ppm
NITROGEN Fruit 480—3,000 ppm
OLEIC-ACID Fruit 810—5,003 ppm
PALMITIC-ACID Fruit 170—1,050 ppm
PALMITOLEIC-ACID Fruit 20—124 ppm
PANTOTHENIC-ACID Fruit 0.7—4 ppm
PECTIN Fruit 40,000 ppm
PHOSPHORUS Fruit 90—1,332 ppm
PHYTOSTEROLS Fruit 80—494 ppm
POTASSIUM Fruit 1,200—11,250 ppm
PROLINE Fruit 110—679 ppm
PROTEIN Fruit 3,690—25,400 ppm
PUFA Fruit 940—5,806 ppm
QUERCETIN Pericarp 28 ppm
QUINIC-ACID Fruit
RIBOFLAVIN Fruit 0.4—2.4 ppm
RUBIDIUM Fruit 1.6—20 ppm
SELENIUM Fruit 0—0.002 ppm
SERINE Fruit 140—865 ppm
SFA Fruit 220—1,359 ppm
SHIKIMIC-ACID Fruit
SILICON Fruit 2—20 ppm
SILVER Fruit 0.015—0.037 ppm
SODIUM Fruit 0—407 ppm
STRONTIUM Fruit 0.45—18.5 ppm
SULFUR Fruit 3—300 ppm
THIAMIN Fruit 0.2—1.2 ppm
THREONINE Fruit 100—618 ppm
TITANIUM Fruit 0.075—7.4 ppm
TYROSINE Fruit 30—185 ppm
URSOLIC-ACID Fruit
VALINE Fruit 140—865 ppm
VITAMIN B6 Fruit 0.1—1.1 ppm
WATER Fruit 817,000—891,000 ppm

ZINC Fruit 0.15—26.6 ppm
ZIRCONIUM Fruit 0.3—1.11 ppm

■ PERSIMMON

Chemical Constituents of *Diospyros virginiana* L. (Ebenaceae)

(E)-2-HEXENAL Fruit
ASCORBIC-ACID Fruit 660—1,855 ppm
ASH Fruit 9,000—25,280 ppm
BENZOTHIAZOLE Fruit
BORNEOL Fruit
BORNYL-ACETATE Fruit
CALCIUM Fruit 270—758 ppm
CARBOHYDRATES Fruit 335,000—941,000 ppm
FAT Fruit 4,000—11,230 ppm
FAT Seed 26,000 ppm
FIBER Fruit 15,000—42,135 ppm
IRON Fruit 25—70 ppm
KILOCALORIES Fruit 1,270—3,567/kg
NERYL-ACETATE Fruit
PALMITIC-ACID Fruit
PHENYLACETALDEHYDE Fruit
PHOSPHORUS Fruit 260—730 ppm
POTASSIUM Fruit 3,100—8,710 ppm
PROTEIN Fruit 8,000—22,470 ppm
PROTEIN Seed 100,000 ppm
SODIUM Fruit 10—28 ppm
WATER Fruit 644,000 ppm

■ PINEAPPLE

Chemical Constituents of *Ananas comosus* L. (Bromeliaceae)

ACETALDEHYDE Fruit 0.61—1.4 ppm
ACETIC-ACID Fruit 0.49 ppm
ACETONE Fruit
ACETOXYACETONE Fruit
ALANINE Fruit 170—1,259 ppm
ALPHA-LINOLENIC-ACID Fruit 620—4,592 ppm

ALPHA-TOCOPHEROL Fruit 1—7 ppm
AMYL-CAPROATE Fruit
ARGININE Fruit 46—1,333 ppm
ASCORBIC-ACID Fruit 148—4,178 ppm
ASH Fruit 2,800—36,000 ppm
ASPARAGINE Fruit 1,251 ppm
ASPARTIC-ACID Fruit 293—4,222 ppm
BETA-CAROTENE Fruit 0—3 ppm
BIACETYL Fruit
BORON Fruit 0.2 ppm
BROMELAIN Fruit
BROMELIN Fruit
BUTYL-FORMATE Fruit
CALCIUM Fruit 62—1,308 ppm
CARBOHYDRATES Fruit 116,000—938,000 ppm
CELLULOSE Fruit 4,300—5,400 ppm
CHAVICOL Fruit 0.27 ppm
CHLORINE Fruit 460 ppm
CITRIC-ACID Fruit 3,200—86,000 ppm
COPPER Fruit 1—8.8 ppm
CYSTINE Fruit 20—148 ppm
DELTA-OCTALACTONE Fruit 0.3 ppm
DIMETHYL-MALONATE Fruit 0.06 ppm
ESTERS Fruit 1—250 ppm
ETHYL-ACRYLATE Fruit 0.77 ppm
ETHYL-ALCOHOL Fruit 60 ppm
ETHYL-BETA-ACETOXYHEXANOATE
    Fruit 0.006 ppm
ETHYL-BETA-HYDROXYHEXANOATE
    Fruit 0.03 ppm
ETHYL-BETA-METHYLTHIOPROPIONATE
    Fruit 0.09 ppm
ETHYL-BUTYRATE Fruit
ETHYL-CAPROATE Fruit 0.77 ppm
ETHYL-CAPRYLATE Fruit
ETHYL-FORMATE Fruit
ETHYL-ISOBUTYRATE Fruit
ETHYL-ISOVALERATE Fruit 0.39 ppm
ETHYL-LACTATE Fruit
ETHYL-PROPIONATE Fruit
FAT Fruit 1,000—42,772 ppm
FERULIC-ACID Plant 200—760 ppm
FIBER Fruit 3,000—45,000 ppm
FRUCTOSE Fruit 6,000—23,000 ppm
GABA Fruit 124 ppm

GAMMA-BUTYROLACTONE Fruit
GAMMA-OCTALACTONE Fruit 0.3 ppm
GLUCOSE Fruit 10,000—32,000 ppm
GLUTAMIC-ACID Fruit 90—3,333 ppm
GLUTAMINE Fruit 256 ppm
GLYCINE Fruit 65—1,259 ppm
HEXOSANS Fruit 1,000—1,500 ppm
HISTIDINE Fruit 48—667 ppm
INODOLE-ACETIC-ACID-OXIDASE Fruit
IODINE Fruit 0—1 ppm
IRON Fruit 3—73 ppm
ISOBUTYL-ACETATE Fruit
ISOBUTYL-FORMATE Fruit
ISOCAPRONIC-ACID Fruit
ISOLEUCINE Fruit 23—963 ppm
ISOPROPYL-ISOBUTYRATE Fruit
L-MALIC-ACID Fruit
LEUCINE Fruit 24—1,407 ppm
LINOLEIC-ACID Fruit 840—6,222 ppm
LYSINE Fruit 46—1,852 ppm
MAGNESIUM Fruit 110—1,075 ppm
MALIC-ACID Fruit 1,000—4,700 ppm
MANGANESE Fruit 12—209 ppm
METHANOL Fruit
METHIONINE Fruit 110—815 ppm
METHYL-ACETATE Fruit
METHYL-BETA-ACETOXYHEXANOATE
    Fruit 0.03 ppm
METHYL-BETA-HYDROXYBUTYRATE
    Fruit 0.006 ppm
METHYL-BETA-HYDROXYHEXANOATE
    Fruit 0.021 ppm
METHYL-BETA-
    METHYLTHIOPROPIONATE Fruit 0.12—
    1.1 ppm
METHYL-BUTYRATE Fruit
METHYL-CAPROATE Fruit
METHYL-CIS-(4)-OCTENOATE Fruit 0.001 ppm
METHYL-ISOBUTYRATE Fruit
METHYL-ISOCAPROATE Fruit 1.4 ppm
METHYL-ISOVALERATE Fruit 0.6 ppm
METHYL-N-PROPYL-KETONE Fruit
MUFA Fruit 480—3,556 ppm
N-VALERIANIC-ACID Fruit
NIACIN Fruit 2—33 ppm

NITRATE Fruit 0—1,200 ppm
NITROGEN Fruit 450—1,150 ppm
OLEIC-ACID Fruit 450—3,333 ppm
OXALIC-ACID Fruit 50—58 ppm
P-AMINOBENZOIC-ACID Fruit 0—1 ppm
P-COUMARIC-ACID Plant 330—730 ppm
PALMITIC-ACID Fruit 190—1,407 ppm
PALMITOLEIC-ACID Fruit 30—220 ppm
PANTOTHENIC-ACID Fruit 1—11 ppm
PECTIN Fruit 600—1,600 ppm
PENTANOL Fruit
PENTOSANS Fruit 3,300—4,300 ppm
PEROXIDASE Fruit
PHENYLALANINE Fruit 40—889 ppm
PHOSPHATASE Fruit
PHOSPHORUS Fruit 60—923 ppm
PHYTOSTEROLS Fruit 60—444 ppm
POTASSIUM Fruit 110—9,932 ppm
PROLINE Fruit 31—963 ppm
PROPANOL Fruit
PROPYL-ACETATE Fruit
PROPYL-FORMATE Fruit
PROTEIN Fruit 4,000—55,000 ppm
PUFA Fruit 1,460—10,815 ppm
RIBOFLAVIN Fruit 0—3 ppm
SERINE Fruit 250—1,852 ppm
SEROTONIN Fruit 19—60 ppm
SFA Fruit 320—2,370 ppm
SILICON Fruit 110—690 ppm
SODIUM Fruit 10—180 ppm
STARCH Fruit 19 ppm
STEARIC-ACID Fruit 110—815 ppm
SUCROSE Fruit 59,000—150,000 ppm
SULFUR Fruit 70 ppm
THIAMIN Fruit 0—7 ppm
THREONINE Fruit 78—859 ppm
TYROSINE Fruit 58—889 ppm
VALINE Fruit 39—1,185 ppm
VANILLIN Fruit
VITAMIN B6 Fruit 0.9—6 ppm
WATER Fruit 812,000—890,000 ppm
ZINC Fruit 0.7—6 ppm

■ PLUM

Chemical Constituents of Prunus domestica L. (Rosaceae)

4-0-METHYL-GLUCURONIC-ACID Fruit
ALANINE Fruit 290—1,959 ppm
ALPHA-TOCOPHEROL Fruit 8—62 ppm
ALUMINUM Fruit 1 - 255 ppm
ARGININE Fruit 130—878 ppm
ARSENIC Fruit 0.001—0.51 ppm
ASCORBIC-ACID Fruit 86—699 ppm
ASH Fruit 3,810—170,000 ppm
ASPARTIC-ACID Fruit 2,490—16,824 ppm
BARIUM Fruit 0.154—25.5 ppm
BETA-CAROTENE Fruit 1.4—43 ppm
BORON Fruit 1—255 ppm
BROMINE Fruit
CADMIUM Fruit 0.001—0.068 ppm
CAFFEIC-ACID Plant
CALCIUM Fruit 38—2,040 ppm
CARBOHYDRATES Fruit 130,100—879,054 ppm
CHLOROGENIC-ACID Fruit
CHROMIUM Fruit 0.005—1.19 ppm
CITRIC-ACID Fruit
COBALT Fruit 0.005—0.34 ppm
COPPER Fruit 0.33—34 ppm
CRYPTOCHLOROGENIC-ACID Fruit
CYANIDIN Plant
CYSTINE Fruit 40—270 ppm
D-GALACTOSE Fruit
D-MANNOSE Fruit
D-XYLOSE Fruit
FAT Fruit 6,000—43,243 ppm
FERULIC-ACID Fruit
FIBER Fruit 6,000—40,540 ppm
FLUORINE Fruit 0.1—0.6 ppm
FOLACIN Fruit 0.019—0.167 ppm
FRUCTOSE 27,000—61,000 ppm
GLUCOSE Fruit 30,000—62,000 ppm
GLUTAMIC-ACID Fruit 370—2,500 ppm
GLYCINE Fruit 120—811 ppm
HEXURONIC-ACID Resin Exudate Sap
HISTIDINE Fruit 130—878 ppm
IRON Fruit 0.8—85 ppm

ISOCHLOROGENIC-ACID Fruit
ISOLEUCINE Fruit 160—1,081 ppm
KILOCALORIES Fruit 550—3,716/kg
LANTHANUM Fruit 1.5—12 ppm
LINOLEIC-ACID Fruit 1,340—9,054 ppm
LITHIUM Fruit 0.088—0.68 ppm
LUTEIN Fruit 2.4—24 ppm
LYSINE Fruit 170—1,149 ppm
MAGNESIUM Fruit 68—3,400 ppm
MALIC-ACID Fruit 15,000 ppm
MANGANESE Fruit 0.22—25.5 ppm
MERCURY Fruit 0—0.013 ppm
METHIONINE Fruit 60—405 ppm
MOLYBDENUM Fruit 0.1—1.7 ppm
MUFA Fruit 4,060—27,432 ppm
NEOCHLOROGENIC-ACID Fruit
NIACIN Fruit 5—34 ppm
NICKEL Fruit 0.03—1.7 ppm
NITROGEN Fruit 960—10,000 ppm
OLEIC-ACID Fruit 4,000—27,027 ppm
P-COUMARIC-ACID Fruit
PALMITIC-ACID Fruit 410—2,770 ppm
PALMITOLEIC-ACID Fruit 50—338 ppm
PANTOTHENIC-ACID Fruit 1.8—13 ppm
PECTIN Fruit 8,000—40,000 ppm
PERSICAXANTHIN Plant
PHENYLALANINE Fruit 170—1,149 ppm
PHOSPHORUS Fruit 70—4,080 ppm
POTASSIUM Fruit 1,677—44,200 ppm
PROLINE Fruit 340—2,297 ppm
PROTEIN Fruit 7,660—55,000 ppm
PUFA Fruit 1,340—9,054 ppm
QUERCETIN Plant
QUINIC-ACID Fruit
RHAMNOSE Fruit
RIBOFLAVIN Fruit 0.9—6.5 ppm
RUBIDIUM Fruit 0.5—15 ppm
SELENIUM Fruit 0—0.013 ppm
SERINE Fruit 200—1,351 ppm
SEROTONIN Fruit
SFA Fruit 490—3,310 ppm
SILICON Fruit 2—62 ppm
SILVER Fruit 0.022—0.51 ppm
SODIUM Fruit 0—54 ppm
STEARIC-ACID Fruit 90—608 ppm
STRONTIUM Fruit 0.33—51 ppm

SUCCINIC-ACID Fruit
SUCROSE Fruit 7,000—48,000 ppm
SUGAR Fruit 100,000—200,000 ppm
SULFUR Fruit 4—400 ppm
TARTARIC-ACID Fruit
THIAMIN Fruit 0.4—2.9 ppm
THREONINE Fruit 160—1,081 ppm
TITANIUM Fruit 0.11—25.5 ppm
TRYPTAMINE Fruit
TYRAMINE Fruit
TYROSINE Fruit 60—405 ppm
VALINE Fruit 190—1,284 ppm
VITAMIN B6 Fruit 0.7—6 ppm
WATER Fruit 840,000—933,000 ppm
ZINC Fruit 0.66—131 ppm
ZIRCONIUM Fruit 0.44—3.4 ppm

■ POMEGRANATE

Chemical Constituents of Punica granatum L.
(Punicaceae)

ARACHIDIC-ACID Seed
ASCORBIC-ACID Fruit 40—636 ppm
ASH Fruit 5,000—35,858 ppm
BORIC-ACID Fruit 50 ppm
CALCIUM Fruit 30—650 ppm
CALCIUM-OXALATE Petiole 40,000 ppm
CARBOHYDRATES Fruit 162,000—927,000
  ppm
CAROTENE Fruit 0—2 ppm
CASUARININ Plant
CEREBROSIDE Seed
CHLOROGENIC-ACID Fruit
CIS-9, TRANS-11, CIS-13-TRIENE-ACID
  Seed
CITRIC-ACID Fruit Juice 8,100—12,300 ppm
COPPER Fruit 2 ppm
CYANIDIN-3,5-DIGLUCOSIDE Fruit
CYANIDIN-3-GLUCOSIDE Fruit
D-MANNITOL Seed
DELPHINIDIN-3,5-DIGLUCOSIDE Pericarp
DELPHINIDIN-3-GLUCOSIDE Fruit
ELAIDIC-ACID Pericarp 5,500 ppm
ESTRADIOL Seed

ESTRONE Seed 17 ppm
FAT Fruit 1,000—38,000 ppm
FAT Seed 50,000—200,000 ppm
FIBER Fruit 2,000—232,000 ppm
FIBER Seed 224,000 ppm
FLAVOGALLOL Pericarp
FRUCTOSE Fruit
GALLIC-ACID Pericarp 900—40,000 ppm
GLUCOSE Fruit
GRANATIN-A Pericarp
GRANATIN-B Pericarp
GUM Petiole 32,000 ppm
INULIN Petiole 10,000 ppm
IRON Fruit 3—16 ppm
ISOQUERCETRIN Pericarp
LINOLEIC-ACID Seed
MAGNESIUM Fruit 120 ppm
MALIC-ACID Fruit
MALTOSE Fruit
MALVIDIN Fruit
MALVIDIN-PENTOSE-GLYCOSIDE Fruit
 Juice
MANNITOL Pericarp 18,000 ppm
MUCILAGE Petiole 6,000—340,000 ppm
NEOCHLOROGENIC-ACID Fruit
NIACIN Fruit 3—50 ppm
OLEIC-ACID Seed
OXALIC-ACID Fruit 140 ppm
P-COUMARIC-ACID Fruit
PALMITIC-ACID Seed
PANTOTHENIC-ACID Fruit 6—31 ppm
PECTIN Fruit 2,700 ppm
PECTIN Pericarp 20,000—40,000 ppm
PELARGONIDIN-3-GLUCOSIDE Seed
PHOSPHATIDYLCHOLINE Seed
PHOSPHATIDYLINOSITOL Seed
PHOSPHATIDYLSERINE Seed
PHOSPHORUS Fruit 80—3,182 ppm
PHYTOSTEROLS Fruit 170—892 ppm
POLYPHENOLS Fruit 2,200—10,500 ppm
POTASSIUM Fruit 1,330—18,950 ppm
PROTEIN Fruit 7,700—73,000 ppm
PROTEIN Seed 25,000 ppm
PROTOCATECHUIC-ACID Fruit
PUNICALAGIN Pericarp
PUNICALIN Pericarp

PUNICIC-ACID Seed 35,000—140,000 ppm
RESINS Pericarp 45,000 ppm
RIBOFLAVIN Fruit 0—4 ppm
SODIUM Fruit 9—350 ppm
SORBITOL Plant
STARCH Seed
STEARIC-ACID Seed
SULFUR Fruit 120 ppm
TANNIN Fruit Juice 1,700 ppm
TANNIN Pericarp 104,000—336,000 ppm
THIAMIN Fruit 0—4 ppm
URSOLIC-ACID Fruit
VITAMIN B6 Fruit 1—5 ppm
WATER Fruit 780,000—823,220 ppm
WATER Seed 350,000 ppm
WAX Pericarp 8,000 ppm

■ QUINCE

Chemical Constituents of Cydonia oblonga
(Rosaceae)

ALDOBIONIC-ACID Seed
AMYGDALIN Seed 4,000 ppm
ASCORBIC-ACID Fruit 100—960 ppm
ASH Fruit 3,000 ppm
ASH Seed 13,000 ppm
BETA-CAROTENE Fruit 0—16 ppm
BORON Fruit 85—160 ppm
CALCIUM Fruit 60—805 ppm
CARBOHYDRATES Fruit 119,000—951,000
 ppm
CELLULOSE Seed
CHLOROGENIC-ACID Fruit
EMULSIN Seed
FAT Fruit 1,000—17,000 ppm
FAT Seed 140,000—192,000 ppm
FERULIC-ACID Fruit
FIBER Fruit 17,000—178,000 ppm
FRUCTOSE Fruit
GALACTOSE Seed
GLUCOSE Fruit
IRON Fruit 6—52 ppm
ISOCHLOROGENIC-ACID Fruit
L-ARABINOSE Seed

LEUCOANTHOCYANIDINE Fruit
LINOLEIC-ACID Seed
LINOLENIC-ACID Seed
MALIC-ACID Seed
MARMELOLACTONE-A Plant
MARMELOLACTONE-B Plant
MUCILAGE Seed 200,000—220,000 ppm
MYRISTIC-ACID Seed
NEOCHLOROGENIC-ACID Fruit
NIACIN Fruit 2—22 ppm
OLEIC-ACID Seed
P-COUMARIC-ACID Fruit
PECTIN Fruit
PHOSPHORUS Fruit 150—1,049 ppm
POTASSIUM Fruit 1,970—12,160 ppm
PROTEIN Fruit 3,000 ppm
PROTOPECTIN Fruit
RIBOFLAVIN Fruit 0.3—1.9 ppm
ROSEOSIDE Plant
SACCHAROSIDE Fruit
SODIUM Fruit 247 ppm
SUGARS Fruit 96,000 ppm
TANNIN Seed
TARTARIC-ACID Seed
THIAMIN Fruit 0.2—1.9 ppm
WATER Fruit 824,000—857,000 ppm

■ RED RASBERRY

Chemical Constituents of Rubus idaeus L. (Rosaceae)

1-PENTANOL Fruit
1-PENTEN-3-OL Plant
2-HEXEN-4-OLIDE Plant
3-METHYL-2-BUTEN-1-OL Plant
5-METHYL-FURFURAL Fruit
ACETIC-ACID Plant
ACETOIN Fruit
ALPHA-CAROTENE Fruit 0.13—0.6 ppm
ALPHA-FURANCARBONIC-ACID Plant
ALPHA-TOCOPHEROL Fruit 9—56 ppm
ALUMINUM Leaf 392 ppm
ASCORBIC-ACID Leaf 3,670 ppm
ASCORBIC-ACID Seed 300 ppm

ASH Leaf 80,000 ppm
BENZALDEHYDE Plant
BENZOIC-ACID Plant
BETA-CAROTENE Fruit 0.06—0.3 ppm
BETA-CAROTENE Leaf 114 ppm
BETA-IONONE Plant
BETA-PHENYLETHYLALCOHOL Fruit
BORON Fruit 1—13 ppm
BUTRYIC-ACID Fruit
CAFFEIC-ACID Fruit
CALCIUM Leaf 12,100 ppm
CAPRONIC-ACID Fruit
CAPRYLIC-ACID Fruit
CARBOHYDRATES Leaf 790,000 ppm
CHROMIUM Leaf 13 ppm
CINNAMYL-ALCOHOL Plant
CIS-HEXEN-3-OL Plant
COBALT Leaf 34 ppm
CYANIDIN-3-GLUCOSIDE Plant
CYANIDIN-3-GLUCOSYLRUTINOSIDE
    Plant
CYANIDIN-3-RUTINOSIDE Plant
CYANIDIN-3-SOPHOROSIDE Plant
CYANIDIN-5-MONOGLYCOSIDE Plant
CYANIN Fruit
DAMASCENE Plant
DEXTROSE Fruit 35,000 ppm
DIACETYL Fruit
DIHYDRO-BETA-IONONE Plant
ELLAGIC-ACID Leaf
EPOXY-BETA-IONONE Plant
ETHANOL Plant
ETHYL-ACETATE Plant
FARNESOL Plant
FAT Leaf 17,000 ppm
FAT Seed 145,000—240,000 ppm
FERULIC-ACID Fruit
FIBER Leaf 82,000 ppm
FORMIC-ACID Fruit
FURFURAL Fruit
GALLIC-ACID Leaf
GERANIOL Fruit
HEXEN-2-ACID Fruit
HEXEN-3-ACID Fruit
IRON Leaf 1,010 ppm
ISOAMYL-ALCOHOL Fruit

ISOBUTYRIC-ACID Fruit
ISOVALERIANIC-ACID Fruit
KAEMPFEROL-3-BETA-GLUCURONIDE
Plant
KILOCALORIES Leaf 2,750/kg
LACTIC-ACID Leaf
LEVULOSE Fruit 35,000 ppm
LUTEIN Fruit 0.76—4 ppm
MAGNESIUM Leaf 3,190 ppm
MALIC-ACID Fruit
MALTOL Fruit
MANGANESE Fruit 16—18 ppm
MANGANESE Leaf 146 ppm
NIACIN Leaf
O-PHTHALIC-ACID Plant
ORGANIC-ACIDS Plant 15,000—20,000 ppm
OXYBENZOIC-ACID Fruit
P-CRESOL Plant
P-ETHEYL-PHENOL Plant
P-HYDROXYPHENYLETHYLALCOHOL
Plant
PECTIN Fruit 14,500 ppm
PELARGONIN-3,2-
GLUCOSYLRUTINOSIDE Fruit
PELARGONIN-3,5-DIGLYCOSIDE Fruit
PHOSPHORUS Leaf 2,340 ppm
POTASSIUM Leaf 13,400 ppm
PROPIONIC-ACID Fruit
PROTEIN Leaf 113,000 ppm
QUERCETIN-3-BETA-GLUCURONIDE Plant
RIBOFLAVIN Leaf
SALICYCLIC-ACID Fruit
SELENIUM Leaf
SILICON Leaf 13 ppm
SODIUM Leaf 77 ppm
SUCCINIC-ACID Fruit
SUCCINIC-ACID Leaf
TANNIN Fruit 6,200 ppm
TANNIN Leaf 100,000—120,000 ppm
THEASPIRANE Plant
THIAMIN Leaf 3.4 ppm
TRANS-2-PHENYLBUTANONE Plant
VALERIANIC-ACID Fruit
WATER Leaf 831,000 ppm
ZINC Leaf

■ STRAWBERRY

Chemical Constituents of Fragaria spp (Rosaceae)

ALANINE Fruit 310—3,677 ppm
ALPHA-LINOLENIC-ACID Fruit 780—9,253
ppm
ALPHA-TOCOPHEROL Fruit 1—54 ppm
ALUMINUM Fruit 3—70 ppm
ARGININE Fruit 260—3,084 ppm
ARSENIC Fruit
ASCORBIC-ACID Fruit 400—6,948 ppm
ASH Fruit 3,900—52,065 ppm
ASPARTIC-ACID Fruit 1,380—16,370 ppm
BETA-CAROTENE Fruit 0.089—7 ppm
BORON Fruit 1—160 ppm
BROMINE Fruit
CADMIUM Fruit 0.004—0.18 ppm
CAFFEIC-ACID Fruit 15—34 ppm
CALCIUM Fruit 135—2,900 ppm
CARBOHYDRATES Fruit 70,200—850,000
ppm
CATECHIN Fruit
CATECHOL Fruit
CHLOROGENIC-ACID Fruit
CHROMIUM Fruit 0.005—0.18 ppm
CITRIC-ACID Fruit 3,500—8,000 ppm
COBALT Fruit 0.004—2 ppm
COPPER Fruit 0.4—17 ppm
CYSTINE Fruit 50—593 ppm
ELLAGIC-ACID Fruit 430—8,430 ppm
ELLAGIC-ACID Seed 1,370—21,650 ppm
FAT Fruit 2,350—59,893 ppm
FAT Seed 190,000 ppm
FIBER Fruit 5,300—181,000 ppm
FLUORINE Fruit 0.03—0.9 ppm
FOLACIN Fruit 0.1—0.2 ppm
GALLIC-ACID Fruit 80—121 ppm
GALLOCATECHIN Fruit
GENTISIC-ACID Fruit
GLUTAMIC-ACID Fruit 900—10,676 ppm
GLYCINE Fruit 240—2,847 ppm
HISTIDINE Fruit 120—1,423 ppm
IRON Fruit 3—100 ppm
ISOLEUCINE Fruit 140—1,661 ppm

KAEMPFEROL-3-BETA-
MONOGLUCOSIDE Fruit
KEAMPFEROL-7-MONOGLUCOSIDE Fruit
KILOCALORIES Fruit 300—3,559/kg
LECITHIN Fruit 620 ppm
LEUCINE Fruit 310—3,667 ppm
LINOLEIC-ACID Fruit 1,080—12,811 ppm
LINOLEIC-ACID Seed 153,900 ppm
LINOLENIC-ACID Seed 9,975 ppm
LUTEIN Fruit 0.3—3 ppm
LYSINE Fruit 250—2,966 ppm
MAGNESIUM Fruit 98—1,545 ppm
MALIC-ACID Fruit 3,500—8,000 ppm
MALVIDIN-3,5-DIGLUCOSIDE Fruit
MANGANESE Fruit 1.4—125 ppm
MERCURY Fruit 0—0.009 ppm
METHIONINE Fruit 10—119 ppm
METHYL-FURFURAL Plant
MOLYBDENUM Fruit
MUFA Fruit 520—6,168 ppm
NEOCHLOROGENIC-ACID Fruit
NIACIN Fruit 2.3—27 ppm
NICKEL Fruit 0.03—0.36 ppm
NICOTINIC-ACID Plant 2 ppm
NITROGEN Fruit 880—10,000 ppm
OLEIC-ACID Fruit 510—6,050 ppm
OLEIC-ACID Seed 9,975 ppm
P-COUMARIC-ACID Fruit 63—125 ppm
P-HYDROXUYBENZOIC-ACID Fruit 19—
108 ppm
PALMITIC-ACID Fruit 140—1,661 ppm
PALMITOLEIC-ACID Fruit 10—119 ppm
PANTOTHENIC-ACID Fruit 3.4—40 ppm
PECTIN Fruit 5,400 ppm
PELARGONIDIN-3-MONOGLUCOSIDE
Fruit
PHOSPHORUS Fruit 185—3,191 ppm
PHYTOSTEROLS Fruit 120—1,423 ppm
PROLINE Fruit 190—1,898 ppm
PROTEIN Fruit 5,840—85,000 ppm
PROTOCATECHUIC-ACID Fruit
PUFA Fruit 1,860—22,064 ppm
QUERCETIN-3-BETA-GLUCURONIDE Fruit
QUERCETIN-3-BETA-MONOGLUCOSIDE
Fruit
RIBOFLAVIN Fruit 0.7—8 ppm

RUBIDIUM Fruit 0.2—6.5 ppm
SALICYLIC-ACID Fruit
SELENIUM Fruit 0.002 ppm
SERINE Fruit 230—2,728 ppm
SFA Fruit 200—2,372 ppm
SILICON Fruit 10—270 ppm
SODIUM Fruit 8—106 ppm
STEARIC-ACID Fruit 40—475 ppm
SULFUR Fruit 77—1,270 ppm
THIAMIN Fruit 0.2—4 ppm
THREONINE Fruit 190—2,254 ppm
TRYPTOPHAN Fruit 70—830 ppm
VALINE Fruit 180—2,135 ppm
VANILLIC-ACID Fruit 3—25 ppm
VITAMIN B6 Fruit 0.6—7 ppm
WATER Fruit 870,000—917,000 ppm
ZINC Fruit 1.1—17 ppm

■ STRAWBERRY GUAVA

Chemical Constituents of Psidium Cattleianum
(Myrtaceae)

ALANINE Fruit 290—1,500 ppm
ARGININE Fruit 150—775 ppm
ASCORBIC-ACID Fruit 150—2,100 ppm
ASH Fruit 5,000—44,000 ppm
ASPARTIC-ACID Fruit 370—1,915 ppm
BETA-CAROTENE Fruit 0—9 ppm
CALCIUM Fruit 210—3,400 ppm
CARBOHYDRATES Fruit 145,000—939,000
ppm
CYANIDIN Plant
ELLAGIC-ACID Plant
FAT Fruit 3,000—33,000 ppm
FIBER Fruit 52,000—352,000
GLUTAMIC-ACID Fruit 760—3,930 ppm
GLYCINE Fruit 290—1,500 ppm
HISTIDINE Fruit 50—260 ppm
IRON Fruit 2—82 ppm
ISOLEUCINE Fruit 210—1,085 ppm
KAEMPFEROL Plant
KILOCALORIES Fruit 560—3,570 ppm
LEUCINE Fruit 390—-2,015 ppm
LINOLEIC-ACID Fruit 1,820—9,410 ppm

LINOLENIC-ACID Fruit 710—3,670 ppm
LYSINE Fruit 160—825 ppm
MAGNESIUM 170—880 ppm
METHIONINE Fruit 40—205 ppm
MUFA Fruit 550—2,845 ppm
MYRISTIC-ACID Fruit 120—620 ppm
NIACIN Fruit 3—38 ppm
OLEIC-ACID Fruit 520—2,690 ppm
PALMITIC-ACID Fruit 1,440—7,445 ppm
PHENYLALANINE Fruit 10—50 ppm
PHOSPHORUS Fruit 170—2,305 ppm
POTASSIUM Fruit 2,890—15,880 ppm
PROLINE Fruit 180—930 ppm
PROTEIN Fruit 4,000—55,000 ppm
PUFA Fruit 2,530—13,080 ppm
QUERCETIN Plant
RIBOFLAVIN Fruit 0.2—1.9 ppm
SERINE Fruit 170—880 ppm
SFA Fruit 1,720—8,900 ppm
SODIUM Fruit 40—1,915 ppm
STEARIC-ACID Fruit 160—825 ppm
THIAMIN Fruit 0.2—1.9 ppm
THREONINE Fruit 220—1,140 ppm
TRYPTOPHAN Fruit 50—260 ppm
TYROSINE Fruit 70—360 ppm
VALINE Fruit 200—1,035 ppm
WATER Fruit 783,200—843,000 ppm

■ STRAWBERRY PEAR

Chemical Constituents of Hylocerues undatus (Cactaceae)

ASCORBIC-ACID Fruit 80—515 ppm
ASH Fruit 6,000—38,460 ppm
BETA-CAROTENE Fruit
CALCIUM Fruit 100—640 ppm
CARBOHYDRATES Fruit 43,300—846,150 ppm
FAT Fruit 1,700—25,640 ppm
FIBER Fruit 11,200—141,025 ppm
IRON Fruit 13—83 ppm
KILOCALORIES Fruit 540—3,460 ppm
NIACIN Fruit 3—19 ppm
PHOSPHORUS Fruit 260—1,665 ppm

PROTEIN Fruit 4,800—89,745 ppm
RIBOFLAVIN Fruit 0.4—2.6 ppm
THIAMIN Fruit 0.4—2.6 ppm
WATER Fruit 844,000—922,000 ppm

■ SUGAR APPLE

Chemical Constituents of Annona squamosa L. (Annonceae)

ANNONACIN Seed
ANNONACIN-A Seed
ANNONASTATIN Seed
ANNONIN-I Seed
ANNONIN-VI Seed
ANOLOBINE Root
ANONAINE Seed
ARGININE Fruit
ASCORBIC-ACID Fruit 340—1,600 ppm
ASH Fruit 7,000—40,000 ppm
ASIMCIN Seed
CALCIUM Fruit 216—1,335 ppm
CAMPHOR Plant
CARBOYDRATES Fruit 200,000—904,000 ppm
CITRULLINE Fruit
FAT Fruit 2,000 21,000 ppm
FAT Seed 140,000—490,000
FIBER Fruit 12,000—71,000 ppm
FRUCTOSE Fruit
GABA Fruit
GLUCOSE Fruit 72,900—272,500 ppm
IRON Fruit 6—66 ppm
KILOCALORIES Fruit 780—3,530/kg
LIMONENE Plant
LYSINE Fruit 550—2,055 ppm
MAGNESIUM Fruit 210—785 ppm
METHIONINE Fruit 70—260 ppm
NEOANNON Seed
NIACIN Fruit 8—36 ppm
ORNITHINE Fruit
PANTOTHENIC-ACID fruit 2—8 ppm
PHOSPHORUS Fruit 260—1,600 ppm
POTASSIUM Fruit 2,200—13,290
PROTEIN Fruit 14,000—86,590 ppm

RIBOFLAVIN Fruit 1—5 ppm
SODIUM Fruit 50—457 ppm
SQUAMOCIN Seed
SUCROSE Fruit 72,900—272,500 ppm
SUGAR Fruit 145,800 ppm
THIAMIN Fruit 1—5 ppm
TRYPTOPHAN Fruit 100—375 ppm
VITAMIN B6 Fruit 2—8 ppm
WATER Fruit 728,000—775,000 ppm

■ WATERMELON

Chemical Constituents of Citrullus lanatus (Cucurbitaceae)

ALANINE Fruit 2,000 ppm
ALANINE Seed 15,000 ppm
ARGININE Fruit 6,949 ppm
ARGININE Seed 46,600 ppm
ASH Fruit 30,600 ppm
ASH Seed 62,000 ppm
ASPARTIC-ACID Fruit 4,594 ppm
ASPARTIC-ACID Seed 25,500 ppm
BETA-CAROTENE Fruit 2—48 ppm
BORON Fruit 1—4 ppm
CALCIUM Fruit 100—3,400 ppm
CALCIUM Seed 1,294—1,300 ppm
CAPRIC-ACID Seed 2,200—4,840 ppm
CAPRYLIC-ACID Seed 400—880 ppm
CARBOHYDRATES Fruit 3,800—859,000 ppm
CARBOHYDRATES Seed 44,000—48,000 ppm
CIS,CIS-3,6-NONADIEN-1-OL Fruit
CITRULLIC-ACID Plant
CITRULLINE Fruit 1,627 ppm
CITRULLOL Fruit
COPPER Fruit 4 ppm
CUCURBITACIN-E Fruit
CYSTEINE Fruit 236 ppm
CYSTEINE Seed 5,742 ppm
FAT Fruit 200—89,000 ppm
FAT Seed 200,000—571,000 ppm
FIBER Fruit 35,300—257,000 ppm
FIBER Seed 67,000—316,000 ppm

FOLACIN Fruit 0.259 ppm
GLOBULIN Seed
GLUTAMIC-ACID Fruit 7,420 ppm
GLUTAMIC-ACID Seed 53,000 ppm
GLUTELIN Seed
GLYCINE Fruit 1,178 ppm
HENTRIACONTANE Fruit
HISTIDINE Fruit 707 ppm
HISTIDINE Seed 7,018 ppm
HYDROXYPROLINE Fruit
IRON Fruit 2—143 ppm
IRON Seed 75 ppm
ISOLEUCINE Fruit 2,238 ppm
ISOLEUCINE Seed 12,100 ppm
KILOCALORIES Fruit 3,513/kg
KILOCALORIES Seed 6,500/kg
L-(+)-ISOLEUCINE Plant
L-(-)-PHENYLALANINE Plant
L-(-)-THREONINE Plant
L-(-)-TYROSINE Plant
L-BETA-(PYRAZOL-1-YL)-ALANINE Fruit
L-BETA-(PYRAZOL-1-YL)-ALANINE Seed
L-GLUTAMIC-ACID Seed
LAURIC-ACID Seed 1,600—3,250 ppm
LEUCINE Fruit 2,210 ppm
LEUCINE Seed 21,100 ppm
LINOLEIC-ACID Seed 52,000—210,280 ppm
LUTEIN Fruit 0.14—3 ppm
LYCOPENE Fruit 45—900 ppm
LYSINE Fruit 7,303 ppm
LYSINE Seed 8,932 ppm
MAGNESIUM Fruit 1,081—1,500 ppm
MANGANESE Fruit 4 ppm
METHIONINE Fruit 707 ppm
METHIONINE Seed 5,742 ppm
MYRISTIC-ACID 400—800 ppm
N-COTACOSANOL Fruit
NEOLYCOPENE Fruit
NEUROSPORIN Fruit
NIACIN Fruit 15—27 ppm
OLEIC-ACID Seed 71,000—189,000 ppm
OXYSILVINE Seed
PALMITIC-ACID Seed 15,200—55,000 ppm
PANTOTHENIC-ACID Fruit 25 ppm
PECTIN Fruit
PHENYLALANINE Fruit 1,767 ppm

PHENYLALANINE Seed 16,600 ppm
PHOSPHORUS Fruit 1—2,900 ppm
PHOSPHORUS Seed 8,300—14,600 ppm
PHYSETOLIC-ACID Plant
PHYTOFLUIN Fruit
PHYTOIN Fruit
PHYTOSTEROLS Fruit 236 ppm
POLY-CIS-LYCOPENE Fruit
POTASSIUM Fruit 13,514—18,000 ppm
PRO-BETA-CAROTENE Fruit
PROLINE Fruit 2,827 ppm
PROLINE Seed 11,800 ppm
PRONEUROSPORIN Fruit
PROTEIN Fruit 1,000—100,000 ppm
PROTEIN Seed 198,000—343,000 ppm
RIBOFLAVIN Fruit 2—8 ppm
RIBOFLAVIN Seed 1 ppm
SERINE Fruit 1,885 ppm
SERINE Seed 13,700 ppm
SODIUM Fruit 135—236 ppm
STEARIC-ACID Seed 12,200—66,000 ppm
THIAMIN Fruit 4—9 ppm
THREONINE Fruit 3,180 ppm
THREONINE Seed 15,300 ppm
TRYPTOPHAN Fruit 825 ppm
TYROSINE Fruit 1,413 ppm
TYROSINE Seed 10,200 ppm
UREASE Seed
VALINE Fruit 1,885 ppm
VALINE Seed 10,200 ppm
WATER Fruit 915,100—957,000 ppm
WATER Seed 71,000—81,000 ppm
ZINC Fruit 8 ppm

■ YELLOW PLUM

Chemical Constituents of Spondias pinnata L. (Anacardiaceae)

ASCORBIC-ACID Fruit 210—2,165 ppm
ASH Fruit 5,000—52,000 ppm
BETA-CAROTENE Fruit 2—28 ppm
CALCIUM Fruit 360—3,170 ppm
CARBOHYDRATES Fruit 55,000—567,000 ppm
FAT Fruit 30,000—309,000 ppm
FIBER Fruit 10,000—103,000 ppm
FRUCTOSE Fruit 18,000 ppm
GLUCOSE Fruit 17,000 ppm
IODINE Fruit 0.04—0.61 ppm
IRON Fruit 39—400 ppm
KILOCALORIES Fruit 218—4,180/kg
NIACIN Fruit 3—31 ppm
PHOSPHORUS Fruit 110—1,135 ppm
POTASSIUM Fruit
PROTEIN Fruit 7,000—72,000 ppm
RIBOFLAVIN Fruit 0.2—2.1 ppm
SODIUM Fruit
SUCROSE Fruit 29,000 ppm
THIAMIN Fruit 0.2—2.1 ppm
WATER Fruit 903,000 ppm

VEGETABLE/PHYTOCHEMICALS

■ ALFALFA

Chemical Constituents of Medicago sativa L. (Fabaceae)

11,12-DIMETHYOXY-7-HYDROXYCOUMESTIN Plant
1-METHYLPROPANOL Essential Oil
3'-METHOXYCOUMESTROL Plant
3-METHYLBUTANOL Essential Oil
4-0-METHYLCOUMESTROL Plant
4-AMINO-BUTYRIC-ACID Root
ACETONE Essential Oil
ADENINE Plant
ADENOSINE Plant
ALFALFONE Plant
ALPHA-SPINASTEROL Plant
ALPHA-TOCOPHEROL Plant 26—257 ppm
ALUMINUM Plant 135 ppm
AMYLASE Plant
ARABINOSE Plant
ASCORBIC-ACID Plant 1,470—9,364 ppm
ASH Plant 14,000—100,000 ppm
ASH Seed 44,000—49,830 ppm
BETA-CAROTENE Leaf 0.06—394 ppm
BETA-SITOSTEROL Plant
BETAINE Plant
BIOCHANIN-A Plant
BIOTIN Plant 0.18 ppm
BORON Leaf 25 ppm
BORON Plant 17—45 ppm
BORON Stem 14 ppm

BUTANONE Essential Oil
CALCIUM Plant 120—17,200 ppm
CAMPESTEROL Plant
CARBOHYDRATES Plant 95,000—717,000 ppm
CARBOHYDRATES Seed 401,000—454,135 ppm
CHLOROPHYLLIDE-A Plant
CHOLINE Plant
CHROMIUM Plant 9 ppm
CITRIC-ACID Plant
COAGULASE Plant
COBALT Plant 115 ppm
COUMESTROL Plant
CRYPTOXANTHIN Plant
CYCLOARTENOL Plant
CYTIDINE Plant
DAIDZEN Plant
DAPHNORETIN Plant
EREPSIN Plant
FAT Plant 4,000—43,000 ppm
FAT Seed 101,000—123,000 ppm
FIBER Plant 31,000—423,000 ppm
FIBER Seed 81,000—91,732 ppm
FOLACIN Plant
FORMONONETIN Plant
FRUCTOSE Plant
FUMARIC-ACID Plant
GENISTEIN Leaf
GENISTEIN Plant
GUANINE Plant
GUANOSINE Plant
HEDERAGENIN Plant
HENTRIACONTANE Plant

HYDROGEN-CYANIDE Plant
HYPOXANTHINE Plant
INOSINE Plant
INOSITOL Plant
INVERTASE Plant
IRON Plant 54—333 ppm
ISOCYTOSINE Plant
L-HOMOSTACHYDRINE Seed
L-STACHYDRINE Hay 1,400 ppm
LIMONENE Essential Oil
LUCERNOL Plant
LUTEIN Plant
MAGENSIUM Plant 2,300—4,400 ppm
MALIC-ACID Plant
MANGANESE Plant 25.3 ppm
MEDICAGENIC-ACID Plant
MEICAGOL Plant
MOLYBDENUM Leaf 0.028 ppm
MOLYBDENUM Stem 0.015 ppm
MYRISTONE Plant
NEOXANTHIN Plant
NIACIN Plant
OCTACOSANOL Plant
OXALIC Plant
PANTOTHENIC Plant
PECTIN Plant
PECTINASE Plant
PENTANAL Essential Oil
PEROXIDASE Plant
PHAEOPHORBIDE-A Plant
PHOSPHORUS Plant 510—3,100 ppm
POTASSIUM Plant 12,000—20,300 ppm
PROPANAL Plant
PROTEIN Leaf 60,000—347,000 ppm
PROTEIN Seed 332,000—385,000 ppm
PYRIDOXINE Plant
QUINIC-ACID Plant
RIBOFLAVIN Plant 1.4—16.1 ppm
RIBOSE Plant
SAPONIN Plant 5,000—20,000 ppm
SATIVOL Plant
SELENIUM Leaf 0.026 ppm
SELENIUM Plant
SELENIUM Stem 0.015 ppm
SHIKIMIC-ACID Plant
SILICON Plant

SODIUM Plant 170 ppm
SOYASAPOGENOLS Plant
STACHYDRINE Seed
STARCH Plant 30,000—80,000 ppm
STIGMASTEROL Plant
SUCCINIC-ACID Plant
SUCROSE Plant
TANNIN Hay 27,000—28,000 ppm
THIAMIN Plant 1.3—7.5 ppm
TIN Plant
TRIACONTANOL Plant
TRICIN Plant
TRIFOLIOL Plant
TRIGONELLINE Plant
TIMETHYLAMINE Plant
TRYPTOPHAN Plant
VIOLAXANTHIN Plant
VITAMIN E Plant
VITAMIN K Plant
WATER Plant 812,000—827,000 ppm
XANTHOPHYLLS Plant
XYLOSE Plant
ZEAXANTHIN Plant
ZINC Plant

■ ARTICHOKE

Chemical Constituents of Cynara scolymus L. (Asteraceae)

1,3-DI-O-CAFFEOYLQUINIC-ACID Flower
1,4-DICAFFEOYLQUINIC-ACID Flower
1,5-DI-O-CAFFEOYLQUINIC-ACID Flower
1-CAFFEOYLQUINIC-ACID Flower
3-CAFFEOYLQUINIC-ACID Flower
4-CAFFEOYLQUINIC-ACID Flower
5-CAFFEOYLQUINIC-ACID Flower
ASCORBIC-ACID Flower 0—828 ppm
ASH Flower 10,600—106,000 ppm
BETA-CAROTENE Flower 1—20 ppm
BETA-SELINEENE Essential Oil
BORON Flower 2—5 ppm
CAFFEIC-ACID Flower
CAFFEOYL-4-QUINIC-ACID Flower
CALCIUM Flower 120—5,286 ppm

CARBOHYDRATES Flower 105,000—755,000 ppm
CARYOPHYLLENE Essential Oil
CHLOROGENIC-ACID Flower
COPPER Flower 2—24 ppm
CYANIDOL-3-CAFFEYLGLUCOSIDE Plant
CYANIDOL-3-CAFFEYLSOPHOROSIDE Plant
CYANIDOL-5-GLUCOSIDE-3-CAFFEYLSOPHOROSIDE Plant
CYANIDOL-DICAFFEYLSOPHOROSIDE Plant
CYANIDOL-GLUCOSIDE Plant
CYANIDOL-SOPHORISIDE Plant
CYNARATRIOL Flower
CYNAROLIDE Plant
DECANAL Essential Oil
EUGENOL Essential Oil
FAT Flower 1,000—20,000 ppm
FERULIC-ACID Plant
FIBER Flower 11,400—224,000 ppm
FLAVONOIDS Flower 1,000—10,000 ppm
FOLACIN Flower 0.7—4.7 ppm
GLYCERIC-ACID Flower
GLYCOLIC-ACID Flower
HETEROSIDE-B Flower
HEX-1-EN-3-ONE Flower
INULIN Flower
IRON Flower 11—101 ppm
ISOAMERBOIN Plant
KILOCALORIES Flower 470—3,120/kg
LAURIC-ACID Flower 20—135 ppm
LINOLEIC-ACID Flower 460—3,055 ppm
LINOLENIC-ACID Flower 170—1,130 ppm
LUTEOLIN-4-BETA-D-GLUCOSIDE Flower
LUTEOLIN-7-BETA-D-GLUCOSIDE Flower
LUTEOLIN-7-BETA-RUTINOSIDE Flower
LUTEOLIN-7-RUTINOSIDE-4'-GLUCOSIDE Plant
MAGNESIUM Flower 2—17 ppm
MUCILAGE Plant
MUFA Flower 50—330 ppm
MYRISTIC-ACID Flower 20—135 ppm
NEOCHLOROGENIC-ACID Plant
NIACIN Flower 10—82 ppm
NON-TRANS-2-ENAL Flower

O-DIPHENOLICS Flower 20,000 ppm
OCT-1-EN-3-ONE Flower
OLEIC-ACID Flower 50—330 ppm
PALMITIC-ACID Flower 290—1,925 ppm
PANTOTHENIC-ACID Flower 3—23 ppm
PHENYLACETALDEHYDE Flower
PHOSPHORUS Flower 860—6,240 ppm
POTASSIUM Flower 3,500—29,780 ppm
PROTEIN Flower 31,000—276,000 ppm
PUFA Flower 630—4,185 ppm
RIBOFLAVIN Flower 0.6—7 ppm
SCOLYMOSIDE Flower
SFA Flower 350—2,325 ppm
SODIUM Flower 850—6,840 ppm
STEARIC-ACID Flower 30—200 ppm
TANNIN Plant
THIAMIN Flower 0.7—6 ppm
VITAMIN B6 Flower 1—8 ppm
WATER Flower 773,000—854,870 ppm
ZINC Flower 4—36 ppm

■ ASPARAGUS

Chemical Constituents of Asparagus officinalis L. (Liliaceae)

22-SPIROSTAN-3-BETA-OL Shoot
4-VINYLGUAICOL Shoot
4-VINYLPHENOL Shoot
ALANINE Seed 1,440—18,581 ppm
ALPHA-AMINODIMETHYL-GAMMA-BUTYROTHETIN Rhizome
ALPHA-CAROTENE Plant
ALPHA-LINOLENIC-ACID Shoot 50—645 ppm
ALUMINUM Shoot 13—700 ppm
ARGININE Shoot 1,430—18,452 ppm
ARSENIC Shoot 0.005—0.006 ppm
ASCORBIC-ACID Shoot 100—5,714 ppm
ASH Shoot 6,000—171,000 ppm
ASPARAGINE Shoot
ASPARAGOSIDES Shoot
ASPARAGUSIC-ACID Shoot
ASPARASAPONINS Plant
ASPARTIC-ACID Shoot 3,550—45,805 ppm

BARIUM Shoot 2—70 ppm
BETA-CAROTENE Shoot 0.3—120 ppm
BORON Shoot 6—104 ppm
CADMIUM Shoot 0.018—0.07 ppm
CALCIUM Shoot 160—3,840 ppm
CARBOHYDRATES Shoot 36,000—602,000 ppm
CHROMIUM Shoot 0.135—0.7 ppm
COBALT Shoot 0.09—0.12 ppm
CONIFERIN Shoot
COPPER Shoot 1—24 ppm
CYANIDIN-3,5-DIGLUCOSIDE Shoot
CYANIDIN-3-MONOGLUCOSIDE Shoot
CYANIDIN-3-RHAMNOSYLGLUCOSIDE Shoot
CYANIDIN-3-RHAMNOGYLGLUCOSYLGLUCOSIDE Shoot
CYSTINE Shoot 360—4,645 ppm
DIOGENIN Shoot
FAT Shoot 2,000—41,000 ppm
FIBER Shoot 7,000—141,000 ppm
FOLACIN Shoot 1—18 ppm
GLUCOSE Shoot
GLUTAMIC-ACID Shoot 5,010—64,645 ppm
GLYCINE Shoot 990—12,774 ppm
GUAIACOL Shoot
HISTIDINE Shoot 470—6,065 ppm
INOSITOL Shoot
INULIN Root
IRON Shoot 6—240 ppm
ISOLEUCINE Shoot 1,120—14,452 ppm
JAMOGENIN Shoot
KAEMPFEROL Root
KILOCALORIES Shoot 210—3,130/kg
LAURIC-ACID Shoot 10—129 ppm
LEAD Shoot 1.5—30 ppm
LEUCINE Shoot 1,330—17,161 ppm
LINOLEIC-ACID Shoot 910—11,742 ppm
LITHIUM Shoot 0.36—0.6 ppm
LUTEIN Plant
LYSINE Shoot 1,450—18,710 ppm
M-CRESOL Shoot
MAGNESIUM Shoot 165—7,000 ppm
MANGANESE Shoot 2—100 ppm
MERCURY Shoot 0.001—0.001 ppm

METHIONINE Shoot 290—3,742 ppm
MOLYBDENUM Shoot 0.63—1.8 ppm
MUFA Shoot 70—903 ppm
MYRISTIC-ACID Shoot 10—129 ppm
NIACIN Shoot 11—366 ppm
NICKEL Shoot 0.9—1.8 ppm
O-CRESOL Shoot
OFFICINALISIN-II Root
OLEIC-ACID Shoot 60—774 ppm
P-CRESOL Shoot
PAEONIDIN-3-GLUCOSYLRHAMNOSYLGLUCOSIDE Shoot
PAEONIDINRHAMNOSYLGLUCOSIDE Shoot
PALMITIC-ACID Shoot 450—5,806 ppm
PALMITOLEIC-ACID Shoot 10—129 ppm
PANTOTHENIC-ACID Shoot 2—22.4 ppm
PENTOSANS Shoot 70,000 ppm
PHENOL Shoot
PHENYLALANINE Shoot 720—9,290 ppm
PHILOTHION Shoot
PHOSPHORUS Shoot 390—10,244 ppm
PHYTOSTEROLS Shoot 246—3,097 ppm
POTASSIUM Shoot 2,210—55,200 ppm
PROLINE Shoot 1,620—20,903 ppm
PROTEIN Shoot 22,000—394,840 ppm
PSEUDOASPARAGOSE Rhizome
PUFA Shoot 960—12,387 ppm
QUERCETIN Root
RHAMNOSE Shoot
RIBOFLAVIN Shoot 1—36 ppm
RUTIN Root
SARSAPOGENIN Shoot
SELENIUM Shoot 0.041—0.078 ppm
SERINE Shoot 1,160—14,968 ppm
SFA Shoot 500—6,452 ppm
SILVER Shoot 0.09—0.12 ppm
SODIUM Shoot 18—685 ppm
STEARIC-ACID Shoot 30—387 ppm
STRONTIUM Shoot 19—200 ppm
SUCCINIC-ACID Shoot
SUCROSE Rhizome
SUGAR Shoot 15,000 ppm
SULFUR Shoot 56—864 ppm
THIAMIN Shoot 1—26 ppm

THREONINE Shoot 850—10,968 ppm
TITANIUM Shoot 0.45—180 ppm
TOCOPHEROL Shoot 19.8—256 ppm
TRYPTOPHAN Shoot 300—3,871 ppm
TYROSINE Shoot 480—6,194 ppm
VALINE Shoot 1,180—15,226 ppm
VANADIUM Shoot 0.3—2 ppm
WATER Plant 914,000—950,000 ppm
ZEAXANTHIN Plant
ZINC Shoot 12—124 ppm
ZIRCONIUM Shoot 1.8—2.4 ppm

■ ASPARAGUS PEA

Chemical Constituents of Psophocarpus tetra-gonolobus L. (Fabaceae)

ALANINE Seed 10,400—11,346 ppm
ALPHA-LINOLENIC-ACID Seed 230—2,858 ppm
ARGININE Seed 18,860—20,576 ppm
ASCORBIC-ACID Fruit 190 ppm
ASCORBIC-ACID Seed
ASH Seed 6,120—80,863 ppm
ASPARTIC-ACID Seed 31,870—34,770 ppm
BETA-CAROTENE Seed 0.78—6 ppm
CALCIUM Seed 567—8,586 ppm
CARBOHYDRATES Seed 43,100—455,051 ppm
COPPER Seed 28—33 ppm
CYSTINE Seed 5,450—5,946 ppm
ERUCIC-ACID Seed 20—154 ppm
FAT Seed 5,430—180,020 ppm
FIBER Seed 21,980—227,005 ppm
FOLACIN Seed 0.4—0.5 ppm
GADOLEIC-ACID Seed 3,030—3,306 ppm
GLUTAMIC-ACID Seed 40,100—43,749 ppm
GLYCINE Seed 11,400—12,437 ppm
IRON Seed 15—158 ppm
ISOLEUCINE Seed 14,680—16,016 ppm
KILOCALORIES Seed 490—4,462/kg
LEUCINE Seed 24,970—17,242 ppm
LINOLEIC-ACID Seed 1,640—44,381 ppm
LYSINE Seed 21,360—23,304 ppm
MAGNESIUM Seed 340—2,623 ppm

MANGANESE Seed 34—44 ppm
METHIONINE Leaf 640—2,765 ppm
METHIONINE Seed 3,560—3,884 ppm
MUFA Seed 2,500—65,590 ppm
MYRISTIC-ACID Seed 10—305 ppm
NIACIN Seed 9—69 ppm
OLEIC-ACID Seed 2,480—61,684 ppm
PALMITIC-ACID Seed 660—13,692 ppm
PHENYLALANINE Seed 14,290—15,590 ppm
PHOSPHORUS Seed 334—5,058 ppm
POTASSIUM Seed 2,014—18,873 ppm
PROLINE Seed 19,240—20,991 ppm
PROTEIN Seed 39,760—765,738 ppm
PROTEIN Tuber 116,000—272,300 ppm
PUFA Seed 1,860—47,240 ppm
RIBOFLAVIN Seed 1—7.7 ppm
SERINE Seed 12,350—13,474 ppm
SFA Seed 2,380—25,125 ppm
SODIUM Seed 31—429 ppm
STEARIC-ACID Seed 7,450—8,128 ppm
THIAMIN Seed 1.4—11.2 ppm
THREONINE Seed 11,790—12,863 ppm
TRYPTOPHAN Seed 7,620—8,313 ppm
TYROSINE Seed 14,570—15,896 ppm
VALINE Seed 15,300—16,692 ppm
VITAMIN B6 Seed 1.1—8.7 ppm
WATER Seed 79,780—882,930 ppm
ZINC Seed 43—51 ppm

■ AVOCADO

Chemical Constituents of Persea americana (Lauraceae)

ALANINE Fruit 960—4,625 ppm
ALPHA-CAROTENE Fruit 0.19—1 ppm
ALPHA-TOCOPHEROL Fruit 13—49 ppm
ARGININE Fruit 470—2,293 ppm
ASCORBIC-ACID Fruit 65—994 ppm
ASH Fruit 6,000—56,000 ppm
ASPARTIC-ACID Fruit 2,270—11,000 ppm
BETA-CAROTENE Fruit 0.3—27 ppm
BIOTIN Fruit 0.1—0.4 ppm
BORON Fruit 5 - 13 ppm

CAFFEIC-ACID Fruit
CALCIUM Fruit 60—964 ppm
CAMPESTEROL Plant
CARBOYDRATES Fruit 8,000—629,000 ppm
CHLOROGENIC-ACID Fruit
CHOLESTEROL Plant
COPPER Fruit 2—11 ppm
CRYPTOXANTHIN Fruit 0.38—2 ppm
CYCLOARTENOL Plant
CYSTINE Fruit 170—816 ppm
D-ERYTHRO-D-GALACTO-OCTITOL Fruit
D-ERYTHRO-L-GLUCO-NONULOSE Fruit
D-GLYCERO-D-GALACTO-HEPTITOL Fruit
D-GLYCERO-D-GALACTO-HEPTOSE Fruit
D-GLYCERO-D-GALACTO-OCTULOSE
  Fruit
D-GLYCERO-D-MANNO-OCTULOSE Fruit
D-MANNOHEPTULOSE Fruit
D-MONNOKEPTOHEPTOSE Fruit
D-TALOHEPTULOSE Fruit
DOPAMINE Fruit
EO Leaf 5,000 ppm
FAT Fruit 61,000—864,000 ppm
FIBER Fruit 10,000—106,000 ppm
FOLACIN Fruit 0.3—2.4 ppm
FOLACIN Fruit 0.5—2.8 ppm
GLUTAMIC-ACID Fruit 1,660—8,045 ppm
GLYCEROL Fruit
GLYCINE Fruit 660—3,226 ppm
HENTRIACOSANE Fruit
HEPTACOSANE Fruit
HISTIDINE Fruit 230—1,127 ppm
IRON Fruit 6—71 ppm
ISOLEUCINE Fruit 570—2,759 ppm
ISOLUTEIN Fruit
KILOCALORIES Fruit 940—6,700/kg
LECITHIN Fruit
LEUCINE Fruit 990—4,780 ppm
LINOLEIC-ACID Fruit 24,340—505,440 ppm
LINOLENIC-ACID Fruit 245—28,510 ppm
LUTEIN Fruit 3.2—16 ppm
LYSINE Fruit 750—3,653 ppm
MAGNESIUM Fruit 370—1,740 ppm
MANGANESE Fruit 2—10 ppm
METHIONINE Fruit 290—1,438 ppm
METHYL-CHAVICOL Leaf

MUFA Fruit 96,080—373,400 ppm
MYOINOSITOL Fruit
NIACIN Fruit 14—101 ppm
NONACOSANE Fruit
OLEIC-ACID Fruit 27,450—691,200 ppm
P-COUMARIC-ACID Fruit
P-COUMARYLQUINIC-ACID Fruit
PALMITIC-ACID Fruit 4,270—266,000 ppm
PALMITOLEIC-ACID Fruit 6,430—25,000
  ppm
PANTOTHENIC-ACID Fruit 8—37.7 ppm
PENTACOSANE Fruit
PERSEITOL Seed 89,000 ppm
PHENYLALANINE Fruit 540—2,643 ppm
PHYTOSTEROLS Fruit
POTASSIUM Fruit 2,780—27,470 ppm
PROLINE Fruit 620—2,993 ppm
PROTEIN Fruit 11,000—81,000 ppm
PUFA Fruit 19,550—76,000 ppm
PYRIDOXINE Fruit 6—23 ppm
RIBOFLAVIN Fruit 1—7.7 ppm
SERINE Fruit 810—3,148 ppm
SEROTONIN Fruit
SFA Fruit 24,370—94,700 ppm
SODIUM Fruit 20—520 ppm
STEARIC-ACID Fruit 120—4,320 ppm
TARTARIC-ACID Fruit 200 ppm
THIAMIN Fruit 0.5—4.2 ppm
THREONINE Fruit 530—2,565 ppm
TRIACOSANE Fruit
TRYPTOPHAN Fruit
TYRAMINE Fruit
TYROSINE Fruit 390—1,904 ppm
VALINE Fruit 970—3,770 ppm
VIOLAXANTHIN Fruit
VITAMIN B6 Fruit 10.9 ppm
VITAMIN D Fruit
WATER Fruit 716,000—830,000 ppm
ZINC Fruit 4—16 ppm

■ BASIL

Chemical Constituents of Ocimum basilicum L.
(Lamiaceae)

(-)-LINALOOL Plant 30—300 ppm
1,8-CINEOLE Plant 776 ppm
1-EPI-BICYCLOSESQUIPHELLANDRENE
  Plant
1-OCTEN-3-OL Plant
2-EPI-ALPHA-CEDRENE Plant
3-OCTANONE Plant
ACETIC-ACID Essential Oil
AESCULETIN Leaf
AESCULIN Leaf
ALANINE Leaf 7,470 ppm
ALPHA-AMORPHENE Plant
ALPHA-BERGAMOTENE Essential Oil
ALPHA-BISABOLOL Essential Oil
ALPHA-CADINENE Plant
ALPHA-CEDRENE Plant
ALPHA-CUBEBENE Plant
ALPHA-FARNESENE Plant
ALPHA-FENCHENE Essential Oil
ALPHA-GUAIENE Plant
ALPHA-HUMULENE Plant 47—313 ppm
ALPHA-MUUROLENE Plant
ALPHA-P-DIMETHYLSTYRENE Plant
ALPHA-PINENE Plant 2—180 ppm
ALPHA-SANTALENE Essential Oil
ALPHA-SELINENE Plant
ALPHA-TERPINENE Plant 1—10 ppm
ALPHA-TERPINEOL Plant 36—239 ppm
ALPHA-TERPINYL-ACETATE Plant
ALPHA-THUJONE Plant
ANETHOLE Plant
APIGENIN Plant
ARGININE Leaf 6,620 ppm
ASCORBIC-ACID Leaf 27—612 ppm
ASPARTIC-ACID Leaf 16,960 ppm
BENZYL-ACETATE Leaf 17—163 ppm
BENZYL-ALCOHOL Essential Oil
BETA-BOURBONENE Plant
BETA-CADINENE Plant
BETA-CADINOL Essential Oil
BETA-CAROTENE Leaf 4—333 ppm
BETA-CARYOPHYLLENE Plant 0—377 ppm
BETA-CEDRENE Plant
BETA-CUBEBENE Plant
BETA-CYMENE Plant 5—36 ppm
BETA-ELEMENE Essential Oil

BETA-MYRCENE Plant
BETA-OCIMENE Plant 1 - 435 ppm
BETA-PINENE Plant 3—160 ppm
BETA-SANTALENE Essential Oil
BETA-SELINENE Plant
BETA-SITOSTEROL Flower 1,051 ppm
BETA-SITOSTEROL Leaf 896—1,705 ppm
BETA-SITOSTEROL Root 408 ppm
BETA-SITOSTEROL Sprout Seedling 230 ppm
BETA-SITOSTEROL Stem 230 ppm
BETA-THUJONE Plant
BORNEOL Plant
BORNEOL-ACETATE Plant 90—900 ppm
BORON Plant 18—31 ppm
BUTYRIC-ACID Essential Oil
CAFFEIC-ACID Leaf 19,000 ppm
CAFFEIC-ACID-N-BUTYL-ESTER Leaf 252
  ppm
CALAMENE Plant
CALCIUM Leaf 20,148—22,112 ppm
CAMPHENE Plant 0—400 ppm
CAMPHOR Plant 2—31 ppm
CAPROIC-ACID Essential Oil
CARBOHYDRATES Leaf 70,000—61,000
  ppm
CARVONE Plant
CARYOPHYLLENE Plant 18—3,196 ppm
CARYOPHYLLENE-OXIDE Essential Oil
CHAVICOL-METHYL-ESTER Essential Oil
CHAVICOL-METHYL-ESTER Plant 500—
  5,658 ppm
CINEOLE Plant
CINNAMIC-ACID-METHYL-ESTER Essen-
  tial Oil
CIS-3-HEXENOL Plant
CIS-ALLOOCIMENE Plant
CIS-ANETHOLE Plant
CIS-CINNAMIC-ACID-METHYL-ESTER
  Plant 67—900 ppm
CIS-LIMONENE Plant 30—933 ppm
CIS-OCIMENE Plant 3—252 ppm
CIS-SABINENE-HYDRATE Plant
CITRAL Plant 560—7,000 ppm
CITRONELLOL Plant 3—2,419 ppm
COPAENE Plant 20 ppm
COPPER Leaf 14 ppm

CYCLOSATIVENE Plant
CYSTINE Leaf 1,590 ppm
D-ARABINOSE Seed
D-GALACTOSE Seed
D-GALACTURONIC-ACID Seed
D-GLUCOSE Seed
D-MANNOSE Seed
D-MANNURONIC-ACID Seed
DELTA-GUAIENE Plant
ELEMOL Essential Oil
EO Plant 1,500—10,000 ppm
ERIODICTYOL Leaf
ERIODICTYOL-7-O-GLUCOSIDE Leaf
ESTRAGOLE Plant 35—9,000 ppm
EUGENOL Leaf 35—8,575 ppm
EUGENOL-METHYL-ETHER Plant 375—
    2,500 ppm
FARNESOL Plant
FAT leaf 35,752—43,680 ppm
FENCHONE Plant
FENCHYL-ACETATE Plant 1—60 ppm
FENCHYL-ALCOHOL Plant 9—951 ppm
FIBER Leaf 145,790—154,290 ppm
FURFURAL Plant
GAMMA-CADINENE Plant
GAMMA-GURJUNENE Plant
GAMM-MUUROLENE Plant
GAMMA-TERPINENE Plant 1—10 ppm
GERANIAL Plant 560—3,750 ppm
GERANIOL Plant 1—1,000 ppm
GERANYL-ACETATE Leaf 11—84 ppm
GLUTAMIC-ACID Leaf 15,650 ppm
GLYCINE Leaf 6,900 ppm
HISTIDINE Leaf 2,870 ppm
HUMULENE Essential Oil
HYDROXY-BENZOIC-ACID-4-BETA-D-
    GLUCOSIDE Leaf
IRON Leaf 362—478 ppm
ISOCARYOPHYLLNENE Plant
ISOEUGENOL Plant 8—95 ppm
ISOEUGENOL-METHYL-ETHER Plant
ISOLEUCINE Leaf 5,880 ppm
ISOQUERCETIN Leaf
JUVOCIMENE-I Plant 0.007—0.05 ppm
JUVOCIMENE-II Plant 0.007—0.05 ppm
KAEMPFEROL Leaf

KAEMPFEROL3-O-BETA-D-RUTINOSIDE
    Leaf
L-RHAMNOSE Seed
LEDENE Plant
LEUCINE Leaf 10,780 ppm
LIMONENE Plant 2—934 ppm
LINALOOL Plant 5—8,730 ppm
LINALYL-ACETATE Plant 15—240 ppm
LINOLEIC-ACID Seed
LINOLENIC-ACID Seed
LUTEOLIN Plant
LYSINE Leaf 6,180 ppm
MAGNESIUM Leaf 4,100—4,340 ppm
MANGANESE Leaf 32 ppm
MENTHOL Plant 4—32 ppm
MENTHONE Plant 1 ppm
METHIONINE Leaf 2,020 ppm
METHYL-CHAVICOL Plant 238—8,780 ppm
METHYL-CINNAMATE Plant 1—2,800 ppm
METHYL-EUGENOL Plant 13—1,400 ppm
MUCILAGE Seed 93,000 ppm
MYRCENE Leaf 2—80 ppm
NEROL Plant 15—300 ppm
NEROLIDIOL Essential Oil
NEROLIDOL Essential Oil
NIACIN Leaf 8—69 ppm
OCTANOL Plant
OLEANOLIC-ACID Flower 1,300 ppm
OLEIC-ACID Seed
ORIENTIN Plant
P-COUMARIC-ACID Leaf 760 ppm
P-CYMENE Plant 1—16 ppm
P-METHOXYCINNAMALDEHYDE Flower
    Essential Oil 1,000—4,000 ppm
PALMITIC-ACID Seed
PHELLANDRENE Plant
PHENYLETHYL-ALCOHOL Plant 18—136
    ppm
PHOSPHORUS Leaf 4,632—5,168 ppm
PHYTOSTEROLS Leaf 1,060 ppm
PLANTEOSE Seed
POTASSIUM Leaf 32,321—42,900 ppm
PROLINE Leaf 5,880 ppm
PROPIONIC-ACID Essential Oil
PROTEIN Leaf 118,550—169,850 ppm
QUERCETIN Leaf

QUERCETIN-3-O-DIGLUCOSIDE Leaf
RIBOFLAVIN Leaf 3—4 ppm
ROSMARINIC-ACID Plant 1,000—1,300 ppm
ROSMARINIC-ACID Shoot 19,000 ppm
RUTIN Leaf
SABINENE Plant
SAFROLE Plant 60—400 ppm
SALICYLIC-ACID-2-BETA-D-GLUCOSIDE
  Leaf
SAMBULENE Leaf
SERINE Leaf 5,610 ppm
SESQUITHUJENE Plant
SODIUM Plant 294—386 ppm
STEARIC-ACID Seed
STIGMASTEROL Plant
SUCCINIC-ACID Plant
SYRINGIC-ACID-4-BETA-D-GLUCOSIDE
  Leaf
SYRINGOYL-GLUCOSE Leaf
TANNIN Tissue Culture
TERPINEN-4-OL Plant 2—120 ppm
TERPINOLENE Plant 1—22 ppm
THIAMIN Leaf 1 ppm
THREONINE Leaf 5,880 ppm
THYMOL Leaf 1,415 ppm
TRANS-ALLOOCIMENE Plant
TRANS-AMTHEOLE Plant 11—74 ppm
TRANS-CINNAMIC-ACID Plant 350—7,000
  ppm
TRANS-CINNAMIC-ACID-METHYL-ESTER
  Plant 350—7,000 ppm
TRANS-OCIMENE Plant 8—161 ppm
TRANS-SABINENE-HYDRATE Plant
TRICYLCLENE Essential Oil
TRYPTOPHAN Leaf 2,210 ppm
TYROSINE Leaf 4,320 ppm
UNDECYLALDEHYDE Plant
URSOLIC-ACID Flower 1,740 ppm
URSOLIC-ACID Leaf 413—1,143 ppm
URSOLIC-ACID Sprout Seedling 63 ppm
URSOLIC-ACID Stem 845 ppm
VALERIC-ACID Essential Oil
VALINE Leaf 7,170 ppm
VANILLIC-ACID-4-BETA-D-GLUCOSIDE
  Leaf
VICENIN-2 Leaf

XANTHOMICROL Leaf 350 ppm
XI-BULGARENE Plant
XYLOSE Seed
ZINC Leaf 5—6 ppm

■ BEET

Chemical Constituents of Beta vulgaris L. (Chenopodiaceae)

3-HYDROXYTYRAMINE Root
ACETAMIDE Root
ACONITIC-ACID Plant
ADENINE Root
ADIPIC-ACID Root
ALANINE Root 560—4,338 ppm
ALLANTOIN Root
ALPHA-LINOLENIC-ACID Leaf 316—3,160
  ppm
ALPHA-LINOLENIC-ACID Root 40—315
  ppm
ALPHA-SPINASTERYLGLUCOSIDE Root
ALPHA-TOCOPHEROL Leaf 321—439 ppm
ALPHA-TOCOPHEROL Root 0.5—3.6 ppm
ALUMINUM Root 1—420 ppm
ARGININE Root 380—2,997 ppm
ARSENIC Root 0.01—0.08 ppm
ASCORBIC-ACID Leaf 120—3,696 ppm
ASCORBIC-ACID Root 50—868 ppm
ASH Root 7,600—140,000 ppm
ASPARTIC-ACID Root 1,060—8,360 ppm
BARIUM Root 17—70 ppm
BETA-CAROTENE Root 0—438 ppm
BETA-INDOLEACETIC-ACID Root
BETA-SITOSTEROL Leaf
BETAINE Root
BETANIDINE Root
BETANIN Root
BORON Root 1—80 ppm
BROMINE Root 2—16 ppm
CADMIUM Root 0.01—0.33 ppm
CAFFEIC-ACID Leaf
CALCIUM Leaf 700—17,368 ppm
CALCIUM Root 120—4,200 ppm

CARBOHYDRATES Leaf 36,000—609,000 ppm
CARBOHYDRATES Root 95,000—794,000 ppm
CHLOROGENIC-ACID Leaf
CHROMIUM Root 0.001—0.33 ppm
CITRIC-ACID Root
COBALT Root 0.001—0.42 ppm
CONIFERIN Plant
CONIFERIN Seed
COPPER Root 0.6—17 ppm
CYSTINE Root 180—1,420 ppm
D-ALPHA-OXYGLUTARIC-ACID Root
D-RIBULOSE Leaf
DAUCIC-ACID Plant
DIOXYMALONIC-ACID Root
FARNESOL Root Essential Oil
FAT Leaf 2,000—58,000 ppm
FAT Root 1,000—16,000 ppm
FAT Seed 28,000—70,000 ppm
FERULIC-ACID Leaf
FIBER Leaf 4,000—279,000 ppm
FIBER Root 8,000—90,000 ppm
FOLACIN Root 0.8—8 ppm
FORMALDEHYDE Root
GABA Root
GALACTOSE Root
GLUCOSE Root
GLUTAMIC-ACID Root 3,930—30,994 ppm
GLUTARIC-ACID Root
GLYCINE Root 290—2,287 ppm
GLYCOCEREBROSIDE Root
GLYCOXALIC-ACID Sprout Seedling
GUANINE Root
GUANOSINE Root
HETEROXANTHIN Root
HEXOSANS Root
HISTIDINE Root 200—1,575 ppm
HOMOGENTISINIC-ACID Root
HYDANTOIN Sprout Seedling
HYDROCAFFEIC-ACID Root
HYPOXANTHIN Root
INVERTASE Root
IRON Leaf 7—392 ppm
IRON Root 5—165 ppm
ISOLEUCINE Root 440—3,470 ppm

KAEMPFEROL Plant
KAEMPFEROL-GLYCOSIDE Leaf
KILOCALORIES Leaf 210—3,310/kg
KILOCALORIES Root 430—3,610/kg
L-ARABINOSE Root
LEAD Root 0.01—3.5 ppm
LEUCINE Root 630—4,968 ppm
LINOLEIC-ACID Root 460—3,628 ppm
LITHIUM Root 0.36—0.6 ppm
LYSINE Root 530—4,180 ppm
MAGNESIUM Root 130—4,200 ppm
MANGANESE Root 3—90 ppm
MELILOTIC-ACID Root
MERCURY Root 0—0.016 ppm
METHIONINE Root 170—1,341 ppm
MOLYBDENUM Root
MUFA Root 270—2,219 ppm
NEOBETANIN Plant
NIACIN Leaf 4—68 ppm
NIACIN Root 2—32 ppm
NICKEL Root 0—2.5 ppm
NITROGEN Root 2,600—35,830 ppm
OLEANOLIC-ACID-3-O-BETA-D-GLUCOPYRANOSIDE Root
OLEIC-ACID Root 404 ppm
OXYCITRONIC-ACID Root
P-COUMARIC-ACID Plant
P-HYDROXYBENZOIC-ACID Root
PALMITIC-ACID Root 210—1,656 ppm
PANTOTHENIC-ACID Root 1.5—11.8 ppm
PENTOSANS Root
PHENYLALANINE Root 420—3,312 ppm
PHOSPHORUS Leaf 290—5,946 ppm
PHYTOSTEROLS Root 250—1,972 ppm
POTASSIUM Leaf 4,380—61,798 ppm
POTASSIUM Root 3,033—50,000 ppm
PRAEBETANINE Root
PROLINE Root 380—2,997 ppm
PROTEIN Leaf 16,000—270,000 ppm
PROTEIN Root 12,850—143,000 ppm
PROTEIN Seed 110,000—150,000 ppm
PROTOPORPHYRIN Root
PUFA Root 500—3,943 ppm
QUERCETIN Plant
QUERCETIN-GLUCOSIDE Leaf
QUINIC-ACID Leaf

RAFFINOSE Root
RAPHANOL Plant
RAPHANOL Root
RAPHANOL Seed
RIBOFLAVIN Leaf 1.7—26 ppm
RIBOFLAVIN Root 0.2—3.9 ppm
RUBIDIUM Root 0.76—32 ppm
SALICYLIC-ACID Root
SEDOHEPTULOSE Leaf
SELENIUM Root
SERINE Root 540—4,259 ppm
SFA Root 220—1,735 ppm
SILICON Root 1—83 ppm
SODIUM Leaf 1,300—16,571 ppm
SODIUM Root 590—6,705 ppm
STEARIC-ACID Root 10—79 ppm
STRONTIUM Root 16—70 ppm
SUCROSE Root 270,000 ppm
SULFUR Root 130—2,000 ppm
SYRINGIC-ACID Root
TARTARIC-ACID Root
THIAMIN Leaf 0.6—14 ppm
THIAMIN Root 0.1—2.4 ppm
THREONINE Root 440—3,470 ppm
TIN Root 0.8—2.8 ppm
TITANIUM Root 0.5—9.8 ppm
TRICARALLYL-ACID Leaf
TRYPTOPHAN Root 170—1,341 ppm
TYROSINE Root 350—2,760 ppm
VALINE Root 520—4,100 ppm
VANILLIC-ACID Leaf
VANILLIN Root
VITAMIN B6 Root 0.5—3.6 ppm
VULGAXANTHIN-1 Plant
VULGAXANTHIN-II Plant
WATER Leaf 864,000—926,000 ppm
WATER Root 865,000—881,340 ppm
XYLOSE Leaf
ZINC Root 3—70 ppm
ZIRCONIUM Plant

■ BELL PEPPER

Chemical Constituents of Capsicum annuum L.
(Solanaceae)

1-HEXANOL Fruit
1-O-CAFFEOYL-BETA-D-GLUCOSE Fruit
1-O-FERRULOYL-BETA-D-GLUCOSE Fruit
2,3,5-TRIMETHYLPYRANZINE Fruit
2,3-BUTANEDIOL Fruit
2,3-DIMETHYLPYRAZINE Fruit
2-BUTANONE Fruit
2-HEXANOL Fruit
2-HEXANONE Fruit
2-METHOXY-3-ISOBUTYLPYRAZINE Fruit
2-METHYL-5-ETHYLPYRAZINE Fruit
2-METHYL-BUTAN-1-OL Fruit
2-METHYL-BUTAN-2-OL Fruit
2-METHYL-BUTANAL Fruit
2-METHYL-BUTYRIC-ACID Fruit
2-METHYL-PENTAN-2-OL Fruit
2-METHYL-PROPIONIC-ACID Fruit
2-PENTYLFURAN Fruit
2-PENTYLPYRIDINE Fruit
24-(R)-ETHYL-LOPHENOL Seed
24-METHYL-LANOST-9(11)-EN-3-BETA-
   OL Seed
24-METHYL-LOPHENOL Seed
24-METHYLENE-CYCLOARTANOL Seed
3,6-EPOXIDE-5-HYDROXY-5,6-DIHYDRO-
   ZEAXANTHIN Fruit
3-(SEC-BUTYL)-2-METHOXYPYRAZINE
   Fruit
3-HEXANOL Fruit
3-HYDROXY-ALPHA-CAROTENE Fruit
3-ISOBUTYL-2-METHOXYPYRAZINE Fruit
3-ISOPROPYL-2-METHOXYPYRAZINE
   Fruit
3-METHYL-1-PENTYL-3-METHYL-
   BUTYRATE Fruit
3-METHYL-BUTANAL Fruit
3-METHYL-BUTYRIC-ACID Fruit
3-METHYL-PENTAN-3-OL Fruit
31-NOR-LANOST-8-EN-3-BETA-OL Seed
31-NOR-LANOST-9(11)-EN-3-BETA-OL
   Seed
31-NOR-LANOSTEROL Seed
31-NORCYCLOARTANOL Seed
4-ALPHA-14-ALPHA-24-TRIMETHYL-
   CHOLESTA-8(24)-DIEN-3-BETA-OL Seed

4-ALPHA-24-DIMETHYL-CHOLESTA-
7,24-DIEN-3-BETA-OL Seed
4-ALPHA-METHYL-5-ALPHA-CHOLEST-
8(14)-EN-3-BETA-OL Seed
4-METHY-1-PENTYL-2-METHYL-
BUTYRATE Fruit
4-METHY-3-PENTEN-2-ONE Fruit
4-METHYL-HEPTADECANE Fruit
4-METHYL-HEXADECANE Fruit
4-METHYL-PENTANOIC-ACID Fruit
4-METHYLPENTADECANE Fruit
4-METHYLTETRADECANE Fruit
4-METHYLTRIDECANE Fruit
5,6-DIHYDROXY-5,6-DIHYDRO-
ZEAXANTHIN Fruit
5-HYDROXY-CAPSANTHIN-5,6-EPOXIDE
Fruit
5-METHYL-2-FURFURAL Fruit
ACETYLCHOLINE Pericarp
ACETYLCHOLINE Seed
ACETYLFURAN Fruit
ALANINE Fruit 350—4,774 ppm
ALPHA-CAROTENE Fruit
ALPHA-COPAENE Fruit
ALPHA-CRYPTOXANTHIN Plant
ALPHA-LINOLENIC-ACID Fruit 220—3,001
ppm
ALPHA-PHELLANDRENE Fruit
ALPHA-PINENE Fruit
ALPHA-TERPINEOL Fruit
ALPHA-THUJENE Fruit
ALPHA-TOCOPHEROL Fruit 22—284 ppm
ALUMINUM Fruit 1—44 ppm
AMMONIA (NH3) Fruit 382 ppm
ANTHERAXANTHIN Fruit
APIIN Fruit
ARACHIDIC-ACID Fruit
ARGININE Fruit 410—5,592 ppm
ARSENIC Fruit 0.004—0.015 ppm
ASCORBIC-ACID Fruit 230—20,982 ppm
ASH Fruit 5,000—122,000 ppm
ASPARAGINE Fruit
ASPARTIC-ACID Fruit 1,200—16,504 ppm
AUROCHROME Fruit
BARIUM Fruit 2—8 ppm
BEHENIC-ACID Fruit

BETA-AMYRIN Seed
BETA-APO-8'-CAROTENAL Fruit
BETA-CAROTENE Fruit 0—462 ppm
BETA-CAROTENE-EPOXIDE Fruit
BETA-CRYPTOXANTHIN Fruit
BETA-PINENE Fruit
BETAINE Fruit
BORON Fruit 1—18 ppm
BROMINE Fruit 0.1—111 ppm
CADMIUM Fruit 0.005—0.33 ppm
CAFFEIC-ACID Fruit 11 ppm
CALCIUM Fruit 36—1,956 ppm
CAMPESTEROL Fruit
CAMPHENE Fruit
CAPSAICIN Fruit 100—4,000 ppm
CAPSANTHIN Fruit
CAPSANTHIN-5,6-EPOXIDE Fruit
CAPSIAMIDE Fruit 20—200 ppm
CAPSIANOSIDE-A Fruit 33—250 ppm
CAPSIANOSIDE-B Fruit 2—18 ppm
CAPSIANOSIDE-C Fruit 35—103 ppm
CAPSIANOSIDE-D Fruit 21—38 ppm
CAPSIANOSIDE-E Fruit 15 ppm
CAPSIANOSIDE-F Fruit 5 ppm
CAPSIANOSIDE-I Fruit 18 ppm
CAPSIANOSIDE-II Fruit 43—138 ppm
CAPSIANOSIDE-III Fruit 15—105 ppm
CAPSIANOSIDE-IV Fruit 9 ppm
CAPSIANOSIDE-V Fruit 2 ppm
CAPSIANSIDE-A Fruit 300 ppm
CAPSIDIOL Fruit 29 ppm
CAPSOCHROME Fruit
CAPSOLUTEIN Fruit
CAPSORUBIN Fruit
CARBOYDRATES Fruit 53,100—813,000 ppm
CARNAUBIC-ACID Seed
CARYOPHYLLENE Fruit
CHLOROGENIC-ACID Fruit
CHOLINE Pericarp 297 ppm
CHOLINE Seed 360 ppm
CHROMIUM Fruit 0—0.546 ppm
CINNAMIC-ACID Tissue Culture
CIS-13'-CAPSANTHIN Fruit
CIS-13-CAPSANTHIN Fruit
CIS-9'-CAPSANTHIN Fruit

CIS-9-10-DIHYDRO-CAPSENONE Tissue
  Culture 1 ppm
CIS-9-CAPSANTHIN Fruit
CITRIC-ACID Fruit
CITROSTADIENOL Seed
CITROXANTHIN Fruit
CITRULLIN Fruit
COBALT Fruit 0.001—0.1 ppm
COPPER Fruit 0.5—20 ppm
CRYPTOCAPSIN Fruit
CRYPTOXANTHIN Fruit
CYCLOARTANOL Seed
CYCLOARTENOL Seed
CYCLOEUCALENOL Seed
CYCLOHEXANONE Fruit
CYCLOPENTANOL Fruit
CYSTINE Fruit 160—2,182 ppm
DECANOIC-ACID-VANILLYLAMIDE Fruit
  1—68 ppm
DEHYDROASCORBIC-ACID Fruit 20,000
  ppm
DELTA-3-CARENE Fruit
DIHYDROCAPSAICIN Fruit 75—1,628 ppm
DIN-N-PROPYL-AMINE Fruit 0.3 ppm
EO Fruit 16,000 ppm
ERIODICTIN Fruit
ETHYL-3-METHYLBUTRYRATE Fruit
EUGENOL Fruit
FAT Fruit 2,000—144,000 ppm
FAT Seed 100,000—150,000 ppm
FIBER Fruit 12,000—351,000 ppm
FLUORINE Fruit 0.05—1 ppm
FOLACIN Fruit 0—3 ppm
FOLIAXANTHIN Fruit
FUNKIOSIDE Root
GALACTOSAMINE Fruit
GALACTOSE Fruit
GAMMA-TERPINENE Fruit
GLUCOSAMINE Fruit
GLUCOSE Fruit
GLUTAMIC-ACID Fruit 1,120—15,277
  ppm
GLUTAMINASE Fruit
GLYCINE Fruit 310—4,228 ppm
GRAMISTEROL Seed
GROSSAMIDE Root 3 ppm

HENEICOSANE Fruit
HEPTADECANE Fruit
HESPERIDIN Fruit
HEXADECANE Fruit
HEXAN-1-AL Fruit
HEXANAL Fruit
HEXANOIC-ACID Fruit
HISTIDINE Fruit 170—2,319 ppm
HOMOCAPSAICIN Fruit 2—90 ppm
HYDROXY-ALPHA-CAROTENE Fruit
HYDROXYBENZOIC-ACID-4-BETA-D-
  GLUCOSIDE Fruit
IRON Fruit 4—286 ppm
ISOHEXYL-ISOCAPROATE Fruit
ISOLEUCINE Fruit 270—3,683 ppm
L-ASPARIGINASE Fruit
LANOST-8-EN-3-BETA-OL Seed
LANOSTEROL Seed
LEAD Fruit 0.004—2 ppm
LEUCINE Fruit 440—6,002 ppm
LIMONENE Fruit
LINALOOL Fruit
LINOLEIC-ACID Fruit 2,190—29,871 ppm
LITHIUM Fruit 0.284—0.4 ppm
LOPHENOL Seed
LUPEOL Seed
LUTEIN Fruit
LYSINE Fruit 380—5,183 ppm
MAGNESIUM Fruit 118—2,340 ppm
MALONIC-ACID Fruit
MALONIC-ACID Leaf
MANGANESE Fruit 0.7—39 ppm
MARGARIC-ACID Fruit
MERCURY Fruit 0.001—0.001 ppm
METHIONINE Fruit 100—1,364 ppm
MOLYBDENUM Fruit 0—15 ppm
MYRCENE Fruit
MYRISTIC-ACID Fruit 10—136 ppm
N-(13-
  METHYLTETRADECYL)ACETAMIDE
  Fruit 300—400 ppm
N-HEXANAL Fruit
N-METHYL-ANILINE Fruit 13.1 ppm
N-NITROSO-DIMETHYLAMINE Fruit
N-NITROSO-PYRROLIDINE Fruit
N-PENTYLAMINE Fruit 3 ppm

N-PROPYLAMINE Fruit 2.3 ppm
NEOXANTHIN Fruit
NIACIN Fruit 4—172 ppm
NICKEL Fruit 0.05—5.5 ppm
NITROGEN Fruit 1,900—23,330 ppm
NONADECANE Fruit
NONANOIC-ACID-VANILLYLAMIDE Fruit 2—45 ppm
NORCAPSAICINE Fruit
NORDIHYDROCAPSAICIN Fruit 15—335 ppm
OBTUSIFOLIOL Seed
OCTANE Fruit
OCTANOIC-ACID Fruit
OLEIC-ACID Fruit 270—3,582 ppm
OLEIC-ACID Seed
OXALIC-ACID Fruit 257—1,171 ppm
P-AMINO-BENZALDEHYDE Root 6 ppm
P-COUMARIC-ACID Fruit 79 ppm
P-CYMENE Fruit
P-XYLENE Fruit
PALMITIC-ACID Fruit 500—6,820 ppm
PALMITIC-ACID Seed
PALMITOLEIC-ACID Fruit 30—409 ppm
PANTOTHENIC-ACID Fruit 0—5 ppm
PENTADECANE Fruit
PENTADECANOIC-ACID Fruit
PHENYLALANINE Fruit 260—3,546 ppm
PHOSPHATIDYL-GLYCEROL Fruit
PHOSPHODIESTERASE Tissue Culture
PHOSPHORUS Fruit 186—3,885 ppm
PHYTOENE Fruit
PHYTOFLUENCE Fruit
PIPERIDINE Fruit 5.2 ppm
POTASSIUM Fruit 1,862—35,000 ppm
PROLINE Fruit 370—5,047 ppm
PROTEIN Fruit 8,000—184,000 ppm
PULEGONE Fruit
PYRROLIDINE Fruit 1.4 ppm
RIBOFLAVIN Fruit 0—19 ppm
RUBIDIUM Fruit 0.38—10 ppm
SABINENE Fruit
SCOPOLETIN Fruit
SELENIUM Fruit 0.001—0.002 ppm
SERINE Fruit 340—4,638 ppm
SILICON Fruit 1—33 ppm

SILVER Fruit 0.071—0.1 ppm
SODIUM Fruit 25—625 ppm
SOLANIDINE Fruit
SOLANINE Fruit
SOLASODINE Fruit
STEARIC-ACID Fruit 160—2,180 ppm
STEARIC-ACID Seed
STIGMASTEROL Fruit
STRONTIUM Fruit 2—12 ppm
SULFOQUINOVOSYL-DIACYL-GLYCEROL Fruit
SULFUR Fruit 190—2,440 ppm
TERPINEN-4-OL Fruit
TERPINOLENE Fruit
TETRADECANE Fruit
TETRAMETHYLPYRAZINE Fruit
THIAMIN Fruit 1—15 ppm
THREONINE Fruit 310—4,228 ppm
TIN Fruit 5 ppm
TITANIUM Fruit 0.355—16 ppm
TOCOPHEROL Fruit 24 ppm
TOLUENE Fruit
TRIGONELLINE Seed 0.6 ppm
TRYPTOPHAN Fruit 110—1,500 ppm
TYROSINE Fruit 180—2,455 ppm
VALINE Fruit 360—4,910 ppm
VANILLOYL-GLUCOSE Fruit
VANILLYL-CAPROYLAMIDE Fruit
VANILLYL-DECANAMIDE Fruit
VANILLYL-OCTANAMIDE Fruit
VIOLAXANTHIN Fruit
VITAMIN B6 Fruit 2 - 22 ppm
WATER Fruit 742,000—937,000 ppm
XANTHOPHYLL-EXPOXIDE Fruit
XYLOSE Fruit
ZEAXANTHIN Fruit
ZETA-CAROTENE Fruit
ZINC Fruit 1—77 ppm
ZIRCONIUM Fruit 1.4—2 ppm

■ BLACK WALNUT

Chemical Constituents of Juglans nigra L. (Juglandaceae)

ALPHA-HYDROJUGLONE-4-GLUCOSIDE
Fruit
ALUMINUM Seed 2.9 ppm
ANTIMONY Seed 0.1 ppm
ARSENIC Seed 0.03 ppm
ASH Seed 23,000—24,000 ppm
BARIUM Seed 8.7 ppm
BETA-CAROTENE Seed 1—2 ppm
BORON Seed 4.7 ppm
BROMINE Seed 2.5 ppm
CADMIUM Seed 0.03 ppm
CALCIUM Seed 668 ppm
CARBOHYDRATES Seed 148,000—153,000
ppm
CERIUM Seed 0.4 ppm
CESIUM Seed 0.1 ppm
CHLORINE Seed 54 ppm
CHROMIUM Seed 1 ppm
COBALT Fruit 36 ppm
COBALT Seed 19 ppm
ELLAGIC-ACID Fruit
EUROPIUM Seed 0.01 ppm
FAT Fruit 52,000 ppm
FAT Seed 593,000—612,000 ppm
FIBER Fruit 162,000 ppm
FIBER Seed 17,000—18,000 ppm
FLUORINE Seed 1.6 ppm
GOLD Seed 0.001 ppm
HAFNIUM Seed 0.1 ppm
IODINE Seed 0.1 ppm
IRON Fruit 455 ppm
IRON Seed 60—73 ppm
LANTHANUM Seed 0.03 ppm
LEAD Seed 0.6 ppm
LUTETIUM Seed 0.02 ppm
MAGNESIUM Fruit 440 ppm
MAGNESIUM Seed 1,794 ppm
MANGANESE Fruit 23 -24 ppm
MANGANESE Seed 30 ppm
MERCURY Seed 0.1 ppm
MOLYBDENUM Seed 0.4 ppm
MYRICETIN Fruit
MYRICITRIN Fruit
NEOSAKURNIN Fruit
NIACIN Fruit
NIACIN Seed 7 ppm

NICKEL Seed 4.8 ppm
PHOPSHORUS Seed 5,700—5,882 ppm
POTASSIUM Seed 4,600—5,154 ppm
PROTEIN Fruit 98,000 ppm
PROTEIN Seed 205,000—212,000 ppm
RIBOFLAVIN Fruit 1 ppm
RIBOFLAVIN Seed 1 ppm
RUBIDIUM Seed 9.3 ppm
SAKURANETIN Fruit
SAKURANIN Fruit
SAMARIUM Seed 0.05 ppm
SCANDIUM Seed 0.004 ppm
SELENIUM Fruit
SELENIUM Seed 0.02 ppm
SILICON Fruit 22 ppm
SILICON Seed 1,387 ppm
SODIUM Seed 3—31 ppm
STRONTIUM Seed 7.1 ppm
SULFUR Seed 2,652 ppm
TANNIN Fruit 147,000 ppm
TANTALUM Seed 0.04 ppm
THIAMIN Fruit 2 ppm
THORIUM Seed 0.4 ppm
TIN Fruit 12 ppm
TIN Seed 1.7 ppm
TITANIUM Seed 2.9 ppm
TUNGSTEN Seed 0.1 ppm
URANIUM Seed 0.04 ppm
VANADIUM Seed 0.03 ppm
WATER Fruit 876,000 ppm
WATER Seed 31,000 ppm
YTTERBIUM Seed 0.1 ppm
ZINC Seed 46 ppm

■ CABBAGE

Chemical Constituents of Brassica oleracea L.
(Brassicaceae)

1-CYANO-2,3-EPITHIOPROPANE Plant
1-CYANO-2-HYDROXY-3-BUTANE Plant
1-CYANO-3,4-EPITHIOBUTANE Plant
1-CYANO-3,4-EPITHIOPENTANE Plant
1-CYANO-3-METHYL-SULFINYL-
PROPANE Plant

1-CYANO-3-METHYL-THIO-PROPANE Leaf
1-CYANO-4-METHYL-SULFINYL-
BUTANE Plant
1-CYANO-4-METHYL-THIO-BUTANE Leaf
1-METHOXY-3-INDOYL-METHYL Plant
1-METHOXYGLUCOBRASSICIN Leaf
1-O-FERULOYL-BETA-D-GLUCOSE Leaf
1-O-P-COUMAROYL-BETA-D-GLUCOSE
Leaf
1-O-SINAPYL-BETA-D-GLUCOSE Leaf
2-HYDROXY-1-CYANO-BUT-3-ENE Leaf
2-HYDROXY-3-BUTENYL-
GLUCOSINOLATE Leaf
2-METHOXY-PHENOL Plant
2-METHYL-THIO-PROPYL-
GLUCOSINOLATE Leaf
2-PHENYL-ETHYL-GLUSOSINOLATE Leaf
2-PROPENYL-GLUCOSINOLATE Plant
3-BUTENYL-GLUCOSINOLATE Leaf
3-BUTENYL-ISOTHIOCYANATE Leaf
3-INDOYL-METHYL-GLUCOSINOLATE
Plant
3-METHYL-SULFINYL-PROPYL-
GLUCOSINOLATE Leaf
3-METHYL-SULFINYL-PROPYL-
ISOTHIOCYANATE Leaf
3-METHYL-THIO-PROPYL-
ISOTHIOCYANATE Leaf
3-O-(2-O-{BETA-D-GLUCOPYRANOSYL}-
6-O-(4-O-{BETA-D-
GLUCOPYRANOSYL}-5-O-BETA-D-
GLUCOPYRANOSYL)...CYANIDIN   Leaf
0.5 ppm
3-O-(2-O-{BETA-D-GLUCOPYRANOSYL}-
6-O-(4-O-{BETA-D-
GLUCOPYRANOZYL}-5-O-BETA-D-
GLUCOPYRANOSYL)...CYANIDIN   Leaf
16 ppm
3-O-(2-O-{BETA-D-GLUCOPYRANOSYL}-
6-O-(4-O-{BETA-D-
GLUCOPYRANOZYL}TRANS-
FERULYL)...CYANIDIN leaf 0.5 ppm
3-O-(2-O-{BETA-D-GLUCOPYRANOSYL}-
6-O-(4-O-{BETA-D-
GLUCOPYRANOZYL}TRANS-P-
COUMARYL)...CYANIDIN Leaf 0.3 ppm

3-O-(6-O-{TRANS-FERULYL)-2-O-BETA-D-
GLUCOPYRANOSYL}...CYANIDIN   Leaf
0.2 ppm
3-O-(6-O-{TRANS-P-COUMAROYL)-2-O-
BETA-D-
GLUCOPYRANOSYL}...CYANIDIN   Leaf
27 ppm
3-O-(6-O-{TRANS-SINAPL}-2-O-(BETA-D-
GLUCOPYRANOSYL)-BETA-D-
GLUCOPYRANOSYL5-O-(BETA-D-
GLUCOPYRANOSYL)-CYANIDIN   Leaf
0.1 ppm
4-CAFFOYLQUINIC-ACID Plant
4-HYDROXY-INDO-3-YL-METHYL-
GLUCOSINOLATE Leaf
4-HYDROXY-INDOYL-3-YL-METHYL-
GLUCOSINOLATE Leaf
4-HYDROXYGLUCOBRASSICIN Leaf
4-METHYL-SULFINYL-BUTYL-
GLUCOSINOLATE Leaf
4-METHYL-SULFINYL-BUTYL-
ISOTHIOCYANATE Leaf
4-METHYL-THIO-BUTYL-
GLUCOSINOLATE Leaf
4-METHYL-THIO-BUTYL-
ISOTHIOCYANATE Leaf
4-P-COUMAROYLQUINIC-ACID Plant
4-PENTENYL-ISOTHIOCYANATE Plant
5-FERULOYLQUINIC-ACID Plant
5-P-COUMAROYLQUINIC-ACID Plant
5-VINYLOXASOLIDINE-2-THIONE Plant
ALANINE Leaf 420—5,615 ppm
ALLYL-CYANIDE Plant
ALLYL-GLUCOSINOLATE Seed
ALLYL-ISOTHIOCYANATE Leaf 20 ppm
ALPHA-LINOLENIC-ACID Leaf 460—6,150
ppm
ALPHA-TOCOPHEROL Leaf 0.4—7 ppm
ALUMINUM Plant
AMMONIA(NH3) Leaf 3,800—11,060 ppm
ANILINE Leaf 1—4 ppm
ANTHERAXANTHIN Leaf
ANTHOXANTHINS Sprout Seedling
ARGININE Leaf 690—9,225 ppm
ARSENIC Leaf 0.004—0.007 ppm
ASCORBIC-ACID Leaf 190—6,774 ppm

ASH Leaf 6,000—98,072 ppm
ASPARTIC-ACID Leaf 1,190—15,910 ppm
BARIUM Leaf 1—87 ppm
BENZYL-GLUCOSINOLATE Leaf
BENZYLAMINE Leaf 2.8—3.3 ppm
BETA-CAROTENE Leaf 0.6—12 ppm
BETA-SITOSTEROL Leaf
BORON Leaf 1—145 ppm
BRASSININ Leaf 1.3 ppm
BROMINE Leaf 0.2—37 ppm
BUTYL-GLUCOSINOLATE Plant
CADMIUM Leaf 0.005—0.39 ppm
CAFFEIC-ACID Leaf 0.5—77 ppm
CAFFEIC-ACID-4-0-BETA-GLUCOSIDE
 Leaf
CALCIUM Leaf 290—7,500 ppm
CARBOHYDRATES Leaf 53,700—717,969
 ppm
CARVONE Plant
CHLOROGENIC-ACID Plant
CHROMIUM Leaf 0.001—8.7 ppm
CITRIC-ACID Leaf
COBALT Leaf 0.001—2.9 ppm
COPPER Leaf 0.3—87 ppm
CROCETIN Leaf
CYANIDIN-3,5-DIGLUCOSIDE Sprout Seed-
 ling 229 ppm
CYANIDIN-3-(DI-P-COUMAROYL)-
 SOPHOROSIDE-5-GLUCOSIDE   Sprout
 Seedling 229 ppm
CYANIDIN-3-(DIFERULYL)-
 SOPHOROSIDE-5-GLUCOSIDE   Sprout
 Seedling 214 ppm
CYANIDIN-3-(DISINAPYL)-
 SOPHOROSIDE-5-GLUCOSIDE   Sprout
 Seedling 257 ppm
CYANIDIN-3-(P-COUMAROYL)-
 SOPHOROSIDE-5-GLUCOSIDE   Sprout
 Seedling 200 ppm
CYANIDIN-3-FERULYL-SOPHOROSIDE-5-
 GLUCOSIDE Sprout Seedling 243 ppm
CYANIDIN-3-MALONYL-SOPHOROSIDE-
 5-GLUCOSIDE Sprout Seedling 171 ppm
CYANIDIN-3-SINAPYL-SOPHOROSIDE-5-
 GLUCOSIDE Sprout Seedling 200 ppm

CYANIDIN-3-SOPHOROSIDE-5-
 GLUCOSIDE Sprout Seedling 257 ppm
CTCLOBRASSININ Leaf 4.3 ppm
CYSTINE Leaf 100—1,337 ppm
DEHYDROASCORBIC-ACID Shoot
DIINDOLYLMETHANE Plant
DIMETHYL-AMINE Leaf 2—2.8 ppm
ERTHRO-1-CYANO-2-HYDROXY-3,4-
 EPITHIOBUTANE Plant
ETHYL-AMINE Leaf 1.3 ppm
ETHYL-METHYL-AMINE Leaf 0.9 ppm
FAT Leaf 1,090—33,559 ppm
FERULIC-ACID Leaf 4—20 ppm
FERULIC-ACID-B-BETA-D-GLUCOSIDE
 Leaf
FIBER Leaf 6,000—106,960 ppm
FLUORINE Leaf 0.02—2.5 ppm
FOLACIN Leaf 0.45—9 ppm
FUMARIC-ACID leaf
GLUCOBRASSICANAPIN Seed
GLUCOBRASSICIN Plant
FLUCOIBERIN Leaf
GLUCORAPAHNIN Leaf
GLUTAMIC-ACID Leaf 2,700—36,099 ppm
GLYCINE Leaf 270—3,610 ppm
GOITRIN Plant
HISTIDINE Leaf 250—3,343 ppm
INDOLE-3-ACETONITRILE Plant
INDOLE-3-CARBONIOL Plant
INDOLE-3-CARBOXALDEHYDE Shoot
INDOYL-3,3'-DIMETHANE Shoot
IRON Leaf 4—151 ppm
ISOLEUCINE Leaf 610—8,156 ppm
ISOMENTHOL Plant
JASMONIC-ACID Leaf
KAEMPFEROL Leaf 100—300 ppm
KAEMPFEROL-3-FERULOYL-
 SOPHOROSIDE Leaf
KAEMPFEROL-3-SINAPOYL-
 SOPHOROSIDE Leaf
KAEMPFEROL-3-SOPHOROSIDE Leaf
KAEMPFEROL-3-SOPHOROSIDE-7-
 GLUCOSIDE Leaf
KAEMPFEROL-7-GLUCOSIDE Leaf
KILOCALORIES Leaf 240—3,209/kg
LANTHANUM Leaf 6.7—20.3 ppm

LEAD Leaf 0.002—5.8 ppm
LEUCINE Leaf 630—8,423 ppm
LINOLEIC-ACID Leaf 350—4,680 ppm
LITHIUM Leaf 0.28—1.4 ppm
LUTEIN Leaf
LYSINE Leaf 570—7,621 ppm
MAGNESIUM Leaf 120—2,228 ppm
MALIC-ACID Leaf
MANGANESE Leaf 1—45 ppm
MENTHOL Plant
MERCURY Leaf 0—0.013 ppm
METHIONINE Leaf 120—1,604 ppm
METHOXYBRASSITIN Leaf 30 ppm
METHYL-AMINE Leaf 3.4—22.7 ppm
MEVALONIC-ACID Leaf
MOLYBDENUM Leaf 0.1—8.7 ppm
N-(1)-METHOXYBRASSININ Leaf 63 ppm
N-METHYL-ANILINE Leaf 0.3 ppm
N-METHYL-BETA-PHENETHYLAMINE
    Leaf 0.5—2 ppm
N-METHYL-PHENETHYLAMINE Leaf 0.5—
    3.7 ppm
N-NONACOSANE Leaf
N-PENTYL-AMINE Leaf 0.6—1.4 ppm
NAPOLEIFERIN Seed
NARCOTINE Leaf
NEOCHLOROGENIC-ACID Plant
NEOGLUCOBRASSICIN Plant
NEOMENTHOL Plant
NEOXANTHIN Leaf
NIACIN Leaf 3—40 ppm
NICKEL Leaf 0.02—8.7 ppm
NITROGEN Leaf 2,100—37,500 ppm
NONACOSAN-15-ONE Leaf
OLEIC-ACID Leaf 130—1,738 ppm
OXALATE Leaf 1,000—13,370 ppm
OXALIC-ACID Leaf 59—350 ppm
P-COUMARIC-ACID Leaf 0.5—9 ppm
P-COUMARIC-ACID-O-BETA-D-
    GLUCOSIDE Leaf
PALMITIC-ACID Leaf 190—2,540 ppm
PANTOTHENIC-ACID Leaf 1.4—19 ppm
PHENETHYL-CYANIDE Leaf
PHENETHYLAMINE Leaf 2.1—8.6 ppm
PHENYLALANINE Leaf 390—5,214 ppm
PHENYLETHYL-ISOTHYIOCYANATE Leaf

PHEOPHYTIN-A Leaf
PHOSPHORUS Leaf 214—6,500 ppm
PHYTOSTEROLS Leaf 110—1,471 ppm
POTASSIUM Leaf 2,368—42,500 ppm
PROGOITRIN Leaf
PROGOITRIN Seed
PROLINE Leaf 2,380—31,821 ppm
PROP-2-ENYL-ISOTHIOCYANATE Plant
PROPYL-GLUCOSINOLATE Plant
PROTEIN LEAF 10,780—179,425 ppm
PROTOCATECHUIC-ACID Plant
QUERCETIN Leaf 2—100 ppm
QUERCETIN-3-GLUCOSIDE Leaf
QUERCETIN-3-SINAPOYL-SOPHOROSIDE
    Leaf
QUERCETIN-3-SOPHOROSIDE Leaf
QUERCETIN-3-SOPHOROSIDE-7-
    GLUCOSIDE Leaf
QUINIC-ACID Leaf
RIBOFLAVIN Leaf 0—4 ppm
RUBIDIUM Leaf 0.4—27.5 ppm
S-METHYL-CYSTEINE-SULFOXIDE Leaf
SEC-BUTYL-ISOTHIOCYANATE Seed
SELENIUM Leaf 0.003—0.25 ppm
SERINE Leaf 710—9,493 ppm
SILICON Leaf 1—25 ppm
SILVER Leaf 0.07—0.58 ppm
SINAPIC-ACID Leaf 13—67 ppm
SINIGRIN Seed
SODIUM Leaf 163—4,510 ppm
SPIROBRASSININ Leaf 35 ppm
STEARIC-ACID Leaf 10—134 ppm
STRONTIUM Leaf 3—870 ppm
SUCCINIC-ACID Leaf
SULFUR Leaf 385—8,750 ppm
THIAMIN Leaf 0.5—10 ppm
THREO-1-CYANO-2-HYDROXY-3,4-
    EPITHIOBUTANE Plant
THREONINE Leaf 420—5,615 ppm
TITANIUM Leaf 0.35—203 ppm
TRYPTOPHAN Leaf 120—1,604 ppm
TYROSINE Leaf 210—2,807 ppm
VALINE Leaf 520—6,952 ppm
VANADIUM Leaf 0.48—14.5 ppm
VIOLAXANTHIN Leaf
VITAMIN B6 Leaf 0.8—14 ppm

VITAMIN U Leaf 2—25 ppm
WATER Leaf 891,000—950,000 ppm
YTTERBIUM Leaf 0.19—8.7 ppm
YTTRIUM Leaf 0.48—29 ppm
ZINC Leaf 2—36 ppm
ZIRCONIUM Leaf 1.4—203 ppm

■ CAPER

Chemical Constituents of Capparis spinosa L. (Capparaceae)

ALKALOIDS Fruit 740 ppm
ALKALOIDS Leaf 200 ppm
ARABINOSE Plant
ASCORBIC-ACID Flower 260—2,300 ppm
ASH Flower 79,000—140,000 ppm
ASH Leaf 132,000 ppm
BETA-SITOSTEROL Plant
BETA-SITOSTEROL-BETA-D-GLUCOSIDE
  Plant
CARBOHYDRATES Leaf 537,000 ppm
CHOLINE Fruit 370 ppm
CHOLINE Leaf 100 ppm
CHOLINE Plant
CITRIC-ACID Plant
COUMARIN Plant
DEXTROSE Flower
FAT Flower 4,700 ppm
FAT Fruit 37,500 ppm
FAT Leaf 7,000—15,000 ppm
FAT Seed 316—346,000 ppm
FIBER Leaf 79,000 ppm
GLUCOCAPANGULIN Plant
GLUCOCAPPARIN Plant
GLUCOCAPPARIN Seed
GLUCOCLEMONIN Plant
GLUCOIBERIN Plant
GLUCOSE Plant
GLUCURONIC-ACID Plant
KAEMPFEROL-3-RUTINOSIDE Plant
L-STACHYDRINE Fruit 370 ppm
L-STACHYDRINE Leaf 100 ppm
LAURIC-ACID Plant
LINOLEIC-ACID Flower 700—2,115 ppm

LINOLEIC-ACID Plant
LINOLENIC-ACID Plant
MUCILAGE Plant
MYRISTIC-ACID Plant
OLEIC-ACID Flower 277—2,162 ppm
OLEIC-ACID Seed 132,720—165,600 ppm
OXALIC-ACID Plant
PALMITIC-ACID Flower 1,123 ppm
PALMITIC-ACID Plant
PECTIC-ACID Plant
PENTOSANS Flower 40,000 ppm
PROTEIN Leaf 138,000 ppm
PROTEIN Seed 190,000—220,000 ppm
QUERCETIN Flower
QUERCETIN-3-RUTINOSIDE Plant
QUERCETIN-7-O-BETA-D-
  GLUCOPYRANOSIDE-BETA-L-
  RHAMNOPYRANOSIDE Plant
RHAMNOSE Flower
RIBOFLAVIN Flower 0.89—2.16 ppm
RUTIC-ACID Plant
RUTIN Flower
RUTIN Plant
RUTINASE Flower
RUTINOSE Flower
SAPONIN Plant
SINIGRIN Plant
STEARIC-ACID Flower 348 ppm
SETARIC-ACID Seed 11,060—16,200 ppm
TANNIN Plant
TARTARIC-ACID Plant
THIAMIN Flower 0.7—0.72 ppm
WATER Flower 696,000—795,000 ppm
WATER Leaf 696,000 ppm

■ CARROT

Chemical Constituents of Daucus carota L. (Apiaceae)

(-)-6-HYDROXY-MELLEIN Root
(-)-6-METHOXY-MELLEIN Root
2-METHOXY-3-SEC-BUTYL-PYRAZINE
  Root
2-OCTANONE Seed

3'-NUCLEOTIDASE Tissue Culture
3,4 DIMETHOXY-ALLYL-BENZENE Root
3-METHOXY-4,5-METHYLENEDIOXY-PROPYL-BENZENE Root
4-BETA-D-GLUCOPYRANOSYL-OXY-BENZOIC-ACID Seed 65 ppm
4-HYDROXYPROLINE Plant
4-METHYL-ISO-PROPENYL-BENZENE Seed
5,7-DIHYDROXY-2-METHYL-CHROMONE Root
6-(GAMMA,GAMMA-DIMETHYL-ALLYL-AMINO)-PURINE Tissue Culture
8-HYDROXY-6-METHOXY-3-METHYL-3,4-DIHYDRO-ISOCOUMARIN Tissue Culture
ACETALDEHYDE Root
ACETONE Root
ACETYLCHOLINE Root
ACORENONE Seed
ALANINE Root 590—4,830 ppm
ALDOLASE Tissue Culture
ALPHA-AMYRIN Root
ALPHA-BERGAMOTENE Root 2,000 ppm
ALPHA-CAROTENE Root 17—25 ppm
ALPHA-CARYOPHYLLENE Root
ALPHA-CURCUMENE Seed
ALPHA-GURJUNEN Seed
ALPHA-HUMULENE Root 12 ppm
ALPHA-IONONE Root
ALPHA-KETOGLUTARIC-ACID Root
ALPHA-LINOLENIC-ACID Seed 270—935 ppm
ALPHA-PHELLANDRENE Root
ALPHA-PINENE Root 48 ppm
ALPHA-PINENE Seed 12—1,300 ppm
ALPHA-PINENE Shoot 12 ppm
ALPHA-TERPINENE Root 28 ppm
ALPHA-TERPINENE Seed 20—40 ppm
ALPHA-TERPINEOL Root 28 ppm
ALPHA-THUJENE Shoot 12 ppm
ALPHA-TOCOPHEROL Leaf 788 ppm
ALPHA-TOCOPHEROL Root 4—36 ppm
ALUMINUM Root 1—1,050 ppm
AMMONIA(NH3) Root 3,970 ppm
AMYLASE Tissue Culture
ANILINE Root 31 ppm

ANTHERAXANTHIN Leaf
APIGENIN Fruit
APIGENIN-4'-O-BETA-D-GLUCOSIDE Seed
APIGENIN-7-O-BETA-D-GALACTOMANNOSIDE Plant
APIGENIN-7-O-BETA-D-GALACTOPYRANOSYL-(1,4)-O-BETA-D-MANN Plant
APIGENIN-7-O-BETA-D-GLUCOSIDE Seed
APIGENIN-7-O-BETA-D-RUTINOSIDE Seed
ARABINOSIDE Root
ARACHIC-ACID Seed 270—936 ppm
ARACHIDONIC-ACID Plant
ARGININE Root 430—3,520 ppm
ARSENIC Root 0.003—1 ppm
ASARALDEHYDE Seed
ASARONE Seed 400 ppm
ASCORBIC-ACID Root 91—775 ppm
ASH Root 56,000—79,000 ppm
ASPARTIC-ACID Root 1,370—11,220 ppm
ASTRAGALIN Seed
AZULENE Seed
BARIUM Root 1.7—150 ppm
BENZOIC-ACID-4-O-BETA-D-GLUCOSIDE Root 11 ppm
BENZYLAMINE Root 2.8 ppm
BERGAMOTENE Seed 200—700 ppm
BERGAPTEN Root 0.3 ppm
BETA-AMYRIN Root
BETA-BISABOLENE Root 116 ppm
BETA-BISABOLENE Seed 100—3,500 ppm
BETA-BISABOLENE Shoot 38 ppm
BETA-CAROTENE Root 27—673 ppm
BETA-CARYOPHYLLENE Seed 55—170 ppm
BETA-CARYOPHYLLENE Shoot 24 ppm
BETA-CRYPTOXANTHIN Root
BETA-ELEMENE Plant
BETA-FARNESENE Root 12 ppm
BETA-GALACTOSIDASE Tissue Culture
BETA-GLUCURONIDASE Tissue Culture
BETA-IONONE Seed 300 ppm
BETA-PHELLANDRENE Shoot 177 ppm
BETA-PINENE Root 4 ppm
BETA-PINENE Seed 50—5,500 ppm
BETA-PINENE Shoot 44 ppm

BETA-SELINENE Seed 118—410 ppm
BETA-SITOSTEROL Root
BETA-SITOSTEROL-GLYCOSIDE Plant
BETAINE Root 35 ppm
BIPHENYL Root 4 ppm
BORNEOL Root
BORNYL-ACETATE Plant
BORNYL-ACETATE Root 24 ppm
BORON Root 1—36 ppm
BROMINE Root 1—36 ppm
BUTYRIC-ACID Root
CADMIUM Root 0.012—0.6 ppm
CAFFEIC-ACID Root
CAFFEIC-ACID-4-O-BETA-D-GLUCOSIDE
    Plant
CAFFEOYLQUINIC-ACID Root
CALCIUM Root 210—5,710 ppm
CAMPESTEROL Root
CAMPHENE Seed 1—70 ppm
CAMPHOR Seed
CAPRIC-ACID Seed 1,360—7,065 ppm
CAR-6-ENE Seed 56—112 ppm
CARBOHYDRATES Root 101,000—850,000
    ppm
CAROTA-1,4-BETA-OXIDE Seed 0.2—0.5
    ppm
CAROTAATOXIN Root
CAROTOL Root 8 ppm
CAROTOL Seed 1,150—8,000 ppm
CAROTOL Shoot 1,450 ppm
CARVONE Seed
CARYOPHYLLENE Root 200 ppm
CARYOPHYLLENE Seed 134—1,000 ppm
CARYOPHYLLENE-OXIDE Root 310—350
    ppm
CARYOPHYLLENE-OXIDE Seed 310—350
    ppm
CHLOROGENIC-ACID Root
CHLOROPHYLL Plant
CHOLESTEROL Leaf
CHOLINE Root 36 ppm
CHOLINE Shoot 73 ppm
CHROMIUM Root 0.005—1.5 ppm
CHRYSIN Seed
CINNAMIC-ACID Tissue Culture
CIS-BETA-BERGAMOTENE Root

CIS-GAMMA-BISABOLENE Root 8 ppm
CITRAL Seed 200 ppm
CITRIC-ACID Root
CITRONELLYL-ACETATE Seed 150—200
    ppm
COBALT Root 0.005—0.058 ppm
COPPER Root 0.3—18 ppm
COSMOSIN Leaf
COUMARIN Root
CROCETIN Leaf
CUMINALDEHYDE Seed
CYANIDIN-3,5-DIGALACTOSIDE Tissue
    Culture
CYANIDIN-3-(SINAPOYL-XYLOSYL-
    GLUCOSYL)-GALACTOSIDE Leaf
CYANIDIN-3-GALACTOSIDE Tissue Culture
CYANIDIN-3-GLUCOGALACTOSIDE Tissue
    Culture
CYANIDIN-3-O-BETA-D-GLUCOSIDE Tis-
    sue Culture
CYANIDIN-DIGLYCOSIDE Root
CYSTEINE Tissue Culture
CYSTEINE Root 80—655 ppm
D-GLUCOSE Root 80,000 ppm
DAUCARIN Seed
DAUCENE Seed 200 ppm
DAUCIC-ACID Root
DAUCINE Plant
DAUCOL Seed 60—1,960 ppm
DAUCOL Shoot 535 ppm
DAUCOSTEROL Root
DEC-2-EN-1-AL Root 1.6 ppm
DECA-TRANS-2-TRANS-4-DIEN-1-AL Plant
DECA-TRANS-2-TRANS-4-DIEN-1-AL Root
DEHYDROASCORBIC-ACID Root
DEHYDROXYDAUCOL Seed
DELTA-3-CARENE Seed 12—120 ppm
DEOXY-RIBONUCLEASE Tissue Culture
DIOSGENIN Root 5,400—6,000 ppm
DIOSGENIN Tissue Culture 5,400—6,000 ppm
DIPENTENE Root
DODECAN-1-AL Root
ELEMICIN Seed 2,000 ppm
EO Root 4,000 ppm
EO Seed 4,000 ppm
EO Shoot 4,000 ppm

EPOXYDIHYDROCARYOPHYLLENE Seed 250—2,000 ppm
EPSILON-CAROTENE Root
ETHANOL Root
ETHYL-METHYL-AMINE Root 7 ppm
ETHYLAMINE Root 1 ppm
ETHYLENE Tissue Culture
EUGENOL Seed 7,000 ppm
FALCARINDIOL Root 88 ppm
FALCARINOL Root 10—47 ppm
FAT Root 1,700—29,000 ppm
FAT Seed 87,000—302,000 ppm
FERULIC-ACID Root
FERULIC-ACID-O-BETA-D-GLUCOSIDE Shoot
FIBER Root 10,000—134,000 ppm
FLUORINE Root 0.03—1.8 ppm
FOLACIN Root 0.1—1.2 ppm
FORMIC-ACID Plant
FRUCTOSE Root
FUMARASE Tissue Culture
FUMARIC-ACID Root
GALACTOSE Root
GAMMA-BISABOLENE Root 264 ppm
GAMMA-CAROTENE Root
GAMMA-DECALACTOSE Seed
GAMMA-DECANOLACTONE Root
GAMMA-LINOLENIC-ACID Seed 540—1,870 ppm
GAMMA-MUUROLENE Root 3,000 ppm
GAMMA-TERPINENE Root 216 ppm
GENTISIC-ACID Tissue Culture
GERANIOL Root 10—8,120 ppm
GERANIOL Seed 10—8,120 ppm
GERANYL-2—METHYL0BUTYRATE Seed 3,000 ppm
GERANYL-ACETATE Shoot 265 ppm
GERANYL-ACETONE Seed 300 ppm
GERANYL-FORMATE Seed
GERANYL-ISOBUTYRATE Seed 500 ppm
GLUTAMATE-OXALACETATE-TRANSAMINASE Tissue Culture
GLTUAMATE-PYRUVATE-TRANSAMINASE Tissue Culture
GLUTAMIC-ACID Root 2,020—16,545 ppm
GLUTAMINE Root

GLYCINE Root 300—2,455 ppm
HCN Root
HEPTAN-1-AL Root 2 ppm
HERACLENIN Root
HISTIDINE Root 160—1,310 ppm
INDOLE-ACETIC-ACID Tissue Culture
INVERTASE Tissue Culture
IONENE Root
IRON Root 3—300 ppm
ISOBUTYRIC-ACID Plant
ISOCHLOROGENIC-ACID Leaf
ISOCITRIC-ACID Root
ISOLEUCINE Root 410—3,360 ppm
ISOPIMPINELLIN Root
ISOPRENE Root
KAEMPFEROL Seed
KAEMPFEROL-3-O-BETA-D-GLUCOSIDE Root
KILOCALORIES Resin Exudate Sap 2,710/kg
KILOCALORIES Root 430—3,520/kg
LAURIC-ACID Root 20—165 ppm
LAURIC-ACID Seed 1,810—6,280 ppm
LEAD Root 0.01—2 ppm
LECITHIN Root
LECITHINASE Plant
LEUCINE Root 430—3,520 ppm
LIMONENE Root 150 ppm
LIMONENE Seed 20—1,500 ppm
LIMONENE Shoot 26 ppm
LINALOOL Root 32 ppm
LINALOOL Seed 4—600 ppm
LINOLEIC-ACID Root 670—5,485 ppm
LINOLEIC-ACID Seed 9,360—43,400 ppm
LINOLENIC-ACID Root 100—820 ppm
LITHIUM Root 0.23—0.6 ppm
LUPEOL Root
LUTEIN Root
LUTEOLIN Plant
LUTEOLIN-4'-O-BETA-D-DIGLUCOSIDE Seed
LUTEOLIN-4'-O-BETA-GLUCOSIDE Seed
LUTEOLIN-7-O-(6"-O-MALONYL)-BETA-D-DIGLUCOSIDE Plant
LUTEOLIN-7-O-BETA-D-DIGLUCOSIDE Seed

LUTEOLIN-7-O-BETA-GLUCOSIDE Root 100 ppm
LUTEOLIN-7-O-BETA-GLUCURONIDE Plant
LUTEOLIN-7-O-BETA-RUTINOSIDE Seed
LYCOPENE Root 80—140 ppm
LYSINE Root 400—3,275 ppm
MAGNESIUM Root 100—1,980 ppm
MALIC-ACID Root
MALTOSE Root
MALVIDIN-3,5-DIGLUCOSIDE Root
MANGANESE Root 1—62 ppm
MANNOSE Root
MERCURY Root 0.001—0.0045 ppm
METHIONINE Root 70—575 ppm
METHYLAMINE Root 3,970 ppm
METHYLPENTOSANS Plant
MEVALONIC-ACID Root 4 ppm
MOLYBDENUM Root 0.1—0.7 ppm
MUFA Root 80—655 ppm
MYRCENE Seed 10—250 ppm
MYRICETIN Fruit
MYRISTIC-ACID Root 10—80 ppm
MYRISTIC-ACID Seed 10,470—36,300 ppm
MYRISTICIN Root 0.5—34 ppm
MYRISTOLEIC-ACID Seed
N-HENTRIACONTANE Seed
N-HEPTACOSANE Seed
N-METHYL-ANILINE Root 0.8 ppm
N-METHYL-BENZLAMINE Root 16 ppm
N-METHYL-PHENETHYLAMINE Root 2 ppm
N-NONACOSANE Seed
N-OCTACOSANE Seed
NEOXANTHIN Leaf
NEUROSPORENE Root
NIACIN Root
NICKEL Root 0—2 ppm
NITROGEN Root 1,400—20,000 ppm
NON-2-EN-1-AL Root 12 ppm
NONAN-1-AL Root 0.8 ppm
NOPOL Root
OCTAN-1-AL Root 8 ppm
OLEIC-ACID Root 60—490 ppm
OLEIC-ACID Seed 55,800—230,300 ppm
OSTHOLE Plant

OXALIC-ACID Root 56 ppm
OXYPEUCEDANIN Root
P-COUMARIC-ACID Root
P-COUMARIC-ACIDO-BETA-D-GLUCOSIDE Shoot
P-CYMEN-8-OL Seed 9,000 ppm
P-CYMENE Root 12 ppm
P-CYMENE Seed 10—160 ppm
P-HYDROXYBENZOIC-ACID Root
P-VINYL-GUAIACOL Seed 4,000 ppm
PALMITIC-ACID Root 230—1,885 ppm
PALMITIC-ACID Seed 3,265—11,500 ppm
PALMITOLEIC-ACID Root 20—165 ppm
PALMITOLEIC-ACID Seed 270—1,725 ppm
PANTOTHENIC-ACID Root 2—17 ppm
PECTIN Root 100,000—188,000 ppm
PECTINESTERASE Root
PENTOSANS Plant
PEROXIDASE Root
PETROXELINIC-ACID Seed 712,000 ppm
PHENYLALANINE Root 320—2,620 ppm
PHENYLALANINE-AMMONIA-LYASE Tissue Culture
PHOSPHATIDYL-CHOLINE Tissue Culture
PHOSPHATIDYL-ETHANOLAMINE Tissue Culture
N-HENTRIACONTANE Seed
N-HEPTACOSANE Seed
N-METHYL-ANILINE Root 0.8 ppm
N-METHYL-BENZYLAMINE Root 16 ppm
N-METHYL-PHENETHYLAMINE Root 2 ppm
N-NONACOSANE Seed
N-OCTACOSANE Seed
NEOXANTHIN Leaf
NEUROSPORENE
NIACIN Root
NICKEL Root 0—2 ppm
NITROGEN Root 1,400—20,000 ppm
NON-2-EN-1-AL Root 12 ppm
NONAN-1-AL Root 0.8 ppm
NOPOL Root
OCTAN-1-AL Root 8 ppm
OLEIC-ACID Root 60—490 ppm
OLEIC-ACID Seed 55,800—230,300 ppm
OSTHOLE Root

OXALIC-ACID Root 56 ppm
OXYPEUCEDANIN Root
P-COUMARIC-ACID Root
P-COUMARIC-ACIDO-BETA-D-
  GLUCOSIDE Shoot
P-CYMEN-8-OL Seed 9,000 ppm
P-CYMENE Root 12 ppm
P-CYMENE Seed 10—160 ppm
P-HYDROXYBENZOIC-ACID Root
P-VINYL-GUAIACOL Seed 4,000 ppm
PALMITIC-ACID Root 230—1,885 ppm
PALMITIC-ACID Seed 270—1,725 ppm
PANTOTHENIC-ACID Root 2—17 ppm
PECTIN Root 100,000—188,000 ppm
PECTINESTERASE Root
PENTOSANS Plant
PEROXIDASE Root
PETROSELINIC-ACID Seed 712,000 ppm
PHENYLALANINE Root 320—2,620 ppm
PHENYLALANINE-AMMONIA-LYASE Tis-
  sue Culture
PHOSPHATIDYL-CHOLINE Tissue Culture
PHOSPHATIDYL-ETHANOLAMINE Tissue
  Culture
PHOSPHATIDYL-GLYCEROL Tissue Culture
PHOSPHATIDYL-INOSITOL Tissue Culture
PHOSPHOFRUCTOKINASE Root
PHOSPHORUS Root 340—5,090 ppm
PHYTIN Root 52,700 ppm
PHYTOENE Plant
PHYTOFLUENCE Root
PHYTOSTEROLS Root 120—980 ppm
PIPECOLIC-ACID Plant
POTASSIUM Root 3,000—46,360 ppm
PROLINE Root 290—2,375 ppm
PROTEIN Root 72,000—106,000 ppm
PSORALEN Root 0.3 ppm
PSORALEN Shoot 0.8 ppm
PUFA Root 770—6,300 ppm
PUTRESCINE Tissue Culture
PYRROLIDINE Plant
QUERCETIN Seed
QUERCETIN-3-O-BETA-GLUCOSIDE Seed
QUERCETRIN Plant
QUINIC-ACID Root
RHAMNOSE Root

RIBOFLAVIN Root 0.6—5 ppm
RIBONUCLEASE Tissue Culture
RUBIDIUM Root 0.42—12.7 ppm
SABINENE Root 160 ppm
SABINENE Seed 50—2,000 ppm
SAKURANETIN Fruit
SCOPOLETIN Root
SELENIUM Root 0.001—0.02 ppm
SERINE Plant
SERINE Root 350—2,865 ppm
SFA Root 300—2,455 ppm
SHIKIMIC-ACID Root
SILICON Root 1—91 ppm
SODIUM Root 340—9,504 ppm
STARCH Root 14,800—25,200 ppm
STEARIC-ACID Root 10—80 ppm
STEARIC-ACID Seed 285—1,240 ppm
STIGMASTEROL Root
STRONTIUM Root 1—148 ppm
SUBERIN Root
SUCCINIC-ACID Root
SUCROSE Root 60,000—339,000 ppm
SULFUR Root 52—1,635 ppm
SYRINGIC-ACID Root
TARAXASTEROL Shoot
TARTARIC-ACID Root
TERPINEN-4-OL Root 28 ppm
TERPINEOL-ACETATE Shoot 746 ppm
TERPINOLENE Root 1,520 ppm
TERPINELONE Seed 10 ppm
TETRADECANOIC-ACID Root
THERMOPSOSIDE Leaf
THIAMIN Root 1—6 ppm
THREONINE Root 380—3,110 ppm
TIGLIC-ACID Seed
TIN Root 0—3 ppm
TITANIUM Root 0.017—30 ppm
TOLUIDENE Root 7.2 ppm
TRANS-1,10-HEPTADECADIENE-5,7-DIYN-
  3-OL Plant
TRANS-2(7)-2,6-DIMETHLOCTA-4,6-
  DIENE Plant
TRANS-BETA-BERGAPTENE Seed 170 ppm
TRANS-CHLOROGENIC-ACID Shoot
TRANS-CINNAMIC-ACID Tissue Culture

TRANS-GAMMA-BISABOLENE Root 268 ppm
TRANS-ISOASARONE Plant
TRYPTOPHAN Root 110-900 ppm
TYROSINE Root 200—1,640 ppm
UBIQUINONE-100 Tissue Culture
UMBELLIFERONE Leaf
UMBELLIFERONE Plant
URONIC-ACID Root
VALINE Root 440- 3,600 ppm
VANILLIC-ACID Tissue Culture
VIOLAXANTHIN Leaf
VITAMIN B6 Root 1—13 ppm
VITAMIN D Plant
VITAMIN E Plant
WATER Root 858,000—907,000 ppm
XANTHOPHYLLS Root 12—16 ppm
XANTHOTOXIN Root 0.3 ppm
XANTHOTOXIN Shoot 1.6 ppm
XYLITOL Root
XYLOSE Root
ZINC Root 2—79 ppm
ZIRCONIUM Root 1—2 ppm
ZOSIMIN Plant

■ CAULIFLOWER

Chemical Constituents of Brassica oleracea L. botrytis L. (Brassicaceae)

3-METHYLSULFINYLPROPYL-GLUCOSINOLATE Flower
3-METHYLTHRIOPROPYL-GLUCOSINOLATE Flower
4-HYDROXY-GLUCOBRASSICIN Flower 7—390 ppm
4-METHOXY-GLUCOBRASSICIN Flower 15—355 ppm
4-METHOXY-INDOL-3-YL-METHYL-GLUCOSINOLATE Flower
4-METHYLSULFINYLBUTYL-GLUCOSINOLATE Flower
4-VINYLGUAIACOL Plant
5-HYDROXY-GLUCOBRASSICIN Tissue Culture

5-METHOXY-GLUCOBRASSICIN Tissue Culture
ABSCISIC-ACID Flower
ACETONE Flower
ALANINE Flower 1,050—13,565 ppm
ALPHA-AMYRIN Flower
ALPHA-TOCOPHEROL Flower 0.3—4 ppm
ALUMINUM Flower 1—150 ppm
AMMONIA(NH3) Flower 6,376 ppm
ANILINE Flower 22 ppm
ARGININE Flower 960—12,400 ppm
ARSENIC Flower
ASCORBIC-ACID Flower 660—9,300 ppm
ASH Flower 6,600—121,250 ppm
BENZYLAMINE Flower 1.4 ppm
BETA-AMYRIN Flower
BETA-CAROTENE Flower 4 ppm
BORON Flower 1—76 ppm
BORON Leaf 36 ppm
BORON Stem 19 ppm
BROMINE Flower
CADMIUM Flower 0.003—0.25 ppm
CAFFEIC-ACID Leaf 9 ppm
CALCIUM Flower 210—4,040 ppm
CARBOHYDRATES Flower 49,200—635,660 ppm
CHROMIUM Flower 0.001—0.125 ppm
CITRIC-ACID Flower
COBALT Flower
COPPER Flower 0.3—8 ppm
CYSTINE Flower 230—2,970 ppm
DIMETHYL-AMINE Flower 14 ppm
DIMETHYL-DISULFIDE Plant
ETHANOL Flower
FAT Flower 1,800—29,400 ppm
FERULIC-ACID Leaf 2 ppm
FIBER Flower 8,000—132,000 ppm
FLUORINE Flower 0.2—2.5 ppm
FUMARIC-ACID Flower
GLUCOBRASSICIN Flower 60—1,670 ppm
GLUCOERUCIN Flower 0—210 ppm
GLUCOIBERIN Flower 0—1,600 ppm
GLUCONAPOLEIFERIN Flower 0—80 ppm
GLUCONASTURTIN Flower
GLUCORAPHANIN Flower 0—990 ppm
GLUCOSINOLATES Flower 20—1,140 ppm

GLUTAMIC-ACID Flower 2,650—34,240 ppm
GLYCINE Flower 640—8,270 ppm
HISTIDINE Flower 400—5,165 ppm
INDOYL-3-METHYL-GLUCOSINOLATE
    Flower
IRON Flower 5—122 ppm
ISOLEUCINE Flower 760—9,820 ppm
KAEMPFEROL Flower 30 ppm
KILOCALORIES Plant 240—3,100/kg
LEAD Flower
LEUCINE Flower 1,160—15,000 ppm
LINOLEIC-ACID Flower 190—2,455 ppm
LINOLENIC-ACID Flower 640—8,270 ppm
LYSINE Flower 1,070 ppm
MAGNESIUM Flower 115—2,250 ppm
MALIC-ACID Flower
MANGANESE Flower 1.5—48 ppm
MERCURY Flower 0—0.025 ppm
METHANOL Flower
METHIONINE Flower 280—3,615 ppm
METHYLAMINE Flower 65 ppm
MOLYBDENUM Flower 0.1 ppm
MOLYBDENUM Leaf 1.65 ppm
MOLYBDENUM Stem 0.98 ppm
MUFA Flower 120—1,550 ppm
N-METHYL-BETA-PHENETHYLAMINE
    Flower 1.6 ppm
N-METHYL-PHENETHYLAMINE Flower 1.6
    ppm
N-PENTYL-AMINE Flower 3.3 ppm
NEOGLUCOBRASSICIN Tissue Culture
NIACIN Flower 5—85 ppm
NICKEL Flower 0.03—12 ppm
NITROGEN Flower 3,100—47,500 ppm
OLEIC-ACID Flower 120—1,550 ppm
OXALIC-ACID Plant
P-COUMARIC-ACID Flower 35 ppm
PALMITIC-ACID Flower 240—3,100 ppm
PANTOTHENIC-ACID Flower 1.4—18 ppm
PHENETHYLAMINE Flower 1.8 ppm
PHENYLALANINE Flower 710—9,175 ppm
PHOSPHORUS Flower 385—7,375 ppm
PHYTOSTEROLS Flower 180—2,325 ppm
POTASSIUM Flower 3,300—49,080 ppm
PROGOITRIN Flower 0—60 ppm
PROLINE Flower 860—11,110 ppm

PROP-2-ENYL-GLUCOSINOLATE Flower
PROTEIN Flower 18,680—300,000 ppm
PUFA Flower 830—10,725 ppm
QUERCETIN Flower 6 ppm
QUINIC-ACID Flower
RIBOFLAVIN Flower 0.3—11 ppm
RUBIDIUM Flower 0.43—11 ppm
SEC-BUTYL-ISOTHIOCYANATE Seed
SELENIUM Flower
SELENIUM Leaf 0.024 ppm
SELENIUM Stem 0.014 ppm
SERINE Flower 1,040—13,440 ppm
SFA Flower 270—3,490 ppm
SILICON Flower 2—125 ppm
SINAPIC-ACID Leaf 20 ppm
SINIGRIN Flower 0—325 ppm
SODIUM Flower 120—2,300 ppm
STEARIC-ACID Flower 30—390 ppm
SUCCINIC-ACID Flower
THIAMIN Flower 0.6—12 ppm
THREONINE Flower 720—9,300 ppm
TRYPTOPHAN Flower 260—3,360 ppm
TYROSINE Flower 430—5,555 ppm
VALINE Flower 1,000—12,920 ppm
VITAMIN B6 Flower 2—30 ppm
WATER Plant 894,000—926,000 ppm
ZINC Flower 3—97 ppm

■ CELERY

Chemical Constituents of Apium graveolens L.
(Apiaceae)

3-BUTYLPHTHALIDE Seed 40—120 ppm
3-ISOBUTYLIDENE-3-A,4-
    DIHYDROPHTHALIDE Seed 133—1,500
    ppm
3-ISOBUTYLIDENE-PHTHALIDE Plant 0.001
    ppm
3-ISOVALERIDENE-3A,4-
    DIHYDROPHTHALIDE Leaf
3-ISOVALERIDINE-PHTHALIDE Leaf
3-ISOVALIDENE-3A,4-
    DIHYDROPHTHALIDE Essential Oil 255
    ppm

3-ISOVALIDENE-3A,4-DIHYDROPHTHALIDE Leaf 0.003 ppm

3-ISOVALIDENE-PHTHALIDE Plant

3-N-BUTYL-4,5-DIHYDROPHTHALIDE Seed

3-N-BUTYL-PHTHALIDE Fruit Essential Oil 108,000 ppm

3-N-BUTYL-PHTHALIDE Leaf Essential Oil 40,000 ppm

3-N-BUTYLPHTHALIDE Seed

4-DIHYDROPHTHALIDE Seed 57—1,500 ppm

5-ALPHA-ANDROST-16-EN-3-ONE Plant 0.009 ppm

5-METHOXY-8-O-BETA-D-GLUCOSYL-OXYPSORALEN Seed 2.9 ppm

5-METHOXYPSORALEN Fruit 0—7 ppm

5-METHOXYPSORALEN Leaf Wax 2 ppm

8-HYDROXY-5-METHOXYPSORALEN Seed 375 ppm

8-METHOXYPSORALEN Leaf 0—1 ppm

ACETALDEHYDE Leaf

ACETIC-ACID Plant

ADENINE Plant

ADENOSINE Plant

ALANINE Petiole 220—4,665 ppm

ALLOOCIMENE-I Leaf Essential Oil 1,000 ppm

ALLOOCIMENE-II Leaf Essential Oil 1,000 ppm

ALPHA-EUDESMOL Seed 76—225 ppm

ALPHA-HUMULENE Leaf 266—2,500 ppm

ALPHA-IONONE Plant

ALPHA-LINOLENIC-ACID Seed 1,600—2,554 ppm

ALPHA-P-DIMETHYL-STYRENE Seed 170—270 ppm

ALPHA-PHELLANDRENE Fruit 2,000 ppm

ALPHA-PINENE Fruit Essential Oil 10,000 ppm

ALPHA-PINENE Leaf Essential Oil 2,000 ppm

ALPHA-PINENE Pericarp Essential Oil 12,000—14,000 ppm

ALPHA-PINENE Root Essential Oil 179,000 ppm

ALPHA-PINENE Seed 38—60 ppm

ALPHA-SELINENE Seed 95—250 ppm

ALPHA-TERPINENE Fruit Essential Oil 1,000 ppm

ALPHA-TERPINENE Leaf

ALPHA-TERPINEOL Fruit Essential Oil 3,000—14,000 ppm

ALPHA-TERPINEOL Leaf Essential Oil 2,000 ppm

ALPHA-TERPINEOL Root Essential Oil 69,000 ppm

ALPHA-TERPINEOL Seed 1 ppm

ALPHA-TERPINYL-ACETATE Leaf

ALPHA-TERPINYL-PROPIONATE Leaf

ALPHA-TOCEPHEROL Petiole 3—67 ppm

ALPHA-TOCEPHEROL Plant 0—64 ppm

ALUMINUM Root 0.3—9 ppm

ANGELIC-ACID Plant

ANILINE Petiole 0.7 ppm

APIGENIN Plant

APIGENIN-7-BETA-APIOSYL-GLUCOSIDE Leaf

APIGRAVIN Seed

APIIN Plant 2,000 ppm

APIOLE Essential Oil

APIUMETIN Seed 12.5 ppm

APIUMETRIN Seed

APIUMOSIDE Seed

ARABINOSE Plant

ARGININE Petiole 200—4,105 ppm

ARSENIC Root 0.01—0.09 ppm

ARSENIC-OXIDE Plant

ASCORBIC-ACID Petiole 58—2,778 ppm

ASCORBIC-ACID Plant 17—129 ppm

ASCORBIC-ACID Seed 171—182 ppm

ASH Petiole 6,000—219,000 ppm

ASH Root 8,300—100,000 ppm

ASH Seed 85,500—106,294 ppm

ASPARAGINE Root

ASPARTIC-ACID Petiole 1,130—23,880 ppm

BENTONITE Plant

BENZOIC-ACID-4-O-BETA-D-GLUCOSIDE Seed 56 ppm

BENZOYL-BENZOATE Leaf

BENZYLAMINE Stem 3.4 ppm

BERGAPTEN Petiole 0.04—0.35 ppm

BERGAPTEN Plant 1—520 ppm

BERGAPTEN Seed 1 ppm
BETA-CAROTENE Petiole 1 - 144 ppm
BETA-CARYOPHYLLENE Fruit Essential Oil 5,000—43,000 ppm
BETA-CARYOPHYLLENE Leaf Essential Oil 5,000 ppm
BETA-CARYOPHYLLENE Seed 95—1,075 ppm
BETA-ELEMENE Fruit Essential Oil 35,000 ppm
BETA-ELEMENE Leaf
BETA-ELEMENE Seed 1—875 ppm
BETA-EUDESMOL Seed 76—225 ppm
BETA-HUMULENE Seed
BETA-PHELLANDRENE Fruit 2,000 ppm
BETA-PINENE Fruit Essential Oil 5—15,000 ppm
BETA-PINENE Seed 57—210 ppm
BETA-SELINENE Fruit Essential Oil 55,000—325,000 ppm
BETA-SELINENE Leaf Essential Oil 30,000 ppm
BETA-SELINENE Seed 209—8,125 ppm
BETA-SELINENE Stem Essential Oil 10,000 ppm
BORON Root 4—103 ppm
BORON Seed 43—61 ppm
BROMINE Root
BUTYLIDINE-NAPHTHALIDE Essential Oil
BUTYLIDINE-PHTHALIDE Fruit Essential Oil 4,000 ppm
BUTYLIDINE-PHTHALIDE Leaf Essential Oil 15,000 ppm
BUTYLIDINE-PHTHALIDE Pericarp Essential Oil 12,000 ppm
BUTYLPHENYL-KETONE Plant
CADMIUM Root 0.001—0.364 ppm
CAFFEIC-ACID Leaf
CALCIUM Petiole 313—11,918 ppm
CALCIUM Root 340—3,635 ppm
CALCIUM Seed 15,814—20,776 ppm
CAMPHENE Leaf Essential Oil 1,000 ppm
CAPRIC-ACID Leaf 200—213 ppm
CAR-3-ENE Essential Oil
CARBOHYDRATES Petiole 36,300—684,980 ppm

CARBOHYDRATES Seed 413,500—439,964 ppm
CAROTENES Leaf 80—145 ppm
CARVEOL-ACETATE Plant
CARVONE Essential Oil 2,000—5,000 ppm
CARVONE Fruit Essential Oil 550,000 ppm
CARVONE Leaf 1 ppm
CARVONE Seed 19—75 ppm
CARVYL-ACETATE Leaf
CELEROIN Seed 13.3 ppm
CELEREOSIDE Seed
CELERIN Seed
CELEROSIDE Seed
CHLOROGENIC-ACID Leaf
CHOLINE Root
CHOLINE-ASCORBATE Leaf
CHROMIUM Root 0.002—0.045 ppm
CHRYSOERIOL-7-APIOSYL-GLUCOSIDE Seed
CIS-1(7),8-DIEN-2-OL Plant
CIS-3-HEXEN-1-YL-PYRUVATE Leaf
CIS-3-HEXENOL Essential Oil
CIS-3-HEXENOL-PYRUVATE Plant
CIS-3-HEXENYL-ACETATE Plant
CIS-CARVEOL Fruit Essential Oil 1,000 ppm
CIS-CARVYL-ACETATE Leaf
CIS-DIHYDRO-ISOCARVONE Fruit Essential Oil 15,000 ppm
CIS-DIHYDROCARVONE Seed 1 ppm
CIS-LIMONENE-OXIDE Seed
CIS-OCIMENE Leaf 2,000—2,500 ppm
CIS-OCIMENE Leaf Essential Oil 145,000 ppm
CIS-OCIMENE Pericarp Essential Oil 78,000 ppm
CIS-OCIMENE Root Essential Oil 68,000 ppm
CIS-P-MENTHA-1(7),8-DIEN-2-YL-ACETATE Plant
CIS-P-MENTHA-2,8-DIEN-1-OL Seed
CITRIC-ACID Petiole
CITRONELLAL leaf
CITRONELLYL-ACETATE Leaf
COPPER Petiole 0.4—7 ppm
COPPER Seed 14 ppm
COUMARIN Plant
CYSTINE Petiole 40—755 ppm
D-SELINENE Seed 2,000—3,000 ppm

DECYL-ACETATE Leaf
DEHYDROASCORBIC-ACID Plant
DI-N-PROPYL-AMINE Petiole 0.9 ppm
DIACETYL Leaf
DIHYDROCARVEOL Fruit Essential Oil 2,000 ppm
DIHYDROCARVEOL Leaf
DIHYDROCARVONE Seed 19—75 ppm
DIHYDROCARVYL-ACETATE Plant
DIHYDRONEOCARVEOL Fruit Essential Oil 1,000 ppm
DIHYDRONEOISOCARVEOL Fruit Essential Oil 2,000 ppm
DIMETHYLAMINE Petiole 5.1 ppm
DODECANAL Leaf
E-BUTYLIDENEPHTHALIDE Plant
E-LIGUSTILIDE Plant 1 ppm
EO Seed 19,000—30,000 ppm
EUDESMOL Fruit Essential Oil 5,000—10,000 ppm
EUGENOL Plant
FALCARINDIOL Root 3.3 ppm
FALCARINONE Root 1.7 ppm
FAT Leaf 1,300—42,000 ppm
FAT Seed 242,730—279,483 ppm
FIBER Petiole 6,900—158,000 ppm
FIBER Seed 106,750—138,586 ppm
FOLAIACIN Petiole 0.3—5.6 ppm
FORMALDEHYDE Plant
FRUCTOSE Plant
FUMARIC-ACID Petiole
GALACTOSE Plant
GALACTURONIC-ACID Plant
GAMMA-SELINENE Plant
GAMMA-TERPINEOL Fruit Essential Oil 3,000—5,000 ppm
GAMMA-TERPINEOL Seed 57—125 ppm
GENTISIC-ACID Leaf
GERANYL-ACETATE Leaf
GERANYL-BUTYRATE Leaf
GLUCOSE Plant
GLUCOSIDASE Plant
GLUTAMIC-ACID Petiole 860—18,285 ppm
GLUTAMINE Root
GLYCINE Petiole 210—4,290 ppm
GLYCOLIC-ACID Root

GRAVEOBIOSIDE-A Seed
GRAVEOBIOSIDE-B Seed
GUAICOL Leaf
GUAICOL Seed
HEPTANAL Leaf
HEPTANOL Leaf
HEXANAL Leaf
HEXANOL Leaf
HISTIDINE Petiole 110—2,425 ppm
HYPOXANTHINE Plant
INDOSTEROL Petiole 300 ppm
INOSINE Plant
INOSITOL Leaf
IRON Petiole 3—347 ppm
IRON Root 3.6—47 ppm
IRON Seed 361—571 ppm
ISOAMYL-ALCOHOL Leaf
ISOBUTYLIDENE Leaf 32 ppm
ISOBUTYLIDENE-3-A,4-DIHYDROPHTHALIDE Fruit Essential Oil 17,000 ppm
ISOBUTYLIDENE-3-A,4-DIHYDROPHTHALIDE Leaf Essential Oil 40,000 ppm
ISOBUTYLIDENE-3-A,4-DIHYDROPHTHALIDE Pericarp Essential Oil 21,000 ppm
ISOBUTYRIC-ACID Leaf
ISOBUTYRIC-ACID Plant
ISOCHLOROGENIC-ACID Leaf
ISOCITRIC-ACID Root
ISOIMPERATORIN Seed
ISOLEUCINE Petiole 200—4,290 ppm
ISOPIMPINELLIN Petiole 0.05—0.41 ppm
ISOPIMPINELLIN Plant 4—122 ppm
ISOQUERCITRIN Seed
ISOVALERIC-ACID Seed 1 ppm
ISOVALERIC-ACID-ETHYL-ESTER Plant
KETO-ALCOHOL Seed 2,140—3,390 ppm
LAURIC-ACID Seed 200—213 ppm
LEAD Root 0.01—2 ppm
LEUCINE Petiole 310—6,530 ppm
LIGUSTILIDE Essential Oil 2,000—5,000 ppm
LIMONENE Fruit Essential Oil 350,000—706,000 ppm
LIMONENE Pericarp Essential Oil 695,000 ppm

LIMONENE Seed 530—24,000 ppm
LINALOOL Seed 1 ppm
LINALYL-ACETATE Leaf
LINASE Plant
LINOLEIC-ACID Leaf 60—1,132 ppm
LINOLEIC-ACID Petiole 690—12,875 ppm
LINOLEIC-ACID Seed 31,310—41,592 ppm
LUTEOLIN Leaf
LUTEOLIN-7-APIOSYL-GLUCOSIDE Fruit
LUTEOLIN-7-O-BETA-GLUCOSIDE Plant
LUTEOLIN-GLYCOSIDE Plant
LYSINE Petiole 260—5,410 ppm
MAGNESIUM Leaf 99—2,650 ppm
MAGNESIUM Seed 4,192—4,903 ppm
MALIC-ACID Petiole
MANGANESE Petiole 1—33 ppm
MANGANESE Seed 76 ppm
MANNITOL Stem 10,000—20,000 ppm
MENTHONE Essential Oil
METHIONINE Petiole 50—1,120 ppm
METHYLAMINE Petiole 6.4 ppm
MUCILAGE Plant
MUFA Petiole 270—5,035 ppm
MYRCENE Fruit Essential Oil 2,000—61,000
  ppm
MYRCENE Leaf Essential Oil 14,000 ppm
MYRCENE Pericarp Essential Oil 18,000 ppm
MYRCENE Root Essential Oil 18,000 ppm
MYRCENE Seed 190—300 ppm
MYRISTIC-ACID Petiole 10—190 ppm
MYRISTIC-ACID Seed 200—213 ppm
MYRISTIC Plant
N-6-BENZYL-ADENINE Seed
N-6-BENZYL-ADENINE-RIBOSIDE Seed
N-6-ISOPENT-2-ENYL-ADENOSINE Seed
N-BUTYLPHTAHLIDE Fruit Essential Oil
  50,000—72,000 ppm
N-BUTYLPHTHALIDE Seed 190—1,800 ppm
N-METHYL-ANILINE Petiole 7 ppm
N-METHYL-PHENETHYLAMINE Petiole 0.5
  ppm
N-PENTYL-AMINE Petiole 7 ppm
N-METHYL-PHENETHYLAMINE Petiole 0.5
  ppm
N-PENTYL-AMINE Petiole 0.8 ppm
N-PENTYL-BENZENE Seed 190—300 ppm

N-PENTYL-CYCLOHEXADIENE Fruit Essential Oil 3,000 ppm
N-PENTYL-CYCLOHEXADIENE Leaf Essential Oil 17,000 ppm
N-PROPYL-AMINE Petiole 2.7 ppm
NEOCNIDILIDE Plant 70—260 ppm
NERAL Leaf
NERYL-ACETATE Leaf
NIACIN Petiole 3—57 ppm
NICKEL Root 0.04—0.9 ppm
NICOTINE Plant
NODAKENETIC Seed
NODAKENIN Seed
OCTANAL Leaf
OLEIC-ACID Petiole 230—4,850 ppm
OLEIC-ACID Seed 146,440—162,560 ppm
OSTHENOL Seed
OXALIC-ACID Plant
P-COUMARIC-ACID Root
P-COUMAROYL-QUINIC-ACID Leaf
P-CYMENE Fruit Essential Oil 2,000—31,000
  ppm
P-CYMENE Pericarp Essential Oil 17,000 ppm
P-CYMENE Seed 190—775 ppm
P-HYDROXYCINNAMIC-ACID Plant
P-MENTH-8(9)-ENE-1,2-DIOL Essential Oil
P-MENTHA-8(9)-EN-1,2-DIOL Seed
P-METHOXY-CINNAMIC-ACID Seed 7.5
  ppm
PALMITIC-ACID Petiole 280—5,970 ppm
PALMITIC-ACID Seed 9,470—17,375 ppm
PALMITOLEIC-ACID Petiole 10—190 ppm
PANTOTHENIC-ACID Petiole 1—36 ppm
PECTIN Leaf 3,000 ppm
PENTOSANE Root 1,600 ppm
PENTYL-BENZENE Fruit Essential Oil 9,000
  ppm
PENTYL-BENZENE Leaf Essential Oil 2,000
  ppm
PERILLALDEHYDE Seed 1 ppm
PEROXIDASE Plant
PETROSELINIC-ACID Seed 2,400—2,554
  ppm
PHENYLALANINE Leaf 190—4,105 ppm
PHOSPHORUS Petiole 201—6,849 ppm
PHOSPHORUS Seed 4,509—6,843 ppm

PHYTOSTEROLS Petiole 60—1,120 ppm
PINOCARVYL-ACETATE Plant
PIPERIDINE Petiole 1 ppm
PIPERITONE Fruit
POTASSIUM Petiole 2,689—57,800 ppm
POTASSIUM Root 3,900—56,360 ppm
POTASSIUM Seed 13,592—15,330 ppm
PROLINE Leaf 170—3,208 ppm
PROPIONALDEHYDE Leaf 3 ppm
PROTEIN Petiole 6,030—194,000 ppm
PROTEIN Seed 170,250—203,385 ppm
PROTOCATECHUIC-ACID Plant
PSORALEN Petiole 0.03—0.15 ppm
PSORALEN Plant
PUFA Petiole 690—12,875 ppm
PYRROLIDINE Petiole 0.4—2.6 ppm
PYRUVIC-ACID Plant
QUERCETIN-3-GALACTOSIDE Plant
QUERCETIN-3-O-BETA-GLUCOSIDE Plant
QUINIC-ACID Petiole
RIBOFLAVIN Petiole 0—34 ppm
RUBIDIUM Root 0.24—9 ppm
RUTARETIN Seed 10 ppm
RUTIN Plant 170 ppm
S-METHYL-METHIONINE Plant
SABINENE Seed
SANTALOL Seed 874—1,150 ppm
SCOPOLETIN Plant
SCOPOLIN Leaf
SEDANENOLIDE Seed 95—900 ppm
SEDANOIC-ACID Plant
SEDANOIC-ALDEHYDE Plant
SEDANOIC-ANHYDRIDE Essential Oil
  30,000—80,000 ppm
SEDANOLIDE Seed
SEDANOLINE Plant
SEDANONIC-ANHYDRIDE Leaf 570—
  15,750 ppm
SELANOLIDE Plant
SELENIUM Root
SERINE Petiole 200—4,105 ppm
SESALIN Seed
SFA Petiole 370—6,900 ppm
SILICON Root 2 ppm
SINAPIC-ACID Plant
SODIUM Petiole 774—17,135 ppm

SODIUM Seed 1,424—1,900 ppm
SPINOSTEROL Plant
STEARIC-ACID Petiole 30—560 ppm
STEARIC-ACID Seed 3,100—5,000 ppm
SUCCINIC-ACID Petiole
SUCCINIC-ACID-DEHYDROGENASE Plant
SUCROSE Plant
SULFUR Root 100—1,000 ppm
TARTARIC-ACID Petiole
TERPINEN-4-OL Leaf Essential Oil 1,000 ppm
TERPINEN-4-OL Seed 1—1,400 ppm
TERPINEOLENE Root Essential Oil 33,000
  ppm
TERPINOLENE Fruit Essential Oil 2,000 ppm
TERPINOLENE Leaf Essential Oil 2,000 ppm
THIAMIN Petiole 0—10 ppm
THREONINE Petiole 190—4,105 ppm
THYMOL Plant
TIGLIC-ACID Plant
TOLUIDINE Petiole 1.1 ppm
TRANS-1,2-EPOXYLIMONENE Seed 1 ppm
TRANS-2-HEXENOL Essential Oil
TRANS-3-HEXENOL Essential Oil
TRANS-ANETHOLE Plant 1 ppm
TRANS-CARVEOL Fruit Essential Oil 1,000
  ppm
TRANS-CARVYL-ACETATE Plant 1 ppm
TRANS-DIHYROCARVONE Fruit Essential
  Oil 14,000 ppm
TRANS-FARNESENE Essential Oil
TRANS-LIMONENE-OXIDE Seed
TRANS-OCIMENE Fruit Essential Oil 3,000
  ppm
TRANS-OCIMENE Leaf
TRANS-OCIMENE Leaf Essential Oil 20,000
  ppm
TRANS-OCIMENE Pericarp Essential Oil
  67,000 ppm
TRANS-OCIMENE Root Essential Oil 201,000
  ppm
TRANS-P-MENTHA-1(7),8-DIEN-2-OL Seed
TRYPTOPHAN Petiole 90—1,865 ppm
TYROSINE Petiole 90—1,865 ppm
UMBELLIFERONE Seed
UNDECANAL Leaf
URONIC-ACID Root

VALERIC-ACID Flower
VALINE Petiole 260—5,600 ppm
VELLEIN Seed
VITAMIN B6 Leaf 0—6 ppm
VITAMIN U Petiole 41—96 ppm
WATER Petiole 927,000—947,000 ppm
WATER Root 890,000 ppm
WATER Seed 60,400 ppm
XANTHOTOXIN Petiole 0.04—0.61 ppm
XANTHOTOXIN Plant 6—183 ppm
XYLOSE Plant
Z-BUTYLIDENEPHTHALIDE Plant
Z-LIGUSTILIDE Plant 1—5 ppm
ZEATIN Seed
ZEATIN-RIBOSIDE Seed
ZINC Leaf 1—44 ppm
ZINC Seed 54—89 ppm

■ CHICORY

Chemical Constituents of Cichorium intybus L. (Asteraceae)

11(S),13-DIHYDRO-8-DEOXYLACTUCIN Root
11(S),13-DINYDROLACTUCIN Root
11(S),13-DIHYDROLACTUCOPICRIN Root
8-DEOXYLACTUCIN Root
ACETOPHENONE Root
AESCULETIN Flower
ALPHA-LINOLENIC-ACID Leaf 60—1,224 ppm
ALPHA-LINOLENIC-ACID Root 130—650 ppm
ARGININE Leaf 730—14,892 ppm
ASCORBIC-ACID Leaf 100—2,040 ppm
ASCORBIC-ACID Root 50—250 ppm
ASH Leaf 6,000—180,000 ppm
ASH Root 8,900—44,500 ppm
BETA-CAROTENE Leaf 0—228 ppm
BETAINE Root
BORON Root 20 ppm
CAFFEIC-ACID Leaf 767 ppm
CALCIUM Root 410—2,050 ppm

CARBOHYDRATES Leaf 32,000—654,000 ppm
CARBOHYDRATES Root 175,100—875,000 ppm
CELLULOSE Root
CHOLINE Root
CICHORIC-ACID Leaf
CICHORIN Flower 1,000—2,000 ppm
ESCULIN Flower
FAT Leaf 1,000—29,000 ppm
FAT Root 2,000—10,000 ppm
FERULIC-ACID Plant
FIBER Plant 9,000—153,000 ppm
FIBER Root 19,500—97,500 ppm
FRUCTOSE Root 45,000—220,000 ppm
GLUCOSE Root 11,000 ppm
HARMAN Root
HISTIDINE Leaf 170—3,468 ppm
INOSITOL Root
INULIN Root 110,000—580,000 ppm
IRON Leaf 5—246 ppm
IRON Root 8—40 ppm
ISOLEUCINE Leaf 600—12,240 ppm
JACQUINELIN Root
KAEMPFEROL Plant
LACTUCIN Latex Exudate
LACTUCIN-P-OXYPHENYLACETICACID-ESTER Root
LACTUCOPICRIN Root
LEUCINE Leaf 440—8,976 ppm
LINOLEIC-ACID Leaf 370—7,548 ppm
LINOLEIC-ACID Root 750—3,750 ppm
LYSINE Leaf 390—7,956 ppm
MAGNESIUM Leaf 130—2,652 ppm
MAGNESIUM Root 220—1,100 ppm
MANNAN Root
MANNITOL Plant
MANNOSE Root
METHIONINE Leaf 60—1,224 ppm
MYRISTIC-ACID Leaf 10—204 ppm
MYRISTIC-ACID Root 30—150 ppm
NIACIN Leaf 5—102 ppm
NIACIN Root 4—20 ppm
NORHARMAN Root
OLEIC-ACID Leaf 20—408 ppm
OLEIC-ACID Root 40—200 ppm

P-HYDROXY-BENZOIC-ACID Leaf 11 ppm
PALMITIC-ACID Leaf 210—4,284 ppm
PALMITIC-ACID Root 410—2,050 ppm
PALMITOLEIC-ACID Root 750—3,750 ppm
PECTIN Root
PENTOSANE Root 47,000—65,000 ppm
PHENYLALANINE Leaf 240—4,896 ppm
PHOSPHORUS Leaf 210—4,284 ppm
PHOSPHORUS Root 610—3,050 ppm
POTASSIUM Leaf 1,820—37,128 ppm
POTASSIUM Root 2,900—14,500 ppm
PROTEIN Leaf 10,000—246,000 ppm
PROTEIN Root 14,000—70,000 ppm
PROTOCATECHUIC-ALDEHYDE Seed
QUERCETIN Plant
RIBOFLAVIN Leaf 1—29 ppm
RIBOFLAVIN Root 0—2 ppm
SCOPOLETIN Flower
SINAPIC-ACID Plant
SODIUM Leaf 70—1,428 ppm
SODIUM Root 500—2,500 ppm
STEARIC-ACID Leaf 10—204 ppm
STEARIC-ACID Root 20—100 ppm
TANNIN Plant
TARAXASTEROL Root
THIAMIN Leaf 1—14 ppm
THIAMIN Root 0—2 ppm
THREONINE Leaf 280—5,712 ppm
TRYPTOPHAN Leaf 180—3,672 ppm
UMBELLIFERONE Flower
VALINE Leaf 450—9,180 ppm
VANILLIC-ACID Leaf 0.5 ppm
WATER Leaf 931,000—951,000 ppm
WATER Root 777,000—800,000 ppm

■ CHINESE CABBAGE

Chemical Constituents of Brassica pekinensis (Brassicaceae)

ALPHA-TOCOPHEROL Leaf 2—56 ppm
ALUMINUM Leaf 28—42 ppm
ARSENIC Leaf 0.038—0.07 ppm
ASH Leaf 190,000—210,000 ppm
BARIUM Leaf 13.3—21 ppm

BORON Leaf 13.3—21 ppm
CADMIUM Leaf 0.038—0.042 ppm
CAFFEIC-ACID Leaf 11 ppm
CALCIUM Leaf 11,780—16,800 ppm
CHROMIUM Leaf 0.285—0.315 ppm
COBALT Leaf 0.19—0.21 ppm
COPPER Leaf 2.85—3.15 ppm
FERULIC-ACID Leaf 6 ppm
IRON Leaf 28.5—63 ppm
LEAD Leaf 3.8—4.2 ppm
LITHIUM Leaf 0.76—0.84 ppm
MAGNESIUM Leaf 2,850—3,150 ppm
MANGANESE Leaf 9.5—10.5 ppm
MERCURY Leaf 0—0.002 ppm
MOLYBDENUM Leaf 1.3—1.47 ppm
NICKEL Leaf 1.9—2.1 ppm
P-COUMARIC-ACID Leaf 7 ppm
PHOSPHORUS Leaf 4,560 ppm—7,560 ppm
POTASSIUM Leaf 74,100—81,900 ppm
SELENIUM Leaf 0.001—0.002 ppm
SILVER Leaf 0.019—0.21 ppm
SINAPIC-ACID Leaf 6 ppm
SODIUM Leaf 1,463—1,932 ppm
STRONTIUM Leaf 190—420 ppm
SULFUR Shoot 1,216—1,365 ppm
TITANIUM Leaf 0.95—1.05 ppm
WATER Leaf 947,000—954,000 ppm
ZINC Leaf 66.5—80 ppm
ZIRCONIUM Leaf 3.8—4.2 ppm

■ CHICK PEA

Chemical Constituents of Cicer arietinum L. (Fabaceae)

ALANINE Seed 8,280—9,360 ppm
ARGININE Seed 11,500—20,560 ppm
ASCORBIC-ACID Seed 30—56 ppm
ASH Seed 24,000—28,900 ppm
ASPARTIC-ACID Seed 22,700—25,660 ppm
BETA-CAROTENE Seed 0.4—0.5 ppm
CALCIUM Seed 1,020—1,220 ppm
CARBOHYDRATES Seed 606,000—685,700 ppm
COPPER Seed 8—10 ppm

CYSTINE Seed 2,470—2,930 ppm
FAT Seed 59,000—69,750 ppm
FIBER Seed 38,900—48,570 ppm
FOLACIN Seed 5—6 ppm
GLUTAMIC-ACID Seed 33,600—38,150 ppm
GLYCINE Seed 8,030—9,075 ppm
HISTIDINE Seed 4,620—6,000 ppm
IRON Seed 61—72 ppm
ISOLEUCINE Seed 8,280—10,320 ppm
KILOCALORIES Seed 2,550—4,114/kg
LEUCINE Seed 11,520—15,530 ppm
LINOLEIC-ACID Seed 25,930—29,310 ppm
LINOLENIC-ACID Seed 1,010—1,140 ppm
LYSINE Seed 12,910—14,595 ppm
MAGNESIUM Seed 1,110—1,348 ppm
MANGANESE Seed 21—26 ppm
METHIONINE Seed 2,320—2,860 ppm
MUFA Seed 13,580—15,350 ppm
MYRISTIC-ACID Seed 90—100 ppm
NIACIN Seed 15—18 ppm
OLEIC-ACID Seed 13,460—15,215 ppm
OXALIC-ACID Seed 24 ppm
PALMITIC-ACID Seed 5,010—5,665 ppm
PALMITOLEIC-ACID Seed 120—135 ppm
PANTOTHENIC-ACID Seed 15—18 ppm
PHENYLALANINE Seed 10,340—12,290 ppm
PHOSPHORUS Seed 3,540—4,275 ppm
PHYTOSTEROLS Seed 350—395 ppm
POTASSIUM Seed 8,460—10,220 ppm
PROLINE Seed 7,970—16,530 ppm
PROTEIN Seed 191,000—220,000 ppm
PUFA Seed 26,940—30,450 ppm
RIBOFLAVIN Seed 2—3 ppm
SERINE Seed 9,730—11,000 ppm
SFA Seed 6,260—7,075 ppm
SODIUM Seed 220—310 ppm
STEARIC-ACID Seed 850—960 ppm
THIAMIN Seed 4—6 ppm
THREONINE Seed 7,160—8,090 ppm
TRYPTOPHAN Seed 1,850—4,970 ppm
TYROSINE Seed 4,790—5,415 ppm
VALINE Seed 8,090—10,150 ppm
VITAMIN B6 Seed
WATER Seed 108,220—122,380 ppm
ZINC Seed 33—50 ppm

■ CHIVES

Chemical Constituents of Allium schoenoprasum
L. (Liliaceae)

1-O-FERULOYL-BETA-D-GLUCOSE Leaf
1-O-P-COUMAROYL-BETA-D-GLUCOSE
  Leaf
2-METHYL-2-BUTENAL Plant
2-METHYL-2-PENTENAL Plant
3,5-DIETHYL-1,2,4-TRITHIOLANE Leaf
ALANINE Leaf 1,260—15,750 ppm
ALLITHIAMINE Plant
ALLYL-DISULFIDE Plant
ALLYL-MERCAPTAN Plant
ALPHA-LINOLENIC-ACID Leaf 130—1,625
  ppm
ARGININE Leaf 2,020—25,250 ppm
ASCORBIC-ACID Leaf 57—9,875 ppm
ASH Leaf 4,000—100,000 ppm
ASPARTIC-ACID Leaf 2,590—32,375 ppm
BETA-CAROTENE Leaf 34—475 ppm
CAFFEIC-ACID Leaf
CALCIUM Leaf 690—10,375 ppm
CARBOHYDRATES Leaf 38,000—667,000
  ppm
CIS-PENTYL-HYDRO-DISULFIDE Essential
  Oil
CIS-PROPENYL-PROPYL-DISULFIDE Plant
CITRIC-ACID Leaf
DESOXYRIBONUCLEIC-ACID Plant
DIPRPYL-DISULFIDE Essential Oil
DOTRIACONTANAL Plant
FAT Leaf 3,000—75,000 ppm
FERULIC-ACID Leaf
FIBER Leaf 7,000—137,500 ppm
FUMARIC-ACID Leaf
GALACTOSE Plant
GAMMA-GLUTAMYL-PEPTIDASE Plant
GAMMA-GLUTAMYL-PEPTIDE Plant
GAMMA-GLUTAMYL-S-
  ALLYLCYSTEINE Plant
GAMMA-GLUTAMYL-TRIPEPTIDE Plant
GAMMA-GLUTAMYL-TRIPEPTIDE Plant
GLUCOSE Plant
GLUTAMIC-ACID Leaf 5,790—72,385 ppm

GLYCINE Leaf 1,390—17,375 ppm
HISTIDINE Leaf 480—6,000 ppm
IRON Leaf 8—200 ppm
ISOLEUCINE Leaf 1,190—14,875 ppm
ISORHAMNETIN-GLYCOSIDE Plant
KAEMPFEROL-DIGLUCOSIDE Plant
KAEMPFEROL-GLUCOSIDE Plant
KAEMPFEROL-TRIGLUCOSIDE Plant
LEUCINE Leaf 1,670—20,875 ppm
LINOLEIC-ACID Leaf 2,220—27,750 ppm
MAGNESIUM Leaf 550—6,875 ppm
MALIC-ACID Leaf
METHIONINE Leaf 300—3,750 ppm
METHYL-ALLYL-ALLITHIAMINE Plant
METHYL-DISULFIDE Plant
METHYL-PENTYL-DISULFIDE Essential Oil
METHYL-PROPYL-DISULFIDE Plant
MYRISTIC-ACID Leaf 30—375 ppm
NIACIN Leaf 5—88 ppm
OCTACOSANOL Plant
OLEIC-ACID Leaf 840—10,500 ppm
OXALIC-ACID Plant
P-COUMARIC-ACID Leaf 21 ppm
PALMITIC-ACID Leaf 910—11,375 ppm
PANTOTHENIC-ACID Leaf 2—22 ppm
PENTYL-HYDRO-DISULFIDE Essential Oil
  25,000 ppm
PHENYLALANINE Leaf 900—11,250 ppm
PHOSPHORUS Leaf 410—6,437 ppm
POTASSIUM Leaf 2,500—31,250 ppm
PROLINE Leaf 1,850—23,125 ppm
PROPYL-ALLYL-ALLITHIAMINE Plant
PROTEIN Leaf 18,000—350,000 ppm
QUERCETIN Leaf 4—9 ppm
QUINIC-ACID Leaf
RIBOFLAVIN Leaf 1—22 ppm
S-(PROPENYL-1-YL)-CYSTEINE-
  SULFOXIDE Plant
SAPONIN Leaf
SCORDININE Plant
SERINE Leaf 1,260—15,750 ppm
SODIUM Leaf 60—750 ppm
STEARIC-ACID Leaf 80—1,000 ppm
SUCCINIC-ACID Leaf
THIAMIN Leaf 1—12 ppm
THREONINE Leaf 1,110—13,875 ppm

TRANS-PENTYL-HYDRO-DISULFIDE
  Essential Oil
TRANS-PROPENYL-PROPYL-DISULFIDE
  Plant
TRIACONTANAL Plant
TRYPTOPHAN Leaf 310—3,875 ppm
TYROSINE Leaf 810—10,125 ppm
VALINE Leaf 1,240—15,500 ppm
VITAMIN B6 Leaf 2—22 ppm
WATER Leaf 913,000—920,000 ppm

■ COLLARDS

Chemical Constituents of Brassica oleracea L.
(Brassicaceae)

ALANINE Leaf 670—10,981 ppm
ALPHA-LINOLENIC-ACID Plant
ARGININE Leaf 800—13,112 ppm
ASCORBIC-ACID Leaf 233—3,819 ppm
ASH Leaf 5,500—90,145 ppm
ASPARTIC-ACID Leaf 1,200—19,668 ppm
BETA-CAROTENE Leaf 20—328 ppm
CALCIUM Leaf 1,170—19,180 ppm
CARBOHYDRATES Leaf 37,600—616,264
  ppm
COPPER Leaf 2—43 ppm
CYSTINE Leaf 160—2,624 ppm
FAT Leaf 2,200—36,058 ppm
FIBER Leaf 5,700—93,423 ppm
FOLACIN Leaf 0.83—2.4 ppm
GLUCOBRASSICANAPIN Seed
GLUCONAPIN Seed
GLUTAMIC-ACID Leaf 1,310 ppm—21,571
  ppm
GLYCINE Leaf 600—9,834 ppm
HISTIDINE Leaf 300—4,917 ppm
IRON Leaf 6—102 ppm
ISOLEUCINE Leaf 640—10,490 ppm
KILOCALORIES Leaf 190—3,112/kg
LEUCINE Leaf 970—15,900 ppm
LINOLEIC-ACID Plant
LYSINE Leaf 750—12,293 ppm
MAGNESIUM Leaf 170—2,786 ppm
MANGANESE Leaf 4—60 ppm

METHIONINE Leaf 210—3,442 ppm
MYRISTIC-ACID Plant
NAPOLEIFERIN Seed
NIACIN Leaf 3.7—61 ppm
OLEIC-ACID Plant
OXALATE Leaf 4,500—73,755 ppm
PALMITIC-ACID Plant
PALMITOLEIC-ACID Plant
PANTOTHENIC-ACID Leaf 0.64—10.5 ppm
PHENYLALANINE Leaf 560—9,178 ppm
PHOSPHORUS Leaf 160—2,622 ppm
PHYTOSTEROLS Plant
POTASSIUM Leaf 1,480—24,257 ppm
PROGOITRIN Seed
PROLINE Leaf 670—10.981 ppm
PROTEIN Leaf 15,700—257,323 ppm
RIBOFLAVIN Leaf 0.6—10.5 ppm
SERINE Leaf 500—8,195 ppm
SINIGRIN Seed
SODIUM Leaf 280—4,589 ppm
STEARIC-ACID Plant
THIAMIN Leaf 0.3—4.75 ppm
THREONINE Leaf 550—9,014 ppm
TRYPTOPHAN Leaf 200—3,278 ppm
TYROSINE Leaf 420—6,884 ppm
VALINE Leaf 770—12,620 ppm
VITAMIN B6 Leaf 0.7—11 ppm
WATER Leaf 932,500—945,500 ppm
ZINC Leaf 10—157 ppm

■ CORN

Chemical Constituents of Zea mays L. (Poaceae)

1,2,3-TRIMETHYL-BENZENE Silk Stigma Style
1,2,4-TRIMETHYL-BENZENE Silk Stigma Styl
1,2-DIMETHYOXY-BENZENE Hull Husk
1,2-DIMETHYL-4-ETHYL-BENZENE Silk Stigma Style
1,3-DIMETHYL-4-ETHYL-BENZENE Silk Stigma Style
1,8-CINEOLE Silk Stigma Style

1-(3-AMINO-PROPYL)-PYRROLINIUM Sprout Seedling
1-P-HYDROXY-TRANS-CINNAMOYL)-GLYCEROL Seed 45 ppm
1.2 Seed
2"-O-ALPHA-RHAMNOSYL-6C-(6-DEOXO-XYLO-HEXOS-4-ULOSYL)-APIGENIN Plant
2"-O-ALPHA-RHAMNOSYL-6C-(6-DEOXO-XYLO-HEXOS-4-ULOSYL)-CHRYSOERIOL Plant
2(3)-BENZOXAZOLINONE Sprout Seedling
2,4-DIHYDROXY-6,7-DIMETHOXY-2H,2,4-BENZOXAZIN-3-ONE Sprout Seedling
2-(2,4-DIHYDROXY-1,4(2H)-BENZOXAZIN-3-ONE Sprout Seedling
2-(2,4-DIHYDROXY-7-METHOXY-1,4-BENZOXAZINE-3-ONE-BETA-D-GLUCOPYRANOSIDE Sprout Seedling
2-(2-HYDROXY-1,4(2H)-BENZOXAZIN-3-(4H)-ON-BETA-D-GLUCOSIDE Sprout Seedling
2-(2-HYDROXY-7-METHOXY-1,4(2H)-BENZOXAZIN-3(4H)-ON-BETA-D-GLUCOSIDE Sprout Seedling
2-ETHYL-1-CYCLOHEXEN-1-YL Essential Oil
2-METHYL-BUTAN-1-AL Silk Stigma Style
2-METHYL-BUTAN-1-OL Silk Stigma Style
2-METHYL-PENT-2-EN-1-AL Silk Stigma Style
2-METHYL-PENTAN-3-ONE Silk Stigma Style
2-METHYL-PROPAN-1-OL Silk Stigma Style
2-O-CAFFEOYLHYDROXY-CITRIC-ACID Shoot
2-O-FERULOYL-HYDROXY-CITRIC-ACID Shoot
2-PENTYL-FURAN Essential Oil 10,000 ppm
2-PENTYL-FURAN Silk Essential Oil 3,000 ppm
24-ETHYLIDENE-LOPHENOL Shoot
24-METHYL-23-DEHYDRO-CHOLESTEROL Seed Oil
24-METHYL-CHOLESTEROL Root

24 METHYLENE-CHOLESTEROL Pollen or Spore
24-METHYLENE-LOPHENOL Shoot
3'-NUCLEOTIDASE Tissue Culture
3'-O-METHYL-MAYSIN Silk Stigma Style
3-METHYL-BUTAN-1-OL Silk Stigma Style
4-ETHYL-GUAIACOL Seed
4-HYDROXYBENZOIC-ACID Tissue Culture
4-METHYL-GUAIACOL Seed
4-VINYL-4-DEETHYL-CHLOROPHYLL-A Plant
4-VINYL-GUAIACOL Seed
4-VINYL-PHENOL Seed
5-DEHYDRO-AVENASTEROL Seed
6-METHOXY-2-(3)-BENZOXAZOLINONE Seed
7-DEHYDRO-AVENASTEROL Seed
ABSCISSIN-II Seed
ACETOIN Plant
ADENINE Seed
ADENOSINE Seed
ALANINE Seed 2,950—12,272 ppm
ALLANTOIN Seed
ALPHA-CAROTENE Seed 0.5—2.5 ppm
ALPHA-LINOLENIC-ACID Seed 160—666 ppm
ALPHA-TERPINEOL Silk Stigma Style
ALPHA-TOCOPHEROL Oil 90—257 ppm
ALPHA-YLANGENE Essential Oil 17,000 ppm
ALPH-ZEIN Seed
ALUMINUM Seed 1—275 ppm
ALUMINUM Silk Stigma Style 213 ppm
AMMONIA(NH3) Seed 1,030 ppm
ANILINE Seed
APIFORAL Silk Stigma Style
APIGENIDIN Silk Stigma Style
ARGININE Seed 1,310—5,450 ppm
ARSENIC Seed 0.001—0.211 ppm
ASCORBIC-ACID Seed 0—85 ppm
ASCORBIC-ACID Silk Stigma Style 11 ppm
ASH Seed 10,000—90,000 ppm
ASH Silk Stigma Style 33,000 ppm
ASPARTIC-ACID Seed 2,440—10,150 ppm
ASTRAGALIN Pollen or Spore
BARIUM Seed 0—14 ppm

BENZALDEHYDE Silk Essential Oil 1,000 ppm
BENZOXAZIONE Sprout Seedling
BENZYLAMINE Seed 3.4 ppm
BETA-AMYRIN Shoot
BETA-CAROTENE Seed 0.5—2.5 ppm
BETA-CAROTENE Silk Stigma Style
BETA-IONONE Plant
BETA-IONONE Silk Essential Oil 1,000 ppm
BETA-PINENE Silk Essential Oil 3,000 ppm
BETA-SITOSTEROL Silk Stigma Style 1,300 ppm
BETA-ZEACAROTENE Plant
BETAINE Shoot 234 ppm
BETAINE Silk Stigma Style
BIOTIN Cob 0.02—0.06 ppm
BIPHENYL Silk Stigma Style
BISABOLOL Essential Oil
BORON Seed 0—15 ppm
BUTAN-1-OL Silk Stigma Style
BUTENYL-ISOTHIOCYANATE Seed
CADMIUM Seed 0—1 ppm
CAFFEIC-ACID Shoot 0.7 ppm
CALCIUM Seed 10—181 ppm
CALCIUM Silk Stigma Style 2,502 ppm
CAMPESTEROL Seed
CARBOHYDRATES Seed 190,209—838,000 ppm
CARBOHYDRATES Silk Stigma Style 825,000 ppm
CARVACROL Seed
CARVACROL Silk Stigma Style 144—216 ppm
CASTASTERONE Pollen or Spore 0.12 ppm
CELLULOSE Plant
CHELIDONIC-ACID Shoot 158 ppm
CHLORINE Fruit 330 ppm
CHOLESTEROL Seed
CHOLINE Seed 430 ppm
CHOLINE Shoot 85 ppm
CHROMIUM Seed 0—1.65 ppm
CHROMIUM Silk Stigma Style 13 ppm
CINNAMIC-ACID-ETHYL-ESTER Silk Stigma Style
COBALT Silk Stigma Style 64 ppm
COPPER Fruit 0—20 ppm
CYANIDIN Silk Stigma Style

CYANIN Cob
CYCLOARTENOL Shoot
CYCLOEUCALENOL Shoot
CYCLOSADOL Seed
CYSTINE Seed 260—1,082 ppm
DAUCOSTEROL Silk Stigma Style 440 ppm
DEC-TRANS-2-CIS-4-DIEN-1-AL Plant
DEC-TRANS-2-CIS-4-DIEN-1-AL Silk Essential Oil 7,000 ppm
DEC-TRANS-2-EN-1-AL Silk Essential Oil 3,000 ppm
DEC-TRANS-2-TRANS-4-DIEN-1-AL Silk Essential Oil 6,000—20,000 ppm
DECAN-1-AL Silk Essential Oil 10,000—90,000 ppm
DECAN-1-OL Silk Stigma Style
DECAN-2-OL Essential Oil 15,000 ppm
DECAN-2-ONE Essential Oil
DELTA-AMINO-LEVULINIC-ACID Sprout Seedling
DIAMINO-PROPANE Sprout Seedling
DIETHYL-AMINE Seed
DIGALACTOSYL-DIGLYCERIDE Seed
DIMETHYL-AMINE Seed 1.1—3.5 ppm
DIOXYCINNAMIC-ACID Plant
DODECAN-1-AL Silk Essential Oil
EO Silk Stigma Style 800—1,200 ppm
ERGOSTEROL Silk Stigma Style
ESTRONE Seed Oil 0.04 ppm
ETHANOL Silk Stigma Style
ETHYL-ACETATE Silk Stigma Style
ETHYL-METHYL-AMINE Seed
ETHYL-PHENYLACETATE Silk Essential Oil 250,000—740,000 ppm
ETHYLAMINE Seed 2.4 ppm
EUGENOL Seed
FAT Seed 10,480—54,579 ppm
FAT Silk Stigma Style 43,000 ppm
FERULIC-ACID Speed 6—27 ppm
FERULIC-ACID Sprout Seedling
FERULOYLQUINIC-ACID Sprout Seedling
FIBER Silk Stigma Style 81,000 ppm
FLUORENE Silk Stigma Style
FOLACIN Fruit 1—2 ppm
FOLACIN Seed 0.142—0.4 ppm
FRIEDELIN Shoot

FRUCTOSE Fruit 1,000—4,000 ppm
GALLIC-ACID Tissue Culture
GAMMA-NONALACTONE Silk Stigma Style
GAMMA-SITOSTEROL Plant
GAMMA-TOCOPHEROL Oil 752 ppm
GEOSMIN Essential Oil 4,000 ppm
GERANIOL Silk Stigma Style
GERANYL-ACETONE Seed
GLOBULIN Seed 4,500—6,000 ppm
GLUCOSE Fruit 2,000—5,000 ppm
GLUTAMIC-ACID Seed 6,360—26,457 ppm
GLUTAMIC-ACID-DECARBOXYLASE Plant
GLUTATHIONE Seed 54—169 ppm
GLUTELIN Fruit 14,685—67,325 ppm
GLYCEROL Plant
GLYCINE Seed 1,270—5,283 ppm
GLYCOLIC-ACID Silk Stigma Style
GUAIACOL Seed
HEMICELLULOSE Cob
HEPT-4-EN-2-ONE Essential Oil 15,000 ppm
HETP-4-EN-OL Essential Oil 120,000 ppm
HEPT-4-EN-OL Plant
HEPT-CIS-4-EN-2-OL Silk Essential Oil 10,000 ppm
HEPTA-TRANS-2-CIS-4-DIEN-1-AL Husk Essential Oil 19,000—21,000 ppm
HEPTA-TRANS-2-CIS-4-DIEN-1-AL Silk Essential Oil 5,000 ppm
HEPTA-TRANS-2-TRANS-4-DIEN-1-AL Silk Essential Oil 3,000 ppm
HEPTAN-1-AL Plant
HEPTAN-1-AL Silk Essential Oil 20,000—50,000 ppm
HEPTAN-1-OL Silk Essential Oil 20,000—30,000 ppm
HEPTAN-2-OL Essential Oil 15,000 ppm
HEPTAN-2-OL Essential Oil 250,000 ppm
HEPTAN-2-OL Silk Essential Oil 10,000—20,000 ppm
HEX-1-EN-3-OL Silk Stigma Style
HEX-CIS-3-EN-1-OL Husk Essential Oil 52,000 ppm
HEX-CIS-3-EN-1-OL Silk Essential Oil 5,000 ppm
HEX-TRANS-2-EN-1-AL Plant

HEX-TRANS-2-TRANS-4-DIEN-1-AL   Silk Essential Oil 3,000 ppm
HEX-TRANS-3-EN-1-OL Silk Essential Oil
HEXADECENOIC-ACID Seed
HEXAN-1-AL Silk Essential Oil 2,000—10,000 ppm
HEXAN-1-OL Plant
HEXAN-1-OL Silk Essential Oil 2,000—10,000 ppm
HEXAN-2-OL Silk Stigma Style
HEXAN-2-ONE Essential Oil
HEXAN-2-ONE Husk Essential Oil
HEXENYL-ISOTHIOCYANATE Seed
HISTIDINE Seed 890—3,702 ppm
HORDENINE Silk Stigma Style
INDOLE Leaf
INDOLE-3-ACETIC-ACID Seed
INDOLE-3-ACETIC-ACID-CELLOSIGLUCAN Seed
INDOLE-3-ACETIC-ACID-MYOINOSITOL Seed
IODINE Seed 0.012 ppm
IRON Seed 5—41 ppm
IRON Silk Sigma Style 504 ppm
ISOAMYL-AMINE Sprout Seedling
ISOBEHENIC-ACID Seed 80 ppm
ISOLEUCINE Seed 1,290—5,366 ppm
ISOPROPYLAMINE Seed 2.3 ppm
ISQUERCETRIN Plant
KILOCALORIES Silk Sigma Style 3,690/kg
LACTIC-ACID Plant
LEAD Seed 0—14 ppm
LEUCINE Seed 3,480—14,477 ppm
LIGNOCERIC-ACID Fruit
LIMONENE Silk Essential Oil 7,000 ppm
LINOLEIC-ACID Seed 5,420—22,547 ppm
LITHIUM Seed 0.048—0.22 ppm
LOPHENOL Shoot
LUTEIN + ZEAXANTHIN Seed 7.3—22 ppm
LUTEOFOROL Silk Stigma Style
LUTEOLINIDIN Silk Stigma Style
LYSINE Seed 1,370—5,699 ppm
MAGNESIUM Seed 100—1,600 ppm
MAGNESIUM Silk Stigma Style 1,790 ppm
MANGANESE Seed 0.84—63 ppm

MANGANESE Silk Stimga Style 34 ppm
MAYSIN Silk Stigma Style 9,000 ppm
MERCURY Seed 0—0.072 ppm
METHIONINE Seed 670—2,787 ppm
METHYL-PHENYLACETATE Silk Essential Oil 30,000—40,000 ppm
METHYLAMINE Seed 27 ppm
MEVALONIC-ACID Seed 14 ppm
MOLYBDENUM Seed 0.084—6.3 ppm
MYRCENE Seed
MYRISTIC-ACID Seed
N-METHYL-BETA-PHENETHYLAMINE Seed 1.1 ppm
N-PROPYL-GALLATE Seed
NAPHTHALENE Silk Essential Oil 3,000 ppm
NIACIN Cob 4—16 ppm
NIACIN Seed 16—71 ppm
NIACIN Silk Stigma Style
NICKEL Seed 0.12—6.3 ppm
NON-CIS-3-EN-1-OL Essential Oil 30,000 ppm
NON-TRANS-2-EN-1-AL Husk Essential Oil 10,000 ppm
NON-TRANS-2-EN-1-AL Silk Essential Oil 10,000 ppm
NONA-TRANS-2-TRANS-4-DIEN-1-AL Silk Essential Oil 3,000 ppm
NONAL-N-2-OL Essential Oil 30,000 ppm
NONAL-1-AL Silk Essential Oil 80,000—28,000 ppm
NONAL-1-OL Essential Oil 30,000 ppm
NONAN-2-OL Essential Oil 260,000 ppm
NONAN-2-OL Silk Essential Oil 2,000 ppm
NONAN-2-ONE Essential Oil 20,000 ppm
O-DIETHYL-PHTHALATE Silk Stigma Style
OBTUSIFOLIOL Shoot
OCT-1-EN-3-OL Silk Essential Oil 1,000 ppm
OCT-TRANS-2-EN-1-AL Plant
OCT-TRANS-2-EN-1-AL Silk Essential Oil 1,000 ppm
OCT-TRANS-2-EN-1-OL Plant
OCTA-3-5-DIENE-2-ONE Silk Stigma Style
OCTA-TRANS-2-TRANS-5-DIEN-2-ONE Silk Essential Oil 2,000 ppm
OCTADECADIENOIC-ACID Seed
OCTADECATRIENOIC-ACID Seed
OCTADECENOIC-ACID Seed

OCTAN-1-OL Silk Essential Oil 5,000—10,000 ppm
OCTAN-2-OL Essential Oil 20,000 ppm
OCTAN-2-OL Plant
OCTAN-2-ONE Essential Oil
OCTAN-2-ONE Husk Essential Oil
OLEIC-ACID Seed 3,470—14,435 ppm
ORIENTIN Silk Stigma Style
OXALIC-ACID Fruit 99 ppm
P-COUMARIC-ACID Seed 4—46 ppm
P-COUMARIC-ACID Shoot 1 ppm
P-HYDROXYBENZALDEHYDE Cob
P-VINYL-GUAIACOL Husk Essential Oil
PALMITIC-ACID Seed 1,710—7,114 ppm
PALMITOLEIC-ACID Fruit
PANTOTHENIC-ACID Cob 3—7 ppm
PANTOTHENIC-ACID Seed 4—34 ppm
PECTIN Leaf 10,000—17,000 ppm
PECTINS Plant 5,900 ppm
PELARGONIDIN Silk Stigma Style
PELARGONIDIN-3-GLUCOSIDE Plant
PENT-1-EN-2-OL Silk Stigma Style
PENTAN-1-OL Silk Stigma Style
PENTAN-2-OL Silk Stigma Style
PENTAN-3-ONE Silk Stigma Style
PEROXIDASE Anther
PHENETHYL-ALCOHOL Silk Stigma Style
PHENYLACETALDEHYDE Plant
PHENYLACETALDEHYDE Silk Essential Oil 1,000 ppm
PHENYLALANINE Seed 1,500—6,240 ppm
PHOSPHOENOL-PYRUVATE Sprout Seedling
PHOSPHOLIPIDS Seed
PHOSPHORUS Seed 600—4,066 ppm
PHOSPHORUS Silk Stigma Style 287 ppm
PHTYOHAEMAGGLUTININ Silk Stigma Style
POTASSIUM Seed 2,400—11,450 ppm
POTASSIUM Silk Stigma Style 12,200 ppm
PROLAMINE Seed 45,000—55,000 ppm
PROLINE Seed 2,920—12,147 ppm
PROLINE Shoot 11 ppm
PROPAN-1-OL Silk Stimga Style
PROTEIN Seed 22,520 ppm
PROTEIN Silk Stigma Style 99,000 ppm
PROTOCATECHUIC-ACID Tissue Culture

PUTRESCINE Sprout Seedling
PYRIDOXINE Cob 1—3 ppm
PYRROLIDINE Seed
RAFFINOSE Fruit
RHAMNOGALACTURONAN-I Tissue Culture
RIBOFLAVIN Cob 1—3 ppm
RIBOFLAVIN Fruit 1—4 ppm
RIBOFLAVIN Silk Stigma Style 1.5 ppm
RIBONCULEASE Tissue Culture
SAPONIN Silk Stigma Style 23,000—32,000 ppm
SELENIUM Seed 0—0.5 ppm
SELENIUM Silk Stigma Style
SERINE Seed 1,530—6,365 ppm
SILICON Silk Stigma Style 237 ppm
SILVER Seed 0.012—0.055 ppm
SODIUM Seed 0—757 ppm
SODIUM Silk Stigma Style 130 ppm
SPERMIDINE Seed
SPERMINE Seed
SQUALINE Seed
STARCH Seed
STEARIC-ACID Seed 110—457 ppm
STIGMASTEROL Seed
STRONTIUM Seed 0.12—14 ppm
SUCROSE Fruit 9,000—19,000 ppm
SULFUR Fruit 6—1,140 ppm
SYRINGALDEHYDE Seed
SYRINGIC-ACID Tissue Culture
TEASTERONE Pollen or Spore 0.041 ppm
THIAMIN Fruit 2—8 ppm
THIAMIN Silk Stigma Style 2.1 ppm
THREONINE Seed 1,290—5,366 ppm
THYMOL Seed
THYMOL Silk Stigma Style
TIN Seed 1—1.8 ppm
TIN Silk Stigma Style
TITANIUM Seed 0.06—63 ppm
TOCOPHEROLS Seed 900—1,000 ppm
TRANS-24-METHYL-23-DEHYDRO-LOPHENOL Seed
TRIDECAN-1-AL Husk Essential Oil
TRIGONELLINE Seed 4 ppm
TRYPTOPHAN Seed 230—957 ppm
TYPHASTEROL Pollen or Spore 0.066 ppm
TYROSINE Seed 1,230—5,117 ppm

UNDEC-TRANS-2-EN-1-AL Silk Essential Oil 2,000 ppm
UNDECAN-1-AL Husk Essential Oil
UNDECAN-2-OL Essential Oil 45,000 ppm
UNDECAN-2-OL Husk Essential Oil
UNDECAN-2-ONE Husk Essential Oil
URDINE Seed
VALINE Seed 1,850—7,696 ppm
VANADIUM Seed 0.05—1.35 ppm
VANILLIC-ACID Sprout Seedling
VANILLIN Seed 4—31 ppm
VITAMIN B6 Seed
VITEXIN Silk Stigma Style
WATER Seed 100,000—885,000 ppm
WATER Silk Stigma Style 620,000 ppm
XYLENE Husk Essential Oil
YTTERBIUM Seed 0.02—4.5 ppm
ZEANIN Seed
ZEANOSIDE-B Seed
ZEANOSIDE-C 1.2 ppm
ZEATIN Plant 0.014 ppm
ZINC Seed 4—20 ppm
ZIRCONIUM Seed 0.2—1.8 ppm

■ CUCUMBER

Chemical Constituents of Cucumis sativus L. (Cucurbitaceae)

1,3-DIAMINO-PROPANE Seed
22-DIHYDRO-SPINASTEROL Leaf
22-DIHYDROBRASSICASTEROL Seed
24(R)-14ALPHA-METHYL-24-ETHYL-5ALPH-CHOLES-9(11)-EN-3BETA-OL Plant
24-BETA-ETHYL-25(27)-DEHYDROLATHOSTEROL Seed
24-EPSILON-ETHYL-25(27)-DEHYDROLOPHENOL Seed
24-EPSILON-ETHYL-31-NORLANOSTA-8,25(27)-DIEN-3-BETA-OL Seed Oil 11 ppm
24-ETHYL-5ALPHA-CHOLESTA-7,22-DIEN-3BETA-OL Plant
24-ETHYLCHOLESTA-5-EN-7BETA-OL Plant

24-METHYL-25(27)-DEHYDROCYCLOARTANOL Seed
24-METHYL-CHOLEST-7-EN-3-BETA-OL Seed
24-METHYL-LATHOSTEROL Seed
24-METHYLENE-24-DIHYDRO-LANOSTEROL Seed
24-METHYLENE-24-DIHYDRO-PARKEOL Seed
24-METHYLENE-CHOLESTEROL Seed
24-METHYLENECYCLOARTENOL Seed
24-METHYLENEPOLLINASTEROL Plant
25(27)-DEHYDRO-CHONDRILLASTEROL Seed
25(27)-DEHYDRO-FUNGISTEROL Seed
25(27)-DEHYDRO-PORIFERASTEROL Seed
7,22-STIGMASTADIEN-3BETA-OL Plant
7-DEHYDROAVENASTEROL Seed
7-STIGMASTEN-3BETA-OL Plant
ALANINE Fruit 180—4,557 ppm
ALPHA-AMYRIN Seed
ALPHA-LINOLENIC-ACID Fruit 290—7,342 ppm
ALPHA-SPINASTEROL Leaf
ALPHA-TOCOPHEROL Fruit 0.4—38 ppm
ALUMINUM Fruit 0.4—21,000 ppm
ARGININE Fruit 340—8,608 ppm
ARSENIC Fruit 0.003—0.25 ppm
ASH Fruit 3,670—140,000 ppm
ASPARTIC-ACID Fruit 320—8,101 ppm
AVENASTEROL Seed
BARIUM Fruit 2—70 ppm
BETA-AMYRIN Fruit
BETA-CAROTENE Fruit 0.3—8 ppm
BETA-PYRAZOL-1-YL-ALANINE Seed
BETA-SITOSTEROL Fruit
BORON Fruit
BUTYRIC-ACID Seed 1,200—1,700 ppm
CADMIUM Fruit 0.001—0.56 ppm
CAFFEIC-ACID Fruit
CALCIUM Fruit 129—10,000 ppm
CAMPESTEROL Seed
CARBOHYDRATES Fruit 29,100—736,709 ppm
CHLOROGENIC-ACID Fruit
CHROMIUM Fruit 0.002—0.98 ppm

CITRULLINE Fruit 146 ppm
CLADOCHROMES Sporut Seedling
COBALT Fruit 0—0.14 ppm
COPPER Fruit 0.3—42 ppm
CUCURBITACIN-A Fruit
CUCURBITACIN-B Fruit
CUCURBITACIN-C Fruit
CUCURBITACIN-D Fruit
CUCURBITACIN-E Fruit
CUCURBITACIN-I Sprout Seedling
CUCURBITIN Seed
CYCLOARTENOL Seed
CYCLOEUCALENOL Seed
CYSTINE Fruit 30—759 ppm
D-GLUCOSE Petiole
EUPHOL Seed
FAT Fruit 900—43,037 ppm
FAT Seed 300,000—425,000 ppm
FERULIC-ACID Fruit
FIBER Fruit 6,000—151,896 ppm
FLUORINE Fruit
FOLACIN Fruit 0.12—4 ppm
GAMMA-GLUTAMYL-BETA-PYRAZOL-1-
  YL-ALANINE Seed
GLUTAMIC-ACID Fruit 1,540—38,987 ppm
GLYCINE Fruit 190—4,810 ppm
GRAMISTEROL Seed
HEXANAL Fruit
HEXEN-2-AL-1 Fruit
HISTIDINE Fruit 80—2,025 ppm
IRON Fruit 2.6—420 ppm
ISOLEUCINE Fruit 170—4,303 ppm
ISOMULTIFLORINEOL Seed
ISOORIENTIN Leaf
LEAD Fruit 0.002—2.8 ppm
LEUCINE Fruit 230—5,822 ppm
LINOLEIC-ACID Cotyledon 35,100—486,700
  ppm
LINOLEIC-ACID Fruit 220—5,570 ppm
LINOLEIC-ACID Seed 66,900—170,468 ppm
LINOLEIC-ACID Cotyledon 312,200 ppm
LITHIUM Fruit 0.236—0.56 ppm
LUPEOL Seed
LYSINE Fruit 220—5,570 ppm
LYSOLECITHIN Seed
MAGNESIUM Fruit 101—7,000 ppm

MANGANESE Fruit 0.5—98 ppm
MELOSIDE-A Leaf
MERCURY Fruit 0—0.05 ppm
METHIONINE Fruit 40—1,012 ppm
MEVALONIC-ACID Fruit 3 ppm
MOLYBDENUM Fruit 0.1—2.8 ppm
MUFA Fruit 30—759 ppm
MULTIFLORINEOL Seed
MYRISTIC-ACID Fruit 10—253 ppm
NIACIN Fruit 3—76 ppm
NICKEL Fruit 0.01—1.25 ppm
NITROGEN Fruit 1,400—80,000 ppm
NON-TRANS-2-EN-AL Fruit
NONA-TRANS-2-CIS-6-DIEN-1-AL Plant
NONADIEN-2,6-AL-1 Fruit
NONADIEN-2,6-OL-2 Fruit
NONEN-2-AL-1 Fruit
OBTUSIFOLIOL Seed
OLEIC-ACID Cotyledon 55,200—241,000 ppm
OLEIC-ACID Fruit 20—506 ppm
OLEIC-ACID Seed 116,100—180,000 ppm
PALMITIC-ACID Cotyledon 213,200—
  504,700 ppm
PALMITIC-ACID Fruit 270—6,835 ppm
PALMITIC-ACID Seed 12,420—20,400 ppm
PANTOTHENIC-ACID Fruit 2.5—63 ppm
PENTADEC-CIS-8-EN-1-AL Fruit
PHOSPHATIDIC-ACID Seed
PHOSPHATIDYL-CHOLINE Seed
PHOSPHATIDYL-ETHANOLAMINE Seed
PHOSPHATIDYL-GLYCEROL Seed
PHOSPHATIDYL-INOSITOL Seed
PHOSPHORUS Fruit 158—12,600 ppm
PHYTOSTEROLS Fruit 14—3,544 ppm
PL Plant
POTASSIUM Fruit
PROLINE Fruit 120—3,038 ppm
PROPANAL Fruit
PROTEIN Fruit 5,120—142,772 ppm
PUFA Fruit 510—12,911 ppm
RIBOFLAVIN Fruit 0.2—5.1 ppm
RUBIDIUM Fruit 0.4—19 ppm
SELENIUM Fruit 0.001—2.8 ppm
SERINE Fruit 160—4,051 ppm
SFA Fruit 330—8,354 ppm
SILICON Fruit 10—1,000 ppm

SILVER Fruit 0.01—0.14 ppm
SODIUM Fruit 16—714 ppm
SPERMIDINE Seed
SQUALENE Fruit
STEARIC-ACID Cotyledon 28,800—59,100 ppm
STEARIC-ACID Fruit 30—759 ppm
STEARIC-ACID Seed 11,100—69,785 ppm
STELLASTEROL Seed
STIGMAST-7,22,25-TRIEN-3-BETA-OL Seed
STIGMAST-7,25-DIEN-3-BETA-OL Seed
STIGMAST-7-EN-3-BETA-OL Leaf
STIGMASTEROL Plant
STRONTIUM Fruit 4—98 ppm
SUGAR Fruit 10,000 ppm
SULFOQUINOVOSYL-DIACYL-GLYCEROL Petiole
SULFUR Fruit 140—5,250 ppm
TARAXEROL Seed
THIAMIN Fruit 0.3—7.6 ppm
THREONINE Fruit 150—3,797 ppm
TIRUCALLOL Seed
TITANIUM Fruit 0.3—18 ppm
TRYPTOPHAN Fruit 40—1,012 ppm
TYROSINE Fruit 90—2,278 ppm
VITAMIN B6 Fruit 0.5—13 ppm
WATER Fruit 944,000—971,000 ppm
ZINC Fruit 2—157 ppm
ZIRCONIUM Fruit 1.18—2.8 ppm

■ EGGPLANT

Chemical Constituents of Solanum melongena L. (Solanaceae)

5-HYDROXYTRYPTAMINE Fruit
9-OXONEROLIDOL Plant
ALANINE Fruit 420—6,815 ppm
ALPHA-LINOLENIC-ACID Fruit 70—867 ppm
ALUMINUM Fruit 10—16 ppm
ARACHIDIC-ACID Seed
ARGININE Fruit 610—7,559 ppm
ARSENIC Fruit
ASCORBIC-ACID Fruit 13—947 ppm

ASCORBIC-ACID Leaf 790—5,809 ppm
ASH Fruit 5,000—80,000 ppm
ASH Leaf 20,000—147,000 ppm
ASPARTIC-ACID Fruit 1,770—21,933 ppm
AUBERGENONE Plant
BARIUM Fruit 3.5—5.6 ppm
BETA-AMINO-4-ETHYL-GLYOXALINE Fruit
BETA-CAROTENE Fruit 0—6 ppm
BORON Fruit 1—8 ppm
CADMIUM Fruit 0.3—0.44 ppm
CAFFEIC-ACID Fruit
CALCIUM Fruit 120—5,706 ppm
CALCIUM Leaf 2,540—18,676 ppm
CARBOHYDRATES Fruit 56,000—811,000 ppm
CARBOHYDRATES Leaf 66,000—485,000 ppm
CHLORINE Fruit 520 ppm
CHROMIUM Fruit 0.1—0.12 ppm
COBALT Fruit 0.07—0.08 ppm
COPPER Fruit 0.6—20 ppm
CYANIDIN Fruit
CYSTINE Fruit 60—743 ppm
DELPHINIDIN Fruit
DELPHINIDIN-3-RUTINOSIDE-3-(4'-COUMAROYLRUTINOSIDE)5-GLUC Plant
DELPHINIDIN-P-COUMAROYL-MONORHAMNOSIDE-DIGLUCOSIDE Fruit
ETHYL-CAFFEATE Root
FAT Fruit 1,000—38,000 ppm
FAT Leaf 4,000—29,000 ppm
FAT Seed 198,300—212,000 ppm
FERULIC-ACID Root
FIBER Fruit 9,000—137,000 ppm
FOLACIN Fruit 0.1—2.6 ppm
GABA Fruit
GAMMA-HYDROXYGLUTAMIC-ACID Fruit
GLUTAMIC-ACID Fruit 2,010—24,907 ppm
GLYCINE Fruit 320—5,452 ppm
GLYCOALKALOIDS Fruit 280—470 ppm
HCN Fruit
HISTIDINE Fruit 240—3,098 ppm

IRON Fruit 3—137 ppm
IRON Leaf 155—1,140 ppm
ISOLEUCINE Fruit 480—5,948 ppm
ISOSCOPOLETIN Root
KILOCALORIES Fruit 250—3,370/kg
KILOCALORIES Leaf 150—2,790/kg
LEAD Fruit 1.4—1.6 ppm
LEUCINE Fruit 570—8,550 ppm
LINOLEIC-ACID Fruit 350—4,337 ppm
LITHIUM Fruit 0.28—0.32 ppm
LUBIMEN Plant
LYCOPENE Fruit
LYCOXANTHIN Fruit
LYSINE Fruit 510—6,320 ppm
MAGNESIUM Fruit 85—1,563 ppm
MANGANESE Fruit 1.4—40 ppm
MERCURY Fruit 0.001—0.001
METHIONINE Fruit 60—1,487 ppm
MOLYBDENUM Fruit 0.5—0.56 ppm
MUFA Fruit 90—1,152 ppm
N-TRANS-FERULOYL-OCTOPAMINE Root
N-TRANS-FERULOYL-TYRAMINE Root
N-TRANS-P-COUMAROYL-OCTOPAMINE
 Root
N-TRANS-P-COUMAROYL-TYRAMINE
 Root
NASUNIN Fruit
NEOCHLOROGENIC-ACID Fruit
NIACIN Fruit 0.9—98 ppm
NICKEL Fruit 0.7—0.8 ppm
NITROGEN Fruit 5,400—10,250 ppm
OLEIC-ACID Fruit 80—991 ppm
OXALIC-ACID Fruit 291 ppm
PALMITIC-ACID Fruit 140—1,735 ppm
PALMITOLEIC-ACID Fruit 1-—124 ppm
PANTOTHENIC-ACID Fruit 0.8—10 ppm
PECTIN Fruit 110,000 ppm
PHENYLALANINE Fruit 430—5,700 ppm
PHOSPHORUS Fruit 189—5,836 ppm
PHOSPHORUS Leaf 380—2,794 ppm
PHYTOSTEROLS Fruit—867 ppm
PIPECOLIC-ACID Fruit
POTASSIUM Fruit 620—32,000 ppm
PROLINE Fruit 460—5,700 ppm
PROTEIN Fruit 10,000—200,000 ppm
PROTEIN Leaf 46,000—338,000 ppm

PUFA Fruit 420—5,204 ppm
RIBOFLAVIN Fruit 0.2—8.8 ppm
SCOPOLETIN Fruit
SELENIUM Fruit 0.001—0.002 ppm
SERINE Fruit 410—5,576 ppm
SFA Fruit 200—2,478 ppm
SILVER Fruit 0.07—0.18 ppm
SODIUM Fruit 20—2,150 ppm
SOLAMARGINE Fruit
SOLANIDINE Fruit
SOLANINE Fruit
SOLASODINE Fruit
SOLASONINE Fruit
STEARIC-ACID Fruit 50—620 ppm
STRONTIUM Fruit 2—5.6 ppm
SUCROSE Fruit
SUGAR Fruit 20,000—30,000 ppm
SULFUR Fruit 126—152 ppm
TANNIN Fruit 2,000 ppm
THIAMIN Fruit 0.4—10 ppm
THREONINE Fruit 380—4,957 ppm
TITANIUM Fruit 0.35—0.4 ppm
TRIGONELLINE Fruit
TRYPTAMINE Fruit
TRYPTOPHAN Fruit 100—1,239 ppm
TYRAMINE Fruit
TYROSINE Fruit 250—3,593 ppm
VALINE Fruit 550—7,063 ppm
VANILLIN Root
VITAMIN B6 Fruit 0.9—11.6 ppm
WATER Fruit 905,000—932,000 ppm
WATER Leaf 864,000 ppm
ZINC Fruit 18—25.6 ppm
ZIRCONIUM Fruit 1.4—1.6 ppm

■ ELEPHANT GARLIC

Chemical Constituents of Allium ampeloprasum
L. (Liliaceae)

1-O-CAFFEOYL-BETA-D-GLUCOSE Plant
3,4-DIMETHYL-2,5-DIOXO-2,5-
 DIHYDROTHIOPHENE Plant
3,5-DIALKYLTRITHIOLANES Plant
4-HYDROXY-PROLINE Plant

ACETYL-SYNTHETASE Plant
ADENYLIC-ACID Plant
AECULETIN Plant
ALANINE Plant
ALCOHOL-DEHYDROGENASE Plant
ALLIN Plant
ALLITHIAMINE Plant
ALLYL Plant
ALLYL-MONOSULFIDE Plant
ALLYL-SULFIDE Plant
ALPHA-TOCOPHEROL Plant
ALUMINUM-PHOSPHATE Plant
ARGINASE Plant
ARGININE Plant
ASCORBIC-ACID Flower 400—2,367 ppm
ASCORBIC-ACID Leaf 170—3,019 ppm
ASCORBIC-ACID Root 170—1,241 ppm
ASCORBIC-ACID-OXIDASE Plant
ASH Flower 4,000—24,000 ppm
ASH Leaf 8,000—75,000 ppm
ASH Root 9,000—66,000 ppm
ASPARAGINE Plant
ASPARTIC-ACID Plant
BETA-CAROTENE Flower 25—151 ppm
BETA-CAROTENE Leaf 0.2—230 ppm
BETA-CAROTENE Root 0.2—1.8 ppm
BETA-SITOSTEROL Plant
BUTYL-SULFIDE Plant
CAFFEIC-ACID Plant
CALCIUM Flower 230—1,361 ppm
CALCIUM Leaf 520—5,472 ppm
CALCIUM Root 520—3,796 ppm
CARBOHYDRATES Flower 105,000—621,000 ppm
CARBOHYDRATES Leaf 70,000—767,000 ppm
CARBOHYDRATES Root 103,000—752,000 ppm
CATALASE Plant
CELLULOSE Plant
CHLOROGENIC-ACID Plant
CYCLOALLIN Plant
CYTIDYLIC-ACID Plant
DEHYDROASCORBIC-ACID Plant
DEOXYRIBONUCLEIC-ACID Plant
DI-PROPYL-THIOSULFINATES Plant

DIALLYL-SULFIDE Plant
DIKETOGLUCONIC-ACID Plant
DIMETHYL-DISULFIDE Plant
ESTERASE Plant
ETHYL-SULFIDE Plant
ETHYLENE-BIS-DIETHIO-CARBAMATE Plant
FAT Flower 5,000—30,000 ppm
FAT Leaf 3,000—47,000 ppm
FAT Root 3,000—22,000 ppm
FERRIC-PHOSPHATE Plant
FERULIC-ACID Plant
FIBER Flower 11,000—65,000 ppm
FIBER Leaf 10,000—94,000 ppm
FOLACIN Plant
FRUCTOSE Plant
FRUCTOSYLSUCROSE Plant
GALACTOSE Plant
GLUCOFRUCTAN Plant
GLUCOSE Plant
GLUTAMATE-DEHYDROGENASE Plant
GLUTAMIC-ACID Plant
GLUTAMINE Plant
GUANYLIC-ACID Plant
HEMICELLULOSE Plant
HISTIDINE Plant
HISTONES Plant
IRON Flower 9—53 ppm
IRON Leaf 11—255 ppm
IRON Root 11—80 ppm
ISOCHLOROGENIC-ACID Plant
ISOLEUCINE Plant
KAEMPFEROL-3-BETA-D-GLUCOSIDE Plant
KAEMPFEROL-3-XYLOSYL-BETA-D-GLUCOSIDE Plant
KAEMPFEROL-HETEROSIDE Plant
KILOCALORIES Flower 550—3,250/kg
KILOCALORIES Leaf 350—3,560/kg
KILOCALORIES Root 450—3,280/kg
LACTATE-DEHYDROGENASE Plant
LEUCINE Plant
LIGNIN Plant
LIGNOCERIC-ACID Plant
LINOLEIC-ACID Plant
LINOLENIC-ACID Plant

LYSINE Plant
MALTOSE Plant
MANNITOL Plant
METHIONINE Plant
METHYL-ALLIN Plant
METHYL-SULFIDE Plant
MYOINOSITOL Plant
NIACIN Flower 9—53 ppm
NIACIN Leaf 5—57 ppm
NICOTINIC-ACID Plant
ODORIN Plant
OXALATE-DEHYDROGENASE Plant
OXALIC-ACID Plant
P-COUMARIC-ACID Plant
PALMITIC-ACID Plant
PECTINS Plant
PEROXIDASE Plant
PHENATHRENE Plant
PHENOL-OXIDASE Plant
PHENYLALANINE Plant
PHOSPHORUS Flower 380—2,249 ppm
PHOSPHORUS Leaf 480—4,528 ppm
PHOSPHORUS Root 500—3,650 ppm
POLYPHENOLS Plant
POTASSIUM Leaf 3,160—29,811 ppm
PROLINE Plant
PROPANE-THIOSULFINATE Plant
PROPYL-DISULFIDE Plant
PROPYLOALLIN Plant
PROTEIN Flower 55,000—325,000 ppm
PROTEIN Leaf 22,000—217,000 ppm
PROTEIN Root 22,000—161,000 ppm
QUERCETIN-3-GLUCOSIDE Plant
RAFFINOSE Plant
RIBOFLAVIN Flower 1.9—11.2 ppm
RIBOFLAVIN Leaf 0.6—9.4 ppm
RIBONUCLEIC-ACID Plant
S-2,2-PROPENYL-AMINO-ACID-
    SULFOXIDE Plant
SAPONINS Plant
SCOPOLETIN Plant
SERINE Plant
SIDERAMINES Plant
SILICON-DIOXIDE Plant
SINAPIC-ACID Plant
SODIUM Leaf 50—472 ppm

STACHYOSE Plant
STEARIC-ACID Plant
SUCCINC-DEHYDROGENASE Plant
SUCROSE Plant
SULFUR Leaf 600—700 ppm
SULFUR-TRIOXIDE Plant
THIAMIN Flower 1.4—8.3 ppm
THIAMIN Leaf 0.9—8.5 ppm
THIAMIN Root 1.1—8 ppm
THIAMIN-PYROPHOSPHATE Plant
THREONINE Plant
TRYPTOPHAN Plant
TYROSINE Plant
UMBELLIFERONE Plant
URIDYLIC-ACID Plant
VALINE Plant
VITAMIN U Plant
WATER Flower 831,000 ppm
WATER Leaf 854,000—894,000 ppm
WATER Root 863,000 ppm
ZINC Plant

ENDIVE

Chemical Constituents of Cichorium endiva L. (Asteraceae)

ALANINE Leaf 620—9,984 ppm
ALPHA-LINOLENIC-ACID Leaf 130—2,093
    ppm
ALUMINUM Leaf 60—168 ppm
ARGININE Leaf 620—9,984 ppm
ARSENIC Leaf 0.04—0.048 ppm
ASCORBIC-ACID Leaf 462—9,302 ppm
ASH Leaf 13,590—240,000 ppm
ASPARTIC-ACID Leaf 1,300—20,934 ppm
BARIUM Leaf 14—24 ppm
BETA-CAROTENE Leaf 9.6—241 ppm
BETA-LACTUCEROL Latex Exudate
BORON Leaf 1—24 ppm
CADMIUM Leaf 0.2—0.24 ppm
CAFFEIC-ACID Leaf
CALCIUM Leaf 462—10,080 ppm
CAOUTCHOUC Latex Exudate

CARBOHYDRATES Leaf 33,500—539,452 ppm
CHROMIUM Leaf 0.3—0.48 ppm
COBALT Leaf 0.2—0.24 ppm
COPPER Leaf 1—16.8 ppm
CYSTINE Leaf 100—1,610 ppm
FAT Leaf 2,000—32,200 ppm
FIBER Leaf 9,000—144,927 ppm
FOLACIN Leaf 1.2—25 ppm
GLUTAMIC-ACID Leaf 1,660—26,731 ppm
GLYCINE Leaf 580—9,340 ppm
HISTIDINE Leaf 230—3,704 ppm
HYDROXYCINNAMIC-ACID Leaf
INULIN Root
IRON Leaf 6—360 ppm
ISOLEUCINE Leaf 720—11,594 ppm
KAEMPFEROL-3-GLUCOSIDE Leaf
KEAMPFEROL-GLYCOSIDES Plant
KILOCALORIES Leaf 170—2,737/kg
LEAD Leaf 4—4.8 ppm
LEUCINE Leaf 980—15,781 ppm
LINOLEIC-ACID Leaf 750—12,077 ppm
LITHIUM Leaf 0.8—0.96 ppm
LYSINE Leaf 630—10,145 ppm
MAGNESIUM Leaf 95—2,400 ppm
MANGANESE Leaf 4—72 ppm
MERCURY Leaf 0.002—0.002 ppm
METHIONINE Leaf 140—2,254 ppm
MOLYBDENUM Leaf 1.4—1.68 ppm
MUFA Leaf 40—644 ppm
MYRISTIC-ACID Leaf 30—483 ppm
NIACIN Leaf 4—64 ppm
NICKEL Leaf 2—2.4 ppm
OLEIC-ACID Leaf 40—644 ppm
PALMITIC-ACID Leaf 410—6,602 ppm
PANTOTHENIC-ACID Leaf 9—145 ppm
PHENOLICS Leaf 32,000 ppm
PHENYLALANINE Leaf 530—8,535 ppm
PHOSPHORUS Leaf 242—5,760 ppm
POTASSIUM Leaf 2,915—96,000 ppm
PROLINE Leaf 590—9,500 ppm
PROTEIN Leaf 12,000—209,300 ppm
PUFA Leaf 870—14,010 ppm
QUERCETIN Leaf
RIBOFLAVIN Leaf 0.7—13 ppm
SELENIUM Leaf 0.008—0.024 ppm

SERINE Leaf 490—7,890 ppm
SFA Leaf 480—7,729 ppm
SILVER Leaf 0.2—0.24 ppm
SODIUM Leaf 179—4,560 ppm
STEARIC-ACID Leaf 20—322 ppm
STRONTIUM Shoot 140—240 ppm
SULFUR Shoot 740—912 ppm
TARAXASTEROL Latex Exudate
THIAMIN Leaf 0.7—14 ppm
THREONINE Leaf 500—8,051 ppm
TITANIUM Leaf 1—1.2 ppm
TRYPTOPHAN Leaf 50—805 ppm
TYROSINE Leaf 400—6,441 ppm
VALINE Leaf 630—10,145 ppm
VITAMIN B6 Leaf 0.2—3.2 ppm
WATER Leaf 934,000—943,800 ppm
ZINC Leaf 8—146 ppm
ZIRCONIUM Leaf 4—4.8 ppm

■ GARLIC

Chemical Constituents of Allium sativum L. (Liliaceae)

1,2-(PROP-2-ENYL)-DISULFANE Bulb
1,2-DIMERCAPTOCYCLOPENTANE Bulb 2.4 PPM
1,2-EPITHIOPROPANE Bulb 0.1—1.66 ppm
1,3-DITHIANE Bulb 0.08—3 ppm
1-HEXANOL Bulb 0.23 ppm
1-METHYL-1,2-(PROP-2-ENYL)-DISULFANE Bulb
1-METHYL-2-(PROP-2-ENYL)-DISULFANE Bulb
1-METHYL-3-(PROP-2-ENYL)-TRISULFANE Bulb
2,3,4-TRITHIAPENTANE Bulb
2,5-DIMETHYL-TETRAHYDROTHIOPHENE Bulb 0.6 ppm
2-METHYLBENZALDEHYDE Bulb 0.1 ppm
2-PROPEN-1-OL Bulb 0.1—121 ppm
2-VINYL-4H-1,3-DITHIN Bulb 2—29 ppm
24-METHYLENE-CYCLOARTENOL Plant
3,5-DIETHYL-1,2,4-TRITHIOLANE Bulb 0.15—43 ppm

3-METHYL-2-CYCLOPENTENE-1-THIONE
Bulb 0.16—1.6 ppm
3-VINYL-4H-1,2-DITHIN Bulb 0.34—10.65
ppm
4-METHYL-5-VINYLTHIAZOLE Bulb 0.75
ppm
5-BUTYL-CYSTEINE-SULFOXIDE Bulb
ADENOSINE Bulb
AJOENE Bulb
ALANINE Bulb 1,320—3,168 ppm
ALLICIN Bulb 1,500—27,800 ppm
ALLIIN Bulb 5,000—10,000 ppm
ALLINASE Bulb
ALLISTATIN-I Bulb
ALLISTATIN-II Bulb
ALLIXIN Bulb
ALLYL-METHYL-DISULFIDE Bulb
ALLYL-METHYL-TRISULFIDE Bulb
ALLYL-PROPYL-DISULFIDE Bulb 36—216
ppm
ALPHA-PHELLANDRENE Bulb
ALPHA-PROSTAGLANDIN-F-1 Bulb
ALPHA-PROSTAGLANDIN-F-2 Bulb
ALPHA-TOCOPHEROL Bulb
ALUMINUM Bulb 52 ppm
ANILINE Bulb 10 ppm
ARACHIDONIC-ACID Bulb
ARGININE Bulb 6,340—15,216 ppm
ASCORBIC-ACID Bulb 100—788 ppm
ASCORBIC-ACID Flower 440—3,793 ppm
ASCORBIC-ACID Leaf 390—2,868 ppm
ASCORBIC-ACID Shoot 420—1,883 ppm
ASH Bulb 10,000—395,000 ppm
ASH Flower 6,000—52,000 ppm
ASH Leaf 10,000—74,000 ppm
ASH Shoot 7,000—31,000 ppm
ASPARTIC-ACID Bulb 4,890—11,736 ppm
BETA-CAROTENE Bulb 0—0.17 ppm
BETA-CAROTENE Flower 0.6—5 ppm
BETA-CAROTENE Leaf 9—68 ppm
BETA-CAROTENE Shoot 2—9 ppm
BETA-PHELLANDRENE Bulb
BETA-SITOSTEROL Plant
BETA-TOCOPHEROL Bulb
BIOTIN Bulb 22 ppm
BORON Bulb 3—6 ppm

CAFFEIC-ACID Bulb 20 ppm
CALCIUM Bulb 180—4,947 ppm
CALCIUM Flower 250—2,155 ppm
CALCIUM Leaf 580—4,265 ppm
CALCIUM Shoot 120—538 ppm
CALCIUM-OXALATE Bulb
CARBOHYDRATES Bulb 274,000—851,000
ppm
CARBOHYDRATES Flower 94,000—810,000
ppm
CARBOHYDRATES Leaf 95,000—699,000
ppm
CARBOHYDRATES Shoot 201,000—91,000
ppm
CHLOROGENIC-ACID Plant
CHOLINE Bulb
CHROMIUM Bulb 2.5—15 ppm
CIS-AJOENE Bulb
CITRAL Bulb
COBALT Bulb 0.5—100 ppm
COPPER Bulb 4.8—9.7 ppm
CYCLOALLIIN Bulb
CYSTINE Bulb 650—1,560 ppm
DESGALACTOTIGONIN Root 400 ppm
DESOXYRIBONCULEASE Bulb
DIALLYL-DISULFIDE Bulb 16—613 ppm
DIALLYL-SULFIDE Bulb 2—99 ppm
DIALLYL-TETRASULFIDE Bulb
DIALLYL-TRISULFIDE Bulb 10—1,061 ppm
DIGALACTOSYL-DIGLYCERIDE Bulb
DIMETHYL-DIFURAN Bulb 5—30 ppm
DIMETHYL-DISULFIDE Bulb 0.6—2.5 ppm
DIMETHYL-SULFIDE Bulb
DIMETHYL-TRISULFIDE Bulb 0.8—19 ppm
EICOSAPENTAENOIC-ACID Bulb
EO Bulb 600—3,600 ppm
FAT Bulb 2,000—12,000 ppm
FAT Flower 2,000—17,000 ppm
FAT Leaf 5,000—37,000 ppm
FAT Shoot 3,000—13,000 ppm
FERULIC-ACID Bulb 27 ppm
FIBER Bulb 7,000—39,000 ppm
FIBER Flower 8,000—69,000 ppm
FIBER Leaf 18,000—132,000 ppm
FIBER Shoot 17,000—76,000 ppm
FOLIACIN Bulb 1 ppm

FRUCTOSE Bulb
GAMMA-L-GLUTAMYL-ISOLEUCINE Bulb
GAMMA-L-GLUTAMYL-L-LEUCINE Bulb
GAMMA-L-GLUTAMYL-L-PHENYLALANINE Bulb
GAMMA-L-GLUTAMYL-L-VALINE Plant
GAMMA-L-GLUTAMYL-METHIONINE Bulb
GAMMA-L-GLUTAMYL-S-(2-CARBOXY-1-PROPYL)-CYSTEINEGLYCINE Plant
GAMMA-L-GLUTAMYL-S-ALLYL-CYSTEINE Bulb
GAMMA-L-GLUTAMYL-S-ALLYL-MERCAPTO-CYSTEINE Bulb
GAMMA-L-GLUTAMYL-S-BETA-CARBOXY-BETA-METHYL-ETHYL-CYSTEINYL-GLYCINE Bulb
GAMMA-L-GLUTAMYL-S-METHYL-L-CYSTEINE-SULFOXIDE Bulb
GAMMA-L-GLUTAMYL-S-PROPYL-L-CYSTEINE Bulb
GERANIOL Bulb
GERMANIUM Bulb
GIBBERELLIN-A-3 Bulb
GIBBERELLIN-A-7 Bulb
GITONIN Root 300 ppm
GLUCOSE Bulb
GLUTAMIC-ACID Bulb 8,050—19,320 ppm
GLUTATHIONE Bulb
GLYCEROL-SULFOQUINOVOSIDE Bulb
GLYCINE Bulb 2,000—4,800 ppm
GUANOSINE Bulb
HEXA-1,5-DIENYL-TRISULFIDE Bulb
HEXOKINASE Bulb
HISTIDINE Bulb 1,130—2,712 ppm
IODINE Bulb
IRON Bulb 15—129 ppm
IRON Flower 9—78 ppm
IRON Leaf 6—44 ppm
IRON Shoot 17—76 ppm
ISOBUTYL-ISOTHIOCYANATE Bulb 0.14—25 ppm
ISOLEUCINE Bulb 2,170—5,208 ppm
KAEMPFEROL Plant
KILOCALORIES Bulb 1,170—3,630 ppm
KILOCALORIES Flower 390—3,366/kg

KILOCALORIES Leaf 440—3,240/kg
KILOCALORIES Shoot 760—3,410/kg
LEUCINE Bulb 3,050—7,392 ppm
LINALOOL Bulb
LINOLENIC-ACID Plant
LYSINE Bulb 2,730—6,552 ppm
MAGNESIUM Bulb 240—1,210 ppm
MANGANESE Bulb 5.4—15.3 ppm
METHIONINE Bulb 760—1,824 ppm
METHYL-ALLYL-DISULFIDE Bulb 6—104 ppm
METHYL-PROPYL-DISULFIDE Bulb 0.03—0.66 ppm
METHYLALLYL-SULFIDE Bulb 0.5—4.6 ppm
METHYLALLYL-TRISULFIDE Bulb 6—279 ppm
MONOGALACTOSYL-DIGLYCERIDE Bulb
MYROSINASE Bulb
NIACIN Bulb 4—17 ppm
NIACIN Flower 4—34 ppm
NIACIN Leaf 6—44 ppm
NIACIN Shoot 5—22 ppm
NICKEL Bulb 1.5—1.7 ppm
NICOTINIC-ACID Bulb 4.8 ppm
OLEANOLIC-ACID Plant
OLEIC-ACID Plant
ORNITHINE Leaf
P-COUMARIC-ACID Bulb 58 ppm
P-HYDROXYBENZOIC-ACID Plant
PEROXIDASE Bulb
PHENYLALANINE Bulb 1,830—4,392 ppm
PHLOROGLUCINOL Plant
PHOSPHATIDYL-CHOLINE Bulb
PHOSPHATIDYL-ETHANOLAMINE Bulb
PHOSPHATIDYL-INOSITOL Bulb
PHOSPHATIDYLSERINE Bulb
PHOSPHORUS Bulb 880—5,220 ppm
PHOSPHORUS Flower 460—3,382 ppm
PHOSPHORUS Leaf 460—3,382 ppm
PHOSPHORUS Shoot 520—2,332 ppm
PHYTIC-ACID Plant
POTASSIUM Bulb 3,730—13,669 ppm
POTASSIUM Leaf 3,260—23,971 ppm
POTASSIUM Shoot 2,730—12,242 ppm
PROLINE Bulb 1,000—2,400 ppm

PROP-2-ENYL-DISULFANE Bulb
PROPENE Bulb 0.01—6 ppm
PROPENETHIOL Bulb 1—41 ppm
PROSTAGLANDIN-A-1 Bulb
PROSTAGLANDIN-A-2 Bulb
PROSTAGLANDIN-B-1 Bulb
PROSTAGLANDIN-B-2 Bulb
PROSTAGLANDIN-E-1 Bulb
PROSTAGLANDIN-E-2 Bulb
PROTEIN Bulb 35,000—179,000 ppm
PROTEIN Flower 14,000—121,000 ppm
PROTEIN Leaf 26,000—191,000 ppm
PROTEIN Shoot 12,000—54,000 ppm
PROTODEGALACTOTIGONIN Bulb 10 ppm
PROTOERUBOSIDE-B Bulb 10 ppm
PROTODEGALACTOTIGONIN Bulb 10 ppm
PROTOERUBOSIDE-B Bulb 100 ppm
PSEUDOSCORIDININE-A Bulb
PSEUDOSCORIDININE-B Bulb
QUERCETIN Bulb 200 ppm
QUERCETIN-3-O-BETA-D-GLUCOSIDE
    Plant
RAFFINOSE Bulb
RIBOFLAVIN Bulb 0.5—3 ppm
RIBOFLAVIN Bulb 0.6—5.2 ppm
RIBOFLAVIN Leaf 1.4—10.3 ppm
RIBOFLAVIN Shoot 0.6—2.7 ppm
RUTIN Plant
S-(2-CARBOXY-PROPYL)-GLUTATHIONE
    Bulb 92.5 ppm
S-ALLO-MERCAPTO-CYSTEINE Bulb 2 ppm
S-ALLYL-CYSTEINE Bulb 10 ppm
S-ALLYL-CYSTEINE-SULFOXIDE Bulb
S-ETHYL-CYSTEINE-SULFOXIDE Bulb
S-METHYL-CYSTEINE-SULFOXIDE Bulb
S-METHYL-L-CYSTEINE-SULFOXIDE Bulb
S-PROPENYL-CYSTEINE Bulb
S-PROPYL-CYSTEINE-SULFOXIDE Bulb
SAPONIN Bulb
SATIVOSIDE-B-1 Bulb 30 ppm
SATIVOSIDE-R-1 Root 500 ppm
SATIVOSIDE-R-2 Root 300 ppm
SCORDINE Bulb 250 ppm
SCORDIN-A Bulb 39,000 ppm
SCORODININ-A-1 Bulb 67—30,000 ppm
SCORODININ-A-2 Bulb 250—8,000 ppm

SCORODININ-B Bulb 800 ppm
SCORODININE-A-3 Bulb 333 ppm
SCORODOSE Bulb
SELENIUM Bulb
SERINE Bulb 1,900—4,560 ppm
SILICON Bulb
SINAPIC-ACID Plant 27 ppm
SODIUM Bulb 158—559 ppm
SODIUM Leaf 40—294 ppm
STIGMASTEROL Plant
SUCCINIC-ACID Plant
SUCROSE Bulb
TAURINE Plant
THIAMACORNINE Bulb
THIAMAMIDINE Bulb
THIAMIN Bulb 2—8 ppm
THIAMIN Flower 1.1—9.5 ppm
THIAMIN Leaf 1.1—8.1 ppm
THIAMIN Shoot 1.4—6.3 ppm
THREONINE Bulb 1,570—3,768 ppm
TIN Bulb 6 ppm
TRANS-1-PROPENYL-METHYL-
    DISULFIDE Bulb 0.9 ppm
TRANS-AJOENE Bulb 268 ppm
TRANS-S-(PROPENYL-1-YL)-CYSTEINE-
    DISULFIDE Bulb
TRYPTOPHAN Bulb 660—1,584 ppm
TYROSINASE Bulb
TYROSINE Bulb 810—1,944 ppm
URANIUM Bulb
VALINE Bulb 2,910—6,984 ppm
VITAMIN U Plant
WATER Bulb 585,000—678,000 ppm
WATER Flower 884,000 ppm
WATER Leaf 864,000
WATER Shoot 777,000 ppm
ZINC Bulb 15.3 ppm

■ GREENBEAN

Chemical Constituents of Phaseolus vulgaris L.
(Fabaceae)

12-DICARONIC-ACID Hull Husk
2-HYDROXYGENISTEIN Fruit

2-METHOXYPHASEOLINISOFLAVAN
Sprout Seedling
ALANINE Fruit 840—8,633 ppm
ALANINE Seed 9,050—10,171 ppm
ALANINE Sprout Seedling 1,740—18,710 ppm
ALLANTOIC-ACID Fruit 360—3,700 ppm
ALPHA-LINOLENIC-ACID Fruit 360—3,700 ppm
ALPHA-LINOLENIC-ACID Seed 2,780—3,124 ppm
ALPHA-LINOLENIC-ACID Sprout Seedling 1,690—18,172 ppm
ALPHA-TOCOPHEROL Fruit 0.2—14 ppm
ALPHA-TOCOPHEROL Leaf 698—719 ppm
ALUMINUM Fruit 1—1,050 ppm
ALUMINUM Seed 5—73 ppm
APIGENIN Plant
ARGININE Fruit 730—7,503 ppm
ARGININE Seed 13,370—15,026 ppm
ARGININE Sprout Seedling 2,280—24,516 ppm
ARSENIC Fruit 0.003—0.01
ARSENIC Seed 0.002—0.002 ppm
ASCORBIC-ACID Fruit 10—2,389 ppm
ASCORBIC-ACID Leaf 1,100—8,333 ppm
ASCORBIC-ACID Seed 0—177 ppm
ASCORBIC-ACID Sprout Seedling 387—4,161 ppm
ASH Fruit 6,000—156,000 ppm
ASH Leaf 26,000—177,000 ppm
ASH Seed 17,000—62,000 ppm
ASH Sprout Seedling 5,000—53,763 ppm
ASPARAGINE Fruit
ASPARTIC-ACID Fruit 2,550—26,208 ppm
ASPARTIC-ACID Seed 26,130—29,366 ppm
ASPARTIC-ACID Sprout Seedling 5,460—58,710 ppm
BARIUM Fruit 0.4—45 ppm
BARIUM Seed 0.1—7.3 ppm
BETA-CAROTENE Fruit 2.2—66 ppm
BETA-CAROTENE Leaf 32.4—245.5 ppm
BETA-CAROTENE Seed 0.1—9.8 ppm
BETA-CAROTENE Sprout Seedling
BORON Fruit 0.1—45 ppm
BORON Seed 0.1—9.8 ppm
BROMINE Fruit 2—20 ppm

CADMIUM Fruit 0.002—0.2 ppm
CADMIUM Seed 0.007—0.039 ppm
CALCIUM Fruit 356—18,000 ppm
CALCIUM Leaf 2,740—20,758 ppm
CALCIUM Seed 510—3,295 ppm
CALCIUM Sprout Seedling 170—1,828 ppm
CARBOHYDRATES Fruit 56,000—733,778 ppm
CARBOHYDRATES Leaf 66,000—500,000 ppm
CARBOHYDRATES Seed 278,000—701,039 ppm
CARBOHYDRATES Sprout Seedling 41,000—440,860 ppm
CEREBROSIDE Fruit
CHOLINE Fruit
CHROMIUM Fruit 0.005—1.5 ppm
CHROMIUM Seed 0.051—4.9 ppm
COBALAMINE Root
COBALT Fruit 0—10.5 ppm
COBALT Seed 0.034—1.05 ppm
COPPER Fruit 0.62—45 ppm
COPPER Seed 2—15 ppm
CYSTINE Fruit 180—1,850 ppm
CYSTINE Seed 2,350—2,641 ppm
CYSTINE Sprout Seedling 480—5,161 ppm
DEC-2-EN Hull Husk
FAT Fruit 2,000—47,000 ppm
FAT Leaf 4,000—54,000 ppm
FAT Seed 3,000—24,000 ppm
FAT Sprout Seedling 5,000—53,763 ppm
FERULIC-ACID Plant
FIBER Fruit 10,000—159,000 ppm
FIBER Leaf 28,000—212,000 ppm
FIBER Seed 37,000—88,700 ppm
FLUORINE Fruit 0.1—2 ppm
FOLACIN Seed 4.1—5.3 ppm
FOLACIN Sprout Seedling 0.3—4.1 ppm
GENISTEIN Fruit
GIBBERELIN-A-37 Plant
GIBBERELIN-A-38 Plant
GLUCOKININ Fruit
GLUTAMIC-ACID Fruit 1,870—19,219 ppm
GLUTAMIC-ACID Seed 32,940—37,019 ppm
GLUTAMIC-ACID Sprout Seedling 5,120—55,054 ppm

GLUTATHIONE Root
GLYCINE Fruit 650—6,680 ppm
GLYCINE Seed 8,430—9,474 ppm
GLYCINE Sprout Seedling 1,440—15,484 ppm
HISTIDINE Fruit 340—3,494 ppm
HISTIDINE Seed 6,010—6,754 ppm
HISTIDINE Sprout Seedling 1,180—12,688 ppm
INOSITOL Fruit
IRON Fruit 6—1,050 ppm
IRON Leaf 92—697 ppm
IRON Seed 24—147 ppm
IRON Sprout Seedling 8—87 ppm
ISOLEUCINE Fruit 660—6,783 ppm
ISOLEUCINE Seed 9,540—10,722 ppm
ISOLEUCINE Sprout Seedling 1,860—20,000 ppm
KAEMPFEROL-3-GLUCYRONIDE Leaf
KILOCALORIES Fruit 280—3,830/kg
KILOCALORIES Leaf 360—2,730/kg
KILOCALORIES Seed 3,230—3,832/kg
KILOCALORIES Sprout Seedling 290—3,118/kg
LEAD Fruit 0.01—10.5 ppm
LEAD Seed 0.7—1 ppm
LEUCINE Fruit 1,120—11,511 ppm
LEUCINE Sprout Seedling 3,020—32,473 ppm
LIGNIN Seed 4,100—10,800 ppm
LINOLEIC-ACID Fruit 230—2,364 ppm
LINOLEIC-ACID Seed 3,320—3,731 ppm
LINOLEIC-ACID Sprout Seedling 1,070—11,505 ppm
LITHIUM Fruit 0.216—2.7 ppm
LITHIUM Seed 0.136—2.45 ppm
LUTEOLIN Plant
LYSINE Fruit 880—9,044 ppm
LYSINE Seed 14,830—16,667 ppm
LYSINE Sprout Seedling 2,390—25,700 ppm
MAGNESIUM Fruit 210—18,000 ppm
MAGNESIUM Sprout Seedling 210—2,258 ppm
MALONIC-ACID Fruit
MANGANESE Fruit 1—150 ppm
MANGANESE Seed 2—24 ppm
MERCURY Fruit 0—0.02 ppm
METHIONINE Fruit 220—2,261 ppm

METHIONINE Seed 3,250—3,653 ppm
METHIONINE Sprout Seedling 440—4,731 ppm
MOLYBDENUM Fruit 0—20 ppm
MOLYBDENUM Seed 0.5—14 ppm
MUFA Fruit 50—514 ppm
MUFA Seed 1,230—1,382 ppm
MUFA Sprout Seedling 390—4,194 ppm
NIACIN Fruit 5—77 ppm
NIACIN Leaf 13—98 ppm
NIACIN Seed 15—38 ppm
NIACIN Sprout Seedling 29—312 ppm
NICKEL Fruit 0—15 ppm
NICKEL Seed 0.5—7 ppm
NITROGEN Fruit 3,600—41,000 ppm
OLEIC-ACID Fruit 40—411 ppm
OLEIC-ACID Seed 1,230—1,382 ppm
OLEIC-ACID Sprout Seedling 390—4,194 ppm
OXALIC-ACID Fruit 312 ppm
P-COUMARIC-ACID Plant
PALMITIC-ACID Fruit 220—2,261 ppm
PALMITIC-ACID Seed 3,430—3,855 ppm
PALMITIC-ACID Sprout Seedling 640—6,882 ppm
PANTOTHENIC-ACID Fruit 0.9—10 ppm
PANTOTHENIC-ACID Seed 9—10 ppm
PHASELIC-ACID Plant
PHASEOLIDES Plant
PHASEOLLIDIN Plant
PHASEOLLIN Plant
PHASEOLLIN-ISOFLAVONE Plant
PHENYLALANINE Fruit 670—6,886 ppm
PHENYLALANINE Seed 11,680—13,127 ppm
PHENYLALANINE Sprout Seedling 2,120—22,796 ppm
PHOSPHORUS Fruit 370—13,500 ppm
PHOSPHORUS Leaf 750—5,682 ppm
PHOSPHORUS Seed 2,130—5,880 ppm
PHOSPHORUS Sprout Seedling 370—3,978 ppm
PHYTIC-ACID Seed 4,800 ppm
PHYTOSTEROLS Seed
PIPECOLIC-ACID Fruit
POTASSIUM Fruit 1,960—58,500 ppm
POTASSIUM Seed 9,840—21,070 ppm

POTASSIUM Sprout Seedling 1,870—20,108 ppm
PROLINE Fruit 680—6,989 ppm
PROLINE Seed 9,160—10,294 ppm
PROLINE Sprout Seedling 1,690—18,172 ppm
PROTEIN Fruit 17,700—224,000 ppm
PROTEIN Leaf 36,000—297,000 ppm
PROTEIN Seed 98,000—394,000 ppm
PROTEIN Sprout Seedling 42,000—451,613 ppm
PUFA Fruit 590—6,064 ppm
PUFA Seed 6,100—6,855 ppm
PUFA Sprout Seedling 2,760—29,677 ppm
PYRROLIDINONCARBONIC-ACID Fruit
QUERCETIN-3-GLUCURONIDE Leaf
RIBOFLAVIN Fruit 1—12 ppm
RIBOFLAVIN Leaf 0.6—4.5 ppm
RIBOFLAVIN Seed 1.2—3 ppm
RIBOFLAVIN Sprout Seedling 2.5—27 ppm
RUBIDIUM Fruit 0.47—7 ppm
SELENIUM Fruit 0.001—0.008 ppm
SELENIUM Seed 0—0.01 ppm
SERINE Fruit 990—10,175 ppm
SERINE Seed 11,750—13,205 ppm
SERINE Sprout Seedling 2,240—24,086 ppm
SFA Fruit 260—2,672 ppm
SFA Seed 3,660—4,113 ppm
SFA Sprout Seedling 720—7,742 ppm
SILICON Fruit 80—1,200 ppm
SILVER Fruit 0—0.3 ppm
SILVER Seed 0.034—0.147 ppm
SODIUM Fruit 5.4—707 ppm
SODIUM Seed 0.85—112 ppm
STEARIC-ACID Fruit 40—411 ppm
STEARIC-ACID Seed 220—247 ppm
STEARIC-ACID Sprout Seedling 90—968 ppm
STRONTIUM Fruit 2—105 ppm
STRONTIUM Seed 0.7—34 ppm
SUCCINIC-ACID Fruit
SULFUR Fruit 54—875 ppm
SULFUR Seed 54—137 ppm
THIAMIN Fruit 0.5—8.8 ppm
THIAMIN Leaf 1.8—13.6 ppm
THIAMIN Seed 3.7—10 ppm
THIAMIN Sprout Seedling 3.7—40 ppm
THREONINE Fruit 790—8,119 ppm

THREONINE Seed 9,090—10,216 ppm
THREONINE Sprout Seedling 1,760—18,925 ppm
TITANIUM Fruit 0.1—105 ppm
TITANIUM Seed 0.17—7.4 ppm
TRAUMATINIC-ACID Hull Husk
TRIGONELLINE Fruit
TRYPTOPHAN Fruit 190—1,953 ppm
TRYPTOPHAN Seed 2,560—2,877 ppm
TRYPTOPHAN Sprout Seedling 440—4,731 ppm
TYROSINE Fruit 420—4,317 ppm
TYROSINE Seed 6,080—6,833 ppm
TYROSINE Sprout Seedling 1,440—15,484 ppm
VALINE Fruit 900—9,250 ppm
VALINE Seed 11,300—12,699 ppm
VALINE Sprout Seedling 2,160—23,226 ppm
VANADIUM Fruit 0.24—105 ppm
VITAMIN B6 Fruit 0.74—7.6 ppm
VITAMIN B6 Seed 2.8—3.3 ppm
WATER Fruit 688,000—942,000 ppm
WATER Leaf 868,000 ppm
WATER Seed 63,000—604,000 ppm
WATER Sprout Seedling 907,000 ppm
ZINC Fruit 2—150 ppm
ZINC Seed 19—50 ppm
ZIRCONIUM Fruit 1—22 ppm
ZIRCONIUM Seed 0.68—1.47 ppm

■ LENTIL

Chemical Constituents of Lens culinaris (Fabaceae)

ALANINE Seed 11,720—13,200 ppm
ALANINE Sprout Seedling 3,560—11,865 ppm
AMYLASE Seed
ARGININE Seed 21,680—24,400 ppm
ARGININE Sprout Seedling 6,110—20,365
ASCORBIC-ACID Seed 42—70 ppm
ASCORBIC-ACID Sprout Seedling 148—605 ppm
ASH Seed 21,000—30,875
ASH Sprout Seedling 14,330—47,765 ppm

BETA-CAROTENE Seed 16 ppm
BETA-CAROTENE Sprout Seedling 0.3—1 ppm
BIOTIN Seed 132 ppm
CALCIUM Seed 386—604 ppm
CALCIUM Sprout Seedling 0.3—1 ppm
CARBOHYDRATES Seed 597,000—642,800 ppm
CARBOHYDRATES Sprout Seedling 221,400 ppm
CHLORINE Seed 636 ppm
COPPER Seed 8—9 ppm
COPPER Sprout Seedling 3.3—12 ppm
CYSTINE Seed 3,680—4,145 ppm
CYSTINE Sprout Seedling 3,340 ppm
ESCULIN Seed
FAT Seed 7,000—11,800 ppm
FAT Sprout Seedling 5,200—19,335 ppm
FERULIC-ACID Plant
FIBER Seed 49,000—61,675 ppm
FIBER Sprout Seedling 21,900—106,333 ppm
FOLACIN Seed 1.1 ppm
FOLACIN Sprout Seedling 1—4 ppm
GADOLEIC-ACID Seed 40—45 ppm
GLUTAMIC-ACID Seed 43,500—49,000 ppm
GLUTAMIC-ACID Sprout Seedling 12,580—41,935 ppm
GLYCINE Sprout Seedling 3,190—10,635 ppm
HERMICELLULOSE Seed
HISTIDINE Seed 7,900—8,900 ppm
HISTIDINE Sprout Seedling 2,570—8,565 ppm
INOSITOL Seed 1,300 ppm
IODINE Seed 0.025—0.03 ppm
IRON Seed 22—106 ppm
ISOLEUCINE Seed 12,120—13,650 ppm
ISOLEUCINE Sprout Seedling 3,260—10,865 ppm
KAEMPFEROL-3-O-ALPHA-L-RHAMNOSIDE-BETA-D-GLUCOSYL...PL Plant
KAEMPFEROL-3-RUTINOSYL-7-O-ALPHA-L-RHAMNOSIDE Plant
KAEMPFEROL-7-O-BETA-D-GLUCOSIDE-O-ALPHA-L-RHAMNOSYL...PL Plant
KILOCALORIES Seed 3,380—3,805/kg

KILOCALORIES Sprout Seedling 1,060—3,533/kg
LEUCINE Seed 20,340—22,900 ppm
LEUCINE Sprout Seedling 6,280—20,935 ppm
LINOLEIC-ACID Seed 3,510—3,950 ppm
LINOLEIC-ACID Sprout Seedling 1,810—6,035 ppm
LINOLEIC-ACID Seed 960—1,080 ppm
LINOLEIC-ACID Sprout Seedling 380—1,265 ppm
LYSINE Seed 19,570—22,035 ppm
LYSINE Sprout Seedling 7,120—23,735 ppm
MAGNESIUM Seed 765—1,280 ppm
MAGNESIUM Sprout Seedling 345—1,323 ppm
MANGANESE Sprout Seedling 5—18 ppm
METHIONINE Sprout Seedling 1,050—3,500 ppm
MUFA Seed 1,630—1,835 ppm
MUFA Sprout Seedling 1,040—3,465 ppm
MYRISTIC-ACID Seed 30—34 ppm
NIACIN Seed 17—30 ppm
NIACIN Sprout Seedling 10—40 ppm
OLEIC-ACID Seed 1,570—1,770 ppm
OLEIC-ACID Sprout Seedling 1,040—3,465 ppm
OXALIC-ACID Seed 212 ppm
P-COUMARIC-ACID Plant
PALMITIC-ACID Seed 1,160—1,300 ppm
PALMITIC-ACID Sprout Seedling 520—1,733 ppm
PALMITOLEIC-ACID Seed 20—23 ppm
PANTOTHENIC-ACID Seed 16—22 ppm
PANTOETHNIC-ACID Sprout Seedling 5—20 ppm
PARAGALACTOARABAN Seed
PHENYLALANINE Seed 13,830—15,575 ppm
PHOSPHATASE Seed
PHOSPHORUS Seed 2,420—5,275 ppm
PHOSPHORUS Sprout Seedling 1,610—6,165 ppm
PHYTASE Seed
POTASSIUM Seed 6,730—10,440 ppm
POTASSIUM Sprout Seedling 3,000—11,495 ppm
PROLINE Seed 11,720—13,200 ppm

PROLINE Sprout Seedling 3,560—11,865 ppm
PROTEIN Seed 251,000—349,000 ppm
PROTEIN Sprout Seedling 83,500—316,667 ppm
PUFA Seed 4,470—5,035 ppm
PUFA Sprout Seedling 2,190—7,300 ppm
PYRIDOXINE Seed 4.9 ppm
RIBOFLAVIN Seed 2 —3 ppm
RIBOFLAVIN Sprout Seedling 4,450—14,835 ppm
SFA Seed 1,350—1,520 ppm
SFA Sprout Seedling 570—1,900 ppm
SODIUM Seed 76—360 ppm
SODIUM Sprout Seedling 56—545 ppm
STACHYOSE Seed
STARCH Seed 285,000 ppm
STEARIC-ACID Seed 140—160 ppm
STEARIC-ACID Sprout Seedling 60—200 ppm
SULFUR Seed 1,220 ppm
THIAMIN Seed 2.6—6 ppm
THIAMIN Sprout Seedling 2—8 ppm
THREONINE Seed 10,060—11,325 ppm
THREONINE Sprout Seedling 3,280—10,935 ppm
TOCOPHEROL Seed 20 ppm
TRYPTOPHAN Seed 2,510—2,826 ppm
TYROSINE Sprout Seedling 2,520—8,400 ppm
VALINE Seed 13,920—15,675 ppm
VALINE Sprout Seedling 3,990—13,300 ppm
VITAMIN B6 Seed 5—6 ppm
VITAMIN B6 Sprout Seedling 2—6.6 ppm
VITAMIN K Seed 2.5 ppm
WATER Seed 111,900—124,000 ppm
WATER Sprout Seedling 650,000—700,000 ppm
ZINC Seed 37—42 ppm
ZINC Sprout Seedling 14—54 ppm

■ LETTUCE

Chemical Constituents of Lactuca sativa L. (Asteraceae)

ALANINE Leaf 560—9,333 ppm
ALPHA-LACTUCEROL Plant
ALPHA-LINOLENIC-ACID Leaf 1,130—18,833 ppm
ALPHA-TOCOPHEROL Fruit 6—139 ppm
ALUMINUM Leaf 3—126 ppm
ARGININE Leaf 710—11,833 ppm
ARSENIC Leaf 0.001—0.58 ppm
ASCORBIC-ACID Leaf 180—3,000 ppm
ASH Leaf 7,700—290,000 ppm
ASPARTIC-AID Leaf 1,420—23,667 ppm
BARIUM Leaf 0.126—145 ppm
BETA-CAROTENE Leaf 11—190 ppm
BETA-LACTUCEROL Plant
BORON Leaf 0.9—87 ppm
BROMINE Leaf
CADMIUM Leaf 0.01—4 ppm
CAFFEIC-ACID Plant
CALCIUM Leaf 360—19,140 ppm
CAMPESTEROL Seed
CAOUTCHOUC Latex Exudate 400—1,400 ppm
CARBOHYDRATES Leaf 35,000—583,333 ppm
CERYL-ALCOHOL Leaf
CHLORINE Leaf 395 ppm
CHOLINE Leaf
CHROMIUM Leaf 0.005—20 ppm
CITRIC-ACID Leaf 500 ppm
COBALT Leaf 0.002—0.87 ppm
COPPER Leaf 0.36—29 ppm
CYSTINE Leaf 160—2,677 ppm
DELTA-5-AVENASTEROL Seed
DELTA-7-AVENASTEROL Seed
ERGOSTEROL Leaf
FAT Leaf 3,000—50,000 ppm
FERULIC-ACID Plant
FIBER Leaf 7,000—116,667 ppm
FLUORINE Leaf 0.02—8 ppm
FOLACIN Leaf
GALLIUM Stem 0.18—7 ppm
GLUTAMIC-ACID Leaf 1,820—30,333 ppm
GLYCINE Leaf 570—9,500 ppm
GUM Leaf 26,000 ppm
HISTIDINE Leaf 220—3,667 ppm
HYOSCYAMINE Plant
IRON Leaf 5—176 ppm
ISOLEUCINE Leaf 840—14,000 ppm

KAEMPFEROL Plant
LACTUCAXANTHIN Plant
LACTUCIN Plant
LACTUCOPICRIN Plant
LANTHANUM Leaf 1.26—20.3 ppm
LEAD Leaf 0.02—6 ppm
LEUCINE Leaf 790—13,167 ppm
LINOLEIC-ACID Leaf 470—7,833 ppm
LITHIUM Leaf 0.07—2.6 ppm
LUTEOLIN Plant
LYSINE Leaf 840—14,000 ppm
MAGNESIUM Leaf 110—8,700 ppm
MALIC-ACID Leaf 600 ppm
MANGANESE Leaf—240 ppm
MANNITOL Plant
MERCURY Leaf 0—0.04 ppm
METHIONINE Leaf 160—2,667 ppm
MOLYBDENUM Leaf 0.1—2 ppm
MUFA Leaf 120—2,000 ppm
N-HEXACOSYLALCHOL Leaf
NIACIN Leaf 4—67 ppm
NICKEL Leaf 0.18—28 ppm
NITROGEN Leaf 2,200—54,000 ppm
OLEIC-ACID Leaf 90—1,500 ppm
OXALIC-ACID Leaf 110—136 ppm
P-COUMARIC-ACID Plant
PALMITIC-ACID Leaf 350—5,833 ppm
PALMITOLEIC-ACID Leaf 30—500 ppm
PANTOTHENIC-ACID Leaf 2—33 ppm
PECTINS Leaf 40,000 ppm
PHENYLALANINE Leaf 550—9,167 ppm
PHOSPHORUS Leaf 108—13,920 ppm
PHYTOSTEROLS Leaf 380—6,333 ppm
POTASSIUM Leaf 2,900—121,800 ppm
PROLINE Leaf 480—8,000 ppm
PROTEIN Leaf 13,000—216,667 ppm
PUFA Leaf 1,590—26,500 ppm
QUERCETIN Plant
SELENIUM Leaf 0—0.058 ppm
SERINE Leaf 390—6,500 ppm
SILICON Leaf 10—800 ppm
SILVER Leaf 0.018—0.58 ppm
SITOSTEROL Seed
SODIUM Leaf 28—18,560 ppm
STEARIC-ACID Leaf 40—667 ppm
STIGMAST-7-EN-3BETA-OL Seed

STIGMASTEROL Seed
STRONTIUM Shoot 2—580 ppm
SUGAR Leaf 65,000 ppm
SULFUR Shoot 29—3,800 ppm
TARAXASTEROL Plant
THIAMIN Leaf 0.5—8.3 ppm
THREONINE Leaf 590—9,833 ppm
TITANIUM Leaf 0.09—870 ppm
TRYPTOPHAN Leaf 90—1,500 ppm
TYROSINE Leaf 320—5,333 ppm
VALINE Leaf 700—11,667 ppm
VANADIUM Leaf 0.27—20.3 ppm
VITAMIN B6 Leaf 0.6—9.2 ppm
VITAMIN E Leaf
VITAMIN G Leaf
VITAMIN K Leaf
WATER Leaf 920,000—971,000 ppm
YTTERBIUM Leaf 0.036—0.87 ppm
YTTRIUM Leaf 0.36—8.7 ppm
ZINC Leaf 2.7—974 ppm
ZIRCONIUM Leaf 0.36—87 ppm

■ LIMA BEAN

Chemical Constituents of Phaseolus lunatus L. (Fabaceae)

ALANINE Seed 2,600—12,190 ppm
ALPHA-LINOLEIC-ACID Seed 950—4,570 ppm
ALUMINUM Seed 0.44—3,000 ppm
AMYGDALIN Seed
ARGININE Seed 4,580—15,390 ppm
ASCORBIC-ACID Seed 0—952 ppm
ASCORBIC-ACID Sprout Seedling 70—194 ppm
ASH Fruit 40,000 ppm
ASH Seed 15,000—100,000 ppm
ASH Sprout Seedling 22,000—61,000 ppm
ASPARTIC-ACID Seed 7,350—30,802 ppm
BARIUM Seed 1—30 ppm
BETA-CAROTENE Seed 0—9.8 ppm
BETA-CAROTENE Sprout Seedling 0.3—0.8 ppm
BORON Seed 1— 30 ppm

CALCIUM Leaf 80—2.857 ppm
CALCIUM Seed 250—8,600 ppm
CALCIUM Sprout Seedling 1,090—3,028 ppm
CARBOHYDRATES Fruit 766,000 ppm
CARBOHYDRATES Seed 201,000—731,000 ppm
CARBOHYDRATES Sprout Seedling 200,000—556,000 ppm
CHROMIUM Seed 0—5 ppm
COBALT Seed 0—1 ppm
COPPER Seed 3—15 ppm
CYSTINE Seed 830—2,789 ppm
FAT Fruit 6,000 ppm
FAT Leaf 0—48,000 ppm
FAT Seed 1,000—28,898 ppm
FAT Sprout Seedling 2,900—22,000 ppm
FIBER Fruit 175,000 ppm
FIBER Leaf 111,000 ppm
FIBER Seed 10,000—84,500 ppm
FIBER Sprout Seedling 6,000—17,000 ppm
GLUTAMIC-ACID Seed 8,810—33,820 ppm
GLUTAMYL-5-METHYLCYSTEINE Plant
GLYCINE Seed 2,7400—10,090 ppm
HISTIDINE Seed 2,320—7,796 ppm
IRON Seed 22—1,000 ppm
IRON Sprout Seedling 13—228 ppm
ISOLEUCINE Seed 4,400—14,785 ppm
KILOCALORIES Leaf 80—2,860/kg
KILOCALORIES Seed 1,130—3,840/kg
KILOCALORIES Sprout Seedling 100—3,060/kg
LEAD Seed 0.4—5 ppm
LEUCINE Seed 5,380—20,595 ppm
LIGNIN Seed 3,400—6,400 ppm
LINOLEIC-ACID Seed 2,150—9,509 ppm
LYSINE Seed 4,520—19,010 ppm
MAGNESIUM Seed 580—7,000 ppm
MANGANESE Seed 8—100 ppm
METHIONINE Seed 680—3,017 ppm
MOLYBDENUM Seed 0—15 ppm
MUFA Seed 500—1,680 ppm
MYRISTIC-ACID Seed 20—67 ppm
NIACIN Seed 10—49.5 ppm
NIACIN Sprout Seedling 8—56 ppm
NICKEL Seed 0.3—7 ppm
OLEIC-ACID Seed 500—1,680 ppm

PALMITIC-ACID Seed 1,180—5,813 ppm
PANTOTHENIC-ACID Seed 2.3—16 ppm
PHASEOLUNATIN Seed
PHENYLALANINE Seed 3,370—13,760 ppm
PHOSPHORUS Seed 1,130—9,000 ppm
PHOSPHORUS Sprout Seedling 3,820—10,611 ppm
POTASSIUM Seed 2,950—39,000 ppm
PROLINE Seed 1,020—10,855 ppm
PROTEIN Fruit 188,000 ppm
PROTEIN Seed 68,400—287,000 ppm
PROTEIN Sprout Seedling 130,000—361,000 ppm
PUFA Seed 3,090—14,079 ppm
RIBOFLAVIN Seed 0.3—5.1 ppm
RIBOFLAVIN Sprout Seedling 1.4—3.9 ppm
S-METHYLCYSTEINE Plant
SERINE Seed 4,270—15,900 ppm
SFA Seed 1,620—6,653 ppm
SODIUM Seed 5—269 ppm
STEARIC-ACID Seed 220—739 ppm
STRONTIUM Seed 1—100 ppm
THIAMIN Seed 1.6—7.4 ppm
THIAMIN Sprout Seedling 0.1—4.7 ppm
THREONINE Seed 2,900—10,320 ppm
TITANIUM Seed 0—20 ppm
TRYPTOPHAN Seed 900—3,024 ppm
TYROSINE Seed 2,200—8,450 ppm
VALINE Seed 4,270—14,370 ppm
VANADIUM Seed 0.22—3 ppm
VITAMIN B6 Seed 2—7.2 ppm
WATER Seed 46,900—702,400 ppm
WATER Sprout Seedling 640,000 ppm
ZINC Seed 7—100 ppm
ZIRCONIUM Seed 0.9—7 ppm

■ MUNG BEAN

Chemical Constituents of Vigna radiata L. (Fabaceae)

ADENOSINE-5'-MONOPHOSPHATE Sprout Seedling
ADENOSINE-DIPHOSPHATE Sprout Seedling

ADENOSINE-DIPHOSPHATE-D-RIBOSE Sprout Seedling

ADENOSINE-TRIPHOSPHATE Sprout Seedling

ALANINE Seed 10,500—11,545 ppm

ALANINE Sprout Seedling 990—10,399 ppm

ALPHA-LINOLENIC-ACID Seed 270—297 ppm

ALPHA-LINOLENIC-ACID Sprout Seedling 160—1,681 ppm

ARACHIDIC-ACID Seed 117—135 ppm

ARGININE Seed 16,720—18,383 ppm

ARGININE Sprout Seedling 1,970—20,693 ppm

ARSENIC Seed 0.09 ppm

ASCORBIC-ACID Seed 48—53 ppm

ASCORBIC-ACID Sprout Seedling 113—1,506 ppm

ASCORBIGEN Seed 24—26 ppm

ASH Seed 32,210—37,609 ppm

ASH Sprout Seedling 3,750—53,025 ppm

ASPARAGINE Seed

ASPARTIC-ACID Seed 27,560—30,302 ppm

ASPARTIC-ACID Sprout Seedling 4,790—50,315 ppm

BEHENIC-ACID Seed 312—360 ppm

BETA-CAROTENE Seed 0.9—1.2 ppm

BETA-CAROTENE Sprout Seedling 0.1—1.4 ppm

BIOCHANIN-A Plant

CADMIUM Seed 0.165 ppm

CALCIUM Seed 1,183—1,602 ppm

CALCIUM Sprout Seedling 59,300—622,899 ppm

CARBOHYDRATES Seed 626,200—688,510 ppm

CARBOHYDTATES Sprout Seedling 59,300—622,899 ppm

CEROTIC-ACID Seed 819—945 ppm

CHLORINE Seed 1,670—1,856 ppm

COPPER Seed 9—13 ppm

COPPER Sprout Seedling 1—23 ppm

COUMESTROL Sprout Seedling

CYSTINE Seed 2,100—2,309 ppm

CYSTINE Sprout Seedling 170—1,786 ppm

CYTIDINE-5'-MONOPHOSPHATE Sprout Seedling

DAIDZEIN Plant

FAT Seed 10,600—14,234 ppm

FAT Sprout Seedling 1,350—23,625 ppm

FIBER Seed 44,950—66,495 ppm

FIBER Sprout Seedling 7,200—94,500 ppm

FLAVADENINE-DINUCLEOTIDE Sprout Seedling

FOLACIN Seed 1.4—1.6 ppm

FOLACIN Seed 5.8—7.3 ppm

FOLACIN Sprout Seedling 0.539—7.105 ppm

FORMONONETIN Plant

FUCOSE Seed

GALACTOSE Seed

GENISTEIN Plant

GLUCOSE Seed

GLUTAMIC-ACID Seed 42,640—46,883 ppm

GLUTAMIC-ACID Sprout Seedling 1,610—16,912 ppm

GLUTATHIONE Sprout Seedling

GLYCINE Seed 9,540—10,489 ppm

GLYCINE Sprout Seedling 930—6,618 ppm

GUANOSINE-5'-MONOPHOSPHATE Sprout Seedling

HEMICELLULOSE Seed

HISTIDINE Seed 6,950—7,642 ppm

HISTIDINE Sprout Seedling 700—7,353 ppm

HOMOGLUTATHIONE Sprout Seedling

HYDROXYGENISTEIN Leaf Diffusate

HYDROXYLAMINE Root

IMIDAZOLEACRYLIC-ACID Sprout Seedling

INOSITOL Seed

IODINE Seed 0.034—0.037 ppm

IRON Seed 58—84 ppm

IRON Sprout Seedling 5.6—132 ppm

ISOLEUCINE Sprout Seedling 1,320—13,866 ppm

KILOCALORIES Seed 3,340—3,815/kg

KILOCALORIES Sprout Seedling 3,151/kg

LEAD Seed 1.57 ppm

LEUCINE Seed 18,470—20,308 ppm

LEUCINE Sprout Seedling 1,750—18,382 ppm

LINOLEIC-ACID Seed 3,570—4,890 ppm

LINOLEIC-ACID Sprout Seedling 420—4,412 ppm

LINOLENIC-ACID Seed 1,872—2,160 ppm
LYSINE Seed 16,640—18,269 ppm
LYSINE Sprout Seedling 1,666—17,437 ppm
MAGNESIUM Seed 1,777—2,203 ppm
MAGNESIUM Sprout Seedling 176—2,560 ppm
MANGANESE Seed 9.6—12.2 ppm
MANGANESE Sprout Seedling 1.4—25 ppm
MANNOSE Seed
MERCURY Seed 0.036 ppm
METHIONINE Seed 2,860—3,145 ppm
METHIONINE Sprout Seedling 1.4—25 ppm
METHIONINE Sprout Seedling 340—3,571 ppm
MUFA Seed 1,610—1,770 ppm
MUFA Sprout Seedling 220—2,311 ppm
MYRISTIC-ACID Sprout Seedling
NARINGENIN Plant
NIACIN Seed 21—27 ppm
NIACIN Sprout Seedling 6.8—85 ppm
NICKEL 3.456 ppm
OLEIC-ACID Seed 832—11,770 ppm
OLEIC-ACID Sprout Seedling 220—2,311 ppm
P-COUMARIC-ACID Seed 2,500—4,215 ppm
PALMITIC-ACID Sprout Seedling 320—3,361 ppm
PANTOTHENIC-ACID Seed 18—22 ppm
PANTOTHENIC-ACID Sprout Seedling 2.9—48 ppm
PECTIN Seed
PHENYLALANINE Seed 14,430—15,865 ppm
PHENYLALANINE Sprout Seedling 1,170—12,290 ppm
PHOSPHORUS Seed 3,260—4,500 ppm
PHOSPHORUS Sprout Seedling 455—6,560 ppm
PHYTIN-PHOSPHORUS Seed 1,480—2,322 ppm
PHYTOSTEROLS Seed 230—253 ppm
PHYTOSTEROLS Sprout Seedling 150—1,576 ppm
POTASSIUM Seed 12,038—14,170 ppm
POTASSIUM Sprout Seedling 1,256—18,092 ppm
PROLINE Seed 10,950—12,090 ppm
PROTEIN Seed 234,890—266,541 ppm

PROTEIN Sprout Seedling 25,740—368,130 ppm
PUFA Seed 3,840—4,222 ppm
PUFA Sprout Seedling 580—6,092 ppm
PYRIDOXINE Seed
QUINIC-ACID Seed
RAFFINOSE Seed 8,000 ppm
RHAMNOSE Seed
RIBOFLAVIN Seed 2.1—2.8 ppm
RIBOFLAVIN Sprout Seedling 1—15 ppm
RIBOSE Seed
ROBININ Plant
SERINE Seed 11,760—12,930 ppm
SERINE Sprout Seedling 330—3,466 ppm
SFA Seed 3,480—3,826 ppm
SFA Sprout Seedling 460—4,831 ppm
SHIKIMIC-ACID Seed
SODIUM Seed 129—311 ppm
SODIUM Sprout Seedling 45—782 ppm
STACHYOSE Seed 25,000 ppm
STEARIC-ACID Seed 710—1,170 ppm
STEARIC-ACID Sprout Seedling 80—840 ppm
STIGMASTEROL Seed 230 ppm
SUCROSE Seed 18,000 ppm
SULFUR Seed 1,880—2,378 ppm
THIAMIN Seed 5.4—7.7 ppm
THIAMIN Sprout Seedling 0.7—10.3 ppm
THREONINE Seed 7,820—8,598 ppm
THREONINE Sprout Seedling 370—3,886 ppm
TYROSINE Seed 7,140—7,850 ppm
TYROSINE Sprout Seedling 520—5,462 ppn
URIDINE-5'-MONOPHOSPHATE Sprout Seedling
URIDINE-DIPHOSPHATE Sprout Seedling
URIDINE-DIPHOSPHATE-GALACURONIC-ACID Sprout Seedling
URIDINE-DIPHOSPHATE-GLUCURONIC-ACID Sprout Seedling
URIDINE-DIPHOSPHATE-N-ACETYL-GLUCOSAMINE Sprout Seedling
UROCANIC-ACID Sprout Seedling
VALINE Seed 12,370—13,600 ppm
VALINE Sprout Seedling 1,300—13,655 ppm
VERBASCOSE Seed 38,000 ppm
VITAMIN B12 Seed
VITAMIN B6 Seed 3.7—4.3 ppm

VITAMIN B6 Sprout Seedling 0.8—11 ppm
WATER Seed 86,100—94,890 ppm
WATER Sprout Seedling 888,140 ppm
XYLOSE Seed
ZINC Seed 26—31 ppm
ZINC Sprout Seedling 3.5—48 ppm

■ MUSTARD GREENS

Chemical Constituents of Brassica juncea L. (Brassicaceae)

24-METHYLENE-25-
    METHYLCHOLESTEROL Plant
ALLYL-ISOTHIOCYANATE Seed
ASH Leaf 10,000—108,695 ppm
ASH Seed 53,000—56,500 ppm
CALCIUM Leaf 512—14 ppm
COPPER Leaf 1.3—14 ppm
CROTONYL-ISOTHIOCYANATE Seed
EO Seed 4,500—30,900 ppm
FAT Leaf 12,700—138,000 ppm
FAT Seed 300,000—380,000 ppm
FIBER Seed 80,000—85,300 ppm
GLYCOLIPIDS Plant 3,225—35,055 ppm
IRON Leaf 16—174 ppm
MAGNESIUM Leaf 353—3,837 ppm
OXALIC-ACID Leaf 1,287 ppm
PHOSPHOLIPIDS Plant 5,588—60,740 ppm
PROTEIN Leaf
WATER Leaf 908,000 ppm
WATER Seed 62,000 ppm
ZINC Leaf 6—65 ppm

■ OATS

Chemical Constituents of Avena sativa L. (Poaceae)

1,3,4-PENTANE-TRICARBOXYLIC-ACID-
    TRIMETHYL-ESTER Pericarp 1.3 ppm
1-(3-AMINO-PROPYL)-PYRROLINIUM
    Sprout Seedling
2,2,6-TRIMETHYL-CYCLOHEXONE Seed

2-METHY-HEPT-2-EN-6-ONE Seed
26-DESGLUCOAVENACOSIDES Plant
3,4-DIMETHOXY-ACETOPHNONE Petiole
4,5-DIHYDROXY-7-METHOXY-8-C-
    GLUCOSYL-O-RHAMNOSIDE Leaf
4-VINYL-GUAIACOL Seed
5-HYDROXY-3',5'-DIMETHOXY-
    GLUCOSIDE Leaf
5-HYDROXY-N-HENTRIACONTAN-14,16-
    DIONE Seed
6-HYDROXY-N-HENTRIACONTAN-14, 16-
    DIONE Seed
7-HYDROXY-N-HENTRIACONTAN-14, 16
    DIONE Seed
7-METHOXY-VITEXIN-O-RHAMNOSIDE
    Leaf
ACETIC-ACID Plant
AEGILOPSIN Hull Husk
ALANINE Seed 4,000 ppm
ALPHA-KETO-GLUTARIC-ACID Petiole
ALPHA-TOCOPHEROL Seed 4.4—10.1 ppm
ALUMINUM Plant
APIGENIN-6,8-DI-C-GLUCOSIDE Leaf
APIGENIN-6-C-GLUCOSIDE Leaf
APIGENIN-6-C-GLUCOSYL-
    ARABINOSIDE Leaf
APIGENIN-8-C-ARABINOSYLHEXOSIDE
    Leaf
APIGENIN-8-C-RHAMNOSYLGLUCOSIDE
    Leaf
ARGININE Seed 3,000—13,000 ppm
ASH Plant 22,000—210,000 ppm
ASH Seed 19,000—96,000 ppm
ASPARTIC-ACID Seed 7,000 ppm
AVENACINS Root
AVENACOSIDE-A Seed
AVENACOSIDE-B Seed
AVENATHRAMIDES Seed
AVENARIN Plant
AVENIC-ACIDS Root
AVENIN Root
BENZALDEHYDE Seed
BETA-CAROTENE Plant 0—75 ppm
BETA-CYCLOCITRAL Seed
BETA-HYDROXY-BETA-METHYL-
    GLUTARIC-ACID Petiole

BETA-IONONE Seed
BETA-SITOSTEROL Plant
BETAINE Root 11.7 ppm
BETAINE Shoot 234 ppm
BIOTIN Seed 0.132—1.4 ppm
BORON Seed 2—7 ppm
BRASSICASTEROL Seed
BUTENYL-ISOTHIOCYANATE Seed
CAFFEIC-ACID Plant
CAFFEIC-ACID-ESTER Seed
CALCIUM Plant 1,300—14,300 ppm
CALCIUM Seed 400—4,800 ppm
CAMPESTEROL Seed
CARBOHYDRATES Plant 265,000—861,000 ppm
CARBOHYDRATES Seed 562,000—775,000 ppm
CAROTENE Plant 2.6—702 ppm
CAROTENE Seed 0—0.22 ppm
CARYOPHYLLENE Seed
CELLULOSE Hull Husk 350,000 ppm
CELLULOSE Plant 305,000 ppm
CHLORINE Plant 1,000—1,900 ppm
CHLOROPHYLL-A Plant
CHLOROPHYLL-B Plant
CHOLESTEROL Seed
CHOLINE Root 24 ppm
CHOLINE Seed 134—1,712 ppm
CHOLINE Shoot 37 ppm
CHROMIUM Plant 39 ppm
CITRIC-ACID Petiole
COBALT Plant 0.03—0.224 ppm
COBALT Seed 0—0.32 ppm
COLAMINE Seed
COPPER Plant 4 ppm
COPPER Seed 2.4—25.7 ppm
CYSTINE Seed 1,000—5,000 ppm
DEC-TRANS-2-EN-1-AL Seed
DEC-TRANS-2-TRANS-4-DIEN-1-AL Seed
DELTA-5-AVENASTEROL Seed
DELTA-7-AVENASTEROL Seed
DELTA-7-STIGMASTEROL Seed
DELTA-AMINO-LEVULINIC-ACID   Sprout
    Seedling
DIADENOSINE-TETRAPHOSPHORIC-ACID
    Sprout Seedling

DIAMINO-PROPANE Sprout Seedling
DIMETHOXY-BUTYL-BENZENE Petiole
ERGOTHIONEINE Seed
FAT Plant 19,000—39,000 ppm
FAT Seed 11,000—97,000 ppm
FERULIC-ACID Seed
FERULIC-ACID-ESTER Seed
FIBER Plant 122,000—417,000 ppm
FIBER Seed 10,000—289,000 ppm
FOLACIN Seed 0—0.75 ppm
FORMALDEHYDE Seed
FRUCTOSE Plant
FUR-2-ALDEHYDE Seed
FURFURAL Hull Husk 100,000 ppm
GAMMA-MUUROLENE Seed
GERANIOL-ACETONE Seed
GLUCOSE Plant
GLUCOVANILLIN Hull Husk
GLUTAMIC-ACID Plant 19,000 ppm
GLUTAMIC-ACID Seed 29,000—31,000 ppm
GLUTARIC-ACID Petiole
GLYCINE Seed 2,000 ppm
GRAMININE Rhizome
GUANINE Plant
HEPTAN-1-AL Seed
HEPTANAL Seed
HEX-CIS-3-EN-1-OL Seed
HEX-TRANS-3-ENYL-ACETATE Seed
HEXANAL Seed
HEXYL-ACETATE Seed
HISTIDINE Seed 1,000—6,000 ppm
HYPOXANTHIN Plant
INDOLE-3-ACETIC-ACID-
    GLUCOPROTEIN Shoot
IODINE Plant 0.154 ppm
IRON Plant 110—990 ppm
IRON Seed 20—300 ppm
ISOLEUCINE Plant 13,000 ppm
ISOLEUCINE Seed 4,000—9,000 ppm
ISOORIENTIN Leaf
ISOORIENTIN-2"-O-ARABINOSIDE Leaf
ISOORIENTIN-2"-O-BETA-D-
    DIGLYCOSIDE Leaf
ISOORIENTIN-7-O-BETA-D-GLYCOSIDE
    Leaf

ISOSWERTISIN-2"-O-ALPHA-L-
RHAMNOSIDE Leaf
ISOSWERTISIN-2"-RHAMNOSIDE Leaf 16
ppm
ISOVITEXIN Plant
ISOVITEXIN-2"-O-ALPHA-L-
ARABINOSIDE Shoot
ISOVITEXIN-2"-O-ARABINOSIDE Leaf
ISOVITEXIN-2"-O-RHAMNOSIDE Stem
KILOCALORIES Plant 4,529—4,540/kg
KILOCALORIES Seed 3,740—4,710/kg
LEUCINE Plant 18,000 ppm
LEUCINE Seed 6,000—14,000 ppm
LICHENIN Seed
LIGNIN Hull Husk 100,000—150,000 ppm
LIGNIN Plant 85,000 ppm
LIMONENE Seed
LOPHENOL Seed
LUTEOLIN-6-C-GLUCOSIDE Leaf
LUTEOLIN-6-C-GLUCOSYL-
ARABINOSIDE Leaf
LYSINE Plant
LYSINE Seed 2,000—7,000 ppm
MAGNESIUM Plant 300—14,800 ppm
MAGNESIUM Seed 300—2,900 ppm
MALIC-ACID Petiole
MALONIC-ACID Petiole
MANGANESE Plant 5—168 ppm
MANGANESE Seed 20—204 ppm
METHIONINE Plant 2,000 ppm
METHIONINE Seed 1,000—4,000 ppm
METHOXY-MALIC-ACID Petiole
MYRCENE Seed
NIACIN Seed 6—44 ppm
NICOTIANAMINE Sprout Seedling
NONA-TRANS-2-TRANS-4-DIENAL Seed
NONAN-1-AL Seed
NONAN-1-OL Seed
O"RHAMNOSYL-8-C-D-
GLUCOPYRANOSYLGENKWANIN
Sprout Seedling
OCT-1-EN-3-OL Seed
OCT-TRANS-2-EN-1-OL Seed
OCTAN-1-AL Seed
OCTAN-1-OL Seed
OCTANAL Seed

OXALIC-ACID Plant 400 ppm
P-COUMARIC-ACID Seed
P-HYDROXYBENZOIC-ACID Seed
PANTOTHENIC-ACID Plant 3.5—45.3 ppm
PANTOTHENIC-ACID Seed 4.4—28.3 ppm
PENTOSANS Hull Husk 320,000—360,000
ppm
PHAEOPHROBIDE Sprout Seedling
PHENYLALANINE Seed 4,000—10,000 ppm
PHOSPHORUS Plant 1,600—8,800 ppm
PHOSPHORUS Seed 500—10,200 ppm
POTASSIUM Plant 2,000—78,900 ppm
POTASSIUM Seed 2,200—8,900 ppm
PROLINE Root 276 ppm
PROLINE Shoot 150 ppm
PROPANAL Seed
PROTEIN Plant 14,000—424,000 ppm
PROTEIN Seed 74,000—232,000 ppm
PUTRESCINE Leaf
PYRIDOXINE Plant 1.76—3.08 ppm
PYRIDOXINE Seed 0.22—2.4 ppm
QUERCETIN Hay 310 ppm
RIBOFLAVIN Plant 4.6—26 ppm
RIBOFLAVIN Seed 0.66—11.66 ppm
SALICYLIC-ACID-METHYL-ESTER Seed
SCOPOLETIN Root 10 ppm
SCOPOLIN Sprout Seedling
SECALOSE Plant
SELENIUM Plant
SERINE Seed 4,000 ppm
SILICON Plant 183 ppm
SILICON-OXIDE Ash
SINAPIC-ACID Seed
SODIUM Plant 700—9,400 ppm
SODIUM Seed 100—1,600 ppm
SPERMIDINE Leaf 14 ppm
SPERMINE Leaf 13 ppm
STARCH Seed 500,000—600,000 ppm
STIGMASTADIENOL Seed
STIGMASTEROL Seed
SUCROSE Plant
SUGARS Plant 30,000—93,000 ppm
SUGARS Seed 20,000—50,000 ppm
SULFUR Plant 800—4,100 ppm
SULFUR Seed 1,500—3,100 ppm
TARTARIC-ACID Petiole

THIAMIN Plant 0.9—4 ppm
THIAMIN Seed 2.6—12.1 ppm
THREONINE Plant 16,000 ppm
THREONINE Seed 3,000—7,000 ppm
TIN Plant
TRANS-BETA-OCIMENE Seed
TRANS-HEPT-2-ENAL Seed
TRANS-NON-2-ENAL Seed
TRICIN Leaf
TRICIN-4',7-DI-O-BETA-D-GLYCOSIDE
    Inflorescence
TRICIN-4'-O-ALPHA-L-ARABINOSIDE
    Inflorescence
TRICIN-4'-O-BETA-D-GLYCOSIDE Leaf
TRICIN-7-O-ALPHA-L-RHAMNOSYL-
    HEXOSIDE Stem
TRICIN-7-O-BETA-D-GLYCOSIDE Leaf
TRYPTOPHAN Plant 2,000 ppm
TRYPTOPHAN Seed 0—3,000 ppm
TYROSINE Seed 2,000—14,000 ppm
URONIC-ACIDS Plant
VALINE Plant 12,000 ppm
VALINE Seed 4,000—11,000 ppm
VANILLIC-ACID Seed
VANILLIN Plant
VITEXIN-2''-RHAMNOSIDE Leaf
VITEXIN-O-GLUCOSIDE Sprout Seedling
WATER Plant 792,000 ppm
WATER Seed 48,000—213,000 ppm
WAX Seed 9,000 ppm
XANTHPHYLL-EPOXIDE Sprout Seedling
ZINC Plant

■ OKRA

Chemical Constituents of Abelmoschus esculen-
tus L. (Malvaceae)

12,13-EPOXYOLEIC-ACID Seed
9-HEXADECANOIC-ACID Seed
ALANINE Fruit 730—7,300 ppm
ALPHA-TOCOPHEROL Oil 310 ppm
ARGININE Fruit 840—8,450 ppm
ASCORBIC-ACID Plant 190—2,340 ppm
ASH Fruit 7,000—70,000 ppm

ASH Seed 47,400 ppm
ASPARTIC-ACID Fruit 1,450—14,820 ppm
CALCIUM Fruit 810—8,100 ppm
CALCIUM Seed 2,100 ppm
CARBOHYDRATES Fruit 76,300—760,000
    ppm
COPPER Fruit 1—9 ppm
CYANIDIN-3-GLUCOSIDE-4'-GLUCOSIDE
    Flower
CYANIDIN-4'-GLUCOSIDE Flower
CYSTINE Fruit 180—1,900 ppm
FAT Fruit 1,000—10,000 ppm
FAT Seed 160,000—220,000 ppm
FIBER Fruit 9,400—94,000 ppm
FIBER Seed 210,200 ppm
FOLACIN Fruit 0.7—10 ppm
GAMMA-TOCOPHEROL Oil 430 ppm
GLUTAMIC-ACID Fruit 2,710—27,100 ppm
GLYCINE Fruit 440—4,400 ppm
GOSSYPETIN Flower
GOSSYPOL Seed 70 ppm
HISTIDINE Fruit 310—3,100 ppm
IRON Fruit 8—150 ppm
ISOLEUCINE Fruit 550—6,900 ppm
KILOCALORIES Fruit 180—3,800/kg
LEUCINE Fruit 1,050—10,500 ppm
LINOLEIC-ACID Seed 32,575—44,790 ppm
LYSINE Fruit 810—8,100 ppm
MAGNESIUM Fruit 380—6,000 ppm
MANGANESE Fruit 10—100 ppm
METHIONINE Fruit 210—2,100 ppm
MUFA Fruit 170—1,700 ppm
MYRISTIC-ACID Seed 1,120—1,540 ppm
NIACIN Fruit 10—100 ppm
OLEIC-ACID Seed 72,864—100,190 ppm
OXALIC-ACID Fruit 103 ppm
PALMITIC-ACID Seed 33,920—46,640 ppm
PANTOTHENIC-ACID Fruit 2—24 ppm
PECTIN Fruit
PECTIN Seed 21,500 ppm
PENTOSANS Seed 142,700 ppm
PHENYALANINE Fruit 650—6,500 ppm
PHOSPHORUS Fruit 630—6,300 ppm
PHOSPHORUS Seed 7,900 ppm
PHYTOSTEROLS Fruit 240—2,400 ppm
POTASSIUM Fruit 2,200—32,500 ppm

POTASSIUM Seed 8,200 ppm
PROLINE Fruit 450—14,930 ppm
PROTEIN Fruit 2,000—122,000 ppm
PROTEIN Seed 193,800 ppm
PUFA Fruit 270—2,700 ppm
QUERCETIN Flower
RIBOFLAVIN Fruit 0.6—7 ppm
SERINE Fruit 440—4,510 ppm
SFA Fruit 260—2,600 ppm
SODIUM Fruit 10—1,000 ppm
STARCH Seed 89,200 ppm
STEARIC-ACID 7,360—10,120 ppm
SUGAR Seed 40,300 ppm
SULFUR Fruit 140—1,400 ppm
THIAMIN Fruit 0.8—20 ppm
THREONINE Fruit 650—6,500 ppm
TRYPTOPHAN Fruit 170—1,710 ppm
TYROSINE Fruit 480—8,700 ppm
VALINE Fruit 910—9,100 ppm
VITAMIN B6—Fruit 2—22 ppm
WATER Fruit 880,000—895,000 ppm
WATER Seed 98,900 ppm
ZINC Fruit 6—60 ppm

■ OLIVE

Chemical Constituents of Olea europaea L.
(Oleaceae)

(+)-CYCLO-OLIVIL Branches
1-CAFFEYL-GLUCOSE Fruit
3,4-DIHYDROXYPHENYLETHANOL-4-
    DIGLUCOSIDE Fruit
3,4-DIHYDROXYPHENYLETHANOL-4-
    MONOGLUCOSIDE Fruit
3,4-
    DIHYDROXYPHENYLETHYLALCOHOL
    Fruit
AESCULETIN Stem
AESCULIN Stem
ALPHA-TOCOPHEROL Oil 119 ppm
APIGENIN Leaf
APIGENIN-7-DI-O-XYLOXIDE Leaf
APIGENIN-7-GLUCOSIDE Leaf
ARABINOSE Fruit

ARACHIDIC-ACID Fruit 300—800 ppm
ASH Fruit 64,000—294,000 ppm
ASH Leaf 61,000 ppm
ASH Twig 85,000 ppm
BETA-AMYRIN Leaf
BETA-CAROTENE Fruit 1.8—8.3 ppm
BETA-SITOSTEROL-GLUCOSIDE Leaf
BORON Fruit 1—4 ppm
CAFFEIC-ACID Fruit
CALCIUM Fruit 610—2,798 ppm
CALCIUM Leaf 11,800 ppm
CARBOHYDRATES   Fruit   13,000—60,000
    ppm
CARBOHYDRATES Leaf 735,000 ppm
CARBOHYDRATES Twig 765,000 ppm
CATECHIN Fruit
CATECHOL-MELANIN Fruit
CHOLINE Leaf
CHRYSOERIOL-7-O-GLUCOSIDE Leaf
CINCHONIDINE Leaf
CRATAEGOLIC-ACID Fruit
CYANIDIN-3-GLUCOSIDE Fruit
CYANIDIN-3-MONOGLUCOSIDE Pericarp
CYANIDIN-3-
    RHAMNOSYLGLUCOSYLGLUCOSIDE
    Fruit
CYANIDIN-3-RUTINOSIDE Fruit
D-1-ACETOXPINORESINOL-4"-O-
    METHYL-ETHER Stem
D-1-ACETOXPINORESINOL-4'-BETA-D-
    GLUCOSIDE Stem
D-1-HYDROXYPINORESINOL Stem
D-1-HYDROXYPINORESINOL-4"-O-
    METHYL-ETHER Stem
D-ACETOXPINORESINOL Stem
DEMETHYLOLEOEUROPEIN Leaf
DIHYDROCINCHONINE Leaf
DIHYDROXYPHENYLPROPANE Leaf
ELENOLIDE Fruit
ERYTHRODIOL Pericarp
ESCULIN Stem
ESTRONE Seed
FAT Fruit 127,000—583,000 ppm
FAT Leaf 73,000 ppm
FAT Seed 300,000 ppm
FAT Twig 61,000 ppm

FIBER Fruit 13,000—60,000 ppm
FIBER Leaf 177,000 ppm
FIBER Twig 289,000 ppm
FRUCTOSE Fruit
GALACTOSE Fruit
GALACTYRONIC-ACID Fruit
GAMMA-TOCOPHEROL Oil 13 ppm
GLUCOSE Fruit
IRON Fruit 16—73 ppm
KAEMPFEROL Stem
KILOCALORIES Fruit 1,160—5,310/kg
L-OLIVIL Resin Exudate Sap
LIGUSTROLIDE Fruit
LINOLEIC-ACID Fruit 10,500—28,000 ppm
LUTEOLIN Leaf
LUTEOLIN-4'-O-GLUCOSIDE Leaf
LUTEOLIN-5-O-GLUCOSIDE Fruit
LUTEOLIN-7-O-GLUCOSIDE Leaf
LUTEOLINTETRAGLUCOSIDE Leaf
MANNITOL Leaf
MASLINIC-ACID Petiole
METHYL-DELTA-MASLINATE Leaf
MYRISTIC-ACID Petiole
OLEIC-ACID Fruit 122,400—326,400 ppm
OLEOSIDE Leaf
OLEOSIDE-7-METHYL-ESTER Bark
OLEUROPEIC-ACID Root Bark
OLEUROPEIN Plant
OLIVIN Leaf
OLIVIN-4'-DIGLUCOSIDE Leaf
P-COUMARIC-ACID Fruit
PAEONIDIN-3-GLUCOSIDE Fruit
PAEONIDIN-3-
    RHAMNOSYLGLUCOSYLGLUCOSIDE
    Fruit
PALMITIC-ACID Fruit 14,250—38,000 ppm
PECTIN Fruit
PHOSPHORUS Fruit 170—780 ppm
PHOSPHORUS Leaf 900 ppm
POTASSIUM Fruit 550—2,523 ppm
PROTEIN Fruit 14,000—64,000 ppm
PROTEIN Leaf 131,000 ppm
PROTEIN Twig 89,000 ppm
PROTECATECHUIC-ACID Fruit
QUERCETIN Stem
QUERCETIN-3-O-RHAMNOSIDE Pericarp

QUERCETIN-3-RUTINOSIDE Pericarp
QUINONE Fruit
RHAMNOSE Fruit
RUTIN Pericarp
SODIUM Fruit 24,000—110,092 ppm
SQUALENE Fruit
STEARIC-ACID Fruit 2,100—5,600 ppm
TANNINS Leaf
UVAOL Pericarp
VERBASCOSIDE Fruit
WATER Fruit 782,000 ppm

■ ONION

Chemical Constituents of Allium cepa L. (Liliaceae)

1(F)-BETA-FRUCTOSYL-SUCROSE Bulb
1-(METHYLSULFINYL)-PROPYL-
    METHYL-DISULFIDE Bulb
1-METHYLDITHIO-PROPANE Essential Oil
1-METHYLTRITHIO-PROPANE Essential Oil
1-O-CAFEOYL-BETA-D-GLUCOSE Leaf
1-O-FERULOYL-BETA-D-GLUCOSE Leaf
1-O-P-COUMAROYL-BETA-D-GLUCOSE
    Leaf
1-PROPYLTRITHIO-PROPANE Essential Oil
2,3-DIMETHYL-(DL)-BUTANE-CIS-1-CIS-
    DITHIAL-S,S'-DIOXIDE Bulb
2,3-DIMETHYL-5,6-DITHIA-
    BICYCLO(2,2,1)HEXANE-5-OXIDE Bulb
2,3-DIMETHYLTHIPHENE Bulb
2,4-DIMETHYLTHIPHENE Bulb
2,5-DIMETHYLTHIPHENE Bulb
2-METHYL-BUT-2-EN-1-AL Bulb
2-METHYL-BUTYR-2-ALDEHYDE Bulb
2-METHYL-PENT-2-EN-1-AL Essential Oil
24-METHYLENE-CYCLOARTENOL Bulb
28-ISOFUCOSTEROL Bulb
3,4-DIMETHYL-2,5-DIOXO-2,5-
    DIHYDROTHIOPHENE Bulb
3,4-DIMETHYLTHIOPHENE Bulb
31-NORCYCLOARTENOL Bulb
31-NORLANOSTENOL Bulb
4-ALPHA-METHYL-ZYMOSTENOL Bulb

5-DEHYDRO-AVENASTEROL Seed
5-HEXYL-CYCLOPENTA-1,3-DIONE Bulb
5-OCTYL-CYCLOPENTA-1,3-DIONE Bulb
6(G)-BETA-FRUCTOSYL-SUCROSE Bulb
9,12,13-TRIHYDROXY-OCTADEC-10-
    ENOIC-ACID Bulb
9,10,13-TRIHYDROXY-OCTADEC-11-
    ENOIC-ACID Bulb
ABSCISSIC-ACID Bulb
ACETAL Bulb
ACETIC-ACID Bulb
ALANINE Bulb 330—8,597 ppm
ALLICIN Bulb
ALLIIN Bulb
ALLIOFUROSIDE-A Pericarp 220 ppm
ALLIOSPIROSIDE-A Pericarp 4,600 ppm
ALLIOSPIROSIDE-B Fruit 500 ppm
ALLIOSPIROSIDE-C Fruit 491 ppm
ALLIOSPIROSIDE-D Fruit 71 ppm
ALLYLPROPYL-DISULFIDE Bulb
ALPH-AMYRIN Bulb
ALPHA-SITOSTEROL Bulb
ALPHA-TOCOPHEROL Bulb 0.4—30 ppm
ALUMINUM Bulb 0.3—385 ppm
ARABINOSE Bulb
ARACHIDIC-ACID Seed
ARGININE Bulb 1,580—17,222 ppm
ARSENIC Bulb 0.002—0.076 ppm
ASCORBIC-ACID Bulb 60—2,703 ppm
ASCORBIC-ACID Leaf 390—5,000 ppm
ASH Bulb 4,000—63,000 ppm
ASH Leaf 7,000—90,000 ppm
ASPARAGINE Bulb
ASPARTIC-ACID Bulb 640—6,967 ppm
BARIUM Bulb 4—28 ppm
BENZYL-ISOTHIOCYANATE Bulb
BETA-CAROTENE Bulb 0—52 ppm
BETA-CAROTENE Flower 28 ppm
BETA-CAROTENE Leaf 12—158 ppm
BETA-SITOSTEROL Bulb
BETA-TOCOPHEROL Seed
BORON Bulb 1—45 ppm
BRASSICASTEROL Seed
BROMINE Bulb 1—15 ppm
CADMIUM Bulb 0.005—0.38 ppm
CAFFEIC-ACID Bulb

CALCIUM Bulb 200—3,008 ppm
CALCIUM Leaf 420—5,385 ppm
CALCIUM-OXALATE Bulb
CAMPESTEROL Bulb
CARBOHYDRATES Bulb 73,200—798,000
    ppm
CARBOHYDRATES Leaf 47,000—603,000
    ppm
CATECHOL Bulb
CEPAENES Bulb
CEPOSIDE-D Seed
CHOLEST-7-EN-3-BETA-OL Bulb
CHOLESTEROL Bulb
CHOLINE Bulb 830 ppm
CHROMIUM Bulb 0.057—4 ppm
CHROMIUM Seed 4.8 ppm
CIS-1-(PROPENYL-DITHIO)-PROPANE
    Essential Oil
CIS-2,3-DIMETHYL-5,6-DITHIA-
    CYCLO(2,2,1)HEPTANE-5-OXIDE Bulb
CIS-3,5-DIETHYL-1,2,4-TRITHIOLANE Leaf
CIS-PROPANETHIOL-S-OXIDE Bulb
CITRIC-ACID Bulb
COBALT Bulb 0.001—0.2 ppm
COBALT Seed 2.5 ppm
COPPER Bulb 0.3—11 ppm
COPPER Seed 18.2 ppm
CYANIDIN-3-O-BETA-D-DIGLYCOSIDE
    Bulb
CYANIDIN-3-O-LAMINARIBIOSIDE Bulb
CYANIDIN-BIOSIDE Bulb
CYANIDIN-DIGLYCOSIDE Bulb
CYANIDIN-MONOGLYCOSIDE Bulb
CYCOLALLIIN Bulb
CYCLOARTENOL Bulb
CYCLOEUCALENOL Bulb
CYSTEINE Bulb
CYSTINE Bulb 210—2,289 ppm
D-MANNITOL Bulb
DIALLYL-DISULFIDE Essential Oil
DIALLYL-SULFIDE Essential Oil
DIHYDROALLIIN Bulb
DIMETHYL-DISULFIDE Bulb
DIMETHYL-SULFIDE Essential Oil
DIMETHYL-TRISULFIDE Essential Oil
DIPHENYLAMINE Bulb 14—11,000 ppm

DIPROPYL-DISULPHIDE Bulb
DIPROPYL-TRISULFIDE Bulb
EICOSEN-1-OL Seed
EO BULB 50—150 ppm
ETHANOL Bulb
FAT Bulb 1,000—36,079 ppm
FAT Leaf 6,000—77,000 ppm
FERULIC-ACID Bulb
FIBER Leaf 11,000—141,000 ppm
FLUORINE Bulb 0.04—0.8 ppm
FRUCTOSAN Bulb
FRUCTOSE Bulb 65,600—162,600 ppm
FUMARIC-ACID Bulb
GAMMA-GLUTAMYL-LEUCINE Bulb
GAMMA-GLUTAMYL-PHENYLALANINE
  Bulb
GAMMA-GLUTAMYL-PHENYLALANINE-
  ETHYL-ESTER Bulb
GAMMA-GLUTAMYL-S-METHYL-
  CYSTEINE Plant
GAMMA-L-GLUTAMYL-ARGININE Bulb
GAMMA-L-GLUTAMYL-CYSTEINE Bulb
GAMMA-L-GLUTAMYL-ISOLEUCINE Bulb
GAMMA-L-GLUTAMYL-S(2-CARBOXY-N-
  PROPYL)L-CYSTEINE Bulb
GAMMA-L-GLUTAMYL-S-(1-
  PROPENYL)L-CYSTEINE-SULFOXIDE
  Bulb
GAMMA-L-GLUTAMYL-S-(2-CARBOXY-
  BETA-METHYL-ETHYL)-CYSTEINYL-
  GLYCINE Bulb
GAMMA-L-GLUTAMYL-S-(2-CARBOXY-
  BETA-METHYL-ETHYL)-CYSTEINYL-
  GLYCINE- ETHYL-ESTER Bulb
GAMMA-L-GLUTAMYL-VALINE Bulb
GIBBERELLIN-A-4 Root
GLUCOFRUCTAN Bulb
GLUCOSE Bulb 102,000—158,600 ppm
GLUTAMINE Bulb
GLUTAN Bulb
GLYCINE Bulb 490—5,341 ppm
GLYCOLIC-ACID Bulb
GRAMISTEROL Bulb
HEXADECEN-1-OL Seed
HISTIDINE Bulb 190—2,071 ppm
IRON Bulb 2—135 ppm

IRON Leaf 34—436 ppm
IRON Seed 235 ppm
ISOLEUCINE Bulb 420—4,578 ppm
KAEMPFEROL Bulb
KAEMPFEROL-3,4'-DI-O-BETA-D-
  GLUCOSIDE Bulb
KAEMPFEROL-4',7-DI-O-BETA-D-
  GLUCOSIDE Bulb
KAEMPFEROL-4'-O-BETA-D-GLUCOSIDE
  Bulb
KILOCALORIES Bulb 380—3,750/kg
KILOCALORIES Leaf 260—3,330/kg
LEAD Bulb 0.01—1.4 ppm
LEUCINE Bulb 410—4,469 ppm
LINOLEIC-ACID Seed Oil
LITHIUM Bulb 0.152—0.324 ppm
LOPHENOL Bulb
LYSINE Bulb 560—6,104 ppm
MAGNESIUM Bulb 76—1,230 ppm
MALIC-ACID Bulb
MALIC-ACID Leaf
MANGANESE Bulb 1—38 ppm
MANGANESE Seed 19.4 ppm
MERCURY Bulb 0—0.001 ppm
METHANOL Bulb
METHIONINE Bulb 100—1,090 ppm
METHIONINE-METHYLSULFONIUM Plant
METHIONINE-SULFONE Bulb
METHYL-ALLIIN Bulb
METHYL-CIS-PROPENYL-DISULFIDE Bulb
METHYLPROPYL-DISULFIDE Bulb
METHYLPROPYL-TRISULFIDE Bulb
MEVALONIC-ACID Bulb 0.5 ppm
MOLYBDENUM Bulb 0.1—2.3 ppm
MUFA Bulb 230—2,230 ppm
MYRISTIC-ACID Bulb 10—100 ppm
MYROSINASE Bulb
N-PROPYL-MERCAPTAN Bulb
NIACIN Bulb 1—75 ppm
NIACIN Leaf 7—90 ppm
NICKEL Bulb 0.05—2.5 ppm
NICKEL Seed 0.03—4 ppm
NITROGEN Bulb 1,700—17,690 ppm
NONADECANOIC-ACID Bulb
OLEANOLIC-ACID Bulb
OLEIC-ACID Bulb 230—2,230 ppm

OLEIC-ACID Bulb 230—2,230 ppm
OLEIC-ACID Seed Oil
OXALIC-ACID Bulb 10 ppm
P-COUMARIC-ACID Bulb
P-HYDROXYBANZOIC-ACID Bulb 107 ppm
PAEONIDIN-GLYCOSIDE Bulb
PALMITIC-ACID Bulb 240—2,325 ppm
PANTOTHENIC-ACID Bulb 1 —16 ppm
PECTIN Bulb
PELARCONIDIN-MONOGLYCOSIDE Bulb
PENTOSAN Bulb
PEROXIDASE Bulb
PHENYLALANINE Bulb 300—3,270 ppm
PHLOROGLUCINOL Bulb 100 ppm
PHLOROGLUCINOL-CARBOXYLIC-ACID
   Bulb 100 ppm
PHOSPHORUS Bulb 275—4,038 ppm
PHOSPHORUS Leaf 310—5,513 ppm
PHYTOHORMONE Bulb
PHYTOSTEROLS Bulb 150—1,455 ppm
POTASSIUM Bulb 1,514—22,164 ppm
PROLINE Bulb 370—4,033 ppm
PROP-CIS-ENYL-PROPYL-DISULFIDE Bulb
PROP-CIS-ENYL-PROPYL-TRISULFIDE
   Bulb
PROP-TRANS-ENYL-PROPYL-DISULFIDE
   Bulb
PROP-TRANS-ENYL-PROPYL-
   TRISULFIDE Bulb
PROPAN-1-OL Bulb
PROPANE-1-THIOL Bulb
PROPIONAL Bulb
PROPIONALDEHYDE Bulb
PROSTAGLANDIN-A-1 Bulb 1 ppm
PROTEIN Bulb 10,940—162,000 ppm
PROTEIN Leaf 18,000—231,000 ppm
PROTOCATECHUIC-ACID   Bulb   4,500—
   17,540 ppm
PUFA Bulb 620—6,005 ppm
PYROCATECHOL Bulb
PYRUVIC-ACID Fruit 1,034 ppm
QUERCETIN Bulb 0—48,100 ppm
QUERCETIN-3,4'-DI-O-BETA-D-
   GLUCOSIDE Bulb 1,700—5,600 ppm
QUERCETIN-3-0-BETA-D-GLUCOSIDE
   Bulb 0—40 ppm

QUERCETIN-4',7-DI-O-BETA-D-
   GLUCOSIDE Bulb 0—160 ppm
QUERCETIN-4-O-BETA-D-GLUCOSIDE
   Bulb 100—800 ppm
QUINIC-ACID Bulb
RAFFINOSE Bulb
RHAMNOSE Bulb
RIBOFLAVIN Bulb 0.4—15 ppm
RIBOSE Bulb
RUBIDIUM Bulb 0.14—6.6 ppm
RUTIN Bulb
S-(2-CARBOXY-PROPYL)-GLUTATHIONE
   Bulb 125 ppm
S-(BETA-CARBOXYBETA-METHYL-
   ETHER)-CYSTEINE Bulb
S-ALLYL-CYSTEINE Bulb
S-METHYLCYSTEINE Bulb
S-METHYLCYSTEINE Bulb
S-METHYLCYSTEINE-SULFOXIDE Bulb
S-PROP-1-ENYL-CYSTEINE-S-OXIDE   Bulb
   26 ppm
S-PROPYL-CYSTEINE-SULFOXIDE Bulb
SAPONIN Bulb
SELENIUM Bulb 0.001—0.003 ppm
SELENO-HOME-CYSTINE Plant
SELENO-METHIONINE Bulb
SELENO-METHYL-SELENOCYSTEINE
   Bulb
SELENO-METHYL-SELENOMETHIONINE
   Bulb
SELENOSIDE Plant
SERINE Bulb 350—3,815 ppm
SFA Bulb 260—2,520 ppm
SILICON Bulb 1—75 ppm
SILVER Bulb 0.038—0.054 ppm
SINAPIC-ACID Bulb
SODIUM Bulb 8—2,052 ppm
SPIRAEOSIDE Bulb 10,000—11,300 ppm
STEARIC-ACID Bulb 20—195 ppm
STIGMASTEROL Bulb
STRONTIUM Bulb 57—162 ppm
SUCCINIC-ACID Bulb
SUCROSE Bulb 82,600—145,900 ppm
SULFUR Bulb 80—4,075 ppm
TARTARIC-ACID Bulb
THIAMIN Bulb 0.3—6 ppm

THIAMIN Leaf 0.5—6.4 ppm
THIOPROPANAL-S-OXIDE Bulb
THIOPROPANAL-S-OXIDE Bulb
THREONINE Bulb 280—3,052 ppm
TITANIUM Bulb 0.38—11 ppm
TRANS-1-(PROPENYL-DITHIO)-PROPANE
  Essential Oil
TRANS-2,3-DIMETHYL-5,6-DITHIA-
  CYCLO(2,2,1)HEPTANE-5-OXIDE Bulb
TRANS-3,5-DIETHYL-1,2,4-TRITHIOLANE
  Leaf
TRANS-S-(1-PROPENYL)-CYSTEINE-
  SULFOXIDE Bulb
TRANS-S-(1-PROPENYL)CYSTEINE-
  SULFOXIDE Bulb
TRIGONELLINE Seed 13 ppm
TRYPTOPHAN Bulb 170—1,853 ppm
TSEPOSIDES Seed
TULIPOSIDE-A Root
TULIPOSIDE-B Root
TYROSINE Bulb 290—3,161 ppm
VALINE Bulb 270—2,943 ppm
VANILLIC-ACID Bulb 258 ppm
VITAMIN B6 Bulb 1—18 ppm
WATER Bulb 866,000—918,000 ppm
WATER Leaf 922,000 ppm
XYLITOL Bulb
XYLOSE Bulb
ZINC Bulb 2—53 ppm
ZINC Seed 34 ppm
ZIRCONIUM Bulb 0.76—1 ppm.

■ PAK CHOI

Chemical Constituents of Brassica chinensis L.
(Brassicaceae)

ALANINE Leaf 860—18,378 ppm
ALPHA-LINOLENIC-ACID Leaf 510—10,899
  ppm
ALPHA-TOCOPHEROL Leaf 2—56 ppm
ARGININE Leaf 840—17,951 ppm
ASCORBIC-ACID Leaf 450—9,713 ppm
ASH Leaf 8,000—170,960 ppm
ASPARTIC-ACID Leaf 1,080—23,080 ppm

BETA-CAROTENE Leaf 18—385 ppm
CALCIUM Leaf 1,050—22,400 ppm
CARBOHYDRATES Leaf 21,800—465,866
  ppm
CYSTINE Leaf 170—3,633 ppm
FAT Leaf 2,000—42,740 ppm
FIBER Leaf 6,000—128,220 ppm
GLUTAMIC-ACID Leaf 3,600—76,932 ppm
GLYCINE Leaf 430—9,189 ppm
HISTIDINE Leaf 260—5,556 ppm
IRON Leaf 8—171 ppm
ISOLEUCINE Leaf 850—18,164 ppm
KILOCALORIES Leaf 130—2,778/kg
LEUCINE Leaf 880—18,806 ppm
LINOLEIC-ACID Leaf 390—8,334 ppm
LYSINE Leaf 890—19,019 ppm
MAGNESIUM Leaf 106—5,844 ppm
METHIONINE Leaf 90—1,923 ppm
NIACIN Leaf 5—107 ppm
OLEIC-ACID Leaf 140—2,992 ppm
PALMITIC-ACID Leaf 220—4,701 ppm
PHENYLALANINE Leaf 440—9,402 ppm
PHOSPHORUS Leaf 370—7,907 ppm
POTASSIUM Leaf 1,804—69,143 ppm
PROLINE Leaf 310—6,652 ppm
PROTEIN Leaf 15,000—320,550 ppm
RIBOFLAVIN Leaf 0.7—15 ppm
SERINE Leaf 480—10,258 ppm
SODIUM Leaf 295—21,477 ppm
STEARIC-ACID Leaf 10—214 ppm
THIAMIN Leaf 0.4—9 ppm
THREONINE Leaf 490—10,471 ppm
TRYPTOPHAN Leaf 150—3,206 ppm
TYROSINE Leaf 290—6,197 ppm
VALINE Leaf 660—14,104 ppm
WATER Leaf 950,000—956,400 ppm

■ PARSLEY

Chemical Constituents of Petroselinum crispum
(Apiaceae)

0-METHYLBENZYL-ACETATE Leaf 0.36
  ppm
1,3,8-P-MENTHATRIENE Leaf 63 ppm

1,3,8-P-MENTHATRIENE Seed 87 ppm

1-ALLYL-2,3,4,5-TETRAMETHOXYBENZENE Seed 5—26,600 ppm

1-METHYL-4-ISOPROPENYLBENZENE Plant

2,3-DIOXA-1-METHYL-4-(METHYL-ETHENYL)-BICYCLO-(2,2,2)-OCT-5-ENE Plant

2-(P-TOLUYL)-PROPAN-2-OL Plant

2-ALPHA-TOLYL-PROPENE Leaf

2-PENTYL-FURAN Leaf

3,8-DIOXA-4-METHYL-7(METHYL-ETHENYL)-TRICYCLO-(5,1,0)-OCTANE Leaf

3-N-BUTYL-PHTHALIDE Seed

4-BETA-D-GLUCOPYRANOSYL-OXYBENZOIC-ACID Seed 165 ppm

4-ISOPROPENYL-1-METHYL-BENZENE Leaf 27 ppm

4-ISOPROPENYL-1-METHYL-BENZENE Seed 87 ppm

4-ISOPROPYL-CYCLOHEX-2-ENONE Leaf 0.42 ppm

4-PROPAN-1-AL-2-YL-TOLUENE Leaf

4-PROPAN-2-OL-2-YL-TOLUENE Leaf

5-METHOXYPSORALEN Fruit 0—12 ppm

5-METHOXYPSORALEN Leaf 10 ppm

6,7-DIHYDRO-8,8-DIMETHYL-2(H),8(H)BENZO-(1,2B,5,4B'-DIPYRAN-2-6-DIONE Seed 12 ppm

6-ACETYL-7-HYDROXY-COUMARIN Seed 5 ppm

7-OCTADECANOIC-ACID Seed

8-METHOXYPSORALEN Fruit 0—5 ppm

ALPHA-CADINOL Leaf 0.18 ppm

ALPHA-COPAENE Leaf 7.92 ppm

ALPHA-CUBEBENE Leaf 1.86 ppm

ALPHA-ELEMENE Leaf

ALPHA-GURJUNENE Leaf 4.92 ppm

ALPHA-NEROLIDOL Leaf 0.18 ppm

ALPHA-PHELLANDRENE Leaf 4.3 ppm

ALPHA-PHELLANDRENE Seed 0.6—210 ppm

ALPHA-PINENE Seed 1—31,080 ppm

ALPHA-TERPINENE Leaf 0.24 ppm

ALPHA-TERPINEOL Leaf 2.7 ppm

ALPHA-TERPINEOL Seed 22 ppm

ALPHA-THUJENE Leaf 0.1 ppm

ALPHA-THUJENE Seed 4—490 ppm

ALPHA-TOCOPHEROL Leaf 36—252 ppm

ALUMINUM Plant 6—390 ppm

APIGENIN Plant

APIGENIN-7-0-BETA-D-GLUCOSIDE Plant

APIGENIN-7-GLUCOAPIOSIDE Plant

APIIN Seed

APIOLE Leaf 0.36—22 ppm

APIOLE Seed 19,650—36,580 ppm

APIOSE Plant

ARSENIC Plant 0.01—0.21 ppm

ASCORBIC-ACID Plant

ASH Plant

BARIUM Plant 28—40 ppm

BENZALDEHYDE Leaf

BENZOIC-ACID4-O-BETA-D-GLUCOSIDE Shoot 3 ppm

BERGAPTEN Root

BERGAPTEN Seed

BERGAPTEN Shoot 21—2,000 ppm

BETA-BISABOLENE Leaf 2.76 ppm

BETA-BISABOLENE Seed 22 ppm

BETA-CAROTENE Plant 15—267 ppm

BETA-CARYOPHYLLENE Leaf 2.46 ppm

BETA-CARYOPHYLLENE Seed 6.6—770 ppm

BETA-ELEMENE Leaf 5.4 ppm

BETA-FARNESENE Leaf 3.9 ppm

BETA-FARNESENE Seed 25 ppm

BETA-PHELLANDRENE Leaf 60 ppm

BETA-PHELLANDRENE Seed 43—4,970 ppm

BETA-PHENYLETHANOL Seed

BETA-PINENE Seed 1—26,460 ppm

BETA-SELINENE Leaf 1.68 ppm

BICYCLOGERMACRENE Leaf 5.16 ppm

BIS-NORYANGONIN Tissue Culture

BORON Plant 4—54 ppm

BROMINE Plant 3—21 ppm

CADMIUM Plant 0.01—0.57 ppm

CAFFEIC-ACID Stem

CALCIUM Plant 1,000—16,850 ppm

CAMPHENE Leaf 0.24 ppm

CAMPHENE Seed 3—490 ppm

CARBOHYDRATES Plant 69,100—590,805 ppm
CARVEOL Leaf 3.9 ppm
CHALCONE-FLAVONOID-ISOMERASE Tissue Culture
CHALCONE-SYNTHASE Tissue Culture
CHLOROGENIC-ACID Stem
CHROMIUM Plant 0.06—0.7 ppm
CHRYSOERIOL-7-O-BETA-D-GLUCOSIDE Seed
CIS-3-HEXEN-1-OL Leaf 18.6 ppm
CIS-3-HEXEN-1-OL Plant
CIS-BETA-OCIMENE Plant
CIS-BETA-OCIMENE Plant
CIS-LIGUSTILIDE Root
COBALT Plant 0.001—0.2 ppm
COPPER Plant 1—12 ppm
CRYPTONE Leaf
DELTA-3-CARENE Leaf 0.12 ppm
DELTA-CADINENE Leaf 1.38 ppm
DELTA-CADINENE Seed 109 ppm
DELTA-CADINOL Leaf
DIMETHYL-BENZOFURAN Leaf
DIMETHYL-SULFIDE Leaf
E0 Leaf 600 ppm
ELEMICIN Leaf 18 ppm
ELEMICIN Seed 821 ppm
EO Plant 500—3,000 ppm
EO Root 500—1,000 ppm
EO Seed 15,500—70,000 ppm
ERIODICTYOL Plant
ESTRAGOLE Leaf 1.6 ppm
ETHANOL Plant
FALCARINONE Root
FAT Plant 3,000—53,218 ppm
FAT Seed 130,000—330,000 ppm
FIBER Plant 12,000—202,464 ppm
FLAVANONE-SYNTHASE Tissue Culture
FLUORINE Plant 0.6—7.8 ppm
FOLACIN Plant 2—17 ppm
GAMMA-CADINENE Leaf
GAMMA-ELEMENE Leaf
GAMMA-TERPINENE Leaf 0.42 ppm
GAMMA-TERPINENE Seed 3—1,120 ppm
GERANIOL Leaf 1.26 ppm
GERMACRENE-D-Leaf 6.9 ppm

GLYCOLIC-ACID Root
GLYCOLIC-ACID Seed
GRAVEOLONE Tissue Culture
HERACLENOL Seed 3.7 ppm
HEX-3-EN-1-YL-ACETATE Plant
HEX-CIS-3-EN-1-YL-ACETATE Plant
HEXADECENOIC-ACID Leaf 0.24 ppm
HEXAN-1-AL Leaf
IMPERATORIN Fruit 1—6 ppm
IMPERATORIN Leaf 0.53 ppm
INOSITOL Plant
IRON Plant 25—250 ppm
ISOIMPERATORIN Fruit 0—6 ppm
ISOIMPERATORIN Root
ISOPIMPINELLIN Shoot 0l.3—79 ppm
JASMONIC-ACID Leaf
KAEMPFEROL Plant
LEAD Plant 0.08—4 ppm
LF Plant
LIMONENE Leaf 16 ppm
LIMONENE Seed 6—1,470 ppm
LINALOOL Leaf 0.12 ppm
LITHIUM Plant 0.76—0.792 ppm
LUTEIN Plant
LUTEOLIN-7-APIOSYLGLUCOSIDE Seed
LUTEOLIN-7-DIGLUCOSIDE Plant
LYSINE Plant 2,190—18,724 ppm
M-XYLENE Leaf
MAGNESIUM Plant 290—5,577 ppm
MANGANESE Plant 2—375 ppm
MERCURY Plant 0.004—0.37 ppm
METHANOL Leaf
METHIONINE Plant 150—1,282 ppm
METHYL-DISULFIDE Plant
MOLYBDENUM Plant 0.1—14 ppm
MUCILAGE Root
MYRCENE Leaf 18 ppm
MYRCENE Seed 168—1,680 ppm
MYRISTIC-ACID Seed
MYRISTICIN Leaf 131 ppm
MYRISTICIN Plant 425—2,550 ppm
MYRISTICIN Seed
MYRISTICIN Seed 14,785—19,800 ppm
MYRISTOLIC-ACID Seed
N-HEXANAL Leaf 0.4 ppm
N-HEXANOL Leaf 0.2 ppm

NARINGENIN Plant
NEOXANTHIN Shoot
NERAL Leaf 2.9 ppm
NIACIN Plant 5—87 ppm
NICKEL Plant 0.1—8.5 ppm
NICOTINAMIDE Plant
NICOTINIC-ACID Sprout Seedling
NICOTINIC-ACID-BETA-D-GLUCOSIDE
 Tissue Culture
NICOTINIC-ACID-N-ALPHA-L-
 ARABINOSIDE Tissue Culture
NITROGEN Leaf 4,900—40,700 ppm
OLEIC-ACID Seed 53,000 ppm
OSTHOLE Plant 840—3,975 ppm
OXYPEUCEDANIN Fruit 7—26 ppm
OXYPEUCEDANIN Leaf 100 ppm
P-COUMARIC-ACID Stem
P-CYMENE Leaf 1.44 ppm
P-CYMENE Seed 34 ppm
P-CYMENE-8-OL Leaf 4.38 ppm
P-CYMENE-8-OL Seed 28 ppm
P-MENTHATRIENE Leaf 0.36 ppm
P-MENTHATRIENOLE Leaf 0.84—18.3 ppm
P-MENTHYL-ACETOPHENONE Leaf 3.66
 ppm
P-MENTHYL-ACETOPHENONE Seed 31 ppm
P-XYLENE Leaf
PALMITIC-ACID Seed 5,000 ppm
PANTOTHENIC-ACID Plant 3—26 ppm
PENTATRIACONTANE Leaf 0.18 ppm
PETROSELINIC-ACID Seed 715,000 ppm
PHENYLALANINE-AMMONIA-LYSASE
 Tissue Culture
PHENYLACETALDEHYDE Leaf
PHOSPHORUS Plant 405—6,425 ppm
POTASSIUM Plant 4,425—53,833 ppm
PROTEIN Plant 20,000—254,096 ppm
PROTEIN Seed 191,000 ppm
PROTOCATECHUIC-ACID Stem
PSORALEN Fruit 1—10 ppm
PSORALEN Leaf 2.5 ppm
QUERCETIN Plant
RIBOFLAVIN Plant 2 —14 ppm
ROSMARINIC-ACID Plant
RUBIDIUM Leaf 2.2—65 ppm
RUTIN Leaf 30,000 ppm

SABINENE Leaf 0.54 ppm
SABINENE Seed 1—140 ppm
SEDANENOLIDE Seed
SELENIUM Plant 0.001—0.021 ppm
SENKYUNOLIDE Root 5 ppm
SESQUIPHELLANDRENE Leaf
SILICON Leaf 60—1,425 ppm
SILVER Plant 0.19—0.2 ppm
SODIUM Plant 213—5,569 ppm
STEARIC-ACID Seed
STRONTIUM Plant 285—396 ppm
SUCCINIC-ACID Plant
SULFUR Plant 380—4,700 ppm
TAURINE Plant
TERPINEN-4-OL Leaf 0.72 ppm
TERPINOLENE Leaf 33 ppm
TERPINOLENE Seed 6—700 ppm
TETRADECANAL Leaf 3.84 ppm
THIAMIN Plant 0 - 7 ppm
TITANIUM Plant 1—2 ppm
TOLUENE Leaf
TRANS-2-HEXENAL Leaf 12.5 ppm
TRANS-2-HEXENOL Leaf 0.2 ppm
TRANS-BETA-OCIMENE Plant
TRIGONELLINE Tissue Culture
VITAMIN B6 Plant 2—14 ppm
WATER Plant 73,000—889,450 ppm
XANTHOTOXIN Shoot 3—289 ppm
ZINC Plant 7—164 ppm
ZIRCONIUM Plant 3.8—4 ppm

■ PARSNIP

Chemical Constituents of Pastinaca sativa L.
(Apiaceae)

5-ALPHA-ANDROST-16-EN-3-ONE Root
5-METHOXYLPSORALEN Root 7.3 ppm
ALPHA-LINOLENIC-ACID Root 30—145
 ppm
ALPHA-PHELLANDRENE Root
ALPHA-TERPINENE Root
ALPHA-THUJENE Root
ALUMINUM Root 1—35 ppm
ANGELICIN Root 34 ppm

APTERIN Root
ARSENIC Root 0.01 ppm
ASCORBIC-ACID Root 160—830 ppm
ASH Root 9,800—90,000 ppm
ASH Seed 12,000 ppm
BERGAPTEN Root 3.2—3,800 ppm
BERGAPTEN Seed
BETA-BISABOLENE Root
BETA-CAROTENE Root 0.2—1 ppm
BETA-PHELLANDRENE Root
BETA-PINENE Root
BETA-TRANS-FARNESENE Root
BORON Root 4—25 ppm
BROMINE Root
CADMIUM Root 0.01—0.4 ppm
CALCIUM Root 315—3,525 ppm
CAMPHENE Root
CARBOHYDRATES Root 17,500—902,000 ppm
CHROMIUM Root 0.01—0.01 ppm
CIS-ALLOOCIMENE Root
CIS-BETA-OCIMENE Root
COBALT Root
COPPER Root 0.8—12 ppm
FAT Root 3,000—24,000 ppm
FAT Seed 173,000—288,000 ppm
FIBER Root 15,000—97,700 ppm
FLUORINE Root 0.1 ppm
FOLACIN Root 0.6—3.6 ppm
GAMMA-TERPINENE Root
IMPERATORIN Leaf
IMPERATORIN Root 1,700 ppm
IMPERATORIN Seed
IRON Root 4—112 ppm
ISOBERGAPTEN Plant
ISOIMPERATORIN Seed
ISOPIMPINELLIN Seed
ISORHAMNETIN Leaf
ISORHAMNETIN-3-GLUCOSIDE-4-RHAMNOSIDE Plant
KAEMPFEROL Seed
KILOCALORIES Root 650—3,664 ppm
LEAD Root 0.01—0.1 ppm
LIMONENE Root
LINOLEIC-ACID Root 410—2,000 ppm
LINOLEIC-ACID Seed 36,330 ppm

MAGNESIUM Root 230—2,100 ppm
MANGANESE Root 2- 33 ppm
MERCURY Root 0.001—0.002 ppm
MOLYBDENUM Root 0.1—0.5 ppm
MUFA Root 1,120—5,470 ppm
MYRCENE Root
MYRISTIC-ACID Root 30—145 ppm
MYRISTICIN Root Essential Oil 183,000—662,000 ppm
N-HEPTACOSANE Seed
N-HEXACOSANE Seed
N-NONACOSANE Seed
N-NONADECONE Seed
N-OCTACOSANE Seed
N-OCTADECANE Seed
N-TRIACONTANE Seed
NIACIN Root 2—34 ppm
NICKEL Root 0.04—1.6 ppm
NITROGEN Root 3,000—33,160 ppm
OCTYL-BUTYRATE Plant
OCTYL-PROPIONATE Plant
OLEIC-ACID Seed 1,020—158,000 ppm
OXALIC-ACID Root 205 ppm
P-CYMENE Root
PALMITIC-ACID Root 300—1,730 ppm
PALMITIC-ACID Seed 1,730—2,880 ppm
PALMITOLEIC-ACID Root 30—145 ppm
PANTOTHENIC-ACID Root 6—29 ppm
PASTINACIN Seed
PETROSELINDIOLEIN Seed
PETROSELINIC-ACID Seed 79,580—132,500 ppm
PETROSELINOLEIN Seed
PHOSPHORUS Root 400—7,365 ppm
PIMPINELLIN Plant
POTASSIUM Root 3,300—40,000 ppm
PROTEIN Root 12,000—85,000 ppm
PROTEIN Seed 150,000—155,000 ppm
PSORALEN Root 7.1—10.5 ppm
PUFA Root 470—2,300 ppm
PYRUVIC-CARBOXYLASE Root
QUERCETIN Leaf
QUERCETIN-3-O-BETA-D-GLUCOSIDE Leaf
QUERCETIN-3-RHAMNOGLUCOSIDE Leaf
RIBOFLAVIN Root 0.5—4 ppm

RUBIDIUM Root 0.6—10 ppm
RUTIN Plant
SABINENE Root
SELINIUM Root 0.001—0.002 ppm
SFA Root 500—2,445 ppm
SILICON Root 2—50 ppm
SODIUM Root 100—575 ppm
SPHONDIN Root
STEARIC-ACID Root 140—685 ppm
SUBERIN Root
SULFUR Root 270—11,050 ppm
TERPINOLENE Root Essential Oil 253,000—
    666,000 ppm
THIAMIN Root 0.8—11.4 ppm
TRANS-BETA-OCIMENE Root
TRIPESTROSELINENE Seed
UMBELLIFERONE Plant
VITAMIN B6 Root 0.9—4.4 ppm
WATER Root 724,000—810,000 ppm
WATER Root 724,000—812,000 ppm
XANTHOTOXIN Leaf 800 ppm
XANTHOTOXIN Root 26—1,000 ppm
XANTHOTOXOL Plant
ZINC Root 5—70 ppm

■ PEA

Chemical Constituents of Pisum sativum L.
(Fabaceae)

(R)-DIHYDRO-MALEIMIDE Shoot 67 ppm
(R)-DIHYDRO-MALEIMIDE-BETA-D-
    GLUCOSIDE Shoot 62 ppm
1-3-(4,5-DIHYDRO-FURANONE)-5-
    (HYDROXY-METHYL)-PYRROLE-2-
    CARBOXYALDEHYDE Cotyledon
1-O-FERULOYL-BETA-D-GLUCOSE Petiole
1-O-P-COUMAROYL-BETA-D-GLUCOSE
    Petiole
1-O-SINAPOYL-BETA-D-GLUCOSE Petiole
14-HENTRIACONTANOL Wax
15-HENTRIACONTANOL Wax
16-HENTRIACONTANOL Wax
2,3,9-TRIMETHOXYPTEROCARPAN
    Embryo

24-METHYLENE-CHOLESTEROL Seed
3-HYDROXY-2,9-
    DIMETHOXYPTEROCARPAN Embryo
4,4'-DIHYDROXY-2'-METHOXY-
    CHALCONE Plant
4-HYDROXY-2,3,9-
    TRIMETHOXYPTEROCARPAN Embryo
5'-O-(6-O-MALONYL-BETA-D-
    GLYCOPYRANOSYL)-PYRIDOXINE
    Sprout Seedling
5'-O-(6-O-{3-HYDROXY-3-METHYL-4-
    CARBOXY-BUTANOYL}-BETA-D- GLY-
    COPYRANOSYL)PYRIDOXINE   Sprout
    Seedling 39 ppm
5'-O-BETA-D-GLUCOPYRANOSYL-
    PYRIDOXINE Sprout Seedling
ABSCISIC-ACID Seed
ALANINE Fruit 580—5,737 ppm
ALANINE Seed 2,400—11,353 ppm
ALANINE Shoot 313 ppm
ALLANTOIN Shoot
ALPHA-AMINO-ADIPIC-ACID Seed
ALPHA-AMYRIN Seed
ALPHA-CAROTENE Seed
ALPHA-LINOLENIC-ACID Fruit 130—1,286
    ppm
ALPHA-LINOLENIC-ACID Seed 350—1,656
    ppm
ALUMINUM Seed 1— 24 ppm
ARACHIDIC-ACID Seed
ARGININE Fruit 1,340—13,254 ppm
ARGININE Seed 4,280—20,246 ppm
ARSENIC Seed 0.01—0.04 ppm
ASCORBIC-ACID Fruit 600—5,935 ppm
ASCORBIC-ACID Seed 44—1,892 ppm
ASH Fruit 5,600—55,391 ppm
ASH Plant 60,000—191,000 ppm
ASPARTIC-ACID Fruit 2,280—22,552 ppm
ASPARTIC-ACID Seed 4,950—23,415 ppm
ASPARTIC-ACID Shoot 22 ppm
BETA-AMYRIN Seed
BETA-CAROTENE Fruit 0.8—8.3 ppm
BETA-CAROTENE Seed 3.6—18.2 ppm
BETA-CRYPTOXANTHIN Seed
BETA-SITOSTEROL Seed
BETAINE Root 59 ppm

BETAINE Shoot 94 ppm
BIOTIN Seed 82 ppm
BORON Seed 2—23 ppm
BROMINE Seed 0.2—12 ppm
CADMIUM Seed 0.001—0.3 ppm
CAFFEIC-ACID Plant
CAFFEIC-ACID-4-O-BETA-D-GLUCOSIDE
  Fruit
CALCIUM Fruit 430—4,253 ppm
CALCIUM Seed 230—1,700 ppm
CALCIUM-OXALATE Fruit
CAMPESTEROL Seed
CARBOHYDRATES Fruit 75,600—747,774
  ppm
CARBOHYDRATES Seed 144,600—684,000
  ppm
CELLULOSE Seed 74,000—96,000 ppm
CEPHALIN Seed
CHLORINE Seed 200—590 ppm
CHOLESTEROL Seed
CHOLINE Fruit 1,970—2,800 ppm
CHOLINE Seed 1,970—2,800 ppm
CHOLINE Shoot 121 ppm
CHROMIUM Seed 0.005—0.17 ppm
CIS-SINAPIC-ACID Seed
CITRIC-ACID Seed
COBALT Seed 0.002—0.24 ppm
COPPER Seed 2—10 ppm
COUMESTROL Fruit 300 ppm
COUMESTROL Seed 0.6 ppm
CRYPTOXANTHIN Seed 0.09—0.9 ppm
CYCLOARTENOL Sprout Seedling
CYSTINE Fruit 320—3,165 ppm
CYSTINE Seed 320 —1,,514 ppm
DEHYDROASCORBICACID Seed 1—7 ppm
DELPHINIDIN Flower
DIHYDROFOLATE-SYNTHESASE   Sprout
  Seedling
FAT Fruit 2,000—19,782 ppm
FAT Seed 3,670—20,481 ppm
FERULIC-ACID Seed
FIBER Fruit 25,000—247,280 ppm
FIBER Seed 22,100—104,541 ppm
FLUORINE Seed 0.1—1 ppm
FOLACIN Seed 0.6—3 ppm
GABA Shoot 153 ppm

CAMMA-HYDROXY-HOMOARGININE
  Sprout Seedling 100 ppm
GENISTEIN Shoot
GENTISTIC-ACID Seed
GIBBERELLINS Seed
GLUTAMIC-ACID Fruit 4,480—44,313 ppm
GLUTAMIC-ACID Seed 7,400—35,005 ppm
GLUTAMIC-ACID Shoot 70 ppm
GLYCINE Fruit 720—7,122 ppm
GLYCINE Seed 1,840—8,704 ppm
GLYCOLIC-ACID Seed
HENTRIACONTANE Wax 500,000 ppm
HISTAMINE Shoot
HISTIDINE Fruit 170—1,682 ppm
HISTIDINE Seed 1,070—5,061 ppm
HOMOSERINE Shoot 733 ppm
INOSITOL Seed 1,500 ppm
IODINE Seed 0.009 ppm
IRON Fruit 21—206 ppm
IRON Seed 14—90 ppm
ISOLEUCINE Fruit 1,610—15,925 ppm
ISOLEUCINE Seed 1,950—9,224 ppm
ISOXAZOLIN-5-ONE-2-BETA-D-
  GLUCOSIDE Sprout Seedling
JASMONIC-ACID Fruit
KAEMPFEROL Tissue Culture 500 ppm
KILOCALORIES Fruit 420—4,154/kg
KILOCALORIES Seed 810—3,832/kg
L-(+)-2-AMINOBUTRYIC-ACID Plant
L-(+)-HOMOSERINE Sprout Seedling
L-THREO-ALPHA-AMINO-BETA-CHLORO-
  BUTYRIC-ACID Juice
LEAD Seed 0—0.5 ppm
LECITHIN Seed
LEGUMIN Seed
LEGUMINELIN Seed
LEUCINE Fruit 2,280—22,552 ppm
LEUCINE Seed 3,230—15,279 ppm
LEUCINE Shoot 35 ppm
LINOLEIC-ACID Fruit 1,750—7,418 ppm
LINOLEIC-ACID Seed 1,520—7,190 ppm
LUPEOL Sprout Seedling
LYSINE Fruit 2,020—19,980 ppm
LYSINE Seed 3,170—14,995 ppm
M-XYLOHYDROQUINONE Seed
MAGNESIUM Fruit 218—2,591 ppm

MAGNESIUM Seed 319—1,700 ppm
MALIC-ACID Seed
MANGANESE Seed 3—21 ppm
MERCURY Seed 0.001—0.024 ppm
MESOXALIC-ACID Sprout Seedling
METHIONINE Fruit 110—1,088 ppm
METHIONINE Seed 820—3,879 ppm
METHYL-4-CHLORO-INODYL-3-
    ACETATE Seed
MOLYBDENUM Seed 0.1—3 ppm
MUFA Fruit 210—2,077 ppm
MUFA Seed 350—1,656 ppm
MYOINOSITOL Seed 1,000 ppm
MYRISTIC-ACID Fruit 20—198 ppm
NEO-BETA-CAROTENE-B Seed
NEO-BETA-CAROTENE-U Seed
NIACIN Fruit 6—59 ppm
NIACIN Seed 20—105 ppm
NICKEL Seed 0.2—3 ppm
NICOTINAMIDE Sprout Seedling 0.7 ppm
NICOTINIC-ACID Seed 18 ppm
NICOTINIC-ACID Sprout Seedling 18 ppm
NITROGEN Seed 11,000—50,000 ppm
O-ACETYL-HOMOSERINE Shoot 433 ppm
O-COUMARIC-ACID Seed
OLEIC-ACID Fruit 210—2,077 ppm
OLEIC-ACID Seed 350—1,656 ppm
ONONITOL Root 3.23 ppm
OXALIC-ACID Fruit 60 ppm
P-COUMARIC-ACID Seed
P-HYDROXYBENZOIC-ACID Seed
PAEONIDIN Flower
PALMITIC-ACID Fruit 330—3,264 ppm
PALMITIC-ACID Seed 640—3,027 ppm
PALMITOLEIC-ACID Fruit
PANTOTHENIC-ACID Fruit 7.5—74 ppm
PANTOTHENIC-ACID Seed 1—5 ppm
PARAGLACTAN Seed
PECTIN Seed 25,000 ppm
PHENYLALANINE Fruit 900—8,902 ppm
PHENYLALANINE Seed 2,000—9,460 ppm
PHOSPHORUS Fruit 530—5,240 ppm
PHOSPHORUS Seed 1,038—6,250 ppm
PHYTIC-ACID Seed
PHYTOHEMAGGLUTININ Seed
PHYTOPRECIPITIN Seed

PENITOL Seed 500 ppm
PISATIN Sprout Seedling
POTASSIUM Fruit 1,701—22,737 ppm
POTASSIUM Seed 2,273—15,830 ppm
PROLINE Fruit 630—6,231 ppm
PROLINE Seed 2,273—15,830 ppm
PROLINE Shoot 23 ppm
PROTEIN Fruit 28,000—276.954 ppm
PROTEIN Seed 52,800—262.042 ppm
PUFA Fruit 890—8,803 ppm
PUFA Seed 1,870—8,846 ppm
PUTRESCINE Leaf
PYRIDOXINE Seed 1.4 ppm
PYRROLINE Sprout Seedling
QUERCITRIN Seed
QUINIC-ACID Seed
RAFFINOSE Seed 6,000 ppm
RIBOFLAVIN Fruit 0.8—8 ppm
RIBOFLAVIN Seed 1.2—6.7 ppm
RUBIDIUM Seed 0.77—10 ppm
S-4-CHLORO-TRYPTOPHAN Seed
SALICYLIC-ACID Plant
SELENIUM Seed 0.001—0.002 ppm
SERINE Fruit 1,250—12,364 ppm
SERINE Seed 1,810—8,562 ppm
SFA Fruit 390—3,857 ppm
SFA Seed 710—3,350 ppm
SILICON Seed 2—59 ppm
SODIUM Fruit 22—578 ppm
SODIUM Seed 37—297 ppm
SOYASAPONIN-I Seed
SQUALENE Sprout Seedling
STACHYOSE Seed 20,000 ppm
STARCH Seed 329,000—434,000 ppm
STEARIC-ACID Fruit 30—297 ppm
STEARIC-ACID Seed 70—331 ppm
STIGMASTEROL Seed
SUCCINIC-ACID Seed
SUCROSE Seed 22,500—280,000 ppm
SUGAR Seed 41,000—59,000 ppm
SULFUR Seed 410—2,290 ppm
SYRINGIC-ACID Seed
THIAMIN Fruit 1.5—15 ppm
THIAMIN Seed 2.4—13.9 ppm
THREONINE Fruit 990—9,792 ppm
THREONINE Seed 2,030—9,603 ppm

TOCOPHEROL Seed 0.3—22 ppm
TRANS-SINAPIC-ACID Seed
TRIGONELLINE Fruit 6—203 ppm
TRIGONELLINE Seed 128—227 ppm
TRIGONELLINE Shoot 55 ppm
TRIGONELLINE Sprout Seedling 91 ppm
TRIGONELLINE Stem 1—24 ppm
TRYPTOPHAN Fruit 270—2,671 ppm
TRYPTOPHAN Seed 370—1,750 ppm
TYROSINE Fruit 990—9,792 ppm
TYROSINE Seed 1,130—5,345 ppm
VALINE Fruit 2,730—27,003 ppm
VALINE Seed 2,350—11,116 ppm
VALINE Shoot 33 ppm
VANILLIC-ACID Seed
VERBASCOSE Seed 31,000 ppm
VICILIN Seed
VITAMIN B12 Seed 0.004 ppm
VITAMIN B6 Fruit 1.6—16 ppm
VITAMIN B6 Seed 1.6—8.6 ppm
WATER Fruit 880,000—897,750 ppm
WATER Seed 760,000—793,670 ppm
XANTHOPHYLL Seed
ZINC Seed 11—60 ppm

■ PEANUT

Chemical Constituents of Arachis hypogaea L.
(Fabaceae)

4-METHYLENEPROLINE Seed
ALANINE Seed 10,390—12,137 ppm
ALPHA-CEPHALIN Seed
ALPHA-KETOGLUTARIC-ACID Seed
ALPHA-LINOLENIC-ACID   Seed   30—110
  ppm
ALPHA-TOCOPHEROL Oil 89 ppm
ALPHA-TOCOPHEROL Seed 83—116 ppm
ALUMINUM Seed 14 ppm
ARACHIDIC-ACID Seed 11,803—12,644 ppm
ARACHIN Seed
ARGININE Seed 31,280—37,022 ppm
ASCORBIC-ACID Seed 0—190 ppm
ASH Seed 16,000—28,000 ppm
ASPARTIC-ACID Seed 31,900—36,968 ppm

BEHENIC-ACID Seed 15,246—16,332 ppm
BETA-CAROTENE Seed 0—0.34 ppm
BIOTIN Seed
BORON Seed 5—18 ppm
CADMIUM Seed 0.03 ppm
CAFFEIC-ACID Seed 11 ppm
CALCIUM Seed 560—969 ppm
CARBOHYDRATES Seed 161,800—377,000
  ppm
CELLULOSE Seed 20,000—50,000 ppm
CHLOROGENIC-ACID Seed 12 ppm
CHOLINE Seed
CHROMIUM Seed 0.08 ppm
CHRYSOERIOL Plant
COBALT Seed 0.02—0.08 ppm
CONARACHIN Seed
CONGLUTIN Seed
COPPER Seed 8.6—11 ppm
CYSTINE Seed 3,290—3,580 ppm
DELTA-TOCOPHEROL Seed
FAT Seed 194,800—526,834 ppm
FERULIC-ACID Seed 45 ppm
FIBER Seed 11,900—52,383 ppm
FOLACIN Seed 1—3 ppm
FUMARASE Seed
GADOLEIC-ACID Seed 5,230—5,585 ppm
GAMMA-METHYLENE-ALPHA-
  KETOGLUTARIC-ACID Seed
GAMMA-TOCOPHEROL Oil 35 ppm
GENTISIC-ACID Seed 14 ppm
GLUTAMIC-ACID Seed 54,650—65,281 ppm
GLUTATHIONE Seed
GLYCINE Seed 15,760—18,993 ppm
HISTIDINE Seed 6,610—8,013 ppm
IRON Seed 21—42 ppm
ISOCHLOROGENIC-ACID Seed 3 ppm
ISOCITRATYLLASE Seed
ISOFERULIC ACID Seed 0.2 ppm
ISOLEUCINE Seed 9,200 ppm
KILOCALORIES Seed 3,030—6,074/kg
LEAD Seed 0.07 ppm
LECITHIN Seed 5,000—7,000 ppm
LEUCINE Seed 16,960—20,653 ppm
LEUCOYANIDIN Seed
LEUCODELPHINIDIN Seed
LIGNOCERIC-ACID Seed 5,409—5,795 ppm

LINOLEIC-ACID Seed 155,300—183,655 ppm
LYSINE Seed 9,390—10,627 ppm
MAGNESIUM Seed 1,700—2,110 ppm
MANGANESE Seed 11—30 ppm
MERCURY Seed
METHIONINE Seed 2,630—3,430 ppm
MUFA Seed 223,280—261,265 ppm
MYRISTIC-ACID Seed 250—300 ppm
NIACIN Seed 141—182 ppm
NITROGEN Seed 40,000 ppm
NONADECENOIC-ACID Plant
NONAHEXADECANOIC-ACID Plant
NONAHEXEDECANOIC-ACID Plant
O-COUMARIC-ACID Seed 20 ppm
P-HYDROXYBENZOIC-ACID Seed 14 ppm
PALMITIC-ACID Seed 51,450—60,615 ppm
PALMITOLEIC-ACID Seed 90—4,806 ppm
PANTOTHENIC-ACID Seed 17—30 ppm
PHENYLALANINE Seed 13,560—15,715 ppm
PHLORETIC-ACID Plant
PHOSPHOLIPASE-D Seed
PHOSPHORIC-ACID-
  MONOESTERHYDROLASE Seed
PHOSPHORUS Seed 2,450—4,248 ppm
POTASSIUM Seed 4,210—7,681 ppm
PROLINE Seed 11,540—15,362 ppm
PROTEIN Seed 150,000—275,000 ppm
PROTOCATECHUIC ACID Seed 4 ppm
PUFA Seed 155,340—183,785 ppm
RIBOFLAVIN Seed 1.3—3.1 ppm
RUBIDIUM Seed 13 ppm
SALICYLIC-ACID Seed 18 ppm
SARKOSIN Seed
SELENIUM Seed 0.02 ppm
SERINE Seed 12,710—15,362 ppm
SFA Seed 68,230—81,740 ppm
SINAPIC-ACID Seed 14 ppm
SODIUM Seed 40—260 ppm
SPHINGOGLYCOLIPID Seed
STEARIC-ACID Seed 10,980—13,760 ppm
STIZOLAMINE Seed
SULFUR Seed 2,100 ppm
SYRINGIC-ACID Seed 51 ppm
THIAMIN Leaf 2.3—11 ppm
THIAMIN Seed 6—17 ppm
THREONINE Seed 7,430—9,570 ppm

TRYPTOPHAN Seed 2,540—3,321 ppm
TYROSINE Seed 10,630—13,198 ppm
VALINE Seed 10,970—12,437 ppm
VANILLIC ACID Seed 43 ppm
VITAMIN B6 Seed 2.96—3.7 ppm
WATER Seed 56,000—422,000 ppm
ZINC Seed 31—35 ppm

■PECAN

Chemical Constituents of Carya illinoensis (Juglandaceae)

ALUMINUM Seed 11 ppm
ANTIMONY Seed 0.2 ppm
ARSENIC Seed 0.02 ppm
ASCORBIC ACID Seed 20—21 ppm
ASH Seed 16,000—17,000 ppm
BARIUM Seed 14 ppm
BETA-CAROTENE Seed 0.13—0.83 ppm
BORON Seed 6.5—7.6 ppm
BROMINE Seed 1.5 ppm
CADMIUM Seed 0.03 ppm
CALCIUM Seed 618—763 ppm
CARBOHYDRATES Seed 130,000—191,637
  ppm
CARYATIN Plant
CESIUM Seed 0.3 ppm
CHLORINE Seed 46 ppm
CHROMIUM Seed 0.3 ppm
COBALT Seed 0.4 ppm
COPPER Seed 15 ppm
EUROPIUM Seed 0.02 ppm
FAT Seed 712,000—753,000 ppm
FIBER Seed 22,000—24,000 ppm
FLUORINE Seed 1.6 ppm
GOLD Seed 0.001 ppm
HAFNIUM Seed 0.1 ppm
IODINE Seed 0.1 ppm
IRON Seed 24—73 ppm
KILOCALORIES Seed 6,670—7,180/kg
LANTHANUM Seed 0.02 ppm
LEAD Seed 0.3 ppm
LUTETIUM Seed 0.01 ppm
MAGNESIUM Seed 980 ppm

MANGANESE Seed 30 ppm
MERCURY Seed 0.1 ppm
NIACIN Seed 8.9—9.3 ppm
NICKEL Seed 1.6 ppm
PANTOTHENIC ACID Seed 17—18 ppm
PHOSPHORUS Seed 2,890—3,340 ppm
POTASSIUM Seed 3,971—6,242 ppm
PROTEIN Seed 92,000—97,000 ppm
QUERCETIN-3,5-DIMETHYLETHER Plant
QUERCETIN-3-GLUCOSIDE Plant
QUERCETIN-5-METHYLETHER Plant
RIBOFLAVIN Seed 1.1—1.3 ppm
RUBIDIUM Seed 22 ppm
SAMARIUM Seed 0.06 ppm
SCANDIUM Seed 0.004 ppm
SELENIUM Seed 0.02 ppm
SILICON Seed 200 ppm
SODIUM Seed 0—31 ppm
STRONTIUM Seed 2.5 ppm
SULFUR Seed 800 ppm
TANTALUM Seed 0.1 ppm
THIAMIN Seed 7.2—8.9 ppm
THORIUM Seed 0.1 ppm
TIN Seed 1.8 ppm
TITANIUM Seed 2.8 ppm
TUNGSTEN Seed 0.05 ppm
VANDIUM Seed 0.01 ppm
VITAMIN B6—Seed 1.8—2 ppm
WATER Seed 30,000—50,540 ppm
YTTERBIUM Seed 0.03 ppm
ZINC Seed 56 ppm

■ POTATO

Chemical Constituents of Solanum tuberosum L.
(Solanaceae)

(25S)-BAROGENIN Tuber 9.5 ppm
11-HYDROXY-11-METHYL-ETHYL-6,10-
    DIMETHYL-SPIRO-(4,5)-DEC-6-EN-8-
    ONE Tuber 81 ppm
2'CHLORO-DIAZEPAM Tuber
2'CHLORO-N-DEMETHYL-DIAZEPAM
    Tuber
2-(1',2'DIHYDROXY-1'-METHYL-ETHYL)-
6,10-DIMETHYL-9-HYDROXY-SPIRO-
    (4,5)-DEC-6-EN- 8-ONE Tuber
2-(12-O-BETA-D-GLUCOSYL-11-
    HYDROXY-11-METHYL-ETHYL)-6,10-
    DIMETHYL-SPIRO-4,5)-   DEC-6-EN-8-
    ONE Tuber 262 ppm
2-ALPHA-ETHOXY-DIHYDRO-
    PHYTUBERIN Tuber
2-BETA-ETHOXY-DIHYDRO-
    PHYTUBERIN Tuber
24-METHYLENECYCLOARTENOL Fruit
3,4,DICAFFEOYL-QUINIC-ACID   Tuber   3
    ppm
3,5,DICAFFEOYL-QUINIC-ACID Tuber
3-HYDROXY-2'CHOLORO-N-DEMTHYL-
    DIAZEPAM Tuber
5-ALPHA-CHOLESTANE Tuber
6,10-DIMETHYL-SPIRO-(4,5)-DEC-6-EN-
    2,8-DIONE Tuber
6-(3-METHYL-2-BUTENYL-
    AMINO)PURINE Tuber
ACETYL-DEHYDRO-RISHITINOL Tuber
ACONITIC-ACID Plant
ACROLEIN Essential Oil
ALANINE Tuber 1,140—5,700 ppm
ALPHA-CHACONINE Tuber 0.5—635 ppm
ALPHA-GLUCOSIDASE Tuber
ALPHA-SOLANINE Tuber 5—125,100 ppm
ALPHA-TOCOPHEROL Tuber 0.5—2.8 ppm
ALUMINUM Tuber 3.9—255 ppm
ARGININE Tuber 950—6,850 ppm
ARSENIC Tuber 0.001—0.6 ppm
ASCORBIC-ACID Tuber 170—990 ppm
ASH Tuber 8,100—85,000 ppm
ASPARTIC-ACID Tuber 4,340—24,050 ppm
BARIUM Tuber 0.078—60 ppm
BEHENYL-FERULATE Tuber
BETA-2-CHACONINE Tuber
BETA-ANHYDROORUTUNDOL Tuber
BETA-CAROTENE Tuber 1 ppm
BETA-CHACONINE Tuber
BORON Tuber 1—8 ppm
BROMINE Tuber 0.2—30 ppm
CADMIUM Tuber 0.004—0.455 ppm
CAFFEIC-ACID Tuber 280 ppm
CALCIUM Tuber 34—2,550 ppm

CAPRIC-ACID Tuber 10—48 ppm
CARBOHYDRATES Tuber 171,000—862,000 ppm
CAROTENOIDS Tuber 3 ppm
CHLORINE Tuber 16 ppm
CHLOROGENIC ACID Tuber 22—71 ppm
CHOLINE Tuber 330—1,000 ppm
CHROMIUM Tuber 0.002—1.4 ppm
CITRIC ACID Tuber 2,000 ppm
COBALT Tuber 0.02—0.3 ppm
COPPER Tuber 0.48—14 ppm
CRYPTOCHLOROGENIC-ACID Tuber 11 ppm
CYCLOARTENOL Tuber
CYCLODEHYDROISOLUBIMIN Tuber 0.7 ppm
CYCLOLAUDENOL Fruit
CYSTINE Tuber 230—1,235 ppm
DEACETYL-PHYTUBERIN Tuber 36 ppm
DEMISSIDINE Tuber
DEMISSINE Tuber
DIAZEPAM Tuber
EICOSYL-FERULATE Tuber
EO Plant 2 ppm
EPILUBIMEN Tuber
FAT Tuber 1,000—9,000 ppm
FERULIC-ACID Tuber 28 ppm
FIBER Tuber 3,000—27,000 ppm
FLUROINE Tuber 0.06—1 ppm
FOLACIN Tuber 0.074 ppm
FUMARIC-ACID Tuber
GAMMA-CHACONINE Tuber
GIBBERELLINS Tuber
GLUCINOL Tuber
GLUTAMIC ACID Tuber 3,470—24,150 ppm
GLYCINE Tuber 620—5,700 ppm
HEXACOSYL FERULATE Tuber
HEXADECYL FERULATE Tuber
HISTIDINE Tuber 450—2,140 ppm
IRON Tuber 5—128 ppm
ISOBUTYRALDEHYDE Essential Oil
ISODITYROSINE Tissue Culture
ISOFRAXIDIN-7-O-BETA-D-GLUCOSIDE Tuber 19 ppm
ISOLEUCINE Tuber 840—5,700 ppm
ISOLUBIMIN Tuber

ISOVALERALDEHYDE Essential Oil
JASMONIC ACID Tuber
KAEMPFEROL-3-SOPHOROSIDE Seed
KAEMPFEROL-3-SOPHOROSIDE-RHAMNOSIDE
KILOCALORIES Tuber 780—3,755/kg
LAURIC ACID Tuber 30—143 ppm
LEAD Tuber 0.01—4.2 ppm
LEUCINE Tuber 1,240—7,100 ppm
LIGNOCERYL-FERULATE Tuber
LINOLEIC ACID Tuber 320—1,520 ppm
LINOLEIC ACID Tuber 100—475 ppm
LITHIUM Tuber 0.104—0.28 ppm
LORMETAZEPAM Tuber
LUBIMINOL Tuber
LYCOPHENOL Fruit
LYSINE Tuber 1,260—6,800 ppm
MAGNESIUM Tuber 190—4,250 ppm
MALIC ACID Tuber 1,120 ppm
MANGANESE Tuber 1.3—22 ppm
MERCURY Tuber 0—0.05 ppm
METHIONINE Tuber 310—1,568 ppm
MEVALONIC ACID Tuber
MOLYBDENUM Tuber 0.1—2.1 ppm
MUFA Tuber 20—95 ppm
MYRISTIC ACID Tuber 10—48 ppm
N-BUTYRALDEHYDE Essential Oil
N-DEMETHYL-DIAZEPAM Tuber
NEOCHLOROGENIC ACID Tuber 7 ppm
NIACIN Tuber 148—74 ppm
NICKEL Tuber 0.02—2.6 ppm
NICOTINIC ACID Tuber 12 ppm
NITROGEN Tuber 2,200—17,000 ppm
NORADRENALIN Fruit
NOREPINEPHRINE Tuber
OCTACOSYL-FERULATE Tuber
OCATDECYL-FERULATE Tuber
OXYLEPILUBIMIN Tuber
OXYGLUTINOSONE Tuber
OXYLUBIMIN Tuber
P-COUMARIC-ACID Tuber 4 ppm
P-COUMAROYL-GLUCOSE Fruit
PAEONANIN Plant
PALMITIC ACID Tuber 160—760 ppm
PALMITOLEIC-ACID Tuber 10—48 ppm
PANTOTHENIC ACID Tuber 3—18 ppm

PATATIN Tuber
PECTIN Leaf 21,000—73,000 ppm
PECTIN Tuber 18,000—33,000 ppm
PHENYLALANINE Tuber 920—5,550 ppm
PHOSPHORUS Tuber 320—4,200 ppm
PHYTOSTEROLS Tuber 50—240 ppm
PHYTBERIN Tuber
POTASSIUM Tuber 2,470—30,000 ppm
PROLINE Tuber 740—6,700 ppm
PROTEIN Tuber 10,000—127,000 ppm
PUFA Tuber 430—2,043 ppm
QUINIC ACID Tuber
RIBOFLAVIN Tuber 0.4—1.9 ppm
RIBOFURANOSYL-CIS-ZEATIN Tuber
RIBOFURANOSYL-TRANS-ZEATIN Tuber
RISHITIN Tuber 11 ppm
RISHITINONE Tuber 0.4 ppm
RUBIDIUM Tuber 0.64—23 ppm
SCOPOLETIN Tuber Epidermis
SCOPOLIN Tuber 98 ppm
SELENIUM Tuber 0—0.01 ppm
SERINE Tuber 90—5,250 ppm
SFA Tuber 260—1,235 ppm
SILICON Tuber 1—10 ppm
SILVER Tuber 0.026—0.07 ppm
SINAPIC ACID Tuber 3 ppm
SODIUM Tuber 2.6—323 ppm
SOLAMINE Sprout Seedling
SOLANIDINE Tuber
SOLANOLONE Tuber 2.2 ppm
SOLANTHRENE Tuber
SOLASODINE Tuber
SOLAVETIVONE Tuber 6—83 ppm
SPIROVETIVA-1(10),11,DIEN-2-ONE Tuber
SPIROVETIVA-1(10),3,11,   TRIEN-2-ONE
   Tuber
STARCH Tuber 150,000—800,000 ppm
STEARIC ACID Tuber 40—190 ppm
STRONTIUM Tuber 0.39—60 ppm
SUBERIN Tuber
SULFUR Tuber 16—1,900 ppm
THIAMIN Tuber 1—5 ppm
THREONINE Tuber 750—4,300 ppm
TITANIUM Tuber 0.13—17 ppm
TOLATID-5-EN-3BETA-OL Plant
TOMATIDINE Tuber

TOMATINE Tuber
TRANS-N-FEROLOYL-PUTRESCINE Tuber
TRANS-ZEATIN Tissue Culture
TRYPTOPHAN Tuber 320—2,250 ppm
TYRAMINE Fruit
TYROSINE Tuber 770—3,900 ppm
UMBELLIFERONE Tuber
VALINE Tuber 117—6,450 ppm
VITAMIN B6 Tuber 700,000—800,000 ppm
ZINC Tuber 1.9—44.1 ppm

■ PUMPKIN

Chemical Constituents of Cucurbita pepo L.
(Cucurbitaceae)

(+)-CIS-ABSCISIC-ACID Plant
(+)-DEHYDROVOMIFOLIOL Plant
(+)-TRANS-ABSCISIC-ACID Plant
(+)-VOMIFOLIOL Plant
24-ETHYL-5-ALPHA-CHOLESTRA-7,22,25-
   TRIEN-3-BETA-OL Seed
24-ETHYL-5-ALPHA-CHOLESTRA-7,25-
   DIEN-3-BETA-OL Seed
24-ALPHA-ETHYLLATHASTEROL Plant
5-ALPHA-STIGMASTA-7,25-DIEN-3BETA-
   OL Plant
ADENINE Flower
ADENOSINE Flower
ALANINE Fruit 280—3,333 ppm
ALANINE Seed 11,580—12,441 ppm
ALPHA-KETO-BETA-METHYL-BUTYRIC-
   ACID Juice 100 ppm
ALPHA-KETO-BETA-METHYL-
   VALERAINIC-ACID Juice 180 ppm
ALPHA-LINOLENIC-ACID Flower 20—410
   ppm
ALPHA-LINOLENIC-ACID Fruit   30—357
   ppm
ALPHA-LINOLEINC-ACID   Seed   1,810—
   1,945 ppm
ALPHA-SPINASTEROL Seed
ALPHA-TOCOPHEROL Fruit 10—119 ppm
ALUMINUM Seed 11 ppm
ARACHIDIC ACID Seed 200 ppm

ARGININE Fruit 370—6,429 ppm
ARGININE Seed 40,330—43,328 ppm
ASCORBIC ACID Fruit 90—1,071 ppm
ASH Fruit 7,500—95,238 ppm
ASH Seed 47,530 ppm
ASPARTIC ACID Fruit 1,020—12,143 ppm
ASPARTIC ACID Seed 24,770—26,612 ppm
BETA-CAROTENE Fruit 9.6—114 ppm
BETA-CAROTENE Seed 2—2.5 ppm
BETA-HYDROXYBUTYRIC-ACID Fruit
BETA-SITOSTEROL Seed
BORON Fruit 1 ppm
CALCIUM Fruit 210—2,500 ppm
CALCIUM Seed 418—474 ppm
CARBOHYDRATES Fruit 65,000—773,809 ppm
CARBOHYDRATES Seed 178,100—191,341 ppm
CHROMIUM Seed 17 ppm
COBALT Seed 143 ppm
COPPER Seed 14—15 ppm
CUCURBITAXANTHIN Fruit
CUCURBITIN Seed 16,600—66,300 ppm
CUCURBITOL Seed
CYSTINE Fruit 30—700 ppm
CYSTINE Seed 3,010—3,234 ppm
DEHYDROASCORBIC ACID Seed
DL-CITRULLIN Seed
EDESTINE Seed
FAT Flower 700—14,430 ppm
FAT Fruit 1,000—11,905 ppm
FAT Seed 384,500—520,000 ppm
FERULIC ACID Plant
FIBER Fruit 11,000—130,952 ppm
FIBER Seed 19,690—26,538 ppm
FLAVOXANTHIN Juice
GABA Seed
GLUTAMIC ACID Fruit 1,840—35,000 ppm
GLUTAMIC ACID Seed 43,150—46,358 ppm
GLYCINE Fruit 270—8,000 ppm
GLYCINE Seed 17,960—19,295 ppm
GLYCOXALIC ACID Juice 200 ppm
GUANOSINE Sprout Seedling
HISTIDINE Fruit 140—1,905 ppm
HISTIDINE Seed 6,810—7,316 ppm
HYDROXYBRNZTRAUBEN ACID Fruit

IRON Seed 86—172 ppm
ISOLEUCINE Fruit 310—3,690 ppm
ISOLEUCINE Seed 12,640—13,580 ppm
KILOCALORIES Fruit 220—3,095/kg
KILOCALORIES Seed 2,730—5,812/kg
LAURIC ACID Fruit 10—119 ppm
LAURIC ACID Seed 440—472 ppm
LECITHIN Seed 4,000 ppm
LEUCINE Fruit 460—5,476 ppm
LINOLEIC ACID Fruit 20—238 ppm
LINOLEIC ACID Seed 209,040—222,411 ppm
LYSINE Fruit 470—6,429 ppm
LYSINE Seed 18,330—19,693 ppm
M-CARBOXYPHENYLALANINE Seed
MAGNESIUM Fruit 120—1,429 ppm
MANGANESE Seed 40 ppm
MANNITOL Fruit 150,000—200,000 ppm
METHIONINE Fruit 110—1,310 ppm
METHIONINE Seed 5,510—5,920 ppm
MUFA Flower 90—1,855 ppm
MYRISTIC ACID Fruit 60—714 ppm
MYRISTIC ACID Seed 200—559 ppm
NIACIN Fruit 6 ppm
NIACIN Seed 14—22 ppm
OLEIC ACID Fruit 60—714 ppm
OLEIC ACID Juice 400 ppm
OXYCEROTINIC ACID Seed
PALMITIC ACID Fruit 370—4,405 ppm
PALMITIC ACID Seed 56,120—60,292 ppm
PALMITOLEIC ACID Fruit 60—714 ppm
PALMITOLEIC ACID Seed 990—1,064 ppm
PHENYLALANINE Fruit 300—3,810 ppm
PHENYLALANINE Seed 12,220—13,128 ppm
PHOSPHOLIPIDS Seed
PHOSPHORUS Fruit 440—5,238 ppm
PHOSPHORUS Seed 10,600—12,982 ppm
PHYTIC ACID Seed 15,000—22,000 ppm
PHYTOSTEROLS Fruit 120—1,428 ppm
POTASSIUM Fruit 3,400—40,476 ppm
POTASSIUM Seed 5,540—8,670 ppm
PROLINE Fruit 260—17,100 ppm
PROLINE Seed 10,000—10,743 ppm
PROTEIN Fruit 10,000—140,000 ppm
PROTEIN Seed 86,000—271,797 ppm
PUFA Fruit 50—595 ppm
PUFA Seed 209,040—224,581 ppm

RIBOFLAVIN Flower 0.7—15 ppm
RIBOFLAVIN Fruit 1.1—13.1 ppm
RIBOFLAVIN 2.7—4.9 ppm
SALICYLIC ACID Seed
SELENIUM Seed
SERINE Fruit 440—6,100 ppm
SERINE Seed 11,480—12,333 ppm
SFA Fruit 520—6,190 ppm
SFA Seed 86,740—93,180 ppm
SILICON Seed
SODIUM Fruit 10—119 ppm
SODIUM Seed 180—193 ppm
STEARIC ACID Fruit 30—357 ppm
STEARIC ACID Seed 28,110—30,200 ppm
SUCROSE Seed 14,000 ppm
THIAMIN Fruit 0.5—5.9 ppm
THIAMIN Seed 1.9—3.7 ppm
THREONINE Fruit 250—3.452 ppm
THREONINE Seed 9,030—9,701 ppm
TIN Seed 23 ppm
TRIGONELLINE Sprout Seedling
TRYPTOPHAN Fruit 120—1,800 ppm
TRYPTOPHAN Seed 4,310—4,6230 ppm
TYROSINE Fruit 130—5,000 ppm
TYROSINE Seed 10,190—10,948 ppm
UREASE Seed
VALINE Fruit 350—4,167 ppm
VALINE Seed 19,720—21,186 ppm
WATER Fruit 916,000 ppm
WATER Seed 65,200—73,110 ppm
ZINC Seed 74—83 ppm

■ RADISH

Chemical Constituents of Raphanus sativus L.
(Brassicaceae)

4-METHYLSULFOXIDEBUTEN-(3)-YL-
CYANIDE Seed 200 ppm
ALANINE Root 220—4,265 ppm
ALUMINUM Root 6—185 ppm
ARGININE Plant
ARSENIC Root
ASCORBIC ACID Fruit 690—7,822 ppm
ASCORBIC ACID Leaf 810—7,043 ppm

ASCORBIC ACID Root 226—6,216 ppm
ASH Root 10,000—185,700 ppm
ASPARTIC ACID Root 480—9,300 ppm
BETA-CAROTENE Fruit 0.3—26.2 ppm
BETA-CAROTENE Leaf 24.7—214 ppm
BETA-CAROTENE Root 0—1 ppm
BETA-HEXYLALDEHYDE Seed
BORON Root 0.6—64 ppm
BROMINE Root
CADMIUM Root 0.005—0.57 ppm
CAFFEIC ACID Root 91 ppm
CALCIUM Fruit 260—10,130 ppm
CALCIUM Leaf 2,380—19,130 ppm
CALCIUM Root 190—8,570 ppm
CALCIUM Seed 3,670 ppm
CARBOHYDRATES Fruit 54,000—701,000
ppm
CARBOHYDRATES Leaf 57,000—496,000
ppm
CARBOYHDRATES Root 36,000—757,000
ppm
CHROMIUM Root 0.01—0.14 ppm
COBALT Root
COPPER Root 0.3—8 ppm
COPPER Seed 6 ppm
CYSTINE Root 50—970 ppm
DIALLYLSULFIDE Root
ERUCIC ACID Seed
FAT Fruit 3,000—50,000 ppm
FAT Leaf 6,000—52,000 ppm
FAT Root 1,000—187,000 ppm
FAT Seed 298,000—410,000 ppm
FERULIC ACID Root 16 ppm
FIBER Fruit 11,000—147,000 ppm
FIBER Leaf 11,000—96,000 ppm
FIBER Root 5,200—176,000 ppm
FLUORINE Root
FOLACIN Root 0.3—5.8 ppm
GLUCOBRASSICIN Plant
GLUCOCAPPARIN Seed
GLUCLEPIDIIN Seed
GLUCOPUTRANJIVIN Root
GLUCORAPHANIN Root
GLUTAMIC ACID Root 1,320—25,580 ppm
GLYCEROL SINAPATE Seed
GLYCINE Root 220—4,265 ppm

HISTIDINE Root 130—2,520 ppm
INDOLEACETIC ACID Root
INDOLEACETONITRILE Root
IRON Fruit 4—295 ppm
IRON Leaf 41—357 ppm
IRON Root 2—189 ppm
IRON Seed 120 ppm
ISOBUTYRALDEHYDE Leaf
ISOLEUCINE Root 300—5,815 ppm
KILOCALORIES Fruit 340—3,370/kg
KILOCALORIES Leaf 330—2,870/kg
KILOCALORIES Root 170—3,510/kg
L-SULFORAPHENE Root
LEAD Root 0.01—0.57 ppm
LEUCINE Root 370—7,170 ppm
LINOLEIC ACID Root 160—3,100 ppm
LINOLENIC ACID Root 290—5,620 ppm
LYSINE Root 350—6,785 ppm
MAGNESIUM Root 85—3,570 ppm
MAGNESIUM Seed 3,960 ppm
MANGANESE Root 0.5—20 ppm
MANGANESE Seed 40 ppm
MERCURY Root 0—0.014 ppm
METHIONINE Root 70—1,355 ppm
MEHTYL MERCAPTAN Seed
MOLYBDENUM Root
MUFA Root 170—3,295 ppm
MYRISTIC ACID Root
N-BUTYRALDEHYDE Leaf
NIACIN Fruit 2—59 ppm
NIACIN Leaf 40—348 ppm
NIACIN Root 3—68 ppm
NICKEL Root 0.01—0.71 ppm
NITROGEN Root 2,000—38,570 ppm
OLEIC ACID Root 160—3,100 ppm
OXALIC ACID Root 92 ppm
P-COUMARIC ACID Root 91 ppm
PALMITIC ACID Root 260—5,040 ppm
PANTOTHENIC ACID Root 0.8—18 ppm
PHYLALANINE Root 230—4,455 ppm
PHOSPHORUS Fruit 240—10,526 ppm
PHOSPHORUS Leaf 300—2,609 ppm
PHOSPHORUS Root 160—5,850 ppm
PHYTOSTEROLS Root 70—1,355 ppm
POTASSIUM Fruit 2,070—20,495 ppm
POTASSIUM Leaf 5,000—43,478 ppm

POTASSIUM Root 2,215—85,700 ppm
PROLINE Root 180—3,490 ppm
PROTEIN Root 13,000—257,000 ppm
PROTEIN Leaf 33,000—287,000 ppm
PROTEIN Root 5,260—182,000 ppm
PROTEIN Seed 236,000—336,000 ppm
PUFA Root 450—8,720 ppm
PUTRESCINE Leaf
RAPHANIN Seed
RAPHANUSIN-A Root
RAPHANUSIN-B Root
RAPHANUSIN-C Root
RAPHANUSIN-D Root
RIBOFLAVIN Fruit 0.3—5.3 ppm
RIBOFLAVIN Leaf 2.6—24 ppm
RIBOFLAVIN Root 0.3—9.3 ppm
RUBIDIUM Root 0.44—15.7 ppm
S-METHYL-L-CYSTEINSULFOXIDE Root
SELENIUM Root
SERINE Root 210—4,070 ppm
SILICON Root 10—425 ppm
SINAPIC ACID Root
SINIGRIN Seed
SODIUM Fruit 50—495 ppm
SODIUM Leaf 1,100—9,565 ppm
SODIUM Root 100—5,020 ppm
SODIUM Seed 134 ppm
SPERMINE Leaf
SPERMINIDINE Leaf
STEARIC ACID Root 40—775 ppm
SULFUR Root 350—6,140 ppm
THIAMIN Fruit 0.3—7.9 ppm
THIAMIN Leaf 1.4—7 ppm
THIAMIN Root 0.3—9.7 ppm
THREONINE Root 290—5,620 ppm
TRIACONTANE Seed
TRYPTOPHAN Root 40—775 ppm
TYROSINE Root 130—2,520 ppm
VALINE Root 320—6,200 ppm
VITAMIN B6 Root 0.7—14.5 ppm
WATER Fruit 899,000—923,000 ppm
WATER Leaf 856,000 ppm
WATER Root 926,000—945,000 ppm
ZINC Root 2—72 ppm
ZINC Seed 29 ppm

■ RICE

Chemical Constituents of Oryzra sativa L. (Poaceae)

(+)-DEHYDROVOMIFOLIOL Petiole 1 ppm
1-RHAMNONO-1,4-LACTONE Plant
12(S),13(S)-EPOXY-11(R)-HYDROXY-OCTADECA-CIS-9,CIS15-DIEN-1-OIC-ACID Shoot 0.9 ppm
12(S),13(S)-EPOXY-11(S)-HYDROXY-OCTADECA-CIS-9,CIS15-DIEN-1-OIC-ACID Shoot 0.4 ppm
15,16-DIHYDROCORONARIC-ACID Shoot 0.8 ppm
2,4-DINITROPHENYLHYDRAZONE Seed
2-C-HYDROXY-METHYL-D-ERYTHRONO-1,4-LACTONE Plant
2-C-METHYL-D-ERYTHRONO-1,4-LACTONE Plant
2-DEOXY-D-LYXONO-1,4-LACTONE Plant
24-METHYL-24-METHOXYCYCLOARTANOL Plant
24-METHYLENE-CYCLOARTANOL Plant
25-EHTOXY-24-METHOXYCYLCOARTANOL Plant
25-HYDROXY-24-METHOXYCYCLOARTANOL Plant
3-DEOXY-D-ARABINO-HEXONO-1,4-LACTONE Plant
5'O-(BETA-D-GLUCOPYRANOSYL)-PYROXIDINE Fruit
9,10-DIOXYSTEARIC-ACID Plant
ACETALDEHYDE Plant
ACETONE Plant
ADENINE Seed
ALLANTOIN Seed
ALPHA-GLUCAN Tissue Culture
ALPHA-TOCOPHEROL Seed
AMYLOSE Seed 0—131,075 ppm
ANTHERAXANTHIN Plant
ARABINOSE Seed
ARACHIDIC ACID Seed
ARSENIC Seed 0.211 ppm
ARUNDOIN Shoot
ASCORBIC ACID Seed

ASH Plant 75,000—185,000 ppm
ASH Seed 7,000—57,000 ppm
ASPARAGINE Juice
ASPARTIC ACID Hay
BEHENIC ACID Seed
BETA-CAROTENE Seed
BETA-CYCLOORYSTENOL Seed
BETA-SITOSTEROL Juice
BETA-SITOSTEROL Sprout Seedling
BUTANAL Plant
CADMIUM Seed 0.18 ppm
CALCIUM Plant 1,900—3,300 ppm
CALCIUM Seed 71—364 ppm
CAMPESTEROL Plant
CARBOHYDRATES Plant 420,000—478,000 ppm
CARBOHYDRATES Seed 734,000—892,000 ppm
CARLINOSIDE Leaf
CELLOPENTAOSYLSITOSTEROL Plant
CELLOTETRAOSYLSITOSTEROL Plant
CELLULOSE Petiole 190,000—210,000 ppm
CELLULOSE Plant 340,000—534,600 ppm
CERAMIDE Shoot 15 ppm
CERYL-CEROTATE Fruit
CHOLINE Seed 880 ppm
CHRYSANTHEMIN Plant
COPROSTAN Plant
CORONARIC ACID Shoot 0.1 ppm
CYANIDIN-5-GLYCOSIDE Leaf
CYANIDIN-DIGLYCOSIDE Leaf
CYANIDIN-MONOGLYCOSIDE Leaf
CYANIN Plant
CYCLOARTANOL Plant
CYCLOARTENOL Plant
CYCLOBRANOL Plant
CYCLOEUCALENOL Seed
CYLINDRIN Shoot
CYSTEINE Plant
D-ALANYL-D-ALANINE Leaf
D-ALANYL-GLYCINE Leaf
D-ARABINO-1,4-LACTONE Plant
D-ERYTHRONO-1,4-LACTONE Plant
D-LYXONO-1,4-LACTONE Plant
DESOXYCORTICOSTEROL Plant
DEXTRIN Seed 15,600—20,500 ppm

DIGLYCOSYL-CERAMIDE Shoot 2 ppm
DIHYDRO-BETA-SITOSTEROL Petiole
DIMETHYLAMINE Seed
DNA-POLYMERASE Tisse Culture
ERGOSTEROL Sprout Seedling
ESTERASE Plant
FAT Plant 9,000—15,000 ppm
FAT Seed 8,000—121,000 ppm
FURFURAL Petiole 90,000—100,000 ppm
GAMMA-SITOSTEROL Sprout Seedling
GAMMA-TOCOPHEROL Seed
GLUCOSE Seed 14,500—26,500 ppm
GLUCOTRICIN Plant
GLUTAMIC ACID Hay
GLYCINE Plant
GUANIDINE Seed
GUANINE Seed
HEXANAL Plant
HEXANOL Plant
HYPOXANTHINE Plant
INDOLE-3-ACETIC-ACID-MYOINOSITOL
    Seed 4.5 ppm
INEKETONE Petiole 0.003 ppm
IRON Seed 14—85 ppm
ISOARBORINOL Shoot
ISOCERYL-ISOCEROTATE Fruit
ISOEUGENOL Plant
ISOLEUCINE Hay
ISOSCOPARIN-2"-GLUCOSIDE Plant
ISOSCOPARIN-2"-GLUCOSIDE-6"-
    FERULIC-ESTER Plant
ISOSCOPARIN-2"-GLUCOSIDE-6"-P-
    COUMARIC-ESTER Plant
KERACYANIN Plant
KILOCALORIES Seed 3,410—4,100/kg
LEAD Seed 0.9 ppm
LECITHIN Play
LEUCINE Hay
LIGNIN Plant 45,000—255,300 ppm
LIGNOCERIC ACID Seed
LINOLEIC ACID Seed 6,600—11,880 ppm
LINOLENIC-ACID Seed
LUTEIN Play
LYSINE Hay
LYSOLECETHIN Seed
MAGNESIUM Plant 1,100—2,200 ppm

MERCURY Seed 0.167 ppm
METHIONINE Plant
MOMILACTONE-A Petiole 4 ppm
MOMILACTONE-B Petiole 1 ppm
MOMILACTONE-C Plant
MONOGLYCOSYL-CERAMIDE Shoot 250
    ppm
MYRICYL-CEROTATE Fruit
NAPHTHALINE Sprout Seedling
NEOCARLINOSIDE Plant
NEOSCHAFTOSIDE Leaf
NEOXANTHIN Plant
NIACIN Seed 40—65 ppm
NICKEL Seed 1.632 ppm
NICOTIANAMINE Sprout Seedling
OLEIC ACID Seed 4,500—8,100 ppm
ORYZABRANS Seed
ORYZALEXIN-A Leaf 1—1.4 ppm
ORYZALEXIN-B Leaf 0.6 ppm
ORYZALEXIN-C Leaf 5.4 ppm
ORYZALEXIN-D Leaf
ORYZANOL-A Seed
ORYZANOL-B Seed
ORYZANOLE Plant
ORYZARANS Root
ORYZAROL Stem
ORYZENIN Seed
OXALIC ACID Seed 46 ppm
P-AMINOBENZOIC ACID Plant
P-COUMARIC ACID Petiole 0.9 ppm
P-HYDROXYBENZOIC ACID Plant
PALMITIC ACID Seed 1,800—3,240 ppm
PANGAMIC ACID Petiole
PANTOTHENIC ACID Seed 6—17 ppm
PELARGONIC ACID Plant
PENTANAL Plant
PENTOSANS Plant 209,000 ppm
PHOSPHORUS Plant 600—3,478 ppm
PHOSPHORUS Seed 528—5,588 ppm
PHYTIN Seed
PHYTIN-PHOSPHORUS Seed 211—2,235
    ppm
PHYTOCEREBROSIDE Plant
POTASSIUM Plant 12,000—12,600 ppm
POTASSIUM Seed 1,000—2,431 ppm
PRIMULIN Seed

PROPANAL Plant
PROTEIN Hay
PROTEIN Plant 34,000—45,000 ppm
PROTEIN Seed 58,000—85,000 ppm
PYRIDOXINE Seed 4—10 ppm
QUINIC-ACID Leaf
RHAMNOGALACTURONAN-I Tissue Culture
RIBOFLAVIN Seed 0.5—0.7 ppm
RIBOTIDE-CIS-ZEATIN Root
SATIVIC ACID Sprout Seedling
SCHAFTOSIDE Leaf
SERINE Plant
SHIKIMIC ACID Leaf
SILICA Plant 140,000 ppm
SILICIC ACID Leaf
SODIUM Plant 3,500 ppm
SODIUM Seed 90—939 ppm
SQUALENE Seed
STARCH Seed 722,000—749,000 ppm
STEARIC ACID Seed 150—270 ppm
STIGMASTEROL Juice
SUCROSE Seed 3,000—4,800 ppm
SULFUR Plant 1,000 ppm
TARXANTHIN Plant
THIAMIN Seed 2.2—3.9 ppm
THREONINE Hay
TOCOPHEROL Wax
TRANS-ACONITIC-ACID Shoot
TRIACONTANOL-(1) Sprout Seedling
TRICIN Petiole 0.066 ppm
TRICIN Plant
TRICIN-5-GLUCOSIDE Plant
TRICIN-5-O-BETA-D-GLUCOSIDE Plant
TRIGLYCOSYL-CERAMIDE Shoot 1 ppm
TRIGONELLINE Sprout Seedling
TRIMETHYLAMINE Seed
TYROSINE Plant
UNDECYLIC ACID Plant
URACIL Seed
VALINE Hay
VANILLIC ACID Plant
VERNOLIC ACID Shoot 0.1 ppm
VIOLANTHIN Plant
VIOLAXANTHIN Plant
WATER Seed 103,000 ppm
XANTHINE Plant

XANTHOPHYLL Plant
XYLOSE Seed

■ RYE

Chemical Constituents of Secale cereale L. (Poaceae)

ALANINE Seed 7,110—7,985 ppm
ARGININE Seed 8,130—9,130 ppm
ASH Seed 18,000—24,650 ppm
ASH Seed 54,750 ppm
ASPARTIC ACID Seed 11,770—13,215 ppm
CALCIUM Seed 315—685 ppm
CARBOHYDRATES Leaf 848,850 ppm
CARBOHYDRATES Seed 697,600—824,720 ppm
COPPER Seed 4—5 ppm
CYSTINE Seed 3,290—3,695 ppm
FAT Leaf 23,000 ppm
FAT Seed 14,000—40,425 ppm
FIBER Leaf 23,000 ppm
FIBER Seed 15,000—20,470 ppm
GADOLEIC ACID Seed 130—145 ppm
GLUTAMIC ACID Seed 36,610—41,110 ppm
GLYCINE Seed 7,010—7,870 ppm
HISTIDINE Seed 3,670—4,120 ppm
IODINE Seed 0.07—0.08 ppm
ISOLEUCINE Seed 5,490—6,165 ppm
KILOCALORIES Seed 3,350—3,760/kg
LEUCINE Seed 9,800—11,000 ppm
LINOLEIC ACID Seed 9,580—10,760 ppm
LINOLENIC ACID Seed 1,570—1,765 ppm
LYSINE Seed 6,050—6,795 ppm
MAGNESIUM Seed 1,185—1,740 ppm
MANGANESE Seed 25—30 ppm
METHIONINE Seed 2,480—2,785 ppm
MUFA Seed 3,030—3,400 ppm
MYRISTIC ACID Seed 30—35 ppm
NIACIN Seed 10—11 ppm
OLEIC ACID Seed 2,800—3,145 ppm
PALMITIC ACID Seed 2,710—3,045 ppm
PALMITOLEIC ACID Seed 100—110 ppm
PANTOTHENIC ACID Seed 10—11 ppm
PECTINS Seed 11,300 ppm

PENTOSANS Seed
PHENYLALANINE Seed 6,740—7,570 ppm
PHOSPHORUS Leaf 1,970 ppm
PHOSPHORUS Seed 3,725—4,225 ppm
POTASSIUM Leaf 11,500 ppm
POTASSIUM Seed 2,500—5,090 ppm
PROLINE Seed 14,910—16,745 ppm
PROTEIN Leaf 73,385 ppm
PROTEIN Seed 120,000—196,500 ppm
PUFA Seed 11,150—12,520 ppm
RAFFINOSE Seed
RIBOFLAVIN Seed 1—2 ppm
SERINE Seed 6,810—7,645 ppm
SFA Seed 2,870—3,225 ppm
SODIUM Seed 45—70 ppm
STEARIC ACID Seed 90—100 ppm
SULFUR Seed 1,460—1,640 ppm
THIAMIN Seed 3—3 ppm
THREONINE Seed 5,320—5,975 ppm
TOCOPHEROLS Seed 800 ppm
TRYPTOPHAN Seed 1,540—1,730 ppm
TYROSINE Seed 3,390—3,800 ppm
VALINE Seed 7,470—8,390 ppm
VITAMIN B6 Seed 3 ppm
WATER Seed 100,000—110,000 ppm
ZINC Seed 35—45 ppm

■ SOYBEAN

Chemical Constituents of Glycine max L. (Fabaceae)

(6AR,11AR)-3-6(A)-9-
  TRIHYDROXYPTEROCARPAN Cotyledon
1-DODECENE Plant
1-HEXANOL Plant
1-O-FERULOYL-BETA-D-GLUCOSE Sprout
  Seedling
1-O-PARA-COUMAROYLE-BETA-D-
  GLUCOSE Sprout Seedling
2,4-HEXADIEN-1-OL Plant
2-HEXENAL Plant
24-METHYLENE-CYCLOARTENOL Seed
3,5,5,TRIMETHYL-2-HEXENE Seed
3-HEXENAL-1-OL Plant

3-HYDROXY-LINOLEIC ACID Tissue Culture
3-HYDROXY-OLEIC ACID Tissue Culture
4'-5-7-TRIACETOXYISOFLAVONE Shoot
4'-5-7-TRIMETHOXYISOFLAVONE Shoot
4'-7-DIACETOXYLISOFLAVONE Shoot
4'7-DIMETHOXYISOFLAVONE Shoot
4-HEXENYLOL-ACETATE Plant
4-HYDROXY-BENZOIC ACID Root
5"-O-ACETYL-DAIDZIN Seed 0—145 ppm
6"-O-ACETYL-DAIDZIN Seed 0—80 ppm
6"-O-ACETYL-GENISTIN Seed 17—145 ppm
6,8-DI-HEXOSYL-GENKWANIN Root
6-(4-O-BETA-D-GLUCOSYL-3-METHYL-
  TRANS-BUT-2-ENYL-AMINO)PURINE
  Tissue Culture 6-CARBOXY-PTERIN Seed
  0.087 ppm
6-HYDROXY-METHYL-PTERIN Plant
7-DEHYDROAVENASTEROL Seed
ABSCISIC ACID Seed
ACETALDEHYDE Plant
ACETIC ACID Seed
ACETONE Plant
ACETYL-SOYASAPONIN-A-1 Seed 410 ppm
ACETYL-SOYASAPONIN-A-2 Seed 110 ppm
ACETYL-SOYASAPONIN-A-3 Seed 30 ppm
ACETYL-SOYASAPONIN-A-4 Seed 378 ppm
ACETYL-SOYASAPONIN-A-5 Seed 89 ppm
ACETYL-SOYASAPONIN-A-6 Seed 50 ppm
ACID-PHOSPHATASE Plant
ADENINE Seed 210—500 ppm
ADENINE Sprout Seedling
ADENOSINE Sprout Seedling
ADENYLIC ACID Sprout Seedling
ALANINE Seed 17,190—18,795 ppm
ALCOHOL-DEHYDROGENASE Plant
ALLANTOIN Seed
ALLANTIONASE Seed
ALPHA-AMYLASE Seed
ALPHA-AMYRIN Sprout Seedling
ALPHA-KETOGLUTARIC ACID Seed
ALPHA-LINOLENIC ACID Seed 13,300—
  14,540 ppm
ALPHA TOCOPHEROL Oil 95 ppm
ALPHA TOCOPHEROL Seed 8—19 ppm
ALUMINUM Seed 2—60 ppm
AMMONIA Seed 8,600 ppm

AMYLASE Seed
ANTHOCYANIN Seed
ARABINOGALACTAN Seed
ARABINOSE Seed
ARACHIDONIC ACID Seed
ARGININE Seed 28,310—30,950 ppm
ASCORBIC ACID Fruit 290—942 ppm
ASCORBIC ACID Seed 0—849 ppm
ASCORBIC ACID Sprout Seedling 100—949 ppm
ASCORBICASE Seed
ASH Fruit 16,000—52,000 ppm
ASH Plant 55,000—119,000 ppm
ASH Seed 17,000—61,000 ppm
ASH Sprout Seedling 8,000—58,000 ppm
ASPARAGIC ACID Seed
ASPARTATE-AMINO-TRANSFERASE Plant
ASPARTIC ACID Seed 45,890—50,175 ppm
BARIUM Seed 1—90 ppm
BETA-AMYLASE Seed
BETA-AMYRIN Sprout Seedling
BETA-CAROTENE Fruit 4.1—13.4 ppm
BETA-CAROTENE Plant 0.3 ppm
BETA-CAROTENE Seed 0—11.3 ppm
BETA-CAROTENE Sprout Seedling 0.2—3.5 ppm
BETA-CONGLYCIN Seed
BETA-INDOLACETIC ACID Shoot
BETA-NEOCAROTENE Seed
BETA-SITOSTEROL Seed 900 ppm
BETA-TOCOPHEROL Seed
BETAINE Seed
BIOCHANIN-C Seed
BIOTIN Seed 750 ppm
BORON Seed 4—18 ppm
BOWMAN-BIRK-INHIBITOR Seed 500—3,000 ppm
BUTYROSPERMOL Seed
CADAVERINE Seed
CAFFEIC-ACID Seed 1- 4 ppm
CALCIUM Fruit 670—2,200 ppm
CALCIUM Plant 9,400—13,000 ppm
CALCIUM Seed 780—4,440 ppm
CALCIUM Sprout Seedling 480—3,504 ppm
CAMPESTEROL Seed
CANAVANINE Seed

CARBOHYDRATES Fruit 132,000—429,000 ppm
CARBOHYDRATES Plant 658,000—781,000 ppm
CARBOHYDRATES Seed 53,000—432,000 ppm
CARBOXYLASE Seed
CATALASE Seed
CEPHALIN Seed 4,650—7,750 ppm
CHIROINOSITOL Root 620 ppm
CHLORINE Seed 200 ppm
CHLOROGENIC ACID Shoot
CHLOROPHYLL Seed
CHOLESTEROL Seed
CHOLINE Seed 2,490 ppm
CICERITOL Seed 230—800 ppm
CINNAMIC-ACID-4-HYDROXYLASE Tissue Culture
CIS-ACONTIC-ACID Root
CITRIC ACID Seed 8,000—13,000 ppm
COBALT Seed 0—0.78 ppm
COPPER Seed 4.3—18 ppm
COPROPORPHYRIN Tissue Culture
COUMESTROL Seed 1.2 ppm
COUMESTROL Shoot
CYANIDIN-3-GLUCOSIDE Seed
CYANIDIN-3-MONOGLUCOSIDE Seed
CYCLOARTENOL Sprout Seedling
CYCLOLAUDENOL Sprout Seedling
CYSTEINE Seed 5,880—6,430 ppm
D-GALACTOSE Seed
D-PINITOL Seed
D-PINITOL Stem
DAIDZEIN Cotyledon 14—28 ppm
DAIDZEIN Hypocotyl 140—190 ppm
DAIDZEIN Seed 8—328 ppm
DAIDZEIN Testa 7—10 ppm
DAIDZIN Cotyledon 375—1,028 ppm
DAIDZIN Hypocotyl 7,599—10,315 ppm
DAIDZIN Seed 129—8,100 ppm
DAIDZIN Testa 66—86 ppm
DELPHINIDIN-3-MONOGLUCOSIDE Seed
DELTA-TOCOPHEROL Seed
DI-GALACTOSYL-GLYCEROL Seed 100—170 ppm
DIAPHORASE Plant

DIHYDRO-BETA-SITOSTEROL Seed
DIMETHYLAMINE Seed 8 ppm
ERGOST-4-EN-3-6-DION Tissue Culture
ERGOST-4-EN-3-ONE Tissue Culture
ERGOSTEROL Seed
ERUCIC ACID Seed
ERYTHRO-NEOPTERIN Seed 0.014 ppm
ESTERASE Plant
ETHANOL Plant
ETHYLAMINE Seed 0.5 ppm
ETHYLENE Tissue Culture
ETHYLVINYLKETONE Seed
FAT Fruit 51,000—160,000 ppm
FAT Plant 25,000—62,000 ppm
FAT Seed 45,000—218,000 ppm
FAT Sprout Seedling 14,000—102,000 ppm
FERULIC ACID Plant 1—4 ppm
FERULIC ACID Seed 1—4 ppm
FIBER Fruit 14,000—45,000 ppm
FIBER Plant 281,000—355,000 ppm
FIBER Seed 19,000—63,000 ppm
FIBER Sprout Seedling 7,000—58,000 ppm
FLAZIN Seed 10 ppm
FLUORINE Seed 0.06 ppm
FOLACIN Seed 0.3—4 ppm
FORMOMONETIN Plant
FUMARIC ACID Seed
GALACT0PINITOL-A Seed 1,520—4,280 ppm
GALACT0PINITOL-B Seed 500—1,800 ppm
GALACTINOL Seed 120—230 ppm
GALACTOMANNAN Seed
GALLIC ACID Leaf 0.1—2.9 ppm
GAMMA-CONGLYCIN Seed
GAMMA-COUMARIC ACID Seed
GAMMA-SITOSTEROL Seed
GAMMA-TOCOPHEROL Oil 699 ppm
GAMMA-TOCOPHEROL Seed 140 ppm
GENISTEIN Cotyledon 28—59 ppm
GENISTEIN Endosperm 267 ppm
GENISTEIN Hypocotyl 242—247 ppm
GENISTEIN Seed 20—46 ppm
GENISTEIN Testa 5—15 ppm
GENISTIN Cotyledon 1,139—2,058 ppm
GENISTIN Hypocotyl 53—91 ppm
GENISTIN Seed 522—13,400 ppm
GENSITIN Testa 28—74 ppm

GENTISTIC ACID Seed
GLUCOSAMINE Seed
GLUCOSE Seed
GLUCURONIC ACID Seed
GLUTAMATE-OXALOACETIC-TRANSAMINASE Plant
GLUTAMIC ACID Seed 70,680—77,280 ppm
GLUTAMYL-ALANINE Seed
GLUTAMYL-TYROSINE Seed
GLYCEOLLIN-I Sprout Seedling
GLYCEOLLIN-II Sprout Seedling
GLYCEOLLIN-III Sprout Seedling
GLYCEOLLIN-IV Cotyledon
GLYCINE Seed 16,870—18,445 ppm
GLYCININE Seed 345,000—388,880 ppm
GLYCITIEN Hypocotyl 93—118 ppm
GLYCITEIN Seed 13—30 ppm
GLYCITEIN Testa 15 ppm
GLYCITEIN-7-O-BETA-D-GLUCOSIDE Cotyledon 16—17 ppm
GLYCITIN Seed
GLYCITIN-7-BETA-GLUCOSIDE Cotyledon 16—17 ppm
GLYCITIN-7-BETA-GLUCOSIDE Hypocotyl 5,888—6,641 ppm
GLYCITIN-7-BETA-GLUCOSIDE Seed 95—159 ppm
GLYCOLIC ACID Seed
GLYCOLIC ACID Sprout Seedling
GOSSYPOL Seed 60 ppm
GUANIDINE Seed
HEXAN-1-AL Plant
HISPIDINIC-ACID Sprout Seedling
HISPIDOL Seed
HISTIDINE Seed 9,840—10,770 ppm
HISTIDINE Sprout Seedling
HYDROXYPHASEOLIN Seed
HYPOGEIC ACID
HYPOXANTHINE Sprout Seedling
INDOLE-3-ACETIC ACID Root
INOSITOL Sprout Seedling
INOSITOL-HEXAPHOSPHATE Seed 14,000 ppm
INVERTASE Tissue Culture
IODINE Seed 0.5—16 ppm
IRON Fruit 28—91 ppm

IRON Plant 210 ppm
IRON Seed 38—180 ppm
IRON Sprout Seedling 10—73 ppm
ISOCAPRIC ACID Seed
ISOCITRATE-DEHYDROGENASE Plant
ISOCOUMARIC ACID Plant
ISOFERULIC ACID Seed
ISOVLAVONES Seed 3,010—10,000 ppm
ISOFUCOSTEROL Seed
ISOLEUCINE Seed 19,353 ppm
ISOLIQUIRITIGENIN Seed
ISOPROPYL-AMINE Seed
ISOVALERIANIC ACID Seed
ISOXANTHOPTERIN Seed 0.062 ppm
JASMONIC ACID Petiole
KAEMPFEROL Plant
KAEMPFEROL-3-0-BETA-D-RUTINOSIDE
    Plant
KILOCALORIES Fruit 1,340—4,350/kg
KILOCALORIES Seed 1,390—4,548/kg
KILOCALORIES Sprout Seedling 460—3,360/
    kg
KUNITZ-TRYPSIN-INHIBITOR Seed 500 ppm
LECITHIN Seed 15,000—25,000 ppm
LECTIN,SOYBEAN(SBL) Seed 0—9,760 ppm
LEGUMELIN Seed
LEUCINE Seed 29,720—32,500 ppm
LEUCINE-AMINO-PEPTIDASE Plant
LIGNIN Tissue Culture
LINOLEIC ACID Seed 70,335—126,082 ppm
LIPASE Seed
LIPOXIDASE Seed
LIPOXYGENASE Sprout Seedling
LIPOXYGENASE Plant
LUMAZINE Seed
LUPEOL Seed
LUTEIN Leaf
LYSINE Seed 24,290—26,560 ppm
MAGNESIUM Seed 430—3,160 ppm
MALATE-DEHYDROGENASE Plant
MALIC ACID Seed 700—1,000 ppm
MALTOSE Sprout Seedling
MANGANESE Seed 8—60 ppm
MANNOSE-6-PHOSPHATE-ISOMERASE
    Plant
METHANOL Plant

METHIONINE Seed 4,920—5,380 ppm
METHYLAMINE Seed 0.5—50 ppm
METHYLGENISTEIN Seed
MOLYBDENUM Seed 0—4 ppm
MUFA Seed 44,040—48,150 ppm
MYRISTIC ACID Seed 550—600 ppm
N-ACYL-PHOSPHATIDYL-
    ETHANOLAMINE Sprout Seedling
N-BUTYL-AMINE Seed 1 ppm
N-CAPRIC-ACID Seed
N-CAPRYLIC-ACID Seed
N-METHYL-PHENETHYLAMINE   Seed   50
    ppm
N-NONANOIC ACID Seed
N-VALERIANIC ACID Seed
NAPD-ACTIVE-ISOCITRATE-
    DEHYDROGENASE Plant
NARINGENIN Leaf
NEOCHLOROGENIC ACID Plant
NEOXANTHIN Leaf
NEURAMINIC ACID Seed
NH3 Seed 8,600 ppm
NIACIN Fruit 14—46 ppm
NIACIN Seed 13—32 ppm
NIACIN Sprout Seedling 8—58 ppm
NICKEL Seed 1— 30 ppm
NICOTIFLORIN Leaf
NITROGENASE Tissue Culture
O-COUMARIC-ACID Seed
OCTADECA-2,9,12-TRIENOIC ACID Tissue
    Culture
OCTADECA-2,9-DIENOIC ACID Tissue Cul-
    ture
OCTADECA-9,12-DIENOIC ACID Tissue Cul-
    ture
OLEIC-ACID Seed 40,230—72,116 ppm
ONONIN Plant
OXALIC ACID Seed 770 ppm
P-COUMARIC ACID Seed 1—4 ppm
P-HYDROXYBENZOIC ACID Seed 0.7—2.7
    ppm
PALMITIC ACID Seed 14,895—26,862 ppm
PALMITOLEIC ACID Seed 550—600 ppm
PANTOTHENIC ACID Seed 6—12 ppm
PENTANAL Plant
PANTANE Plant

PERLOLIDIN Seed
PEROXIDASE Seed
PHASEOL Leaf
PHASEOLIN Seed
PHASIN Seed
PHENYLALANINE Seed 19,050—20,830 ppm
PHENYLALANINE-AMMONIA-LYASE Tissue Culture
PHOSPHATIDES Seed 1,350—7,260 ppm
PHOSPHATIDIC ACID Sprout Seedling
PHOSPHATIDYL-CHOLINE Seed
PHOSPHATIDYL-ETHANOLAMINE Sprout Seedling
PHOSPHATIDYL-GLYCEROLE Sprout Seedling
PHOSPHATIDYL-INOSITOL Sprout Seedling
PHOSPHOGLUCOMUTASE Plant
PHOSPHOGLUCOSE-ISOMERASE Plant
PHOSPHORUS Fruit 2,250—7,305 ppm
PHOSPHORUS Plant 2,400—5,410 ppm
PHOSPHORUS Seed 1,580—8,040 ppm
PHOSPHORUS Sprout Seedling 580—4,891 ppm
PHYSETOLIC ACID Seed
PHYTASE Seed
PHYTIC ACID Seed
PHYTOHEMAGGLUTININ Seed
PHYTOSTEROLS Seed 1,610—1,760 ppm
PINITOL Seed 2,000—2,980 ppm
PIPERIDINE Seed
POLYSACCHARIDES Seed 120,000 ppm
POTASSIUM Plant 10,600 ppm
POTASSIUM Seed 4,100—27,600 ppm
POTASSIUM Sprout Seedling 2,790—15,081 ppm
PROLINE Seed 21,350—23,344 ppm
PROPANAL Plant
PROPIONIC ACID Seed
PROTEASE Seed
PROTEIN Fruit 109,000—354,000 ppm
PROTEIN Plant 139,000—166,000 ppm
PROTEIN Seed 130,000—409,000 ppm
PROTEIN Sprout Seedling 62,000—453,000 ppm
PROTOCATECHUIC ACID Plant 0.2—0.5 ppm

PTERIN Seed 0.052 ppm
PUFA Seed 112,550—123,060 ppm
PYRIDOXINE Seed 6.4 ppm
PYROGLUTAMIC ACID Seed 1,000—3,000 ppm
QUERCETIN Plant
QUERCETIN-3-O-BETA-D-2-GLUCOSYL-RUTINOSIDE Leaf
QUERCETIN-3-O-BETA-O-SOPHOROSIDE Leaf
QUERCETRIN Leaf
RAFFINOSE Seed 5,000—15,000 ppm
RIBOFLAVIN Fruit 1.6—5 ppm
RIBOFLAVIN Seed 1.7—13 ppm
RIBOFLAVIN Sprout Seedling 1.5—15 ppm
RIBOSE-1,5-DIPHOSPHATE-CARBOXYLASE Tissue Culture
ROTENOIDS Seed 1,000 ppm
RUTIN Shoot
SALICYLIC ACID Seed
SAPOGENOL-C Sprout Seedling
SAPONINS Seed 50,000 ppm
SELENIUM Seed 0.04—1.25 ppm
SERINE Plant
SERINE Seed 21,150—23,125 ppm
SFA Seed 14,850—32,670 ppm
SILICON Seed
SINAPIC ACID Seed
SODIUM Seed 9—3,800 ppm
SODIUM Sprout Seedling 300—1,622 ppm
SOJAGOL Plant
SOPHORAFLAVNOLOSIDE Leaf
SOYASAPOGENOL-A Seed
SOYASAPOGENOL-B Seed
SOYASAPOGENOL-B-1 Seed
SOYASAPOGENOL-C Seed
SOYASAPONIN-A Seed
SOYASAPONIN-A-1 Seed 239—400 ppm
SOYASAPONIN-A-2 Embryo
SOYASAPONIN-A-3 Seed 100 ppm
SOYASAPONIN-A-4 Seed
SOYASAPONIN-A-5 Seed
SOYASAPONIN-A-6 Seed
SOYASAPONIN-B Seed
SOYASAPONIN-C Seed
SOYASAPONIN-D Seed

SOYASAPONIN-E Seed
SOYASAPONIN-I Cotyledon 300—3,000 ppm
SOYASAPONIN-I Hypocotyl 5,000—19,000 ppm
SOYASAPONIN-I Pericarp 100—2,500 ppm
SOYASAPONIN-I Root 600—3,300 ppm
SOYASAPONIN-I Seed 139—1,200 ppm
SOYASAPONIN-II Seed 47—150 ppm
SOYASAPONIN-III Seed 10—22 ppm
SOYASAPONIN-IV Seed 140—160 ppm
SOYASAPONIN-V Seed
SQUALENE Seed
STACHYOSE Seed 22,300—51,050 ppm
STARCH Seed 10,000 ppm
STEARIC ACID Seed 4,320—7,785 ppm
STIGMAST-4-EN-3-6-DIONE Tissue Culture
STIGMAST-4-EN3-ONE Tissue Culture
STIGMASTA-4-22-DIEN-3-6-DIONE Tissue Culture
STIGMASTA-4-22-DIEN-3-ONE Tissue Culture
STIGMASTEROL Seed
STRONTIUM Seed 3—42 ppm
SUCCINIC ACID Root
SUCCINIC ACID Seed
SUCCINIC ACID Sprout Seedling
SUCROSE Seed 27,950—71,700 ppm
SUGARS Seed 125,000 ppm
SULFUR Seed 4,066 ppm
SYRINGIC ACID Root 4.1—4.7 ppm
SYRINGIC ACID Seed
TATOIN Seed
TETRAMETHYLPYRAZINE Seed
THIAMIN Fruit 4.4—14 ppm
THIAMIN Seed 4—10 ppm
THIAMIN Sprout Seedling 1.9—17 ppm
THREONEOPTERIN Seed 0.017 ppm
THREONINE Seed 15,850—17,330 ppm
TITANIUM Seed 0—12 ppm
TRANS-OCIMENE Plant
TRIGONELLINE Fruit 3.7—16.2 ppm
TRIGONELLINE Seed 19.7—71.8 ppm
TRIGONELLINE Seed 1.5—7.6 ppm
TRYPTOPHAN Seed 5,300—5,795 ppm
TYROSINE Seed 13,800—15,090 ppm
UNDYLIC ACID Sprout Seedling

UREASE Seed
URICASE Seed
UROPORPHYRIN Tissue Culture
VALINE Seed 18,210—19,910 ppm
VANILLIC ACID Root 1—4 ppm
VANILLIC ACID Seed
VERBACOSE Seed 280—410 ppm
VERBACOSE Seed 3,000 ppm
VITAMIN B6 Seed 3—6 ppm
VITAMIN D Seed
VITAMIN E Seed
VITAMIN K Seed
VITEXIN Root
WATER Fruit 692,000 ppm
WATER Seed 83,980—682,000 ppm
WATER Sprout Seedling 815,000—863,000 ppm
XANTHINE Sprout Seedling
XYLOGALACTOMANNAN Seed
XYLOSE Seed
ZINC Seed 22—90 ppm
ZIRCONIUM Seed 0.8—2.4 ppm

■ SPINACH

Chemical Constituents of Spinacia oleraceae L. (Chenopodiaceae)

3-HYDROXYTYRAMINE Leaf
6-(HYDROXYMETHYL)-LUMAZINE Leaf
7-STIGMASTEROL Leaf
ACETYLCHOLINE Leaf
ALANINE Plant 1,420—16,864 ppm
ALPHA-LINOLENIC ACID Plant 480—13,657 ppm
ALPHA-TOCOPHEROL Leaf 12—419 ppm
ALUMINUM Leaf 5—270 ppm
ARGININE Plant 1,620—19,239 ppm
ARSENIC Leaf 0.02—0.29 ppm
ASCORBATE Plant 212—4,450 ppm
ASCORBIC ACID Plant 239—7,595 ppm
ASH Plant 16,850—285,700 ppm
ASPARTIC ACID Plant 2,400—28,502 ppm
BETA-CAROTENE Plant 4—690 ppm
BORON Leaf 2.4—40 ppm

BROMINE Leaf 4 ppm
CADMIUM Leaf 0.05—5 ppm
CALCIUM Plant 730—15,700 ppm
CARBOHYDRATES Plant 35,000—415,660 ppm
CEPHALIN Leaf
CHLORINE Plant 540—6,835 ppm
CHOLESTEROL Leaf
CHROMIUM Flower 0.01—0.42 ppm
COBALT Plant 0.001—1.2 ppm
COLAMINE Leaf
COPPER Plant 0.1—24 ppm
CYSTINE Plant 350—4,157 ppm
DIGALACTOSYLDIACYLGLYCEROL Plant
FAT Plant 3,070—46,672 ppm
FERULIC ACID Leaf 16 ppm
FIBER Plant 6,000—111,634 ppm
FLUORINE Leaf 0.3—5.7 ppm
FOLACIN Plant 1.2—15 ppm
FOLACIN Plant 1.59—27.13 ppm
GLUTAMIC ACID Plant 3,430—40,735 ppm
GLUTATHIONE Plant 90—1,065 ppm
GLYCINE Plant 1,340—15,914 ppm
HEXADECA-7,10,13-TRIENOIC ACID Leaf
HEXOSAMINE Seed 380 ppm
HISTIDINE Plant 640—7,601 ppm
IODINE Plant 0.2 ppm
IRON Plant 0.2 ppm
ISOLEUCINE Plant 1,470—17,458 ppm
KAEMPFEROL Plant
KILOCALORIES Plant 220—2,613/kg
LEAD Leaf 0.03—3 ppm
LECITHIN Leaf
LEUCINE Plant 2,230—26,483 ppm
LINOLEIC ACID Plant 104—2,613 ppm
LYSINE Plant 1,740—20,664 ppm
MAGNESIUM Plant 420—11,000 ppm
MANGANESE Plant 3—485 ppm
MERCURY Leaf 0.003—0.11 ppm
METHIONINE Plant 530—6,294 ppm
MOLYBDENUM Plant 0.06—0.8 ppm
MONOGALACTOSYLDIACTYLGLYC-
EROL Plant
MYRISTIC ACID Plant 1—950 ppm
N,N-DIMETHYLHISTAMINE Leaf
N-ACETYLHISTAMINE Leaf

NIACIN Plant 6.9—89.8 ppm
NICKEL Plant
NITROGEN Leaf 3,200—45,700 ppm
OLEIC ACID Plant 18—475 ppm
OXALIC ACID leaf 6,580 ppm
P-COUMARIC ACID Leaf 133 ppm
PALMITIC ACID Plant 106—4,869 ppm
PALMITOLEIC ACID Plant 21—475 ppm
PANTOETHNIC ACID Plant 0.57—8.7 ppm
PATULETIN Leaf
PHENYLALANINE Plant 1,290—15,320 ppm
PHOSPHATIDYLCHOLINE Plant
PHOSPHATIDYLETHANOLAMINE Plant
PHOSPHATIDYLGLYCEROL Leaf
PHOSPHATIDYLINOSITOL Leaf
PHOSPHATIDYLSERINE Leaf
PHOSPHORUS Plant 250—6,232 ppm
PHYTOSTEROLS Plant 90—1,800 ppm
POLYPHENOL OXIDASE Leaf
POTASSIUM Plant 2,060—69,077 ppm
PROLINE Plant 1,120—13,301 ppm
PROTEIN Plant 27,480—352,954 ppm
QUERCETIN Leaf 19 ppm
RIBOFLAVIN Plant 1.8—23.4 ppm
RUBIDIUM Leaf 0.9—90 ppm
RUTIN Leaf 170 ppm
SELENIUM Leaf 0—0.057 ppm
SERINE Plant 1,040—12,351 ppm
SILICON Leaf 1—855 ppm
SODIUM Plant 585—10,669 ppm
SPINASAPONINS Plant
SPINASTEROL Leaf
STEARIC ACID Plant 7—356 ppm
STRONTIUM Plant 0.06—0.77 ppm
SULFOLIPIDS Plant
SULFUR Plant 270—5,700 ppm
THIAMIN Plant 0.7—10.2 ppm
THREONINE Plant 1,220—14,489 ppm
TRIMETHYLHISTAMINE Leaf
TRYPOTPHAN Plant 390—4,632 ppm
TYROSINE Plant 1,080—12,826 ppm
VALINE Plant 1,610—19,120 ppm
VITAMIN B6 Plant 1.9—24 ppm
WATER Plant 913,120—930,000 ppm
ZINC Plant 4—185 ppm

■ SUMMER SQUASH

Chemical Constituents of Cucurbita spp (Cucurbitaceae)

ALANINE Fruit 620—9,810 ppm
ARGININE Fruit 500—7,910 ppm
ASCORBIC-ACID Fruit 148—2,340 ppm
ASH Fruit 5,550—96,045 ppm
ASPARTIC ACID Fruit 1,440—22,785 ppm
BETA-CAROTENE Fruit 0.12—1.9 ppm
CALCIUM Fruit 200—3,165 ppm
CARBOHYDRATES Fruit 43,500—688,300 ppm
COPPER Fruit 0.7—12 ppm
CYSTINE Fruit 120—1,900 ppm
FAT Fruit 2,100—33,230 ppm
FIBER Fruit 6,000—94,935 ppm
FOLACIN Fruit 0.2—4.6 ppm
GLUTAMIC ACID Fruit 1,260—19,935 ppm
GLYCINE Fruit 440—6,962 ppm
HISTIDINE Fruit 250—3,955 ppm
IRON Fruit 4—73 ppm
ISOLEUCINE Fruit 420—6,645 ppm
KILOCALORIES Fruit 200—3,165/kg
LAURIC ACID Fruit 10—160 ppm
LEUCINE Fruit 690—10,920 ppm
LINOLEIC ACID Fruit 330—5,220 ppm
LINOLENIC ACID Fruit 560—8,860 ppm
LYSINE Fruit 650—10,285 ppm
MAGNESIUM Fruit 230—3,640 ppm
MANGANESE Fruit 1— 27 ppm
METHIONINE Fruit 170—2,690 ppm
MUFA Fruit 160—2,530 ppm
MYRISTIC ACID Fruit 10—160 ppm
NIACIN Fruit 5—85 ppm
OLEIC ACID Fruit 140—2,215 ppm
PALMITIC ACID Fruit 380—6,015 ppm
PALMITOLEIC ACID Fruit 10—169 ppm
PANTOTHENIC ACID Fruit 1—18 ppm
PECTIN Fruit 6,000—94,935 ppm
PHENYLALANINE Fruit 410—6,485 ppm
PHOSPHORUS Fruit 350—5,540 ppm
POTASSIUM Fruit 1,950—30,855 ppm
PROLINE Fruit 370—5,855 ppm
PROTEIN Fruit 11,800—186,700 ppm

PUFA Fruit 890—14,080 ppm
RIBOFLAVIN Fruit 0.4—6 ppm
SERINE Fruit 480—7,595 ppm
SFA Fruit 440—6,960 ppm
SODIUM Fruit 20—315 ppm
STEARIC ACID Fruit 40—635 ppm
THIAMIN Fruit 0.6—10 ppm
THREONINE Fruit 280—4,430 ppm
TRYPTOPHAN Fruit 110—1,740 ppm
TYROSINE Fruit 310—4,905 ppm
VALINE Fruit 530—8,385 ppm
VITAMIN B6 Fruit 1—18 ppm
WATER Fruit 936,800 ppm
ZINC Fruit 2—41 ppm

■ POTATO

Chemical Constituents of Ipomoea batatas L. (Convolvulaceae)

ALANINE Root 300—3,314 ppm
ALPHA-LINOLENIC ACID Root 200—736 ppm
ALUMINUM Root 8 ppm
ARGININE Root 520—2,835 ppm
ASCORBIC ACID Leaf 210—4,234 ppm
ASCORBIC ACID Root 201—1,186 ppm
ASH Leaf 12,000—259,000 ppm
ASH Root 7,000—36,064 ppm
ASPARTIC ACID Root 2,730—10,383 ppm
BATATIC ACID Root
BETA-CAROTENE Root 0.1—476 ppm
BORON Root 0.8—20 ppm
CAFFEIC ACID Root
CALCIUM Root 203—2,300 ppm
CALCIUM-OXALATE Root 320 ppm
CARBOHYDRATES Leaf 80,000—620,000 ppm
CARBOHYDRATES Root 242,800—925,000 ppm
CAROTENOIDS Root 30—350 ppm
CHLORINE Root 850 ppm
CHLOROGENIC ACID Root
COPPER Root 1.5—7 ppm

CYANIDIN-3-(CAFFEOYLSOPHOROSIDE)-5-GLUCOSIDE Root
CYANIDIN-3-DICAFFEOYLSOPHOROSIDE-5-GLUCOSIDE Plant
CYSTINE Root 130—760 ppm
FAT Leaf 2,000—58,000 ppm
FAT Root 1,400—14,000 ppm
FIBER Root 8,000—32,000 ppm
FOLACIN Root 0.1—0.6 ppm
FURAN-BETA-CARBONIC ACID Root
GLUTAMIC ACID Root 1,590—6,360 ppm
GLYCINE Root 580—2,725 ppm
HISTIDINE Root 300—1,200 ppm
IODINE Root 0.045 ppm
IPOMOEAMARONE Root
IPOMOEANINE Root
IRON Root 4—64 ppm
ISOCHLOROGENIC ACID Root
ISOLEUCINE Root 580—3,019 ppm
ISQUERCITRIN Root
KILOCALORIES Root 990—3,920/kg
LEUCINE Root 890—4,455 ppm
LINOLEIC ACID Root 1,110—4,087 ppm
LYSINE Root 810—3,280 ppm
MAGNESIUM Root 95—710 ppm
MANGANESE Root 1—15 ppm
METHIONINE Root 230—1,510 ppm
MUFA Root 110—405 ppm
NEOCHLOROGENIC ACID Root
NIACIN Root 6—26 ppm
OLEIC ACID Root 110—405 ppm
OXALATE Leaf 3,700 ppm
OXALIC ACID Root 1,000 ppm
PAEONIDIN-3-(CAFFEOYLSOPHOROSIDE)-5-GLUCOSIDE Root
PALMITIC ACID Root 580—2,135 ppm
PANTOTHENIC ACID Root 580—2,135 ppm
PANTOTHENIC ACID Root 5—24 ppm
PECTIN Root 30,000 ppm
PEONIDIN Plant
PHENYLALANINE Root 720—3,645 ppm
PHOSPHORUS Root 261—2,000 ppm
PHYTIN Root 10,500 ppm
PHYTOENE Root 0.8—9 ppm

PHYTOFLUENE Root 0.6—7 ppm
PHYTOSTEROLS Root 120—442 ppm
POTASSIUM Leaf 5,300—42,256 ppm
POTASSIUM Root 1,970—15,740 ppm
PROLINE Root 710—2,840 ppm
PROTEIN Root 10,000—65,982 ppm
PUFA Root 1,320—4,860 ppm
QUERCETIN Root
RIBOFLAVIN Root 0.3—7 ppm
SCOPOLIN Root
SERINE Root 850—3,400 ppm
SFA Root 640—2,356 ppm
SKIMMINE Root
SODIUM Root 10—1,229 ppm
SQUALENE Root
STARCH Root 118,000—201,000 ppm
STEARIC ACID Root 60—221 ppm
SUGAR Root 23,800—97,000 ppm
SULFUR Root 130—610 ppm
THIAMIN Root 0.6—5.1 ppm
THREONINE Root 720—3,019 ppm
TOCOPHEROL Root 40 ppm
TRANS-CINNAMIC ACID Root
TRYPTOPHAN Root 200—800 ppm
TYROSINE Root 460—2,504 ppm
URONIC ACID Root 18,000 ppm
VALINE Root 830—3,967 ppm
VITAMIN B6 Root 2—10 ppm
WATER Root 682,000—806,000 ppm
ZETA CAROTENE Root 0.5—6 ppm
ZINC Root 2—11 ppm

■ TOMATO

Chemical Constituents of Lycopersicon esculentum (Solanaceae)

1',2'-EPOXY-1',2'-DIHYDRO-BETA-EPSILON-PSEUDOCAROTENE Fruit
1',2'-EPOXY-1',2'-DIHYDRO-BETA-PSI-CAROTENE Fruit
1,2,-EPOXY-1,2-DIHYDRO-PSI,PSI-CAROTENE Fruit
1-BUTYL-2-THIAZOL Fruit
1-O-FERULOYL-BETA-D-GLUCOSE Fruit

1-O-P-COUMAROYL-BETA-D-GLUCOSE Fruit
10,16-DIHYDROXY-DECANOIC-ACID Fruit
10,16-DIHYDROXY-HEXADECANOIC-ACID Fruit
16-HYDROXYHEXADECANOIC-ACID Fruit
2,7-DIMETHYL-OCT-4-ENEDIOIC-ACID Shoot 1.2 ppm
2,7-DIMETHYL-OCTA-2,4-DIENOIC-ACID Shoot 1.8 ppm
2-BUTANONE Fruit
2-PENTANONE Fruit
2-PROPANE Fruit
24-(R)-ETHYL-LOPHENOL Seed
24-METHYL-31-NOR-LANOST-9(11)-EN-3-BETA-OL Seed
24-METHYL-LOPHENOL Seed
24-METHYLENE-CYCLOARTANAL Seed
24-METHYLENE-CYCLOARTENAL Plant
3-BETA-HYDROXY-5-ALPHA-PREG-16-EN-20-ONE Shoot
3-O-FERULOYL-QUINIC-ACID Leaf
31-NOR-LANOST-8-EN-3-BETA-OL Seed
31-NOR-LANOST-9(11)-EN-3-BETA-OL Seed
31-NORCYYCLOARTENAL Seed
4-ALPHA-24-DIMETHYL-CHOLESTA-7,24-DIEN-3-BETA-OL Seed
4-ALPHA-METHYL-24-ETHYL-CHOLESTA-7,24-DIEN-3-BETA-OL Seed
4-VINYL-GUAIACOL Leaf
4-VINYL-GUAIACOL Seed
5,6-EPOXY-5,6-DIHYDRO-PSEUDO-PSEUDOCAROTENE Fruit
5-HYDROXYTRYPTAMINE Fruit
5ALPHA-FUROSTANE-3BETA,22,26TRIOL-3-O-BETA-D-GLUCOPYRANSOYL Plant
9,10,16-TRIHYDROXYHEXADECANOIC ACID Fruit
9,10,18-TRIHYDROXYOCTADECANOIC ACID Fruit
ABCISIC ACID-1',4'-TRANS-DIOL Fruit
ABCISIC ACID-1',4'-TRANS-DIOL Leaf
ABCISIC ACID-1'O-BETA-D-GLUCOPYRA-NOSIDE Stem
ACETALDEHYDE Fruit

ACETIC ACID Fruit
ACETONE Fruit
ADENOSINE Flower
ALANINE Fruit 30—4,132 ppm
ALPHA-AMYRIN Fruit
ALPHA-CAPROLACTONE Fruit
ALPHA-IONENE Fruit
ALPHA-IONENE Fruit
ALPHA-KETOGLUTARIC ACID Fruit
ALPHA-LINOLENIC ACID Fruit 30—496 ppm
ALPHA-NONALACTONE
ALPHA-OCTALACTONE
ALPHA-OXOGLUTARIC ACID Fruit
ALPHA-PINENE Fruit
ALPHA-TOCOPHEROL Fruit 7—143 ppm
ALUMINUM Fruit 0.3—1,700 ppm
ARABIC ACID Fruit
ARGININE Fruit 1—3,637
ARSENIC Fruit 0.003—0.043 ppm
ASCORBIC ACID Fruit 50—2,952 ppm
ASH Fruit 5,700—105,461 ppm
ASPARAGINE Fruit 300 ppm
ASPARTIC ACID Fruit 1,230—20,332 ppm
AUROXANTHIN Fruit
BARIUM Fruit 0—60 ppm
BENZALDEHYDE Fruit
BENZYL-ALCOHOL Fruit
BETA-AMYRIN Fruit
BETA-CAROTENE Fruit 7—113 ppm
BETA-D-GLUCOPYRANOSYL-PHASEIC ACID Plant
BETA-IONENE Fruit
BETA-SITOSTEROL Fruit
BETAINE Root 23 ppm
BETAINE Shoot 69 ppm
BIOTIN Fruit
BORON Fruit 0—96 ppm
BUTANOL-2-ON-3 Fruit
BUTANOLS Fruit
BUTYROLACTONE Fruit
CADMIUM Fruit 0.005—1.7 ppm
CAFFEIC ACID Fruit 6 ppm
CAFFEIC ACID-4-O-BETA-D-GLUCOSIDE Fruit
CALCIUM Fruit 60—2,400 ppm

CALCIUM Leaf 60,800 ppm
CAMPESTEROL Fruit
CAPRYLIC ACID Fruit
CARBOHYDRATES Fruit 43,400—717,400 ppm
CABOXYLIC ACID Leaf
CELLULASE Fruit
CELLULOSE Fruit
CERIUM Fruit 7—60 ppm
CHLORINE Fruit 510 ppm
CHLOROGENIC ACID Fruit 18 ppm
CHLOROPHYLL Fruit 18 ppm
CHLOROPHYLL-A Fruit
CHLOROPHYLL-B Fruit
CHOLINE Root 36 ppm
CHOLINE Shoot 48 ppm
CHROMIUM Fruit 0—3 ppm
CINNAMALDEHYDE Fruit
CIS-3-HEXENOL-1 Fruit 4—40 ppm
CIS-5'-BETA-PSEUDOCAROTENE Fruit
CIS-5'-EPSILON-PSEUDOCAROTENE Fruit
CIS-5'-NEUROSPORENE Fruit
CIS-5,CIS-5'-LYCOPENE Fruit 1—20 ppm
CIS-HEXEN-3-AL Fruit
CITRAL Fruit
CITRIC ACID Fruit
CITROSTADIENOL Seed
COBALT Fruit 0—1.4 ppm
COPPER Fruit 0.4—100 ppm
CUTIN Fruit
CYCLOARTANOL Seed
CYCLOARETNOL Seed
CYCLOEUCALENOL Seed
CYCLOHEXANOL Fruit
CYSTINE Fruit 120—1,984 ppm
DAMASCENONE Fruit
DECADIEN-TRANS-2,TRANS-4-AL Fruit
DIACETYL Fruit
DIHYDROXYTARTARIC ACID Fruit
DIHYDROZEATIN Flower
EPOXY-5,6-IONENE Fruit
EPOXY-LUTEIN Fruit
ETHANOL Fruit
ETHYL-PHENOL Fruit
ETHYLENE Fruit
EUGENOL Fruit

FALCARINDIOL Seed
FALCARINOL Seed
FARNESAL Fruit
FARNESYL-ACETONE Fruit
FAT Fruit 1,330—47,441 ppm
FAT Seed 150,000—250,000 ppm
FERULIC ACID Fruit
FERULIC ACID-O-BETA-D-GLUCOSIDE Fruit
FIBER Fruit 4,700—77,691 ppm
FLUORINE Fruit 0.02—1.7 ppm
FOLACIN Fruit 0—2 ppm
FORMIC ACID Fruit
FRUCTOSE Fruit 11,700 ppm
FUMARIC ACID Fruit
FURFURAL Fruit
GABA Fruit 220—480 ppm
GAMMA-CAROTENE Fruit
GENTISIC ACID Leaf
GERANYL-ACETONE Fruit
GIBBERELLINS Fruit
GLUCOSE Fruit 16,300 ppm
GLUTAMIC ACID Fruit 90—54,053 ppm
GLYCERIC ACID Fruit
GLYCINE Fruit 23—3,637 ppm
GLYCOLIC ACID Fruit
GLYOXAL Fruit
GRAMISTEROL Seed
GUAIACOL Fruit
HEMICELLULOSE Fruit
HEPTADIEN-TRANS-2,CIS-4-AL Fruit
HEPTADIEN-TRANS-2,CIS TRANS-4-AL Fruit
HEPTULOSE Fruit
HEXADIEN-TRANS-2-,TRANS-4-AL Fruit
HEXANOLS Fruit
HISTIDINE Fruit 30—2,149 ppm
HYDROCINNAMALDEHYDE Fruit
I-VALERALDEHYDE Fruit
I-VALERIC ACID Fruit
INDOLE-3-ACETIC ACID Root
IODINE Fruit
IRON Fruit 1—800 ppm
ISOAMYLOL Fruit 7—40 ppm
ISOLEUCINE Fruit 210—3,471 ppm
ISOPENTENYL-ADENINE Root
ISOPENTENYL-ADENOSINE Root
ISOVALERALDEHYDE Fruit 0.006 ppm

JSGGALACTURONIC ACID Fruit
KAEMPFEROL Seed
KETOHEPTOSE Fruit
LACTIC ACID Fruit
LANOSTEROL Seed
LEAD Fruit 0.003—60 ppm
LEUCINE Fruit 330—5,455 ppm
LEUCINES Fruit 1—90 ppm
LEUCIONPINE Tissue Culture
LEUCIONPINE-LACTAM Tissue Culture
LINALOOL Fruit
LINOLEIC ACID Fruit 830—13,720 ppm
LIONLENIC ACID Fruit
LITHIUM Fruit 0.28—0.68 ppm
LOPHENOL Seed
LUPEOL Plant
LUTEIN Fruit
LUTEIN-5,6-EPOXIDE Fruit
LUTEIN-EPOXIDE Fruit
LYCOPENE Fruit 1—20 ppm
LYCOPERSICONOL Root
LYCOPERSICONOLIDE Root 6.7 ppm
LYCOPHYLL Fruit
LYCOXANTHIN Fruit
LYSINE Fruit 20—5,455 ppm
MAGNESIUM Fruit 70—6,000 ppm
MAGNESIUM Leaf 4,300 ppm
MALIC ACID Fruit
MANGANESE Fruit 0.6—100 ppm
MERCURY Fruit 0.001—0.002 ppm
METHANOL Fruit
METHIONINE Fruit 16—1,322 ppm
METHYL-2-BUTYRIC ACID Fruit
METHYL-6-HEPTEN-5-ON-2 Fruit
METHYL-GLYOXAL Fruit
METHYL-SALICYLATE Fruit
MEVALONIC ACID Fruit 3—4 ppm
MOLYBDENUM Fruit 0—6 ppm
MYRISTIC ACID Fruit
N(6)-ISOPENT-2-ENYL-ADENINE Flower
N-DOTRIACONTANE Fruit
N-HENTRIACONTANE Fruit
N-HEXANOL Fruit
N-PENTANOL Fruit 7—40 ppm
N-TETRATIACONTANE Fruit
N-TRITRIACONTANE Fruit

N-NARCOTINE Fruit
NARINGENIN Fruit
NEO-BETA-CAROTENE-B Fruit
NEO-BETA-CAROTENE-U Fruit
NEO-CHLOROGENIC ACID Leaf
NEODYMIUM Fruit 2—30 ppm
NEOLYCOPENE-A Fruit
NEOLYCOPENE-B Fruit
NEOTIGOGENIN Tissue Culture 300—1,500 ppm
NEOXANTHIN Fruit
NESTIGOGENIN Fruit
NEUROSPORINE Fruit
NIACIN Fruit 6—99 ppm
NICKEL Fruit 0.01—5 ppm
NICOTIANAMINE Leaf
NITROGEN Fruit 1,300—23,330 ppm
NITROGEN Leaf 26,000 ppm
NONACOSANE Fruit
O-CRESOL Fruit
O-HYDROXY-ACETOPHENONE Fruit
OBTUSIFOLIOL Seed
OLEIC ACID Fruit 310—5,124 ppm
OXALIC ACID Fruit 36—263 ppm
P-COUMARIC AICD Fruit
P-COUMARIC ACID-O-BETA-D-GLUCOSIDE Fruit
P-HYDROXYBENZALDEHYDE Plant
PALMITIC ACID Fruit 210—3,471 ppm
PALMITOLEIC ACID Fruit 10—165 ppm
PANTOTHENIC ACID Fruit 1—61 ppm
PECTIN Fruit 100—31,000 ppm
PECTINESTERASE Fruit
PENTANOLS Fruit
PENTEN-1-OL-3 Fruit
PHENOL Fruit
PHENOLICS Fruit 27—570 ppm
PHENYL-2-ETHANOL Fruit
PHENYLACETALDEHYDE Fruit
PHENYLACETONITRILE Fruit
PHENYLALANINE Fruit 72—3,801 ppm
PHOSPHATIDYL-GLYCEROL Leaf
PHOSPHORUS Fruit 110—8,400 ppm
PHOSPHORUS Leaf 5,500 ppm
PHYTOENE Fruit
PHYTOENE-1,2-OXIDE Fruit

PHYTOFLUENE Fruit
PHYTOSTEROLS Fruit 70—1,157 ppm
PIPECOLIC ACID Fruit
POLYGALACTURONASE Fruit
POTASSIUM Fruit 780—58,800 ppm
POTASSIUM Leaf 47,000 ppm
PROLINE Fruit 170—2,810 ppm
PROLINE Root 541 ppm
PROLINE Root 725 ppm
PROLYCOPENE Fruit
PROPANOLS Fruit
PROPIONIC ACID Fruit
PROTEIN Fruit 8,790—148,935 ppm
PROTOPECTIN Fruit 11,700—24,200 ppm
PYRUVIC ACID Fruit
QUERCETIN Fruit
QUERCETIN-3-RHAMNOSIDE Fruit
QUERCETRIN Fruit
RIBOFLAVIN Fruit 1—8 ppm
RISHITIN Plant
RUBIDIUM Fruit 0.3—22 ppm
RUTIN Fruit
RUTIN Leaf 24,000 ppm
RUTINOSIDE Fruit
S-METHYL-METHIONINE Fruit 16—35 ppm
SALICYLALDEHYDE Fruit
SELENIUM Fruit 0.001—0.034 ppm
SERINE Fruit 57—3,967 ppm
SILICON Fruit
SILVER Fruit 0—1.4 ppm
SODIUM Fruit 10—6,600 ppm
SOLADULCIDINE Shoot
SOLANINE Fruit
SQUALENE Fruit
STARCH Fruit 120—10,000 ppm
STEARIC ACID Fruit 80—1,322 ppm
STIGMASTEROL Fruit
STRONTIUM Fruit 0—140 ppm
SUCCINIC ACID Fruit
SUCROSE Fruit
SUGARS Fruit 15,000—45,000 ppm
SULFOQUINOVOSYL-DIACYL-
  GLYCEROL Leaf
SULFUR Fruit 107—2,330 ppm
SYRINGALDEHYDE Plant
TARTARIC ACID Fruit

TETRA-DECA-CIS-6-ENE-1,3-DIYNE-5,8-
  DIOL Stem
THIAMIN Fruit 1—10 ppm
THREONINE Fruit 65—3,637 ppm
TITANIUM Fruit 0—140 ppm
TOMATIDA-3,5-DIENE Shoot
TOMATIDINE Plant
TOMATINE Flower
TOMATINE Leaf 6—8 ppm
TOMATOSIDE-A Seed
TRANS-ACONITIC-ACID Fruit
TRANS-METHYL-6-HEPTADIENE-3,5-ON-
  2 Plant
TRIACONTANE Fruit
TRICODECAN-3-ONE Leaf
TRIDECAN-2-ONE Leaf
TRIDECAN-3-ONE Leaf
TRIGONELLINE Root 14 ppm
TRIGONELLINE Root 69 ppm
TRIMETHYL-2,6,6-HYDROXY-2-
  CYCLOHEXANONE Fruit
TRYPTAMINE Fruit
TRYPTOPHAN Fruit 1—1,157 ppm
TYRAMINE Fruit
TYROSINE Fruit 38—2,479 ppm
UBIQUINONE-10 Tissue Culture 60 ppm
VALINE Fruit 1—3,801 ppm
VANADIUM Fruit 0—6 ppm
VANILLIN Plant
VIOLAXANTHIN Fruit
VITAMIN B6 Fruit 0—9 ppm
WATER fruit 910,000—982,000 ppm
XANTHOPHYLL Fruit
YTTRIUM Fruit 0—6 ppm
ZEATIN Fruit
ZEATIN-GLUCOSIDE Flower
ZEATIN-RIBOSIDE Flower
ZEAXANTHIN Fruit
ZETA-CAROTENE Fruit

■ TURNIP

Chemical Constituents of Brassica rapa L. rapa
(Brassicaceae)

(+)-CYSTEINE Root
(+)-S-METHYL-L-CYSTEINE-SULFOXIDE Root
4ALPHA,7ALPHA,24-TRIMETHYL-5ALPHA-CHOLESTA-8,24-DIEN-3BETA-OL Plant ALANINE Root 350—4,305 ppm
ALLANTOIC ACID Root
ALLANTOIN Root
ALUMINUM Root 2—10 ppm
ARGININE Root 240—2,950 ppm
ARSENIC Root
ASCORBIC ACID Root 210—2,580 ppm
ASH Root 7,000—86,000 ppm
ASPARTIC ACID Root 630—7,750 ppm
BETA-CAROTENE Root
BORON Root 2—20 ppm
BRASSICASTEROL Plant
BROMINE Root
CADMIUM Root 0.01—0.1 ppm
CALCIUM Root 300—3,690 ppm
CAMPESTEROL Plant
CARBOHYDRATES Root 62,300—766,290 ppm
CHROMIUM Root 0.005—0.05 ppm
COBALT Root
COPPER Root 0.4—4 ppm
CYSTINE Root 50—615 ppm
FAT Root 1,000—12,300 ppm
FIBER Root 9,000—110,700 ppm
FLUORINE Root
FOLACIN Root 0.14—2 ppm
GLUTAMIC ACID Root 1,300—15,990 ppm
GLYCINE Root 250—3,075 ppm
HISTIDINE Root 140—1,720 ppm
IRON Root 2—37 ppm
ISOLEUCINE Root 360—4,425 ppm
KILOCALORIES Root 270—3,321/kg
LEAD Root 0.02—0.2 ppm
LEUCINE Root 330—4,060 ppm
LINOLEIC ACID Root 120—1,475 ppm
LINOLENIC ACID Root 400—4,920 ppm
LYCOPENE Root
LYSINE Root 360—4,425 ppm
MAGNESIUM Root 110—2,000 ppm
MANGANESE Root 0.6—7 ppm
MERCURY Root 0.001—0.01 ppm

METHIONINE Root 110—1,350 ppm
MOLYBDENUM Root 0.1—1 ppm
MUFA Root 60—740 ppm
NIACIN Root—49 ppm
NICKEL Root 0.01—0.1 ppm
NITROGEN Root 1,800—18,000 ppm
OLEIC ACID Root 60—740 ppm
PALMITIC ACID Root 100—1,230 ppm
PLAMITOLEIC ACID Root 10—120 ppm
PANTOTHENIC ACID Root 2—25 ppm
PHENYLALANINE Root 170—2,090 ppm
PHOSPHORUS Root 270—5,000 ppm
POTASSIUM Root 1,700—30,000 ppm
PROTEIN Root 9,000—110,700 ppm
PUFA Root 530—6,520 ppm
RAPIN Root
RIBOFLAVIN Root 0.3—4 ppm
RUBIDIUM Root 1—10 ppm
SELENIUM Root
SERINE Root 290—3,565 ppm
SFA Root 110—1,350 ppm
SILICON Root 120—1,200 ppm
SODIUM Root 400—11,600 ppm
STEARIC ACID Root 10—120 ppm
SULFUR Root 510—5,100 ppm
THIAMIN Root 0.4—5 ppm
THREONINE Root 250—3,075 ppm
TRYPTOPHAN Root 90—1,100 ppm
TYROSINE Root 130—1,600 ppm
VALINE Root 300—3,690 ppm
VITAMIN B6 Root 1—11 ppm
WATER Root 900,000—921,120 ppm
ZINC Root 2—23 ppm

■ WATER CHESTNUT

Chemical Constituents of Eleocharis dulcis (Cyperaceae)

ASCORBIC ACID Tuber 40—317 ppm
ASH Tuber 11,000—60,000 ppm
BETA-CAROTENE Tuber
CALCIUM Tuber 40—265 ppm
CARBOHYDRATES Tuber 161,000—876,000 ppm

FAT Tuber 2,000—16,000 ppm
FIBER Tuber 6,000—39,000 ppm
IRON Tuber 6—37 ppm
KILOCALORIES Tuber 680—3,640/kg
NIACIN Tuber 10—53 ppm
PHOSPHORUS Tuber 650—4,075 ppm
POTASSIUM Tuber 4,810—25,450 ppm
PROTEIN Tuber 14,000—85,000 ppm
PUCHIIN Tuber
RIBOFLAVIN Tuber 0.2—9 ppm
SODIUM Tuber 100—920 ppm
STARCH Tuber 70,000—400,000 ppm
SUCROSE Tuber 63,500—317,500 ppm
THIAMIN Tuber 0.3—6 ppm
WATER Tuber 773,000—811,000 ppm

■ WATERCRESS

Chemical Constituents of Nasturtium officinale R. (Brassicaceae)

ALANINE Herb 1,370—27,400 ppm
ARGININE Herb 1,500—30,000 ppm
ASCORBIC ACID Herb 430—13,690 ppm
ASH Herb 13,000—179,000 ppm
ASPARTIC ACID Herb 1,870—37,400 ppm
BETA-CAROTENE Herb 28—560 ppm
BIOTIN Plant
CALCIUM Herb 1,200—24,000 ppm
CARBOHYDRATES Herb 12,900—25,800 ppm
COPPER Plant
CYSTINE Herb 70—1,400 ppm
DIASTASE Plant

EO Plant 600—660 ppm
FAT Herb 1,000—20,000 ppm
FIBER Herb 700—77,670 ppm
FOLACIN Plant
GLUCONASTURTIN Plant
GLUTAMIC ACID Herb 1,900—38,000 ppm
GLYCINE Herb 1,120—22,400 ppm
HISTIDINE Herb 400—8,000 ppm
IRON Herb 2—262 ppm
ISOLEUCINE Herb 530—10,600 ppm
KILOCALORIES Herb 300—2,915/kg
LEUCINE Herb 1,660—33,200 ppm
LYSINE Herb 1,340—26,800 ppm
MAGNESIUM Herb 210—4,200 ppm
METHIONINE Herb 200—4,000 ppm
NIACIN Herb 2—113 ppm
PANTOTHENIC ACID Plant 3—62 ppm
PHENYLALANINE Herb 1,140—22,800 ppm
PENYLETHYL-ISOTHIOCYANATE Plant
PHOSPHORUS Herb 600—12,000 ppm
POTASSIUM Herb 3,300—66,000 ppm
PROLINE Herb 960—19,200 ppm
PROTEIN Herb 23,000—460,000 ppm
RIBOFLAVIN Herb 1—25 ppm
SERINE Herb 600—12,000 ppm
SODIUM Herb 410—8,200 ppm
THIAMIN Herb 1—18 ppm
THREONINE Herb 1,330—26,600 ppm
TRYPTOPHAN Herb 300—6,000 ppm
TYROSINE Herb 630—12,600 ppm
VALINE Herb 1,370—27,400 ppm
VITAMIN B6 Herb 1—26 ppm
WATER Herb 897,000—951,000 ppm
ZINC Plant

PHYTOCHEMICAL/ACTIVITIES

(+)-CATECHIN: Anticoagulant; Anticomplementary ; Antimutagenic; Antioxidant; Antiperoxidant; Antiradicular; Cancer-Preventive; Cardiotonic; Dermatitigenic; Hemostat; Hepatoprotective; Immunostimulant; Phagocytotic; Vasocontstrictor; cAMP-Phosphdiesterase-Inhibitor.

(-)-EPICATECHIN: Allelochemic; Anti-EBV; Antianaphylactic; Antidiabetic; Antihpatitic; Antileukemic; Antimutagenic; Antioxidant; Antiperoxidant; Antiviral; Bactericide; Cancer-Preventive; Cardiotonic; Choline-Sparing; Hypocholesterolemic; Hypoglycemic; Insulinogenic; Lipoxygenase-Inhibitor; Pancreatogenic; Pesticide; Xanthine-Oxidase-Inhibitor.

1,4-DICAFFEOYLQUINIC-ACID: Choleretic.

1,8-CINEOLE: AchE-Inhibitor; Allelopathic; Allergenic; Anesthetic; Anthelmintic; Antiallergic; Anti-alzheimeran; Antibronchitic; Anticatarrh; Anticholinesterase; Antihalitosic; Antilaryngitic; Antipharyngitic; Antirhinitic; Antiseptic; Antitussive; Bactericide; CNS-Stimulant; Choleretic; Counterirritant; Dentifrice; Expectorant; Fungicide; Hepatotonic; Herbicide; Hypotensive; Insectifuge; Nematicide; Pesticide; Rubefacient; Sedative.

2-VINYL-4H-1,3-DITHIN: Antiaggregant; Antithrombotic; Pesticide.

3-N-BUTYKPHTHALIDE: Antitumor 60 mg/mus/6 days.

3',4',5,6,7,8-HEXAMETHOXYFLAVONE: Cancer-Preventive.

4-HYDROXYCINNAMIC-ACID: Cancer-Preventive.

5-HEXYL-CYCLOPENTA-1,3-DIONE: Antiseptic; Pesticide.

5-HYDROXYTRYPTAMINE: Antidepressant; Antidote (Manganese) to 3 g/man/day; Antimutilation; Antiparkinsonian; Antitourette 400 mg/4xday/orl/man; Cancer-Preventive; Cerebrophilic; Hypertensive; Insecticide; Pesticide; Secretogogue; Spasmogenic; Ulcerogenic; Vasoconstrictor.

5-METHOXYPSORALEN: Antipsoriac; Cancer-Preventive; Carcinogenic.

5-OCTYL-CYCLOPENTA-1,3-DIONE: Antiseptic; Pesticide.

5,7-DIHYDROXYCHROMONE: Antifeedant; Bactericide; Herbicide; Pesticide.

8-METHOXYPSORALEN: Antialopecic; Antilymphomic; Antimycotic 20-50 mg/man/day; Antipsoriac 20-50 mg/man/day; Antitumor; Antiviral; Bactericide; Fungicide; Lymphocytogenic; Mitogenic; Mutagenic; Pesticide; Phototoxic; Viricide.

24-METHYLENE-CYCLOARTANOL: Cancer-Preventive.

ABCISSIC-ACID: Juvabional; Pesticide; Phytohormonal.

ACETIC-ACID: Acidulant; Antiotitic; Antivaginitic 1-2%; Bactericide 5,000 ppm; Expectorant; Fungicide; Keratitigenic; Mucolytic; Osteolytic; Pesticide; Protisticide; Spermicide; Ulcerogenic; Verrucolytic.

ACETYLCHOLINE: Allergenic; Antiamblyopic; Antidiuretic; Antiileus; Antitachycardic; Cardiodepressant; Cerebrostimulant; Histaminic; Hypotensive; Miotic; Myocontractant; Myopic; Myotonic; Neurotransmitter; Parasympathomimetic; Peristaltic; Sialogogue; Spasmogenic; Vasodilator.

ACETYLDEHYDE: Fungicide; Pesticide; Respiraparalytic.

ACTINIDIN: Proteolytic.

ADENINE: Antianemic 1.5 g/day; Antigranulocytopenic; Antiviral; CNS-Stimulant; Diuretic; Hyperuricemic; Insectifuge; Lithogenic; Myocardiotonic; Pesticide; Vasodilator; Viricide.

ADENOSINE: Antiaggregant; Antiarrhythmic; Antiendotoxic 500 mg/kg ipr mus; Antilipolytic; Antitachycardic 50-250 ug/kg/ivn; Arteriodilator; Hypoglycemic; Insulinic; Respirastimulant; Secretomotor; Vasodilator.

ADENOSINE-TRIPHOSPHATE: Antienzymatic; Antirheumatic; Antitachycardic; Myotonic.

AESCULETIN: Analgesic; Anti-Capillary-Fragility; Antiarrhythmic; Antiasthmatic; Antidysentric; Antiinflammatory.

AESCULIN: Anti-Capillary-Fragility; Antiarthritic; Antihistaminic; Cardiotonic; Diuretic; Hypertensive; Lipoxygenase-Inhibitor; Sunscreen.

AJOENE: Antiaggregant; Antimalarial 50 mg/kg; Antimutagenic; Antithrombotic; Fungicide; Hypocholesterolemic; Lipoxygenase-Inhibitor; Pesticide; Prostaglandin-Inhibitor.

ALANINE: Antioxidant; Cancer-Preventive; Oxidant.

ALFALFONE: Plant.

ALLANTOIN: Antidandruff; Anti-inflammatory; Antipeptic 30-130 mg/man/day; Antipsoriac 2%; Antiulcer; Immunostimulant; Keratolytic; Sunscreen; Suppurative; Vulnerary.

ALLICIN: Amebidice 30 ug/ml; Antiaggregant; Antibiotic; Antidiabetic; Antihypertensive; Antimutagenic; Antiprostaglandin; Antitumor; Bactericide; Candidicide; Fungicide; Hypocholesterolemic; Hypoglycemic; Insecticide; Insulin-Sparing 100 mg/kg/man; Larvicide; Lipoxygenase-Inhibitor; Mucokinetic; Pesticide; Trichomonicide; Vibriocide.

ALLIIN: Antiaggregant; Antibiotic; Antihepatoxic; Antioxidant; Antiradicular; Antithrombotic; Bactericide; Hypocholosterolemic; Pesticide.

ALLISTATIN-I: Bactericide; Pesticide.

ALLISTATIN-II: Bactericide, Pesticide.

ALLYL-ISOTHIOCYANATE: Allergenic; Antiasthmic; Antifeedant; Antimutagenic; Antiseptic; Cancer-Preventive; Counterirritant; Decongestant; Embryotoxic; Herbicide; Insectiphile; Mutagenic; Nematiovistat 50 ug/ml; Pesticide.

ALLYL-MERCAPTAN: Acantholytic; Pemphigenic; Spice.

ALLYL-SULFIDE: Acantholytic; Allergenic; Bactericide; Pemphigenic; Pesticide; Respiradepressant.

ALPHA-AMYRIN: Antitumor; Cytotoxic.

ALPHA-BISABOLOL: Antiarthritic; Antiburn; Antiinflammatory; Antipyretic; Antiseptic; Antispasmodic; Antitubercular; Antiulcer; Bactericide; Candidicide; Cosmetic; Fungicide; Musculotropic; Pesticide; Protisticide; Spasmolytic; Vulnerary.

ALPHA-CHACONINE: Antialzheimeran; Antifeedant; Cholinesterase-inhibitor; Fungicide; Memranolytic; Nematistat; Pesticide; Teratogenic.

ALPHA-CURCUMENE: Antiinflammatory; Antitumor.

ALPHA-HUMULENE: Antitumor.

ALPHA-LINOLENIC-ACID: Antimenorrhagic; Antiprostatitic; Cancer-Preventive.

ALPHA-PHELLANDRENE: Dermal; Insectiphile; Irritant; Pesticide.

ALPHA-PINENE: Allelochemic; Allergenic; Antiflu; Antiinflammatory; Antiviral; Bactericide; Cancer-Preventive; Coleoptiphile; Expectorant; Herbicide; Insectifuge; Pesticide; Sedative; Tranquilizer.

ALPHA-SOLANINE: Antifeedant; Fungicide; Pesticide.

ALPHA-TERPINEOL: Anticariogenic; Antiseptic; Bactericide; Motor-Depressant; Nematicide; Pesticide; Sedative; Termiticide.

ALPHA-TOCOPHEROL: Antimutagenic.

ALUMINUM: Antisilicotic; Antivaginitic; Candidicide; Encephalopathic; Pesticide.

AMYGDALIN: Antiinflammaotry; Antitussive; Cancer-Preventive; Cyanogenic; Expectorant.

ANETHOLE: Allergenic; Antihepatotic; Antiseptic; Bactericide; Cancer-Preventive; Carminative; Dermatitogenic; Digestive; Estrogenic; Expectorant; Fungicide; Gastrostimulant; Immunostimulant; Insecticide; Lactagogue; Leucocytogenic; Pesticide; Spasmolytic.

ANISALDEHYDE: Antimutagenic; Insecticide; Pesticide.

ANNONACIN: Antimalarial; Artemicide; Cytotoxic; Larvicide; Nematicide; Pesticide.

ANONAINE: Antiseptic; Bactericide; Candidicide; Cytotoxic; Dopamine-Adenylate-Cyclase-Inhibitor; Fungicide; Hypotensive; Insecticide; Mycoplasmicide; Pesticide.

ANTHOCYANINS: Antimyopic 600 mg/man/orl; Antinyctalopic 600 mg/man/orl; Goitrogenic; Pesticide; Viricide.

ANTHRANILIC-ACID: Antiarthritic; Antifeedant; Antiinflammatory; Insulinase-inhibitor; Insulinotonic.

APIGENIN: Antiaggregant; Antiallergic; Antiarrhythmic; Antidermatitic; Antiestrogenic; Antiherpetic; Antihistamine; Antiinflammatory; Antimutagenic; Antioxidant; Antispasmodic; Antithyroid; Antiviral; Bactericide; Calcium-Blocker; Cancer-Preventive; Choleretic; Cytotoxic; Deiodinase-Inhibitor;

Diuretic; Hypotensive; Musculotropic; Myorelexant; Nodulation-Signal; Pesticide; Sedative; Spasmolytic; Vasodilator.

APIIN: Aldose-Reductase-Inhibitor; Antiarrhythmic; Antibradykinic; Spasmolytic.

APIOLE: Abortifacient; Antipyretic; Diuretic; Emmenagogue; Hepatotoxic; Insecticide; Intoxicant; Pesticide; Secretolytic; Spasmolytic; Synergist; Uterotonic.

ARABINOGALACTAN: Anticomplementary; Antileishmanic 250 ug/ml; Immunostimulant 3.7-500 ug/ml; Infereronogenic 3.7-500; Mitogenic; Phagocytotic.

ARACHIDONIC-ACID: Antidermatitic; Antieczemic; Antipsoriatic; Cancer-Preventive; Hepatoprotective; Insulinogenic; Insulin-Sparing; Pesticide; Urinary-Antiseptic.

ARBUTIN: Allelochemic; Antiseptic 60-200 mg/man; Antitussive; Artemicide; Bactericide; Candidicide; Diuretic 60-200 mg.

ARGININE: Antidiabetic; Antiencephalopathic; Antihepatic; Antiinfertility 4 g/day; Antioxidant; Diuretic; Hypoammonemic; Spermigenic 4 g/day.

ASARONE: Anticonvulsant; Antielleptic; CNS-Depressant; Cardiodepressant; Emetic; Febrifuge; Fungicide; Hypothalmic-Depressant; Myorelaxant; Pesticide; Psychoactive; Sedative; Tranquilizer.

ASCORBIC-ACID: Acidulant; Analgesic 5-10 g per day; AntiChron's 50-100 mg/day/or/man; Antiarthritic 1 g per day; Antiasthmatic 1,000 mg per day; Antiatherosclerotic; Anticataract 350 mg/day; Anticold 1-2 g/man/day; Antidecubtic 500 mg/man/2x/day; Antidepressant 2,000 mg/day; Antidote (Aluminum); Antidote (Cadmium); Antidote (Lead); Antidote (Paraquat); Antieczemic 3.5-5 g/day; Antiedemic 1 g/man/day; Antiencephalitic; Antigingivitic; Antiglaucomic 2 g/day; Antihemorrhagic 1 g/man/day; Antihepatic 2-6 g/man/day; Antihepatoxic; Antiherpetic; 1-5 g/day; Antihistaminic; Antiinfertility 1 g/day; Antiinflammatory; Antilepric 1.5 g/man/day; Antimeasles; Antimigraine; Antimutagenic; Antinitrosic 1 g/man/day; Antiobesity; 1 g/3xday; Antiorchitic; Antiosteoarthritic 1 g/2xday; Antiosteoporotic 500 mg day; Antioxidant 100 ppm; Antiparkinsonian 1 g/2xday; Antiparotitic; Antiperiodontitic 1 g/2xday; Antipneumonic; Antipodriac; Antipoliomyeltic; Antiscorbutic 10 mg/man/day; Antiseptic; Antishingles; Antiulcer; Antiviral 1-5 g/day; Asthma-preventive 1,000 mg/day/orl; Bactericide; Cancer-Preventive; Cold-Preventive; 1-2 g/day; Detoxicant; Diuretic 700 mg/man/orl; Febrifuge; Fistula Preventive; Hypocholesterolemic 300-1,000 mg/day; Hypotensive; 1,000 mg/man/day; Inteferonogenic; Lithogenic; Mucolytic 1 g/woman/day; Pesticide; Uricosuric 4 g/man/day; Urinary-Acidulant; Viricide; Vulnerary.

ASIATIC-ACID: Collagenic.

ASIMICIN: Antifeedant; Antimalarial; Aphicide; Artemicide; Cytotoxic; Larvicide; Nematicide; Pesticide.

ASPARAGINE: Antisickling; Diuretic.

ASPARAGUSIC-ACID: Allelopathic; Nematicide 50 ug/ml; Nemativoistat 50 ug/ml; Pesticide.

ASPARTIC-ACID: Antimorphinic; Neuroexcitant; Roborant.

ASTRAGALIN: Aldose-Reductase-Inhibitor; Antileukemic; Expectorant; Hypotensive; Immunostimulant.

AUBERGENONE: Phytoalexin.

AURAPTEN: Antiaggregant; Spasmolytic.

AUREUSIDIN: Iodothyronine-Deiodinase-Inhibitor.

AVENIN: Neuromyostiumant.

AVICULARIN: Aldose-Reductase-Inhibitor; Antibiotic; Diuretic; Pesticide.

AZULENE: Antiallergic; Antiinflammatory; Antiseptic; Antiulcer; Bactericide 500 ppm; Febrifuge; Pesticide.

BENZALDEHYDE: Allergenic; Anesthetic; Antipeptic; Antiseptic; Antispasmodic; Antitumor; Insectifuge 50 ppm; Motor-Depressant; Narcotic; Nematicide; Pesticide; Sedative.

BENZOIC-ACID: Allergenic; Anesthetic; Antiotitic; Antspetic; Bactericide; Cholerertic; Expectorant; Febrifuge; Fungicide; Insectifiuge; Pesticide; Phytoalexin; Uricosuirc; Vulnerary.

BENZYL-ALCOHOL: Allergenic; Anesthetic; Antiodontalgic; Antipruritic; Antiseptic; Pesticide; Sedative.

BENZYL-BENZOATE: Acaricide; Allergenic; Antiasthmatic; Antidysmenorrheic; Antispasmodic; Antitumor; Artemicide; CNS-Stimulant; Hypotensive; Myorelaxant; Pediculicide; Pesticide; Scabicide.

BENZYL-ISOTHIOCYANATE: Allergenic; Antiasthmatic; Antimutagenic; Antineoplastic; Antitumor; Bactericide; Fungicide; Herbicide; Laxative; Pesticide.

BERGAPTEN: Antiapertif; Anticonvulsant; Antihistamine; Antiinflammatory; Antijet-lag; Antileukodermic; Antimitotic; Antipsoriatic; Antitumor; Calcium-Antagonist; Cancer-Preventive 5-25 ug/ml; Clastogenic; DME-Inhibitor; Hypotensive; Insecticide; Molluscicide; Mutagenic; Pesticide; Phototoxic; Piscicide; Spasmolytic.

BETA-BISABOLENE: Abortifacient; Antirhonoviral; Antiulcer; Antiviral.

BETA-CAROTENE: Allergenic; Androgenic; AntiPMS; Anticarcinomic; Anticoronary 50 mg/man/2 days; Antihyperkeratotic; Antiichysthoyotic; Antileukoplakic; Antilupus 150 mg/man/day/2mos; Antimastitic; Antimutagenic; Antioxidant; Antiozenic; Antiphotophobic 30-300 mg man/day; Antipsoriac; Antiradicular; Antistress; Antitumor; Antiulcer 12 mg/3xday/man/orl; Antixeropththalmic; Cancer-Preventive 22 ppm; Immunostimulant 180 mg/man/day/orl; Mucogenic; Phagocytotic; Thymoprotective; Ubiquiot.

BETA-ELEMENE: Anticancer (Cervix).

BETA-EUDESMOL: Antianoxic; Antipeptic; CNS-Inhibitor; Hepatoprotective.

BETA-IONONE: Anticariogenic; Antitumor; Bactericide; Cancer-Preventive; Fungicide; Hypocholesterolemic; Nematicide.

BETA-MYRCENE: Cancer-Preventive.

BETA-PHELLANDRENE: Expectorant.

BETA-PINENE: Allergenic; Flavor; Herbicide; Insectifuge; Pesticide.

BETA-SANTALENE: Antiinflammatory.

BETA-SESQUIPHELLANDRENE: Antirhinoviral; Antiulcer; Pesticide.

BETA-SITOSTEROL: Androgenic; Anorexic; Antiadenomic; Antiandrogenic; Antiestrogenic; Antifeedant; Antifertility; Antigonadotrophic; Antihyperlipoproteinaemic; Antiinflammatory; Antileukemic; Antimutagenic 250 ug/ml; Antiophidic 2.3 mg mus; Antiprogestational; Antiprostatadenomic; Antiprostatitic; Antitumor; Antiviral; Artemicide; Bactericide; Cancer-Preventive; Candidicide; Estrogenic; Gonadotrophic; Hepatoprotective; Hypoglycemic; Hypolipidemic; Pesticide; Spermicide; Ubiquiot; Viricide.

BETA-SITOSTEROL-D-GLUCOSIDE: Antitumor; CNS-Depressant; CNS-Stimulant; Convulsant; Hypoglycemic; Spasmolytic.

BETA-SOLAMARINE: Antisarcomic; Antitumor.

BETAINE: Abortifacient; Antigastric; Antihomocystinuric; Antimyoatrophic; Bruchiphobe; Emmenagogue; Hepatoprotective; Lipotropic.

BETULINIC-ACID: AntiHIV; Anticarcinomic; Antiinflammatory; Antimelanomic; Antitumor; Antiviral, Cytotoxic.

BIOCHANIN-A: Antimutagenic; Antiprostatedenomic; Cancer-Preventive; Estrogenic; Fungicide; Fungistat; Herbicide-Safener; Hypocholesterolemic; Hypolipidemic; Pesticide; VAM-simulant.

BIOTIN: Antialopecic; Antidermatitic 3 mg/2x/day; Antiseborrheic 3 mg/2x/day.

BORNEOL: Analgesic; Antibronchitic; Antiinflammatory; CNS-Toxic; Febrifuge; Flavor; Hepatoprotectant; Herbicide; Insectifuge; Nematicide; Pesticide; Spasmolytic.

BORNYL-ACETATE: Antifeedant; Bactericide; Expectorant; Insectifuge; Pesticide; Sedative; Spasmolytic; Viricide.

BORON: Androgenic 3 mg/man/day; Antiosteoarthritic; Antiosteoporotic 3 mg/man/day; Estrogenic 3 mg/man/day.

BOWMAN-BIRK-INHIBITOR: Antinutrient; Antitrypsic; Antitumor; Cancer-Preventive.

BROMELAIN: Antiaggregant; Antianginal 1,500 mg/day; Antiappetant; Antiarthritic; Antibronchitic; Anticellulitic; Antidysmenorrheic; ; Antidyseptic; Antiecchymotic; Antiedemic; Antiepisiotomic; Antiinfective; Antiinflammatory; Antiluekemic; Antimetastatic; Antiplaque; Antipneumonic; Antiprostaglandin; Antiradiation; Antisclerodermic; Antisinusitic; Antithrombophlebitic; Antithrombotic 60-800 mg; Antitumor; Antitisussive; Antiulcer; Bactericide; Chemopreventive; Digestive; Emetic; Fibrinolytic; Hypotensive; Laxative; Lipolytic; Mucolytic; Myorelaxant; Nematicide; Pesticide; Proteolytic 400-600 mg/3xdaily/; Spasmolytic; Vermifuge; Vulnerary.

BULLATACINE: Antileukemic; Aphicide; Artemicide; Cytotoxic; Larvicide.

BULLATACINONE: Artemicide; Cytotoxic; Pesticide.

BUTYLIDENE-PHTHALIDE: Abortifacient; Antiinflammatory; Antispasmodic; Emmenagogue; Spasmolytic.

BUTYRIC-ACID: Anticancer; Bruchifuge; Nematistat 880 ug/ml; Pesticide.

BYAKANGELICIN: Antiestrogenic; Antigonadotropic.

CADAVERINE: Phytohormonal.

CADMIUM: Hypertensive; Lithogenic; Nephrotoxic.

CAFFEIC-ACID: Allergenic; Analgesic; Anti-Tumor-Promoter; AntiHIV; Antiadenoviral; Antiaggregant; Anticarcinogenic; Antidedemic; Antiflu; Antigonadotropic; Antihemolytic 25 uM; Antihepatotoxic; Antiherpectic 50 ug/ml; Antihypercholesterolemic; Antiinflammatory; Antimutagenic; Antinitrosaminic; Antioxdixant; Antiperoxidant; Antiradicular 10 uM; Antiseptic; Antispasmodic; Antistomatitic; Antithiamin; Antithyroid; Antitumor; Antiulcerogenic; Antivaccinia; Antiviral; Bactericide; CNS-Active; Cancer-Preventive; Cholagogue; Choleretic; Clastogenic; DNA-Active; Diuretic; Fungicide; Hepatoprotective; Hepatotropic; Histamine-Inhibitor; Insectifuge; Leukotriene-Inhibitor; Lipoxygenase-Inhibitor; Metal-Chelatory; Ornithine-Decarboxylase-Inhibitor; Pesticide; Prostaglandigenic; Sedative 500 mg; Spasmolytic; Sunscreen; Tumorigenic; Viricide; Vulnerary.

CAFFEINE: Analeptic 200 scu mus; Antiapneic; Antiasthmatic 5-10 mg/kg/orl/man; Anticarcinogenic; Antidermatic; Antiemetic; Antifeedant; Antiflu; Antiherpetic; Antihypotensive 250 mg/day/orl/man; Antinarcotic; Antiobesity; Antioxidant; Antirhinitic 140 mg/day/orl/man; Antiserotonergic; Antitumor; Antivaccinia; Antiviral; CNS-Stimulant; Cancer-Preventive; Cardiotonic; Catabolic; Choleretic; Diuretic; Ergotamine-Enhancer; Flavor; Herbicide; Hypertensive; Hypoglycemic; Insecticide; Neurotoxic; Pesticide; Respirastimulant; Stimulant; Teratogenic; Vasodilator; Viricide; Phosphodeiesterase-Inhibitior.

CALCIUM: AntiPMS 1 g per day; Antiallergenic 500 mg per day; Antianxiety; Antiatherosclerotic 500 mg per day; Antidepressant; Antidote (Aluminum); Antidote (Lead); Antihyperkinetci; Antiinsomniac; Antiosteoporotic 500 mg/day; Antiperiodontitic; 750 mg/day; Antitic; Hypocholesterolemic 500 mg/day; Hypotensive 1 g/day.

CAMPHENE: Antilithic; Antioxidant; Hypocholesterolemic; Insectifuge; Pesticide; Spasmogenic.

CAMPHOR: Abortifacient; Allelopathic; Analgesic; Anesthetic; Antiacne; Antiemetic 100-200 mg/man/orl; Antifeedant; Antifibrositic; Antineuralgic; Antipruritic; Antiseptic; CNS-Stimulant; Cancer-Preventive; Carminative; Convulsant; Counterirritant; Decogestant; Deliriant; Ecbolic; Emetic; Expectorant; Fungicide; Herbicide; Insectifuge; Irritant; Nematicide; Occuloirritant; Pesticide; Respirainhibitor; Respirastimulant; Rubefacient; Spasmolytic; Stimulant; Verrucolytic.

CANAVANINE: Allelochemic; Antifeedant; Antiflu; Antimetabolic; Antitumor; Antiviral; Bactericide; Cytotoxic; Fungicide; Herbicide; Juvabional; Lupus-Generating; Mitogenic; Pesticide.

CAPRYLIC-ACID: Candidicide 300 mg/man/12xday/; Fungicide; Irritant; Pesticide.

CAPSAICIN: 5-Lipoxygenase-Inhibitor; Analgesic; Anaphylactic; Anesthetic; Antiaggregant; Antico-lonospasmic.

CAPSIDOL: Fungicide; Pesticide; Phytoalexin.

CARPAINE: Amebicide; Antitubercular; Antitumor; Bactericide; CNS-Depressant; Cardiodepressant; Cardiotonic; Diuretic; Hypotensive; Paralytic; Pesticide; Respiradepressant; Trichuridicde; Vasocon-strictor; Vermicide.

CARPOSIDE: Anthelminthic; Antienteritic; Cardiac; Pesticide.

CARVACROL: AchE-Inhibitor; Allergenic; Anesthetic; Anthelminithic; Antialzheimeran; Anticholin-esterase; Antidiuretic; Antiinflammatory; Antimelanomic; Antioxidant; Antiplaque; Antiradicular; Antiseptic; Bactericide; Carminative; Enterorelxant; Expectorant; Fungicide; Nematicide; Pesticide; Prostaglandin; Inhibitor; Spasmoyltic; Tracheorelaxant; Vermifuge.

CARVEOL: SNS Stimulant.

CARVONE: Allergenic; Antiseptic; CNS-Stimulant; Cancer-Preventive; Carminative; Insecticide; Insectifuge; Motor-Depressant; Nematicide; Pesticide; Sedative; Vermicide.

CARYOPHYLLENE: Anticariogenic; Antiedemic; Antifeedan 500 ppm; Antiinflammatory; Antitu-mor; Bactericide; Insectifuge; Pesticide; Spasmolytic; Termitifuge.

CARYOPHYLLEN-OXIDE: Antiedemic; Antifeedant; Antiinflammatory; Antitumor; Insecticide; Pes-ticide.

CASUARIN: Antiperoxidant; Lipoxygenase-Inhibitor; Xanthine-Oxidase-Inhibitor.

CATALASE: Antioxidant.

CATECHIN: Allelochemic; Antialcoholic 2,000 mg/man/day; Antiarthritic; Anticariogenic; Antie-demic; Antiendotoxic; Antifeedant.

CATECHOL: 5-Lipoxygenase-Inhibitor; Allelochemic; Allergenic; Antigonadotropic; Antioxidant; Antiseptic; Antistomatitic; Antithiamin; Antithyreotropic; Antiviral; Cancer-Preventive; Convulsant; Dermatitigenic; Pesticide.

CELLULOSE: Hemostat.

CEPHALIN: Hemostat.

CHARANTIN: Abortifacient; Antidiabetic; Antitesticular; Hypoglycemic 50 mg/kg/orl/rbt.

CHAVICOL: Fungicide; Nematicide; Pesticide.

CHELIDONIC-ACID: Antiwart; Irritant.

CHLORINE: Antiherpetic; Antiseptic; Bactericide; Candidicide; Fungicide; Pesticide; Viricide.

CHLOROGENIC-ACID: Allergenic; Analgesic; Anti-EBV; AntiHIV; Antifeedant; Antigonadotropic; Antihemolytic; Antihepatotoxic; Antiherpectic; Antihypercholesterolemic; Antiinflammatory; Antimutagenic; Antinitrosaminic; Antioxidant; Antiperoxidant; Antipolio; Antiradicular; Antiseptic; Antithyroid; Anti-Tumor-Promoter; Antiulcer; Antiviral; Bactericide; CNS-Active; CNS-Stimulant; Cancer-Preventive; Cholagogue; Choleretic; Clastogenic; Diuretic; Fungicide; Hepatoprotective; Histamine-Inhibitor; Immunostimulant; Insectifuge; Interferon-Inducer; Juvabional; Larvistat; Leukotriene-Inhibitor; Lipoxygenase-Inhibitor; Metal-chelator; Ornithine-Decarboxylase-Inhibitor; Oviposition-Stimulant; Pesticide.

CHLOROPHYLL: Antidecubitic; Antihalitosic; Antimenorrhagic 25 mg/day/wmn/orl; Antimutagenic; Antioxidant.

CHOLINE: Antialzheimeran 5-16 g/man/day; Antichoreic; Anticirrhotic 6,000 mg/man/day; Anticystinuric; Antidiabetic; Antidyskinetic 150-200 mg.

CHROMIUM: Anmphiglycemic; Antiatherosclerotic 20 ug/day; Anticorneotic; Antidiabetic; Antidote (Lead); Antiglycosuric; Antitriglyceride 20 ug/day; Hypocholesterolemic 20 ug/day; Insulinogenic.

CHRYSIN: Antiaggregant; Antiallergic; Antimutagenic; Antispasmodic; Antithrombic; Anxiolytic; Cancer-Preventive; Cyclooxygenase-Inhibitor; Fungicide; Myorelaxant; Pesticide; Termitifuge.

CHRYSOERIOL: Aldose-Reductase-Inhibitor; Antimutagenic; Antirhinoviral; Antiviral; Cancer-Preventive.

CICHORIC-ACID: Antiflu; Antistomatitic; Antiviral; Immunostimulant 10-100 ug/ml; Pesticide; Phagocytotic 10-100 ug/ml; Viricide.

CICHORIIN: Antiaggregant; Antifeedant.

CINCHONINE: Antimalarial; Pesticide.

CINNAMALDEHYDE: Allelochemic; Allergenic; Antiaggregant; Antiherpetic; Antimutagenic; Antiulcer 500 mg/kg/orl; Antiviral; CNS-Depressant; CNS-Stimulant; Cancer-Preventive; Choleretic 500 mg/kg/orl; Chronotropic; Circulostimulant; Cytotoxic; 5-60 ug/ml; Febrifuge; Fungicide; Herbicide; Histaminic; Hypoglycemic; Hypotensive; Hypothermic; Inotropic; Insecticide; Mutagenic; Nematicide; Pesticide; Sedative; Spasmolytic; Sprout-Inhibitor; Teratogenic; Tranquilizer.

CINNAMIC-ACID: Allergenic; Anesthetic; Antiinflammatory; Antimutagenic; Bactericide; Cancer-Preventive; Chloretic; Dermatitigenic; Fungicide; Herbicide; Laxative; Lipoxygenase-Inhibitor; Pesticide; Spasmolytic; Vermifuge.

CINNAMIC-ACID-ETHYL-ESTER: Cancer-Preventive.

CINNAMYL-ALCOHOL: Allelochemic; Antimutagenic; Herbicide; Nematicide; Pesticide.

CIS-3,5,4'-TRIHYDROXY-4-ISOPENTENYLSTILBENE: Fungicide; Pesticide.

CITRAL: Allergenic; Antiallergic; Antihistamine; Antiseptic; Antishock; Bactericide; Bronchorelaxant; Cancer-Preventive; Expectorant; Fungicide; Herbicide; Nematicide; Pesticide; Sedative; Teratogenic.

CITRANTIN: Antifertiliy; Contraceptive.

CITRIC-ACID: Allergenic; Antiaphthic 20,000 ppm; Anticalculic; Anticoagulant; Antimutagenic; Antioxidant Synergist; Antiseborrheic; Antitumor; Disinfectant; Hemostat; Laxative; Litholytic; Refrigerant.

CITRONELLAL: Allergenic; Antiseptic; Bactericide; Embryotoxic; Insectifige; Motor Depressant; Mutagenic; Nematicide; Pesticide; Sedative; Teratogenic.

CITRONELLOL: Allergenic; Bactericide; Candidicide; Fungicide; Herbicide; Nematicide; Pesticide; Sedative.

CITRULLINE: Antiasthenic 180 mg/kg/day; Antihepatotic; Antiosteoporotic; Diuretic

CNIDILIDE: Abortifacient; Antiinflammatory; Emmenagogue; Fungicide; Pesticide; Spasmolytic.

COBALT: Cardiomyopathogenic; Erythrocytogenic

COPPER: Antiarthritic; Antidiabetic 2-4 mg/day; Antiinflammatory; Antinociceptive; Contraceptive; Hypocholesterolemic; Schizophrenic.

COREXIMINE: Antihypertensive; Respirastimulant.

CORILAGEN: ACE-Inhibitor; Antiallergic; Antiasthmatic; Xanthine-Oxidase-Inhibitor.

CORYDINE: Antitumor; CNS-Depressant; Cardiodepressant; Hypnotic; Respirodepressant; Sedative.

COSMOSIIN: Aldose-Reductase-Inhibitor; Bactericide; Candidicide.

COUMARIN: Allelochemic; Antiaggregant; Antiandrogenic; Antibrucellosic; Antiedemic; Antiinflammatory; Antimelanomic; Antimitotic; Antimutagenic; Antisporiac; Antitumor; Bruchiphobe; Cancer-Preventive; Cardiodepressant; DME-Inhibitor; Emetic; Fungicide; Hemorrhagic; Hepatotoxic; Hypnotic; Hypoglycemic; Immunostimulant; Juvabional; Lymphocytogenic 100 mg/day; Ovicide; Pesticide; Phagocytogenic; Piscicide; Rodenticide; Sedative.

COUMESTROL: Antimicrobial; Estrogenic; Fungicide; Nematicide; Nematistat 5-25 ug/ml; Peroxidase-Inhibitor; Pesticide; Phytoalexin.

CROCETIN: Antihypoxic; Antimutagenic; Choleretic 100 mg/kg; Hypocholesterolemic; Lipolytic.

CUCURBITACIN-B: Antihepatotoxic; Antiinflammatory; Cancer-Preventive; Cytotoxic.

CUCURBITACIN-E: Antigibberellin; Antihepatotoxic; Antitumor; Cytotoxic.

CUCURBITACIN-I: Anticarcinomic; Anticarcinomic; Antileukemic.

CUCURBITAN: Antihelminthic; Pesticide; Schistosomicide.

CUMINALDEHYDE: Bactericide. Fungicide; Larvicide; Pesticide.

CYANIDIN: Allelochemic; Antioxidant; Pesticide; Pigment.

CYANIN: Antipolio; Antiviral; Emetic; Pesticide.

CYNARIN: Cholagogue; Choleretic 200-250 mg/3xday; Cholesterolytic; Diuretic; Hepatoprotective 100 mg/kg; Hyperemic; Hypocholesterolemic 500 mg/man; Hypolipidemic.

CYCLOALLIIN: Lachrymatory.

CYCLOARTENOL: Antiinflammatory; Ubiquet.

CYSTEINE: Antiaddisonian; Anticataract; Anticytotoxic; Antiophthalmic; Antioxidant; Antitumor; Antiulcer; Cancer-Preventitive; Detoxicant; Opthalmic-Antialkalin; Pesticide.

CYSTINE: Adjuvant; Antihomocystinuric; Anticoagulant; Cancer-Preventive; Cardiotonic; Vasoconstrictor.

D-AFZELECHIN: Allelopathic.

D-CATECHIN: Anticoagulant; Cancer-Preventive; Cardiotonic; Vasoconstrictor.

D-LIMONENE: Anti-Tumor-Promoter; Anticancer (Breast); Antimelanomic; Cancer-Preventive; Hypochlosterolemic; Litholytic; Pesticide.

DAIDZEIN: Antialcoholic; Antiarrhythmic; Antidipsomanic 150 mg/kg/day; Antihemolytic; Antiinflammatory.; Antileukemic; Antimicrobial; Antimutagenic; Antioxidant; Antispasmodic; Coronary-Dilator; Estrogenic; Fungicide; Hypotensive; Lipase-Inhibitor; Spasmolytic.

DAIDZIN: Antialcoholic; Antidipsomanic 150 mg/kg/day, Antioxidant; Antispasmodic; Cancer-Preventive; Estrogenic; Fungicide; Hypotensive; Lipase-Inhibitor; Pesticide; Spasmolytic.

DAPHNORETIN: Anticarcinomic; Antitumor.

DAUCOSTEROL: Antileukemic; Antitumor; Hypoglycemic; Spasmolytic.

DECAN-1-AL: Cancer-Preventive.

DELPHINIDIN: Allelochemic; Allergenic; Antioxidant; Cancer-Preventive; Pesticide.

DELTA-3-CARENE: Allergenic; Antiinflammatory; Bactericide; Dermatitigenic; Insectifuge.

DELTA-CADINENE: Anticariogenic; Bactericide; Pesticide.

DIALLYL-SULFIDE: Antimutagenic; Antitumor; Cancer-Preventive (Esophagus) 200 mg/kg; Hypocholesterolemic; Occuloirritant; Pesticide.

DIALLYL-TRISULFIDE: Antiseptic; Hypocholesterolemic; Hypoglycemic; Insecticide; Larvicide; Pesticide.

DIAZEPAM: Amnesigenic; Anesthetic 1-40 mg/man; Antialcoholic; Anticonvulsant; Antiepileptic; Antimyocarditic; Antischizophrenic.

DIHYDROCAPSAICIN: Hypocholesterolemic.

DIMETHYL-DISULFIDE: Antithyroid.

DIOSGENIN: Antifatigue; Antiinflammatory; Antistress; Estrogenic; Hypocholesterolemic.

DIOSMETIN: Aldose-Reductase-Inhibitor; Antimutagenic; Antirhinoviral; Cancer-Preventive.

DIOSMIN: Anti-Capillary-Fragility 300 mg/2x/day/woman; Antihemorrhoidal; Antiinflammatory; Antimetrorrhagic.

DIPENTENE: Antiviral; Bactericide; Expectorant; Pesticide; Sedative; Viricide.

DOPA: Antiparkinsonian.

DOPAMINE: Adreneric; Antilactagogue; Antimyocontractant; Antineurogenic; Antiparkinsonian; Antishock; Antithyreotropic; Cardiotonic; Hypertensive; Inotropic; Myocontractant; Neurotransmitter; Sympathomimetic; Teratogenic; Vasoconstrictor; Vasodilator.

ELEMICIN: Antiaggregant; Antidepressant; Antifeedant; Antihistaminic; Antiserotonic; Antistress; DNA-Binding; Hallucinogenic; Hypotensive; Insecticide; Insectifuge; Neurotoxic; Pesticide; Schistosomicide.

ELLAGIC-ACID: ACE-Inhibitor; Aldose-Reductase-Inhibitor; AntHIV; Anticataract; Antimutagenic.

ELLAGITANNIN: AntHIV; Antiallergic; Antioxidant; Antitumor; Cardiotoxic; Immunostimulant; Interferon-Stimulant; Rt-Inhibitor.

EPICATECHIN: Allelochemic; Antidiabetic; AntiEBV; Anticomplementary; Antiinflammatory; Antileukemic; Bactericide; Hepatotropic; Pesticide.

EPSILON-VINIFERIN: Fungicide; Pesticide.

ERIODICTYOL: Antifeedant; Cancer-Preventive; Expectorant; Pesticide.

ERUCIC-ACID: Antitumor.

ESCULIN: Anti-Capillary-Fragility; Antiarthritic; Antidermatotic; Antifeedant; Antihistaminic; Antiinflammatory; Antioxidant; Bactericide; Cancer-Preventive; Cardiotonic; Choleretic; Diuretic; Expectorant; Hypertensive; Juvabional; Lipoxygenase-Inhibitor; Pesticide; Sunscreen.

ESTRAGOLE: Antiaggregant; Cancer-Preventive; DNA-Binder; Hepatocarginogenic; Hypothermic; Insecticide; Insectifuge.

ESTRONE: Aphrodisiac; Antiimpotency; Antimenopausal 0.7-2.8 mg/day/orl/wmn; Antiprostatadenomic; Antivaginitic; Estrogenic.

ETHANOL: Anesethetic; Antihydrotic; Antipruritic; Antiseptic; Bactericide; CNS-Depressant; Hepatotoxic; Hypnotic; Hypocalcemic; Neurolytic; Pesticide; Rubefacient; Sclerosant; Teratogenic; Tremorilytic; Ulcerogenic.

ETHYL-ACETATE: Antispasmotic; CNS-Depressant; Carminative; Spasmolytic; Stimulant.

ETHYLENE: Anesthetic.

EUGENOL: Analgesic; Anesthetic; Antiaggregant; Anticonvulsant; Antidemic; Antifeedant; Antiinflammatory; Antimitotic; Antimutagenic; Antinitrosating; Antioxidant; Antiprostaglandin; Antiradicular; Antiseptic 3 ml/man/day; Antithromboxane; Antitumor; Antiulcer; Apifuge; Bactercide; CNS-Depressant; Cancer-Preventive; Candidicide; Carcinogenic; Carminative; Choleretic; Cytotoxic; 25 ug/ml; Dermatitigenic; Enterorelaxant; Febrifuge 3 ml/man/day; Fungicide; Herbicide; Insecticide; Insectifuge; Irritant; Juvabional; Larvicide; Motor-Depressant; Nematicide; Neurotoxic; Pesticide; Sedative; Spasmolytic; Trichomonistat; Trypsin-Enhancer; Ulcerogenic; Vermifuge.

EUGENOL-METHYL-ETHER: CNS-Despressant; Cancer-Preventive; DNA-Binding; Hypothermic; Myorelaxant.

EUPHOL: Abortifacient.

FALCARINDIOL: Analgesic; Bactericide; Fungicide; Pesticide; Phytoalexin.

FARNESOL: Antimelanomic; Nematicide; Juvabional; Pesticide.

FENCHONE: AchE-Inhibitor; Antialzheimeran; Anticholinesterase; Counterirritant; Secretolytic.

FERULIC-ACID: Allelopathic; Analgesic; Anti-Tumor-Promoter; Antiaggregant; Antidysmenorrheic; Antiestrogenic; Antiinflammatory; Antimitotic; Antimutagenic; Antinitrosamine; Antioxidant 3,000 uM; Antioxidant; Antiserotonin; Antitumor; Antiviral; Arteriodilator; Bactericide; Cancer-Preventive; Candidicide; Cardiac; Cholagogue; Choleretic; Fungicide; Hepatotrophic; Herbicide; Hydrocholerectic; Immunostimulant; Insectifuge; Metal-Chelator; Ornithine-Decarboxylase-Inhibitor; Pesticide; Phagocytotic; Preservative; Prostaglandigenic; Spasmolytic; Sunscreen; Uterosedative.

FIBER: Antidiabetic; Antiobesity; Antitumor; Antiulcer; Cancer-Preventive; Cardioprotective; Hypocholesterolemic; Hypotensive 10 g/man/day; Laxative.

FICIN: Antiinflammatory; Dermatitigenic; Irritant; Pesticide; Proteolytic; Pruritogenic; Trichuricide; Vermifuge.

FISETIN: 5-Lipoxygenase-Inhibitor; Antihistamine; Antimutagenic; Antioxidant; Antiviral; Cyclooxy-genase-Inhibitor; Iodothyronine-Deiodinase-Inhibitor; Lipoxygenase-Inhibitor; Oxidase; Inhibitor; Pesticide.

FLUORIDE: Anticariogenic; Antiosteoporotic; Antiosteosclerotic.

FOLACIN: Anti-spina-bifida; Antianemic 5-20 mg/man/day; Anticervicaldysplasic 8-30 mg/wmn/day/orl; Anticheilitic; Antidepressant; Antigingivititic 2-5 mg/day/man; Antiglossitic; Antimyelotoxic 5 mg/day/orl/man; Antineuropathic; Antiperiodontitic; Antiplaque; Antipsychotic; Hematopoietic; Uricosuric; Xanthine-Oxidase-Inhibitor.

FORMALDEHYDE: Anesthetic; Anticystitic; Antiplantar; Antiseptic; Antiviral; Fungicide; Irritant; Neoplastic; Pesticide; Scolicide; Viricide.

FORMIC-ACID: Antiseptic; Antisyncopic; Astringent; Counterirritant; Fungitoxic; Pesticide.

FORMONONETIN: Abortifacient; Antifeedant; Antiulcer; Cancer-Preventive; Estrogenic; Fungicide; Herbicide-Safener; Hypocholosterolemic; Hypolipidemic; Pesticide; VAM-Stimulant.

FRIEDELIN: Antiinflammatory 30 mg/kg; Diuretic.

FRUCTOSE: Antialcoholic; Antidiabetic; Antihangover; Antiketotic; Antinauseant; Neoplastic.

FUMARIC-ACID: Acidulant; Antidermatatic; Antipsoriatic; Antihepatocarcinogenic; Antioxidant, Antitumor.

FURFURAL: Antiseptic; Fungicide; Insecticide; Pesticide.

GABA: Analeptic; Anticephalgic; Antichoreic 1-32 g/man/day; Antiinsomniac; Antitinnitic; Diuretic; Hypotensive 1,000 — 4,000 mg/day; Neuroinhibitor; Neurotransmitter; Tranquilizer.

GALACTOSE: Sweetener.

GALLIC-ACID: ACE-Inhibitor; Anti HIV; Antiadenovirus; Antiallergenic; Antianaphylactic; Anti-asthmatic; Antibacterial; Antibronchitic; Anticarcinomic; Antifibrinolytic; Antiflu; Antihepatotoxic; Antiherpetic; Antiinflammatory; Antimutagenic; Antinitrosaminic; Antioxidant; Antiperoxidant; Antipolio; Antiseptic; Antitumor; Antiviral; Astringent; Bacteristatic; Bronchodilator; Cancer-Preventive; Carcinogenic; Choleretic; Cycloosygenase-Inhibitor; Floral-Inhibitor; Hemostat; Immuno-suppressant; Insulin-Sparing; Myorelaxant; Nephrotoxic; Pesticide; Styptic; Viricide; Xanthine-Oxidase-Inhibitor.

GAMMA-DECALACTONE: Cancer-Preventive.

GAMMA-LINOLENIC-ACID: AntiMS; AntiPMS; Antiacne; Antiaggregant; Antialcoholic; Antiarthritic 540 mg/day; Antiatherosclerotic; Antieczemic; Antimenorrhagic; Antiobesity; Antiprostatic; Antitumor; Hypotensive.

GAMMA-TERPINENE: Antioxidant; Insectifuge; Pesticide.

GENTISIC-ACID: Analgesic; Antifeedant; Antiinflammatory; Antirheumatic; Bactericide; Pesticide; Viricide.

GERANIAL: Bactericide; Pesticide.

GERANIIN: ACE-Inhibitor; Adrenocorticotrophic; AntiHIV; Antiallergenic; Antiasthmatic; Antiherpetic; Antihypertensive; Antilipolytic; Antiradicular; Antimutagenic; Antioxidant; Antiperoxidant; Antiradicular; Antiviral; Juvabional; Larvistat; Pesticide; Vasodilator; Viricide; Xanthine-Oxidase-Inhibitor.

GERANIOL: Anticariogenic; Antimelanomic; Antiseptic; Antitumor; Bactericide; Cancer-Preventive; Candidicide; Embryotixic; Emetic; Fungicide; Insectifuge; Nematicide; Pesticide; Sedative; Spasmolytic.

GERMACRENE-D: Pesticide; Pheromone.

GLAUCINE: Adrenalytic; Antisuperoxidgogenic; Antitussive; Hypoglycemic; Hypotensive; Respiradepressant; Spasmolytic.

GLUCOSE: Acetylcholinergic; Antiedemic; Antihepatoxic; Antiketotic; Antivaricose; Hyperglycemic; Memory-Enhancer.

GLUCURONIC-ACID: Detoxicant.

GLUTAMIC-ACID: Antalkali 500-1,000 mg/day/orl/man; Antiepilpetic; Antihyperammonenic; Antilithic; Antiretardation; Anxiolytic; Neurotoxic.

GLUTAMINE: Antialcoholic 1,000 mg/man/day/orl; Antisickling; Antiulcer 1,600 mg/man/day/orl; Antidepressant.

GLUTATHIONE: Anticytoxic; Antidote (Heavy Metals); Antieczemic; Antihepatitic; Antioxidant; Cancer-Preventive.

GLYCERIC-ACID: Antalakali 500-1,000 mg/day/orl/man; Antiepileptic; Antihyperammonemic; Anti-lithic; Antiretardation; Anxiolytic; Cholesterolytic; Diuretic; Hepatotoxic.

GLYCINE: Antiacid; Antialdosteronic; Antidote (Hypoglycin-A); Antiencephalopathic; Antigastric; Antiprostatic; Antipruritic; Antisickling; Antiulcer; Cancer-Preventive; Neuroinhibitor; Uricosuric.

GLYCITEIN: Antioxidant; Cancer-Preventive; Estrogenic; Fungicide; Pesticide.

GLYCOLIC-ACID: Cholesterolytic; Diuretic; Hepatotonic; Irritant.

GOITRIN: Antithyroid; Goitrogenic.

GOLD: Antiarthritic; Antiulcer; Nephrotoxic.

GOSSYPETIN: Antimutagenic; Antioxidant; Bactericide; Lipoxygenase-Inhibitor; Pesticide.

GOSSYPOL: Amebicide; Anaphrodisiac; Antibiotic; Anti-Corpus-Luteum; AntiHIV; Antibiotic; Anti-cancer; Antiencephalitic; Antiestrogenic; Antifeedant; Antifertility 30 mg/kg; Antiflu; Antiherpetic; Antimplantation; Antikeratitic; Antimalarial; Antioxidant; Antiprogesterone; Antiproliferant; ; Anti-rabies; Antispermatogenic; Antistomatitic; Antitestosterone; Antitumor; Antiviral; Avicide; Bacteri-cide; Contraceptive (Male) 10 mg/man/day; Cytotoxic 25 uM; Fungicide; Hepatotoxic; Hypokalemic; Immunostimulant; Insectifuge; Interferon-Inducer; Larvicide; Libidolytic; Mutagenic; Nematistant 125 ug/ml; Paralytic; Pesticide; Plasmodicide; Prostaglandigenic; Spermicide 0.2-100 uM; Trypanoc-ide; Trypanosomicide; Tumorigenic; Viricide.

GUAIACOL: Anesthetic; Antidermatitic; Antieczemic; Antiesophagitic; Antiseptic; Antitubercular; Bactericide; Expectorant 0.3-0.6 ml/man; Insectifuge; Pesticide.

GUAIAZULENE: Antiallergic; Antiinflammatory; Antileprotic; Antipeptic; Antipyretic; Antiulcer.

HCN: Antiasthmatic; Antidote (Amyl Nitrate); Antitussive; Bronchosedative; Insecticide; Pesticide; Respirastimulant; Rodenticide; Vasomotor-Stimulant.

HARDWICKIC-ACID: Antiseptic; Bactericide; Fungicide; Pesticide.

HERACLENIN: Anticoagulant; Antiinflammatory.

HESPERIDIN: Anti-DNA; Anti-RNA; Antiallergenic; Antibradykinic; Antiflu; Antiinflammatory 100 mg/kg; Antioxidant; Antistomatitic; Antivaccinia; Antiviral; Capillariprotective; Catabolic; Chlorec-tic; Pesticide; Vasopressor.

HESPERETIN: Antifeedant; Antilipidolytic; Bactericide; Cancer-Preventive; Fungistatic; Hepatoprotective; Pesticide; Viricide.

HETEROSIDE-B: Choleretic; Hepatotonic.

HEXANAL: Pesticide.

HIGENAMINE: Antiarrhythmic; Antithrombic; Antitussive; Cardiotonic.

HISTAMINE: Antichiliblain; Antimeniere's; Antimigraine; Bronchostimulant; Cardiovascular; Gastrostimulant; Histaminic; Hypotensive; Myostimulan; Radioprotective; Secretogogue; Spasmogenic; Tachycardic; Vasodilator.

HISTIDINE: Antiarteriosclerotic; Antinephritic; Antioxidant; Antiulcer; Antiuremic.

HORDENINE: Antiasthmatic; Antidiarrheic; Antifeedant; Bronchorelaxant; Cardiotonic; Hepatoprotective; Pesticide; Vasoconstrictor.

HYDROQUINONE: Allelochemic; Allergenic; Antilithic; Antimalarial; Antimelanomic; Antimelasmic; Antimenorrhagic; Antinephritic; Antioxidant; Antipertussic; Antiseptic; Antithyreotropic; Antitumor; Astringent; Bactericide; Carcinogenic; Co-carcinogenic; Convulsant; Cytotoxic; Depigmentor; Emetic 1 g/orl; Herbicide; Hypertensive; Pesticide; Trypanosomicide.

HYDROXYPHASEOLIN: Fungicide; Pesticide.

HYDROXYPROLINE: Vulnerary.

HYOSCYAMINE: Analgesic; Anticholinergic 150-300 ug/4xday/man; Antidote (Anticholinesterase); Antiemetic; Antiherpetic; Antimeasles; Antimuscarinic; Antineuralgic; Antiparkinsonian; Antipolio; Antisialogogue; Antispasmodic; Antiulcer; Antivertigo; Antivinous; Bronchodilator; Bronchorelaxant; CNS-Depressant; CNS-Stimulant; Cardiotonic; Mydriatic; Pesticide; Photophobigenic; Psychoactive; Sedative; Spasmolytic; Viricide.

HYPERIN: Aldose-Reductase-Inhibitor; Antiinflammatory; Antihepatotoxic; Antiinflammatory; Antioxidant; Antitussive; Antiviral; Capillarifortificant; Capillarigenic; Diuretic; Hepatoprotective; Hypotensive; Pesticide; Viricide.

HYPEROSIDE: Anti-Capillary-Fragility; Antidermatitic; Antiflu; Antiinflammatory; Antiviral; Bactericide 250-500 ug/ml; Cancer-Preventive; Capillarifortificant; Capillarigenic; Diuretic; Hypotensive; Pesticide; Viricide; cAMP-Inhibitor.

IMPERATORIN: Anti-Tumor-Promotor; Antialopecic; Anticonvulsant; Antiinflammatory; Antileukodermic; Antimutagenic; Antivitiligic; Calcium-Antagonist; DME-Inhibitor; Hepatotoxic; Molluscicide.

INDOLE: Anticariogenic; Bactericide; Cancer-Preventive; Insectiphile; Nematicide.

INDOLE-3-ACETIC-ACID: Allelochemic; Cancer-Preventive; Herbicide; Hypoglycemic; Insulinase-Inhibitor; Insulinotonic.

INDOLE-3-CARBINOL: Antitumor; Cancer-Preventive.

INOSITOL: Antialopeic; Anticirrhotic; Antidiabetic; Cholestoerlytic 200 mg/man/day; Lipotropic.

INULIN: Antidiabetic; Immunostimulant.

IODINE: Acnegenic; Antigoiter; Antithyrotoxic; Dermatitigenic; Goitrogenic; Thyrotropic.

IRON: Antiakathisic; Antianemic; Anticheilitic; Antimenorrhagic 100 mg/day/wmn/orl.

ISOCHLOROGENIC-ACID: Antioxidant; Antisepetic; Cancer-Preventive; Pesticide.

ISOFERULIC-ACID: Hypothermic.

ISOFRAXIDIN: Antileukemic; Antimalarial; Cancer-Preventive; Choleretic.

ISOIMPERATORIN: Anti-Tumor-Promoter; Artemicide; DME-Inhibitor; Pesticide.

ISOLEUCINE: Antiencephalopathic; Antipellagric; Essential.

ISOLIQUIRITIGENIN: Aldose-Reductase-Inhibitor; Antiaggregant; Antidepressant; Antidiabetic; Antiulcer; Cancer-Preventive; MAO-Inhibitor; Spasmolytic.

ISOORIENTIN: Larvistat; Pesticide.

ISOPIMPINELLIN: Antiappetant; Antifeedant; Antiinflammatory 100 ppm; Antitubercular; Calcium-Antagonist; Diuretic 125 mg/kg; Insecticide; Molluscicide; Mutagenic; Pesticide.

ISOQUERCITRIN: Aldose-Reductase-Inhibitor; Antifeedant; Antioxidant; Bactericide; Cancer-Preventive; Capillarigenic; Diuretic 10 ppm; Hypotensive; Insectiphile; Pesticide.

ISORHAMNETIN: Antihistaminic; Antiinflammatory; Antioxidant; Bactericide; Cancer-Preventive; Hepatoprotective; Pesticide; Spasmolytic.

ISORHAMNETIN-3-GLUCOSIDE: Hepatoprotective.

ISOVALERIC-ACID—ETHYL-ESTER: Cancer-Preventive.

ISOVITEXIN: Antioxidant; Cancer-Preventive.

JASMONE: Anticariogenic 800-1,600 ug/ml; Bactericide 800-1.600 ug/ml; Cancer-Preventive; Insectiphile; Nematicide; Pesticide.

JUGLONE: Allelochemic; Antidermatophytic; Antifeedant; Antiparasitic; Antimenorrhagic 100 mg/day/wmn/orl; Antiseptic; Antitumor; Antiviral; Bactericide; Fungicide 500 ug/ml; Keratolytic; Pesticide; Sedative; Sternutatory.

KAEMPFERITRIN: Antiinflammatory.

KAEMPFEROL: 5-Lipoxygenase-Inhibitor; Antiallergic; Anti-Tumor-Promoter; Antifertility 250 mg/kg/60 days/orl; Antihistaminic; Antiimplantation; Antiinflammatory 20 mg/kg; Antileukemic 3.1 ug/ml; Antilymphocytic; Antimutagenic; Antioxidant; Antiradicular; Antispasmodic; Antitumor-Promoter; Antiulcer; Antiviral; Bactericide; Cancer-Preventive; Choleretic; Cyclooxygenase-Inhibitor; Diaphoretic; Diuretic; HIV-RT-Inhibitor; Hypotensive; Iodothyronine-Deiodinase-Inhibitor; Lipoxygense-Inhibitor; Mutagenic; Natriuretic; Spasmolytic; Teratologic; Viricide; cAMP-Phosphodiesterase-Inhibitor.

KAEMPFEROL-3-GLUCOSIDE: Choleretic.

KAEMPFEROL-3-RHAMNOSIDE: Aldose-Reductase-Inhibitor.

LACTIC-ACID: Antileukorrheic; Antivaginitic; Antixerotic; Keratolytic.

LANOSTEROL: Cancer-Preventive.

LECITHIN: AntiTourette's 20-50 g/man/day/orl; Antialzheimeran 40-100 g/man/day/orl; Antiataxic; Anticirrhotic; Antidementic; Antidyskinetic 40-80 g/man/day/orl; Antieczemic; Antilithic; Antimanic; Antimorphinistic; Antioxidant Synergist; Antipsoriac; Antisclerogermic; Antiseborrheic; Antisprue; Cholinogenic; Hepatoprotective; Hypocholesterolemic 20-30 g/man/day; Lipotropic.

LEPTINE: Antifeedant; Insecticide; Pesticide.

LEUCINE: Antiencephalopathic.

LEUCOANTHOCYANIN: Antioxidant.

LEVULOSE: Sweetener.

LIGNIN: AntiHIV; Anticancer; Anticoronary; Antidiarrheic; Antinitrosamine; Antioxidant; Antiviral; Bactericide; Chelator; Hypocholesterolemic; Laxative; Pesticide; Viricide.

LIGNOCERIC-ACID: Antihepatotoxic.

LIGUSTILIDE: Antiasthmatic; Spasmolytic.

LIMONENE: AchE-Inhibitor; Allergenic; Antialzheimeran; Anticancer; Antiflu; Antilithic; Antimutagenic; Antitumor; Antiviral; Bactericide; Cancer-Preventive; Candistat; Enterocontractant; Expectorant; Fungiphilic; Fungistat; Herbicide; Insecticide; Insectifuge; Irritant; Nematicide; Pesticide; Sedative; Spasmolytic; Viricide.

LIMONIN: Anticataleptic; Antifeedant; Antimalarial; Antileukemic; Pesticide.

LINALOOL: Allergenic; Antiallergenic; Anticariogenic; Antihistamine; Antiseptic; Antishock; Antiviral; Bactericide; Bronchorelaxant; Cancer-Preventive; Candistat; Expectorant; Fungicide; Insectifuge; Motordepressant; Nematicide; Pesticide; Sedative; Spasmolytic; Termitifuge; Tumor-Promoter; Viricide.

LINALYL-ACETATE: Sedative; Spasmolytic.

LINARIN: Aldose-Reductase-Inhibitor.

LINOLEIC-ACID: AntiMS; Antianaphylactic; Antiarteriosclerotic; Antiarthritic; Anticoronary; Antieczemic; Antifibrinolytic; Antigranular; Antihistaminic; Anitinflammatory; Antimenorrhagic; Antiprostatic; Cancer Preventive; Carcinogenic; Hepatoprotective; Immunomodulator; Insectifuge; Metastatic; Nematicide.

LIRIODENINE: Analgesic; Antidermatophytic; Antitumor; Bactericide; Candidicide; Cytotoxic; Fungicide; Sedative.

LITHIUM: AntiPMS; Antidepressant; Antihyperthyroid; Antimanic; Antipyschotic; Antischizophrenic; Deliriant; Nephrotoxic.

LUPEOL: Antirheumatic; Antitumor; Antiurethrotic; Cytotoxic 50-500 ppm.

LUTEOLIN: Aldose-Reductase-Inhibitor; Anticataract; Antidermatic; Antifeedant; Antiherpetic; Anti-histaminic; Antiinflammatory; Antimutagenic; Antioxidant; Antipolio; Antispasmodic; Antitussive; Antiviral; Bactericide; Cancer-Preventive; Choleretic; Deiodinase-Inhibitor; Diuretic; Iodothyronine-Deiodinase-Inhibitor; Spasmolytic; Xanthine-Oxidase-Inhibitor.

LUTEOLIN-7-O-BETA-GLUCOSIDE: Cancer-Preventive; Cholagogue.

LYCOPENE: Antioxidant; Antiradicular; Antitumor; Cancer-Preventive.

LYSINE: Antialkalotic; Antiherpetic 2,000 — mg/man/day; Hypoarginanemic; 250 mg/kg.

MAGNESIUM: AntiPMS 400-800 mg/day/wmn/orl; Antiaggregant; Antianorectic; Antianxiety 400 mg/day; Antianginal 400 mg/day; Antiarrhythmic; Antiarthritic; Antiasthmatic; Antiatherosclerotic 400 mg/day; Anticonvulsant; Antidepressant; Antidiabetic 400 mg/day; Antidysmenorrheic 100 mg/4xday; Antiepileptic 450 mg/day; Antihyperkinetic; Antihypoglycemic; Antiinflammatory 100 mg/4xday; Antiinsomniac; Antilithic; Antimastalgic; Antimigraine 200 mg/day; Antineurotic; Antiosteo-porotic 500-1,000 mg/day/wmn/oral; Antispasmophilic 500 mg/day; CNS-depressant; Calcium-Antagonist; Hypocholesterolemic 400 mg/day; Hypotensive 260-500 mg/day; Myorelaxant 100 mg/4xday; Uterorelaxant 100 mg/4xday; Vasodilator.

MALIC-ACID: Bacteristat; Bruciphobe; Hemopoietic; Laxative; Pesticide; Sialogogue.

MALTOSE: Sweetener.

MANGANESE: Antialcoholic; Antianemic; Antidiabetic; Antidiscotic; Antidyskinetic; Antiepileptic 450 mg/day; Antiotic.

MANNITOL: Allergenic; Anthelminthic; AntiReye's; Antiglaucomic; Antiinflammatory; Antimuta-genic; Antinephritic; Antioxidant; Antiradicular; Diuretic; Emetic; Laxative; Nephrotoxic; Pesticide; Spasmolytic.

MASLINIC-ACID: Antihistaminic; Antiinflammatory.

MAYSIN: Juvabional; Larvistat; Pesticide.

MEDICAGENIC-ACID: Aphicide; Candidicide; Fungicide 7.5-25 ppm; Molluscicide 7.5-25 ppm; Pesticide.

MEDICAGOL: Fungicide; Pesticide.

MENTHOL: Analgesic; Anesthetic; Antiaggregant; AntiAllergic; Antibronchitic; Antidandruff; Antihalitosic; Antihistaminic; Antiinflammatory; Antineuralgic; Antiodontalgic; Antipruritic; Antirheumatic; Antiseptic; Antisinusitic; Bactericide; Bradycardic 65 mg/3xday/woman; Bronchomucolytic; Bronchomucotropic; Bronchorrheic; CNS-Stimulant; CNS-Depressant; Calcium-Antagonist; Carminative; Ciliotoxic; Congestant; Convulsant; Counterirritant; Decongestant; Dermatitigenic; Diaphoretic; Enterorelaxant; Expectorant; Gastrosedative; Myorelaxant; Nematicide; Neurodepressant; Neuropathogenic; Nociceptive; Pesticide; Refrigerant; Rubefacient; Spasmolytic; Vibriocide.

MENTHONE: Analgesic; Antiseptic; Cancer-Preventive; Sedative; Spasmolytic.

METHIONINE: Anticataract; Antidote (Acetominaphen) 10 g/6hr/man/orl; Antidote (Paracetamol) 10 g/16 hr/man/orl; Antieczemic; Antihepatotic; Antioxidant; Antiparkinsonian 1-5 g/day; Cancer-Preventive; Emetic; Essential; Glutathionigenic; Hepatoprotective; Lipotropic; Urine-Acidifier 200 mg/3xday/man/orl; Urine-Deodorant.

METHYL-GALLATE: Antileukemic; Antiseptic; Antitumor; Bactericide; Pesticide; Reverse-Transcriptase-Inhibitor; Xanthine-Oxidase-Inhibitor.

METHYL-SALICYLATE: Allergenic; Analgesic; Antiinflammatory; Antipyretic; Antiradicular; Antirheumatalgic; Cancer-Preventive; Carminative; Counterirritant; Dentifrice; Insectifuge.

MOLYBDENUM: Anticancer.

MUCILAGE: Cancer-Preventive; Demulcent.

MYRCENE: Allergenic; Analgesic; Antimutagenic; Antinociceptive 10-20 mg/kg ipr mus; Antinociiceptive 20-40 mg/kg scu mus; Antioxidant; Bactericide; Fungicide; Insectifuge; Pesticide; Spasmolytic.

MYRICETIN: Allelochemic; Antiallergenic; Antifeedant; Antigastric; Antigonadotrophic; Antihistamine; Antiinflammatory; Antimutagenic; Antioxidant; Bactericide; Cancer-Preventive; Candidicide; Diuretic; Hypoglycemic; Larvistat; Lipoxygenase-Inhibitor; Mutagenic; Oxidase-Inhibitor; Pesticide; Tyrosine-Kinase-Inhibitor.

MYRISTIC-ACID: Cancer-Preventive; Nematicide.

MYRISTICIN: Amphetaminagenic; Anesthetic; Antiaggregant; Antidepressant; Antiinflammatory; Antioxidant 25-100 mg/kg/orl; Antistress; Cancer-Preventive 10 mg/mus/orl/day; Hypnotic; Hypotensive; Insecticide; Insecticide-Synergist; MAO-Inhibitor; Neurotoxic; Oxytoxic; Paralytic; Pesticide; Psychoactive; Sedative; Serotinergic; Spasmolytic; Tachycardic; Uterotonic.

N-BUTYLPHTHALIDE: Anticonvulsant.

N-HENTRIACONTANE: Antiinflammatory; Diuretic.

N-HEXACOSANE: Bacteristat; Pesticide.

N-METHYL-TYRAMINE: Cancer-Preventive.

NARCOTINE: Analgesic; Antitussive; Sedative.

NARINGENIN: Alsdose-Reductase-Inhibitor; Antiaggregant; Antihepatotoxic; Antiherpetic; Antiinflammatory 20 ppm; Antileukemic 10 ug/ml; Antimutagenic; Antioxidant; Antiperoxidant; Antispasmodic; Antiulcer; Antiviral; Bactericide 500 ug/ml; Cancer-Preventive; Choleretic; Decarboxylase-Inhibitor; Fungicide; Fungistatic; Pesticide; Serotonin-Inhibitor; cAMP-Phosphodiesterase-Inhibitor.

NARINGIN: Antidermatitic; Antiinflammatory; Antioxidant; Antiviral; Cancer-Preventive; Pesticide.

NEOANNONIN: Larvicide 72-70 ppm diet; Ovicide 62-70 ppm diet.

NERAL: Bactericide; Pesticide.

NEROL: Bactericide, Pesticide.

NIACIN: AntiMeniere's; Antiacrodynic; Antiallergenic 50 mg/2xday/; Antiamblyopic; Antianginal; Antichilblain; Anticonvulsant 3 g/day; Antidermatic; Antidysphagic; Antieleptic 3 g/day; Antihistaminic 50 mg/2x/day; Antihyperactivity 1.5-6 g/day; Antineuralgic; Antiinsomniac; Antineuralgic; Antiparkinsonian 100 mg day; Antipellagric; Antiscotomic; Antispasmodic 100 mg/2xday; Antivertigo; Cancer-Preventive; Hepatoprotective; Hypoglycemic; Hypolipidemic; Sedative; Serotenergic; Vasodilator.

NICKEL: Antiadrenaline; Anticirrhotic; Insulin-Sparing.

NICOTINE: ANS-Paralytic; ANS-Stimulant; Antifeedant; Cholinergic; Dopaminigenic; Ectoparasiticde; Herbicide; Insecticide; Pesticide.

NICOTINAMIDE: Cancer-Preventive; Depressant.

NOBILETIN: Antiallergic; Antihistamine; Antiproliferative; Cancer-Preventive; Chloinergic; Fungicide; Fungistatic; Pesticide.

NODAKENIN: Antiaggregant.

NONACOSANE: Antimutagenic 250 ug/ml; Antiviral.

NOOTKATONE: Antiulcer.

NORADRENALIN: Adrenergic; Antishock; Hypertensive; Inotropic; Neurotransmitter; Sympathomimetic; Vasoconstrictor.

NORHARMAN: Tremorogenic.

O-CRESOL: Allelochemic; Antimutagenic; Antiseptic; Cancer-Preventive; Pesticide; Rodenticide.

OBACUNONE: Anticataleptic; Antifeedant; Pesticide.

OCTACOSANOL: Antiviral; Hypolipidemic.

ODORIN: Bactericide; Pesticide.

OLEANOLIC-ACID: Abortifacient; Anticariogenic; Antifertility; Antihepatotoxic; Antiinflammatory; Atioxidant; Antisarcomic; Cancer-Preventive; Cardiotonic; Diuretic; Hepatoprotective; Uterotonic.

OLEANIC-ACID-METHYL-ESTER: Hemolytic.

OLEIC-ACID: Anemiagenic; Cancer-Preventive; Choleretic 5 ml/man; Dermatigenic; Insectifuge; Percutaneostimulant.

OLEUROPEIN: Antiarrhthmic; Antihypertensive; Bacteristat; Coronary-Dilator; Hypotensive; Spasmolytic; Vasodilator.

ORIENTIN: Antiinflammatory; Cancer-Preventive; cAMP-Phosphodiesterase-Inhibitor.

ORNITHINE: Anticholesteremic; Antiencephalopathic; Hypoammonemic; Hyparginanemic.

OSTHOLE: Antimalarial; Juvabional; Pesticide.

OXYPEUCEDANIN: Anti-Tumor-Promoter; Calcium-Antagonist; DME-Inhibitor.

OXYPEUCEDANIN-HYDRATE: Calcium-Antagonist.

P-AMINOBENZOIC-ACID: Antineoplastic; Antirickettsial; Bactericide; Cancer-Preventive; Choleretic; Lipoxygenase-Inhibitor; Pesticide; Sunscreen.

P-COUMARIC-ACID: Allelopathic; Antifertility; Antineoplastic; Antihepatotoxic; Antioxidant; Antiperoxidant; Antitumor; Bactericide; Cancer-Preventive; Choloretic; Lipoxygenase-Inhibitor; Pesticide; Prostaglandin-Synthesis-Inhibitor.

P-CRESOL: Allelochemic; Antimutagenic; Antiseptic; Cancer-Preventive; Parasiticide; Pesticide; Rodenticide.

P-CYMENE: Analgesic; Antiflu; Antirheumatalgic; Antiviral; Bactericide; Fungicide; Herbicide; Insectifuge; Pesticide; Viricide.

P-HYDROXYCINNAMIC-ACID: Antioxidant.

P-HYDROXYBENZALDEHYDE: Antifeedant.

P-HYDROXYBENZOIC-ACID: Antimutagenic; Antioxidant; Antisickling; Bactericide; Cancer-Preventive; Fungistat; Immunosuppressant; Pesticide; Phytoalexin; Prostaglandigenic; Ubiquiot.

PALMITIC-ACID: Antifibrinolytic; Hemolytic; Nematicide; Pesticide.

PANGAMIC-ACID: Antifibrinolytic; Hepatoprotective.

PANTOTHENIC-ACID: Antiallergenic; Antiarthritic; Anticephalagic; Anticlaudificant; Antidermatic; Antihypercholestorlemic; Antifatigue; Antiielus; Antiinsomniac; Antirheumatic; Cancer-Prevention.

PARAFFIN: Antihemoorhoidal; Antiproctalgic; Emollient; Laxative 45 ml/day/orl/man.

PATULETIN: Cholagogue; Spasmolytic.

PECTIN: Antiatheromic 15 g /man/day; Antidiabetic 10 g/man/day/orl; Antidiarrheic; Antitumor; Antitussive; Antiulcer; Bactericide; Cancer-Preventive; Demulcent; Hemostat; Hypocholesterolemic; Pesticide.

PECTINASE: Pectinolytic.

PELARGONIDIN: Antiherpetic; Antiviral; Cancer-Preventive.

PELLETIERINE: Anthelminic; Cestodicine; Emetic; Hypertensive; Mydriatic; Oxyuricide; Pesticide; Taenicide.

PHASEOL: Fungicide; Pesticide.

PHASEOLLIN: Antiseptic 25 ug/ml; Fungicide; Pesticide.

PHELLANDRENE: Hyperthermic; Spasmogenic.

PHELLOPTERIN: Calcium-Antagonist.

PHENETHYLAMINE: Insectifuge; Irritant; Pesticide.

PHENOL: Anesthetic; Anodyne; AntimMS; Antihemorrhoidal; Antihydrocoele; Antiincontinence; Antionychogryphotic; Antiotitic; Antioxidant; Antiprostatitic; Antipyruvetic; Antiseptic; Antisinustic; Antispastic; Antiviral; Antiwrinkle; Bactericide; CNS-Depressant; Cancer-Preventive; Carciongenic; Emetic; Fungicide; Hemolytic; Pesticide; Rodenticide; Vasodilator; Viricide.

PHENYLALANINE: Anti-attention-deficit-disorder 587 mg/day/orl; Antidepressant 50 — 500 mg/day/man; Antiparkinsonian 200 — 500 mg/day/man; Antisickling; Antivitiligic 100 mg/kg/day/orl/man; Monoamine-Precursor; Tremorigenic 1,600-12,600 mg/man/day.

PHLORETIN: Antiallergic; Antifeedant; Bactericide 30 ppm; Lipoxygenase-Inhibitor.

PHLORIZIN: Anticonvulsant; Antifeedant; Antimalarial; Glucosuric 100 ppm; Neuroparalytic; Pesticide; Sedative.

PHOROGLUCINOL: Anti-Tumor-Promoter; Antiseptic; Cancer-Preventive; Decalcifier; Fungicide; Pesiticide.

PHOSPHATIDYL-CHOLINE: Antialzheimeran 25 g/day/orl; Antimanic 15-30 g/man/day/orl.

PHOSPHORUS: Antiosteoporotic; Immunostimulant; Osteogenic.

PHYTIC-ACID: Cancer-Preventive.

PHYTOHAEMAGGLUTININ: Anticancer; Lectin.

PINENE: Antiseptic; Bactericide; Expectorant; Fungicide; Herbicide; Pesticide; Spasmogenic; Spasmolytic.

PIPERIDINE: CNS-Depressant; Insectifuge; Pesticide; Spinoconvulsant.

PINITOL: Antidiabetic; Antifeedant; Expectorant; Insectifuge; Pesticide.

PIPERITONE: Antiasthmatic; Herbicide; Insectifuge; Pesticide.

PISATIN: Bactericide 50 ug/ml; Fungicide; Pesticide.

POTASSIUM: Antiarrhythmic; Antidepressant; Antifatigue; Antihypertensive; Cardiotoxic 18,000 mg/man/day; Spasmolytic.

PROPIONIC-ACID: Fungicide; Pesticide.

PROTOCATECHUIC-ACID: Antiarrhythmic; Antiasthmatic; Antihepatotoxic; Antiherpetic; Antiinflammatory; Antiischemic; Antiophide; Antioxidant; Antiperoxidant; Antispasmodic; Antitussive; Antiviral; Bactericide; Fungicide; Immunostimulant; Pesticide; Phagocytotic; Prostaglandigenic; Ubiquiot; Viricide.

PRUNASIN: Cyanogenic.

PSORALEN: Antileukodermic; Antimitotic; Antimutagenic; Antipsoriac; Antitubercular; Antitumor; Anti-Tumor-Promoter; Antileukemic; Antipsoriac; Antiviral; Artemicide; Bacteriophagicide; Calcium-Antogonist; Cancer-Preventive; Contraceptive; Cytotoxic; Fungicide; Genotoxic; Hypotensive; Mutagenic; Pesticide; Photocarcinogenic; Phototoxic; Phytoalexin; Viricide.

PTEROSTILBENE: Antidiabetic; Bactericide; Hyperglycemic; Hypoglycemic 10-50 mg/kg; Insecticide; Pesticide; Phytoalexin.

PUCHIIN: Bactericide; Pesticide.

PUFA: AntiMS; Antiacne; Antieczemic; Antipolyneuritic.

PULEGONE: AchE-Inhibitor; AntiAlzheimeran; Antihistaminic; Antipyretic; Avifuge; Bactericide; Cancer-Preventive; Candicide; Cerebrotoxic; Encephalopathic; Fungicide; Glutathionalytic; Hepatotoxic; Herbicide; Insecticide; Insectifuge; Nephrotoxic; Neurotoxic; Perfumery; Pesticide; Pulifuge; Pulmonotoxic; Sedative.

PUNICALAGIN: AntiHIV; Pesticide.

PUNICALIN: AntiAIDS; HIV-RT-Inhibitor; Pesticide.

PYRIDOXINE: Anti-carpal-tunnel 100-150 mg/day/12; Anti-morning-sickness; AnitPMS 100 mg/day/orl/wmn; Antiacne; Antiacne; Antiaggregant; Antianemic 50-400 mg/man/day; Antiautistic; Anticheilitic; Antidepresant; Antidermatitic; Antidiabetic; Antidote (Hydrazine) 10 g; Antidyskinetic 250-300 mg/man/4x/day; Antiemetic 20-200 mg/man/day; Antiepileptic; Antiglossitic; Antihyperkinetic; Antinephritic; Antineurotic 150 mg/man/day; Antioxaluric; Antiparkinsonian; Antiprolaactin; Antiradiation; Antischizophrenic 50 mg/man/3xday; Antiseborrheic; Antisickling; Antiulcer; Anti-vertigo; Dopaminergic; Neurotoxic 2-6 g/day for 2-24 months.

PYROGLUTAMIC-ACID: Antilipolytic; Insulinic.

QUERCETIN: 5-Lipoxygenase-Inhibitor; ATPase-Inhibitor; Aldose-Reductase-Inhibitor; Allelochemic; Allergenic; Anti-Tumor-Promoter; Anti-lipo-peroxidant; AntiCrohn's 400 mg/man/3xday; AntiPMS 500 mg/2xday/wmn; Antiaggregant; Antiallergic; Antianaphylactic; Antiasthmatic; Antic-arcinomic (Breast); Anticataract; Anticolitic 400 mg/man/3x/day; Antidermatic 400 mg/man/3x day; Antidiabetic; Antiencephalitic; Antiestrogenic; Antifeedant; Antiflu; Antigastric; Antigonadotropic; Antihepatotoxic; Antiherpetic; Antihistaminic; Antihydrophophic; Antihypertensive; Antiinflammatory; Antileukotrienic; Antimalarial; Antimutagenic; Antimyocarditic; Antioxidant; Antiperiodontal; Antipermeability; Antiperoxidant; Antipharnygitic; Antiplaque; Antipodriac; Antipolio; Antiprostanoid; Antipsoriac; Antiradicular; Antispasmodic; Antithiamin; Antitumor; Antiviral; Bactericide; Bradycardiac; Calmodulin-Antagonist; Cancer-Preventive; Capillariaprotective; Carcinogenic; Catabolic; Cyclooxygenase-Inhibitor; Diaphoretic; HIV-RT-Inhibitor; Hepatomagenic; Hypoglyemic; Insulinogenic; Juvabiol; Larvistat; Lipoxygenase-Inhibitor; Mast-Cell-Stabilizer; Mutagenic; Ornithine-Decarboxylase-Inhibitor; Pesticide; Protein-Kinase-C-Inhibitor; Spasmolytic; Teratologic; Tumorigenic; Tyrosine-Kinase-Inhibitor; Vasodilator; Xanthine-Oxidase-Inhibitor; cAMP-Phosphodiesterase-Inhibitor.

QUERCETIN-3-GALACTOSIDE: Antiinflammatory.

QUERCETIN-3-O-BETA-D-GLUCOSIDE: Antiinflammatory; Cancer-Preventive.

QUERCETIN-3-RHAMNOGLUCOSIDE: Antiinflammatory; Choleretic; Diuretic; Spasmolytic.

QUERCITRIN: Aldose-Reductase-Inhibitor; Antiarrhythmnic; Anticataract; Antiedemic; Antifeedant; Antiflu; Antihemorrhagic; Antihepatotoxic; Antiherpetic; Antiinflammatory; Antimutagenic; Antioxidant; Antipurpuric; Antispasmodic; Antithombogenic; Antitumor; Antiulcer; Antiviral; Bactericide; CNS-Depressant; Cancer-Preventive; Cardiotonic; Choleretic; Detoxicant; Diuretic; Hemostat; Hepatotonic; Hypoglycemic; Hypotensive; Insectiphile; Paralytic; Pesticide; Spasmolytic; Vasopressor; Viricide.

QUINIC-ACID: Choleretic.

RAPHANIN: Bactericide; Fungicide; Pesitcide.

RESVERATROL: Artemicide; Bactericide; Fungicide; Hypocholesterolemic; Pesticide; Phytoalexin.

RETICULINE: Analgesic; Antidopaminergic; Bactericide; CNS Stimulant; Convulsant; Hyperthermic; Spasmolytic.

REYNOUTRIN: Aldose-Reductase-Inhibitor.

RHOIFOLIN: Aldose-Reductase-Inhibitor; Antiarrhthmic.

RIBOFLAVIN: Antiarabiflavinotic 2-10 mg/oral/day; Anticarpal-Tunnel 50 mg/day; Anticheilotic; Anticataract 15 mg/day; Anticheilitic; Antidecubitic; Antiglossitic; Antikeratitic; Antimigraine; Antipellagric; Antiphotophobic; Cancer-Preventive.

RIBONUCLEASE: Analgesic; Antiarthritic.

RIBONUCLEIC-ACID: Antiasthenic; Antidementic; Memorigenic.

RICINOLEIC-ACID: Carcinogenic; Spermicide.

RISHITIN: Pesticide; Phytoalexin.

ROSMARINIC-ACID: AchE-Inhibitor; Antianaphylactic 1-100 mg/kg orl; Anticomplementary; Antiedemic 0.316-3.16 mg; Antigonadotropic; Antihemolytic; Antihepatotoxic; Antiherpetic 50 ug/ml; Antiinflammatory; Antileukotrienic; Antilipoperoxidant; Antioxidant; Antipulmonotic; Antiradicular; Antishock; Antithyreotropic; Antithyroid; Antiviral; Bactericide; Cancer-Preventive; Deiodinase-Inhibitor; Pesticide; Viricide.

RUTIN: Aldose-Reductase-Inhibitor; Anti-Capillary-Fragility 20-100 mg orl/man; Anti-Tumor-Promoter; Antiapoplectic; Antiatherogenic; Anticataract; Anticonvulsant; Antidermatitic; Antidiabetic; Antiedemic; Antierythemic; Antifeedant; Antiglaucomic 60 mg/day; Antihmaturic; Antihepatotoxic; Antiherpectic; Antihistaminic; Antihypertensive; Antiinflammatory 20 mg/kg; Antimalarial; Antimutagenic; Antinephritic; Antioxidant; Antipurpuric; Antiradicular; Antithrombogenic; Antitrypanosomic 100 mg/kg; Antitumor; Antivaricosity; Antiviral; Bactericide; Cancer-Preventive; Capillariprotective; Catabolic; Estrogenic; Hemostat; Hypotensive; Insecticide; Insectiphile; Juvabional; Larvistat; Lioxygenase-Inhibitor; Mutagenic; Myorelaxant; Mutagenic; Myorelaxant; Oviposition-Stimulant; Pesticide; Spasmolytic; Vasopressor; Viricide; Phosphdiesterase-Inhibitor.

S-ALLYL-CYSTEINE-SULFOXIDE: Antiatherogenic; Antioxidant; Antiperoxidant; Hypocholesterolemic; Lipolytic.

SAFROLE: Anesthetic; Antiaggregant; Anticonvulsant; Antiseptic; Bactericide; CNS-Depressant; Cancer-Preventive; Carcinogenic; Carminative; DNA-Binder; Hepatoregenerative; Hypothermic; Nematicide; Neurotoxic; Pediculide; Pesticide; Psychoactive; Tremorigenic.

SAKURANETIN: Antiseptic; Bactericide; Fungicide; Pesticide.

SALICYLIC-ACID: Analgesic; Antidermatotic; Anticirrhotic; Anticoronary; Antidandruff; Antidote (Mercury); Antieczemic; Antiichthyosic; Antiinflammatory; Antikeshan; Antineuralgic; Antioncychomycotic; Antioxidant; Antiperiodic; Antipodagric; Antpsoriac; Antipyretic; Antirheumatic; Antiseborrheic; Antiseptic; Antitumor; Antitympanitic; Bactericide; Cancer-Preventive; Comedolytic; Cyclo-Oxygenase-Inhibitor; Dermatitigenic; Febrifuge; Fungicide; Hypoglycemic; Insectifuge; Keratolytic; Pesticide; Tineacide; Ulcerogenic.

SCOLYMOSIDE: Choleretic.

SCOPOLETIN: Allelochemic; Analgesic; Antiasthmatic; Antiedemic; Antifeedant; Antiinflammatory; Antileukotriengoenic; Antiseptic; Antitumor; CNS-Stimulant; Cancer-Preventive; Hypoglycemic; Hypotensive; Myorelaxant; Pesticide; Phytoalexin; Spasmolytic; Uterosedative.

SCUTELLAREN: Aldose-Reductase-Inhibitor; Antihemolytic; Cancer-Preventive; Phospholipase-A1-Inhibitor.

SELENIUM: Analgesic 200 ug/day; Antiacne 200 ug/day; Anorexic; Antiaggregant; Anticirrhotic; Anticoronary 200 ug/day; Antidandruff; Antidote (Mercury); Antikeshan; Antileukotrienic; Antimyalgic 200 ug/day; Antiosteoarthritic; Antioxidant; Antiulcerogenic; Cancer-Preventive; Depressant; Fungicide; Pesticide; Prostaglandin-Sparer.

SELINENE: Expectorant.

SERINE: Cancer-Preventive.

SEROTONIN: Abortifacient; Antiaggregant; Antialzheimeran; Antigastric; Antigastrisecretogogic; Bronchoconstrictor.

SESELIN: Fungicide; Pesticide.

SHIKIMIC-ACID: Bruchifuge; Carcinogenic; Ileorelaxant; Mutagenic; Pesticide; Spasmolytic.

SILICON: Antiarteriosclerotic.

SILVER: Astringent; Bactericide.

SINAPIC-ACID: Antihepatotoxic; Antioxidant; Bactericide; Cancer-Preventive; Fungicide; Pesticide.

SINIGRIN: Cancer-Preventive; Larvicide; Pesticide; Phagostimulant.

SOLAMARGINE: Antitumor; Cytotoxic; Erythrocytolytic; Fungicide; Hepatoprotective; Membranolytic; Pesticide.

SOLANIDINE: Antifeedant; Pesticide.

SOLANINE: Antiasthmatic; Antibronchitic; Antiepileptic; Antiparkinsonian; Cardiodepressant; Cardiotonic; Hemolytic; Memranolytic; Myostimulant; Narcotic; Sedative; Teratogenic.

SOLASODINE: Antiandrogenic 20 mg/kg; Antiinflammatory; Antispermatogenic; Antitumor; Contraceptive; Cytotoxic; Fungicide; Hepatoprotective; Pesticide; Teratogenic.

SOLASONINE: Antitumor; Cardiodepressant; Cardiotonic; Erythroyctolytic; Hemolytic; Hepatoprotective; Insecticide; Memranolytic; Molluscicide; Myostimulant; Pesticide.

SORBITOL: Antidiabetic (Insuling Sparing) 30 g/man/day; Antiketotic; Cathartic; Diuretic; Laxative 5-15 g/man/day; Purgative.

SPIRAEOSIDE: Aldose-Reductase-Inhibitor.

SQUALENE: Antitumor; Bactericide; Cancer-Preventive; Immunostimulant; Lipoxygenase-Inhibitor; Pesticide.

SQUAMOCIN: Cytotoxic; Larvicide; Ovicide.

STACHYDRINE: Cardiotonic; Emmenagogue; Insectifuge; Lactagogue; Oxytocic; Systolic-Depressant.

STARCH: Absorbent; Antidote (Iodine); Antinesidioblastosic; Emollient; Poultice.

STIGMASTEROL: Antihepatotoxic; Antiinflammatory; Antiophidic; Antiviral; Artemicide; Cancer-Preventive; Estrogenic; Hypocholesterolemic; Ovulant; Sedative; Viricide.

SUCCINIC-ACID: Antifeedant; Bruchiphobe; Cancer-Preventive; Pesticide.

SUCROSE: Aggregant; Antihiccup 1 tsp; Antiopthalmic; Antioxidant; Atherogenic; Flatugenic; Hypercholesterolemic.

SULFUR: Acarifuge; Antiacne; Antidandruff; Antigrey; Antiseborrheic; Antiseptic; Comedogenic; Keratolytic; Laxative; Triglycerolytic; Uricogenic; Vulnerary.

SYNEPHRINE: Cancer-Preventive.

SYRINGALDEHYDE: Antidemic; Antiinflammatory; Cancer-Preventive.

SYRINGIN: Adaptogenic; Antistress; Immunostimulant; Neurotropic; Tonic.

TANGERETIN: Antiallergic; Antihistaminic; Antiproliferative; Cancer-Preventive.

TANNIN: Antidiarrheic; Antidysenteric; Antimutagenic; Antinephritic; Antiophidic; Antioxidant; Anti-radicular 500 mg/kg/da/orl; Antirenitic; Antiviral; Bactericide; Cancer-Preventive; Hepatoprotective; Immunosuppressant; Pesticide; Psychotropic; Viricide.

TARTARIC-ACID: Acidifier; Antioxidant; Synergist.

TERPINEN-4-OL: Antiallergic; Antiasthmatic; Antiseptic; Antitussive; Bacteriostatic; Diuretic; Fungicide; Herbicide; Insectifuge; Nematicide; Pesticide; Spermicide; Vulnerary.

TERPINOLENE: Deodorant; Fungicide; Pesticide.

TETRAMETHYLPYRAZINE: Antiaggregant; Antianginal; Anticholinergic; Antidecubitic; Antideliriant; Antidysmenorrheic; Antiembolic; Antiencephalopathic; Antifatigue; Antigastritic; Antiheartburn; Antiherpetic; Antihistaminic 1 mg/kg; Antihypertensive; Antimigraine; Antimyocarditic; Antineuropathic 50 mg; Antipolio; Arteriodilator; Bactericide; Cardiotonic; Diuretic; Hypotensive; Insectifuge 75-150 mg/man/day; Pesticide; Schistosomidice; Spasmolytic; Uterosedative.

THIAMIN: Analgesic 1-4 g/day; Antialcoholic; Antialzheimeran 100-3,000 mg/day; Antianorectic; Antiback-ache 1-4 g/day; Antiberiberi; Anticardiospasmic; Anticolitic; Antidecubitic; Antideliriant; Antiencephalopathic; Antiheartburn; Antiherpetic; Antimigraine; Antimyocarditic; Antineurasthenic; Antineuritic; Antipoliomyelitic; Insectifuge 75-150 mg/man/day; Pesticide.

THYMOL: AchE-Inhibitor; Anesthetic; Anthelminthic; Antiacne; Antiaggregant; Antialzheimeran; Antibronchitic; Antihalitosic; Antiherpetic; Antiinflammatory; Antimelanomic; Antineuritic; Antioxidant; Antiplaque; Aniradicular; Antirheumatic; Antiseptic; Antispasmodic; Antitussive; Bactericide; Carminative; Counterirritant; Dentifrice; Deodorant; Dermatitigenic; Enterorelaxant; Expectorant; Fungicide; Gastroirritant; Larvicide; Myorelaxant; Pesticide; Spasmolytic; Sprout-Inhibitor; Tracheorelaxant; Urinary-Antiseptic; Vermicide.

THREONINE: Antioxidant; Antiulcer.

TIN: Antiacne; Bactericide; Pesticide; Taenicide.

TOLUENE: Encephalopathic.

TOMATIDINE: Antifeedant; Pesticide.

TOMATINE: Antiinflammatory; Bactericide; Fungicide; Molluscicide; Pesticide.

TRANS-BETA-FARNESENE: Insectifuge; Pesticide; Pheromone.

TRANS-FERULIC-ACID: Antioxidant; Cancer-Preventive.

TRANS-ISOASARONE: Bactericide; Bronchospasmolytic; Pesticide; Secretolyic.

TRIACONTANAL: Antihepatotoxic; Hormone; Hypolipidemic.

TRICIN: Antileukemic 6-12 mg/kg; Antioxidant; Antitumor; Estrogenic.

TRIGONELLINE: Anticancer; Antihyperglycemic; Antimigraine; Antiseptic; Hypocholesterolemic; Hypoglcyemic 500-3,000 mg/man/day; Pesticide.

TRIFOLIN: Aldose-Reductase-Inhibitor.

TRYPTAMINE: Hypertensive; Vasopressor.

TRYPTOPHAN: Analgesic 750 mg/4xday/orl/man; Antianxiety 500-1,000 mg/meal; Antidepressant 1-3 g/3xday/orl/man; Antidyskinetic 2-8 g/orl/wmn/day; Antihypertensive; Antiinsomniac 1-3 g/day; Antimanic 12 g/man/day/orl; Animenopausal 6 g/day; Antimigraine 500 mg/man/4xday; Antioxidant; Antiparkinsonian 2 g/3xday; Antiphenylketonuric; Anitpyschotic 12 g/man/day; Antirheumatic; Carcinogenic; Essential; Hypnotic; Hypoglycemic; Hypotensive 3 g/day; Insulinase-Inhibitor; Insulinotonic; Monoamine-Precursor; Prolactinogenic; Sedative 3-10 g/man/day; Serotonigenic 6-12 g/day/orl/man; Tumor-Promoter.

TUBEROSIN: Antistaphylococcic; Antitubercular; Bactericide; Fungicide; Pesticide.

TULIPOSIDE-A: Antiallergic.

TYRAMINE: Adrenergic; Antiaggregant; Insectifuge; Pesticide; Vasopressor.

TYROSINASE: Antihypertensive.

TYROSINE: Antidepressant; Antiencephalopathic; Antiparkinsonian 100 mg/kg/day; Antipheylketonuric; Antiulcer; Cancer-Preventive; Monoamine-Precursor.

UBIQUINONE-10: Anticardotic; Cardioprotective.

UMBELLIFERONE: Allelochemic; Antihistaminic; Antiinflammatory; Antimitotic; Antimutagenic; Antiprostaglandin; Antiseptic; Antispasmodic; Bactericide; Cancer-Preventive; Choleretic; Fungicide; Lipoxygenase-Inhibitor; Pesticide.

URSOLIC-ACID: Antiarthritic; Anticholestatic 28-100 mg/kg orl; Antidiabetic; Antiedemic; Antihepatotoxic 5-20 mg/kg; Antihistaminic; Antiinflammatory; Antileukemic; Antimutagenic; Antiobesity; Antioxidant; Antitumor; Antitumor-Promoter; Antiulcer; CNS-Depressant; Cancer-Preventive; Choleretic 5-20 mg/kg orl; Cytotoxic; Diuretic; Hepatoprotective; Hypoglycemic; Pesticide; Piscicide; Potassium-Sparing; Prostisticide; Sodium-Sparing.

UVAOL: Antitumor; Cytotoxic 100-200 ppm.

VALERIANIC-ACID: Spasmolytic.

VALINE: Antiencephalopathic.

VANADIUM: ATPase-Inhibitor; Antiatherosclerotic; Antiinfertility; Antimanic; Cancer-Preventive; Cardioprotective; Hypocholestorelemic.

VANILLIC-ACID: Anthelminthic; Antifatigue; Antioxidant; Antisickling; Ascaricide; Bactericide; Cancer-Preventive; Choleretic; Immunosuppressant; Laxative; Pesticide; Ubiquiot.

VANILLIN: Allelochemic; Antimutagenic; Antipolio; Antiviral; Cancer-Preventive; Fungicide; Immunosuppressant; Insectifuge; Irritant; Pesticide.

VERBASCOSIDE: Antiseptic; Antitumor; Bactericide; Immunosuppressant; Pesticide.

VICENIN-2: Antiinflammatory.

VITEXIN: Aldose-Reductase-Inhibitor; Antiarrhythmic; Antibradinquinic; Antidermatic; Antihistaminic; Antiinflammatory; Antiserotoninic; Antithyroid; Cancer-Preventive; Goitrogenic; Hypotensive; Thyroid-Peroxidase-Inhibitor; cAMP-Phosphodiesterase-Inhibitor.

XANTHOPHYLL: Bruchifuge; Insectifuge; Pesticide.

XANTHOTOXIN: Anti-Tumor-Promoter; Antidermatitic; Antifeedant; Antihistaminic; Antiinflammatory 20 mg/man/day; Antikerato; Antileucodermic; Antilymphomic 600 ug/kg; Antimitotic 5-25 ug/ml; Antimutagenic; Antimycotic; Antipityriasic; Antipruritic; Antipsoriac; Antiscleromyxoedemic; Antispasmodic; Antitumor-Promoter; Antivitligic 20 mg/man/day; Artemicide; Bactericide; Bufocide; Calcium-Antagonist; Cancer-Preventive; Cytotoxic; Dermatitigenic; Emetic; Fungistat; Herbicide; Hypertrichotic; Insecticide; Pesticide; Phytoalexin; Spasmolytic.

XANTHOTOXOL: Anti-nicotinic; Antihistaminic; Cancer-Preventive.

XANTHOXYYLETIN: Anticonvulsant.

XANTHYLETIN: DME-Inhibitor.

XYLITOL: Anticariogenic; Antiplaque; Diuretic; Hepatoprotective; Hyperuricemic; Laxative; Sweetener.

XYLOSE: Antidiabetic; Diagnostic.

Z-LIGUSTILIDE: Antiasthmatic; Spasmolytic.

ZEATIN: Mitotic.

ZINC: AntiChron's; Antiacne; Antiacrodermatitic 8-34 mg/day/orl/chd; Antialopecic; Antianorexic; Antiarthritic 50 mg/3x/day/orl/man; Anticanker 100 mg/day; Anticataract 30 mg/day; Anticoeliac; Anticold 50 mg; Anticolitic; Antidandruff; Antidote (Cadmium); Antieczemic; Antiencephalopathic; Antiepileptic 100 mg/day; Antifuruncular 45 mg/3x/day; Antiherpetic 25 mg/day; Antiimpotency; Antiinfective 50 mg/day; Antiinfertility 60 mg/day; Antiinsomniac; Antilepric; Antiplaque; Antiprolactin; Antiprostatic 50 mg/man/day/orl; Antirheumatic; Antistomatic 50 mg/man/3x/day; Antitinnitic 60-120 mg/day; Antiulcer 50 mg/3x/day/man; Antiviral; Astringent; Deodarant; Immunostimulant; Immunosuppressant 300 mg/day/6 weeks/orl/man; Mucogenic; Pesticide; Spermigenic 60 mg/day; Testosteronigenic 60 mg/day; Trichomonicide; Vulnerary.

ACTIVITY/PLANTS

ABORTIFACIENT: Chinese Goldthread; Generic Goldthread; Himalayan Mayapple; Huang-Lia; Goldenseal; Henna; Marshmallow; Goldenseal; Malabar Nut; Parsley; Strawberry; Barberry; Strawberry; Calmuba Root; Henna; Clove; Malabar; Scotch Broom; Lambsquarter; Mayapple.

ALLEOPATHIC: Camphor; Lemon; Cardamon; Loomis' Mountain Mint; Boldo; Blue Gum; African Blue Basil; Levant Wormseed; Greek Sage; Bibilical Mint; Tea-Tree; Bay; Indian Bean; Setose Mountain Mint; Rosemary; Qinhghao; Hairy Rosemary; Eastern Hemlock; Spearmint; California Bay.

ANALGESIC: Camu-camu; Sunflower; Opium Poppy; Camphor; Clove; Acerola; White Willow; Broadbean; Coffee; Celery; Chinese Goldthread; Generic Goldthread; Licorice; Huang-Lia; Goldenseal; Chinese Ginseng; Frangipani; Cipo-Ira; Celery; Sunflower.

ANESTHETIC: Parsnip; Sunflower; American Styrax; Camphor; Clove; Oriental Storax; Lemon; Chinese Goldthread; Generic; Goldthread; Licorice; Lemon; Huang-Lia; Goldenseal; Bloodroot; Cardamom; Ajwan; Loomis' Mountain Mint; Lanceleaf Periwinkle; Nude Mountain Mint; Horsemint.

ANTIACNE: Butternut; Sunflower; Brazilnut; Pumpkin; Groundnut; Soybean; Cashew; Pistachio; Avocado; Breadfruit; Black Currant; Evening Primrose; Asparagus Pea; Chickpea; Blackbean; Lettuce; White Lupine; Strawberry; Waxgourd; Kale.

ANTIADD: Sunflower; Buffalo Gourd; Ben Nut; Berro; Blackbean; Black Cumin; Soybean; Pigeonpea; Chaya; Asparagus; Breadfruit; Jew's Mallow; Swamp Cabbage; Watermelon; White Lupine; Pigweed; Green Gram; Groundnut; Asparagus Pea; Lentil.

ANTIAGGREGANT: Parsnip; Sunflower; Evening-Primrose; Clove; White Willow; Lemon; Chinese Goldthread; Generic Goldthread; Sanchi Ginseng; Huang-Lia; Fennel; Tea; Goldenseal; Black Currant; Chinese Skullcap; Ajwan; Mayapple; Onion; Pignut Hickory.

ANTIAGING: Purslane; Indian Mulberry; Garden Sorrel; Luffa; Da-Zao; Vinespinach; Spinach; Carrot;

Nasturtium; Barley; Berro; Roselle; Papaya; Pigweed; Swamp Cabbage; Jew's Mallow; Sweet Potato; Chives; Black Mustard; Bell Pepper.

ANTIALCOHOLIC: Date Palm; Chicory; Onion; Turmeric; Tamarind; Pawpaw; Carob; Black Nightshade; Sour Cherry; Sapodilla; Plum; Apple; Black Currant; Banana/Plantain; Cowberry; Evening-Primrose; Mango; Indian Fig; Apricot; Gooseberry.

ANTIALLERGIC: Sunflower; Grape; Evening-Primrose; Lemon; Licorice; Huaco-Mullo; Crab's Eye; Ramie; Biblical Mint; Cardamon; Lingaloe; Pignut Hickory; Typyical Mountain Mint; Buffalo Gourd; Chih-Shao; Shagbark Hickory; Texas Colubrina; Red Cedar.

ANTIALZHEIMERAN: Brazilnut; Cowage; Dandelion; Opium Poppy; Soybean; Black Gram; Calabash Gourd; Fenugreek; Shepherd's Purse; Flax; Groundnut; Shagbark Hickory; Ben Nut; Pumpkin; Sunflower; Scotch Pine; Pea; Dang Gui; Lentil; Pignut Hickory.

ANTIANEMIC: Red Cedar; Pignut Hickory; Buckbush; Shagbark Hickory; Dandelion; Coneflower; American Styrax; Black Gum; Corn Salad; White Oak; Mugwort; Shortleaf Pine; Red Clover; Northern Red Oak; Ramie; Asian Wild Ginger; Siebold's Wild Ginger; Devil's Claw; Tomatillo; Bilberry.

ANTIANGINAL: Lanceleaf Periwinkle; Pignut Hickory; Sharbark; Hickory; Irish Moss; Purslane; Blackbean; Red Cedar; Opium Poppy; Asparagus; Oats; Cowpea; Ben Nut; Spinach; Purple Tephrosia; Visnaga; Snakeground; Licorice; Black Cherry; Dwarf Sumac; Black Gum.

ANTIANORECTIC: Pignut Hickory; Shagbark Hickory; Irish Moss; Purslane; Red Cedar; Blackbean; Opium Poppy; Oats; Cowpea; Asparagus; Ben Nut; Spinach; Purple Tephrosia; Snakeground; Black Cherry; Dwarf Sumac; Lettuce; Licorice; Black Gum; Buckbush.

ANTIANXIETY: Pignut Hickory; Shagbark Hickory; Huaco-Mullo; Ramie; Red Cedar; Buffalo Gourd; Texas Colubrina; Tomato; Pigweed; Broccoli; Brigham Tea; Chaff Flower; Wolfberry; Luffa; Spiny Pigweed; American Styrax; Red Clover; Valerian; Angel of Death; Da-Zao.

ANTIARRHYTHMIC: Lettuce; Asparagus; Purslane; Chinese Goldthread; Generic Goldthread; Endive; Cowpea; Oats; Black Gram; Radish; Lambsquarter; Pignut Hickory; Chinese Cabbage; Chayote; Dill; Pigweed; Spinach; Cucumber; Huang-Lia; Garland Chrysanthemum.

ANTIARTHRITIC: Cantaloupe; English Walnut; Avocado; Camu-camu; Cucumber; Safflower; Apricot; Great Scarlet Poppy; Sunflower; Butternut; Calabash Gourd; Opium Poppy; Brazilnut; Sesame; Evening Primrose; Pinyon Pine; Marijuana; Canaloupe; Black Cumin; Chilgoza Pine.

ANTIASTHMATIC: Camu-camu; Copaiba; Evening-Primrose; Acerola; Licorice; Horse Chestnut;

Tea; Crab's Eye; Tea; Mango; Emblic; Guarana; Almond; Licorice; Onion; Witch Hazel; Cacao; Chinese Skullcap; Mayapple; Pignut Hickory.

ANTIATHEROSCLEROTIC: Camu-camu; Evening Primrose; Broccoli; Pigweed; Tomato; Pignut Hickory; Luffa; Black Currant; Shagbark Hickory; Purslane; Bitter Melon; European Nettle; Black Cherry; Berro; Groundnut; Chinese Cabbage; Broadbean; Spinach; Lambsquarter.

ANTIBACK-ACHE: Nicaraguan Cacao; Cowpea; Black-Cohosh; Asparagus; Spirulina; Yellow Gentain; Ma Huang; Blackbean; Bael de India; Macambo; Pito; Sunflower; Ben Nut; Shepherd's Purse; Okra; High Mallow; Pokeweed; Buchu; Cerraja.

ANTIBACTERIAL: Chinese Goldthread; Generic Goldthread; Mango; Huang-Lia; Goldenseal; Witch Hazel; Emblic; Pomegranate; Aleppo Oak; Barberry; Huang Po; Prickly Poppy; Strawberry; Rhubarb; Soybean.

ANTIBIOTIC: Chinese Goldthread; Generic Goldthread; Huang-Lia; Goldenseal; Garlic; Indian Tulip Tree; Huang Po; Rosemary; Cotton; Soybean; Watermelon; Indian Fig; Buffalo Gourd; Tepary Bean; Cotton.

ANTIBRONCHITIC: Sunflower; Lemon; Mango; Cardamom; Witch Hazel; Ajwan; Loomis' Mountain Mint; Emblic; Nude Mountain Mint; Boldo; Pomegranate; Aleppo Oak; Horsemint; Blue Gum; Wild Bergamot; Bibilical Mint; Cornmint; Common Thyme; Lavant Wormseed.

ANTIBURN: Annual Camomile; Basil; Aspic.

ANTICANCER: Lemon; Celery; Caraway; Celery; Orange; Cardamom; Fennel; Mandarin; Neroli; Lime; Corn; Bayrum Tree; Mace; Star-Anise; Common Thyme; Sage; Fennel; Cucumber; Carrot; Parsley.

ANTICANKER: Pignut Hickory; Lettuce; Bitter Aloes; Shagbark Hicory; Red Cedar; Chinese Goldthread; Huang-Lia; Generic Goldthread; Asparagus; Sassafras; American Styrax; Black Cherry; Spinach; White Oak; Shortleaf Pine; Parsley; American Persimmon; Brussels-Sprouts.

ANTICARCINOMIC: Mango; Witch Hazel; Asparagus Pea; Emblic; American Dogwood; Pomegranate; Aleppo Oak; Ipecac; Arrow-Poison Tree; Hispid Quabain; Da-Zao; Teak; Ashwagandha; Bogbean; European Squill; Grecian Foxglove; Purslane; Ipecac; Purple Foxglove; Da-Zao.

ANTICARIOGENIC: Grape; Copaiba; Lemon; Licorice; Crab's Eye; Lignaloe; Biblical Min; Typical Mountain Mint; Celery; Common Thyme; Wild Bergamot; Tea; Clove; Agrimony; Cubeb; Camphor; African Blue Basil; Coriander; Winter Savory.

ANTICARPAL-TUNNEL: Angel of Death; Saffron; Pokeweed; Lambsquarter; Asparagus; Ben Nut;

Common Thyme; Nasturtium; Spirulina; Jew's Mallow; Huaca-Mullo; Wheat; Peppermint; Taro; High Mallow; Celery; Cowpea; Ramie; Roselle; Bitter Melon.

ANTICATARACT: Camu-camu; Pansy; Japanese Pagoda Tree; Evening-Primrose; Acerola; Campechy; Buckwheat; Sang-Pai-Pi; Onion; Mayapple; Peegee: Strawberry; Sunflower; Bitter Melon; Purging Croton; American Elder.

ANTICIRRHOTIC: Licorice; Brazilnut; Crab's Eye; Cowage; Chinese Goldthread; Huang-Lia; Goldenseal; Barberry; Dandelion; Opium Poppy; Soybean; Black Gram; Calabash Gourd; Couchgrass; Fenugreek; Autumn Crocus; Shepherd's Purse; Huang Po.

ANTICOAGULANT: Calamansi; Roselle; Pineapple; Cocona; Aveloz; Lemon; Calamansi; Papaya; Black Nightshade; Black Currant; Maracuya; Mangosteen; Cape Gooseberry; Grapefruit; Red Currant; Rose; Carambola; Soybean; Tea; Pomegranate.

ANTICOLD: Camu-camu; Acerola; Bitter Melon; Pokeweed; Emblic; Rose; Bell Pepper; Cayenne; Horseradish; Cashew; English Walnut; Vinespinasch; Guava; Sallow Thorn; Berro; English Walnut; Rosa Mosqueta; Rose Hips; Garden Sorrel; Bitter Melon.

ANTICONVULSANT: Pansy; Japanese Pagoda Tree; Clove; Chinese Godlthread; Generic Goldthread; Huang-Lia; Celery; Buckwheat; Goldenseal; Sang-Pai-Pi; Buckwheat; Levant Berry; Pignut Hickory; Shagbark Hickory; Peegee; Allspice; American Elder.

ANTIDANDRUFF: Sunflower; Cornmint; Comfrey; Broccoli; Dill; Parsnip; Horseradish; Garden Cress; Cabbage; Red Mangrove; Lettuce; Butterbur; Peppermint; European Nettle; Snakeground; Purslane; Radish; Virginia Mountain Mint; Spinach.

ANTIDEPRESSANT: Parsnip; Camu-camu; Acerola; Asparagus; Pignut Hickory; Lettuce; Pigweed; Purslane; Shagbark Hickory; Berro; Lambsquarter; Endive; Spinach; Chinese Cabbage; Broccol; Cowpea; Huaca-Mullo; Tomato; Chayote; Oats.

ANTIDIABETIC: Chicory; Indian Snakeroot; Common Thyme; Two-Flowered Sandspur; Gobo; Red Clover; Da-Zao; Safflower; Kudzu; Maracuya; Indian Fig; Ramie; Dandelion; Rice Paper Tree; Jack Bean; Burn Mouth Vine; Pyrethrum; Desert Date; Flax; Kudzu.

ANTIDIARRHEIC: Red Mangrove; Rowan Berry; Arbutus; Pomegranate; Marshmallow; Canaigre; Babul; Gum Ghatti; Poison Hemlock; Sunflower; Guava; Coconut; Nance; Emblic; Pomegranate; Fenugreek; Winter's Bark; Smooth Sumac; Simaruba Bark; Chinaberry.

ANTIDYSENTERIC: Red Mangrove; Arbutus; Canaigre; Babul; Pomegranate; Gum Ghatti; Guava; Nance; Emblic; Pomegranate; Smooth Sumac; Simaruba Bark; Chinaberry; Betel Nut; Pomengranate; Eastern Hemlock; Japanese Knotweed; California Peppertree; Babul; Black Alder.

ANTIDYSMENORRHEIC: Pignut Hickory; Shagbark Hickory; Irish Moss; Purslane; Blackbean; Red Cedar; Opium Poppy; Oats; Asparagus; Cowpea; Ben Nut; Spinach; Purple Tephrosia; Snakegourd; Licorice; Black Cherry; Dwarf Sumac; Black Gum; Red Mangrove; Buckbush.

ANTIECZEMIC: Butternut; Cantaloupe; Sunflower; Brazilnut; Avocado; Pinyon Pine; English Walnut; Camu-camu; Cucumber; Safflower; Pumpkin; Italian Stone Pine; Apricot; Great Scarlet Poppy; Groundnut; Opium Poppy; Calabash Gourd; Sesame; Evening-Primrose; Soybean.

ANTIEDEMIC: Camu-camu; Copaiba; Date Palm; Turmeric; Mesquite; Tamarind; Sugar-Apple; Horse Chestnut; Pansy; Japanese Pagoda Tree; Licorice; California Peppertree; Clove; Acerola; Pawpaw; Onion; Carob; Crab's Eye; Black Nightshade.

ANTIEPILEPTIC: Asparagus; Carob; Wheat; Ben Nut; White Lupine; Chinese Cabbage; Soybean; Chives; Buffalo Gourd; Groundnut; Butternut; Almond; Opium Poppy; Tomato; Italian Stone Pine; Chaya; Cowpea; Blackbean; Pignut Hickory; White Mustard.

ANTIFATIGUE: Lettuce; Asparagus; Endive; Black Gram; Cowpea; Lambsquarter; Radish; Chayote; Chinese Cabbage; Purslane; Oat; Garland Chrsanthemum; Dill; Dandelion; Pigweed; Cucumber; Kudzu; Spinach; Borage.

ANTIFERTILITY: Himalayan Mayapple; Indian Tulip Tree; Japanese Pagoda Tree; Clove; Indian Bean; Cherimoya; Mayapple; Rosemary; Hawthorn; Cotton Oil; Common Thyme; Hawthorn; Greek Sage; Chinese Skullcap; Aspic; Creeping Thyme; Marjoram.

ANTIFLU: Khasi Pine; Chilgoza Pine; Lemon; Celery; Chir Pine; Horse Chestnut; Evening-Primrose; Longleaf Pine; Tea; Mango; Guarana; Lemon; Orange; Hyssop; Witch Hazel; Emblic; Mayapple; Onion; Cardamom.

ANTIGINGIVITIC: Camu-camu; Acerola; Licorice; Red Mangrove; Crab's Eye; Bitter Melon; Poke-weed; Emblic; Rose; Bell Pepper; Cayenne; Horseradish; Cashew; English Walnut; Vinespinach; Guava; Sallow Thorn; Berro; English Walnut.

ANTIGLAUCOMIC: Camu-camu; Pansy; Japanese Pagoda Tree; Pumpkin; Acerola; Chinese Fox-glove; Buckwheat; Sang-Pai-Pi; Celery; Peegee; Bitter Melon; American Elder; Pokeweed; Parsley; Common Smartweed; Warburghia.

ANTIHALITOSIC: Sunflower; Lemon; Damiana; Cardamom; Ajwan; Loomis Mountain Mint; Nude Mountain Mint; Boldo; Horsemint; Blue Gum; Wild Bergamot; Cornmint; Common Thyme; Levant Wormseed; Biblical Mint; Mate; Greek Sage; Tea-Tree; Bay.

ANTIHEARTBURN: Nicaraguan Cacao; Cowpea; Black-Cohosh; Asparagus; Spirulina; Yellow Gentian; Ma Huang; Blackbean; Bael de India; Macambo; Pito; Sunflower; Ben Nut; Shepherd's Purse; Okra; High Mallow; Pokeweed; Buchu; Cerraja.

ANTIHEMORRHOIDAL: Horse Chestnut; Red Mangrove; Hyssop; Poison Hemlock; Blue Gum; American Pennyroyal; Marjoram; Balm of Gilead; Wall Germander; Buchu; Lemon; Blueberry; Safflower.

ANTIHEPATITIC: Camu-camu; Acerola; Buffalo Gourd; Chinese Foxglove; Bitter Aloes; Sunflower; Italian Stone Pine; Carob; Ben Nut; Black Cumin; Butternut; Asparagus; Chaya; Watermelon; White Lupine; Berro; Pumpkin; Cassie; Groundnut; Bitter Melon.

ANTIHIV: Rowan Berry; Licorice; Posion Hemlock; Sunflower; Coconut; Fenugreek; Winter's Bark; Rice; White Willow; Corn; Giant Reed; Black Locust; Crab's Eye; Cork Oak; Evening-Primrose; Oats; Hull Husk; Lantana; Red Mangrove; Coffee; Mango.

ANTIHYPERACTIVITY: Asparagus; Granadilla; Cassie; Radish; Indian Mulberry; Blackbean; Barbados Gooseberry; Banana Passionfruit; Pokeweed; Tomatillo; Mugwort; Chayote; Cowpea; Ben Nut; Huaco-Mullo; Groundnut; Naranjillo; Susumba; Bell Pepper; Udo.

ANTIHYPERTENSIVE: Pansy; Japanese Pagoda Tree; Evening-Primrose; Lettuce; Asparagus; Endive; Black Gram; Lambsquarter; Cowpea; Radish; Purslane; Chayote; Chinese Cabbage; Oats; Pigweed; Garland Chrysanthemum; Dill; Dandelion; Spinach.

ANTIHYPERTHYROID: Guanique; Shagbark Hickory; Pignut Hickory; Black Oak; White Oak; Common Thyme; Northern Red Oak; Blackbean; Lettuce; Blackbean; Grapefruit; Orange; Cabbage; Asparagus; Buckbush; Endive; Shortleaf; Parsley; Red Cedar.

ANTIIMPOTENCY: Pignut Hickory; Lettuce; Bitter Aloes; Shagbark Hickory; Red Cedar; Chinese Goldthread; Huang-Lia; Generic Goldthread; Asparagus; Sassafras; American Styrax; Black Cherry; Smooth Suman; Spinach; White Oak; Shortleaf Pine; Parsley; American Persimmon; Brussels-Sprouts.

ANTIINFERTILITY: Camu-camu; Acerola; Buffalo Gourd; Chinese Foxgrove; Bitter Aloes; Sunflower; Italian Stone Pine; Carob; Ben Nut; Black Cumin; Butternut; Asparagus; Chaya; Watermelon; White Lupine; Berro; Pumpkin; Cassie; Groundut; Bitter Melon.

ANTIINFLAMMATORY: Chir Pine; Khasi Pine; Chilgoza Pine; Cantaloupe; Parsnip; English Walnut; Avocado; Camu-camu; Apricot; Cucumber; Safflower; Copaiba; Sunflower; Great Scarlet Poppy; Butternut; Calabash Gourd; Opium Poppy; Brazilnut; Sunflower.

ANTIINSOMNIAC: Pignut Hickory; Shagbark Hickory; Huaco-Mullo; Ramie; Red Cedar; Buffalo

Gourd; Texas Colubrina; Tomato; Pigweed; Broccoli; Brigham Tea; Chaff Flower; Wolfberry; Luffa; Spiny Pigweed; American Styrax; Red Clover; Valerian; Angel of Death; Da-Zao.

ANTILEPRIC: Camu-Camu; Bitter Melon; Emblic; Bell Pepper; Cayenne; Horseradish; Cashew; English Walnut; Vinespinach; Guava; Sallow Thorn; Berro; English Walnut; Garden Sorrel; Bitter Melon; Chaya; Calamansi; Broccoli; Black Currant; Cassavra.

ANTILEUKEMIC: Evening-Primrose; Himalayan Mayapple; Mayapple; Onion; Greek Sage; Physic Nut; Orange; Oleander; Tea; Rosemary; Periwinkle; Agrimony; Ipecac; Licorice; Aspic; Common Thyme; Winter Savory; Cherimoya; Autumn Crocus.

ANTILUPUS: Purslane; Wheat; Swamp Cabbage; Indian Mulberry; Nasturtium; Pokeweed; Garland Chrysanthemum; Garden Sorrel; Sensitive Plant; Perejil; Asparagus; Chinese Hibiscus; Da-Zao; Vinespinach; Spinach; Carrot; Barley; Comfrey; Huaco-Mullo.

ANTIMEASLES: Camu-camu; Bitter Melon; Emblic; Bell Pepper; Cayenne; Horseradish; Cashew; English Walnut; Vinespinach; Guava; Sallow Thorn; Berro; English Walnut; Bitter Melon; Garden Sorrel; Chaya; Calamansi; Broccoli; Black Currant; Cassavra.

ANTIMELANOMIC: Grape; Lemon; Himalayab Mayapple; Wild Bergamot; Ajwan; Common Thyme; Asparagus Pea; Nude Mountain Mint; Horsemint; Small-Flowered Oregano; American Dogwood; Tonka Bean; Winter Savory; Portuguese Thyme; Agbo; Waldmeister; Autumn Crocus; Mayapple; Creeping Thyme; Da-Zao.

ANTIMENORRHAGIC: Cantaloupe; English Walnut; Avocado; Cucumber; Safflower; Butternut; Apricot; Great Scarlet Poppy; Sunflower; Calabash Gourd; Flax; Opium Poppy; Brazilnut; Sesame; Evening-Primrose; Pinyon Pine; Marijuana; Cantaloupe; Black Cumin; Chilgoza Pine.

ANTIMIGRAINE: Camu-camu; Bitter Melon; Emblic; Bell Pepper; Cayenne; Berro; Horseradish; Cashew; Evening Primrose; Sunflower; English Walnut; Guava; Sallow Thorn; Chives; Broccoli; Coffee; English Walnut; Chinese Cabbage; Cauliflower.

ANTIMUTAGENIC: Lemon; Celery; Red Mangrove; Camu-camu; Arbutus; Pomegranate; Embric; Canaigre; Babul; Gum Chatti; Guava; Calamansi; Nance; Smooth Sumac; Simarubu Bark; China-berry; Betel Nut.

ANTIOBESITY: Indian Snakeroot; Common Thyme; Two-Flowered Sandspur; Red Clover; Da-Zhao; Camu-camu; Safflower; Kudzu; Maracuya; Indian Fig; Ramie; Rice Paper Tree; Jack Bean; Evening-Primrose; Burn Mouth Vine; Pyrethrum; Desert Date; Flax; Kudzu; Barley.

ANTIOSTEARTHRITIC: Camu-camu; Bitter Melon; Emblic; Bell Pepper; Cayenne; Horseradish;

Cashew; English Walnut; Vinespinach; Guava; Sallow Thorn; Berro; English Walnut; Garden Sorrel; Chaya; Calamansi; Broccoli; Black Currant; Cassava.

ANTIOXIDANT: Parsnip; Pawpaw; Red Mangrove; Camu-camu; Rowan Berry; Pansy; Japanese Pagoda Tree; Arbutus; Date Palm; Pomengranate; Emblic; Canaigre; Vanilla; Babul; Carrot; Licorice; Gum Ghatti; Coffee; Poison Hemlock; Water Chestnut.

ANTIPARKINSONIAN: Camu-camu; Acerola; Broadbean; Ben Nut; Sunflower; Buffalo Gourd; Cowage; Berro; Asparagus; Black Cumin; Blackbean; Spinach; Chaya; Asparagus Pea; Jew's Mallow; Soybean; Vinespinach; Swamp Cabbage; Pigweed.

ANTIPEROXIDANT: Evening-Primrose; Coffee; Mango; Onion; Witch Hazel; Tea; Emblic; Mayapple; Orange; Jalap; Pomegranate; Aleppo Oak; Turmeric; Strawberry; Sunflower; Basil; Pear; Common Thyme; Tarragon.

ANTIPMS: Evening-Primrose; Pignut Hickory; Shagbark Hickory; Huaca-Mullo; Ramie; Red Cedar; Buffalo Gourd; Texas Colubrina; Tomato; Pigweed; Brigham Tea; Black Currant; Chaff Flower; Broccoli; Wolfberry; Luffa; Spiny Pigweed; Onion; American Styrax.

ANTIPNEUMONIC: Camu-camu; Acerola; Chinese Goldthread; Generic Goldthread; Huang-Lia; Goldenseal; Bitter Melon; Pokeweed; Barberry; Emblic; Rose; Bell Pepper; Cayenne; Horseradish; Cashew; English Walnut; Vinespinach; Guava; Sallow Thorn; Berro.

ANTIPSYCHOTIC: Evening-Primrose; Sunflower; Ben Nut; Asparagus Pea; Yellow Gentian; Asparagus; Cretan Culantro; Bonavist Bean; Berro; White Mustard; Buffalo Gourd; Chinese Ginseng; Chickpea; Sesame; Blackbean; Spinach; Pumpkin; Fenugreek.

ANTIRADICULAR: Red Mangrove; Arbutus; Pomengranate; Canaigre; Babul; Gum Ghatti; Guava; Nance; Emblic; Pomengranate; Smooth Sumac; Simaruba Bark; Chinaberry; Betel Nut; Eastern Hemlock; Japanese Knotweed; Pansy; California Peppertree; Japanese Pagoda Tree.

ANTIRHEUMATIC: Sunflower; Licorice; Lemon; White Willow; Crab's Eye; Ajwan; Nude Mountain Mint; Horsemint; Common Thyme; Cornmint; Wild Bergamot; Evening Primrose; Sunflower; Winter Savory; Ben Nut; Autumn Crocus; Asparagus Pea; Yellow Gentian.

ANTISCHIZOPHRENIC: Indian Snakeroot; Licorice; Celandine; Gaunique; Fenugreek; Shagbark Hickory; Avocado; Ajwan; Pea; Spiny Pigweed; Pea; American Ginseng; Pignut Hickory; Wheat; Potato; Barley; Rice; Sesame; Soybean; Black Oak.

ANTISEPTIC: Celery; Grape; Mangosteen; Camu-camu; Cipo-Ira; Lemon; Sunflower; Lambsquarter; Bhutan Pine; Licorice; Camphor; Clove; Acerola; Biblical Mint; Black Pepper; Typical Mountain Mint; Red Mangrove; Karaya.

ANTISHOCK: Grape; Lemon; Sanchi Ginseng; Lignaloe; Lemon; Typical Mountain Mint; Biblical Mint; Self-Heal; Spearmint; Creeping Thyme; Common Thyme; Wild Bergamot; Roesmary; European Bugle; Lemonbalm; Clary Sage; Basil; Marjoram; Sage; Applemint.

ANTISTRESS: Parsnip; Parsley; Fenugreek; Mace; Chinese Ginseng; Black Nightshade; Perilla; Carrot; Eleuthero Ginseng; Purslane; Air Potato; Parsley; Indian Snakeroot; Indian Mulberry; Nasturtium; Pokeweed; Garland Chrysanthemum.

ANTITHROMBOTIC: Horse Chestnut; Chinese Skullcap; Garlic; Marsh Skullcap; Forskohl's Coleus.

ANTITUBERCULAR: Chinese Goldthread; Generic Goldthread; Huang-Lia; Goldenseal; Bitter Aloes; Barberry; Tellicherry Bark; Annual Camomile; Huang Po; Fig; Neem; Frangipani; Papaya; Gotu Kola; Laciniate Cow-parsnip; Prickly Poppy; Parsley; Celery; Basil.

ANTITUMOR: Lemon; Indian Snakeroot; Common Thyme; Celery; Two-Flowered Sandspur; Red Clover; Da-Zao; Safflower; Kudzu; Maracuya; Indian Fig; Ramie; Rice Paper Tree; Jack Bean; Copaiba; Evening Primrose; Burn Mouth Vine; Pyrethrum; Desert Date.

ANTIULCER: Indian Snakeroot; Common Thyme; Two-Flowered Sandspur; Red Clover; Da-Zao; Camu-camu; Safflower; Indian Fig; Kudzu; Maracuya; Ramie; Rice Paper Tree; Jack Bean; Burn Mouth Vine; Pyrethrum; Desert Date; Flax; Kudzu; Evening-Primrose; Barley.

ANTIVIRAL: Khasi Pine; Lemon; Chilgoza Pine; Celery; Red Mangrove; Camu-camu; Rowan Berry; Arbutus; Pomegranate; Emblic; Canaigre; Babul; Gum Ghatti; Poison Hemlock; Guava; Sunflower; Chir Pine; Celery; Coconut.

APHRODISIAC: Broadbean; Lanceleaf Periwinkle; Caper Spurge; Chinese Ginseng; Passionflower; Pomegranate; Apple; Corn.

BACTERICIDE: Lemon; Chir Pine; Khasi Pine; Celery; Chilgoza Pine; Grape; Red Mangrove; Mangosteen; Camu-camu; Copaiba; Hindi Chaulmoogra; Rowan Berry; Arbutus; Pomengranate; Marshmallow; Canaigre; Babul.

CANCER-PREVENTIVE: Avocado; Safflowr; Celery; Khasi Pine; Apricot; Cantaloupe; Common Thyme; Lemon; English Walnut; Marshmallow; Chilgoza Pine; Brazilnut; Karaya; Watermelon; Buffalo Gourd; Indian Snakeroot; Evening-Primrose; Cucumber.

CANDIDICIDE: Clove; Grape; Cowberry; Coconut; Allspice; Garlic; Cucumber; Bayrum Tree; Carrot; Cherimoya; Common Thyme; Basil; Carrot; Clove; Cantaloupe; Allspice; Pignut Hickory; Purslane; Spinach; Oats.

CARDIOTONIC: Tea; Guarana; Chinese Goldthread; Generic Goldthread; Black Pepper; Ouabain;

Huang-Lia; Coffee; Goldenseal; Bloodroot; Cacao; Abata Cola; Yoko; Genipap; Mate; Horse Chestnut; Barberry; Ma Huang; Clove; Cayenne.

CONTRACEPTIVE: Black Nightshade; Fig; Black Cherry; American Styrax; Black Gum; Buckbush; Pignut Hickory; American Persimmon; Sassafras; Tomato; Shagbark Hickory; Cabbage; English Filbert; Sesame; Broccoli; Asparagus.

DECONGESTANT: Camphor; Ma Huang; African Blue Basil; Black Mustard; Sage; Hoary Basil; Hairy Rosemary; Iberian Savory; Montane Mountain Mint; Pakistani Ephedra; Qinghao; Douglas' Savory; Rosemary; African Blue Basil; Greek Sage; Lavender Rosemary; Aspic; Hyssop; Mendizabali's; Horseradish.

DERMATITIGENIC: Avocado; Chir Pine; English Filbert; Macadamia; Peruvian Yellow Oleander; African Oil Palm; Marula; Apricot; Brazilnut; Pistachio; Simaruba; Bark; Andiroba; Candlenut; Caper Spurge; Almond; Olive; Sunflower; Plum; Antler Herb.

FUNGICIDE: Parsnip; Grape; Lemon; Clove; Lemon; Coconut; Potato; Grape; Cardamom; Oats; Coffee; Rice; Common Thyme; Celery; Java-Olive; Bayrum Tree; Winter Savory; Celery; Turmeric; Allspice.

HEPATOPROTECTIVE: Cantaloupe; English Walnut; Red Mangrove; Avocado; Cucumber; Safflower; Arbutus; Brazilut; Apricot; Sunflower; Great Scarlet Poppy; Butternut; Canaigre; Babul; Opium Poppy; Calabash Gourd; Pomegranate; Gum Ghatti; Guava; Sesame.

HYPOCHOLESTEROLEMIC: Indian Snakeroot; Common Thyme; Two-Flowered Sandspur; Red Clover; Da-Zao; Evening Primrose Oil; Rice; Ramie; Camu-camu; Safflower; Kudzu; Maracuya; Barley; Oats; Indian Fig; Burn Mouth Vine; Rice Paper Tree; Jack Bean; Pyrethrum; Desert Date.

HYPOGLYCEMIC: Evening-Primrose; Tea; Chinese Goldthread; Sanchi Ginseng; Gaurana; Greek Sage; Huang-Lia; Onion; Goldenseal; Physic Nut; Mayapple; Coffee; Oleander; Rosemary; Periwinkle; Tonka Bean; Garlic; Cinnamon; Barberry.

HYPOTENSIVE: Indian Snakeroot; Common Thyme; Two-Flowered Sandspur; Parsnip; Red Clover; Da-Zao; Ramie; Camu-camu; Safflower; Kudzu; Maracuya; Indian Fig; Evening-Primrose; Burn Mouth Vine; Rice Paper Tree; Jack Bean; Pyrethrum; Desert Date; Flax; Kudzu.

IMMUNOSTIMULANT: Chicory; Gobo; Elecampane; Dandelion; Licorice; Coneflower; Costus; Leopard's-Bane; Crab's Eye; Coffee; Mugwort; Chinese Goldthread; Generic Goldthread; Java-Olive; Huang-Lia; Goldenseal; Beet; Malangra; Lambsquarter.

LAXATIVE: Indian Snakeroot; Common Thyme; Rice; Red Clover; Da-Zao; Evening Primrose;

Safflower; Kudzu; Maracuya; Indian Fig; Barley; Ramie; Oats; Rice Paper Tree; Jack Bean; Burn Mouth Vine; Pyrethrum; Desert Date; Rowan Berry.

RESPIRASTIMULANT: Camphor; Tea; Guarana; Almond; Bloodroot; Levant Berry; Coffee; Yoko; Abata; Ma Huang; Genipap; Indian Tobacco; Mate; African Blue Basil; Cacao; Sage; Hoary Basil; Hairy Rosemary; Iberian Savory; Montane Mountain Mint.

SEDATIVE: Celery; Lemon; Khasi Pine; Chilgoza Pine; Parsnip; Grape; Chir Pine; Licorice; Biblical Mint; Typical Mountain Mint; Opium Poppy; Clove; Longleaf Pine; White Willow; Muticous Mountain Mint; Virginia Mountain Mint.

SPERMICIDE: Licorice; Prickly Poppy; Indian Tulip Tree; Gum Tragacanth; Cardamom; Cherimoya; Tea Tree; Pericarp Essential Oil; Marjoram; Hawthorn; Paperback Tea Tree; Cacao; Cotton Oil; Hawthorn; Mace; Flax; Sage.

SUNSCREEN: Jalap; Horse Chestnut; Pear; Basil; Common Thyme; Tarragon; Strawberry; Vervain; Creeping Thyme; Betony; Comfrey; Strawberry; Guava; Gobo; Sunflower; Apple; Chia; Chicory.

VIRICIDE: Lemon; Celery; Red Mangrove; Camu-camu; Rowan Berry; Arbutus; Pomegranate; Emblic; Canaigre; Babul; Gum Ghatti; Poison Hemlock; Sunflower; Guava; Coconut; Nance; Fenugreek; Winter's Bark; Grape.

APPENDIX A

ANTIAGING NUTRIENTS

*Cross Referenced

■ ACETYL-L-CARNITINE

Aging

Results of this study showed that the administration of aceteyl-L-carnitine to aged rats for 6 months significantly decreased the percentage of myelinated fibers characterized by age-dependent morphological alterations.

> —C. De Angelis, et al., "Acetyl-L-carnitine Prevents Age-dependent Structural Alterations in Rat Peripheral Nerves and Promotes Regeneration Following Sciatic Nerve Injury in Young and Senescent Rats," *Exp Neurol,* 128(1), July 1994, p. 103-114.

Results of this study showed that aged rats with behavioral impairments receiving acetyl-L-carnitine experienced an enhancement in spatial acquisition in a novel environment.

> —A. Caprioli, et al., "Acetyl-L-Carnitine: Chronic Treatment Improves Spatial Acquisition in a New Environment in Aged Rats," *J Gerontol A Biol Sci Med Sci,* 50(4), July 1995, p. B232-B236.

Results of this study indicated that the administration of 10 mg/kg per day of L-acetylcarnitine for 4 months had both neuroprotective and neurotrophic effects in aging rats.

> —L. Fiore & L. Rampello, "L-acetylcarnitine Attenuates the Age-dependent Decrease of

NMDA-Sensitive Glutamate Receptors in Rat Hippocampus," *Acta Neurol,* 11(5), October 1989, p. 346-350.

Results of this study showed that acetyl-L-carnitine may be effective in ameliorating receptor functionality in the aging rat brain due to its ability to preserve the receptor-mediated functional Ach release response.

—A. Imperato, et al., "In Vivo Probing of the Brain Cholinergic System in the Aged Rat. Effects of Long Term Treatment with Acetyl-L-carnitine," *Annals of the New York Academy of Science,* 621, 1991, p. 90-97.

This study examined the effects of aging and the administration of acetyl-L-carnitine on rat plasma lipid composition and erythrocytes. Aging was found to increase free and esterified levels of cholesterol while fatty acid plasma patterns showed major alterations in aged rats relative to controls. Three hours following acetyl-L-carnitine treatment, results showed such changes were back to normal.

—F.M. Ruggiero, et al., "Effect of Aging and Acetyl-L-carnitine on the Lipid Composition of Rat Plasma and Erythrocytes," *Biochem Biophys Res Commun,* 170(2), July 31, 1990, p. 621-626.

Results of this study indicate acetyl-L-carnitine has a direct action on p75NGFR expression in the central nervous system of aged rodents.

—G. Taglialatela, et al., "Stimulation of Nerve Growth Factor Receptors in PC12 by Acetyl-L-carnitine," *Biochem Pharmacol,* 44(3), August 4, 1992, p. 577-585.

This study examined the effects of acetyl-L-carnitine administration for 37 weeks on lipopigment in the Purkinje neurons of rats. Results showed acetyl-L-carnitine to have prophylactive effects against adverse effects of cerebral aging.

—J.H. Dowson, et al., "The Morphology of Lipopigment in Rat Purkinje Neurons after Chronic Acetyl-L-carnitine Administration: A Reduction in Aging-related Changes," *Biol Psychiatry,* 32(2), July 15, 1992, p. 179-187.

Results of this study showed that acetyl-L-carnitine administered in 50-100 mg/kg daily doses improved neuronal bioenergetic mechanisms in rats

—C. Bertoni-Freddari, et al., "Dynamic Morphology of the Synaptic Junctional Areas During Aging: The Effect of Chronic Acetyl-L-carnitine Administration," *Brain Research,* 656(2), September 12, 1994, p. 359-366.

Results of this double-blind, placebo-controlled study indicated that the administration of 1500 mg per day of acetyl-L-carnitine to elderly patients with mild mental impairments proved to be beneficial against cognitive and emotional-affective mental impairment.

—C. Cipolli & G. Chiari, [Effects of L-acetylcarnitine on Mental Deterioration in the Aged: Initial Results], *Clin Ter,* 132(6 Suppl), March 31, 1990, p. 479-510.

This study examined the effects of treatment with 75 mg/kg per day for 11 months on the optic nerve and brain morphology in rats. Results showed that treatment improved the structural organization of the cerebral areas in questions and increased the volume densities of pyramidal neurons of the prefrontal cortex layers. Results also showed the treatment reduced the level of impairment of myelination of the pyramidal tract and optic nerve.

—M.T. Ramacci, et al., ''Effect of Long-term Treatment with Acetyl-L-carnitine on Structural Changes of Aging Rat Brain,'' *Drugs Exp Clin Res,* 14(9), 1988, p. 593-601.

This single-blind, placebo-controlled study examined the effects of 1500 mg per day of acetyl-L-carnitine for 90 days on elderly subjects with mild mental impairment. Results showed the treatment to be effective with respect to improvements on cognitive performance, and behavioral measures.

—G. Salvioli & M. Neri, ''L-acetylcarnitine Treatment of Mental Decline in the Elderly,'' *Drugs Exp Clin Res,* 20(4), 1994. p. 169-176.

This study examined the effects of acetyl-L-carnitine on brain adenylate cyclase activity in rats. Results showed that the treatment enhanced receptor-stimulated AC response in the frontal cortex of rats of all ages.

—T. Florio, et al., ''Effect of Acetyl-L-carnitine Treatment on Brain Adenylate Cyclase Activity in Young and Aged Rats,'' *European Neuropsychopharmacology,* 3(2), June 1993, p. 95-101.

Results of this study found that acetyl-L-carnitine increased nerve growth factor levels and utilization in aged rats' central nervous systems.

—G. Taglialatela, et al., ''Acetyl-L-carnitine Treatment Increases Nerve Growth Factor Levels and Choline Acetyltransferase Activity in the Central Nervous System of Aged Rats,'' *Exp Gerontol,* 29(1), January-February 1994, p. 55-66.

This study examined the effects of acetyl-L-carnitine on NMDA receptors in aged rats. Results showed significant reductions of NDMA in old rats relative to young were attenuated by treatment with acetyl-L-carnitine for 6 months. Single-dose treatment increased the Bmax value in old rats by 35%.

—M. Castorina, et al., ''A Cluster Analysis Study of Acetyl-L-carnitine Effect on NMDA Receptors in Aging,'' *Exp Gerontol,* 28(6), November-December 1993, p. 537-548.

This study examined the effects of aging and the administration of acetyl-L-carnitine on the activity of cytochrome oxidase and adenine nucleotide translocase in the heart mitochondria of rats. In aged rats, 30% reductions were found for the activity of both mitochondrial proteins systems with acetyl-L-carnitine totally reversing such effects.

—G. Paradies, et al., ''Effect of Aging and Acetyl-L-carnitine on the Activity of Cytochrome Oxidase and Adenine Nucleotide Translocase in Rat Heart Mitochondria,'' *FEBS Letters,* 350(2-3), August 22, 1994, p. 213-215.

Results of this study showed that the administration of acetyl-L-carnitine significantly improved the acquisition and retention of avoidance responses in aged rats.

—C. Valerio, et al., ''The Effects of Acetyl-l-carnitine on Experimental Models of Learning and Memory Deficits in the Old Rat,'' *Funct Neurol,* 4(4), October-December 1989, p. 387-390.

Results of this double-blind, placebo-controlled study showed that the administration of 3 g per day of acetyl-L-carnitine for 30-60 days significantly reduced the severity of symptoms associated with depression relative to controls in senile subjects between the ages of 60-80.

> —R. Bella, et al., "Effect of Acetyl-L-carnitine on Geriatric Patients Suffering from Dysthymic Disorders," *International Journal of Clinical Pharmacology Research,* 10(6), 1990, p. 355-360.

Results of this double-blind, placebo-controlled study showed that the administration of 2 g per day of acetyl-L-carnitine for three months led to significant improvements in elderly patients suffering from mental impairment.

> —M. Passeri, et al., "Acetyl-L-carnitine in the Treatment of Mildly Demented Elderly Patients," *International Journal of Clinical Pharmacology Research,* 10(1-2), 1990, p. 75-79.

Results of this study showed that 80 mg per day of acetyl-L-carnitine attenuated age related cognitive deficits in rats when administered long term.

> —A.L. Markowska & D.S. Olton, "Dietary Acetyl-L-carnitine Improves Spatial Behaviour of Old Rats," *International Journal of Clinical Pharmacology Research,* 10(1-2), 1990, p. 65-68.

This study examined the effects of L-carnitine and acetyl-L-carnitine on cell proliferation in peripheral blood lymphocytes from donors varying in age. Results found that phytohaemagglutinin-induced peripheral blood lymphocyte proliferation increased significantly in L-carnitine- or acetyl-L-carnitine-preloaded lymphocytes from subject of all ages, but with the strongest increases seen in older subjects.

> —C. Franceschi, et al., "Immunological Parameters in Aging: Studies on Natural Immunomo-dulatory and Immunoprotective Substances," *International Journal of Clinical Pharmacology Research,* 10(1-2), 1990, p. 53-57.

Results of this study showed that the administration of acetyl-L-carnitine had positive effects on age-related changes in the dopaminergic system of mice.

> —H. Sershen, et al., "Effect of Acetyl-L-carnitine on the Dopaminergic System in Aging Brain," *Journal of Neuroscience Research,* 30(3), November 1991, p. 555-559.

Results of this study showed that the administration of acetyl-L-carnitine for 7 months had positive effects on age-related changes in the hippocampus of rats.

> —F.R. Patacchioli, et al., "Acetyl-L-carnitine Reduces the Age-dependent Loss of Glucocorti-coid Receptors in the Rat Hippocampus: An Autoradiographic Study," *Journal of Neuroscience Research,* 23(4), August 1989, p. 462-466.

Results of this study showed that the administration of acetyl-L-carnitine ameliorated age-induced cognitive deficits in rats.

> —L. Angelucci, et al., "Nerve Growth Factor Binding in Aged Rat Central Nervous System: Effect of Acetyl-L-carnitine," *Journal of Neuroscience Research,* 20(4), August 1988, p. 491-496.

This review article cites studies supporting the efficacy of acetyl-L-carnitine in counteracting negative age-induced effects on physiological and pathological brain modifications in rats.

   —M. Castorina & L. Ferraris, ''Acetyl-L-carnitine Affects Aged Brain Receptorial System in Rodents,'' *Life Science,* 54(17), 1994, p. 1205-1214.

This study examined the effects of aging and the administration of 50 mg/kg per day of acetyl-L-carnitine on the bioenergetics and cholinergic metabolism in non-synaptic mitochondria and synaptosomes isolated from the cerebral cortex, hippocampus and striatum of rats. Results showed that acetyl-L-carnitine increased the high-affinity choline uptake in rat cerebral cortex as well as increased cytochrome oxidase activity in the hippocampus.

   —D. Curti, et al., ''Effect of Aging and Acetyl-L-carnitine on Energetic and Cholinergic Metabolism in Rat Brain Regions,'' *Mech Ageing Development,* 47(1), January 1989, p. 39-45.

Results of this study showed that the administration of acetyl-L-carnitine for 6 months improved memory performance in aged rats relative to controls.

   —C.A. Barnes, et al., ''Acetyl-1-carnitine. 2: Effects on Learning and Memory Performance of Aged Rats in Simple and Complex Mazes,'' *Neurobiological Aging,* 11(5), September-October 1990, p. 499-506.

Results of this study showed that the in vivo administration of L-acetylcarnitine reduced the enzyme activities associated with Krebs' cycle of synaptic rat mitochondria and increased the cytochrome oxidase activity of synaptic and non-synaptic mitochondria.

   —R.F. Villa & A. Gorini, ''Action of L-acetylcarnitine on Different Cerebral Mitochondrial Populations from Hippocampus and Striatum During Aging,'' *Neurochem Research,* 16(10), October 1991, p. 1125-1132.

Results of this study showed that treatment with acetyl-L-carnitine via drinking water led to significant reductions in the decline in the number of hippocampus NMDA receptors in the frontal cortex and striatum of rats relative to controls.

   —M. Castornia, et al., ''Age-dependent Loss of NMDA Receptors in Hippocampus, Striatum, and Frontal Cortex of the Rat: Prevention by Acetyl-L-carnitine,'' *Neurochem Research,* 19(7), July 1994, p. 795-798.

This review article notes that studies have confirmed acetyl-L-carnitine's ability to counteract the age-dependent reduction of several receptors in rodent central nervous systems.

   —M. Castorina & L. Ferraris, ''Acetyl-L-carnitine Affects Aged Brain Receptorial System in Rodents,'' *Life Science,* 54(17), 1994, p. 1205-1214.

Results of this study showed that the administration of acetyl-L-carnitine led to significant improvements in discrimination learning tasks in rats relative to controls.

   —O. Ghirardi, et al., ''Effect of Acetyl-1-carnitine Chronic Treatment on Discrimination Models in Aged Rats,'' *Physiol Behavior,* 44(6), 1988, p. 769-773.

Results of this study showed that the long-term administration of acetyl-L-carnitine antagonized the deterioration of learning ability in old rats due to aging.

—A. Caprioli, et al., "Age-dependent Deficits in Radial Maze Performance in the Rat: Effect of Chronic Treatment with Acetyl-L-Carnitine," *Prog Neuropsychopharmacol Biol Psychiatry,* 14(3), 1990, p. 359-369.

Results of this study showed that the administration of acetyl-L-carnitine for 8 months antagonized the deterioration the acquisition ability of a spatial learning task in old rats due to aging.

—O. Ghirardi, et al., "Long-term Acetyl-L-carnitine Preserves Spatial Learning in the Senescent Rat," *Prog Neuropsychopharmacol Biol Psychiatry,* 13(1-2), 1989, p. 237-245.

AIDS/HIV

Results of this study showed that 6 g per day of L-carnitine for two weeks was effective in ameliorating lipid metabolism as well as immune response in AIDS patients receiving AZT.

—C. De Simone, et al., "High Dose L-carnitine Improves Immunologic and Metabolic Parameters in AIDS Patients," *Immunopharmacol Immunotoxicol,* 15(1), January 1993, p. 1-12.

Alcoholism

Results of this double-blind, placebo-controlled indicated that acetyl-L-carnitine may have beneficial effects with respect to the cognitive dysfunctions associated with chronic alcoholism.

—E. Tempesta, et al., "Role of Acetyl-L-carnitine in the Treatment of Cognitive Deficit in Chronic Alcoholism," *International Journal of Clinical Pharmacology Research,* 10(1-2), 1990, p. 101-107.

Alzheimer's Disease

This double-blind, placebo-controlled study examined the effects of 2.5 g per day of acetyl levocarnitine hypochloride for 3 months followed by 3 g for 3 months on mild to moderately demented Alzheimer's patients. Results showed those receiving the treatment experienced significantly less deterioration in timed cancellation tasks and digit span.

—M. Sano, et al., "Double-blind Parallel Design Pilot Study of Acetyl Levocarnitine in Patients with Alzheimer's Disease," *Arch Neurol,* 49(11), November 1992, p. 1137-1141.

This double-blind, placebo-controlled study examined the effects of acetyl-L-carnitine treatment administered to patients with Alzheimer's disease for one year. Results found the treatment significantly slowed the rate of deterioration relative to controls.

—A. Spagnoli, et al., "Long-term Acetyl-L-carnitine Treatment in Alzheimer's Disease," *Neurology,* 41(11), November 1991, p. 1726-1732.

This review article argues that acetyl-L-carnitine possesses numerous pharmacologic properties which offer protection against neurodegeneration due to aging and thus it may be effective in reducing the development of Alzheimer's disease.

—A. Carta & M. Calvani, "Acetyl-L-carnitine: A Drug Able to Slow the Progress of Alzheimer's Disease?," *Annals of the New York Academy of Science,* 640, 1991, p. 228-232.

Results of this double-blind, placebo-controlled study found that treatment with 2 g of acetyl-L-carnitine per day for 24 weeks had beneficial short-term memory effects on patients with Alzheimer-type dementia.

> —G. Rai, et al., "Double-blind, Placebo Controlled Study of Acetyl-l-carnitine in Patients with Alzheimer's Dementia," *Curr Med Res Opin,* 11(10), 1990, p. 638-647.

Results of this study showed that the oral and intravenous administration of acetyl-L-carnitine increased CSF and plasma concentrations in Alzheimer's patients.

> —L. Parnetti, et al., "Pharmacokinetics of IV and Oral Acetyl-L-carnitine in a Multiple Dose Regimen in Patients with Senile Dementia of Alzheimer Type," *European Journal of Clinical Pharmacology,* 42(1), 1992, p. 89-93.

Results of this double-blind, placebo-controlled study found that patients treated with acetyl-L-carnitine experienced significantly less deterioration in mental status than controls.

> —J.W. Pettegrew, et al., "Clinical and Neurochemical Effects of Acetyl-L-carnitine in Alzheimer's Disease," *Neurobiol Aging,* 16(1), January-February 1995, p. 1-4.

Amenorrhea

In this study, hypothalamic amenorrhea patients received 2 g per day of acetyl-L-carnitine for 6 months. Results showed the treatment had a significant, positive impact on menstruation.

> —A.D. Genazzani, et al., "Acetyl-l-carnitine as Possible Drug in the Treatment of Hypothalamic Amenorrhea," *Acta Obstet Gynecol Scand,* 70(6), 1991, p. 487-492.

Cancer

Results of this study showed that the addition of 100 microM L-acetylcarnitine to P19 teratoma cells in an N2 synthetic, serum free medium, enhanced cell survival by slowing DNA fragmentation and nuclear condensation.

> —G. Galli & M. Fratelli, "Activation of Apoptosis by Serum Deprivation in a Teratocarcinoma Cell Line: Inhibition by L-acetylcarnitine," *Exp Cell Res,* 204(1), January 1993, p. 54-60.

Cardiovascular/Coronary Heart Disease

Results of this study showed that the administration of acetyl-L-carnitine (2 mg/kg iv plus 1 mg/kg/min for 30 min) to aged rats led to restoration of cardiolipin levels to levels of young rats as well as a decrease in age-induced reductions in phosphate carrier activity in rat heart mitochondria.

> —G. Paradies, et al., "The Effect of Aging and Acetyl-L-carnitine on the Activity of the Phosphate Carrier and on the Phospholipid Composition in Rat Heart Mitochondria," *Biochim Biophys Acta,* 1103(2), January 31, 1992, p. 324-326.

This study administered 3 mg per day of acetyl-L-carnitine intravenously to five patients undergoing aortic reconstructive surgery prior to ischemia induction. Results indicated acetyl-L-carnitine may have positive effects on the amelioration of human skeletal muscle damage induced by ischemia-reperfusion.

> —C. Adembri, et al., "Ischemia-reperfusion of Human Skeletal Muscle During Aortoiliac Surgery: Effects of Acetylcarnitine," *Histol Histopathol,* 9(4), October 1994, p. 683-690.

Dementia

Results of this study showed acetyl-L-carnitine administration for 10 weeks led to significant behavioral improvements in dementia patients relative to controls.

> —E. Sinforiani, et al., "Neuropsychological Changes in Demented Patients Treated with Acetyl-L-Carnitine," *International Journal of Clinical Pharmacology Research*, 10(1-2), 1990, p. 69-74.

This double-blind, placebo-controlled study examined the effects of 1000 mg per day of L-acetylcarnitine on the senile human brain. Results showed treatment led to significant improvements relative to controls with few side effects.

> —E. Bonavita, "Study of the Efficacy and Tolerability of L-acetylcarnitine Therapy in the Senile Brain," *International Journal of Clinical and Pharmacol Ther Toxicol*, 24(9), September 1986, p. 511-516.

Depression

Results of this double-blind, placebo-controlled study found that the administration of 1500 mg per day of acetyl-L-carnitine led to significant improvements in patients between the ages of 70 and 80 suffering from symptoms of depression.

> —G. Garzya, et al., "Evaluation of the Effects of L-acetylcarnitine on Senile Patients Suffering from Depression," *Drugs Exp Clin Res*, 16(2), 1990, p. 101-106.

Results of this study showed the administration of acetyl-L-carnitine to be significantly effective relative to controls in reducing depressive symptoms among elderly patients hospitalized for depression.

> —G. Garzya, et al., "Evaluation of the Effects of L-acetylcarnitine on Senile Patients Suffering from Depression," *Drugs Exp Clin Res*, 16(2), 1990, p. 101-106.

Diabetes

Results of this study found an association between metabolic and functional abnormalities related to diabetic polyneuropathy in rats and imbalances in carnitine metabolism. Treatment with acetyl-L-carnitine prevented such abnormalities.

> —Y. Ido, et al., "Neural Dysfunction and Metabolic Imbalances in Diabetic Rats. Prevention by Acetyl-L-carnitine," *Diabetes*, 43(12), December 1994, p.p. 1469-1477.

Results of this study showed that the administration of acetyl-L-carnitine to rats prevented acute Na+/-K+— ATPase defect and had corrective effects on PGE1 in diabetic nerves.

> —A.A. Sima, et al., "Primary Preventive and Secondary Interventionary Effects of Acetyl-L-Carnitine on Diabetic Neuropathy in the Bio-breeding Worcester Rat," *Journal of Clinical Investigations*, 97(8), April 15, 1996, p. 1900-1917.

This study examined the effects of acetyl-L-carnitine and proprionyl-L-carnitine on motor and sensory nerve conduction in diabetic rats. Results showed that treatment for 2 months following diabetes induction significantly attenuated the development of sciatic motor nerve conduction velocity deficits.

> —M.A. Cotter, et al., "Effects of Acetyl- and Proprionyl-L-carnitine on Peripheral Nerve

Function and Vascular Supply in Experimental Diabetes,'' *Metabolism,* 44(9), September 1995, p. 1209-1214.

This case-control study examined the effects of 50 mg/kg per day on the diminished nerve conduction velocity (NCV) of streptozotocin-induced hyperglycemic rats. Results showed an association between acetyl-L-carnitine and a decrease in the content of diabetic sciatic nerve which indicated a reduction in lipid peroxidation.

—S. Lowitt, et al., ''Acetyl-L-carnitine Corrects the Altered Peripheral Nerve Function of Experimental Diabetes,'' *Metabolism,* 44(5), May 1995, p. 677-680.

Results of this study showed that treatment with acetyl-L-carnitine or sorbinil reduced structural, functional and biochemical changes in the myelin sheath of rats due to hypoglycemia.

—J.I. Malone, et al., ''The Effects of Acetyl-L-carnitine and Sorbinil on Peripheral Nerve Structure, Chemistry, and Function in Experimental Diabetes,'' *Metabolism,* 45(7), July 1996, p. 902-907.

Results of this study showed that the oral administration of 250 mg/kg of acetyl-L-carnitine to diabetic rats led to improvements in nerve conduction velocity after 6 weeks of treatment.

—E. Morabito, et al., ''Acetyl-L-carnitine Effect on Nerve Conduction Velocity in Streptozotocin-diabetic Rats,'' *Arzneimittelforschung,* 43(3), March 1993, p. 343-346.

Results of this study showed that acetyl-alpha-carnitine had a more pronounced effect on hypoglycemic action than did chloropropamide in diabetic rabbits. In addition, results showed that acetyl-alpha-carnitine significantly enhanced chloropropamide's effects.

—E.K. Kim, et al., [A Comparative Evaluation of the Hypoglycemic Activity of Acetyl-alpha-carnitine and Chlorpropamide in Experimental Diabetes], *Eksp Klin Farmakol,* 57(4), July-August 1994, p. 52-53.

Results of this study indicated acetyl-L-carnitine can prevent reductions in levels of substance P and methionine-enkephalin in the intestine, making it a promising treatment for autonomic neuropathies associated with diabetes.

—A. Gorio, et al., ''Peptide Alterations in Autonomic Diabetic Neuropathy Prevented by Acetyl-L-Carnitine,'' *International Journal of Clinical Pharmacology Research,* 12(5-6), 1992, p. 225-230.

Down's Syndrome

Results of this study showed significant improvement in visual memory and attention in Down's Syndrome patients relative to controls following treatment with acetyl-L-carnitine for 90 days.

—F.A. De Falco, et al., [Effect of the Chronic Treatment with L-acetylcarnitine in Down's Syndrome], *Clin Ter,* 144(2), February 1994, p. 123-127.

Neurological Function

Results of this double-blind, placebo-controlled study found that the oral administration of 3 g per day of acetyl-L-carnitine coupled with 50 mg of methylprednisolone for 14 days led to significant functional recovery of the nerves in patients suffering from idiopathic facial paralysis.

—C. Mezzina, et al., ''Idiopathic Facial Paralysis: New Therapeutic Prospects with Acetyl-

L-carnitine," *International Journal of Clinical Pharmacology Research,* 12(5-6), 1992, p. 299-304.

Results of this study showed that the administration of acetyl-L-carnitine significantly increased rat sensory neuron survival time in primary cultures for up to 40 days.
— A. Formenti, et al., "Effects of Acetyl-L-carnitine on the Survival of Adult Rat Sensory Neurons in Primary Cultures," *International Journal of Dev Neuroscience,* 10(3), June 1992, p. 207-214.

This study examined the effects of 10-50 microM of acetyl-L-carnitine administered for 10 days on primary cell cultures from hippocampal formation and cerebral cortex of 17-day-old rat embryos. Results showed the treatment had neuroprotective effects.
— G. Forloni, et al., "Neuroprotective Activity of Acetyl-L-carnitine: Studies in Vitro," *Journal of Neuroscience Research,* 37(1), January 1994, p. 92-96.

Results of this study showed that the administration of acetyl-L-carnitine for 10 months had positive neuroprotective effects on aged rats.
— S. Davis, et al., "Acetyl-L-carnitine: Behavioral, Electrophysiological, and Neurochemical Effects," *Neurobiol Aging,* 14(1), January-February 1993, p. 107-115.

Results of this study indicated that pre-ischemic administration of acetyl-L-carnitine in gerbils had neuroprotective effects.
— A. Shuaib, et al., "Acetyl-L-carnitine Attenuates Neuronal Damage in Gerbils with Transient Forebrain Ischemia Only When Given Before the Insult," *Neurochem Research,* 20(9), September 1995, p. 1021-1025.

This study assayed the in vitro effects of acetyl-L-carnitine on spontaneous and induced lipoperoxidation in rat skeletal muscle. Results showed that 10-40 mM of acetyl-L-carntine present in the medium produced significant reductions in MDA and conjugated diene formation in rat skeletal muscle.
— C. Di Giacomo, et al., "Effect of Acetyl-L-carnitine on Lipid Peroxidation and Xanthine Oxidase Activity in Rat Skeletal Muscle," *Neurochem Research,* 18(11), November 1993, p. 1157-1162.

Results of this study indicated that the administration of L-acetylcarnitine had positive effects on sciatic nerve regeneration in rats.
— E. Fernandez, et al., "Effects of L-carnitine, L-acetylcarnitine and Gangliosides on the Regeneration of the Transected Sciatic Nerve in Rats," *Neurol Research,* 11(1), March 1989, p. 57-62.

This study examined the effects of intravenous L-acetylcarnitine on Renshaw cell activity in spastic paraparesis patients. Results showed L-acetylcarnitine significantly increased recurrent inhibition levels.
— R. Mazzocchio, et al., "Enhancement of Recurrent Inhibition by Intravenous Administration of L-Acetylcarnitine in Spastic Patients," *Journal of Neurol Neurosurg Psychiatry,* 53(4), April 1990, p. 321-326.

Results of this study involving a canine model of global cerebral ischemia and reperfusion showed that the postischemic administration of acetyl-L-carnitine potentiated the normalization of brain energy metabolites and produced marked improvements in neurological outcome.

—R.E. Rosenthal, et al., ''Prevention of Postischemic Canine Neurological Injury through Potentiation of Brain Energy Metabolism by Acetyl-L-carnitine,'' *Stroke,* 23(9), September 1992, p. 1312-1317.

Results of this study showed that the administration of acetyl-L-carnitine led to significant reductions in lipofuscin accumulation within pyramidal neurons of the prefontal cortex and hippocampus of rats.

—F. Amenta, et al., ''Reduced Lipofuscin Accumulation in Senescent Rat Brain by Long-term Acetyl-L-carnitine Treatment,'' *Arch Gerontol Geriatr,* 9(2), September-October 1989, p. 147-153.

Parkinson's Disease

Results of this study indicated that the administration of either 1 g or 2 g per day for seven days of acetyl-L-carnitine led to improvements in H response, sleep stages and spindling activity in Parkinson's disease patients.

—F.M. Puca, et al., ''Clinical Pharmacodynamics of Acetyl-L-carnitine in Patients with Parkinson's Disease,'' *International Journal of Clinical Pharmacology Research,* 10(1-2), 1990, p. 139-143.

Results of this study showed monkeys pretreated with acetyl-L-carnitine did not exhibit symptoms of Parkinsonism normally associated with exposure to 1-methyl, 4-phenyl- 1,2,3,6-tetrahydropyridine (MPTP).

—I. Bodis-Wollner, et al., ''Acetyl-levo-carnitine Protects Against MPTP-induced Parkinsonism in Primates,'' *Journal of Neural Transm Park Dis Dement Sect,* 3(1), 1991, p. 63-72.

Reproductive Function

This study examined the effects of L-acetyl-l-carnitine on the male reproductive functions of rats made oligoasthenospermic with dibromochloropropane (DBCP). Results showed that one injection of L-acetyl-l-carnitine led to sperm count recovery and that L-acetyl-l-carnitine stimulated the production of testosterone.

—S. Palmero, et al., ''The Effect of L-acetylcarnitine on Some Reproductive Functions in the Oligoasthenospermic Rat,'' *Horm Metab Res* (1990 Dec) 22(12):622-6.

Senility

Results of this study showed that acetyl-L-carnitine administered at high levels can have positive effects on the release of amino acids as well as neurotransmitters such as dopamine and acetylcholine in the brain of rats.

—E. Toth, et al., ''Effect of Acetyl-L-carnitine on Extracellular Amino Acid Levels in Vivo in Rat Brain Regions,'' *Neurochem Research,* 18(5), May 1993, p. 573-578.

Stroke

Results of this double-blind, placebo-controlled study showed that acetyl-L-carnitine had significant positive effects on memory and cognitive performance tasks in elderly patients with cerebrovascular insufficiency.

> —A. Arrigo, et al., "Effects of Acetyl-L-carnitine on Reaction Times in Patients with Cerebrovascular Insufficiency," *International Journal of Clinical Pharmacology Research,* 10(1-2), 1990, p. 133-137.

Results of this study showed that the intravenous administration of 1.5 g of acetyl-L-carnitine led to improvements in cerebral blood flow in cerebrovasular disease patients who had suffered from a stroke at least 6 months prior to treatment.

> —A. Postiglione, et al., "Cerebral Blood Flow in Patients with Chronic Cerebrovascular Disease: Effect of Acetyl L-Carnitine," *International Journal of Clinical Pharmacology Research,* 10(1-2), 1990, p. 129-132.

Results of this study found that the intravenous administration of 1500 mg of acetyl-L-carnitine had beneficial effects on 4 out of 10 patients suffering from brain ischaemia.

> —G. Rosadini, et al., "Acute Effects of Acetyl-L-carnitine on Regional Cerebral Blood Flow in Patients with Brain Ischaemia," *International Journal of Clinical Pharmacology Research,* 10(1-2), 1990, p. 123-128.

This study examined the effects 1.5 g of intravenous L-acetyl-l-carnitine on cerebral blood flow in patients with chronic cerebrovascular disease. Results showed the treatment led to significant enhancements in cerebral blood flow.

> —A. Postiglione, et al., "Effect of Acute Administration of L-acetyl Carnitine on Cerebral Blood Flow in Patients with Chronic Cerebral Infarct," *Pharmacology Research,* 23(3), April 1991, p. 241-246.

■ ALPHA-LIPOIC ACID

AIDS/HIV

Results of this study indicated alpha-lipoic acid exhibited anti-HIV activity both in vitro and in vivo.

> —A. Baur, et al., "Inhibition of HIV-infectivity and Replication by Alpha-lipoic Acid," *International Conference on AIDS,* 7(1), June 16-21, 1991, p. 110.

Results of this study indicated alpha-lipoic acid inhibited HIV-1 replication in vitro.

> —A. Baur, et al., "Alpha-lipoic Acid is an Effective Inhibitor of Human Immuno-deficiency Virus (HIV-1) Replication," *Klin Wochenschr,* 69(15), October 2, 1991, p. 722-724.

Cancer

Results of this study showed that the ALPHA-lipoic acid derivatives 1,2-dithiocyclo pentane-4- semicarbazone (Ph 800/l), 1,2-dithio cyclopentane-3,5-dicarboxylic acid (Ph 800/8) and 1,2-dithiocyclopentane-

4-thiosemicarbazone (Ph 800/18) inhibited the growth of mouse Ehrlich carcinoma cells in vitro and of Ehrlich ascites carcinoma in vivo.

—J. Kieler & B. Biczowa, "The Effects of Structural Analogues of the Effect of Structural Analogues of Alpha-Lipoic Acid on the Growth and Metabolism of L-Firboblasts and Ehrlic Cells," *Arch Immunol Ther Exp,* 15(1), 1967, p. 106-111.

Cerebral Ischemia

Results of this study showed that alpha-lipoic acid was effective in improving survival and protecting the rat brain from cerebral ischemia-induced reperfusion injury.

—M. Panigrahi, et al., "Alpha-Lipoic Acid Protects Against Reperfusion Injury Following Cerebral Ischemia in Rats," *Brain Research,* 717(1-2), April 22, 1996, p. 184-188.

Results of this study showed that intraperitoneal injections of alpha-lipoic acid provided neuroprotective effects against ischemia/reperfusion evoked cerebral injury in gerbils.

—X. Cao & J.W. Phillis, "The Free Radical Scavenger, Alpha-Lipoic Acid, Protects Against Cerebral Ischemia-Reperfusion Injury in Gerbils," *Free Radical Research,* 23(4), October 1995, p. 365-370.

Diabetes

Results of this study showed that antioxidant therapy including 600 mg of alpha-lipoic acid or 100 mcg of sodium selenite per day or 1200 IE of D-alpha-tocopherol over a period of 3 months led to improvements in symptoms of distal symmetric neuropathy in patients suffering from long-term diabetic late syndrome.

—W. Kahler, et al., "Diabetes Mellitus—a Free Radical-Associated Disease. Results of Adjuvant Antioxidant Supplementation," *Z.Gesamte Inn Med,* 48(5), May 1993, p. 223-232.

Results of this study showed that lipoic acid improved symptoms associated with streptozotocine-induced diabetic neuropathy in rats.

—N. Nagamatsu, et al., "Lipoic Acid Improves Nerve Blood Flow, Reduces Oxidative Stress, and Improves Distal Nerve Conduction in Experimental Diabetic Neuropathy," *Diabetes Care,* 18(8), August 1995, p. 1160-1167.

Results of this study showed that the parenteral administration of alpha-lipoic acid significantly enhanced the capacity of the insulin-stimulatable glucose transport system and of both oxidative and nonoxidative pathways of glucose metabolism in insulin-resistant rat skeletal muscle.

—S. Jacob, et al., "The Antioxidant Alpha-lipoic Acid Enhances Insulin-stimulated Glucose Metabolism in Insulin-resistant Rat Skeletal Muscle," *Diabetes,* 45(8), August 1996, p. 1024-1029.

Results of this double-blind, placebo-controlled study indicated that the administration of 1000 mg of alpha-lipoic acid significantly increased insulin stimulated glucose disposal in NIDDM patients.

—S. Jacob, et al., "Enhancement of Glucose Disposal in Patients with Type 2 Diabetes by Alpha-lipoic Acid," *Arzneimittelforschung,* 45(8), August 1995, p. 872-874.

Results of this double-blind, placebo-controlled study showed that the intravenous administration of 600 mg per day of alpha-lipoic acid over a period of 3 weeks reduced symptoms associated with diabetic peripheral neuropathy in NIDDM patients.

> —D. Ziegler, et al., "Treatment of Symptomatic Diabetic Peripheral Neuropathy with the Anti-oxidant Alpha-lipoic Acid. A 3-week Multicentre Randomized Controlled Trial," *Diabetologia,* 38(12), December 1995, p. 1425-1433.

Results of this study indicated that the oral administration of thiotic acid at doses of either 2 x 50 mg or 2 x 100 mg per day proved to be a successful treatment for diabetic neuropathy in human patients.

> —W. Klein, [Treatment of Diabetic Neuropathy with Oral Alpha-lipoic Acid], *MMW Munch Med Wochenschr,* 117(22), May 30, 1975, p. 957-958.

General

Results of this study showed that alpha-lipoic acid counteracted glycollate-induced free radical toxicity in rats.

> —R. Sumathi, et al., "Effect of DL Alpha-lipoic Acid on Tissue Lipid Peroxidation and Antioxidant Systems in Normal and Glycollate Treated Rats," *Pharmacol Res,* 27(4), May-June 1993, p. 309-318.

Results of this study showed that the administration of 600 mg of lipoic acid per day for one month led to increases in available brain energy levels and skeletal muscle energy levels in a woman affected by chronic progressive external opthalmoplegia and muscle mitochondria DNA deletion.

> —B. Barbirolli, et al., "Lipoic (thiotic) Acid Increases Brain Energy Availability and Skeletal Muscle Performance as Shown by in Vivo 31P-MRS in a Patient with Mitochondrial Cytopathy," *Journal of Neurology,* 242(7), July 1995, p. 472-477.

Glaucoma

Results of this study found that the administration of 0.15 g per day of lipoic acid for 1 month led to improvements of biochemical parameters, visual function, and of the coefficient of efficacy of liquid discharge in patients with stages I and II open-angle glaucoma. Positive effects were most frequent among stage II patients.

> —A.A. Filina, et al., "Lipoic Acid as a Means of Metabolic Therapy of Open-Angle Glaucoma," *Vestn Oftalmol,* 111(4), Oct-Dec 1995, p. 6-8.

Memory

Results of this study showed that alpha-lipoic acid improved memory in aged mice.

> —S. Stoll, et al., "The Potent Free Radical Scavenger Alpha-lipoic Acid Improves Memory in Aged Mice: Putative Relationship to NMDA Receptor Deficits," *Pharmacol Biochem Behav,* 46(4), December 1993, p. 799-805.

■ COENZYME Q10

AIDS/HIV

This article reports on two ARC patients who have survived 4 to 5 years with no symptoms of adenopathy or infection while taking CoQ10 continuously. The authors also report results on 14 newly found normal subjects that experienced increased T4/T8 ratios in response to CoQ10 administration.

—K. Folkers, et al., "Coenzyme Q10 Increases T4/T8 Ratios of Lymphocytes in Ordinary Subjects and Relevance to Patients Having the AIDS Related Complex," *Biochem Biophys Res Commun,* 176(2), April 30, 1991, p. 786-791.

Results of this study showed that AIDS patients had a significantly blood deficiency of CoQ10 relative to controls and relative to ARC patients. ARC patients showed a significant deficiency relative to controls as well, as did patients infected with HIV. Results found that CoQ10 deficiency increased with the increased severity of the disease. When 7 AIDS patients were treated with CoQ10, 5 survived and were symptomatically better after 4-7 months.

—K. Folkers, et al., "Biochemical Deficiencies of Coenzyme Q10 in HIV-infection and Exploratory Treatment," *Biochem Biophys Res Commun,* 153(2), June 16, 1988, p. 888-896.

Cancer

This study examined the effects of CoQ10 on the cardiotoxicity of adriamycin in cultures of beating heart cells from neonatal rats. After 12 hours of exposure, results found that cultures treated with CoQ10 showed beating activities comparable to those of untreated controls, while adriamycin-treated cultures exhibited either arrhythmias or lacked beating activity. Cultures treated concurrently with adriamycin and CoQ10 continued to beat normally.

—A.B. Combs, et al., "Prevention by Coenzyme Q10 of the Cardiotoxicity of Adriamycin in Cultured Heart Cells," *IRCS Med Sci: Cancer,* 4(8), 1976, p. 403.

Results of this study showed that mice pretreated with CoQ10 experienced significant reductions in the lethality of antitumor antibioitc anthramycin as well as its ability to decrease ventricular weights.

—W.C. Lubawy, et al., "Protection Against Anthramycin-induced Toxicity in Mice by Coenzyme Q10," *Journal of the National Cancer Institute,* 64(1), January 1980, p. 105-109.

Results of this placebo-controlled study showed that CoQ10 treatment helped to prevent liver damage in mitomycin C-induced sarcoma 10 solid type-tumor-bearing mice.

—S. Yamada, et al., [Experimental Research on Coenzyme Q10 Treatment for Liver Damage Induced by Antibeoplastic Drugs," *Nippon Kagaku Ryoho Gakkai Zasshim,* 27(4), 1979, p. 675-680.

This article cites numerous clinical and case studies supporting the use of CoQ10 in the treatment of breast cancer. Results of one study in particular found that 390 mg per day proved effective in 3 subjects monitored over a 3-5 year period.

—K. Lockwood, et al., "Progress on Therapy of Breast Cancer with Vitamin Q10 and the Regression of Metastases," *Biochem Biophys Res Commun,* 212(1), July 6, 1995, p. 172-177.

In this study, 6 of 32 patients at high risk for breast cancer who were treated with 90 mg of CoQ10 in addition to other antioxidants and fatty acids showed partial tumor regression. When 1 of these 6 patients increased dosage to 390 mg of CoQ10 per day the tumor was no longer palpable after one month and, following another month, mammagrophy indicated an absence of tumor. When yet another case was given 300 mg of CoQ10 per day there was no residula tumor three months following the start of treatment.

> —K. Lockwood, et al., "Partial and Complete Regression of Breast Cancer in Patients in Relation to Dosage of Coenzyme Q10," *Biochem Biophys Res Commun,* 199(3), March 30, 1994, p. 1504-1508.

This review article notes that studies have shown that CoQ10 can overcome adriamycin-induced inhibition in vitro when supplemented at high levels and has been shown to overcome cardiotoxicity in intact rabbits and isolated rabbit hearts.

> —T. Kishi & K. Folkers, "Prevention by Coenzyme Q10 (NSC-140865) of the Inhibition by Adriamycin (NSC-123127) of Coenzyme Q10 Enzymes," *Cancer Treat Rev,* 60(3), 1976, p. 223-224.

This study examined the effects of CoQ10 administered intravenously at doses of 1 mg/kg per day on the prevention of adriamycin and dauborubicin-induced side effects in malignant lymphoma patients. Results showed the degree of alopecia, fever, nausea and vomiting, the incidences of diarrhea and stomatitis were significantly reduced in the CoQ10-treated patients relative to controls.

> —K. Tsubaki, et al., [Investigation of the Preventive Effect of CoQ10 Against the Side-effects of Anthracycline Antineoplastic agents], *Gan To Kagaku Ryoho,* 11(7), July 1984, p. 1420-1427.

Results of this study found that the administration of CoQ10 may prevent some electrocardiographic changes induce by adriamycin in humans.

> —K. Okuma, et al., [Protective Effect of Coenzyme Q10 in Cardiotoxicity Induced by Adriamycin], *Gan To Kagaku Ryoho,* 11(3), March 1984, p. 502-508.

Results of this study indicated the usefulness of CoQ10 in the enhancement of cancer immunochemotherapy in rats using masked compounds in combination with immunopotentiators and exhibited no side effects.

> —T. Kokawa, et al., [Coenzyme Q10 in Cancer Chemotherapy—experimental Studies on Augmentation of the Effects of Masked Compounds, Especially in the Combined Chemotherapy with Immunopotentiators], *Gan To Kagaku Ryoho,* 10(3), March 1983, p. 768-774.

This study examined the effects of BCG, CoQ10, or the two together on the cell-mediated immune response in tumor-bearing mice. Results found that depressed oligomycin-sensitive ATPase activity significantly recovered by treatment with BCG or coenzyme Q10.

> —I. Kawase, et al., [The Enhancing Effect of Coenzyme Q10 on Immunorecovery with BCG in Tumor Bearing Mice: In Realtion to Changes in Coeznymes Q Content and ATP-ASE Activity in Spleen Lymphocytes of Tumor-Bearing Rats," *Gan To Kagaku Ryoho,* 6(2), 1979, p. 281-288.

Results of this study showed that the combined treatment of CoQ10 and BCG led to improvement of depressed bioenergetic in tumor-bearing rat lymphocytes.

—H. Niitani, et al., "Combined Effect of BCG and Coenzyme Q10 on ATP-ase Activity and Coenzyme Q Content in spleen Lymphocytes of Tumor-bearing Rats," *Gann*, 70(3), June 1979, p. 315-322.

Results of this study showed that CoQ10 enhanced immunorestoration with BCG in tumor-bearing mice.

—I. Kawase, et al., "Enhancing Effect of Coenzyme, Q10 on Immunorestoration with Mycobacterium Bovis BCG in Tumor-bearing Mice," *Gann*, 69(4), August 1978, p. 493-497.

Cardiovascular/Coronary Heart Disease

This double-blind, placebo-controlled study examined the effects of 150 mg per of CoQ10 for 4 weeks on exercise performance in middle age, stable angina pectoris patients. Results indicated CoQ10 to be an effective and safe treatment for the condition.

—T. Kamikawa, et al., "Effects of Coenzyme Q10 on Exercise Tolerance in Chronic Stable Angina Pectoris," *American Journal of Cardiology*, 56(4), August 1, 1985, p. 247-251.

Results of this study found that the administration of CoQ10 to rats significantly improved the functional recovery during reperfusion by enhancing the recovery of high-energy phosphates and preventing overload of Ca2+.

—O. Hano, et al., "Coenzyme Q10 Enhances Cardiac Functional and Metabolic Recovery and Reduces Ca2+ Overload During Postischemic Reperfusion," *American Journal of Physiology*, 266(6 Pt 2), June 1994, p. H2174-81.

Results of this case-control study found that 30-60 mg per day of CoQ10 administered orally for 6 days preoperatively significantly increased heart tolerance to ischemia during aortic clamping in humans.

—J. Tanaka, et al., "Coenzyme Q10: The Prophylactic Effect on Low Cardiac Output Following Cardiac Valve Replacement," *Annals of Thoracic Surgery*, 33(2), February 983, p. 145-151.

Results of this case-control study found that elective coronary artery bypass patients pretreated with 150 mg per day of CoQ10 for 7 days prior to surgery showed a significantly lower incidence of ventricular arrhythmias during the recovery period than controls.

—M. Chello, et al., "Protection by Coenzyme Q10 from Myocardial Reperfusion Injury During Coronary Artery Bypass Grafting," *Annals of Thoracic Surgery*, 58(5), November 1994, p. 1427-1432.

In this study, mongrel dogs experienced an hour of carioplegic solution-induced cardiac arrest under cardiopulmonary bypass. One of three types of cardioplegic solution was used: clinical potassium cardioplegic solution (K+, 22.31 mEq/L), potassium cardioplegic solution with coenzyme Q10 added (coenzyme Q10, 30 mg/500 ml of solution), and cardioplegic solution with coenzyme Q10 solvent. Results showed that exogenous coenzyme Q10 containing solution provided significantly high myocardial stores of adenosine triphosphate and creatine phosphate and a low level of lactate during induced ischemia and reperfusion while recovery percentage of the aortic flow was significantly greater relative to the other two solutions as well. Results also found that CoQ10 added to potassium cardioplegia improved myocardial oxygen utilization and accelerated recovery of myocardial energy metabolism following circulation reestablishment.

> —F. Mori & H. Mohri, "Effects of Coenzyme Q10 Added to a Potassium Cardioplegic Solution for Myocardial Protection During Ischemic Cardiac Arrest," *Annals of Thoracic Surgery*, 39(1), January 1985, p. 30-36.

Results of this study showed that rabbits pretreated with CoQ10 experienced a recovery of cardiac contractile force and of myocardial ATP content upon reoxygenation, while the release of creatine phosphokinase from hearts during hypoxia and reoxygenation was totally inhibited by pretreatment. Results also showed that UV absorbance of the perfusate changes indicated that CoQ10 decreased loss of ATP metabolites from hypoxic hearts.

> —S. Takeo, et al., "Possible Mechanism by which Coenzyme Q10 Improves Reoxygenation-Induced Recovery of Cardiac Contractile Force After Hypoxia," *Journal of Pharmacol Exp Ther*, 243(3), December 1987, p. 1131-1138.

Results of this case-control study found that pretreatment with 30 mg per day CoQ10 administered for 7 days effectively decreased aortic cross clamping-induced ischemic injury in rats.

> —R. Tominaga, et al., "Effects of Pretreatment with Coenzyme Q10 on Myocardial Preservation During Aortic Cross Clamping," *Journal of Surg Res*, 34(2), February 1983, p. 111-117.

Results of this double-blind, placebo-control study found that pretreatment with CoQ10 was effective in preventing myocardial injury during preservation and subsequent reperfusion in dogs.

> —T. Matsushima, et al., "Protection by Coenzyme Q10 of Canine Myocardial Reperfusion Injury After Preservation," *Journal of Thoracic Cardiovascular Surgery*, 103(5), May 1992, p. 945-951.

In this case control study, isolated hearts from rats pretreated with either coenzyme Q10, 20 mg/kg intramuscularly and 10 mg/kg intraperitoneally 24 and 2 hours before the experiment were subjected to 15 minutes of equilibration, 25 minutes of ischemia, and 40 minutes of reperfusion. Results found that Coenzyme Q10 pretreatment improved myocardial function after ischemia and reperfusion.

> —J.A. Crestanello, et al., "Elucidation of a Tripartite Mechanism Underlying the Improvement in Cardiac Tolerance to Ischemia by Coenzyme Q10 Pretreatment," *Journal of Thoracic Cardiovasc Surgery*, February 1996, 111(2), p. 443-450.

Results of this study found that the administration of CoQ10 prior to reoxygenation inhibited oxygen mediated myocardial injury in piglets caused by reoxygenation of the hypoxemic immature heart on cardiopulmonary bypass.

> —K. Morita, et al., "Studies of Hypoxemic/reoxygenation Injury: Without Aortic Clamping. VII. Counteraction of Oxidant Damage by Exogenous Antioxidants: Coenzyme Q10," *Journal of Thoracic Cardiovascular Surgery*, 110(4 Pt 2), October 1995, p. 1221-1227.

Results of this study found that CoQ10 administered to dogs intravenously prior to reperfusion enhanced the role of substrate-enriched blood cardioplegic solution in salvaging ischemic myocardium to make way for recovery.

> —F. Okamoto, et al., "Reperfusate Composition: Supplemental Role of Intravenous and

Intracoronary Coenzyme Q10 in Avoiding Reperfusion Damage," *Journal of Thoracic Cardiovascular Surgery,* 92(3 Pt 2), September 1986, p. 573-582.

Results of this study found that brain ischemia/reperfusion injury in dogs can result from oxygen-derived free radicals and abnormal energy metabolism and that the administration of CoQ10 can provide protection against such damage by improving cerebral metabolism
— Z. Ren, et al., "Mechanisms of Brain Injury with Deep Hypothermic Circulatory Arrest and Protective Effects of Coenzyme Q10," *Journal of Thoracic Cardiovascular Surgery,* 108(1), July 1994, p. 126-133.

Results of this double-blind, placebo-controlled study found patients pretreated with CoQ10 had less left atrial pressure, a decreased incidence of low cardiac output, a wider pulse pressure, and a better preserved right and left ventricular myocardial ultrastructure relative to controls.
— Y.F. Chen, et al., "Effectiveness of Coenzyme Q10 on Myocardial Preservation During Hypothermic Cardioplegic Arrest," *Journal of Thoracic Cardiovascular Surgery,* 107(1), January 1994, p. 242-247.

This case-control study examined the effects of CoQ10 on mice inoculated with the M variant of encephalomyocarditis virus. Results showed significantly higher rates of survival in mice receiving the CoQ10 than controls.
— C. Kishimoto, et al., "The Protection of Coenzyme Q10 Against Experimental Viral Myocarditis in Mice," *Japanese Circulatory Journal,* 48(12), December 1984, p. 1358-1361.

Results of this study found that the administration of CoQ10 for 8 weeks preserved left ventricular function and attenuated cardiomyopathy progression in hamsters.
— S. Momomura, et al., "Coenzyme Q10 Attenuates the Progression of Cardiomyopathy in Hamsters," *Japanese Heart Journal,* 32(1), January 1991, p. 101-110.

Results of this study showed that the administration of CoQ10 provided protection against chlorpromzine-induced injury in the myocardial cells of rats.
— M. Chiba, "A Protective Action of Coenzyme Q10 on Chlorpromazine-induced Cell Damage in the Cultured Rat Myocardial Cells," *Japanese Heart Journal,* 25(1), January 1984, p. 127-137.

This study examined CoQ10's electrophysiological and inotropic effects on isoproterenol or barium-induced slow responses in ventricular papillary muscle depolarized by high K+ concentration under hypoxia. Results showed significant reversing effects on hypoxia-induced deterioration of the slow response.
— M. Arita, et al., "Electrophysiological and Inotropic Effects of Coenzyme Q10 on Guinea Pig Ventricular Muscle Depolarized by Potassium Under Hypoxia," *Japanese Heart Journal,* 23(6), November 1982, p. 961-974.

Results of this study found that the combined treatment of vitamin B2-butyrate for lipid peroxidation reduction and CoQ10 for restoring deficiency can prevent adriamycin-induced cardiotoxicity in rats during cancer chemotherapy.
— T. Katsuki, [Experimental Studies on the Combination Use of Vitamin B2-butyrate and

Coenzyme Q10 to Protect Against Adriamycin-Induced Cardiac Mitochondrial Disorders],
Kurume Igakkai Zasshi, 44(12), 1981, p. 869-883.

Results of this study showed that Vitamin B2-butyrate and CoQ10 inhibited lipid peroxide production
in Ehrlich ascites tumor cells treated with adriamycin.

—M. Chinami, et al., [Effect of Coenzyme Q10 and Vitamin B-2 Butyrate to Anticancer
Ability and Lipid Peroxidation of Adriamycin," *Kurume Igakkai Zasshi,* 44(9/10), 1981, p.
678-683.

This review article cites studies showing the CoQ10 may be an effective treatment for ischemic heart
disease, congestive heart failure, toxin-induced cardiotoxicity, and hypertension.

—S.M. Greenberg & W.H. Frishman, "Coenzyme Q10: A New Drug for Myocardial Ischemia?" *Medical Clinics of North America,* 72(1), January 1988, p. 243-258.

This article reports on the single case of a patient with mitochondrial encephalomyopathy and cytochrome c oxidase deficiency who took high doses of CoQ10 for 2 years. Results showed that such
treatment led to decreases in abnormal elevation of the serum lactate per pyruvate ratio and the
increased concentration of serum lactate plus pyruvate induced by exercise. Results also showed that
CoQ10 improved impaired central and peripheral nerve conductivities.

—Y. Nishikawa, et al., "Long-term Coenzyme Q10 Therapy for a Mitochondrial Encephalomyopathy with Cytochrome C Oxidase Deficiency: A 31P NMR Study," *Neurology,* 39(3),
March 1989, p. 399-403.

Results of this study showed that the administration of 60 to 120 mg per day of CoQ10 for 3 months
to a patient with Kearns-Sayre syndrome led to the normalization of lactate and pyruvate serum levels
and improvement of occular movement and atriventricular block.

—S. Ogasahara, et al., "Improvement of Abnormal Pyruvate Metabolism and Cardiac Conduction Defect with Coenzyme Q10 in Kearns-Sayre Syndrome," *Neurology,* 35(3), March 1985,
p. 372-373.

Results of this study showed that the administration of CoQ10 led to the preservation of hepatic
ischemia-induced cellular damages in rats and that such preservation was likely due to the protection
of cellular and subcellular membranes from lipid peroxidation.

—S. Marubayashi, et al., "Preservation of Ischemic Rat Liver Mitochondrial Functions and
Liver Viability with CoQ10," *Surgery,* 91(6), June 1982, p. 631-637.

Results of this study showed that pretreatment of donor rats with 10 mg/kg of CoQ10 intravenously
increased survival time following warm ischemic damage of rat liver grafts.

—K. Sumimoto, et al., "Ischemic Damage Prevention by Coenzyme Q10 Treatment of
the Donor Before Orthotopic Liver Transplantation: Biochemical and Histologic Findings,"
Surgery, 102(5), November 1987, p. 821-827.

Results of this study showed that CoQ10 administration exhibited protective effects on hypertrophied
ischemic myocardium in dogs.

—F. Okamoto, et al., "Effect of Coenzyme Q10 on Hypertrophied Ischemic Myocardium

During Aortic Cross Clamping for 2 Hr, from the Aspect of Energy Metabolism,'' *Adv Myocardiol*, 4, 1983, p. 559-566.

This review article cites numerous double-blind studies and case histories supporting the efficacy and safety of using CoQ10 in the treatment of heart failure.
—K. Folkers, et al., ''Therapy with Coenzyme Q10 of Patients in Heart Failure Who Are Eligible or Ineligible for a Transplant,'' *Biochem Biophys Res Commun*, 182(1), January 15, 1992, p. 247-253.

Results of this study showed that the administration of CoQ10 can prevent or inhibit the cardiomyopathy of doxorubican in rabbits.
—N. Domae, et al., ''Cardiomyopathy and Other Chronic Toxic Effects Induced in Rabbits by Doxorubicin and Possible Prevention by Coenzyme Q10,'' *Cancer Treat Rep*, 65(1-2), January-February 1981, p. 79-91.

Results of this study indicated that pretreatment with 5 mg/kg administered intravenously of CoQ10 was effective in the prevention of left ventricular depression in early reperfusion and in minimizing myocardial cellular injury during coronary artery bypass grafting followed by reperfusion in humans.
—M. Sunamori, et al., ''Clinical Experience of Coenzyme Q10 to Enhance Intraoperative Myocardial Protection in Coronary Artery Revascularization,'' *Cardiovasc Drugs Ther*, 5 Suppl 2, March 1991, p. 297-300.

This study examined the effects of CoQ10 on the ischaemic myocardium following constriction of left anterior descending coronary artery in open-chest mongrel dogs. Results showed that dogs premedicated with 20 mg/kg of intravenous CoQ10 had a significantly higher ATP content in ischaemic myocardium relative to controls.
—Y. Nakamura, et al., ''Protection of Ischaemic Myocardium with Coenzyme Q10,'' *Cardiovascular Research*, 16(3), March 1982, p. 132-137.

Results of this study found that CoQ10 improved recovery of the left ventricular peak systolic pressure and the coronary sinus flow in rats.
—T. Konishi, et al., ''Improvement in Recovery of Left Ventricular Function During Reperfusion with Coenzyme Q10 in Isolated Working Rat Heart,'' *Cardiovascular Research*, 19(1), January 1985, p. 38-43.

Results of this study showed the administration of CoQ10 supported cardiovascular hemodynamics and prevented free radical mediated lipid peroxidation during E. coli septic shock in dogs.
—J.L. Lelli, et al., ''Effects of Coenzyme Q10 on the Mediator Cascade of Sepsis,'' *Circ Shock*, 39(3), March 1993, p. 178-187.

This study examined the efficacy and safety of adjunctive treatment with 50-100 mg of CoQ10 per day for 3 months in congestive heart failure patients. Results showed the patient improvement rates after three months of treatment were: cyanosis 81%, edema 76.9%, pulmonary rates, 78.4%, enlargement of the liver area 49.3%, jugular reflux 81.5%, dyspnea 54.2%, palpitations 75.7%, sweating 82.4%, arrhythmia 62%, insomnia 60.2%, vertigo 73%, and nocturia 50.7%.
—E. Baggio, et al., ''Italian Multicenter Study on the Safety and Efficacy of Coenzyme Q10

as Adjunctive Therapy in Heart Failure (interim analysis). The CoQ10 Drug Surveillance Investigators,'' *Clinical Investigations,* 71(8 Suppl), 1993, p. S145-149.

Results of this case control study of patients suffering from symptoms commonly preceding congestive heart failure showed that the administration of CoQ10 led to improvement in all patients, high blood pressure reduction in 80%, improved diastolic function all; reduction in myocardial thickness in 53% of hypertensives and 36% of the combined prolapse and fatigue syndrome groups; and reduction in fractional shortening in those high at control and an increase in those initially low.
 —P.H. Langsjoen, et al., ''Isolated Diastolic Dysfunction of the Myocardium and its Response to CoQ10 Treatment,'' *Clinical Investigations,* 71(8 Suppl), 1993, p. S140-144.

Results of this double-blind, placebo-controlled, year-long study showed that 2mg/kg per day of CoQ10 coupled with conventional therapy in chronic congestive heart failure patients significantly decreased hospitalization rates for heart failure worsening and complication incidence.
 —C. Morisco, et al., ''Effect of Coenzyme Q10 Therapy in Patients with Congestive Heart Failure: A Long-term Multicenter Randomized Study,'' *Clinical Investigations,* 71(8 Suppl), 1993, p. S134-S146.

Results of this study showed that the administration of 50 mg per day of CoQ10 for 4 weeks coupled with conventional therapy led to improvements in dyspnea at rest, exertional dyspnea, palpitation, cyanosis, hepatomegaly, pulmonary rates, ankle edema, heart rate, and both systolic and diastolic blood pressure in patients with chronic heart failure.
 —M. Lampertico & S. Comis, ''Italian Multicenter Study on the Efficacy and Safety of Coenzyme Q10 as Adjuvant Therapy in Heart Failure,'' *Clinical Investigations,* 71(8 Suppl), 1993, p. S129-S133.

This review article cites numerous studies supporting the efficacy of CoQ10 in the treatment of heart disease.
 —S.A. Mortensen, ''Perspectives on Therapy of Cardiovascular Diseases with Coenzyme Q10 (Ubiquinone),'' *Clinical Investigations,* 71(8 Suppl), 1993, p. S116-S123.

Results of this placebo-controlled study found that pretreatment with CoQ10 provided protection of the ischemic myocardium in an open-chest swine model.
 —D. Atar, et al., ''Coenzyme Q10 Protects Ischemic Myocardium in an Open-chest Swine Model,'' *Clinical Investigations,* 71(8 Suppl), 1993, p. S103-S11.

Results of this study showed that 100 mg per day of CoQ10 proved to be an effective therapeutic agent in case of advanced chronic heart failure.
 —S.A. Mortensen, et al., ''Long-term Coenzyme Q10 Therapy: A Major Advance in the Management of Resistant Myocardial Failure,'' *Drugs Exp Clin Res,* 11(8), 1985, p. 581-593.

In this double-blind, crossover study, CoQ10 was administered to 19 chronic myocardial disease patients. Results showed that 18 experienced improved activity tolerance with replacement therapy.

Results also found significant improvements among patients in stroke volume measured by impedance cardiography, and ejection fractions calculated from systolic time intervals.

—P.H. Langsjoen, et al., "Effective Treatment with Coenzyme Q10 of Patients with Chronic Myocardial Disease," *Drugs Exp Clin Res,* 11(8), 1985, p. 577-579.

Results of this study showed that the administration of 3.0-3.4 mg per day (average) of CoQ10 was effective against cardiac dysfunction in patients with mitral valve prolapse and improved stress-induced cardiac dysfunction.

—T. Oda, "Effect of Coenzyme Q10 on Stress-induced Cardiac Dysfunction in Paediatric Patients with Mitral Valve Prolapse: A Study by Stress Echocardiography," *Drugs Exp Clin Res,* 11(8), 1985, p. 557-576.

This study examined the effects of carnitine and CoQ10 on doxorubicin cardiotoxicity in rats. Results showed that the drugs proved most effective when administered together and in doses of 200 mg/kg per day or carnitine and 10 mg/kg per day of CoQ10.

—S. Ronca-Testoni, et al., "Effect of Carnitine and Coenzyme Q10 on the Calcium Uptake in Heart Sarcoplasmic Reticulum of Rats Treated with anthracyclines," *Drugs Exp Clin Res,* 18(10), 1992, p. 437-442.

This study examined the effects of L-carnitine, coenzyme Q10 and their combined administration on haemodynamic and metabolic variables in isolated perfused working rat hearts after 10 min of global normothermic ischaemia followed by 60 min of reperfusion. Results showed a lower purine release in the perfusate of the hearts of the rats treated with both compounds.

—A. Bertelli, et al., "L-carnitine and Coenzyme Q10 Protective Action Against Ischaemia and Reperfusion of Working Rat Heart," *Drugs Exp Clin Res,* 18(10), 1992, p. 431-436.

This study examined the relationship between CoQ10 serum levels and cardiac performance in patients suffering from either hyperthyroidism, hypothyroidism, or normal subjects. Results found a significant inverse association between thyroid hormones and Coenzyme Q10 levels. Based on their findings, the authors concluded that CoQ10 has therapeutic value for thyrotoxicosis-induced congestive heart failure

—H. Suzuki, et al., "Cardiac Performance and Coenzyme Q10 in Thyroid Disorders," *Endocrinol Jpn,* 31(6), December 1984, p. 755-761.

This study examined adriamycin-induced cardiotoxicity and the effects on it by CoQ10 in rabbits. Results showed CoQ10 injections provided protection against the cardiotoxicity.

—M. Tajima, [Chronic Cardiotoxicity of Anthracycline Derivatives and Possible Prevention by Coenzyme Q10], *Gan No Rinsho,* 30(9 Suppl), July 1984, p. 1211-1216.

Results of this study found that pretreatment with CoQ10 exhibited protection against the isolated ventricular muscle subjected to hypoxia action potential and contraction induced deterioration in guinea pigs.

—M. Aomine & M. Arita, "Pretreatment with Coenzyme Q10 Protects Guinea Pig Ventricular Muscle From Hypoxia-induced Deterioration of Action Potentials and Contraction," *Gen Pharmacol,* 16(2), 1985, p. 91-96.

Results of this study found that the administration of CoQ10 provided protection against biochemical derangements in the thyrotoxic heart in rabbits.

—C. Kotake, et al., "Protective Effect of Coenzyme Q10 on Thyrotoxic Heart in Rabbits," *Heart Vessels,* 3(2), 1987, p. 84-90.

Results of this study showed that CoQ10 administered in doses of 60 mg per day for two months reduced blood viscosity in patients with ischemic heart disease.

—T. Kato, et al., "Reduction in Blood Viscosity by Treatment with Coenzyme Q10 in Patients with Ischemic Heart Disease," *Int J Clin Pharmacol Ther Toxicol,* 28(3), March 1990, p. 123-126.

This study examined the effects of 100 mg per day of CoQ10 for 2 months on dilated cardiomyopathy patients. Results indicated that CoQ10 deficiency could be reversed through supplementation and that CoQ10 treatment may be effective when coupled with conventional treatment in patients with chronic cardiac failure.

—U. Manzoli, et al., "Coenzyme Q10 in Dilated Cardiomyopathy," *International Journal of Tissue React,* 12(3), 1990, p. 173-178.

Results of this study found that 100 mg of CoQ10 per day administered orally to be an effective treatment for chronic cardiomyopathy.

—P.H. Langsjoen, et al., "A Six-year Clinical Study of Therapy of Cardiomyopathy with Coenzyme Q10," *International Journal of Tissue React,* 12(3), 1990, p. 169-171.

Results of this study found that treatment with CoQ10 fed to highly significant increases in survival rates in patients with cardiomyopathy.

—P.H. Langsjoen, et al., "Pronounced Increase of Survival of Patients with Cardiomyopathy when Treated with Coenzyme Q10 and Conventional Therapy," *International Journal of Tissue React,* 12(3), 1990, p. 163-168.

Diabetes

This article reports on the case of a 71-year-old man diagnosed with diabetic amyotrophy who experienced relief in symptoms of the legs, fatigue, and residual urine in the bladder following the administration of CoQ10.

—Y. Suzuki, et al., "A Case of Diabetic Amyotrophy Associated with 3243 Mitochondrial tRNA(leu; UUR) Mutation and Successful Therapy with Coenzyme Q10," *Endocr Journal,* 42(2), April 1995, p. 141-145.

General

Results of this study found that a combination of CoQ10 and nicotinamide attenuated mild to moderate experimentall induced neurotoxicity.

—J.B. Schulz, et al., "Coenzyme Q10 and Nicotinamide and a Free Radical Spin Trap Protect Against MPTP Neurotoxicity," *Exp Neurol,* 132(2), April 1995, p. 279-283.

In this study, weaning rats fed a Torula yeast-based diet either unsupplemented or supplemented with 30 mg beta-carotene/kg, 30 IU vitamin E/kg, 1 mg selenium/kg or 30 mg coenzyme Q10/kg. Results showed CoQ10 and beta-carotene act as antioxidants in ways similar to selenium and vitamin E.

> —R. Zamora, et al., ''Comparative Antioxidant Effectiveness of Dietary Beta-carotene, Vitamin E, Selenium and Coenzyme Q10 in Rat Erythrocytes and Plasma,'' *Journal of Nutrition,* 121(1), January 1991, p. 50-56.

Results of this study found that dietary CoQ10 supplementation proved active against tertbutyl hydroperoxide-induced lipid peroxidation in rats.

> —B. Leibovitz, et al., ''Dietary Supplements of Vitamin E, Beta-carotene, Coenzyme Q10 and Selenium Protect Tissues Against Lipid Peroxidation in Rat Tissue Slices,'' *Journal of Nutrition,* 120(1), January 1990, p. 97-104.

This study examined the effects of CoQ10 on lipid peroxidation and survival time of mice treated with adriamycin. Results found that CoQ10 exhibited protective effects against a adriamycin-induced subacute toxicity, with mice administered 10 mg/kg of CoQ10 showing the most prolonged survival time.

> —S. Shinozawa, et al., ''Effect of CoQ10 on the Survival Time and Lipid Peroxidation of Adriamycin (doxorubicin) Treated Mice,'' *Acta Med Okayama,* 38(1), February 1984, p. 57-63.

Hearing Loss

Results of this study found that CoQ10 promoted recovery auditory hair damage in guinea pigs and prevented respiratory metabolic impairment of hair cell caused by hypoxia.

> —K. Sato, ''Pharmacokinetics of Coenzyme Q10 in Recovery of Acute Sensorineural Hearing Loss Due to Hypoxia,'' *Acta Otolaryngol Suppl,* 458, 1988, p. 95-102.

Immune Enhancement

In this study, CoQ10 and vitamin B6 were administered together and independently to three groups of subjects. Results showed that blood levels of IgG increased significantly when CoQ10 and B6 were administered together as well as when CoQ10 was administered alone. T4-lymphocyte blood levels increased significantly when CoQ10 and B6 were administered together and independently. T4/T8 lymphocytes ratio increased significantly when CoQ10 and B6 were administered together and independently.

> —K. Folkers, et al., ''The Activities of Coenzyme Q10 and Vitamin B6 for Immune Responses,'' *Biochem Biophys Res Commun,* 193(1), May 28, 1993, p. 88-92.

This review article cites numerous studies noting the beneficial effects of CoQ10 and concludes that CoQ10 is a key factor in the optimal immune system functioning.

> —K. Folkers & A. Wolaniuk, ''Research on Coenzyme Q10 in Clinical Medicine and in Immunomodulation,'' *Drugs Exp Clin Res,* 11(8), 1985, 539-545.

Kearns-Sayre Syndrome

Results of this study showed that the administration of 120 to 150/mg of CoQ10 per day led to an improvement in abnormal metabolism of pyruvate and NADH oxidation in the skeletal muscle of

Kearns-Sayre Syndrome patients. CoQ10 also decreased the concentration of CSF protein and CSF lactate/pyruvate ratio, while improvement were seen in neurologic symptoms and ECG abnormalities as well.

> —S. Ogasahara, et al., ''Treatment of Kearns-Sayre Syndrome with Coenzyme Q10,'' *Neurology,* 36(1), January 1986, p. 45-53.

Liver Damage

Results of this double-blind, placebo-controlled study showed that pretreatment with CoQ10 can inhibit acetaminophen-induced hepatic injury in mice.

> —T. Amimoto, et al., ''Acetaminophen-induced Hepatic Injury in Mice: The Role of Lipid Peroxidation and Effects of Pretreatment with Coenzyme Q10 and Alpha-tocopherol,'' *Free Radic Biol Med,* 19(2), August 1995, p. 169-176.

Results of this study indicated that CoQ10 exhibited direct antioxidative effects against CC14 hepatoxicity in rats.

> —T. Yoshikawa, et al., ''The Protection of Coenzyme Q10 Against Carbon Tetrachloride Hepatotoxicity,'' *Gastroenterol Jpn,* 16(3), 1981, p. 281-285.

Results of this study found that the administration of CoQ10 and L-carnitine together decreased hepatic damage brought on by hyperbaric oxygen and chronic alcohol poisoning in rats.

> —A. Bertelli, et al., ''Protective Action of L-carnitine and Coenzyme Q10 Against Hepatic Triglyceride Infiltration Induced by Hyperbaric Oxygen and Ethanol,'' *Drugs Exp Clin Res,* 19(2), 1993, p. 65-68.

Lung Disease

Results of this study showed that oral administration of 90 mg per day of CoQ10 for 8 weeks had significant beneficial effects on muscular energy metabolism in chronic lung disease patients suffering from hypoxemia either during exercise or at rest.

> —S. Fujimoto, et al., ''Effects of Coenzyme Q10 Administration on Pulmonary Function and Exercise Performance in Patients with Chronic Lung Diseases,'' *Clinical Investigations,* 71, 1993, (8 Suppl), p. S162-S166.

Muscular Injury

This study examined the effects of CoQ10 on muscular injury due to exercise in rats. Results found that CoQ10 provided protection against exercise-induced injury in skeletal muscles.

> —Y. Shimomura, et al., ''Protective Effect of Coenzyme Q10 on Exercise-induced Muscular Injury,'' *Biochem Biophys Res Commun,* 176(1), April 15, 1991, p. 349-355.

This study examined the effects of CoQ10 on continuous electric field stimulation-induced muscular injury in cultured cells obtained from neonatal rat femoral muscles. Results showed that administration of 5 microM CoQ10 provided protection for the cells against biochemical changes after the stimulation, indicating one of the causal mechanisms of muscular injury is an increase in [Ca2+] due to the excess entry of extracellular Ca2+, and that CoQ10 can protect skeletal muscle cells against it.

> —T. Okamoto, et al., ''Protective Effect of Coenzyme Q10 on Cultured Skeletal Muscle Cell

Injury Induced by Continuous Electric Field Stimulation,'' *Biochem Biophys Res Commun,* 216(3), November 22, 1995, p. 1006-1012.

This article reports on the results from 2 double-blind, placebo-controlled studies supporting the use of CoQ10 in the treatment of Duchenne, Becker, and limb-girdle dystrophies, myotonic dystrophy, Charcot-Marie-Tooth disease, and the Welander disease.
—K. Folkers & R. Simonsen, ''Two Successful Double-blind Trials with Coenzyme Q10 (vitamin Q10) on Muscular Dystrophies and Neurogenic Atrophies,'' *Biochim Biophys Acta,* 1271(1), May 24, 1995, p. 281-286.

Stroke

This study examined the effects of long-term CoQ10 administration on membrane lipid alterations in the kidney of stroke-prone spontaneously hypertensive rats. Results found that CoQ10 attenuated the elevation of blood pressure, the membranous phospholipid degradation, and the enhanced phospholipase A2 activity.
—H. Okamoto, et al., ''Effect of CoQ10 on Structural Alterations in the Renal Membrane of Stroke-prone Spontaneously Hypertensive Rats,'' *Biochem Med Metab Biol,* 45(2), April 1991, p. 216-226.

■ CONJUGATED LINOLEIC ACID

Cancer

This review article notes that studies have shown conjugated linoleic acid to be a powerful anticarcinogen against mammary tumors on a rat model.
—C. Ip, et al., ''Conjugated Linoleic Acid. A Powerful Anticarcinogen from Animal Fat Sources,'' *Cancer,* 74(3 Suppl), August 1, 1994, p. 1050-1054.

Results of this study showed that synthetic conjugated linoleic acid inhibited DMBA-induced mammary tumors in rats.
—C. Ip, et al., ''Mammary Cancer Prevention by Conjugated Dienoic Derivative of Linoleic Acid,'' *Cancer Research,* 51(22), November 15, 1991, p. 6118-6124.

Results of this study showed that synthetic conjugated linoleic acid inhibited DMBA-induced forestomach tumors in rats.
—Y.L. Ha, et al., ''Inhibition of Benzo(a)pyrene-induced Mouse Forestomach Neoplasia by Conjugated Dienoic Derivatives of Linoleic Acid,'' *Cancer Research,* 50(4), February 15, 1990, p. 1097-1101.

Results of this study showed that conjugated linoleic acid inhibited DMBA-induced mammary tumors in rats.
—C. Ip, et al., ''Conjugated Linoleic Acid Suppresses Mammary Carcinogenesis and Proliferative Activity of the Mammary Gland in the Rat,'' *Cancer Research,* 54(5), March 1, 1994, p. 1212-1215.

Results of this study showed that synthetic conjugated linoleic acid inhibited DMBA-induced foresto-mach tumors in rats.

—H. Benjamin, et al., "TPA-Mediated Induction of Ornithine Decarboxylase Activity in Mouse Forestomach and Its Inhibition by Conjugated Dienoic Derivatives of Linoleic Acid," *FASEB Journal,* 4(3), 1990, p. A508.

Results of this study showed that dietary conjugated linoleic acid significantly suppressed subcutane-ously injected human breast cancer cell growth in mice.

—S. Visonneau, et al., "Conjugated Linoleic Acid (CLA) Suppresses Growth of Human Breast Carcinoma MDA-MB468 in SCID Mice," *FASEB Journal,* 9(4), 1995, p. A869.

Results of this study found that both linoleic acid and conjugated linoleic acid exhibited cytotoxic and cystostatic effects against human cancer cell in vitro.

—W.R. Seaman, et al., "Differential Inhibitory Response to Linoleic Acid and Conjugated Dienoic Derivatives of Linoleic Acid in Cultures of Human Cancer Cells," *FASEB Journal,* 1992, 6(4), p. A1396.

Results of this study showed that conjugated linoleic acid suppressed human cancer cell growth in vitro by inhibiting protein and nucleotide biosynthesis.

—T.D. Shultz, et al., "Inhibitory Effect of Conjugated Dienoic Derivatives of Linoleic Acid and Beta-carotene on the in Vitro Growth of Human Cancer Cells," *FASEB Journal,* 6(4), 1992, p. A1396.

Results of this study showed that the oral administration of conjugated linoleic acid inhibited TPA-induced forestomach tumors in rats.

—H. Benjamin, et al., "The Effect of Conjugated Dienoic Derivatives of Linoleic Acid (CLA) on Mouse Forestomach Protein Kinase C (PKC)-like Activity," *FASEB Journal,* 6(4), 1992, p. A1396.

Results of this study found that conjugated linoleic acid exhibited cytotoxic effects against human breast cancer cells in vitro.

—T.D. Shultz, et al., "Differential Stimulatory and Inhibitory Responses of Human MCF-7 Breast Cancer Cells to Linoleic Acid and Conjugated Linoleic Acid in Culture," *Anticancer Research,* 12(6B), November-December 1992, p. 2143-2145.

Results of this study found that conjugated linoleic acid exhibited inhibitory effects against human breast, colorectal, and malignant melanoma cancer cells in vitro.

—T.D. Shultz, et al., "Inhibitory Effect of Conjugated Dienoic Derivatives of Linoleic Acid and Beta-Carotene on the in Vitro Growth of Human Cancer Cells," *Cancer Letters,* 63(2), April 15, 1992, p. 125-133.

Results of this study found that conjugated linoleic acid inhibited TPA-induced skin tumor promotion in mice.

—M.A. Belury, et al., "Dietary Conjugated Linoleic Acid Modulation of Phorbol Ester Skin Tumor Promotion," *Nutr Cancer,* 26(2), 1996, p. 149-157.

Cardiovascular/Coronary Heart Disease

Results of this study found that 12 weeks administration of conjugated linoleic acid significantly reduced LDL cholesterol and triglyceride levels in rabbits. Significant reductions were also found in the LDL cholesterol to HDL cholesterol ratio as well total cholesterol to HDL cholesterol ratio.

—K.N. Lee, et al., "Conjugated Linoleic Acid and Atherosclerosis in Rabbits," *Atherosclerosis,* 108(1), July 1994, p. 19-25.

■ CURCUMIN/TURMERIC

AIDS/HIV

This study examined curcumin's effects on purified HIV-1 integrase. Results showed that curcumin had an inhibitory concentration 50 (IC50) for strand transfer of 40 microM and suggest that HIV-1 integrase inhibition might be involved in curcumin's antiviral effects study.

—A. Mazumder, et al., "Inhibition of Human Immunodeficiency Virus type-1 integrase by Curcumin," *Biochem Pharmacol,* 49(8), April 18, 1995, p. 1165-1170.

This article notes that curcumin is a modest inhibitor of HIV-1 (IC50 = 100 microM) and HIV-2 (IC50 = 250 microM) proteases.

—Z. Sui, et al., "Inhibition of the HIV-1 and HIV-2 proteases by Curcumin and Curcumin Boron Complexes," *Bioorg Med Chem,* 1(6), December 1993, p. 415-422.

Antifungal Activity

Results of this study found that turmeric oil exhibited antifungal activity against tichophyton-induced dermatophytosis in guinea pigs.

—A. Apisariyakul, et al., "Antifungal Activity of Turmeric Oil Extracted from Curcuma Longa (Zingiberaceae)," *Journal of Ethnopharmacology,* 49(3), December 15, 1995, p. 163-169.

Antiinflammatory Effects

Results of this placebo-controlled study showed that phenylbutazone and curcumin exhibited anti-inflammatory effects in patients with postoperative inflammation.

—R.R. Satoskar, et al., "Evaluation of Anti-inflammatory Property of Curcumin (Diferuloyl Methane) in Patients with Postoperative Inflammation," *International Journal of Clinical Pharmacology Ther Toxicol,* 24(12), December 1986, p. 651-654.

Cancer

Results of this study showed that curcumin exhibited inhibitory effects on TPA-induced tumor promotion in the epidermis of mice.

—M.T. Huang, et al., "Inhibitory Effects of Curcumin on in Vitro Lipoxygenase and Cyclooxygenase Activities in Mouse Epidermis," *Cancer Research,* 51(3), February 1, 1991, p. 813-819.

Results of this study indicated that the topical application of curcumin inhibited TPA-induced epidermal ornithine decarboxylase activity in female mice. In addition to these findings, the topical application of curcumin coupled with TPA twice a week over a period of 20 weeks to mice previously exposed to DMBA significantly inhibited the number of TPA-induced tumors.

> —M.T. Huang, et al., "Inhibitory Effect of Curcumin, Chlorogenic Acid, Caffeic Acid, and Ferulic Acid on Tumor Promotion in Mouse Skin by 12-O-tetradecanoylphorbol-13-acetate," *Cancer Research,* 48(21), November 1, 1988, p. 5941-5946.

This study examined the chemopreventive effects of curcumin on azoxymethane-induced colon cancer in rats. Results showed that the curcumin significantly reduced the incidence of colon adenocarcinomas, the multiplicity of both invasive and noninvasive adenocarcinomas, and suppressed colon tumor volume relative to controls.

> —C.V. Rao, et al., "Chemoprevention of Colon Carcinogenesis by Dietary Curcumin, a Naturally Occurring Plant Phenolic Compound," *Cancer Research,* January 15, 1995, p. 55(2), p. 259-266.

This study examined the effects of curcumin on experimentally-induced tumorigenesis in the forestomach, duodenum, and colon of mice. Results found that curcumin inhibited the number of tumors per mouse, tumor size, and the percentage of mice with tumors.

> —M.T. Huang, et al., "Inhibitory Effects of Dietary Curcumin on Forestomach, Duodenal, and Colon Carcinogenesis in Mice," *Cancer Research,* 54(22), November 15, 1994, p. 5841-5847.

Results of this study showed that an aqueous extract of turmeric suppressed the mutagenicity of both direct- and indirect-acting mutagen, benzo(a)pyrene (B(a)P) in Salmonella typhimurium strains TA98 and TA100. In addition to these findings, aqueous turmeric extracts reduced incidence and multiplicity of B(a)P-induced forestomach tumors in mice, and curcumin was shown to inhibit B(a)P- DNA-adduct formation and B(a)P-induced strand breaks.

> —M.A. Azuine, et al., "Mechanisms of Chemoprevention of Cancer by Turmeric," *Third International Conference on Mechanisms of Antimutagenesis and Anticarcinogenesis, May 5-10, 1991, Lucca, Italy,* 1991, p. 59.

Results of this study found that the topical administration of curcumin exhibited inhibitory effects on TPA-induced tumorigenesis in the skin of mice.

> —A.H. Conney, et al., "Inhibitory Effect of Curcumin and Some Related Dietary Compounds on Tumor Promotion and Arachidonic Acid Metabolism in Mouse Skin," *Adv Enzyme Regul,* 31, 1991, p. 385-396.

Results of this study showed that curcumin induced apoptotic cell death in promyelocytic leukemia HL-60 cells at concentrations as low as 3.5 micrograms/ml.

> —M.L. Kuo, et al., "Curcumin, An Antioxidant and Anti-tumor Promoter, Induces Apoptosis in Human Leukemia Cells," *Biochim Biophys Acta,* 1317(2), November 15, 1996, p. 95-100.

Results of this study found that the administration of curcumin in mice inhibited AOM-induced colonic neoplasia in mice.

> —M.T. Huang, et al., "Effect of Dietary Curcumin and Ascorbyl Palmitate on Azoxymethanol-

induced Colonic Epithelial Cell Proliferation and Focal Areas of Dysplasia,'' *Cancer Letters,* 64(2), June 15, 1992, p. 117-121.

Results of this study inhibited the DNA synthesis of human umbilical vein endothelial cells in vitro, pointing to its potential as a useful new therapy for cancer.
> —A.K. Singh, et al., ''Curcumin Inhibits the Proliferation and Cell Cycle Progression of Human Umbilical Vein Endothelial Cell,'' *Cancer Letters,* 107(1), October 1, 1996, p. 109-115.

Results of this study showed that curcumin exhibited inhibitory effects on TPA-induced skin cancer in mice.
> —S.S. Kakar & D. Roy, ''Curcumin Inhibits TPA Induced Expression of C-fos, C-jun and C-myc Proto-Oncogenes Messenger RNAs in Mouse Skin,'' *Cancer Letters,* 87(1), November 24, 1995, p. 85-89.

Results of this showed that the i.p. administration of 100 mg/kg and 200 mg/kg of curcumin significantly reduced the number of palpable DMBA-induced mammary tumors and mammary adenocarcinomas in rats.
> —K. Singletary, et al., ''Inhibition of 7,12-dimethylbenz[a]anthracene (DMBA)-induced Mammary Tumorigenesis and DMBA-DNA Adduct Formation by Curcumin,'' *Cancer Letters,* 103(2), June 5, 1996, p. 137-141.

Results of this study showed that a tumeric extract inhibited cell growth in Chinese Hamster Ovary cells and was cytotoxic to lymphocytes and Dalton's lymphoma cells.
> —R. Kuttan, et al., ''Potential Anticancer Activity of Turmeric,'' *Cancer Letters,* 29(2), November 1985, p. 197-202.

Results of this study showed the curcumin inhibited xanthine oxidase in vitro, xanthine oxidase being one a causative factor in PMA-mediated tumor promotion.
> —J.K. Lin & C.A. Shih, ''Inhibitory Effect of Curcumin on Xanthine Dehydrogenase/oxidase Induced by Phorbol-12-myristate-13-acetate in NIH3T3 Cells,'' *Carcinogenesis,* 15(8), August 1994, p. 1717-1721.

Results of this study found that the administration of curcumin mediated a dose-dependent inhibition of the incidence and multiplicity of AOM-induced colon adenomas in rats relative to controls.
> —M.A. Pereira, et al., ''Effects of the Phytochemicals, Curcumin and Quercetin, Upon Azoxymethane Induced Colon Cancer and 7,12-dimethylbenz[a]anthracene-induced Mammary Cancer in Rats,'' *Carcinogenesis,* 17(6), June 1996, p. 1305-1311.

Results of this study showed that curcumin had inhibitory effects on TPA-induced tumor promotion in DMBA-initiated mouse skin.
> —M.T. Huang, et al., ''Effects of Curcumin, Demethoxycurcumin, Bisdemethoxycurcumin and Tetrahydrocurcumin on 12-O-tetradecanoylphorbol-13- Acetate-induced Tumor Promotion,'' *Carcinogenesis,* 16(10), October 1995, p. 2493-2497.

Results of this study showed that the topical application of 3 or 10 mumol of curcumin 5 min prior to the application of 20 nmol [3H]B[a]P inhibited the formation of [3H]B[a]P-DNA adducts in the epidermis of mice and inhibited the incidence and number of DMBA-induced skin tumors.

> —M.T. Huang, et al., "Inhibitory Effects of Curcumin on Tumor Initiation by Benzo[a]pyrene and 7,12-dimethylbenz[a]anthracene," *Carcinogenesis,* 13(11), November 1992, p. 2183-2186.

Results of this study showed that the oral administration of betel-leaf extract combined with turmeric had inhibitory effects on chemical-induced carcinogenesis in hamsters.

> —M.A. Azuine & S.V. Bhide, "Protective Single/combined Treatment with Betel Leaf and Turmeric Against Methyl (acetoxymethyl) Nitrosamine-induced Hamster Oral Carcinogenesis," *International Journal of Cancer,* 51(3), May 28, 1992, p. 412-415.

Results of this study showed that curcumin I inhibited benzopyrene- (BP) induced forestomach tumors and DMBA-induced TPA-promoted skin tumors in female mice, while curcumin III inhibited DMBA—induced skin tumors in bald mice.

> —M. Nagabhushan & S.V. Bhide, "Curcumin as an Inhibitor of Cancer," *Journal of the American College of Nutrition,* 11(2), April 1992, p. 192-198.

Results of this study showed that an aqueous turmeric extract and its constituents, curcumin-free aqueous turmeric extract and curcumin exhibited chemopreventive effects in female mice.

> —M.A. Azuine, et al., "Protective Role of Aqueous Turmeric Extract Against Mutagenicity of Direct-Acting Carcinogens as Well as Benzo [alpha] pyrene-induced Genotoxicity and Carcinogenicity," *Journal of Cancer Research and Clinical Oncology,* 118(6), 1992, p. 447-452.

Results of this study found that turmeric and catechin exhibited chemopreventive effects in golden hamsters and in mice.

> —M.A. Azuine & S.V. Bhide, "Adjuvant Chemoprevention of Experimental Cancer: Catechin and Dietary Turmeric in Forestomach and Oral Cancer Models," *Journal of Ethnopharmacology,* 44(3), December 1994, p. 211-217.

Results of this study showed turmeric to be an effective antimutagen in smokers, pointing to its potential as a chemopreventive agent.

> —K. Polasa, et al., "Effect of Turmeric on Urinary Mutagens in Smokers," *Mutagenesis,* 7(2), March 1992, p.p. 107-109.

Results of this study showed that curcumin I, II, and III inhibited mutagenesis and croton oil-induced tumor promotion in mice.

> —R.J. Anto, et al., "Antimutagenic and Anticarcinogenic Activity of Natural and Synthetic Curcuminoids," *Mutation Research* (1996 Sep 13) 370(2), September 13, 1996, p. 127-131.

Results of this study showed that curcumin suppressed UV irradiation-induced mutagenesis in Salmonella typhimurium and Eschericia coli strains in vitro.

> —Y. Oda, "Inhibitory Effect of Curcumin on SOS Functions Induced by UV Irradiation." *Mutation Research,* 348(2), October 1995, p. 67-73.

Results of this study showed that turmeric inhibited DMBA-induced skin tumors and BP-induced forestomach tumors in mice.

—M.A. Azuine & S.V. Bhide, ''Chemopreventive Effect of Turmeric Against Stomach and Skin Tumors Induced by Chemical Carcinogens in Swiss Mice,'' *Nutr Cancer,* 17(1), 1992, p. 77-83.

Results of this study showed that curcumin induced cell shrinkage, chromatin condensation, and DNA fragmentation, characteristics of apoptosis, in immortalized mouse embryo fibroblast NIH 3T3 erb B2 oncogene-transformed NIH 3T3, mouse sarcoma S180, human colon cancer cell HT-29, human kidney cancer cell 293, and human hepatocellular carcinoma Hep G2 cells.

—M.C. Jiang, et al., ''Curcumin Induces Apoptosis in Immortalized NIH 3T3 and Malignant Cancer Cell Lines,'' *Nutr Cancer,* 26(1), 1996, p. 111-120.

Results of this study found that the oral administration of curcumin inhibited benzo[a]pyrene (B[a]P)-induced forestomach tumorigenesis, ENNG-induced duodenal tumorigenesis, and AOM-induced colon tumorigenesis in mice.

—M.T. Huang, et al., ''Inhibitory Effect of Dietary Curcumin on Gastrointestinal Tumorigenesis in Mice,'' *Proceedings of the Annual Meeting of the American Association of Cancer Researchers,* 34, 1993, p. A3305.

Results of this study indicated that commercial, purified, and demethoxy—curcumin exhibited inhibited TPA-induced skin tumors in mice previously exposed to DMBA.

—M.T. Huang, et al., ''Effects of Derivatives of Curcumin on 12-O-Tetradecanolyphorbol-13-Acetate (TPA)-Induced Tumor Promotion in Mouse Epidermis and-Independent Growth of Cultured JB6 Cells,'' *Proceedings of the Annual Meeting of the American Association of Cancer Researchers,* 33, 1992, p. A994.

Results of this study found that patients with external cancerous lesions experienced significant relief following treatment with an ethanol turmeric extract and a curcumin ointment.

—R. Kuttan, et al., ''Turmeric and Curcumin as Topical Agents in Cancer Therapy,'' *Tumori,* 73(1), February 28, 1987, p. 29-31.

Cardiovascular/Coronary Heart Disease

Results of this study showed that ischaemia-induced changes in cat hearts were prevented by both curcumin and quinidine.

—M. Dikshit, et al., ''Prevention of Ischaemia-induced Biochemical Changes by Curcumin & Quinidine in the Cat Heart,'' *Indian Journal of Medical Research,* January 1995, p. 101.

Results of this study showed that the administration of 500 mg per day of curcumin for 7 days significantly reduced the level of serum lipid peroxides, increased HDL cholesterol, and decreased total serum cholesterol in healthy human subjects.

—K.B. Soni & R. Kuttan, ''Effect of Oral Curcumin Administration on Serum Peroxides and Cholesterol Levels in Human Volunteers,'' *Indian J Physiol Pharmacol,* 36(4), October 1992, p. 273-275.

Results of this study showed that oral curcumin significantly reduced increased lipid peroxidation in different mouse organs including the brain, liver, lung, and kidney. Curcumin significantly reduced serum and tissue cholesterol levels in mice as well.

—K.K. Soudamini, et al., "Inhibition of Lipid Peroxidation and Cholesterol Levels in Mice by Curcumin," *Indian Journal of Physiol Pharmacol*, 36(4), October 1992, p. 239-243.

Results of this study showed that curcumin inhibited arachidonate, adrenaline, and collagen-induced platelet aggregation in human blood.

—K.C. Srivastava, et al., "Curcumin, A Major Component of Food Spice Turmeric (Curcuma longa) Inhibits Aggregation and Alters Eicosanoid Metabolism in Human Blood Platelets," *Prostaglandins Leukot Essent Fatty Acids*, 52(4), April 1995, p. 223-227.

Cataracts

Results of this in vitro study found that curcumin provided protection against lipid peroxidation-induced cataractogenesis in rat lenses.

—S. Awasthi, et al., "Curcumin Protects Against 4-hydroxy-2-trans-nonenal-induced Cataract Formation in Rat Lenses," *American Journal of Clinical Nutrition*, 64(5), November 1996, p. 761-766.

Diabetes

Results of this study indicated that dietary curcumin over an 8 week period led to an enhanced metabolic status across numerous diabetic conditions in albino rats relative to controls.

—P.S. Babu & K. Srinivasan, "Influence of Dietary Curcumin and Cholesterol on the Progression of Experimentally Induced Diabetes in Albino Rat," *Mol Cell Biochem*, 152(1), November 8, 1995, p. 13-21.

Gallstones

Results of this study found that mice fed a lithogenic diet supplemented with 0.5 per cent curcumin over a period of 10 weeks experienced a significantly decreased incidence of gallstone formation relative to controls as well as a significant reduction in biliary cholesterol concentration.

—M.S. Hussain & N. Chandrasekhara, "Effect on Curcumin on Cholesterol Gall-stone Induction in Mice," *Indian Journal Medical Research*, 96, October 1992, p. 288-291.

General

This study compared the ability of the natural curcuminoids (curcumin (CAS 458-37-7), demethoxycurcumin, bisdemethoxycurcumin) and acetylcurcumin to scavenge superoxide radicals and to interact with 1,1-diphenyl-2-picryl-hydrazyl (DPPH) stable free radicals. The results found curcumin to be the most potent scavenger of superoxide radicals.

—N. Sreejayan & M.N. Rao, "Free Radical Scavenging Activity of Curcuminoids," *Arzneimittelforschung*, 46(2), February 1996, p. 169-171.

Results of this study showed that turmeric reduced lipid peroxidation in male rats by enhancing antioxidant enzyme activities.

—A.C. Reddy & B.R. Lokesh, "Effect of Dietary Turmeric (Curcuma longa) on Iron-induced Lipid Peroxidation in the Rat Liver," *Food Chem Toxicol*, 32(3), March 1994, p. 279-283.

Results of this study showed that demethoxycurcumin, bisdemethoxycurcumin and acetylcurcumin were equally effective in their ability to inhibit iron-stimulated lipid peroxidation in rat brain homogenate and rat liver microsomes.

—Sreejayan & M.N. Rao, "Curcuminoids as Potent Inhibitors of Lipid Peroxidation," *Journal of Pharm Pharmacol,* 46(12), December 1994, p. 1013-1016.

Results of this study showed that curcumin and an aqueous extract of turmeric were effective inhibitors of lipid peroxidation.

—V.K. Shalini & L. Srinivas, "Lipid Peroxide Induced DNA Damage: Protection by Turmeric (Curcuma longa)," *Mol Cell Biochem,* 77(1), September 1987, p. 3-10.

Liver Damage

Results of this study showed that 30 mg/kg body weight of curcumin administered over a period of 10 days reduced the iron-induced liver damage in male rats by lowering lipid peroxidation.

—A.C. Reddy & B.R. Lokesh, "Effect of Curcumin and Eugenol on Iron-induced Hepatic Toxicity in Rats," *Toxicology,* 107(1), January 22, 1996, p. 39-45.

■ DEPRENYL

Aging

Results of this study showed that the administration of deprenyl significantly prolonged lifespan in aging rats.

—K. Kitani, et al., "Chronic Treatment of (-)deprenyl Prolongs the Life Span of Male Fischer 344 Rats. Further Evidence," *Life Science,* 52(3), 1993, p. 281-288.

Results of this study found that the combined therapy of Dinh lang root extract and (-)deprenyl significantly increased memory performance and the lifespan of aged mice.

—T.T. Yen & J. Knoll, "Extension of Lifespan in Mice Treated with Dinh Lang (Policias fruticosum L.) and (-)deprenyl," *Acta Physiol Hung,* 79(2), 1992, 119-124.

Results of this study showed that the administration of deprenyl significantly prolonged lifespan in aging male rats.

—K. Kitani, et al., "Upregulation of Antioxidant Enzyme Activities by Deprenyl. Implications for Life Span Extension," *Annals of the New York Academy of Sciences,* 786, June 15, 1996, p. 391-409.

Results of this study showed that (-)-Deprenyl significantly prevented oxidative damage produced during aging in older rats.

—C.P. de la Cruz, et al., "Protection of the Aged Substantia Nigra of the Rat Against Oxidative Damage by (-)-deprenyl," *British Journal of Pharmacology,* 117(8), April 1996, p. 1756-1760.

Results of this study showed that the administration of deprenyl beginning after the second year of life prolonged lifespan and increased sexual performance in male rats.

—J. Knoll, et al., "Striatal Dopamine, Sexual Activity and Lifespan. Longevity of Rats Treated with (-)Deprenyl," *Life Science,* 45(6), 1989, p. 525-531.

Results of this study showed that the administration of deprenyl beginning after the 8th month of life prolonged lifespan in male rats with low sexual performance.

—J. Knoll, et al., "Sexually Low Performing Male Rats Die Earlier than their High Performing Peers and (-)deprenyl Treatment Eliminates this Difference," *Life Sciences,* 54(15), 1994, p. 1047-1057.

Results of this study found that L-Deprenyl reduced expression of some microanatomical changes associated with aging in the rat brain.

—Y.C. Zeng, et al., "Influence of Long-term Treatment with L-deprenyl on the Age-dependent Changes in Rat Brain Microanatomy," *Mech Ageing Dev,* 73(2), February 1994, p. 113-126.

Results of this study showed that the administration of L-Deprenyl enhanced cognitive function in aging rats.

—R. Brandeis, et al., "Improvement of Cognitive Function by MAO-B Inhibitor L-deprenyl in Aged Rats," *Pharmacol Biochem Behav,* 39(2), June 1991, p. 297-304.

Results of this study showed that L-deprenyl administration improved spatial memory in aged dogs.

—E. Head, et al., "The Effects of L-deprenyl on Spatial Short Term Memory in Young and Aged Dogs," *Prog Neuropsychopharmacol Biol Psychiatry,* 20(3), April 1996, p. 515-530.

Alzheimer's Disease

Results of this double-blind, placebo-controlled study showed that the addition of 5 mg b.i.d of oral L-Deprenyl to the normal treatment of Alzheimer's patients taking tacrine or physostigmine over a period of 4 weeks led to significant improvement.

—L.S. Schneider, et al., "A Double-blind Crossover Pilot Study of l-deprenyl (Selegiline) Combined with Cholinesterase Inhibitor in Alzheimer's Disease," *American Journal of Psychiatry,* 150(2), February 1993, p. 321-323.

Results of this double-blind, placebo-controlled study found that the administration of L-Deprenyl over a period of 6 months led to significant improvements of memory and learning skills in patients suffering from Alzheimers.

—G. Finali, et al., "L-deprenyl Therapy Improves Verbal Memory in Amnesic Alzheimer Patients," *Clinical Neuropharmacology,* 14(6), December 1991, p. 523-536.

Results of this double-blind, placebo-controlled study found that the administration of 10 mg per day of L-Deprenyl over a period of 6 months led to significant improvements of cognitive function in patients suffering from dementia of the Alzheimer's type.

—G.L. Piccinin, et al., "Neuropsychological Effects of L-deprenyl in Alzheimer's Type Dementia," *Clinical Neuropharmacology,* 13(2), April 1990, p. 147-163.

Results of this study showed that the administration of (-) deprenyl over a period of between 3-6 months led to significant improvements in elderly females patients suffering from senile dementia of Alzheimer type.

> —E. Martini, et al., "Brief Information on an Early Phase-II Study with Deprenyl in Demented Patients," *Pharmacopsychiatry,* 20(6), November 1987, p. 256-257.

Results of this double-blind, placebo-controlled study found that the administration of 10 mg per day of L-Deprenyl significantly improved episodic memory, sustained consciousness, and performance on complex learning tasks in patients suffering from dementia of the Alzheimer's type.

> —P.N. Tariot, et al., "Cognitive Effects of L-deprenyl in Alzheimer's Disease," *Psychopharmacology,* 91(4), 1987, p. 489-495.

Aphrodisiac

Results of this study showed that (-)deprenyl exhibited long-lasting aphrodisiac effects on male rats.

> —T.T. Yen, et al., "The Aphrodisiac Effect of Low Doses of (-) Deprenyl in Male Rats," *Pol Journal Pharmacol Pharm,* 34(5-6), November-December 1982, p. 303-308.

Cancer

Results of this study found that the administration of deprenyl significantly reduced the incidence of mammary and pituitary tumors in rats relative to controls.

> —S. Thyagarajan, et al., "Deprenyl Reinitiates Estrous Cycles, Reduces Serum Prolactin, and Decreases the Incidence of Mammary and Pituitary Tumors in Old Acyclic Rats," *Endocrinology,* 136(3), March 1995, p. 1103-1110.

Depression

Results of this double-blind, placebo-controlled study found that the administration of 20 mg per day of L-Deprenyl or greater over a period of 6 weeks had beneficial effects in patients suffering from atypical depression.

> —F.M. Quitkin, et al., "l-Deprenyl in Atypical Depressives," *Arch Gen Psychiatry,* 41(8), August 1984, p. 777-781.

Results of this double-blind, placebo-controlled study showed that the administration of 30 mg per day or more of (-)-deprenyl for a minimum of 6 weeks exhibited superior antidepressant effects in depressed outpatients relative to controls.

> —J.J. Mann, et al., "A Controlled Study of the Antidepressant Efficacy and Side Effects of (-)-deprenyl. A Selective Monoamine Oxidase Inhibitor," *Arch Gen Psychiatry,* 46(1), January 1989, p. 45-50.

This study examined the effects of 5-10 mg per day of L-Deprenyl coupled with 250 mg per day of L-phenylalanine in patients suffering from unipolar depression. Results indicated that the oral as well as intravenous administration of both drugs showed beneficial antidepressive effects in 90% of outpatients and 80.5% of inpatients.

> —W. Birkmayer, et al., "L-deprenyl Plus L-phenylalanine in the Treatment of Depression," *Journal of Neural Transmission,* 59(1), 1984, p. 81-87.

Epilepsy

Results of this study found that L-deprenyl exhibited anticonvulsant effects against different kinds of seizure in mice, suggesting it may be effective in the treatment of epilepsy.

> —W. Loscher & H. Lehmann, "L-deprenyl (selegiline) Exerts Anticonvulsant Effects Against Different Seizure Types in Mice," *Journal of Pharmacol Exp Ther,* 277(3), June 1996, p. 1410-1417.

Huntington's Disease

This article reports on the case of a 19-year-old female Huntington's disease patient who experienced significant affective, behavioral, and motoric improvements following combined treatment with fluoxetine and L-Deprenyl.

> —S.V. Patel, et al., "L-Deprenyl Augmentation of Fluoxetine in a Patient with Huntington's Disease," *Annals of Clinical Psychiatry,* 8(1), March 1996, p. 23-26.

Parkinson's Disease

Results of this double-blind, placebo-controlled study found that 10 mg per day of deprenyl delayed the onset of disability associated with early, untreated Parkinson's disease in human subjects.

> —"Effect of Deprenyl on the Progression of Disability in Early Parkinson's Disease. The Parkinson Study Group," *New England Journal of Medicine,* 321(20), November 16, 1989, p. 1364-1371.

This review article notes studies have shown that L-Deprenyl (l-selegiline) to be an effective adjuvant to L-dopa in the treatment of Parkinson's disease.

> —M.B. Youdim & J.P. Finberg, "Pharmacological Actions of l-deprenyl (selegiline) and Other Selective Monoamine Oxidase B Inhibitors," *Clinical Pharmacol Ther,* 56(6 Pt 2), December 1994, p. 725-733.

Results of this double-blind, crossover study showed that the administration of 10 mg per day or on alternate days of (-)-deprenyl prolonged the beneficial effects of levodopa and was effective against mild "on-off" disabilities in patients suffering from idiopathic Parkinson's disease.

> —A.J. Lees, et al., "Deprenyl in Parkinson's Disease," *Lancet,* 2(8042), October 15, 1977, p. 791-795.

Results of this study found that the administration of 10 mg per day of deprenyl over a period of 12 months in patients suffering from mild stages of Parkinson's disease cut the risk of further progression to a stage requiring L-Dopa therapy by half.

> —P.A. LeWitt, "Deprenyl's Effect at Slowing Progression of Parkinsonian Disability: The DATATOP Study. The Parkinson Study Group," *Acta Neurol Scand Suppl,* 136, 1991, p. 79-86.

Results of this double-blind, placebo-controlled study showed that the administration of 5 mg per day of deprenyl for a period of 4 weeks reduced dependence on levodopa in patients suffering from Parkinson's disease.

> —J. Presthus & A. Hajba, "Deprenyl (selegiline) Combined with Levodopa and a Decarboxyl-

ase Inhibitor in the Treatment of Parkinson's Disease,'' *Acta Neurol Scand Suppl,* 95, 1983, p. 127-133.

Results of this study involving 48 patients with Parkinson's disease found that the addition of deprenyl to previous levodopa plus decarboxylase-inhibitor therapy proved beneficial with respect to mild on-off phenomena and end-of-dose akinesia.
　　—F. Gerstenbrand, et al., ''Deprenyl (selegiline) in Combination Treatment of Parkinson's Disease,'' *Acta Neurol Scand Suppl,* 95, 1983, p. 123-126.

This study examined deprenyl's effects in patients with Parkinson's disease experiencing levodopa-induced fluctuations in disease severity. Results showed that the administration of 5-10 mg of deprenyl over a period of 1-3 months significantly decreases such fluctuations in 26 of 45 patients studied.
　　—U.K. Rinne, et al., ''Deprenyl (selegiline) in the Treatment of Parkinson's Disease,'' *Acta Neurol Scand Suppl,* 95, 1993, p. 107-111.

Results of this study found that deprenyl has beneficial effects in the treatment of Parkinson's disease when coupled with levodopa and a peripheral decarboxylase inhibitor.
　　—W. Birkmayer, ''Deprenyl (selegiline) in the Treatment of Parkinson's Disease,'' *Acta Neurol Scand Suppl,* 95, 1983, p. 103-105.

This double-blind study examined the effects of deprenyl coupled with levodopa on patients suffering from Parkinson's disease. Results showed two thirds of cases studied experience significant improvement following treatment.
　　—H. Przuntek & W. Kuhn, ''The Effect of R-(-)-deprenyl in de novo Parkinson Patients on Combination Therapy with Levodopa and Decarboxylase Inhibitor,'' *Journal of Neural Transm Suppl,* 25, 1987, p. 97-104.

Results of this double-blind, placebo-controlled study showed that early administration of 10 mg per day of deprenyl delayed the need for L-Dopa therapy and disease progression in patients suffering from Parkinson's disease.
　　—J.W. Tetrud & J.W. Langston, ''The Effect of Deprenyl (selegiline) on the Natural History of Parkinson's Disease,'' *Science,* 245(4917), August 4, 1989, p. 519-522.

Results of this double-blind, placebo-controlled study found that the administration of 5 mg b.i.d of deprenyl over a period of 6 weeks exhibited moderately beneficial effects in Parkinson's patients with symptoms fluctuations.
　　—L.I. Golbe, et al., ''Deprenyl in the Treatment of Symptom Fluctuations in Advanced Parkinson's Disease,'' *Clin Neuropharmacol,* 11(1), February 1988, p. 45-55.

Results of this study found that combining 10 mg per day of L-Deprenyl with standard L-Dopa treatment significantly reduced the need for L-dopa in patients suffering from Parkinson's Disease.
　　—S. Ruggieri, et al., ''Multicenter Trial of L-Deprenyl in Parkinson Disease,'' *Italian Journal of Neurol Sci,* 7(1), February 1996, p. 133-137.

This article notes that 5-10 mg of deprenyl has been shown to cut the need for levedopa by 20-50% in patients suffering from Parkinson's disease.

—U.K. Rinne, "R-(-)-deprenyl as an Adjuvant to Levodopa in the Treatment of Parkinson's Disease," *Journal of Neural Transm Suppl,* 25, 1987, p. 149-155.

Results of this double-blind, placebo-controlled study found the administration of 5 mg per day of deprenyl over a 6 week period to be useful in the treatment of "on-off" complications common to patients suffering from Parkinson's disease.

—L.I. Golbe & R.C. Duvoisin, "Double-blind Trial of R-(-)-deprenyl for the "on-off" Effect Complicating Parkinson's Disease," *Journal of Neural Transm Suppl,* 25, 1987, p. 123-129.

Results of this double-blind, placebo-controlled study showed (-)deprenyl administered at 20 mg per day had significant beneficial effects in patients suffering from idiopathic Parkinson's disease and reduced their dependence on L-Dopa by an average of 30%.

—P. Giovannini, et al., "(-)Deprenyl in Parkinson's Disease: A Two-year Study in the Different Evolutive Stages," *Journal of Neural Transm Suppl,* 22, 19865, p. 235-246.

Results of this study found that the addition of (-)deprenyl to normal Madopar therapy led to improvements of disability, prolongation of life expectancy, and a reduction of Madopar-induced side effects in patients suffering from Parkinson's disease.

—W. Birkmayer & G.D. Birkmayer, "Effect of (-)deprenyl in Long-term Treatment of Parkinson's Disease. A 10-years Experience," *Journal of Neural Transm Suppl,* 22, 1986, p. 219-225.

Results of this study found that the administration of L-Deprenyl proved to be an effective therapy when coupled with long-term administration of levodopa in the treatment of patients with Parkinson's disease.

—M. Streifler & M.J. Rabey, "Long-term Effects of L-deprenyl in Chronic Levodopa Treated Parkinsonian Patients," *Journal of Neural Transm Suppl,* 19, 1983, p. 265-272.

Results of this study found that patients with Parkinson's disease treated with levodopa plus 10 mg per day of (-)deprenyl live significantly longer than those taking levodopa alone.

—J. Knoll, "The Pharmacological Basis of the Beneficial Effects of (-)deprenyl (selegiline) in Parkinson's and Alzheimer's Disease," *Journal of Neural Transm Suppl,* 40, 1993, p. 69-91.

Postpolio Syndrome

This article reports on the cases of two patients with postpolio syndrome. The first received levodopa/carbidopa combination after developing Parkinson's followed by deprenyl. Results showed the treatment to be effective. The second patient, not suffering from Parkinson's syndrome, received deprenyl by itself and experienced similar improvement.

—C.R. Bamford, et al., "Postpolio Syndrome—Response to Deprenyl (selegiline)," *International Journal of Neuroscience,* 71(1-4), July-August 1993, p. 183-188.

Stroke

Results of this study found that L-Deprenyl was useful as a prophylactic treatment for brain tissue in rats when administered prior to hypoxia/ischemia.

—S. Knollema, et al., "L-deprenyl Reduces Brain Damage in Rats Exposed to Transient Hypoxia-Ischemia," *Stroke*, 26(10), October 1995, p. 1883-1887.

Tourette's Syndrome

Results of this study showed the administration of an average daily dose of 8.1 mg of deprenyl over a period of approximately 7 months was an effective, side effect free treatment for attention deficit associated with Tourette's syndrome in children ranging in age from 6 to 18 years old.

—J. Jankovic, "Deprenyl in Attention Deficit Associated with Tourette's Syndrome," *Arch Neurol*, 50(3), March 1993, p. 286-288.

Ulcer

Results of this study showed that intraperitoneal and intracerebroventricular administration L-Deprenyl significantly attenuated restraint stress-induced gastric ulcers in rats.

—G.B. Glavin, et al., "L-deprenyl Attenuates Stress Ulcer Formation in Rats," *Neuroscience Letters*, 70(3), October 20, 1986, p. 379-381.

■ DHEA

Aging

Results of this study found DHEA to possess beneficial effects among aging subjects with respect to muscle strength, immune function, and overall quality of life.

—S.S. Yen, et al., "Replacement of DHEA in Aging Men and Women. Potential Remedial Effects," *Ann N Y Acad Sci*, 774, December 29, 1995, p. 128-142.

AIDS/HIV

Results of this study showed that DHEA reduced the replication of HIV-1 in vitro.

—E. Henderson, et al., "Dehydroepiandrosterone (DHEA) and Synthetic DHEA Analogs are Modest Inhibitors of HIV-1 IIIB Replication," *AIDS Res Hum Retroviruses*, 8(5), May 1992, p. 625-631.

This article reports on findings showing that high doses of DHEA has shown modest reductions on viral load in patients infected with HIV.

—J.S. James, "DHEA: Modest Viral Load Reduction in Patients," *AIDS Treatment News*, 252, August 2, 1996, p. 7-8.

Results of this study found an inverse association between DHEA levels and increased HIV progression in patients with CD4 counts below 300. Supplemental DHEA to levels greater than 400 mg/dl increased survival in such patients.

—C. Thompson, et al., "Effects of Plasma Dehydroepiandrosterone (DHEA) Levels on HIV RNA Plasma Levels as Measured by PCR," *Int Conf AIDS*, 11(2), July 7-12, 1996, p. 311.

Results of this study showed that the administration of DHEA (300-600 mg po BID) for 28 days, following a 30 day washout period of antivirals, significantly decreased viral load in HIV positive patients with CD4 counts above 50 and below 300.

—P. Salvato, et al., "Viral Load Response to Augmentation of Natural Dehydroepiandrosterone (DHEA)," *Int Conf AIDS*, 11(2), July 7-12, 1996, p. 124.

Results of this study showed that the administration of an average oral dose of 75 mg qd of DHEA coupled with standard antiviral treatment to patients infected with HIV led to significant increases in CD4 and CD8 counts.

—D. Hasheeve, et al., "DHEA: A Potential Treatment for HIV Disease," *International Conference on AIDS*, 10(1), August 7-12, 1994, p. 223.

Results of this study indicated that DHEA modestly inhibited in vitro HIV replication and showed that high risk homosexual males who were HIV-negative had significantly higher DHEA levels than age matched HIV-positive males.

—M.A. Jacobson, et al., "Possible Protective Effect of Dehydroepiandrosterone (DHEA) and/or DHEA-sulfate (DHEA-S) in HIV Infection," *International Conference on AIDS*, 5, June 4-9 1989, p. 560.

Alzheimer's Disease

Results of this study found significantly lower levels of serum DHEA-S in elderly Japanese patients suffering from Alzheimers and/or cerebrovascular dementia relative to age-matched healthy controls.

—T. Yanase, et al., "Serum Dehydroepiandrosterone (DHEA) and DHEA-sulfate (DHEA-S) in Alzheimer's Disease and in Cerebrovascular Dementia," *Endocr Journal*, 43(1), February 1996, p. 119-123.

Cancer

Results of this study showed that DHEA inhibited DMBA-induced skin tumors in mice.

—L.L. Pashko, et al., "Dehydroepiandrosterone (DHEA) and 3 Beta-methylandrost-5-en-17-one: Inhibitors of 7,12-dimethylbenz[a]anthracene (DMBA)-initiated and 12-O-tetradecanoylphorbol-13-Acetate (TPA)-promoted Skin Papilloma Formation in Mice," *Carcinogenesis*, 5(4), April 1984, p. 463-466.

Results of this study showed that DHEA inhibited DMBA binding to hepatic DNA in mice.

—H.R. Prasanna, et al., "Effect of Dehydroepiandrosterone (DHEA) on the Metabolism of 7,12-dimethylbenz[a]anthracene (DMBA) in Rats," *Carcinogenesis*, 10(5), May 1989, p. 953-955.

Results of this study showed that DHEA inhibited lymphopoiesis in mice.

—G. Risdon, et al., "Differential Effects of Dehydroepiandrosterone (DHEA) on Murine Lymphopoiesis and Myelopoiesis," *Exp Hematol*, 19(2), February 1991, p. 128-131.

Results of this study showed DHEA significantly reduced MNU-induced tumor incidence in mice.

—R.A. Lubet, et al., "Effects of Dehydroepiandrosterone (DHEA) on MNU-induced Breast Cancer in Sprague-Dawley Rats," *Proc Annu Meet Am Assoc Cancer Res*, 36, 995, p. A3517.

Results of this study showed that DHEA inhibited MNU-induced mammary carcinogenesis in rats.

—R.C. Moon, et al., "Effects of Intermittent, Delayed or Discontinuous Administration of Dehydroepiandrosterone (DHEA) on MNU-induced Breast Cancer in Rats," *Proc Annu Meet Am Assoc Cancer Res,* 37, 1996, p. 1891.

Cognitive Function

This double-blind, placebo-controlled study examined the effects of a 500 mg oral dose of DHEA on the sleep stages, sleep stage-specific electroencephalogram (EEG) power spectra, and concurrent hormone secretion in 10 healthy young male subjects. Results showed that DHEA significantly increased REM sleep relative to controls, with no changes seen in the other sleep variables. Previous studies have shown REM sleep to be involved in memory storage, thus these findings point to a benefit of DHEA in age- related dementia.

—E. Friess, et al., "DHEA Administration Increases Rapid Eye Movement Sleep and EEG Power in the Sigma Frequency Range," *American Journal of Physiol,* 268(1 Pt 1), January 1995, p. E107-13.

Depression

In this study, 30-90 mg of DHEA per day was administered to six middle-aged and elderly patients over a period of 4 weeks. Results showed significant improvements in symptoms of depression and memory performance.

—O.M. Wolkowitz, et al., "Dehydroepiandrosterone (DHEA) Treatment of Depression," *Biol Psychiatry,* 41(3), February 1, 1997, p. 311-318.

Diabetes

Results of this study found that DHEA had therapeutic effects on diabetic mice by producing a rapid remission of hyperglycemia, a preservation of beta-cell structure and function, and an increased insulin sensitivity as measured by glucose tolerance tests.

—D.L. Coleman, et al., "Therapeutic Effects of Dehydroepiandrosterone (DHEA) in Diabetic Mice," *Diabetes,* 31(9), September 1982, p. 830-833.

Flu

Results of this study showed that treatment with DHEA effectively countered defects in influenza immunity associated with aging in older mice.

—H.D. Danenberg, et al., "Dehydroepiandrosterone (DHEA) Treatment Reverses the Impaired Immune Response of Old Mice to Influenza Vaccination and Protects from Influenza Infection," *Vaccine,* 13(15), 1995, p. 1445-1448.

General

This review article discusses the findings of various studies pointing to the positive effects of DHEA in aging patients with respect to metabolic, immune, and cognitive functions.

—O. Khorram, "DHEA: A Hormone with Multiple Effects," *Curr Opin Obstet Gynecol,* 8(5), October 1996, p. 351-354.

Lupus

Results of this placebo-controlled study showed that the administration of DHEA was beneficial in alleviating symptoms of 50 patients with lupus. DHEA reduced the number of lupus flares when taken over a 3-12 month period.

> —R.F. Van Vollenhoven & J.L. McGuire, "Studies of Dehydroepiandrosterone (DHEA) as a Therapeutic Agent in Systemic Lupus Erythematosus," *Ann Med Interne,* 147(4), 1996, p. 290-296.

Obesity

Results of this study found that DHEA modified food selection in rats leading them to consume diets low in fat.

> —F. Svec & J. Porter, "Effect of DHEA on Macronutrient Selection by Zucker Rats," *Physiol Behav,* 59(4-5), April-May, 1996, p. 721-727.

■ GINKGO BILOBA

Aging

Results of this study indicated that Ginkgo biloba extract had a restorative effect on the neuronal membrane of in aging rats.

> —F. Huguet, et al., "Decreased cerebral 5-HT1A Receptors During Ageing: Reversal by Ginkgo Biloba Extract (EGb 761)," *Journal of Pharm Pharmacol,* 46(4), April 1994, p. 316-318.

Results of this double-blind, placebo-controlled, found that Ginkgo biloba extract proved effective against aging-induced cerebral disorders in humans.

> —J. Taillandier, et al., [Treatment of Cerebral Aging Disorders with Ginkgo Biloba Extract. A Longitudinal Multicenter Double-blind Drug vs. Placebo Study], *Presse Med,* 15(31), September 25, 1986, p. 1583-1587.

This review article cites numerous studies supporting the use of Ginkgo biloba in the treatment of various conditions associated with cerebral aging.

> —M. Allard, [Treatment of the Disorders of Aging with Ginkgo Biloba Extract. From Pharmacology to Clinical Medicine], *Presse Med,* 15(31), September 25, 1986, p. 1540-1545.

Anti-Clastogenic Effects

Results of this study showed that the administration of Ginkgo biloba leaves at doses of 120 mg per day for 2 months reduced plasma clastogenic activity to control levels when measured on the first day following treatment in workers exposed to high levels of radiation from the Chernobyl accident. Such positive effects lasted for a minimum of 7 months.

> —I. Emerit, et al., "Clastogenic Factors in the Plasma of Chernobyl Accident Recovery Workers: Anticlastogenic Effect of Ginkgo Biloba Extract," *Radiat Res,* 144(2), November 1995, p. 198-205.

Results of this study of a small number of Chernobyl workers exposed to radiation showed either regression or total disappearance of plasma clastogenic factors following two months of Gingko biloba extract administered in doses of 120 per day.

> —I. Emerit, et al., "Radiation-induced Clastogenic Factors: Anticlastogenic Effect of Ginkgo Biloba Extract," *Free Radic Biol Med*, 18(6), June 1995, p. 985-991.

Brain Function/Injury

Results of this study found that rats suffering from brain lesions which received treatment with 100 mg/kg Ginkgo biloba extract (GBE) intraperitoneally for 30 days experienced less impairment and a reduction in brain swellings induced by lesions than rats treated with saline or sham controls.

> —M.J. Attella, et al., "Ginkgo Biloba Extract Facilitates Recovery from Penetrating Brain Injury in Adult Male Rats," *Exp Neurol*, 105(1), July 1989, p. 62-71.

This study examined the effects of 100 mg/kg per os of Ginkgo biloba extract for 14 days on electroconvulsive shock induced accumulation of free fatty acids and diacylglycerols in the cerebral cortex and hippocampus of rats. Results found that Ginkgo biloba extract reduced the FFA pool size by 33% and increased the DAG pool by 36% in the hippocampus. A delay of 10 s to 1 min was seen in the rise of DAG content triggered in the cortex and hippocampus by ECS following Gingko biloba treatment, while DAG content showed a more rapid decrease following tonic seizure in rats treated with Gingko biloba relative to sham controls in the hippocampus and cortex.

> —E.B. Rodriguez de Turco, et al., "Decreased Electroconvulsive Shock-induced Diacylglycerols and Free Fatty Acid Accumulation in the Rat Brain by Ginkgo Biloba Extract (EGb 761): Selective Effect in Hippocampus as Compared with Cerebral Cortex," *Journal of Neurochemistry*, 61(4), October 1993, p. 1438-1444.

This study examined the effects of Ginkgo biloba on cerebral edema in rats intoxicated with triethyltin chloride. Results showed severe edema with extensive vacuolization in the cerebral and cerebellar white matter, while significant decrease in these manifestations were seen of the cytotoxic edema when rats received the Ginkgo bilobo extract. Such findings prompted the authors to conclude that Ginkgo biloba extract has a protective effect on cytotoxic edema development in the brain's white matter.

> —M. Otani, et al., "Effect of an Extract of Ginkgo Biloba on Triethyltin-induced Cerebral Edema," *Acta Neuropathol*, 69(1-2), 1986, p. 54-65.

Results of this study found that rats pretreated with a Ginkgo Biloba extract prior to unilateral embolization of the brain experienced suppressed effects of the embolization relative to controls which was due to an apparent increase in the blood flow associated with normalization of cellular energy.

> —L.M. Le Poncin, et al., "Effects of Ginkgo Biloba on Changes Induced by Quantitative Cerebral Microembolization in Rats," *Arch Int Pharmacodyn Ther*, 243(2), February 1980, p. 236-244.

In this double-blind, placebo-controlled study, patients with classical symptoms of organic syndrome were tested for the therapeutic effects of Ginkgo biloba extract administered in doses of 120 mg per day for 8 weeks. Results showed a significant improvement after 4 and 8 weeks of therapy with respect to both saccadic test and the psychometric tests relative to controls.

—B. Hofferberth, [The Effect of Ginkgo Biloba Extract on Neurophysiological and Psychometric Measurement Results in Patients with Psychotic Organic Brain Syndrome. A Double-blind Study Against Placebo], *Arzneimittelforschung,* 39(8), August 1989, p. 918-922.

Results of this meta-analysis involving 7 double-blind, placebo-controlled clinical trials found Ginkgo biloba extract (mean dose of 150 mg per day) significantly effective in reducing clinical symptoms associated with cerebrovascular insufficiency in old age.

—W. Hopfenmuller, [Evidence for a Therapeutic Effect of Ginkgo Biloba Special Extract. Meta-analysis of 11 Clinical Studies in Patients with Cerebrovascular Insufficiency in Old Age], *Arzneimittelforschung,* 44(9), September 1994, p. 1005-1013.

This double-blind, placebo-controlled study examined the effects of 120 mg per day of Ginkgo biloba extract on the central nervous system in geriatric patients with cerebral insufficiency. Results found that chronic Ginkgo biloba extract supplementation led to clear improvement in vigilance as measured in the resting EEG among a subclassification of the subjects.

—B. Gessner, et al., "Study of the Long-term Action of a Ginkgo Biloba Extract on Vigilance and Mental Performance as Determined by Means of Quantitative Pharmaco-EEG and Psychometric Measurements," *Arzneimittelforschung,* 35(9), 1985, p. 1459-1465.

This review article cites numerous studies supporting the effectiveness of Ginkgo biloba extract (mean dose being 120 mg per day for 4-6 weeks) in the treatment of cerebral insufficiency.

—J. Kleijnen & P. Knipschild, "Ginkgo Biloba for Cerebral Insufficiency," *British Journal of Clinical Pharmacology,* 34(4), October 1992, p. 352-358.

Results of this study showed the Ginkgo biloba extract significantly improved the NaNO and memory impaired by scopolamine in mice.

—C. Chen, et al., [Improvement of Memory in Mice by Extracts from Leaves of Ginkgo Biloba L.], *Chung Kuo Chung Yao Tsa Chih,* 16(11), November 1991, p. 681-683.

Results of this double-blind, placebo-controlled study found that elderly subjects with age-related memory impairment experienced significant improvement in the speed of information processing following treatment with either 320 or 600 mg of Ginkgo biloba extract 1 hour prior to performing a dual-code test.

—H. Allain, et al., "Effect of Two Doses of Ginkgo Biloba Extract (EGb 761) on the Dual-coding Test in Elderly Subjects," *Clin Ther,* 15(3), May-June 1993, p. 549-558.

In this double-blind, placebo-controlled study, patients over 50 with some level of memory impairment received treatment with oral doses of 120 mg of Ginkgo biloba per day. Results found that Ginkgo biloba had significant beneficial effects on cognitive function at both 12 and 24 weeks.

—G.S. Rai, et al., "A Double-blind, Placebo Controlled Study of Ginkgo Biloba Extract ('tanakan') in Elderly Outpatients with Mild to Moderate Memory Impairment," *Curr Med Res Opin,* 12(6), 1991, p. 350-355.

Results of this double-blind, placebo-controlled study showed that Ginkgo biloba extract significantly improved memory after 6 weeks of treatment and learning rate after 24 weeks in cerebral insufficiency outpatients.

> —E. Grassel, [Effect of Ginkgo-biloba Extract on Mental Performance: Double-blind Study Using Computerized Measurement Conditions in Patients with Cerebral Insufficiency], *Fortschr Med,* 110(5), February 20, 1992, p. 73-76.

Results of this double-blind, placebo-controlled study of cerebral insufficiency inpatients with depressive mood noted as a leading symptom found that those treated with 160 mg per day of Ginkgo biloba extract experienced a significantly greater degree of clinical improvement than controls.

> —F. Eckmann, [Cerebral Insufficiency—Treatment with Ginkgo-biloba Extract. Time of Onset of Effect in a Double-blind Study with 60 Inpatients], *Fortschr Med,* 108(29), October 10, 1990, p. 557-560.

Results of this randomized, 6-week study of 80 elderly, cererbrovascular disorder patients found that both Ginkgo biloba extract and dihydroergotoxine treatment led to improvements with no significant difference seen between them.

> —G. Gerhardt, et al., [Drug Therapy of Disorders of Cerebral Performance: Randomized Comparative Study of Dihydroergotoxine and Ginkgo Biloba Extract], *Fortschr Med,* 108(19), June 30, 1990, p. 384-388.

In this double-blind, placebo-controlled study, healthy female subjects were given Ginkgo biloba extract in doses of either 120, 240, or 600 mg per day. Results showed significant improvements in memory as measured by the Sternberg technique following treatment with 600 mg of Ginkgo biloba relative to controls.

> —Z. Subhan & I. Hindmarch, ''The Psychopharmacological Effects of Ginkgo Biloba Extract in Normal Healthy Volunteers,'' *International Journal of Clinical Pharmacology Research,* 4(2), 1984, p. 89-93.

Results of this study indicated that Ginkgo biloba extract was effective in aiding recovery of brain function in cats following unilateral vestibular neurectomy.

> —B. Tighilet & M. Lacour, ''Pharmacological Activity of the Ginkgo Biloba Extract (EGb 761) on Equilibrium Function Recovery in the Unilateral Vestibular Neurectomized Cat,'' *Journal of Vestib Research,* 5(3), May-June 1995, p. 187-200.

Results of this study indicated that Ginkgo biloba leaves can decreased increases in oxidative metabolism of rat brain neurons induced by Ca(2+).

> —Y. Oyama, et al., ''Ca(2+)-induced Increase in Oxidative Metabolism of Dissociated Brain Neurons: Effect of Extract of Ginkgo Biloba Leaves,'' *Japanese Journal of Pharmacology,* 61(4), April 1993, p. 367-370.

Results of this study found that visual field damage caused by a chronic lack of blood flow could be reversed by treatment with Ginkgo biloba extract at doses of 160 mg per day for 4 weeks.

> —A. Raabe, et al., [Therapeutic Follow-up Using Automatic Perimetry in Chronic Cerebroretinal Ischemia in Elderly Patients. Prospective Double-blind Study with Graduated Dose Ginkgo

Biloba Treatment (EGb 761)], *Klin Monatsbl Augenheilkd,* 199(6), December 1991, p. 432-438.

Results of this study showed that Ginkgo biloba leaf extract produced reversible inhibition of brain monoamine in rats which the authors argue may be a factor responsible for Ginkgo biloba's reported anxiolytic and antistress activities.

—H.L. White, et al., "Extracts of Ginkgo Biloba Leaves Inhibit Monoamine Oxidase," *Life Sci,* 58(16), 1996, p. 1315-1321.

This study examined the effects of Ginkgo biloba extract on the levels of blood glucose, local cerebral blood flow, and cerebral glucose concentration and consumption. Results found the extract reduced the concentration of cortical glucose and did not changing other substrate levels, indicating Ginkgo biloba can inhibit glucose and may play a role in its capacity to protect brain tissue from hypoxic or ischemic damage.

—J. Krieglstein, et al., "Influence of an Extract of Ginkgo Biloba on Cerebral Blood Flow and Metabolism," *Life Sci,* 39(24), December 15, 1986, p. 2327-2334.

This study examined the effects of Ginkgo biloba extract on the acquisition, performance and retention of mice in an appetite operant condition exercise designed to enhance memory. Results showed that the extract administered at 100 mg/kg per day for a total of 18 weeks enhanced memory processes.

—E. Winter, "Effects of an Extract of Ginkgo Biloba on Learning and Memory in Mice," *Pharmacol Biochem Behavior,* 38(1), January 1991, p. 109-114.

Results of this series of studies involving rats and mice indicated that the antihypoxidotic activity of Ginkgo biloba extract is carried in its non-flavone fraction.

—H. Oberpichler, et al., "Effects of Ginkgo Biloba Constituents Related to Protection Against Brain Damage Caused by Hypoxia," *Pharmacol Res Commun,* 20(5), May 1988, p. 349-368.

Results of this study showed that chronic treatment with Ginkgo biloba extract reduced 3H-dihyroalprenolol binding density as well as in adenulate cyclase activity stimulate by isoproterenol in the cerebral cortex of rats.

—N. Brunello, et al., "Effects of an Extract of Ginkgo Biloba on Noradrenergic Systems of Rat Cerebral Cortex," *Pharmacol Res Commun,* 17(11), November 1985, p. 1063-1072.

Results of this study showed that Panax ginseng and Ginkgo biloba administered in combination improved the retention of learned behavior in rats in a dose-dependent manner.

—V.D. Petkov, et al., "Memory Effects of Standardized Extracts of Panax Ginseng (G115), Ginkgo Biloba (GK 501) and their Combination Gincosan (PHL-00701)," *Planta Med,* 59(2), April 1993, p. 106-114.

The authors of this extensive review article on the clinical psychopharmacology of Gingko biloba extract concluded that the extract appears to be effective in treating vascular disorders, dementia, and cognitive disorders secondary to depression. The authors also suggest that there are no risk associated with taking the drug in doses well above its recommended levels.

—D.M. Warburton, [Clinical Psychopharmacology of Ginkgo Biloba Extract], *Presse Med,* 15(31), September 25, 1986, p. 1595-1604.

Results of this double-blind, placebo-controlled study found that Ginkgo biloba extract administered to patients suffering from senile macular degeneration showed significant improvements in lost distance visual acuity relative to controls.

> —D.A. Lebuisson, et al., [Treatment of Senile Macular Degeneration with Ginkgo Biloba Extract. A Preliminary Double-blind Drug vs. Placebo Study], *Presse Med*, 15(31), September 25, 1986, p. 1556-1558.

Results of this study found the administration of Ginkgo biloba to gerbils with experimentally-induced cerebral ischameia led to significant degrees of normalization of mitochondrial respiration, diminution of cerebral oedema, correlation of the accompanying ionic perturbation, and near complete functional restoration as seen by a normal neurological index.

> —B. Spinnewyn, et al., [Effects of Ginkgo Biloba Extract on a Cerebral Ischemia Model in Gerbils], *Presse Med*, 15(31), September 25, 1986, p. 1511-1555.

This review article notes that Ginkgo biloba extract limits cerebral oedema formation (be if of cytotoxic or vasogenic origin) and suppresses its neurological consequences.

> —A. Etienne, et al., [Mechanism of Action of Ginkgo Biloba Extract in Experimental Cerebral Edema] *Presse Med*, 15(31), September 25, 1986, p. 1506-1510.

Results of this study showed Ginkgo biloba extract given to rats partly reestablished glucose consumption in rats subject to either normobaric hypoxia or catotid clamping.

> —J.R. Rapin, et al., [Cerebral Glucose Consumption. The Effect of Ginkgo Biloba Extract], *Presse Med*, 15(31), September 25, 1986, p. 1494-1497.

Results of this study showed that the chronic administration of Ginkgo biloba extract to aged rats increased the muscarinic receptor population in the hippocampus.

> —J.E. Taylor, [Neuromediator Binding to Receptors in the Rat Brain. The Effect of Chronic Administration of Ginkgo Biloba Extract], *Presse Med*, 15(31), September 25, 1986, p. 149-1493.

Results of this study showed that Ginkgo biloba extract exerts a specific effect on the noradrenergic system and on beta-receptors which suggest central effects of a drug acting on cerebral aging, connected specifically to reactivation of the noradrenergic system in the cerebral cortex.

> —G. Racagni, et al., [Neuromediator Changes During Cerebral Aging. The Effect of Ginkgo Biloba Extract] *Presse Med*, 15(31), September 25, 1986, p. 1488-1490.

Results of this study indicated Ginkgo biloba extract proved beneficial in Parkinsonia patients with additional signs of SDAT.

> —E.W. Funfgeld, ''A Natural and Broad Spectrum Nootropic Substance for Treatment of SDAT—the Ginkgo Biloba Extract,'' *Prog Clin Biol Res*, 317, 1989, p. 1247-1260.

This study notes that rats undergoing simultaneous ligature of both carotid arteries results in certain death and about a 50% fatality rate when ligatures are separated by a four day time period. However, when rats receive extracts of Ginkgo biloba leaves prior to the procedure, dopamine synthesis is increased and survival rate is improved.

—M. Le Poncin-Lafitte, et al., [Cerebral Ischemia after Ligature of Both Carotid Arteries in Rats: Effect of Ginkgo Biloba Extracts,'' *Sem Hop,* 58(7), February 18, 1982, p. 403-406.

Results of this study showed that pretreatment with Ginkgo biloba leaves partially suppressed the effects of unilateral embolization in the brain of rats.

—J.R. Rapin, et al., [Experimental Model of Cerebral Ischemia Preventive Activity of Ginkgo Biloba Extract,'' *Sem Hop,* 55(43-44), December 18-25, 1979, p. 2047-2050.

This review article cites clinical studies supporting efficacy of Ginkgo biloba extracts in the treatment of cerebral insufficiency and atherosclerotic disease of the peripheral arteries.

—A. Z'Brun, [Ginkgo—Myth and Reality], *Schweiz Rundsch Med Prax,* 84(1), January 3, 1995, p. 1-6.

Cardiovascular/Coronary Heart Disease

Results of this study showed that Ginkgo biloba extract improved contractile function following global ischemia in the isolated working heart of rats due its ability to inhibit the formation of oxygen radicals.

—A. Tosaki, et al., "Ginkgo Biloba Extract (EGb 761) Improves Postischemic Function in Isolated Preconditioned Working Rat Hearts," *Coronary Artery Disease,* 5(5), May 1994, p. 443-450.

Results of this showed that the administration of Ginkgo biloba extract over a period of 3 months provided protective effects on the hypoxic myocardium in rats.

—K. Punkt, et al., "Changes of Enzyme Activities in the Rat Myocardium Caused by Experimental Hypoxia With and Without Ginkgo Biloba Extract EGb 761 Pretreatment. A Cytophotometrical Study," *Acta Histochem,* 97(1), January 1995, p. 67-79.

Results of this meta-analysis demonstrated significant therapeutic effects of Ginkgo biloba extract administered to patients suffering from peripheral arterial disease.

—B. Schneider, [Ginkgo biloba extract in peripheral arterial diseases. Meta-analysis of Controlled Clinical Studies], *Arzneimittelforschung,* 42(4), April 1992, p. 428-436.

Results of this single-blind, placebo-controlled study found Ginkgo biloba extract significantly decreased erythrocyte aggregation and increased blood flow in the nail fold capillaries of healthy subjects.

—F. Jung, et al., "Effect of Ginkgo Biloba on Fluidity of Blood and Peripheral Microcirculation in Volunteers," *Arzneimittelforschung,* 40(5), May 1990, p. 589-593.

In this double-blind, placebo-controlled study, patients suffering from peripheral arteriopathy experienced significant improvements in degree of pain free walking distance, maximum walking distance and plethylsmography recordings relative to controls.

—U. Bauer, "6-Month Double-blind Randomised Clinical Trial of Ginkgo Biloba Extract Versus Placebo in Two Parallel Groups in Patients Suffering from Peripheral Arterial Insufficiency," *Arzneimittelforschung,* 34(6), 1984, p. 716-720.

Results of this double-blind, placebo-controlled study showed that the administration of Ginkgo biloba extract for 14 days led to significant improvements in hypoxic hypoxia fixation time of saccadic eye movements and complex choice reaction time in healthy male subjects. The authors argue such findings may be taken as a hypoxia-protective phenomenon.

  —K. Schaffler & P.W. Reeh, [Double Blind Study of the Hypoxia Protective effect of a Standardized Ginkgo Biloba Preparation after Repeated Administration in Healthy Subjects] *Arzneimittelforschung,* 35(8), 1985, p. 1283-1286.

This study examined Ginkgo biloba's cardioprotective effects on myocardial ischemia-reperfusion injury in rabbits. Results showed that 10 mg/kg of Ginkgo biloba injected in the coronary artery significantly inhibited increases in lipid peroxidation relative to rabbits receiving saline perfusion. Treatment with Ginkgo biloba also significantly suppressed decreases in tissue type plasminogen activator and the increase in plasminogen activator inhibitor-1 caused by ischemia-reperfusion.

  —J.G. Shen & D.Y. Zhou, ''Efficiency of Ginkgo Biloba Extract in Antioxidant Protection Against Myocardial Ischemia and Reperfusion Injury,'' *Biochem Mol Biol Int,* 35(1), January 1995, p. 125-134.

Results of this study showed that Ginkgo biloba extract inhibited hypoxia-induced reductions in ATP content in endothelial cells in vitro.

  —D. Janssens, et al., ''Protection of Hypoxia-induced ATP Decrease in Endothelial Cells by Ginkgo Biloba Extract and Bilobalide,'' *Biochem Pharmacol,* 50(7), September 28, 1995, p. 991-995.

Results of this study showed that the water-soluble constituents of Ginkgo biloba episperm 100 or 200 mg/kg po inhibited passive cutaneous allergic response in mice. The same doses administered to rats ip inhibited mast cell degranulation. In guinea pigs, it antagonized the antigen-induced contractile effect of isolated ileum smooth muscles and inhibited the deliverance of SRS-A from anaphylactic lung.

  —H. Zhang, et al., [Anti-anaphylactic Pharmacological Action of Water-soluble Constituents of Ginkgo Biloba L. Episperm], *Chung Kuo Chung Yao Tsa Chih,* 15(8), August 1990, p. 496-497.

Results of this study found that the administration of 240 mg per day of Ginkgo biloba for 12 weeks to patients with a history of elevated fibrinogen levels and plasma viscosity as well as a host of different underlying diseases led to significant improvement in fibrinogen levels and hemorrheological properties.

  —S. Witte, et al., [Improvement of Hemorheology with Ginkgo Biloba Extract. Decreasing a Cardiovascular Risk Factor], *Fortschr Med,* 110(13), May 10, 1992, p. 247-250.

Results of this study showed that a single injection of Ginkgo biloba extract at doses of either 50, 100, 150, or 200 mg had positive effects on whole blood visco-eslasticity and microcirculation in patients with pathological visco-elasticity values.

  —P. Koltringer, et al., [Hemorheologic Effects of Ginkgo Biloba Extract EGb 761. Dose-dependent Effect of EGb 761 on Microcirculation and Viscoelasticity of Blood], *Fortschr Med,* 111(10), April 10, 1993, p. 170-172.

Results of this study found that Ginkgo biloba extract provided protection against cardiac ischemia reperfusion injury in isolated rat hearts.

—N. Haramaki, et al., "Effects of Natural Antioxidant Ginkgo Biloba Extract (EGB 761) on Myocardial Ischemia-reperfusion Injury," *Free Radic Biol Med*, 16(6), June 1994, p. 789-794.

Results of this study showed that Ginkgo biloba extract prevented early ventricular tachycardia by coronary reperfusion in dogs.

—H.M. Lo, et al., "Effect of EGb 761, a Ginkgo Biloba Extract, on Early Arrhythmia Induced by Coronary Occlusion and Reperfusion in Dogs," *Journal of Formos Medical Association*, 93(7), July 1994, p. 592-597.

In this double-blind, placebo-controlled study, arthritis patients received treatment with Ginkgo biloba extract for sixty-five weeks. Results showed that Ginkgo biloba extract provided significantly more pain relief and walking tolerance after 6 months of taking it than placebo.

—U. Bauer, [Ginkgo Biloba Extract in the Treatment of Arteriopathy of the Lower Extremities. A 65-week Trial], *Presse Med*, 15(31), September 25, 1986, p. 1546-1549.

This review article makes the following observations with respect to the vascular impact of Ginkgo biloba extract: Its preferential tissue effect in ischaemic areas is primarily explained its direct impact on both arteries and veins, with the drenergic vasoregulatory system and the vascular endothelium being the preferential targets for arterial impact. The extract reinforces the physiological vasoregulation of the sympathetic nervous system directly, by acting on neuromediator release, and indirectly, by inhibiting their extraneuronal degradation by catechol-orthomethyltransferase. It stimulates the release of endogenous relaxing factors like endothelium-derived relaxing factors and prostacyclin. Its action on the venous system has a venoconstrictor component that maintains the degree of parietal tonus essential to the dynamic clearing of toxic metabolites accumulated during tissue ischaemia.

—M. Auguet, et al., [Pharmacological Bases of the Vascular Impact of Ginkgo Biloba Extract], *Presse Med*, 15(31), September 25, 1986, p. 1524-1528.

Results of this study found that Ginkgo biloba extract injected into rabbits suppressed the vasospasm induced by the topic application of autologous serum on the surface of the brain in a dose dependent manner.

—S. Reuse-Blom & K. Drieu, [Effect of Ginkgo Biloba Extract on Arteriolar Spasm in Rabbits], *Presse Med*, 15(31), September 25, 1986, p. 1520-1523.

Results of this study showed that Ginkgo biloba extract induced a significant reduction in the intensity of ventricular fibrillation during reperfusion stage in an in vitro model of ischaemia-reperfusion. The extract also provided protection action against the ischaemia-induced electrocardiographic disorders on normal or hypertrophied hearts in vivo.

—J.M. Guillon, et al.., [Effects of Ginkgo Biloba Extract on 2 Models of Experimental Myocardial Ischemia], *Presse Med*, 15(31), September 25, 1986, p. 1516-1519.

This article comments on the fact that Ginkgo biloba extract appears to uniformly improve the ultrastructural qualities of vestibular sensorial epithelia when fixed by vascular perfusions. The author suggests that such improvements may be consequential to the effects of the extract on capillary permeability and general microcirculation.

　　—J. Raymond, [Effects of Ginkgo Biloba Extract on the Morphological Preservation of Vestibular Sensory Epithelia in Mice], *Presse Med*, 15(31), September 25, 1986, p. 1484-1487.

This study notes that Ginkgo biloba extract has been found to be capable of partially antagonizing the ability of sodium lactate applied on the pia-mater of rabbits to induce the appearance of venous platelets thrombi.

　　—M.G. Borzeix, et al., [Researches on the Antiaggregative Activity of Ginkgo Biloba Extract], *Sem Hop*, 56(7-8), February 18-25, 1980, p. 393-398.

In this study, 15 patients with arteriosclerotic lesions in the extracranial brain received an infusion of 250 ml physiological NaCl and 25 ml Ginkgo biloba extract while 15 other patients received 250 ml NaCl only. Results showed that significant increases in perfusion in response to Ginkgo biloba extract relative to controls.

　　—P. Koltringer, et al., [Microcirculation in Parenteral Ginkgo Biloba Extract Therapy], *Wien Klin Wochenschr*, 101(6), March 17, 1989, p. 198-200.

Claudication

This review of ten controlled trials on the effects of Ginkgo biloba in the treatment of intermittent claudication concluded the therapy to be effective, but noted the studies reviewed were not of high methodological quality.

　　—E. Erns, [Ginkgo Biloba in Treatment of Intermittent Claudication. A Systematic Research Based on Controlled Studies in the Literature], *Fortschr Med*, 114(8), March 20, 1996, p. 85-87.

Results of this double-blind, placebo-controlled study found 120 mg per day of Gingko biloba extract administered for 3 months led to improvements in some cognitive functions in elderly patients with moderate arterial insufficiency.

　　—H. Drabaek, et al., [The Effect of Ginkgo Biloba Extract in Patients with Intermittent Claudication], *Ugeskr Laeger*, 158(27), July 1, 1986, p. 3928-3931.

Diabetes

This double-blind, placebo-controlled study examined the effects of Ginkgo biloba on early diabetic retinopathy associated with a blue-yellow dyschromatopsia. Results showed statistical improvement among patients receiving the Ginkgo biloba relative to controls.

　　—P. Lanthony & J.P. Cosson, [The Course of Color Vision in Early Diabetic Retinopathy Treated with Ginkgo Biloba Extract. A Preliminary Double-blind Versus Placebo Study], *J Fr Ophtalmol*, 11(10), 1988, 671-674.

Results of this study showed that alloxan-induced diabetic rats treated with Gingko biloba experienced a significantly greater amplitude in electoretinograms than controls.

　　—M. Doly, et al., [Effect of Ginkgo Biloba Extract on the Electrophysiology of the Isolated Retina from a Diabetic Rat], *Presse Med*, 15(31), September 25, 1986, p. 1480-1483.

Edema

Results of this study showed that treatment of women suffering from idiopathic cyclic oedema with Ginkgo biloba extract led to complete correction of the biological anomaly in 10 cases receiving oral and 5 receiving intravenous administration.

> —G. Lagrue, et al., [Idiopathic Cyclic Edema. The Role of Capillary Hyperpermeability and its Correction by Ginkgo Biloba Extract], *Presse Med,* 15(31), September 25, 1986, p. 1550-1553.

General

Results of this study found Ginkgo biloba extract to be a scavenger of nitric oxide in vitro acellular systems.

> —L. Marcocci, et al., "The Nitric Oxide-scavenging Properties of Ginkgo Biloba Extract EGb 761," *Biochem Biophys Res Commun,* 201(2), June 15, 1994, p. 748-755.

Results of this study found that Ginkgo biloba extract can prevent radical mediated damage to human membranes caused by cyclosporin A.

> —S.A. Barth, et al., "Influences of Ginkgo Biloba on Cyclosporin A Induced Lipid Peroxidation in Human Liver Microsomes in Comparison to Vitamin E, Glutathione and N-acetylcysteine," *Biochem Pharmacol,* 41(10), May 15, 1991, p. 1521-1526.

Results of this study found that Ginkgo Biloba extract is an effective peroxyl radical scavenger.

> —I. Maitra, et al., "Peroxyl Radical Scavenging Activity of Ginkgo Biloba Extract EGb 761," *Biochem Pharmacol,* 49(11), May 26, 1995, p. 1649-1655.

Results of this study showed that Ginkgo biloba extract's antioxidant activities provided protection against lipoperoxidation of the retina in rats.

> —M.T. Droy-Lefaix, et al., "Protective Effect of Ginkgo Biloba Extract (EGB 761) on Free Radical-Induced Changes in the Electroretinogram of Isolated Rat Retina," *Drugs Exp Clin Res,* 17(12), 1991, p. 571-574.

This study examined the action of Ginkgo biloba extract against superoxide anion under in vitro conditions. Results showed the extract to have an O2- scavenging effect as well as superoxide dismutase activity.

> —J. Pincemail, et al., "Superoxide Anion Scavenging Effect and Superoxide Dismutase Activity of Ginkgo Biloba Extract," *Experientia,* 45(8), August 15, 1989, p. 708-712.

This study examined Ginkgo biloba extract for the release of activated oxygen species during human neutrophils stimulation by a soluble agonist. Results showed that Ginkgo biloba slowed O2 consumption by its inhibitory action on NADPH-oxidase. Results also found that, because of this action, superoxide anion (O-.2) and hydrogen peroxide production was significantly decreased when the PMNs stimulation was done in the presence of the extract at concentrations of 500, 250 and 125 micrograms/ml, while hydroxyl regeneration was decreased at concentrations as low as 15.6 micrograms Gbe/ml, which indicates that the extract also had activity of myeloperoxidase contained in neutrophils.

> —J. Pincemail, et al., "Ginkgo Biloba Extract Inhibits Oxygen Species Production Generated

by Phorbol Myristate Acetate Stimulated Human Leukocytes, *Experientia,* 43(2), February 15, 1987, p. 181-184.

Results of this study showed that Ginkgo biloba extract provided protection against free radical attack in vitro following the exposure of rat liver microsomes to UV-C irradiation.

—E. Dumont, et al., "UV-C Irradiation-induced Peroxidative Degradation of Microsomal Fatty Acids and Proteins: Protection by an Extract of Ginkgo Biloba (EGb 761), *Free Radic Biol Med,* 13(3), September 1992, p. 197-203.

This review article cites studies supporting the use of Ginkgo biloba in the treatment of hypoxia/ischemia, seizure activity, and peripheral nerve damage.

—P.F. Smith, et al., "The Neuroprotective Properties of the Ginkgo Biloba Leaf: A Review of the Possible Relationship to Platelet-activating Factor (PAF)," *Journal of Ethnopharmacology,* 50(3), March 1996, p. 131-139.

This study examined an extract of Ginkgo biloba's antioxidant activity on healthy human erythrocyte membranes. Results showed that the extract administered at doses of 0, 25, 50, 125, 250 and 500 micrograms/ml indicated its antioxidant potential increased in a dose-dependent manner.

—K. Kose & P. Dogan, "Lipoperoxidation Induced by Hydrogen Peroxide in Human Erythrocyte Membranes. 1. Protective Effect of Ginkgo Biloba Extract (EGb 761)," *Journal of International Medical Research,* 23(1), January-February 1995, p. 1-8.

Results of this case control study showed that Ginkgo biloba extract had a significant protective effect against experimental retinal damage in rabbits.

—S. Pritz-Hohmeier, et al., "Effect of In Vivo Application of the Ginkgo Biloba Extract EGb 761 (Rokan) on the Susceptibility of Mammalian Retinal Cells to Proteolytic Enzymes," *Ophthalmic Research,* 26(2), 1994, p. 80-86.

Results of this study indicated that Ginkgo biloba extract had excitatory effects on the lateral vestibular nuclei neurons in guinea pigs.

—T. Yabe, et al., "Effects of Ginkgo Biloba Extract (EGb 761) on the Guinea Pig Vestibular System," *Pharmacol Biochem Behav,* 42(4), August 1992, p. 595-604.

This study examined the effects of 50 mg/kg ip per day of Ginkgo biloba extract on vestibular compensation in unilateral vestibular neurectomized cats. Results found cats treated with the extract recovered faster than controls and that treatment significantly accelerated postural and locomotor balance recovery.

—M. Lacour, et al., "Plasticity Mechanisms in Vestibular Compensation in the Cat are Improved by an Extract of Ginkgo Biloba (EGb 761)," *Pharmacol Biochem Behav,* 40(2), October 1991, p. 367-379.

This article notes that a flavanol glycosides containing Ginkgo bilob L. extract induces a concentration-dependent relaxation of guinea-pig trachea in vitro and antagonizes in vivo bronchoconstriction induced by various agonists.

—L. Puglisi, et al., "Pharmacology of Natural Compounds. I. Smooth Muscle Relaxant

Activity Induced by a Ginkgo Biloba L. Extract on Guinea-pig Trachea,'' *Pharmacol Res Commun,* 20(7), July 1988, p. 573-589.

Results of this double-blind, placebo-controlled study showed that vertiginous patients treated with Ginkgo biloba extract over 3 months experienced a significant improvement in the intensity, frequency and duration of their condition relative to controls.

—J.P. Haguenauer, et al., [Treatment of Equilibrium Disorders with Ginkgo Biloba Extract. A Multicenter Double-blind Drug vs. Placebo Study], *Presse Med,* 15(31), September 25, 1986, p. 1569-1572.

This article notes that intravenous administration of Ginkgo biloba extract resulted in dramatic recovery in severe cases of hypovolaemic shock related to monoclonal.

—G. Lagrue, et al., [Recurrent Shock with Monoclonal Gammopathy. Treatment in the Acute and Chronic Phases with Oral and Parenteral Ginkgo Biloba Extract], *Presse Med,* 15(31), September 25, 1986, p. 1554-1555.

This review article notes that experimental models of ischaemia, oedema and hypoxia, have shown that Ginkgo biloba extract reduced vascular, tissular and metabolic disturbances along with neurological and behavioral consequences associated with them.

—F. Clostre, [From the Body to the Cell Membrane: The Different Levels of Pharmacological Action of Ginkgo Biloba Extract], *Presse Med,* 15(31), September 25, 1986, p. 1529-1538..

This review article notes that studies have shown Ginkgo biloba to have significant positive effects on the central nervous systems as well as in the treatment of dementia.

—T. Itil & D. Martorano, ''Natural Substances in Psychiatry (Ginkgo Biloba in Dementia),'' *Psychopharmacol Bull,* 31(1), 1995, p. 147-158.

Hair Growth

Results of this study showed that Ginkgo biloba extract promoted hair regrowth in rats.

—N. Kobayashi, et al., [Effect of Leaves of Ginkgo Biloba on Hair Regrowth in C3H Strain Mice], *Yakugaku Zasshi,* 113(10), October 1993, p. 718-724.

Hearing Loss

In this study, patients with idiopathic sudden hearing loss existing no longer than 10 days were given treatment with either Ginkgo EGb 761 (Tebonin) + HAES or Naftidrofuryl (Dusodril)+HAES. Results showed that, after one week of observation, 40% of the patients in both treatment groups experienced a complete remission of hearing loss.

—F. Hoffmann, et al., [Ginkgo Extract EGb 761 (tenobin)/HAES versus Naftidrofuryl (Dusodril)/HAES. A Randomized Study of Therapy of Sudden Deafness], *Laryngorhinootologie,* 73(3), March 1994, p. 149-152.

Results of this double-blind study showed treatment with both Ginkgo biloba extract of nicegoline led to significant recovery in patients with acute cochlear deafness caused by ischemia, with the effects of Ginkgo biloba being markedly stronger.

—C. Dubreuil, [Therapeutic Trial in Acute Cochlear Deafness. A Comparative Study of

Ginkgo Biloba Extract and Nicergoline], *Presse Med,* 15(31), September 25, 1986, p. 1559-1561.

Hepatitis

Results of this study showed that Ginkgo biloba Composita arrested the development of liver fibrosis of chronic hepatitis.

—W. Li, et al., [Preliminary Study on Early Fibrosis of Chronic Hepatitis B Treated with Ginkgo Biloba Composita], *Chung Kuo Chung Hsi I Chieh Ho Tsa Chih,* 15(10), October 1995, p. 593-595.

Intestinal Disorders

Results of this study showed that Ginkgo biloba extract protected the intestinal mucosa of rats against ischaemic damage through the reduction of lipid peroxidation and neutrophil infiltration.

—T. Otamiri & C. Tagesson, "Ginkgo Biloba Extract Prevents Mucosal Damage Associated with Small-Intestinal Ischaemia," *Scandinavian Journal of Gastroenterology,* 24(6), August 1989, p. 666-670.

Neuropathy

In this study, 10 neuropathy patients with an autonomic disregulation of skin were intravenously administered a combination of 87.5 mg of Ginkgo biloba extract standardized to 21.0 mg Flavonglycosids and 3 mg folic acid over a period of 4 days. Results showed significant improvements in nerve function following treatment.

—P. Koltringer, et al., [Ginkgo Biloba Extract and Folic Acid in the Therapy of Changes Caused by Autonomic Neuropathy], *Acta Med Austriaca,* 16(2), 1989, p. 35-37.

PMS

This double-blind, placebo-controlled study examined the effects of Ginkgo biloba extract on congestive symptoms of PMS in a group of 165 women. Results showed the extract proved to be effective in relieving symptoms, particularly those associated with the breasts.

—A. Tamborini & R. Taurelle, [Value of Standardized Ginkgo Biloba Extract (EGb 761) in the Management of Congestive Symptoms of Premenstrual Syndrome], *Rev Fr Gynecol Obstet,* 88(7-9), July-September 1993, p. 447-457.

Pneumocystis Carinii

Results of these in vitro and in vivo studies showed that sesquiterpene bilobalide, extracted from Ginkgo biloba leaves, might be useful for therapy of and prophylaxis against P. carinii infections in humans.

—C. Atzori, et al., "Activity of Bilobalide, A Sesquiterpene from Ginkgo Biloba, on Pneumocystis Carinii," *Antimicrob Agents Chemothe,* 37(7), July 1993, p. 1492-1496.

Spinal Cord Injury

Results of this double-blind study found that Ginkgo biloba had protective effects against ischaemic spinal cord injury in rats due to its antioxidant activities.

—R.K. Koc, et al., "Lipid Peroxidation in Experimental Spinal Cord Injury. Comparison of

Treatment with Ginkgo Biloba, TRH and Methylprednisolone," *Res Exp Med,* 195(2), 1995, p. 117-123.

Stress

This study examined the effects of sub-chronic cold stress on hippocampal 5-HT1A receptors functioning and potential protective effects of Ginkgo biloba extract in old isolated rats. Results showed that the extract prevented the stress-induced desensitization of 5-HT1A.

—F. Bolanos-Jimenez, et al., "Stress-induced 5-HT1A Receptor Desensitization: Protective Effects of Ginkgo Biloba Extract (EGb 761)," *Fundam Clin Pharmacol,* 9(2), 1995, p. 169-174.

Results of this study found that Ginkgo biloba extract enhanced behavioral adaptation in the face of adverse environmental influences in rats. Such findings suggest it may be useful in the treatment of cognitive impairment in humans.

—J.R. Rapin, et al., "Demonstration of the "Anti-stress" Activity of an Extract of Ginkgo Biloba (EGb 761) Using a Discrimination Learning Task," *Gen Pharmacol,* 25(5), September 1994, p. 1009-1016.

Results of this study found that mice administered 50 and 100 mg/kg per day of Ginkgo biloba extract prior to unavoidable shock exposure experienced a reduction in subsequent avoidance deficits in learned helplessness.

—R.D. Porsolt, et al., "Effects of an Extract of Ginkgo Biloba (EGB 761) on "Learned Helplessness" and Other Models of Stress in Rodents," *Pharmacol Biochem Behav,* 36(4), August 1990, p. 963-971.

Tinnitus

Results of this double-blind, placebo-controlled study found that Ginkgo biloba extract treatment led to improvements among patients suffering from tinnitus.

—B. Meyer, [Multicenter Randomized Double-blind Drug vs. Placebo Study of the Treatment of Tinnitus with Ginkgo Biloba Extract], *Presse Med,* 15(31), September 25, 1986, p. 1562-1564.

■ HYDERGINE

Aging

Results of this double-blind, placebo-controlled study found that the long-term administration of ergoloid mesylates had beneficial effects with respect to aging-related symptoms such as tiredness and dizziness and led to improvements in measures of intelligence among healthy, elderly subjects.

—R. Spiegel, et al., "A Controlled Long-term Study with Ergoloid Mesylates (Hydergine) in Healthy, Elderly Volunteers: Results after Three Years," *Journal of the American Geriatric Society,* 31(9), September 1983, p. 549-555.

Results of this study showed that hydergine exhibited modulating effects on the morphological plasticity of dentate gyrus synaptic junctions in aged rats.

> —C. Bertoni-Freddari, et al., "The Effect of Chronic Hydergine Treatment on the Plasticity of Synaptic Junctions in the Dentate Gyrus of Aged Rats," *Journal of Gerontology,* 42(5), September 1987, p. 482-486.

Results of this study showed that hydergine was capable of modifying increased brain MAO activity in some brain regions of aging rats.

> —A. Buyukozturk, et al., "The Effects of Hydergine on the MAO Activity of the Aged and Adult Rat Brain," *Eur Neuropsychopharmacol,* 5(4), December 1995, p. 527-529.

Results of this study showed that the administration of hydergine protected against alcohol-induced effects of aging in mice.

> —T. Samorajski, et al., "Dihydroergotoxine(Hydergine) and Ethanol-induced Aging of C57BL/6J Male Mice," *Pharmacology,* 16 (Suppl 1), 1978, p. 36-44.

Alcohol-Related Encephalopathy

Results of this study found significant improvement following treatment with oral hydergine in symptoms of sleep disturbance, agitation and depression in 7 patients suffering from alcohol-related encephalopathy.

> —K.D. Datta, et al., "Efficacy of Oral Hydergine (Ergoloid Mesylates) in Alcohol Related Encephalopathy," *Prog Neuropsychopharmacol Biol Psychiatry,* 11(1), 1987, p. 87-90.

Asthma

This study examined the effects of hydergine on patients suffering from bronchial asthma. Results showed that 3 to 6 mg per day led to significant improvements in 25% of the patients while 55% showed at least some improvement.

> —S. Kitamura, "The Treatment of Asthmatic Patients Using an Alpha-adrenergic Receptor Blocking Agent, Co-dergocrine Mesylate ('Hydergine')," *Pharmatherapeutica,* 2(5), 1980, p. 330-336.

Cardiovascular/Coronary Heart Disease

Results of this double-blind, placebo-controlled study found that the administration of Hydergine/ Nifedipine (Pontuc) had significant antihypertensive effects in elderly patients with isolated systolic hypertension.

> —P. Dominiak & G. Weidinger, [Therapy Comparison Between the Combination Hydergine/ nifedipine and Nifedipine Alone in Patients with Isolated Systolic Hypertension], *Med Klin,* 86(1), January 15, 1991, p. 15-19.

Results of this double-blind, placebo-controlled study found that patients treated with co-dergocrine experienced significant reductions in platelet deposition relative to controls, suggesting it may be useful in preventing mural thrombus formation, transient ischemic attacks, and atherosclerosis.

> —G. Steurer, et al., "Effects of Hydergine on Platelet Deposition on "active" Human Carotid

Artery Lesions and Platelet Function," *Thromb Research,* 55(5), September 1, 1989, p. 577-589.

Cognitive Function

Results of this double-blind, placebo-controlled study found that the administration of hydergine over a period of 24 weeks led to significant improvements in symptoms of senile mental deterioration among nursing home patients.

—C.M. van Loveren-Huyben, et al., "Double-blind Clinical and Psychological Study of Ergoloid Mesylates (Hydergine) in Subjects with Senile Mental Deterioration," *Journal of American Geriatric Society,* 32(8), August 1984, p. 584-588.

Results of this study found that the administration of 6 mg per day of hydergine over a period of 12 weeks led to significant improvements in memory among elderly outpatients suffering from mild memory impairment.

—O.J. Thienhaus, et al., "A Controlled Double-blind Study of High-dose Dihydroergotoxine Mesylate (Hydergine) in Mild Dementia," *Journal of the American Geriatric Society,* 35(3), March 1987, p. 219-223.

Results of this double-blind, placebo-controlled study found that daily intravenous infusion of 3 mg co-dergocrine mesylate ('Hydergine') for a 14 day period led to significant improvements in symptoms associated with multi-infarct dementia including cognitive dysfunction, depression, fatigue, withdrawal, etc. in elderly patients.

—A. Arrigo, et al., "Effects of Intravenous High Dose Co-dergocrine Mesylate ('Hydergine') in Elderly Patients with Severe Multi-infarct Dementia: A Double-blind, Placebo-controlled Trial," *Curr Med Res Opin,* 11(8), 1989, p. 491-500.

Results of this study showed hydergine enhanced memory function in aging mice.

—J.F. Flood, et al., "Hydergine Enhances Memory in Mice," *Journal Pharmacol,* 16 (Suppl 3), 1985, p. 39-49.

This review article notes that human and animal studies point to the beneficial effects of hydergine in the treatment of elderly patients suffering from senile mental impairment.

—R. Markstein, "Hydergine: Interaction with the Neurotransmitter Systems in the Central Nervous System," *Journal of Pharmacol,* 16 (Suppl 3), 1985, p. 1-17.

Results of this study showed that Co-dergocrine enhances the release of ACh in the hippocampus in a similar manner to both D1 and D2 DA agonists, pointing to its potential has a beneficial therapy in the treatment of dementia associated with Parkinson's disease.

—A. Imperato, et al., "Co-dergocrine (Hydergine) Regulates Striatal and Hippocampal Acetyl-choline Release Through D2 Receptors," *Neuroreport,* 5(6), February 24, 1994, p. 674-676.

Ear Trouble

In this study, patients suffering from problems on the cochlear compartment and/or vestibular level which clinically manifested by perceptive hypoacusia, tinnitus and rotatory vertigo were treated with hydergine doses of 30 drops three time per day, totaling 4.5 mg/day, over a period between 30—90 days. Results showed a global improvement in vertigo symptoms among 93.7% of patients treated. A 57.1% improvement was seen in tinnitus symptoms and 20% improvement with respect to hypoacusia.

>   —N. J. Jimenez-Cervantes & L.M. Amoros Rodriguez, [Hydergine in Pathology of the Inner Ear], *An Otorrinolaringol Ibero Am,* 17(1), 1990. p. 85-98.

General

This article reviewed 26 studies involving the clinical effects of hydergine on numerous conditions associated with aging. Results of such studies showed therapeutic benefits with respect to cognitive dysfunctions, mood depression, and subjective scores of overall well being.

>   —R.J. McDonald, "Hydergine: A Review of 26 Clinical Studies," *Pharmakopsychiatr Neuropsychopharmakol,* 12(6), November 1979, p. 407-422.

Hyperprolactinemia

Results of this double-blind, placebo-controlled study showed that a single oral dose of 2 mg of hydergine exhibited PRL inhibitory activity and proved effective in treating hyperprolactinemic anovulatory patients.

>   —T. Tamura, et al., "Effect of Hydergine in Hyperprolactinemia," *Journal of Clinical Endocrinol Metab,* 69(2), August 1989, p. 470-474.

■ ISOFLAVONES/GENISTEIN

Bone Loss

Results of this study showed that the administration of 1200 mg per day of the isoflavone derivative, Iprivalone, for 15 days followed by 600 mg per day for another 15 days with a washout period in between reduced the biochemical parameters of bone pain and disease activities in patients suffering from Paget's disease.

>   —D. Agnusdei, et al., "Short-term Treatment of Paget's Disease of Bone with Ipriflavone," *Bone Miner,* 19 Suppl 1, October 1992, p. S35-S42.

In this study, primary hyperparathyroidism patients received 1200 mg per day of oral ipriflavone over a period of 21-42 days. Results showed ipriflavone affected bone remodeling by inhibiting bone resorption without affecting bone formation.

>   —G. Mazzuoli, et al., "Effects of Ipriflavone on Bone Remodeling in Primary Hyperparathyroidism," *Bone Miner,* 19 (Suppl 1), October 1992, p. S27-S33

Results of this double-blind, placebo-controlled study found that the administration of ipriflavone over a period of 6 months led to significant increases in the bone mineral density of postmenopausal women relative to controls.

>   —A.B. Kovacs, "Efficacy of Ipriflavone in the Prevention and Treatment of Postmenopausal Osteoporosis," *Agents Actions,* 41(1-2), March 1994, p. 86-87.

Results of this double-blind, placebo-controlled study showed that 600 mg per day of ipriflavone administered for a period of between 3-6 months restrained the bone remodeling processes and prevented rapid bone loss associated with gonadotropin hormone-releasing hormone agonist (GnRH-A)-induced hypogonadism in female patients.

> —M. Gambacciani, et al., ''Ipriflavone Prevents the Bone Mass Reduction in Premenopausal Women Treated with Gonadotropin Hormone-releasing Hormone Agonists,'' *Bone Miner,* 26(1), July 1994, p. 19-26.

In this double-blind, placebo-controlled study, women over the age of 65 suffering from osteoporosis received 600 mg per day of ipriflavone. Results showed a significant increase in bone mineral density at the distal radius relative to controls.

> —M. Passeri, et al., ''Effect of Ipriflavone on Bone Mass in Elderly Osteoporotic Women,'' *Bone Miner,* 19 (Suppl 1), October 1992, p. S57-S62.

Results of this 2-year, multi-center, double-blind, placebo-controlled study found that the administration of 600 mg per day of oral ipriflavone postmenopausal female osteoporosis patients showed a significant increase in bone mineral density among those women in the treatment group after 12 months.

> —D. Agnusdei, et al., ''Effects of Ipriflavone on Bone Mass and Calcium Metabolism in Postmenopausal Osteoporosis,'' *Bone Miner,* 19 (Suppl 1), October 1992, p. S43-S48.

Results of this study found that 12 months of ipriflavone therapy significantly increased bone density of the femoral neck and of the trabecular substructure of Ward's triangle in female patients suffering from bone loss.

> —C.E. Fiore, et al., ''Modification of Cortical and Trabecular Mineral Density of the Femur, Induced by Ipriflavone Therapy, Clinical Results after 12 Months,'' *Clin Ter,* 146(1), January 1995, p. 13-19.

In this double-blind, placebo-controlled study, women with postmenopausal osteoporosis received 600 mg per day of ipriflavone over a period of 6 months. Results showed that ipriflavone facilitated the conservation of bone and significantly improved pain and motility. By contrast, a bone mineral loss was seen among controls.

> —D. Agnusdei, et al., ''Metabolic and Clinical Effects of Ipriflavone in Established Post-Menopausal Osteoporosis,'' *Drugs Exp Clin Res,* 15(2), 1989, p. 97-104.

Results of this study showed that the administration of 200 mg of ipriflavone three times per day over a period of 12 months increased bone mineral density by 5.8% in osteoporotic women.

> —M. Moscarini, et al., ''New Perspectives in the Treatment of Postmenopausal Osteoporosis: Ipriflavone,'' *Gynecol Endocrinol,* 8(3), September 1994, p. 203-207.

Results of this double-blind, placebo-controlled study showed that the combined treatment of ipriflavone and 1 alpha vitamin D significantly reduced postmenopausal bone loss in women.

> —T. Ushiroyama, et al., ''Efficacy of Ipriflavone and 1 Alpha Vitamin D Therapy for the Cessation of Vertebral Bone Loss,'' *International Journal of Gynaecol Obstet,* 48(3), March 1995, p. 283-288.

Results of this study found treatment with Osteochin (ipriflavone) tablets and calcium was an effective therapy of osteoporosis in human subjects.

> —A. Bossanyi & L. Bucsi, ''A New Treatment Possibility for Osteoporosis with Osteochin (Ipriflavone) Tablets,'' *Magy Traumatol Orthop Helyreallito Seb,* 32(2), 1989, p. 109-115.

Results of this study showed that the administration of 600 mg per day of Ipriflavone protected against bone loss in gynecological patients receiving treatment with GnRH.

—M. Pellicano, et al., "Effects of Ipriflavone on Bone Loss Induced by GnRH Analog," *Minerva Ginecol,* 48(10), October 1996, p. 435-439.

Results of this study showed that the administration of Ipriflavone protected against bone loss in gynecological patients receiving treatment with GnRH.

—F. Polatti, et al., "Long-term Assessment of Bone Loss in Patients Treated with GnRH Agonists," *Minerva Ginecol,* 47(5), May 1995, p. 193-196.

Cancer

Results of this study found that genistein inhibited growth of normal and leukaemic haemopoietic progenitors and exerted a direct toxic effect on haemopoietic cells in vitro.

—C. Carlo-Stella, et al., "Effect of the Protein Tyrosine Kinase Inhibitor Genistein on Normal and Leukaemic Haemopoietic Progenitor Cells," *British Journal of Haematol,* 93(3), June 1996, p. 551-557.

Results of this study showed that genistein significantly inhibited the invasion of a highly metastatic subline of a murine mammary carcinoma.

—E.M. Scholar, et al., "Decreased Invasion of Murine Mammary Carcinoma Cells by the Tyrosine Kinase Inhibitor Genistein," *FASEB Journal,* 8(5), 1994, p. A670.

Results of this study showed that genistein inhibited the proliferation of tumor cells in vitro. In addition, genistein excretion in urine of subjects consuming a plant-based diet is in the micromolar range, which is 30 times greater than those eating a more traditional Western diet. Thus such levels of genistein in urine of vegetarians coupled with its tumor-inhibiting effects indicate genistein may contribute to the preventive effect of vegetarian diets on diseases, including cancer.

—T. Fotsis, et al., "Genistein, A Dietary Ingested Isoflavonoid, Inhibits Cell Proliferation and in Vitro Angiogenesis," *Journal Nutr,* 125(3 Suppl), March 1995, p. 790S-797S.

This review article notes that two-thirds of studies involving the effect of genistein-containing soy materials in animal models of cancer have shown significant reductions. Studies with purified genistein have produced similar results.

—S. Barnes, et al., "Effect of Genistein on in Vitro and in Vivo Models of Cancer," *Journal of Nutrition,* 125(3 Suppl), March 1995, p. 777S-783S.

This review article argues that supplementing human diets with various soy products which have been found to suppress cancer in animal studies may reduce the risk of human cancer.

—A.R. Kennedy, "The Evidence for Soybean Products as Cancer Preventive Agents," *Journal of Nutr,* 125(3 Suppl), March 1995, p. 733S-743S.

Results of this study showed that genistein inhibited experimental-induced colon cancer in rats.

—V.E. Steele, et al., "Cancer Chemoprevention Agent Development Strategies for Genistein," *Journal of Nutrition,* 125(3 Suppl), March 1995, p. 713S-716S.

Results of this study showed that genistein inhibited experimental-induced mammary cancer in rats.

—C.A. Lamartiniere, et al., ''Neonatal Genistein Chemoprevents Mammary Cancer,'' *Proc Soc Exp Biol Med,* 208(1), January 1995, p. 120-123.

In this study, human BCP leukemia was treated in a murine model by targeting of genistein to the B cell-specific receptor CD19 with the monoclonal antibody B43. The B43-Gen immunoconjugate bound with high affinity to BCP leukemia cells, selectively inhibited CD19-associated tyrosine kinases, and triggered rapid apoptotic cell death. Greater than 99.999 percent of human BCP leukemia cells were killed, resulting in a 100 percent long-term event-free survival from this fatal form of leukemia.

—F.M. Uckun, et al., ''Biotherapy of B-cell Precursor Leukemia by Targeting Genistein to CD19-associated Tyrosine Kinases,'' *Science,* 267(5199), February 10, 1995, p. 886-891.

Results of this study showed that genistein inhibited human prostate cancer cell proliferation in vitro.

—J.F. Santibanez, et al., ''Genistein Inhibits Proliferation and in Vitro Invasive Potential of Human Prostatic Cancer Cell Lines,'' *Anticancer Research,* 17(2A), March-April, 1997, p. 1199-1204.

Results of this study showed that genistein inhibited human prostate cancer cell proliferation in vitro, but not in vivo.

—H.R. Naik, et al., ''An in Vitro and in Vivo Study of Antitumor Effects of Genistein on Hormone Refractory Prostate Cancer,'' *Anticancer Research,* 14(6B), November-December 1994, p. 2617-2619.

Results of this study showed that genistein inhibited growth of three different human breast cancer cell lines in vitro.

—E. Monti & B.K. Sinha, ''Antiproliferative Effect of Genistein and Adriamycin against Estrogen-Dependent and -independent Human Breast Carcinoma Cell Lines,'' *Anticancer Research,* 14(3A), May-June 1994, p. 1221-1226.

Results of this study showed that the isoflavonoid kievitone strongly inhibited the proliferation of breast cancer cells in vitro.

—R. Hoffman, ''Potent Inhibition of Breast Cancer Cell Lines by the Isoflavonoid Kievitone: Comparison with Genistein,'' *Biochem Biophys Res Commun,* 211(2), June 12, 1995, p. 600-606.

Results of this study showed that genistein inhibited growth of different human breast cancer cell lines in vitro.

—G. Peterson & S. Barnes, ''Genistein Inhibition of the Growth of Human Breast Cancer Cells: Independence from Estrogen Receptors and the Multi-drug Resistance Gene,'' *Biochem Biophys Res Commun,* 179(1), August 30, 1991, p. 661-667.

Results of this study showed that genistein significantly inhibited DMBA-induced mammary cancer in rats.

—W.B. Murrill, et al., ''Prepubertal Genistein Exposure Suppresses Mammary Cancer and Enhances Gland Differentiation in Rats,'' *Carcinogenesis,* 17(7), July 1996, p. 1451-1457.

Results of this study showed that genistein significantly inhibited experimentally-induced mammary cancer in rats.

—C.A. Lamartiniere, et al., "Genistein Suppresses Mammary Cancer in Rats," *Carcinogenesis,* 16(11), November 1995, p. 2833-2840.

Results of this study showed that genistein inhibited the growth of Jurkat T-leukemia cells in vitro.

—F. Spinozzi, et al., "The Natural Tyrosine Kinase Inhibitor Genistein Produces Cell Cycle Arrest and Apoptosis in Jurkat T-leukemia Cells," *Leukemia Research,* 18(6), June 1994, p. 431-439.

Results of this study showed that genistein inhibited the growth of lymphoma cells in vitro.

—A.R. Buckley, et al., "Inhibition by Genistein of Prolactin-induced Nb2 Lymphoma Cell Mitogenesis," *Mol Cell Endocrinol,* 98(1), December 1993, p. 17-25.

Results of this study found that genistein inhibited tumor promoter-induced H2O2 formation both in vivo and in vitro.

—H. Wei, et al., "Inhibition of Tumor Promoter-induced Hydrogen Peroxide Formation in Vitro and in Vivo by Genistein," *Nutr Cancer,* 20(1), 1993, p. 1-12.

Results of this study found genistein inhibited the growth of prostate cancer cells in vitro.

—E. Kyle, et al., "Genistein Inhibits the Growth of Prostate Cancer Cells. What is the Mechanism?" *Proceedings of the Annual Meeting of the American Association of Cancer Researchers,* 36, 1995, p. A2310.

Results of this study showed that genistein inhibited DMBA-induced mammary cancer in rats.

—C.A. Lamartiniere, et al., "Chemoprevention of Mammary Cancer from Neonatal Genistein Treatment," *Proceedings of the Annual Meeting of the American Association of Cancer Researchers,* 35, 1994, p. A3689.

Results of this study found that genistein delayed the onset of DMBA-induced mammary cancer in rats.

—C.A. Lamartiniere, et al., "Chemoprevention of Breast Cancer with the Soy Component, Genistein," *Proceedings of the Annual Meeting of the American Association of Cancer Researchers,* 36, '995, p. A3525.

Results of this study found that genistein might be involved in inhibitory effects of soy protein isolate against DMBA-induced mammary cancer in rats.

—P. Upadhyaya & K. El-Bayoumy, "Effects of Dietary Soy Protein Isolate and Genistein on the Levels of 7,12-dimethylbenz(a)anthracene (DMBA)-DNA Binding in Mammary Glands of female CD Rats," *Proceedings of the Annual Meeting of the American Association of Cancer Researchers,* 36, 1995, p. A3553.

Results of this study found that genistein inhibited TPA-induced skin tumors in mice.

—R. Bowen, et al., "Antipromotional Effect of the Soybean Isoflavone Genistein," *Proceed-*

ings of the Annual Meeting of the American Association of Cancer Researchers, 34, 1993, p. A3310.

Results of this study showed that both genistein and biochanin A inhibited the growth human prostate cancer cells in vitro.
—G. Peterson & S. Barnes, "Genistein and Biochanin A Inhibit the Growth of Human Prostate Cancer Cells but not Epidermal Growth Factor Receptor Tyrosine Autophosphorylation," *Prostate,* 22(4), 1993, p. 335-345.

Results of this study showed that genistein suppressed the proliferation of hepatocarcinoma cells in vitro.
—Y. Mousavi & H. Adlercreutz, "Genistein is an Effective Stimulator of Sex Hormone-binding Globulin Production in Hepatocarcinoma Human Liver Cancer Cells and Suppresses Proliferation of these Cells in Culture," *Steroids,* 58(7), July 1993, p. 301-304.

Herpes

Results of this study showed that genistein inhibited the replication of herpes simplex virus type 1 in vitro.
—Y. Yura, et al., "Inhibition of Herpes Simplex Virus Replication by Genistein, an Inhibitor of Protein-tyrosine Kinase," *Arch Virol,* 132(3-4), 1993, p. 451-461.

Tinnitus

Results of this double-blind study showed ipriflavone administered over a period of 6 months to be effective in controlling tinnitus.
—I. Sziklai, et al., "Double-blind Study on the Effectiveness of a Bioflavonoid in the Control of Tinnitus in Otosclerosis," *Acta Chir Hung,* 33(1-2), 1992-1993, p. 101-107.

■ L-DOPA

AIDS/HIV

Results of this study showed that the administration of levodopa improved symptoms of extrapyramidal dysfunction, including rigidity, stiffness, ambulation difficulties, shuffling gait, dysarthria, drooling, swallowing dysfunction, hypomimetic, inexpressive faces, and bradykinesia in children between the ages of 4-13 years infected with HIV-1.
—M. Mintz, et al., "Levodopa Therapy Improves Motor Function in HIV-infected Children with Extrapyramidal Syndromes," *Neurology,* 47(6), December 1996, p. 1583-1558.

Amenorrhea-Galactorrhea Syndrome

Results of this study showed that the short term administration of L-Dopa had positive effects on women suffering from amenorrhea-galactorrhea syndrome.
—G.P. Koreneva & F.V. Shikaeva, "Endocrine Effect of L-DOPA in Treating the Amenorrhea-Galactorrhea Syndrome," *Probl Endokrinol,* 26(6), 1980, p. 25-28.

Bone Fracture

Results of this study suggested that the administration of 500 mg of L-Dopa per day leading up to 500 mg three times per day over a period of six months accelerated the rate of healing in patients suffering from long bone fractures.

—J.W. Pritchett , "L-dopa in the Treatment of Nonunited Fractures," *Clin Orthop,* 255, June 1990, p. 293-300.

Cardiovascular/Coronary Heart Disease

This review article notes that clinical and experimental studies have shown a high therapeutic activity of L-DOPA in combination with more conventional therapies in the treatment of myocardial infarction patients.

—V.V. Bul'on, et al., "The Use of L-DOPA for Treating Myocardial Infarct Patients," *Eksp Klin Farmakol,* 56(2), March-April 1993, p. 28-30.

Results of this study found that combining L-Dopa to more conventional therapies had positive effects on heart patients suffering from severe dysfunction of the left ventricle when administered over a period of three months.

—P. Leszek, et al., "A Randomized Crossover Trial of Levodopa in Congestive Heart Failure," *Journal of Cardiac Failure,* 2(3), September 1996, p. 163-176.

Craniocerebral Injury

Results of this study found that the administration of L-Dopa had beneficial effects in patients suffering from craniocerebral trauma.

—M.V. Piasetskaia, et al., "Use of L-DOPA in the Complex Treatment of Severe Craniocerebral Injuries," *Zh Nevropatol Psikhiatr,* 87(5), 1987, p. 660-664.

Depression

This article reports on the case of a female patient suffering from bipolar affective disorder who experienced a reduction in manic-depressive cycle length following a double-blind administration of L-Dopa.

—G.N. Ko, et al., "Induction of Rapid Mood Cycling During L-dopa Treatment in a Bipolar Patient," *American Journal of Psychiatry,* 138(12), December 1981, p. 1624-1625.

General

In this study, 25 patients with pathologic laughing and/or crying were administered either levodopa or amantadine hydrochloride. The treatment produced significant improvements in ten patients.

—F. Udaka, et al., "Pathologic Laughing and Crying Treated with Levodopa," *Arch Neurol,* 41(10), October 1984, p. 1095-1096.

Hepatic Encephalopathy

This article reports on the case of a 30-year-old woman with acute hepatic failure in the fifth month of pregnancy who showed significant improvement in levels of both consciousness and electroencephalogram following L-Dopa therapy.

—T. Chajek, et al., "Treatment of Acute Hepatic Encephalopathy with L-dopa," *Postgraduate Medical Journal,* 53(619), May 1977, p. 262-265.

Human Amblyopia

Results of this study showed that one week of daily Levodopa administration improved visual acuity in 70% of the amblyopia patients examined.

—I. Gottlob, et al., "Visual Acuities and Scotomas After One Week Levodopa Administration in Human Amblyopia," *Invest Ophthalmol Vis Sci,* 33(9), August 1992, p. 2722-2728.

Ischemic Optic Neuropathy

Results of this double-blind, placebo-controlled study showed a significant improvement in visual acuity due to visual loss from nonarteritic anterior ischemic neuropathy among subjects receiving low-dose levodopa and carbidopa over a period of 12 weeks.

—L.N. Johnson, et al., "Effect of Levodopa and Carbidopa on Recovery of Visual Function in Patients with Nonarteritic Anterior Ischemic Optic Neuropathy of Longer than Six Months' Duration," *American Journal of Ophthalmology,* 121(1), January 1996, p. 77-83.

Measles Encephalitis

Results of this placebo-controlled study showed that the administration of L-Dopa significantly improved the death rate of patients suffering from measles encephalitis.

—B. Chandra, "Treatment of Disturbances of Consciousness Caused by Measles Encephalitis with Levodopa," *Eur Neurol,* 17(5), 1978, p. 265-270.

Oligozoospermia

Results of this study showed that L-Dopa administered in doses ranging between 500 mg to 750 mg per day for 2 months exhibited stimulatory effects on spermatogenesis in males suffering from primary sterility.

—J.C. Lavieri & A.A. Pierini, "L-dopa and Oligozoospermia," *Andrologia,* 10(1), January-February 1978, p. 74-79.

Parkinson's Disease

This article reports on the case of a Parkinsonian patient with severe motor fluctuations who experienced immediate improvements in sleep disturbance following continuous, nighttime-only levodopa infusions accompanied by daytime oral carbidopa/levodopa use.

—J.I. Sage & M.H. Mark, "Nighttime Levodopa Infusions to Treat Motor Fluctuations in Advanced Parkinson's Disease: Preliminary Observations," *Ann Neurol,* 30(4), October 1991, p. 616-617.

Results of this double-blind study found that the administration of levodopa alone or coupled with a stable dose of amantadine had a beneficial effects in Parkinson's patients lasting three years or more.

—W.H. Timberlake & M.A. Vance, "Four-year Treatment of Patients with Parkinsonism Using Amantadine Alone or with Levodopa," *Ann Neurol,* 3(2), February 1978, p. 119-28.

Results of this study found that the administration of L-Dopa in low or moderate doses reduced pain and related symptoms in all five Parkinsonian patients studied.

—S. Jaradeh & P.J. Dyck, "Hereditary Motor and Sensory Neuropathy with Treatable Extrapyramidal Features," *Arch Neurol,* 49(2), February 1992, p. 175-178.

This article reports on the cases of early onset Parkinson's disease, each of which benefited following treatment with L-Dopa.

    —K.K. Sachdev, et al., "Juvenile Parkinsonism Treated with Levodopa," *Arch Neurol,* 34(4), April 1977, p. 244-245.

This study examined the effects of L-Dopa on the visual contrast sensitivity of Parkinson's patients. Results showed the treatment improved low-frequency contrast and was capable of restoring them to near normal levels in such patients.

    —J.T. Hutton, et al., "Levodopa Improves Spatial Contrast Sensitivity in Parkinson's Disease," *Arch Neurol,* 50(7), July 1993, p. 721-724.

This article reports on the cases of three Parkinson's patients with polycythemia vera present over a period of years before the onset of symptoms associated with Parkinson's. Treatment with L-Dopa plus a decarboxylase inhibitor (Madopar) led to significant improvement in the polycythemia in all three patients.

    —Y. Herishanu & P. Rosenberg, "Effect of L-dopa on Polycythemia," *Journal of the American Geriatric Society,* 25(5), May 1977, p. 218-219.

Results of this study found L-Dopa to be an effective therapy in the treatment of patients with Parkinson's disease when administered over a period of 4-9 months.

    —B. Gilligan & R. Hancock, "Enteric-coated L-dopa (prodopa). A New Approach to L-dopa Therapy in Parkinson's Disease," *Medical Journal of Aust,* 2(22), November 29, 1975, p. 824-826.

Results of this study showed that the continuous administration of levodopa produced immediate benefits in Parkinson's patients.

    —J.I. Sage & M.H. Mark, "The Rationale for Continuous Dopaminergic Stimulation in Patients with Parkinson's Disease," *Neurology,* 42(1 Suppl 1), p. 23-28.

Results of this study found that low doses of levodopa administered on alternate days proved beneficial in patients with early Parkinson's disease and produced fewer side effects than when taken daily.

    —W.C. Koller, "Alternate Day Levodopa Therapy in Parkinsonism," *Neurology,* 32(3), March 1982, p. 324-326.

In this study, Parkinson's patients were administered daily doses of levodopa beginning at a mean of 662.5 mg five times per week and then changing to a mean of 800 mg three times a week after the first year of treatment. Measures of rigidity, tremor, and bradykinesia all improved with the greatest improvement occurring at 12 weeks.

    —J.A. Aarli & N.E. Gilhus, "Sinemet CR in the Treatment of Patients with Parkinson's Disease Already on Long-term Treatment with Levodopa," *Neurology,* 39(11 Suppl 2), November 1989, p. 82-85.

Results of this study found that the oral administration of levodopa led to improvements in swallowing abnormalities among patients suffering from Parkinson's patients.

    —M. Bushmann, et al., "Swallowing Abnormalities and their Response to Treatment in Parkinson's Disease," *Neurology,* 39(10), October 1989, p. 1309-1314.

Results of this double-blind, placebo-controlled study found that the administration of intravenous levodopa led to reductions in anxiety and elevated mood in patients suffering from Parkinson's disease.

—R.A. Maricle, et al., "Dose-response Relationship of Levodopa with Mood and Anxiety in Fluctuating Parkinson's Disease: A Double-blind, Placebo-controlled Study," *Neurology*, 45(9), September 1995, p. 1757-1760.

This study examined the long-duration response to levodopa in Parkinson's patients by measuring changes in tapping rate during 3-5 days of tapping withdrawal. Results showed that "Off" tapping rates deteriorated 22% during the holiday, suggesting that the long-duration response is a key to levodopa's beneficial effects.

—J.G. Nutt, et al., "Long-duration Response to Levodopa," *Neurology*, 45(8), August 1995, p. 1613-1616.

Results of this study showed clinical improvement with respect to visual evoked potential following 3 months of treatment with L-Dopa therapy in Parkinson's patients.

—P.A. Bhaskar, et al., "Effect of L-dopa on Visual Evoked Potential in Patients with Parkinson's Disease," *Neurology*, 36(8), August 1996, p. 1119-1121.

This review article notes that following its introduction in 1979, L-Dopa remains the premier therapy for patients with Parkinson's disease.

—A.J. Lees, "L-dopa Treatment and Parkinson's Disease," *Q J Med*, 59(230), June 1986, p. 535-547.

Results of this study found that the administration of L-Dopa to Parkinson's patients provided its greatest level of benefit after a treatment period of 3 years. Such effects diminished somewhat after five years, but the drug continued to be effective.

—R. Slome, "Levodopa in Parkinsonism," *South African Medical Journal*, 51(11), March 12, 1977, p. 338-340.

In this article, the authors discuss findings from their clinical experience with respect to the treatment of 127 Parkinson's patients with low-dose L-Dopa over a period of 7 years. Approximately 60-65% of patients studied experienced improvements from the therapy while 35-40% either remained unchanged or got worse.

—L. Battistin, et al., "Long-term Treatment of Parkinson's Disease with L-Dopa and Dopa-decarboxylase Inhibitor: Therapeutic Results and Side Effects," *Acta Neurol Scand*, 57(2), February 1978, p. 186-192.

Results of this study found that the administration of 100 mg of L-Dopa plus decarboxylase inhibitor had blood pressure lowering effects on patients with Parkinson's disease.

—S. Iwasaki, et al., "Hypotensive Effect of Long-term Levodopa in Patients with Parkinson's Disease," *Eur Neurol*, 30(4), 1990, p. 194-199.

Results of this study found that the administration of intravenous L-Dopa significantly improved cerebral blood flow problems in patients with idiopathic Parkinson's disease. No such effects were seen in vascular parkinsonian patients.

—M. Oishi, et al., "Effects of Intravenous L-dopa on P300 and Regional Cerebral Blood Flow in Parkinsonism," *International Journal of Neurosci*, 85(1-2), March 1996, p. 147-154.

Results of this study found that the oral administration of L-Dopa significantly improved color discrimination in Parkinson's patients.

—T. Buttner, et al., "L-Dopa Improves Colour Vision in Parkinson's Disease," *Journal of Neural Transm Park Dis Dement Sect,* 7(1), 1994, p. 13-19.

Peptic Ulcer

Results of this study showed that L-Dopa treatment exhibited beneficial effects in patients suffering from duodenal ulcer.

—N.G. Tretiak, "The Hormone Level of Patients with Peptic Ulcer Being Treated with L-dopa," *Vrach Delo,* (7), July 1989, p. 21-23.

Restless Leg Syndrome

Results of this double-blind, placebo-controlled study showed that the administration of levodopa was effective in the treatment of patients suffering from restless leg syndrome.

—C. von Scheele, "Levodopa in Restless Legs," *Lancet,* 2(8504), August 23, 1986, p. 426-427.

Results of this double-blind, placebo-controlled study found L-Dopa to be effective in the treatment of both restless leg syndrome as well as periodic movement syndrome.

—C. Brodeur, et al., "Treatment of Restless Legs Syndrome and Periodic Movements During Sleep with L-dopa: A Double-blind, Controlled Study," *Neurology,* 38(12), December 1988, p. 1845-1848.

Results of this study showed that the administration of levodopa combined with benserazide was effective in the treatment of patients suffering from restless leg syndrome.

—S. Akpinar, "Restless Legs Syndrome Treatment with Dopaminergic Drugs," *Clin Neuropharmacol,* 10(1), 1987, p. 69-79.

Results of this double-blind, placebo-controlled study found that the administration of 100-200 mg per day of L-Dopa had significantly beneficial effects in patients suffering from Restless Leg Syndrome.

—C. Trenkwalder, et al., "L-dopa Therapy of Uremic and Idiopathic Restless Legs Syndrome: A Double-Blind, Crossover Trial," *Sleep,* 18(8), October 1995, p. 681-688.

Schizophrenia

Results of this double-blind, placebo-controlled study found that the administration of up to 1250 mg per day of L-dopa over a period of 6 weeks produced significant improvements in patients suffering from schizophrenia.

—F.H. Buchanan, et al., "Double Blind Trial of L-dopa in Chronic Schizophrenia," *Aust N Z Journal of Psychiatry,* 9(4), December 1975, p. 269-271.

Segawa's Syndrome

This article reports on the case of an 8-year-old boy suffering from walking difficulties caused by Segawa syndrome related dystonia. Treatment with L-Dopa produced an immediate significant improvement.

—O. Puel, et al., "Fluctuating Muscular Dystonia. Segawa's Syndrome. Value of the Treatment with L-Dopa," *Arch Fr Pediatr,* 47(7), August-September 1990, p. 511-512.

Senile Dementia

Results of this double-blind, placebo-controlled showed that the administration of 250 mg per day of L-Dopa over a period of 6 months proved to be a useful treatment in patients suffering from early stages of presenile dementia.

—K. Jellinger, et al., "Levodopa in the Treatment of (pre) Senile Dementia," *Mech Ageing Dev,* 14(1-2), September-October 1980, p. 253-264.

Sleep Disorders

This article reports on the cases of a woman and her son with progressive dystonia and chronic insomnia. Treatment with low dose L-Dopa had significantly beneficial effects over a period of five years with respect to dystonia and insomnia without dyskinesia.

—M. el Alaoui-Faris, et al., "L-dopa-responsive Dystonia: 2 Familial Cases of Adult Onset with Sleep Disorders," *Rev Neurol,* 151(5), May 1995, p. 347-349.

Results of this study found L-Dopa to be effective in controlling periodic movements in sleep in patients suffering from narcolepsy.

—M.A. Bedard, et al., "Effect of L-dopa on Periodic Movements in Sleep in Narcolepsy," *Eur Neurol,* 27(1), 1987, p. 35-38.

Results of this double-blind, placebo-controlled study found that 2 weeks of L-Dopa treatment improved vigilance levels in patients suffering from narcolepsy.

—D.B. Boivin, et al., "The Effects of L-dopa on Excessive Daytime Sleepiness in Narcolepsy," *Neurology,* 41(8), August 1991, p. 1267-1269.

Tardive Dyskinesia

Results of this placebo-controlled study found that one gram per day of L-Dopa reduced the intensity of involuntary movements in patients suffering from tardive dyskinesia.

—I.G. Karniol, et al., "A Double-blind Study of the Effect of L-dopa in Psychotic Patients with Tardive Dyskinesia," *Acta Psiquiatr Psicol Am Lat,* 29(4), December 1983, p. 261-266.

Torsion Dystonia

This article reports on the case of a 36-year old woman who had been able to move from place to place only by crawling being treated with 2.5 g per day of L-DOPA. Within 4 weeks of treatment she experienced a significant improvement in her daily living activities and was able to walk without assistance for the first time in 20 years.

—W. Winkelmann, "Long-term Treatment with L-DOPA in a Case of Torsion Dystonia," *Journal of Neurol,* 208(4), 1975, p. 319-323.

This article reports on the case of a girl suffering from age of 8 years of torsion dystonia associated with athetosis. At age 12, she was unable to stand up, walk or sit up in a chair without arms. The administration of 3,000 mg per day of levodopa for two months led to a total elimination of such symptoms.

—R. Montanini, et al., "Levodopa Treatment of a Case of Torsion Spasm with Athetosis," *Minerva Med,* 70(21), April 30, 1979, p. 1551-1553.

■ LYCOPENE

Cancer

Results of this study found that lycopene exhibited dose-dependent antiproliferative effects against carcinoma cell lines in-vitro.
—S.K. Clinton, et al., "Cis-trans Isomers of Lycopene in the Human Prostate: A Role in Cancer Prevention?" *FASEB Journal,* 9(3), 1995, p. A442.

Results of this study showed that the administration of lycopene normalized changes of intrathymic T cell differentiation caused by tumorigenesis in mice.
—T. Kobayashi, et al., "Effects of Lycopene, a Carotenoid, on Intrathymic T Cell Differentiation and Peripheral CD4/CD8 Ratio in a High Mammary Tumor Strain of SHN Retired Mice," *Anticancer Drugs,* 7(2), February 1996, p. 195-198.

Results of this study showed that the administration of lycopene exhibited chemopreventive effects in a high mammary tumor strain of mice.
—H. Nagasawa, et al., "Effects of Lycopene on Spontaneous Mammary Tumour Development in SHN Virgin Mice," *Anticancer Research,* 15(4), July-August 1995, p. 1173-1178.

Results of this study showed that lycopene exhibited anticancer effects on lung and endometrial cancer cells in vitro.
—J. Levy, et al., "Lycopene, the Major Tomato Carotenoid, Delays Cell Cycle in Breast, Lung and Endometrial Cancer Cells," *Anticancer Research,* 15(5A), 1995, p. 1655.

Results of this study showed that lycopene inhibited the growth of lung and mammary cancer cells in vitro.
—Y. Sharoni, et al., "The Carotenoid Lycopene, Inhibits Cell Proliferation and Interfere with Growth Factor Stimulation in Cancer Cells," *Anticancer Research,* 15(5A), 1995, p. 1654-1655.

Results of this study found that small doses of lycopene exhibited chemopreventive effects against colon cancer in rats.
—T. Narisawa, et al., "Inhibitory Effects of Natural Carotenoids, Alpha-carotene, Beta-carotene, Lycopene and Lutein, on Colonic Aberrant Crypt Foci Formation in Rats," *Cancer Letters,* 107(1), October 1, 1996, p. 137-142.

Results of this study showed that lycopene inhibited endometrial cancer cell proliferation in vitro.
—J. Levy, et al., "Lycopene is a More Potent Inhibitor of Human Cancer Cell Proliferation than Either Alpha-carotene or Beta-carotene," *Nutr Cancer,* 24(3), 1995, p. 257-266.

Results of this study found that lycopene exhibited inhibitory effects against the growth of small cell lung carcinoma cancer cells in vitro.
—M. Danilenko, et al., "Tomato Carotenoid Lycopene Inhibits Cell Growth and Alters Neuropeptide Signaling in Small Cell Lung Carcinoma Cells," *Proc Annu Meet Am Assoc Cancer Research,* 37, 1996, p. A1800.

Results of this study showed that lycopene had radioprotective effects in mice exposed to a lethal dose of 6.5 Gy and which were stronger than such effects exhibited by beta-carotene.

　　　—A.B. Kapitanov, et al., "Radiation-protective Effectiveness of Lycopene," *Radiats Biol Radioecol,* 34(3), May-June 1994, p. 439-445.

■ MELATONIN

Adrenal Function

This study examined the effects treatment with melatonin for 10 days on the adrenal function of male rats. Results indicated melatonin had an inhibitory action on the effect of ACTH on the adrenal gland.

　　　—K. Yamada, "Effects of Melatonin on Adrenal Function in Male Rats," *Research Commun Chem Pathol Pharmacol,* 69(2), August 1990, p. 241-244.

Aging

This article reviews recent findings concerning the role of melatonin in aging. Evidence is cited indicating melatonin may delay the effects of aging by attenuating negative effects associated with free radical-induced neuronal damage.

　　　—R. Sandyk, "Possible Role of Pineal Melatonin in the Mechanisms of Aging," *International Journal of Neuroscience,* 52(1-2), May 1990, p. 85-92.

Results of this study showed that melatonin attenuated decreases in survival rates, testosterone and brain 125I-melatonin binding sites associated with aging in rats.

　　　—S. Oaknin-Bendahan, et al., "Effects of Long-term Administration of Melatonin and a Putative Antagonist on the Ageing Rat," *Neuroreport,* 6(5), March 27, 1995, p. 785-788.

Antiglucocorticoid Effects

Results of this study indicated that melatonin provided significant protection from the damaging effects of a glucocorticoid in adult rats.

　　　—H. Aoyama, et al., "Anti-glucocorticoid Effects of Melatonin on Adult Rats," *Acta Pathol Jpn,* 37(7), July 1987, p. 1143-1148.

Cancer

In this study, 10 mg per day of oral melatonin was administered to patients with metastatic non-small cell lung cancer at 8:00 pm. Results showed that the melatonin coupled with neuroimmunotherapeutic therapy with IL-2 produced beneficial effects and was well tolerated.

　　　—P. Lissoni, et al., "Biological and Clinical Results of a Neuroimmunotherapy with Interleukin-2 and the Pineal Hormone mMelatonin as a First Line Treatment in Advanced Non-small Cell Lung Cancer," *British Journal of Cancer,* 66(1), July 1992, p. 155-158.

This study examined the effects of 20 mg per day of melatonin in metastatic breast cancer patients coupled with tamoxifen treatment. Results showed that the combine therapies induced objective tumor regressions.

　　　—P. Lissoni, et al., "Modulation of Cancer Endocrine Therapy by Melatonin: A Phase II

Study of Tamoxifen Plus Melatonin in Metastatic Breast Cancer Patients Progressing Under Tamoxifen Alone,'' *British Journal of Cancer,* 71(4), April 1995, p. 854-856.

Results of this study showed that melatonin interrupts prolactin-mediated growth signal in human breast cancer cell growth in vitro.
—A. Lemus-Wilson, et al., ''Melatonin Blocks the Stimulatory Effects of Prolactin on Human Breast Cancer Cell Growth in Culture,'' *British Journal of Cancer,* 72(6), December 1995, p. 1435-1440.

Results of this study showed that low dose IL-2 coupled with 50 mg of melatonin per day beginning seven days prior to IL-2 therapy proved to be an effective treatment for advanced digestive tract tumors.
—P. Lissoni, et al., ''Immunotherapy with Subcutaneous Low-dose Interleukin-2 and the Pineal Indole Melatonin as a New Effective Therapy in Advanced Cancers of the Digestive Tract,'' *British Journal of Cancer,* 67(6), June 1993, p. 1404-1407.

In this study, 22 renal cell carcinoma patients were monitored for the effect of a 12 month regimen of 3 mega units of intramuscular human lymphoblastoid interferon 3 times weekly and 10 mg per day of oral melatonin. Results showed 7 remissions and 9 disease stabelizations.
—B. Neri, et al., ''Modulation of Human Lymphoblastoid Interferon Activity by Melatonin in Metastatic Renal Cell Carcinoma: A Phase II Study,'' *Cancer,* 73(12), June 15, 1994, p. 3015-3019.

Results of this study showed that melatonin can improve quality of life and survival time in brain metastases patients.
—P. Lissoni, et al., ''A Randomized Study with the Pineal Hormone Melatonin Versus Supportive Care Alone in Patients with Brain Metastases Due to Solid Neoplasms,'' *Cancer,* 73(3), February 1, 1994, p. 699-701.

Results of this study showed that melatonin inhibited the development of DMBA-induced mammary tumors in rats.
—L. Tamarkin, et al., ''Melatonin Inhibition and Inhibition and Pinealectomy Enhancement of 7,12-Dimethylbenz(a)Anthracene-Induced Mammary Tumors in the Rat,'' *Cancer Research,* 41(11,part1), 1981, p. 4432-4436.

Results of this study showed that melatonin produced a direct, reversible antiproliferative effect on MCF-7 cell growth in vitro.
—S.M. Hill & D.E. Blask, ''Effects of the Pineal Hormone Melatonin on the Proliferation and Morphological Characteristics of Human Breast Cancer Cells (MCF-7) in Culture,'' *Cancer Research,* 48(21), November 1, 1988, p. 6121-6126.

Results of this study showed that melatonin significantly inhibited B16 mouse melanoma growth and led to reductions in adrenal and gonadal weights.
—T. Narita & H. Kudo, ''Effect of Melatonin on B16 Melanoma Growth in Athymic Mice,'' *Cancer Research,* 45(9), September 1985, p. 4175-4177.

This study examined the effects of melatonin on the proliferation and induction of melanogenesis in rodent melanoma cells. Results showed low concentrations of melatonin inhibited cell growth, but had not melanogenesis. High melatonin doses had the exact opposite effect.

—A. Slominski & D. Pruski, "Melatonin Inhibits Proliferation and Melanogenesis in Rodent Melanoma Cells," *Exp Cell Res,* 206(2), June 1993, p. 189-194.

Results of this study found the melatonin injections inhibited growth and increased doubling time of the R3327H Dunning prostatic adenocarcinoma in rats.

—R. Philo & A.S. Berkowitz, "Inhibition of Dunning Tumor Growth by Melatonin," *Journal of Urology,* 139(5), May 1988, p. 1099-1102.

Results of this study showed that 2 mM of melatonin inhibited the growth of ME-180 human cervical cancer cells in vitro after 48 hours of treatment.

—L.D. Chen, et al., "Melatonin's Inhibitory Effect on Growth of ME-180 Human Cervical Cancer Cells is Not Related to Intracellular Glutathione Concentrations," *Cancer Letters,* 91(2), May 8, 1995, p. 153-159.

Results of this study found melatonin antogonoized tumor-promoting actions of estradiol in a rat model of mammary tumorignesis.

—D.E. Blask, et al., "Pineal Melatonin Inhibition of Tumor Promotion in the N-nitroso-N-methylurea Model of Mammary Carcinogenesis: Potential Involvement of Antiestrogenic Mechanisms in Vivo," *Journal of Cancer Res Clin Oncol,* 117(6), 1991, p. 526-532.

Results of this study showed that melatonin modulated mammary epithelium development, thus decreasing the incidence of spontaneous mammary tumor incidence in mice.

—A. Subramanian & L. Kothari, "Melatonin, A Suppressor of Spontaneous Murine Mammary Tumors," *Journal of Pineal Research,* 10(3), April 1991, p. 136-140.

This study examined the effects of 20 mg per day of intramuscular melatonin in cancer patients with metastatic sold tumor. Treatment was followed up with 10 oral mg per day in patients experiencing remission. Results indicated that melatonin had beneficial effects in such patients with respect to PS and quality of life.

—P. Lissoni, et al., "Endocrine and Immune Effects of Melatonin Therapy in Metastatic Cancer Patients," *European Journal of Cancer Clin Oncol,* 25(5), May 1989, p. 789-795.

Results of this study indicated that 20 mg per day of oral melatonin may be a factor involved in the treatment of chemotherapy-induced myelodysplatic syndrome in cancer patients.

—S. Viviani, et al., "Preliminary Studies on Melatonin in the Treatment of Myelodysplastic Syndromes Following Cancer Chemotherapy," *Journal of Pineal Research,* 8(4), 1990, p. 347-354.

Results of this study found melatonin to have antitumor effects on MtT/F4 tumors in rats.

—S. Chatterjee & T.K. Banerji, "Effects of Melatonin on the Growth of MtT/F4 Anterior Pituitary Tumor: Evidence for Inhibition of Tumor Growth Dependent Upon the Time of Administration," *Journal of Pineal Research,* 7(4), 1989, p. 381-391.

This review article examined the effects of melatonin by itself or coupled with interleukin-2 in cancer patients in studies published between 1986-1994. The authors conclude that melatonin offers protection against interleukin-2 and the two agents synergize in their anticancer effects.

—A. Conti & G.J. Maestroni, "The Clinical Neuroimmunotherapeutic Role of Melatonin in Oncology," *Journal of Pineal Research,* 19(3), October 1995, p. 103-110.

In this study, 40 advanced melanoma patients were treated with daily doses of oral melatonin ranging from 5mg/m2 to 700 mg/m2. Results showed partial responses in 6 patients and stable disease in 6 others after 5 weeks of follow-up.

—R. Gonzalez, et al., "Melatonin Therapy of Advanced Human Malignant Melanoma," *Melanoma Research,* 1(4), November-December 1991, p. 237-243.

In this study, human peripheral blood cells were treated increasing concentrations of melatonin (0.5 or 1.0 or 2.0 mM) for 20 min at 37 +/- 1 degrees C and then exposed to 150 cGy gamma-radiation from a 137Cs source. Results showed that lymphocytes pre-treated with melatonin exhibited a significant reduction the frequency of radiation-induced chromosome damage relative to controls.

—Vijayalaxmi, et al., "Melatonin Protects Human Blood Lymphocytes from Radiation-induced Chromosome Damage," *Mutat Research,* 346(1), January 1995, p. 23-31.

This study examined the effects of 20 mg per day of intramuscular melatonin in cancer patients with metastatic solid tumor. Treatment was followed up with 10 oral mg per day in patients experiencing remission. Results indicated that melatonin had beneficial effects in such patients with respect to performance status and quality of life.

—P. Lissoni, et al., "Clinical Results with the Pineal Hormone Melatonin in Advanced Cancer Resistant to Standard Antitumor Therapies," *Oncology,* 48(6), 1991, p. 448-450.

Results of this study indicated that glutathione and glutathione transferase play a direct role in the mechanisms mediating the resistance of estrogen receptor humans breast cancer cells to melatonin.

—D.E. Blask & S.T. Wilson, "Melatonin Suppression of Human Breast Cancer Growth in Vitro Involves Glutathione," *Proceedings of the Annual Meeting of the American Association of Cancer Researchers,* 36, 1995, p. A1514.

Cardiovascular/Coronary Heart Disease

Results of this study showed that the administration of melatonin modulated the functional status of voltage sensitive calcium channels in the heart of rats.

—L.D. Chen, et al., "Melatonin Reduces 3H-nitrendipine Binding in the Heart," *Proceedings of the Society of Exp Biol Medicine,* 207(1), October 1994, p. 34-37.

This study examined the effects of 4 mg injections of melatonin per day over a period of 10-27 days in rats fed regular and high-cholesterol diets. Results showed that the melatonin countered the effects of high-cholesterol diet on plasma lipids and lipoproteins. Melatonin reduced fatty infiltration in the liver of rats on a high-cholesterol diet as well.

—N. Mori, et al., "Anti-hypercholesterolemic Effect of Melatonin in Rats," *Acta Pathol Jpn,* 39(10), October 1989, p. 613-618.

Results of this study showed that melatonin infused i.p. at a dose of 6 mg/rat per day for 5 days exhibited a antihypertensive in spontaneously hypertensive rats.

> —K. Kawashima, et al., "Antihypertensive Action of Melatonin in the Spontaneously Hypertensive Rat," *Clinical Exp Hypertens,* 9(7), 1987, p. 1121-1131.

Results of this study showed that melatonin produced a dose-dependent relaxation of precontracted of the isolated rat aorta and that such actions may be due in part to an interaction with perivascular nerve terminals.

> —L.B. Weekley, "Pharmacologic Studies on the Mechanism of Melatonin-induced Vasorelaxation in Rat Aorta," *Journal of Pineal Research,* 19(3), October 1995, p. 133-138.

Results of this study showed that the administration of melatonin produced a dose-dependent relaxation of precontracted pulmonary vein and artery.

> —L. B. Weekley, "Effects of Melatonin on Isolated Pulmonary Artery and Vein: Role of the Vascular Endothelium," *Pulm Pharmacol,* 6(2), June 1993, p. 149-154.

Colitis

Results of this study showed that the daily administration of intraperitoneal melatonin to mice reduced the severity of dextran sodium-induced colitis.

> —P.T. Pentney & G.A. "Melatonin Reduces the Severity of Dextran-induced Colitis in Mice," *Journal of Pineal Research,* 19(1), August 1995, p. 31-39.

Diabetes

Results of this study showed that melatonin supplementation decreased glucose tolerance in rabbits and most likely influenced blood glucose circadian rhythm via its impact on insulin release by pancreatic B cells.

> —M. Dhar, et al., "Effect of Melatonin on Glucose Tolerance and Blood Glucose Circadian Rhythm in Rabbits," *Indian Journal of Physiol Pharmacol,* 27(2), April-June 1983, p. 109-117.

Encephalitis

This study examined the melatonin's effects on viral encephalitis in mice. Results showed that the daily administration of melatonin beginning 3 days prior and lasting through 10 after exposure to the virus significantly delayed disease onset and death.

> —D. Ben-Nathan, et al., "Protective Effects of Melatonin in Mice Infected with Encephalitis Viruses," *Arch Virol,* 140(2), 1995, p. 223-230.

Epilepsy

Results of this study showed that subcutaneous melatonin had an ameliorative effect on pinealectomy-induce seizures in gerbils.

> —P.K. Rudeen, et al., "Antiepileptic Effects of Melatonin in the Pinealectomized Mongolian Gerbil," *Epilepsia,* 21(2), April 1980, p. 149-154.

Gastric Lesions

Results of this study showed that prior melatonin administration produced a significant reduction in gastric ulceration in rats.

—R. Khan, et al., "The Effect of Melatonin on the Formation of Gastric Stress Lesions in Rats," *Experientia,* 46(1), January 15, 1990, p. 88-89.

Results of this study found that supplemental melatonin protected gastric mucosa from ischemia/reperfusion—induced damage in rats.

—P.C. Konturek, et al., "Melatonin Affords Protection against Gastric Lesions Induced by Ischemia-Reperfusion Possibly Due to its Antioxidant and Mucosal Microcirculatory Effects," *European Journal of Pharmacology,* 322, 1997, p. 73-77.

General

This study looked at the effects of daily melatonin administration on rats with disrupted circadian activity and drinking rhythms under constant light. Results showed that the treatment did either synchronize or at least partly synchronize disrupted circadian patterns.

—M.J. Chesworth, et al., "Effects of Daily Melatonin Injections on Activity Rhythms of Rats in Constant Light," *American Journal of Physiol,* 253(1 Pt 2), July 1987, p. R101-107.

In this study, rats received 10 mg/kg kainate i.p. which produced brain injury of the hippocampus, the amygdala, and the pyriform cortex. 2.5 mg/kg of melatonin was injected into the rats 20 minutes prior to kainate, right after, and 1-2 hours after. Results showed that the cumulative dose of 10 mg/kg of melatonin prevented kainate-induced behavioral and biochemical disturbances and neuronal death.

—P. Giusti, et al., "Neuroprotection by Melatonin from Kainate-induced Excitotoxicity in Rats," *FASEB Journal,* 10(8), June 1996, p. 891-896.

This study examined the effects of melatonin on porphyrins-induced cell damage in the Harderian gland of Syrian hamsters. Results found that melatonin produced cytoprotectives effect by inhibiting the ALA-S gene expression and by raising the mRNA levels for several antioxidant enzymes.

—I. Antolin, et al., "Neurohormone Melatonin Prevents Cell Damage: Effect on Gene Expression for Antioxidant Enzymes," *FASEB Journal,* 10(8), June 1996, p. 882-890.

This study compared the peroxyl radical scavenger ability of melatonin to that of vitamin E, vitamin C and reduced glutathione. Results showed melatonin to be twice as active as vitamin E which is thought to be the most powerful lipophilic antioxidant.

—C. Pieri, et al., "Melatonin: A Peroxyl Radical Scavenger More Effective than Vitamin E," *Life Sci,* 55(15), 1994, p. PL271-PL276.

Results of this study showed that the administration of melatonin provided protection against H_2O_2-induced lipid peroxidation of brain homogenates in vitro.

—E. Sewerynek, et al., "H_2O_2-induced Lipid Peroxidation in Rat Brain Homogenates is Greatly Reduced by Melatonin," *Neurosci Lett,* 195(3), August 11, 1995, p. 203-205.

In this study, mice received intraperitoneally melatonin in doses ranging from 100 to 450 mg/kg. Results showed that such treated proved plasma glucose increase due to alloxan-induced pancreatic toxicity.

—G. Pierrefiche, et al., "Antioxidant Activity of Melatonin in Mice," *Res Commun Chem Pathol Pharmacol,* 80(2), May 1993, p. 211-223.

Immune Enhancement

Results of this study found that exogenous melatonin totally counteracted the effects of acute anxiety-restraint stress on thymus weight and antibody response to sheep red blood cells.

—G.J. Maestroni, et al., "Role of the Pineal Gland in Immunity III. Melatonin Antagonizes the Immunosuppressive Effect of Acute Stress via an Opiatergic Mechanism," *Immunology,* 63(3), March 1988, p. 465-469.

Results of this study showed that melatonin restored the depressed immune function following soft-tissue trauma and hemorrhagic shock in mice.

—M.W. Wichmann, et al., "Melatonin Administration Attenuates Depressed Immune Functions Trauma-Hemorrhage," *Journal of Surgical Research,* 63(1), June 1996, p. 256-262.

Results of this study showed that the chronic injection of melatonin into either young mice or those suffering from aging-induced immunodepression or immunodepression due to treatment with cyclophosphmide enhanced antibody response to a T-dependent antigen.

—M.C. Caroleo, et al., "Melatonin Restores Immunodepression in Aged and Cyclophosphamide-treated Mice," *Annals of the New York Academy of Science,* 719, May 31, 1994, p. 343-352.

Results of this study showed that the chronic injection of melatonin into young or immunodepressed mice can be an effective therapy for immunodepressive conditions.

—M.C. Caroleo, et al., "Melatonin as Immunomodulator in Immunodeficient Mice," *Immunopharmacology,* 23(2), March-April 1992, p. 81-89.

Jet Lag

Results of this double-blind, placebo-controlled study found that 5 mg of melatonin three days prior to flight, during flight, and once a day for three days after flight alleviated jet lag and fatigue in healthy volunteers.

—K. Petrie, et al., "Effect of Melatonin on Jet Lag after Long Haul Flights," *BMJ,* 298(6675), March 18, 1989, p. 705-707.

Results of this double-blind, placebo-controlled study found that 5 mg of melatonin three days prior to flight, during flight, and once a day for three days after flight alleviated jet lag and fatigue in healthy volunteers.

—K. Petrie, et al., "A Double-blind Trial of Melatonin as a Treatment for Jet Lag in International Cabin Crew," *Biological Psychiatry,* 33(7), April 1, 1993, p. 526-530.

Reproductive Function

Results of this study showed that male and female hamsters treated with melatonin experienced a prevention in reproductive organ atrophy associated with the reduced day length of winter.

—R.J. Reiter, et al., "Prevention by Melatonin of Short Day Induced Atrophy of the Reproductive Systems of Male and Female Hamsters," *Acta Endocrinol,* 84(2), February 1977, p. 410-418.

Results of this study showed that melatonin exerted a suppressive effect on baboon dispersed luteal cell P production.

—F.S. Khan-Dawood & M.Y. Dawood, "Baboon Corpus Luteum: The Effect of Melatonin on In Vitro Progesterone Production," *Fertil Steril,* 59(4), April 1993, p. 896-900.

Results of this study showed that melatonin administered in high doses inhibited mammary development in mice.

—E.J. Sanchez-Barcelo, et al., "Influence of Melatonin on Mammary Gland Growth: In Vivo and In Vitro Studies," *Proc Soc Exp Biol Med,* 194(2), June 1990, p. 103-107.

Shock

Results of this study showed that a single melatonin injection protected mice treated from lethal doses of lipolysaccharide, suggesting its usefulness as a potential therapy for septic shock.

—G.J. Maestroni, "Melatonin as a Therapeutic Agent in Experimental Endotoxic Shock," *Journal of Pineal Research,* 20(2), March 1996, p. 84-89.

This study examined the anticonvulsant effects of melatonin in male gerbils. Results showed that daily injection of 25 mg of melatonin for 10 weeks reduced both the incidence and severity of seizures associated with exposure to pentylenetetrazol.

—T.H. Champney & J.A. Champney, "Novel Anticonvulsant Action of Chronic Melatonin in Gerbils," *Neuroreport,* 3(12), December 1992, p. 1152-1154.

Sleep

This article reports on the case of a severely mentally retarded 9-year-old boy with chronic sleep/wake disturbance. Melatonin given at 6:00 pm normalized the sleep/wake pattern and entrained the endogenous rhythm to a normalized 24-hour chronological day.

—L. Palm, et al., "Correction of Non-24-hour Sleep/wake Cycle by Melatonin in a Blind Retarded Boy," *Ann Neurol,* 29(3), March 1991, p. 336-339.

In this double-blind, placebo-controlled study, healthy volunteers received either 0.3 or 1.0 mg of melatonin at 6, 8, or 9 PM. Results showed that either doses given at either time reduced sleep onset latency.

—I.V. Zhdanova, et al., "Sleep-inducing Effects of Low Doses of Melatonin Ingested in the Evening," *Clin Pharmacol Therapy,* 57(5), 1995, p. 552-558.

This double-blind, placebo-controlled study examined the effects of 5 mg of melatonin for four weeks on the sleep/wake cycle in 8 patients with a delayed sleep phase syndrome. Results showed significantly earlier sleep onset time and wake time relative to controls.

> —M. Dahlitz, et al., "Delayed Sleep Phase Syndrome Response to Melatonin," *Lancet,* 337(8750), May 11, 1991, p. 1121-1124.

Results of this double-blind, placebo-controlled study showed that 2 mg per night of controlled-release melatonin for 3 weeks significantly improved sleep quality in elderly subjects.

> —D. Garfinkel, et al., "Improvement of Sleep Quality in Elderly People by Controlled-release Melatonin," *Lancet,* 346(8974), August 26, 1995, p. 541-544.

This article reports on the case of a child with a germ cell tumor involving the pineal region experiencing a melatonin secretion suppression associated with severe insomnia. Supplementation with 3 mg per night for 2 weeks normalized sleep.

> —A. Etzioni, et al., "Melatonin Replacement Corrects Sleep Disturbances in a Child with Pineal Tumor," *Neurology,* 46(1), January 1996, p. 261-263.

This double-blind, placebo-controlled study examined the effects of 75 mg per os of melatonin administered nightly at 10 PM on total sleep time and daytime alertness of chronic insomniacs. Results showed a significant increase in the subjective assessment of total sleep time and daytime alertness relative to controls.

> —J.G. MacFarlane, et al., "The Effects of Exogenous Melatonin on the Total Sleep Time and Daytime Alertness of Chronic Insomniacs: A Preliminary Study," *Biological Psychiatry,* 30(4), August 15, 1991, p. 371-376.

Results of this double-blind, placebo-controlled study showed that 5 mg per night of melatonin had positive effects with respect to sleep and alertness on police officers working successive night shifts.

> —S. Folkard, et al., "Can Melatonin Improve Shift Workers' Tolerance of the Night Shift? Some Preliminary Findings," *Chronobiol Int,* 10(5), October 1993, p. 315-320.

In this study, 15 disabled children with severe, chronic sleep disorders received 2 to 10 mg of oral melatonin. Results showed significant positive effects.

> —J.E. Jan, et al., "The Treatment of Sleep Disorders with Melatonin," *Dev Med Child Neurol,* 36(2), February 1994, p. 97-107.

In this double-blind, placebo-controlled study, 20 healthy volunteers underwent artificially-induced insomnia and were treated with melatonin. Results showed that the administration of melatonin at bedtime reduced the time the subjects were awake before sleep onset, sleep latency, and the number of awakenings during the total sleep period, while it the efficiency of sleep.

> —F. Waldhauser, et al., "Sleep Laboratory Investigations on Hypnotic Properties of Melatonin," *Psychopharmacology,* 100(2), 1990, p. 222-226.

This double-blind, placebo-controlled study examined the hypnotic effects of 5 mg of melatonin in healthy, young adults. Results showed that melatonin significantly increased sleep propensity, the spectral power in the theta, delta and spindles bands, and subjective sleepiness while significantly reducing the power in the alpha and beta bands and oral temperature.

—O. Tzischinsky & P. Lavie, "Melatonin Possesses Time-dependent Hypnotic Effects," *Sleep,* 17(7), October 1994, p. 638-645.

This double-blind, placebo-controlled study examined the effects of melatonin replacement therapy on melatonin-deficient elderly insomniacs. Subject received 2 mg tablets of melatonin for 7 consecutive days 2 hours prior to going to bed. During another phase of the study, subjects received 1 mg of sustained-release melatonin each night at bedtime for 2 months. Results showed that 1-week treatment with 2 mg sustained-release melatonin was effective for sleep maintenance, while sleep initiation was improved by the fast-release melatonin. Such effects were increased following the 2-month 1-mg sustained-release melatonin treatment.

—I, Haimov, et al., "Melatonin Replacement Therapy of Elderly Insomniacs," *Sleep,* 18(7), September 1995, p. 598-603.

Uterine Contraction

Results of this study showed that melatonin administration inhibited carbochol-provoked uterine contraction in rats.

—A.G. Rillo, et al., [Uterine Contraction Induced by Carbachol is Inhibited by Melatonin], *Ginecol Obstet Mex,* 61, February 1993, p. 40-44.

Vision

This study examined the effects of 4 mg/kg per day of melatonin on the formation of cataracts in newborn rats. Results showed that the treatment led to a reduction in cataract formation.

—M. Abe, et al., "Inhibitory Effect of Melatonin on Cataract Formation in Newborn Rats: Evidence for an Antioxidative Role for Melatonin," *Journal of Pineal Research,* 17(2), September 1994, p. 94-100.

Results of this study showed that the administration of melatonin reduced intraocular pressure in human subjects with few side effects.

—J.R. Samples, et al., "Effect of Melatonin on Intraocular Pressure," *Current Eye Research,* 7(7), July 1988, p. 649-653.

■ NAC

Adult Respiratory Distress Syndrome

In this double-blind, placebo-controlled study, 16 patients in the beginning phase of adult respiratory disorder syndrome received NAC. Results showed the treatment, started within eight hours of diagnosis, increased the intracellular GSH in the granulocytes without decreasing spontaneous oxidant production.

—T. Laurent, et al., "Oxidant-antioxidant Balance in Granulocytes During ARDS. Effect of N-cetylcysteine," *Chest,* 109(1), January 1996, p. 163-166.

Results of this study found that NAC administered to sheep significantly attenuated all monitored pathophysiological changes in the endotoxin model of ARDS.

—G.R. Bernard, et al., "Effect of N-acetylcysteine on the Pulmonary Response to Endotoxin in the Awake Sheep and Upon in Vitro Granulocyte Function," *Journal of Clinical Investigation,* 73(6), June 1984, p. 1772-1784.

Results of this series of clinical trials found that ARDS patients experienced relief in common symptoms such as depressed plasma and red cell glutathione concentrations following treatment with intravenous NAC. NAC treatment also showed measurable effects with respect to increase oxygen delivery, improved lung compliance and resolution of pulmonary oedema.

—G.R. Bernard, "Potential of N-acetylcysteine as Treatment for the Adult Respiratory Distress Syndrome," *European Respiratory Journal Supplement,* 11, October 1990, p. 496s-498s.

Results of this study showed that NAC produced significant preventive effects in a microembolism rat model of ARDS.

—T. Wegener, et al., "Effect of N-acetylcysteine on Pulmonary Damage Due to Microembolism in the Rat," *European Journal of Respiratory Disease,* 70(4), April 1987, p. 205-212.

Results of this study showed that the administration of NAC in vivo significantly ameliorated ARDS-like lung injury in rats.

—C.O. Feddersen, et al., [N-acetylcysteine Decreases Functional and Structural, ARDS-typical Lung Changes in Endotoxin-treated Rats], *Med Klin,* 88(4), April 15, 1993, p. 197-206.

AIDS/HIV

Results of this study showed that the oral administration of N-acetylcysteine increased cysteine and glutathione concentrations in mononuclear cells of HIV patients.

—B. de Quay, et al., "Glutathione Depletion in HIV-infected Patients: Role of Cysteine Deficiency and Effect of Oral N-acetylcysteine," *AIDS,* 6(8), August 1992, p. 815-819.

Results of this study indicated that the administration of NAC enhanced the number of CD4+ T cells in patients infected with HIV due to its ability to increase glutathione levels.

—R. Kinscherf, et al., "Effect of Glutathione Depletion and Oral N-acetyl-cysteine Treatment on CD4+ and CD8+ Cells," *FASEB Journal,* 8(6), April 1, 1994, p. 448-451.

This case-control study examined the effects of NAC and glutathione on neutrophil and mononuclear cell cytotoxicity in HIV-infected patients. Results showed that 1 and 5 mM NAC partially reversed BCNU-induced intracellular glutathione depletion and antibody-dependent cellular cytotoxity of neutrophils in both controls and HIV patients.

—R.L. Roberts, et al., "N-acetylcysteine Enhances Antibody-dependent Cellular Cytotoxicity in Neutrophils and Mononuclear Cells from Healthy Adults and Human Immunodeficiency Virus-infected Patients," *Journal of Infectious Disease,* 172(6), December 1995, p. 1492-1502.

This study examined the effects of NAC and GSH on the replication of HIV-1 primary monocyte/macrophages cultured in vitro. Results showed that both GSH and 5-20 mM of NAC significantly reduced HIV infection.

—W.Z. Ho & S.D. Douglas, "Glutathione and N-acetylcysteine Suppression of Human

Immunodeficiency Virus Replication in Human Monocyte/macrophages in Vitro,'' *AIDS Research Hum Retroviruses,* 8(7), July 1992, p. 1249-1253.

This review article cites studies indicating that NAC can block the expression of HIV in infection models as well as replication in normal peripheral blood mononuclear cells.
> —M. Roederer, et al., ''N-acetylcysteine: A New Approach to Anti-HIV Therapy,'' *AIDS Research and Human Retroviruses,* 8(2), February 1992, p. 209-217.

Results of this found NAC to be a more powerful antiviral agent than oxothiazolide with respect to HIV.
> —P.A. Raju, et al., ''Glutathione Precursor and Antioxidant Activities of N-acetylcysteine and Oxothiazolidine Carboxylate Compared in Vitro Studies of HIV Replication,'' *AIDS Research and Human Retroviruses,* 10(8), August 1994, p. 961-967.

This article reports on findings from a Stanford University double-blind, placebo-controlled study of 200 volunteers who were HIV positive. Results showed the administration of NAC increased glutathione levels and, in turn, may have enhanced survival rates.
> —J.S. James, ''NAC: First Controlled Trial, Positive Results,'' *AIDS Treat News,* 250, July 5, 1996, p. 1-3.

This study examined the safety of NAC on patients infected with HIV over a 14 week period. Patients with under 500 CD4 cells/mm3 received either 6 weeks of NAC doses of 3.7, 11, 33 and 100 mg/kg IV tiw or 6 weeks of oral doses of 600, 1200, 2400 and 4800 mg qd. Results showed no major side effects and found NAC to be safe at the doses noted above.
> —R.E. Walker, et al., ''The Safety, Pharmacokinetics, and Antiviral Activity of N-acetylcysteine in HIV-Infected Individuals,'' *International Conference on AIDS,* 8(1), July 19-24, 1992, Mo8.

Results of this study found that NAC enhanced T cell function and growth dramatically in culture.
> —E. Ylar, et al., ''N-acetylcysteine Enhances T Cell Functions and T Cell Growth in Culture,'' *Int Immunol,* 5(1), January 1993, p. 97-101.

This review article notes that N-acetylcysteine has been shown to inhibit inflammatory stimulations such as HIV replication and replinishes glutathione depletion in vivo.
> —M. Roederer, et al., ''N-acetylcysteine: Potential for AIDS Therapy,'' *Pharmacology,* 46(3), 1993, p. 121-129.

Results of this study found that NAC inhibited the tumor necrosis factor alpha- or phorbol ester-stimulated replication of HIV in acutely infected cell cultures, while it also inhibits the cytokine-enhanced HIV long terminal repeat-directed expression of beta-galactosidase in vitro HIV model systems.
> —M. Roederer, et al., ''Cytokine-stimulated Human Immunodeficiency Virus Replication is Inhibited by N-acetyl-L-cysteine,'' *Proceedings of the National Academy of Sciences,* 87(12), June 1990, p. 4884-4888.

Brain Function

Results of this study indicated that treatment with NAC had beneficial effects on oxygen free radical-mediated brain injury in cats.

> —E.F. Ellis, et al., "Restoration of Cerebrovascular Responsiveness to Hyperventilation by the Oxygen Radical Scavenger N-acetylcysteine Following Experimental Traumatic Brain Injury," *Journal of Neurosurg,* 75(5), November 1991, p. 774-749.

Cancer

Results of this study showed that NAC and ascorbic acid each demonstrated protective effects against mutagen-induced chomosomal damage in vitro.

> —Z. Trizna, et al., "Effects of N-acetyl-L-cysteine and Ascorbic Acid on Mutagen-induced Chromosomal Sensitivity in Patients with Head and Neck Cancers," *American Journal of Surgery,* 162(4), October 1991, p. 294-298.

Results of this study showed that NAC administration significantly reduced mtDNA adducts in the liver and lung of rats exposed to cigarette smoke and in the liver of those treated with 2-acetylaminofluorene.

> —R. Balansky, et al., "Induction by Carcinogens and Chemoprevention by N-acetylcysteine of Adducts to Mitochondrial DNA in Rat Organs," *Cancer Research,* 56(7), April 1, 1996, p. 1642-1647.

This review article discusses NAC's role as an antidote to acetaminophen poisoning as well as its chemopreventive properties.

> —N. van Zandwijk, "N-acetylcysteine for Lung Cancer Prevention," *Chest,* 107(5), May 1995, p. 1437-1441.

Results of this study showed that NAC served as an effective adjunct to increase the antitumor activity of IL-2/LAK therapy in mice.

> —C.Y. Yim, et al., "Use of N-acetyl Cysteine to Increase Intracellular Glutathione During the Induction of Antitumor Responses by IL-2," *Journal of Immunology,* 152(12), June 15, 1994, p. 5796-805.

Results of this study found NAC capable of protecting against mutagenic potential of environmental clastogens/mutagens in vitro.

> —R. Barale, et al., "N-Acetylcysteine Inhibits Environmental Pollutant Gentotoxicity in Vitro," *Third International Conference on Mechanisms of Antimutagenesis and Anticarcinogenesis.* May 5-10, 1991, Lucca, Italy, 1991, 12, 1991.

This review article cites studies over the past decade showing NAC inhibits spontaneous mutagenicity and chemical-induced mutagenicity resulting from various sources. NAC has also been shown to significantly reduce the incidence of neoplastic and preneoplastic lesions induced by various chemical carcinogens in rodents.

> —S. De Flora, et al., "N-acetyl-Cysteine for Cancer Chemoprevention: The Experimental Background," *CCPC-93: Second International Cancer Chemo Prevention Conference. April 28-30, 1993, Berlin, Germany,* 1993, 32, 1993.

Results of this study showed that the administration of NAC produced significant protective effects against the cigarette smoke-induced alterations of bronchoalveolar lavage cellularity as well as the increased of miconucleated pulmonary alveolar macrophages, and bone marrow cytotoxicity in rats.

> —R.B. Balansky, et al., "Protection by N-acetylcysteine of the Histopathological and Cytogenetical Damage Produced by Exposure of Rats to Cigarette Smoke," *Cancer Letters,* 64(2), June 15, 1992, p. 123-131.

Results of this study found that NAC had protective effects against DMH carcinogenic activity—reducing intestinal tumor activity in rats, significantly decreasing colic tumor yield colic, and inducing a shift from distal to more proximal sites with respect to location of colon carcinomas.

> —M. Wilpart, et al., "Anti-initiation Activity of N-acetylcysteine in Experimental Colonic Carcinogenesis," *Cancer Letters,* 31(3), June 1986, p. 319-324.

Results of this study showed that NAC protected mice against lipopolysaccharide toxicity as well as inhibited the increase in serum tumor necrosis factor levels in mice treated with lipopolysaccarhides. Results also found NAC inhibited tumor necrosis factor production and hepatotoxicity in lipopolysaccarhides-treated mice in association with a sensitizing dose of Actinomycin D.

> —P. Peristeris, et al., "N-acetylcysteine and Glutathione as Inhibitors of Tumor Necrosis Factor Production," *Cell Immunology,* 140(2), April 1992, p. 390-399.

Results of this study showed that NAC administration had beneficial effects on tumor cell invasion and metastasis of malignant cells in vitro.

> —A. Albini, et al., "Inhibition of Invasion, Gelatinase Activity, Tumor Take and Metastasis of Malignant Cells by N-acetylcysteine," *International Journal of Cancer,* 61(1), March 29, 1995, p. 121-129.

Results of this study indicated that the administration of PZ-51 by itself or coupled with NAC moderated Adriamycin's aerobic toxicity in vitro while having no effect on its hypoxic toxicity.

> —C.A. Pritsos, "Protective Effect of N-acetylcysteine (NAC) and PZ-51 (EBSELEN) Against Adriamycin Toxicity," *Proceedings of the Annual Meeting of the American Association of Cancer Researchers,* 31, 1990, p. A2406.

Results of this study showed that the administration of NAC significantly inhibited chemical-induced lung tumors in mice.

> —S. De Flora, et al., "Metabolic, Desmutagenic and Anticarcinogenic Effects of N-acetylcysteine," *Respiration,* 50(Suppl 1), 1986, p. 43-49.

This study examined the protective effects of NAC on skin reaction in patients receiving radiation therapy. Results showed that those patients receiving NAC required no analgesics for pain, recovered quicker and had less severe reactions relative to controls.

> —J.A. Kim, et al., "Topical Use of N-Acetylcysteine for Reduction of Skin Reaction to Radiation Therapy," *Semin Oncol,* 10(1,Suppl1), 1983, p. 86-88.

Results of this study found NAC capable of inhibiting cyclophosphamide-induced hemorrhagic cystitis without compromising antitumor or immunosuppressive activity in rats and mice.

> —L. Levy & D.L. Vredevoe, "The Effect of N-acetylcysteine on Cyclophosphamide Immunoregulation and Antitumor Activity," *Semin Oncology,* 10(1,Suppl1), 1983, p. 7-16.

Cardiovascular/Coronary Heart Disease

Results of this study found NAC elevated bovine pulmonary artery endothelial cell glutathione following in vitro incubation, prompting the authors to suggest it may be an effective agent for elevating glutathione of the pulmonary vasculature as a means of providing against oxidant stress.

> —D.T. Phelps, et al., "Elevation of Glutathione Levels in Bovine Pulmonary Artery Endothelial Cells by N-acetylcysteine," *American Journal of Respiratory Cell Mol Biol*, 7(3), September 1992, p. 293-299.

Results of this double-blind, placebo-controlled study found that the administration of 150 mg/kg-1 of NAC significantly increased cardiac output and reduced systemic vascular resistance in patients requiring hemodynamic monitoring due to sepsis syndrome.

> —K. Reinhart, et al., "N-acetylcysteine Preserves Oxygen Consumption and Gastric Mucosal pH During Hyperoxic Ventilation," *American Journal of Respiratory Critical Care Medicine*, 151(3 Pt 1), March 1995, p. 773-779.

Results of this study showed that reduced thiol NAC potentiated platelet inhibition by endothelium-derived relaxing factor in bovine aortic endothelial cells.

> —J. Stamler, et al., "N-acetylcysteine Potentiates Platelet Inhibition by Endothelium-derived Relaxing Factor," *Circulatory Research*, 65(3), September 1989, p. 789-795.

Results of this study found that the intravenous administration of 2 g of NAC over 15 minutes followed by 5 mg/kg/hr coupled with intravenous isosorbide denitrate led to partial prevention of antianginal effect tolerance often associated with isosorbide treatment alone in anginal patients.

> —S. Boesgaard, et al., "Preventive Administration of Intravenous N-acetylcysteine and Development of Tolerance to Isosorbide Dinitrate in Patients with Angina Pectoris," *Circulation*, 85(1), January 1992, p. 143-149.

Results of this study showed that the intravenous administration of 100 mg/kg of NAC potentiated nitroglycerin-induced vasodilater effects in patients undergoing cardiac catheterization for chest pain investigation. No such effects were seen among controls.

> —J.D. Horowitz, et al., "Potentiation of the Cardiovascular Effects of Nitroglycerin by N-acetylcysteine," *Circulation*, 68(6), December 1993, p. 1247-1253.

Results of this study found that the administration of NAC prior to reperfusion decreased myocardial stunning following reperfusion in rats.

> —M.B. Forman, et al., "Glutathione Redox Pathway and Reperfusion Injury. Effect of N-acetylcysteine on Infarct Size and Ventricular Function," *Circulation*, 78(1), July 1988, p. 202-213.

In this study, acute myocardial infarction patients were treated with either 15 g of intravenous NAC over a 24 hour period coupled with intravenous nitroglycerin. Results showed the treatment to be a safe and was associated with significant reductions in levels of oxidative controls relative to controls. Results also showed a trend toward improved preservation of the left ventricular function as well more rapid reperfusion.

> —M.A. Arstall, et al., "N-acetylcysteine in Combination with Nitroglycerin and Streptokinase

for the Treatment of Evolving Acute Myocardial Infarction. Safety and Biochemical Effects,'' *Circulation,* 92(10), November 15, 1995, p. 2855-2862.

This double-blind, placebo-controlled study examined the effects of 0.1 microgram/kg per min intravenous nitroglycerin alone and coupled with 2 g of intravenous N-acetylcysteine followed by 5 mg/kg per hour on human veins, peripheral arteries, and microcirculation. Results showed the two agents together potentiated and preserved nitroglycerin-induced venodilation and augmented nitroglycerin's effects on small resistance vessels without influencing the response to nitroglycerin in middle-sized arteries.

> —S. Boesgaard, et al., ''Altered Peripheral Vasodilator Profile of Nitroglycerin During Long-term Infusion of N-acetylcysteine,'' *Journal of the American College of Cardiol,* 23(1), January 1994, p. 163-169.

Results of this study showed that NAC potentiated platelet aggregation inhibition by nitroglycerin in vivo.

> —J. Loscalzo, ''N-Acetylcysteine Potentiates Inhibition of Platelet Aggregation by Nitroglycerin,'' *Journal of Clinical Investigations,* 76(2), August 1985, p. 703-708.

Results of this study found NAC added to cardioplegic solution led to improvements in postarrest recovery of function, increasing the capacity of reperfused myocardium to handle the postischemic burst of free radical production in a rat heart model.

> —P. Menasche, et al., ''Maintenance of the Myocardial Thiol Pool by N-acetylcysteine. An Effective Means of Improving Cardioplegic Protection,'' *Journal of Thoracic Cardiovascular Surgery,* 103(5), May 1992, p. 936-944.

This double-blind, placebo-controlled study examined the effects of pretreatment of cardiac risk patients with the 150 mg/kg NAC on VO2 and other clinical indicators of tissue oxygenation. Results showed that the NAC worked to preserve VO2, oxygen delivery, CI, LVSWI and PvaCO2 during brief hyperoxia and prevented clinical signs of myocardial ischemia.

> —C. Spies, et al., [The Effect of Prophylactically Administered N-acetylcysteine on Clinical Indicators for Tissue Oxygenation During Hyperoxic Ventilation in Cardiac Risk Patients], *Anaesthesist,* 45(4), April 1996, p. 343-350.

This study examined the effects of NAC on percutaneous transluminal angioplasty associated injury in rabbits. Results showed the treatment to be effective in the prevention of vessel damage caused by vessel damage.

> —H. Mass, et al., ''N-acetylcysteine Diminishes Injury Induced by Balloon Angioplasty of the Carotid Artery in Rabbits,'' *Biochem Biophys Res Commun,* 215(2), October 13, 1995, p. 613-618.

This study examined the effects of NAC on vulnerability of heart arrhythmias and mechanical function during reperfusion and ischemia in rats. Results found that the incidences of ischemia-induced ventricular premature beats and ventricular tachycardia decreased from 93% and 67%, among controls to 40% and 27% with 8 microM of NAC, to 33% and 27% with 80 microM NAC, and to 40% and 13% with 2000 microM NAC. Incidence of ventricular fibrillation induced by reperfusion decreased from 93%

to 60%, 67% and 47%, respectively. NAC delayed onset time of arrhthymias during ischemia and reperfusion.

—Y. Qiu, et al., "The Influence of N-acetylcysteine on Cardiac Function and Rhythm Disorders During Ischemia and Reperfusion," *Cardioscience,* 1(1), March 1990, p. 65-74.

Results of this double-blind, placebo-controlled study found that the combination of intravenous NAC (5g 6 hourly) and nitroglycerine and unstable angina pectoris patients augmentes nitroglycerine's clinical benefits primarily by decreased acute myocardial infarction incidence.

—J.D. Horowitz, et al., "Nitroglycerine/N-acetylcysteine in the Management of Unstable Angina Pectoris," *European Heart Journal,* 9 (Suppl A), January 1988, p. 95-100.

This study examined the effects of intravenous glutathione and NAC on the cardiotoxicity of doxorubicinkly in both in vitro and in vivo models. Results showed that both agents prevented doxorubicinkly-induced negative inotropic effects on isolated rat atria.

—F.Villani, et al., "Effect of Glutathione and N-acetylcysteine on in Vitro and in Vivo Cardiac Toxicity of Doxorubicin.," *Free Radic Res Commun,* p. 11(1-3), 1990, p. 145-151.

This study examined the cardioprotective effects of NAC in canines. Results found NAC limited the extent of infarction and significantly decreased incidence of reperfusion ventricular arrhythmias.

—J. Sochman, et al., "Cardioprotective Effects of N-acetylcysteine: The Reduction in the Extent of Infarction and Occurrence of Reperfusion Arrhythmias in the Dog," *International Journal of Cardiology,* 28(2), August 1990, p. 191-196.

Results of this study showed that large doses of NAC increased exercise capacity in isosorbide-5-mononitrate-treated angina pectoris patients.

—J.H. Svendsen, et al., "N-acetylcysteine Modifies the Acute Effects of Isosorbide-5-mononitrate in Angina Pectoris Patients Evaluated by Exercise Testing," *Journal of Cardiovascular Pharmacol,* 13(2), February 1989, p. 320-323.

Results of this study indicated that in vivo NAC potentiation of nitroglycerine responses may have clinically beneficially effects on preventing or reversing the loss of hemodynamic responsiveness to nitroglycerine.

—J. Torresi, et al., "Prevention and Reversal of Tolerance to Nitroglycerine with N-acetylcysteine," *Journal of Cardiovascular Pharmacology,* 7(4), July-August 1985, p. 777-783.

This double-blind, placebo-controlled study examined the effects of a bolus of 100 mg/kg of NAC followed by a continuos infusion of 20mg/kg in the bypass circuit on oxidative response of neutrophils during cardiopulmonary bypass in adult patients. Results showed significantly lower levels of oxidative burst response of neutrophils among those receiving the NAC than controls throughout the bypass.

—L.W. Andersen, et al., "The Role of N-acetylcystein Administration on the Oxidative Response of Neutrophils During Cardiopulmonary Bypass," *Perfusion,* 10(1), 1995, p. 21-26.

Chronic Bronchitis

This double-blind, placebo-controlled study examined the clinical effects of 300 mg b.i.d of NAC on patients suffering from chronic bronchitis. Results showed a significant decrease in number or sick days taken at work following four months of NAC treatment compared to controls.

—J.B. Rasmussen & C. Glennow, "Reduction in Days of Illness after Long-term Treatment with N-acetylcysteine Controlled-release Tablets in Patients with Chronic Bronchitis," *European Respir Journal,* 1(4), April 1988, p. 351-355.

Results of this study showed that the oral administration of NAC inhibited cigarette smoke-induced mucosa cell hyperplasia and epithelial hypertrophy in rats.

—D.F. Rogers & P.K. Jeffery, "Inhibition by Oral N-acetylcysteine of Cigarette Smoke-induced 'Bronchitis' in the Rat," *Exp Lung Research,* 10(3), 1986, p. 267-283.

Results of this study found that daily treatment with 600 mg/kg of NAC of patients with chronic and acute bronchitis was effective and generally free of adverse effects.

—H.H. Gerards & U. Vits, [Therapy of Bronchitis. Successful Single-dosage Treatment with N-acetylcysteine, Results of an Administration Surveillance Study in 3,076 Patients], *Fortschr Medicine,* 109(34), November 30, 1991, p. 707-710.

In this study, atopic children with allergic rhinitis, asthma and maxillary sinusitis received 50-80 mg/kg per day of cefuroxime and 15-25 mg/kg per day of NAC over a 10 day period. Results indicated the treatment to be effective in 95.8% of the patients with 37.5% subsequently able to reduce their treatment for asthma.

—A.L. Boner, et al., "A Combination of Cefuroxime and N-acetyl-cysteine for the Treatment of Maxillary Sinusitis in Children with Respiratory Allergy," *International Journal of Clinical Pharmacol Ther Toxicol,* 22(9), September 1984, p. 511-514.

In this study, 103 children suffering from lower respiratory tract infections received a combination of cefuroxime and NAC. One hundred of the 103 experienced positive results from the treatment. In 58, a total relief of symptoms was reported, while a marked improvement was seen in 42.

—G. Santangelo, et al., "A Combination of Cefuroxime and N-acetyl-cysteine for the Treatment of Lower Respiratory Tract Infections in Children," *International Journal of Clinical Pharmacol Ther Toxicol,* 23(5), May 1985, p. 279-281.

COPD

Results of this study showed that treatment with 10 micrograms/ml of NAC enhanced the antifungal activity of peripheral blood monocyte cells from COPD patients significantly in vitro.

—A. Vecchiarelli, et al., "Macrophage Activation by N-acetyl-cysteine in COPD Patients," *Chest,* 105(3), March 1994, p. 806-811.

Cutaneous Inflammation

Results of this study showed NAC to be an effective treatment of cutaneous inflammation mediated by tumor necrosis factor alpha in mice.

—G. Senaldi, et al., "Protective Effect of N-acetylcysteine in Hapten-induced Irritant and

Contact Hypersensitivity Reactions," *Journal Invest Dermatol,* 102(6), June 1994, p. 934-937.

Diabetes

Results of this study showed that the administration of NAC inhibited reductions in diaphragm contractility in STZ-treated rats without reductions in blood glucose levels.

    —W. Hida, et al., "N-acetylcysteine Inhibits Loss of Diaphragm Function in Streptozotocin-treated Rats," *American Journal of Respiratory Critical Care Medicine,* 153(6 Pt 1), June 1996, p. 1875-1879.

Results of this study found that the administration of NAC suppressed the enhanced tumor necrosis factor production in diabetic rats significantly, suggesting NAC may be an effective means for prevention of tumor necrosis factor mediated pathological conditions associated with the disease.

    —M Sagara, et al., "Inhibition with N-acetylcysteine of Enhanced Production of Tumor Necrosis Factor in Streptozotocin-induced Diabetic Rats," *Clin Immunol Immunopathol,* 71(3), June 1994, p. 333-337.

Results of this study found that the administration of NAC to streptozotocin-induced diabetic rats inhibited the development of functional and structural abnormalities of the peripheral nerve.

    —M. Sagara, et al., "Inhibition of Development of Peripheral Neuropathy in Streptozotocin-induced Diabetic Rats with N-acetylcysteine," *Diabetologia,* 39(3), March 1996, p. 263-269.

Diaphragmatic Function

Results of this study found that NAC exhibited direct temperature-dependent effects on diaphragm function in vitro, consistent with its known antioxidant properties.

    —P.T. Diaz, et al., "Effects of N-acetylcysteine on in Vitro Diaphragm Function are Temperature Dependent," *Journal of Applied Physiology,* 77(5), November 1994, p. 2434-2449.

This study examined the possibility of augmenting diaphragmatic stores of reduced glutathione, thus delay the development of respiratory failure during loaded breathing, via NAC administration. Results showed that the NAC blunted loading-induced decreases in diaphragmatic glutathione levels and led to a decrease in the in vitro fatigability of excised diaphragm muscle strips.

    —G.S. Supinski, et al., "N-acetylcysteine Administration and Loaded Breathing," *Journal of Applied Physiology,* 79(1), July 1995, p. 340-347.

Ear Problems

Results of this study found that NAC decreases inflammation of the middle-ear mucosa and prevented the long-term fibrotic changes in patients suffering from secretory otitis media.

    —T. Ovesen, et al., "Local Application of N-acetylcysteine in Secretory Otitis Media in Rabbits," *Clinical Otolaryngol,* 17(4), August 1992, p. 327-331.

Gallstones

Results of this study showed that NAC accelerated the dissolution of gallstone in vitro significantly.

    —Niu & B.F. Smith, "Addition of N-acetylcysteine to Aqueous Model Bile Systems Accelerates Dissolution of Cholesterol Gallstones,'' *Gastroenterology,* 98(2), February 1990, p. 454-463.

General

Results of this study showed that NAC significantly prevented the immediate effects of both short-term or long-term exposure to ozone on the mucocilary functions of sheep.

—L. Allegra, et al., ''Ozone-induced Impairment of Mucociliary Transport and its Prevention with N-Acetylcysteine,'' *American Journal of Medicine,* 91(3C), September 30, 1991, p. 67S-71S.

This study examined the effects of a 48-hour IV N-acetylcysteine treatment protocol for acute overdose of acetaminophen, consisting of 12 70 mg/kg doses every four hours and a loading dose of 140 mg/kg. Results found the protocol to be effective and equal to oral treatment over a 72-hour period.

—M.J. Smilkstein, et al., ''Acetaminophen Overdose: A 48-hour Intravenous N-acetylcysteine Treatment Protocol,'' *Annals of Emergency Medicine,* 20(10), October 1991, p. 1058-1063.

This study examined the effects of NAC on caustic akaline injury to the esophagus in rats. Results showed that NAC as well as steroids ameliorated tissue reaction to chemical injury and tempered the degree of stenosis formation.

—A.J. Liu & M.A. Richardson, ''Effects of N-acetylcysteine on Experimentally Induced Esophageal Lye Injury,'' *Ann Otol Rhinol Laryngol,* 94(5 Pt 1), September-October 1985, p. 477-482.

This article reports on a single case of acute methylmercury poisoning in which NAC was found to be an effective enhancer of kidney elimination of the toxin.

—M.E. Lund, et al., ''Treatment of Acute Methylmercury Ingestion by Hemodialysis with N-acetylcysteine (Mucomyst) Infusion and 2,3-dimercaptopropane Sulfonate,'' *Journal of Toxicol Clin Toxicol,* 22(1), July 1984, p. 31-49.

This study examined the effects of a 400 mg oral dose of NAC on human blood neutrophil and monocyte function in healthy volunteers. Results showed a significant decrease in neutrophil chemiluminescene response after activation by opsonized zymosan relative to controls.

—T. Jensen, et al., ''Effect of Oral N-acetylcysteine Administration on Human Blood Neutrophil and Monocyte Function,'' *APMIS,* 96(1), January 1988, p. 62-67.

This review article reports on the efficacy of NAC in treating cases of paracetamol intoxication when administered within eight hours of intoxication.

—J. De Groote & W. Van Steenbergen, ''Paracetamol Intoxication and N-acetyl-cysteine Treatment,'' *Acta Gastroenterol Belg,* 58(3-4), May-August 1995, p. 326-334.

Results of this study showed that the administration of N-acetylcysteine before cyclophosphamide prevented hemorrhagic cystitis and lethality resulting from the drug in rats while not diminishing its immunosuppressive or antiproliferative activities.

—L. Levy & R. Harris, ''Effect of N-Acetylcysteine on Some Aspects of Cyclophophsphamide—Induced Toxicity and Immunosuppression,'' *Biochem Pharmacol,* 26(11), 1977, p. 1015-1020.

Results of this single case study indicated that the intravenous administration of N-acetylcysteine can be effective against sulphalazine-induced side effects such as hepatitis, rash, and disseminated intravascular coagulation.

> —C. Gabay, et al., ''Sulphasalazine-related life-threatening Side Effects: is N-acetylcysteine of Therapeutic Value?'' *Clinical Exp Rheumatology,* 11(4), July-August 1993, p. 417-420.

Results of this double-blind, placebo-controlled study found that oral administration of N-acetylcysteine at 0.6 g per day increased mucociliary clearance rates by approximately 35% in healthy human subjects.

> —T. Todisco, et al., ''Effect of N-acetylcysteine in Subjects with Slow Pulmonary Mucociliary Clearance,'' *European Journal of Respir Diseases Suppl,* 139, 1985, p. 136-141.

This study examined the effects of NAC on methyl-mercuric chloride-induced embryotoxicity in mice. Results showed that a single dose of NAC antagonized the embryolethal effects of poisoning by MMC. Palatoschisis incidence was reduced relative to the number of NAC administration. NAC administration improved body weight in fetuses from mothers poisoned with MMC back to normal ranges as well.

> —F. Ornaghi, et al., ''The Protective Effects of N-acetyl-L-cysteine Against Methyl Mercury Embryotoxicity in Mice,'' *Fundam Appl Toxicol,* 20(4), May 1993, p. 437-445.

Results of this study showed that the intravenous administration of N-acetylcysteine led to significant reductions in plasma glutathione S-transferase B1 concentrations in patients suffering from severe paracetamol poisoning.

> —G.J. Beckett, et al., ''Intravenous N-acetylcysteine, Hepatotoxicity and Plasma Glutathione S-Transferase in Patients with Paracetamol Overdosage,'' *Hum Exp Toxicol,* 9(3), May 1990, p. 183-186.

Results of this study showed that the administration of N-acetylcysteine 30 minutes prior to UV irradiation significantly inhibited UVB-induced immunosuppression in mice.

> —L.T. van den Broeke, et al., ''Topically Applied N-acetylcysteine as a Protector Against UVB-induced Systemic Immunosuppression,'' *J Photochem Photobiol B,* 27(1), January 1995, p. 61-65.

Results of this study found that NAC administration protected rats from the effects UVB radiation on epidermal DNA.

> —L.T., van den Broeke, et al., ''The Effect of N-acetylcysteine on the UVB-induced Inhibition of Epidermal DNA Synthesis in Rat Skin,'' *J Photochem Photobiol B,* 26(3), December 1994, p. 271-276.

This review article notes recent findings indicating the ability of early administration of NAC to induce glutathione rescue and recovery, glutathione being an essential protector of biological structure and function.

> —R. Ruffmann & A. Wendel, ''GSH Rescue by N-acetylcysteine,'' *Klin Wochenschr,* 69(18), November 15, 1991, p. 857-862.

Results of this study found that hyperbaric oxygen therapy induces lipid peroxidation and that the simultaneous administration of NAC provides protection against such effects.

> —P. Pelaia, et al., [Assessment of Lipid Peroxidation in Hyperbaric Oxygen Therapy: Protective Role of N-acetylcysteine], *Minerva Anestesiol,* 61(4), April 6, 1995, p. 133-139.

Results of this study showed that the administration of 1000 and 2000 mg kg-1 of NAC 1 hour prior to illumination in patients treated with photodynamic therapy worked to helped ameliorate photosensitivty.

> —P. Baas, et al., ''Partial Protection of Photodynamic-induced Skin Reactions in Mice by N-acetylcysteine: A Preclinical Study,'' *Photochem Photobiol,* 59(4), April 1994, p. 448-454.

This article reports on the cases of two patients with paracetamol overdose who were treated successfully with oral NAC.

> —J. Brahm, et al., [Paracetamol Overdose: A New Form of Suicide in Chile and the Value of N-acetylcysteine Administration], *Rev Med Chil,* 120(4), April 1992, p. 427-499.

Results of this study showed NAC to be effective in the reversal of oligura associated with chromate and borate intoxication in rats, suggesting it to be a good potential chelation agent.

> —W. Banner, Jr., et al., ''Experimental Chelation Therapy in Chromium, Lead, and Boron Intoxication with N-acetylcysteine and Other Compounds,'' *Toxicol Appl Pharmacol,* 83(1), March 30, 1986, p. 142-147.

Results of this study showed that NAC had protected paraquat-intoxicated rats against oxidative lung damage through the delay of inflammation.

> —E. Hoffer, et al., ''N-acetylcysteine Delays the Infiltration of Inflammatory Cells into the Lungs of Paraquat-intoxicated Rats,'' *Toxicol Appl Pharmacol,* 120(1), May 1993, p. 8-12.

Results of this study showed that the administration of NAC to alveolar type II cells incubated with 1 mM paraquat reduced cytoxicity by enhancing glutathione content.

> —E. Hoffer, et al., ''N-acetylcysteine Increases the Glutathione Content and Protects Rat Alveolar Type II Cells Against Paraquat-induced Cytotoxicity,'' *Toxicol Lett,* 84(1), January 1996, p. 7-12.

Results of this study showed that the administration of NAC either 30 minutes before or 6 to 10 hours following carbon tetrachloride administration significantly prevented liver necrosis induced by the hepatotoxin..

> —E.G. Valles, et al., ''N-acetyl Cysteine is an Early but Also a Late Preventive Agent Against Carbon Tetrachloride-induced Liver Necrosis,'' *Toxicol Lett,* 71(1), March 1994, p. 87-95.

Results of this study showed that NAC protected Chinese hamster ovary cells from lead-induced oxidative stress.

> —N. Ercal, et al., ''N-actylcysteine Protects Chinese Hamster Ovary (CHO) Cells from Lead-Induced Oxidative Stress,'' *Toxicology,* 108(1-2), April 15, 1996, p. 57-64.

Glutathione Deficiency

This article reports on the case of a 45-month-old girl with 5-oxoprolinuria (pyroglutamic aciduria), hemolysis, and majorglutathione depletion due to deficiency of glutathione synthetase. Results showed that treatment with 6mmol/kg of NAC and 0.7 mmol/kg ascorbate per day for 1-2 weeks decreased turnover in patients suffering from heriditary glutathione deficiency by increasing the plasma levels of glutathione.

> —A. Jan, et al., "Effect of Ascorbate or N-acetylcysteine Treatment in a Patient with Hereditary Glutathione Synthetase Deficiency," *Journal of Pediatrics,* 124(2), February 1994, p. 229-233.

Results of this study showed that the administration of 15 mg/kg per day of NAC was beneficial in increasing low intracellular concentrations and cysteine availability in patients suffering from a hereditary deficiency in glutathione deficiency.

> —J. Martensson, et al., "A Therapeutic Trial with N-acetylcysteine in Subjects with Hereditary Glutathione Synthetase Deficiency (5-oxoprolinuria)," *Journal of Inherit Metab Dis,* 12(2), 1989, p. 120-130.

Hepatitis

This article reports on the case of a 54-year-old man who developed severe cholestatic jaundice and pure red cell aplasia following treatment with gold sodium thiomalate. The man experienced a complete hematologic recovery following treatment with prednisone and NAC infusions.

> —R.M. Hansen, et al., "Gold Induced Hepatitis and Pure Red Cell Aplasia. Complete Recovery after Corticosteroid and N-acetylcysteine Therapy," *Journal of Rheumatology,* 18(8), August 1991, p. 1251-1253.

Liver Damage

Results of this double-blind, placebo-controlled study found that the administration of NAC to chronic liver disease patients with hepatic failure improved oxygen deliver and consumption, induced mild vasodilation, and reduced base deficit.

> —P.N. Bromley, et al., "Effects of Intraoperative N-acetylcysteine in Orthotopic Liver Transplantation," *British Journal of Anaesth,* 75(3), September 1995, p. 352-354.

Results of this study showed that the injection of 150 mg/kg of NAC into rats increased L-cysteine concentrations within 15 minutes of exposure.

> —H. Nakano, et al., "Protective Effects of N-acetylcysteine on Hypothermic Ischemia-reperfusion Injury of Rat Liver," *Hepatology,* 22(2), August 1995, p. 539-545.

This article reports on the cases of 11 patients at risk of hepatic damage following paracetamol poisoning who received intravenous treatment with NAC. Results showed complete protection against liver failure in all cases with no reported side effects.

> —T.E. Oh & G.M. Shenfield, "Intravenous N-acetylcysteine for Paracetamol Poisoning," *Medical Journal of Australia,* 1(13), June 28, 1980, p. 664-665.

Results of this study showed NAC to be an effective agent for combating alcohol-induced acetaminophen toxicity in mice.

> —E.A. Carter, "Enhanced Acetaminophen Toxicity Associated with Prior Alcohol Consumption in Mice: Prevention by N-acetylcysteine," *Alcohol,* 4(1), January-February 1987, p. 69-71.

Results of this study demonstrated the ability of NAC to rescue mitochondrial glutathione and restore essential mitochondrial functions in rats, pointing to NAC's potential as an effective antidote to oxidative stress-related diseases.

> —J. Traber, et al., "In Vivo Modulation of Total and Mitochondrial Glutathione in Rat Liver. Depletion by Phorone and Rescue by N-acetylcysteine," *Biochem Pharmacol,* 43(5), March 3, 192, p. 9961-9964.

Results of this study indicated NAC coupled with cysteamine can be useful in preventing hepatic necrosis in mice following exposure to acetaminophen at toxic doses.

> —T.C. Peterson and I.R. Brown, "Cysteamine in Combination with N-acetylcysteine Prevents Acetaminophen-induced Hepatotoxicity," *Can J Physiol Pharmacol,* 70(1), January 1992, p. 20-28.

Results of this study showed that the pretreatment of pigs with NAC assists in the maintenance of hepatic glutathione during warm ischemia. NAC proved effective in the replenishment of depleted glutathione stores and was associated with improvements in glutathione homeostasis and bile output.

> —K. Fukuzawa, et al., "N-acetylcysteine Ameliorates Reperfusion Injury after Warm Hepatic Ischemia," *Transplantation,* 59(1), January 15, 1995, p. 6-9.

Results of this study showed that the administration of high doses of NAC to rats undergoing orthotopic liver transport attenuated symptoms associated with microvascular perfusion failure early following reperfusion.

> —T.A. Koeppel, et al., "Impact of N-acetylcysteine on the Hepatic Microcirculation after Orthotopic Liver Transplantation," *Transplantation,* 61(9), May 15, 1996, p. 1397-1402.

Lung Damage

Results of this study showed that the administration of NAC prevents endotoxemia-induced release of granulocyte activating substances from the lung lymph of sheep.

> —W.D. Lucht, et al., "Prevention of Release of Granulocyte Aggregants into Sheep Lung Lymph Following Endotoxemia by N-acetylcysteine," *American Journal of Medical Science,* 294(3), September 1987, p. 161-167.

Results of this study showed that NAC was effective in reducing lung leak, neutrophil influx into lung lavages, and defects in lung history brought on by intratracheal IL-1 administration in rats.

> —J.A. Leff, et al., "Postinsult Treatment with N-acetyl-L-cysteine Decreases IL-1-induced Neutrophil Influx and Lung Leak in Rats," *American Journal of Physiol,* 265(5 Pt 1), November 1993, p. L501-L506.

In this study, intravenous NAC was administered to eight pulmonary fibrosis patients and six controls. Results showed significant increases in bronchoalveolar lavage fluid total glutathione in patients within 3 hours of 1.8 g of NAC administration. No such effects were seen in controls.

> —A. Meyer, et al., "Intravenous N-acetylcysteine and Lung Glutathione of Patients with Pulmonary Fibrosis and Normals," *American Journal of Respiratory Critical Care Medicine,* 152(3), September 1995, p. 1055-1060.

Results of this double-blind, placebo-controlled study found that intravenous administration of 40 mg/kg per day over a period of 72 hours led to improvements in systemic oxygenation and decreases in the requirements for ventilatory support in acute lung injury patients.

> —P.M. Suter, et al., "N-acetylcysteine Enhances Recovery from Acute Lung Injury in Man. A Randomized, Double-blind, Placebo-controlled Clinical Study," *Chest,* 105(1), January 1994, p. 190-194.

This study examined the effects of the stereoisomers of NAC on oxygen-induced lung oedema in rats. Results showed NAC, regardless of stereoconfiguration, protected lungs from oxygen toxicity.

> —B. Sarnstrand, et al., "Effects of N-acetylcysteine Stereoisomers on Oxygen-induced Lung Injury in Rats," *Chem Biol Interact,* 94(2), February 1995, p. 157-164.

This study examined the effects of NAC on acute lung injury in sheep induced by endotoxins. Results indicated the treatment attenuated responses to endotoxemia, and significant reductions of the rise in pulmonary artery pressure.

> —Y. Zhu, [Experimental Study of the Protective Effects of N-acetylcysteine on Endotoxin-induced Acute Lung Injury], *Chung Hua I Hsueh Tsa Chih,* 71(7), July 1991, p. 373-7, 26.

Results of this study showed that NAC offers protection against PMN mediated oxidant injury in lung cells.

> —L.M. Simon & N. Suttorp, "Lung Cell Oxidant Injury: Decrease in Oxidant Mediated Cytotoxicity by N-acetylcysteine," *European Journal of Respiratory Disease Suppl,* 139, 1985, p. 132-135.

This study examined the effects of NAC on tobacco smoke toxicity in vitro. Results showed that concentrations of 1mM of NAC protected cells from toxicity and from glutathione loss.

> —P. Moldeus, et al., "N-acetylcysteine Protection Against the Toxicity of Cigarette Smoke and Cigarette Smoke Condensates in Various Tissues and Cells in Vitro," *European Journal of Respiratory Disease Suppl,* 139, 1985, p. 123-129.

Results of this study showed that the administration of NAC at doses of 400 mg/kg body weight per day to mice produced significant reductions bleomcyin-induced collagen deposition in the lungs.

> —S. Shahzeidi, et al., "Oral N-acetylcysteine Reduces Bleomycin-induced Collagen Deposition in the Lungs of Mice," *European Respiratory Journal,* 4(7), July 1991, p. 845-352.

This study examined the effects of intravenous NAC on O2 toxicity in canine lungs. Results showed the treatment protects against the effects of 100% O2 when measured by both functional and structural criteria.

> —P.D. Wagner, et al., "Protection Against Pulmonary O2 Toxicity by N-acetylcysteine," *European Respiratory Journal,* 2(2), February 1989, p. 116-126.

Results of this study indicated that the administration of 200 mg t.i.d. of NAC over an 8 week period to smokers had beneficial effects on the activity of inflammatory cells in the bronchoalveolar space.
—A. Eklund, et al., "Oral N-acetylcysteine Reduces Selected Humoral Markers of Inflammatory Cell Activity in BAL Fluid from Healthy Smokers: Correlation to Effects on Cellular Variables," *European Respir Journal,* 1(9), October 1988, p. 832-838.

Results of this study found that the administration of 200 mg t.i.d. of NAC over an 8 week period improves the function of alveolar macrophages in healthy smokers.
—M. Linden, et al., "Effects of Oral N-acetylcysteine on Cell Content and Macrophage Function in Bronchoalveolar Lavage from Healthy Smokers," *European Respiratory Journal,* 1(7), July 1988, p. 645-650.

This study examined the effects of oral NAC on oxidant lung injury in rats using a model of acute immunological alveolitis. Results showed a single dose an hour before antigen/antibody treatment prevented pulmonary endothelial cell uptake loss induced by immune complex deposition.
—R. Sala, et al., "Protection by N-acetylcysteine Against Pulmonary Endothelial Cell Damage Induced by Oxidant Injury," *European Respiratory Journal,* 6(3), March 1993, p. 440-446.

Results of this study showed that intratracheal NAC inhibited bleomycin lung toxicity in rats.
—N. Berend, "Inhibition of Bleomycin Lung Toxicity by N-acetyl Cysteine in the Rat," *Pathology,* 17(1), January 1985, p. 108-110.

This review article notes that NAC has been shown to protect human bronchial fibroblasts against tobacco smoke condensates' toxic effects and tobacco smokes' glutathione depleting effects. Studies have also shown NAC can decrease the reactive oxygen intermediate hydrogen peroxide and protect against its toxic effects.
—P. Moldeus, et al., "Lung Protection by a Thiol-containing Antioxidant: N-acetylcysteine," *Respiration,* 50 Suppl 1, 1986, p. 31-42.

This study examined the effects of NAC on the formation of pulmonary edema in isolated perfused rabbits lungs after in vivo phosgene exposure. Results showed that NAC protected against phosgene-induced lung injury by acting as an antioxidant by maintaining protective levels of glutathione, and by decreasing lipid peroxidation as well as the production of arachidonic acid metabolites.
—A.M. Sciuto, et al., "Protective Effects of N-acetylcysteine Treatment after Phosgene Exposure in Rabbits," *American Journal of Respiratory Crit Care Medicine,* 151(3 Pt 1), March 1995, p. 768-772.

Results of this study showed that NAC provided protection to mouse lungs exposed to the adverse effects bleomycin and to hyperbaric oxygen therapy.
—D.D. Jamieson, et al., "Interaction of N-acetylcysteine and Bleomycin on Hyperbaric Oxygen-Induced Lung Damage in Mice," *Lung,* 165(4), 1987, p. 239-247.

Muscle Fatigue

Results of this study showed that pretreatment with 150 mg/kg of NAC improved human limb muscle performance during fatiguing exercise. Such findings, the authors argue, suggest oxidative stress may be an important factor in the fatigue process.

> —M.B. Reid, et al., ''N-acetylcysteine Inhibits Muscle Fatigue in Humans,'' *Journal of Clinical Investigations,* 94(6), December 1994, p. 2468-2474.

Sjogren's Syndrome

In this double-blind, placebo-controlled study, patients suffering from primary or secondary Sjogren's syndrome received oral NAC for four weeks. Results indicated NAC had a true therapeutic effect on the ocular symptoms of such patients relative to controls.

> —M.T. Walters, et al., ''A Double-blind, Cross-over, Study of Oral N-acetylcysteine in Sjogren's Syndrome,'' *Scandinavian Journal of Rheumatol Suppl,* 61, 1986, p. 253-258.

Stroke

Results of this study showed that NAC administration led to improvements in neuronal survival in rats when given before or after ischemia following cerebral ischemia.

> —N.W. Knuckey, et al., ''N-acetylcysteine Enhances Hippocampal Neuronal Survival after Transient Forebrain Ischemia in Rats,'' *Stroke,* 26(2), February 1995, p. 305-311.

■ PHOSPHATIDYLSERINE

Aging

Results of this study showed that chronic phosphatidylserine treatment can improve the release of acetylccholine in aging rats.

> —F. Casamenti, et al., ''Phosphatidylserine Reverses the Age-dependent Decrease in Cortical Acetylcholine Release: A Microdialysis Study,'' *European Journal of Pharmacology,* 194(1), February 26, 1991, p. 11-16.

Results of this study showed that the administration of phosphatidylserine balanced age-altered enzymatic functions in rats.

> —C. Gatti, et al., ''Effect of Chronic Treatment with Phosphatidyl Serine on Phospholipase A1 and A2 Activities in Different Brain Areas of 4 Month and 24 Month Old Rats,'' *Farmaco,* 40(7), July 1985, p. 493-500.

Results of this study showed that phosphatidylserine administered to aging rats can restore acetylcholine by maintaining a sufficient level in the cortical slices.

> —M.G. Vannucchi & G. Pepeu, ''Effect of Phosphatidylserine on Acetylcholine Release and Content in Cortical Slices from Aging Rats,'' *Neurobiol Aging,* 8(5), September-October 1987, p. 403-407.

This study examined the effects of phosphatidylserine in aged rats. Results showed the treatment decreased the number of seizures due to spontaneous EEG bursts by 65% and the length of seizure duration by 70%.

　　—F. Aporti, et al., ''Age-dependent Spontaneous EEG Bursts in Rats: Effects of Brain Phosphatidylserine,'' *Neurobiol Aging,* 7(2), March-April 1986, p. 115-120.

Results of this study showed that the administration of phosphatidylserine to rats led to a reduction in decreases in acetylcholine release due to age by influencing mechanism of stimulus-secretion coupling.

　　—F. Pedata, et al., ''Phosphatidylserine Increases Acetylcholine Release from Cortical Slices in Aged Rats,'' *Neurobiol Aging,* 6(4), Winter 1985, p. 337-339.

Allergic Neuritis

Results of this study found that phosphatidylserine administered in daily intraperitoneal 30 mg/kg injections for a period of 14 days led to a marked reduction in clinical severity and mortality in allergic neuritis rats relative to controls.

　　—Y. Maeda, et al., ''Phosphatidylserine Suppresses Myelin-induced Experimental allergic Neuritis (EAN) in Lewis Rats,'' *Journal of Neuropathology Exp Neurol,* 53(6), November 1994, p. 672-677.

Alzheimer's Disease

Results of this study showed that phosphatidylserine administered in doses of 400 mg per day led to significant, short-term neuropsychological improvements in patients with Alzheimer's disease relative to controls.

　　—W.D. Heiss, et al., ''Long-term Effects of Phosphatidylserine, Pyritinol, and Cognitive Training in Alzheimer's Disease. A Neuropsychological, EEG, and PET Investigation,'' *Dementia,* 5(2), March-April 1994, p. 88-98.

Results of this double-blind, placebo-controlled study showed that the administration of 300 mg per day of phosphatidylserine for 8 weeks led to significant clinical improvements in patients with mild primary degenerative dementia relative to controls.

　　—R.R. Engel, et al., ''Double-blind Cross-over Study of Phosphatidylserine vs. Placebo in Patients with Early Dementia of the Alzheimer Type,'' *Eur Neuropsychopharmacol,* 2(2), June 1992, p. 149-155.

In this double-blind, placebo-controlled study, Alzheimer's patients received 100 mg per day of bovine cortex phosphatidylserine for 12 weeks. Results showed the treatment improved several cognitive measures relative to controls.

　　—T. Crook, et al., ''Effects of Phosphatidylserine in Alzheimer's Disease,'' *Psychopharmacol Bulletin,* 28(1), 1992, p. 61-66.

Antiviral Effects

Results of this study showed that phosphatidylserine binds directly to vesicular stomatitis virus and inhibits its attachment and infectivity on the surface of vero cells.

　　—R. Schlegel, et al., ''Inhibition of VSV Binding and Infectivity by Phosphatidylserine: Is Phosphatidylserine a VSV-binding Site?,'' *Cell,* 32(2), February 1983, p. 639-646.

Behavioral Effects

This study examined the effects of phosphatidylserine administered for 5 days on the behavior of aged rats. Results showed the treatment led to a facilitated acquisition of active avoidance behavior and an improved retention of passive avoidance responses.

> —F. Drago, et al., "Behavioral Effects of Phosphatidylserine in Aged Rats," *Neurobiol Aging,* 2(3), Fall 1981, p. 209-213.

This set of studies examined the effects of phoshatidylserine on the behavior of aged rats. Results showed significant dose-related effects on retention of passive avoidance responses.

> —J. Corwin, et al., "Behavioral Effects of Phosphatidylserine in the Aged Fischer 344 Rat: Amelioration of Passive Avoidance Deficits without Changes in Psychomotor Task Performance," *Neurobiol Aging,* 6(1), Spring 1985, p. 11-15.

Results of this study showed that the administration of 15 mg/kg ip of phosphatidylserine for 30 days led to significant increases in the avoidance performances of rats.

> —A. Zanotti, et al., "Effects of Phosphatidylserine on Avoidance Relearning in Rats," *Pharmacol Res Commun,* 16(5), May 1984, p. 485-493.

Results of this study showed that the administration of phosphatidylserine to mice during the first sixty days of life led to the improvement of cognitive abilities in adulthood.

> —F. Ammassari-Teule, et al., "Chronic Administration of Phosphatidylserine During Ontogeny Enhances Subject-environment Interactions and Radial Maze Performance in C57BL/6 Mice," *Physiol Behav,* 47(4), Apirl 1990, p. 755-760.

Brain Function

Results of this study showed that patients suffering from chronic cerebral decomponensation experienced improvements in mnesic and neuropsychic symtpomatology following phosphatidylserine administration for 60 days.

> —G.F. Lombardi, [Pharmacological Treatment with Phosphatidyl Serine of 40 Ambulatory Patients with Senile Dementia Syndrome], *Minerva Med,* 80(6), June 1989, p. 599-602.

Results of this study showed that the administration of phosphatidlyserine for 21 days led to partial restoration of decreased density of muscarinic cholinergic receptors in aged mouse brains in a dose-dependent manner.

> —C.M. Gelbmann & W.E. Muller, "Chronic Treatment with Phosphatidylserine Restores Muscarinic Cholinergic Receptor Deficits in the Aged Mouse Brain," *Neurobiol Aging,* 13(1), January-February 1992, p. 45-50.

Results of this double-blind, placebo-controlled study showed that age-associated memory impairment patients treated with 100 mg of phosphatidylserine for 12 weeks experienced clinical improvement relevant to controls.

> —T.H. Crook, et al., "Effects of Phosphatidylserine in Age-associated Memory Impairment," *Neurology,* 41(5), May 1991, p. 644-649.

This double-blind, placebo-controlled study examined the effects of 3 x 100 mg of phosphatidylserine on patients hospitalized with dementia. Results showed a significant improvement in the patients receiving phosphatidylserine relative to controls.

>—P.J. Delwaide, et al., "Double-blind Randomized Controlled Study of Phosphatidylserine in Senile Demented Patients," *Acta Neurol Scand,* 73(2), February 1986, p. 136-140.

This double-blind, placebo-controlled study examined the effects of 300 mg per day of phosphatidylserine for 30 days on cognitive, affective and behavioral symptoms of elderly women with depressive disorders. Results showed that patients receiving phosphatidylserine experienced improvements with respect to memory, behavior, and depressive symptoms relative to controls.

>—M. Maggioni, et al., "Effects of Phosphatidylserine Therapy in Geriatric Patients with Depressive Disorders," *Acta Psychiatr Scand,* 81(3), March 1990, p. 265-270.

This double-blind, placebo-controlled study examined the effects of 300 mg per day of phosphatidylserine in cognitive impaired geriatric patients. Results showed the treatment had significant positive cognitive and behavioral effects relative to controls.

>—T. Cenacchi, et al., "Cognitive Decline in the Elderly: A Double-blind, Placebo-controlled Multicenter Study on Efficacy of Phosphatidylserine Administration," *Aging,* 5(2), April 1993, p. 123-133.

Results of this study found that the aged mice treated with 20 mg/kg ip per day of phosphatidylserine over a period of three weeks totally normalized enhanced efficacy and affinity of L-glutamate and glycine and elevated NMDA receptor density by approximately 25%.

>—S.A. Cohen & W.E. Muller, "Age-related Alterations of NMDA-receptor Properties in the Mouse Forebrain: Partial Restoration by Chronic Phosphatidylserine Treatment," *Brain Research,* 584(1-2), July 3, 1992, p. 174-180.

Results of this study indicated that the oral administration of 300 mg per day of soybean transphosphatidylated phosphatidylserine can improve and/or prevent senile dementia in humans.

>—M. Sakai, et al., "Pharmacological Effects of Phosphatidylserine Enzymatically Synthesized from Soybean Lecithin on Brain Functions in Rodents," *Journal of Nutr Sci Vitaminol,* 42(1), February 1996, p. 47-54.

Results of this study showed definite improvements in memory performance in mice treated with bovine brain phosphatidylserine relative to controls.

>—L. Valzelli, et al., "Activity of Phosphatidylserine on Memory Retrieval and on Exploration in Mice," *Methods Find Exp Clin Pharmacol,* 9(10), October 1987, p. 657-660.

Results of this study showed that the postnatal administration of an aqueous suspension of phosphatidylserine led to improvements of memory processes in mice.

>—S. Fagioli, et al., "Phosphatidylserine Administration During Postnatal Development Improves Memory in Adult Mice," *Neurosci Letters,* 101(2), June 19, 1989, p. 229-233.

Results of this study showed that oral administration of 50 mg/kg per day of phosphatidylserine for 12 weeks improved spatial memory and passive avoidance retention of aged impaired rats.

>—A. Zanotti, et al., "Chronic Phosphatidylserine Treatment Improves Spatial Memory and Passive Avoidance in Aged Rats," *Psychopharmacology,* 99(3), 1989, p. 316-321.

Cancer

Results of this study showed that bovine cortex phosphatidylserine significantly reduced experimental autoimmune encephalomyelitis in mice while not inhibiting effector T cells.

> —G. Monastra, et al., "Phosphatidylserine, a Putative Inhibitor of Tumor Necrosis factor, Prevents Autoimmune Demyelination," *Neurology,* 43(1), January 1993, p. 153-163.

Results of this study showed that parental administration of liposomes containing the aminophospholipids phosphatidylserine, and phosphatidylethanolamine is an efficient mode to decrease the endotoxin-induced production of tumor necrosis factor in mice and rabbits.

> —G. Monastra & A. Bruni, "Decreased Serum Level of Tumor Necrosis Factor in Animals Treated with Lipopolysaccharide and Liposomes Containing Phosphatidylserine," *Lymphokine Cytokine Res,* 11(1), February 1992, p. 39-43.

Cardiovascular/Coronary Heart Disease

Results of this study showed that smooth muscle cells expressed phosphatidylserine during apoptosis which partly mediated binding and phagocytosis of dead cells. The authors suggest that these effects could be important in promoting rapid cell removal in the vessel wall.

> —M.R. Bennett, et al., "Binding and Phagocytosis of Apoptotic Vascular Smooth Muscle Cells is Mediated in Part by Exposure of Phosphatidylserine," *Circ Research,* 77(6), December 1995, p. 1136-1142.

Results of this study showed that an anticoagulant containing heparin and phosphatidylserine enhanced rat tolerance to thromboplastin administration to the blood flow. Such effects led to a major decrease in death rate and fibrinogen consumption decrease due to thromboplastin.

> —A. Byshevskii & S.R. Sokolovskii, [Protective Effect of Heparin and Phosphatidylserine in Exogenous Thromboplastinemia], *Biull Eksp Biol Med,* 94(12), December 1982, p. 23-25.

Results of this study found that the intravenous administration of phosphatidylethanol amine-and sphyngomyelin-stabilized phosphatidylserine emulsion produced hypocoagulemia in white mice in a dose dependent manner.

> —M.K. Chabanov, et al., [Effect of an Intravenously Administered Phosphatidylserine Emulsion on Blood Coagulation and Blood System Indices], *Farmakol Toksikol,* 42(3), May-June 1979, p. 257-261.

Results of this study showed that the administration phosphatidylserine into the circulation of rats reduced fibrinogen consumption which was provoked by simultaneous thrombin injection, indicating it phosphatidylserine works as an anticoagulant.

> —A. Byshevskii, et al., [Effect of Phosphatidyl Serine on Conversion of Fibrinogen to Fibrin], *Vopr Med Khim,* 29(4), July-August 1983, p. 16-22.

Results of this study showed that phosphatidylserine containing anticoagulant and heparin mutually increased their anticoagulating activity under conditions of simultaneous treatment both in vitro as well as in vivo.

> —A. Byshevskii & S.R. Sokolovskii, [Potentiation of the Anticoagulant Effects of a Phosphati-

dylserine-Containing Anticoagulant and Heparin], *Vopr Med Khim,* 28(2), March-April 1982, p. 30-34.

Results of this study found that the intravenous administration 30 and 60 mg of phosphatidylserine emulsion led to a rapid reduction in blood coagulation activity in a dose dependent manner.
—O.A. Tersenov & M.K. Chabanov, [Anticoagulant Effect of Phosphatidylserine], *Vopr Med Khim* (1981 Sep-Oct) 27(5), September-October 1981, p. 619-623.

Epilepsy

This study examined the effect of gamma-aminobutyric and phosphatidylserine administered together to drug resistant epilepsy patients. Results showed a dramatic decrease in absence seizures following treatment.
—C. Loeb, et al., "Preliminary Evaluation of the Effect of GABA and Phosphatidylserine in Epileptic Patients," *Epilepsy Research,* 1(3), May 1987, p. 209-212.

General

Results of this study found that both saturated and unsaturated phosphatidylserine inhibited lipid peroxidation induced by ferrous-ascorbate system in the presence of phosphatidylcholine hydroperoxides.
—K. Yoshida, et al., "Inhibitory Effect of Phosphatidylserine on Iron-dependent Lipid Peroxidation," *Biochem Biophys Res Commun,* 179(2), September 16, 1991, p. 1077-1081.

Immune Function

Results of this study showed that phosphatidylserine can upregulate contact hypersensitivy by stimulating the function of APC of epidermal Langerhans cells in mice.
—G. Girolomoni G, et al, "Phosphatidylserine Enhances the Ability of Epidermal Langerhans Cells to Induce Contact Hypersensitivity," *Journal of Immunology,* 150(10), May 15, 1993, p. 4236-4243.

Results of this study showed that phosphatidylserine administered to rats reversed age-induced physiological decline of the humoral immune response. In addition, the same treatment reversed the pharmacological associated depression of specific antibody production in young rats.
—V. Guarcello, et al., "Phosphatidylserine Counteracts Physiological and Pharmacological Suppression of Humoral Immune Response, *Immunopharmacology,* 19(3), May-June 1990, p. 185-195.

Parkinson's Disease

This article notes that clinical and experimental research indicates phosphatidylserine prepared from cow's brain can have positive effects on cerebral changes involved in the symptoms of Alzheimer's type senile dementia among patients with Parkinson's disease.
—E.W. Funfgeld, et al., "Double-blind Study with Phosphatidylserine (PS) in Parkinsonian Patients with Senile Dementia of Alzheimer's Type," *Prog Clin Biol Res,* 317, 1989, p. 1235-1246.

Schizophrenia

This case-control study examined the effects of phosphatidylserine on platelet B-type monoamine oxidase in schizophrenics. Results supported the idea of phosphatidylserine as an allosteric regulator of platelet B-type monoamine oxidase in vivo.

> —K.H. Tachik, et al., "Phosphatidylserine Inhibition of Monoamine Oxidase in Platelets of Schizophrenics," Biological Psychiatry, 21(1), January 1986, p. 59-68.

Stress

This double-blind, placebo-controlled study examined the effects of the administration of 800 mg per day of phosphatidylserine for 10 days on neuroendocrine responses to physical stress in healthy males. Results showed that treatment counteracted activation of the hypothalamo-pituitary-adrenal axis induced by stress.

> —P. Monteleone, et a., "Blunting by Chronic Phosphatidylserine Administration of the Stress-induced Activation of the Hypothalamo-pituitary-adrenal Axis in Healthy Men," *European Journal of Clinical Pharmacology,* 42(4), 1992, p. 385-388.

Results of this study showed that old rats subjected to various stressor that received 20 mg/kg per day of phosphatidylserine for 20 days experienced a normalization of core body temperature relative to controls.

> —F. Drago, et al., Protective Action of Phosphatidylserine on Stress-induced Behavioral and Autonomic Changes in Aged Rats," *Neurobiol Aging,* 12(5), September-October 1991, p. 437-440.

Results of this double-blind, placebo-controlled study showed that healthy males pretreated with both 50 and 75 mg per day of brain cortex-derived phosphatidylserine experienced a significant blunting of the ACTH and cortisol responses to physical stress.

> —P. Monteleone, et al., "Effects of Phosphatidylserine on the Neuroendocrine Response to Physical Stress in Humans," *Neuroendocrinolgy,* 52(3), September 1990, p. 243-248.

■ PIRACETAM

Alcoholism

Results of this double-blind, placebo-controlled study showed that piracetam proved effective in the treatment of alcoholic patients hospitalized due to acute withdrawal syndrome.

> —I. Buranji, et al., "Cognitive Function in Alcoholics in a Double-blind Study of Piracetam," *Lijec Vjesn,* 112(3-4), March-April 1990, p. 111-114.

Results of this double-blind, placebo-controlled study showed that piracetam treatment improved cognitive functions, including short-term memory and concentration, in alcoholic patients suffering from organic mental disorder.

> —C. Barnas, et al., "Treatment of Alcohol Organic Mental Disorder with Piracetam," *Prog Neuropsychopharmacol Biol Psychiatry,* 11(6), 1987, p. 729-737.

Alzheimer's Disease

Results of this study showed that the intravenous administration of 6 g b.i.d. of piracetam over a period of 2 weeks led to significant improvements in most cortical areas of Alzheimer's patients studied.

> —W.D. Heiss, et al., "Effect of Piracetam on Cerebral Glucose Metabolism in Alzheimer's Disease as Measured by Positron Emission Tomography," *Journal of Cerebral Blood Flow Metab,* 8(4), August 1988, p. 613-617.

Results of this placebo-controlled study showed that the administration of 9 g per day to a group of 12 Alzheimer's patients and 2.4 g per day in 16 patients with mild senile dementia led to increases in alertness among patients in both groups.

> —M. Pierlovisi-Lavaivre, et al., [The Significance of Quantified EEG in Alzheimer's Disease. Changes Induced by Piracetam], *Neurophysiol Clin,* 21(5-6), December 1991, p. 411-423.

Burn

Results of this study indicated that piracetam administered twice daily had beneficial effects on burn wounds in rats.

> —P. Germonpre, et al., "Hyperbaric Oxygen Therapy and Piracetam Decrease the Early Extension of Deep Partial-thickness Burns," *Burns,* 22(6), September 1996, p. 468-473.

Cardiovascular/Coronary Heart Disease

Results of this double-blind, placebo-controlled study found that piracetam administration had beneficial effects with respect to clinical improvement of acute circulatory insufficiency and an analgesic effect in myocardial infarct patients.

> —L.A. Leshchinskii, et al., "Therapeutic Use of Piracetam in Myocardial Infarct Patients," *Kardiologiia,* 27(2), February 1987, p. 46-50.

Cerebral Palsy

Results of this study showed that piracetam proved effective in controlling spasticity in 8 of 16 cerebral palsy patients.

> —N.G. Maritz, et al., "Piracetam in the Management of Spasticity in Cerebral Palsy," *South African Medical Journal,* 53(22), June 3, 1987, p. 889-891.

Chronic Bronchitis

Results of this study showed that the intravenous administration of 30 mg/kg bw (10-12 injections per course) of piracetam had beneficial immune enhancing effects on patients suffering from chronic bronchitis.

> —V.P. Sil'vestrov, et al., "Immunological and Metabolic Disorders and the Means for their Correction in Patients with Chronic Bronchitis," *Ter Arkh,* 63(12), 1991, p. 7-11.

Cognitive Function

Results of this double-blind, placebo-controlled study found that the combined administration of 1600 mg 3 times daily of piracetam and 400 mg 3 times daily of pentoxifylline led to improvements in psycho-intellectual performance in elderly patients suffering from recent onset of slight to moderate mental deterioration.

> —L. Parnetti, et al., "Haemorheological Pattern in Initial Mental Deterioration: Results of a Long-term Study Using Piracetam and Pentoxifylline," *Arch Gerontol Geriatr,* 4(2), July 1985, p. 141-155.

Results of this double-blind, placebo-controlled study showed that a single dose of 2400 mg of piracetam exhibited antihypoxidotic effects in healthy male subjects.

> —K. Schaffler & W. Klausnitzer, "Randomized Placebo-controlled Double-blind Cross-over Study on Antihypoxidotic Effects of Piracetam Using Psychophysiological Measures in Healthy Volunteers," *Arzneimittelforschung,* 38(2), February 1988, p. 288-291.

Results of this study showed that the administration of piracetam and oxiracetam prevented damage to the memory processes of rats caused by exposure to microwaves.

> —I.N. Krylov, et al., "Pharmacologic Correction of Learning and Memory Disorders Induced by Exposure to High-frequency Electromagnetic Radiation," *Biull Eksp Biol Med,* 115(3), March 1993, p. 260-262.

This article reviews findings from both animal and human studies supporting the use of piracetam in the treatment of a host of a cognitive disorders.

> —M.W. Vernon & E.M. Sorkin, "Piracetam: An Overview of its Pharmacological Properties and a Review of its Therapeutic Use in Senile Cognitive Disorders," *Drugs Aging,* 1(1), January 1991, p. 17-35.

Results of this 12-week, double-blind, placebo-controlled study found that the administration of either 2.4 or 4.8 g per day of piracetam to elderly psychiatric patients with mild diffuse cerebral impairment led to general improvements, particularly with respect to socialization, cooperation and alertness. Significant improvements were also found with respect to memory performance and IQ scores.

> —G. Chouinard, et al., "Piracetam in Elderly Psychiatric Patients with Mild Diffuse Cerebral Impairment," *Psychopharmacology,* 81(2), 1983, p. 100-106.

Depression

In this study, 200 mg of oral viloxazineand 9 g of oral piracetam a day was administered over a period of 3 months in elderly outpatients suffering from depression. Following the treatment period, such patients then received a maintenance dose of 100 mg viloxazine and 3 g of piracetam per day. Results showed improvements in approximately 75% of the patients with respect to depression psycho-organic syndrome symptoms. Such effects were maintained in approximately 50% over the long term.

> —A. Borromei, et al., [Nonpsychotic Involutional Inhibited Depressions and Psycho-organic Deteriorations: Treatment with Viloxazine and Piracetam], *Minerva Med,* 80(5), May 1989, p. 475-482.

Dyslexia

Results of this double-blind, placebo-controlled study showed that piracetam administered in doses of 3300 mg per day over a period of 12 weeks significantly increased reading speed and number of words written in a timed period among a group of dyslexic boys between 8-13 years old.

> —P. Tallal, et al., "Evaluation of the Efficacy of Piracetam in Treating Information Processing,

Reading and Writing Disorders in Dyslexic Children,'' *International Journal of Psychophysiol,* 4(1), May 1986, p. 41-52.

In this double-blind, placebo-controlled study, dyslexic children between the ages of 7.5 and 13 years old were treated with piracetam. Results showed those receiving the drug experienced significantly improved reading ability and comprehension scores relative to controls.
    —C.R. Wilsher, et al., ''Piracetam and Dyslexia: Effects on Reading Tests,'' *Journal of Clinical Psychopharmacol,* 7(4), August 1987, p. 230-237.

In this double-blind, placebo-controlled study, dyslexic boys between the ages of 8 and 13 years old were treated with piracetam. Results showed those receiving the drug experienced significantly improved reading speed.
    —M. Di Ianni, et al., ''The Effects of Piracetam in Children with Dyslexia,'' *Journal Clinical Psychopharmacol,* 5(5), October 1985, p. 272-278.

In this double-blind, crossover study, 16 dyslexic children were followed through adulthood and then compared to 14 healthy students during a 21 day period of piracetam treatment. Results showed significant increases in verbal learning among dyslexics (15%) and students (8.6%).
    —C. Wilsher, et al., ''Piracetam as an Aid to Learning in Dyslexia. Preliminary Report,'' *Psychopharmacology,* 65(1), September 1979, p. 107-109.

General

Results of this placebo-controlled study found that, of a 100 brain tumor patients studied, significantly more of those administered piracetam were able to maintain near normal consciousness postoperatively relative to controls.
    —A.E. Richardson & F.J. Bereen, ''Effect of Piracetam on Level of Consciousness after Neurosurgery,'' *Lancet,* 2(8048), November 26, 1977, p. 1110-1111.

Result of this study found that piracetam exhibited antihypoxic effects in that it inhibited free-radical lipid peroxidation, retarded the consumption of oxygen in liver mitochondria and enhanced hemoglobin oxygen-binding properties.
    —V.M. Gukasov, et al., [Characteristics of the Antihypoxic Action of Piracetam], *Biull Eksp Biol Med,* 103(6), June 1987, p. 683-685.

Hearing Loss

Results of this study found that the intravenous administration of 10 g per day of piracetam diluted in a 250 ml saline solution over a period of 3 days led to improvements in 6 out of 9 patients suffering from sudden hearing loss.
    —S. Solanellas, et al., ''Sudden Hearing Loss. Treatment with Piracetam,'' *Acta Otorrinolaringol Esp,* 48(1), January-February, 1997, p. 21-25.

Myoclonus

Results of this study showed that 5 of 5 mycoclonus patients treated with 8-9 g per day of oral piracetam experienced significant benefits with no side effects.
    —J.A. Obeso, et al., ''Antimyoclonic Action of Piracetam,'' *Clin Neuropharmacol,* 9(1), 1986, p. 58-64.

Results of this study found that the administration of up to 10 g per day of piracetam to 3 patients suffering from progressive myoclonus epilepsy led to the elimination of photoparoxysmal responses in each.

>—W. Paulus, et al., "Abolition of Photoparoxysmal Response in Progressive Myoclonus Epilepsy," *Eur Neurol,* 31(6), 1991, p. 388-390.

In this patients, 60 myoclonus patients were treated with piracetam. Results found the drug to be effective with respect to gait ataxia, handwriting, motivation, sleep trouble, attention deficit, depression, and convulsions.

>—A. Ikeda, et al., "Clinical Trial of Piracetam in Patients with Myoclonus: Nationwide Multiinstitution Study in Japan. The Myoclonus/Piracetam Study Group," *Mov Disord,* 11(6), November 1996, p. 691-700.

Pain

Results of this study showed that piracetam prevented onset of neuropathic pain syndrome.

>—E.I. Danilova, et al., "The Action of Piracetam and its Complex with Sodium Oxybutyrate in the Neuropathic Pain Syndrome," *Eksp Klin Farmakol,* 59(4), July-August 1996, p. 8-10.

Parkinson's Disease

Results of this case-controlled study found that piracetam improved visuomotor reaction time and accuracy in 6 mildly affected and tracing time in 6 moderately affected Parkinson's patients of the 18 receiving the drug.

>—G. Oepen, et al., "Piracetam Improves Visuomotor and Cognitive Deficits in Early Parkinsonism—A Pilot Study," *Pharmacopsychiatry,* 18(6), November 1985, p. 343-346.

Post-Concussional Syndrome

Results of this double-blind, placebo-controlled study found that the administration of 4,800 mg per day of piracetam over a period of 8 weeks to patients with post-concussional syndrome significantly reduced symptoms associated with the condition including fatigue, sweating, vertigo, headache, reduced alertness, and intense sweating. Side effects were seen in 64% of patients taking the drug as compared to 32% of controls.

>—H. Hakkarainen & L. Hakamies, "Piracetam in the Treatment of Post-concussional Syndrome. A Double-blind Study," *Eur Neurol,* 17(1), 1978, p. 50-55.

Raynaud's Phenomenon

Results of this study established 8 g per of piracetam as the most effective dose of the drug in the treatment of patients suffering from primary as well as secondary Raynaud's syndrome.

>—M. Moriau, et al., "Treatment of the Raynaud's Phenomenon with Piracetam," *Arzneimittelforschung* 43(5), May 1993, p. 526-535.

Sickle Cell Disease

Results of this study showed that 160 mg/kg/day or oral piracetam enhanced HbSS cell deformability in vivo as well as it did in vitro experiments.

>—E.K. Gini & J. Sonnet, "Use of Piracetam Improves Sickle Cell Deformability in Vitro and in Vivo," *Journal of Clin Pathol,* 40(1), January 1987, p. 99-102.

Results of this double-blind, placebo-controlled study showed that the intravenous administration of piracetam to Saudi children suffering from sickle cell disease between the ages of 3-12 years over a 12 month period led to significant reductions in the clinical severity of the disease, hospitalization time, blood transfusion requirements and the number of crises experienced by each child.

> —M.A. el-Hazmi, et al., "Piracetam is Useful in the Treatment of Children with Sickle Cell Disease," *Acta Haematol,* 96(4), 1996, p. 221-226.

Ulcer

Results of this study found piracetam exhibited antiulcerogenic activity stress and protected against aspirin-induced gastric ulcers in rats.

> —R.K. Goel, et al., "Effect of Piracetam, a Nootropic Agent, on Experimental Gastric Ulcers in Rat," *Indian Journal of Exp Biol,* 28(4), April 1990, p. 337-340.

Results of this study showed that piracetam and aevit led to early regression of duodenal ulcer in rats when added to standard antiulcer therapy.

> —L.T. Pimenov, et al., "The Clinico-endoscopic, Psychological and Physical Characteristics of Duodenal Peptic Ulcer Patients Using Piracetam and Aevit," *Ter Arkh,* 69(2), 1997, p. 10-13.

Vertigo

Results of this pilot study found that piracetam proved extremely effective with respect to the pursuit of tracking among 5 of 5 vertigo patients receiving the drug.

> —C.M. Fernandes & J. Samuel, "The Use of Piracetam in Vertigo," *South African Medical Journal,* 68(11), November 23, 1985, p. 806-808.

Results of this study showed that piracetam coupled with ergotoxin proved significantly effective in alleviating symptoms associated with vertigo in vertigo patients and those suffering from related symptoms.

> —C.F. Claussen, et al., "The Treatment of Minocycline-induced Brainstem Vertigo by the Combined Administration of Piracetam and Ergotoxin," *Acta Otolaryngol Suppl,* 468, 1989, p. 171-174.

Results of this study showed that that the combination of piracetam and dihydroergocristine in 55 vertiginous patients administered over a period of 3 months had beneficial effects.

> —H. Ordosgoitia, et al., [Clinical Trial of the Use of the Combination of Piracetam and Dihydroergocristine in Vertigo from Different Causes]," *An Otorrinolaringol Ibero Am,* 16(3), 1989, p. 271-279.

Results of this double-blind, placebo-controlled study showed that piracetam significantly reduced symptoms associated with vertigo in patients suffering from the condition.

> —W.J. Oosterveld, "The Efficacy of Piracetam in Vertigo. A Double-blind Study in Patients with Vertigo of Central Origin," *Arzneimittelforschung,* 30(11), 1980, p. 1947-1949.

Viral Neuroinfections

Results of this study showed that treatment with piracetam had beneficial effects on the depth of consciousness and psychic function in patients suffering from acute viral neuroinfections.

—A.I. Niss, et al., "Efficacy of Piracetam Treatment of Acute Viral Neuroinfections," *Zh Nevropatol Psikhiatr,* 85(2), 1985, p. 189-195.

■ S-ADENOSYLMETHIONINE

Arthritis

Results of this placebo-controlled study showed that weekly intraarticular doses of SAMe significantly reduced the severity of experimentally-induced osteoarthritis in rats.

—D.A. Kalbhen & G. Jansen,'' "Pharmacologic Studies on the Antidegenerative Effect of Ademetionine in Experimental Arthritis in Animals," *Arzneimittelforschung,* 40(9), September 1990, p. 1017-1021.

Cancer

Results of this study showed that the administration of SAMe prevented the development of experimentally-induced liver cancer in rats.

—R.M. Pascale, et al., "Chemoprevention of Rat Liver Carcinogenesis by S-adenosyl-L-methionine: A Long-term Study," *Cancer Research,* 52(18), September 15, 1992, p. 4979-4986.

Results of this study indicated that the administration of SAMe prevents the development of experimentally-induced liver cancer in rats.

—R. Feo, et al., "Molecular Mechanisms of Chemoprevention of Rat Liver Carcinogenesis by S-Adenoysl-L-Methionine," *Third International Conference on Mechanisms of Antimutagenesis and Anticarcinogenesis, Lucca, Italy,* 25, May 5-10, 1991.

Results of this study showed that SAMe had chemopreventive effects against experimentally-induced liver carcinogenesis in rats.

—R.M. Pascale, et al., "Chemoprevention by S-adenosyl-L-methionine of Rat Liver Carcinogenesis Initiated by 1,2-dimethylhydrazine and Promoted by Orotic Acid," *Carcinogenesis,* 16(2), February 1995, p. 427-430.

Results of this study indicated that the administration of SAMe prevents the development of experimentally-induced liver cancer in rats.

—M.M. Simile, et al., "Persistent Chemoprevention by S-adenosyl-L-methionine (SAM) of the Development of Liver Preneoplastic Lesions in Diethylnitrosamine-initiated Rats," *Proceedings of the Annual Meeting of the American Association of Cancer Researchers,* 37, 1996, p. 1881.

Results of this study indicated that the administration of SAMe inhibits experimentally-induced liver cancer in rats.

—R.M. Pascale, et al., "S-adenosyl-L-methionine (SAM) is a Chemopreventive Agent for

1,2- dimethylhydrazine (DMH)-induced Hepatocarcinogenesis in Orotic Acid (OA)-promoted Rats,'' *Proceedings of the Annual Meeting of the American Association of Cancer Researchers,* 36, 1995, p. A727.

Depression

This review article notes that numerous open and double-blind studies have indicated SAMe may possess antidepressant effects.
— M.W. Carney, et al., ''S-adenosylmethionine and Affective Disorder,'' *American Journal of Medicine* 83(5A), November 20, 1987, p. 104-106.

Results of this study showed 7 of 9 patients receiving treatment with SAMe for depression experienced improvement or total remission of symptoms.
— J.F. Lipinski, et al., ''Open Trial of S-adenosylmethionine for Treatment of Depression,'' *American Journal of Psychiatry,* 141(3), March 1994, p. 448-550.

Results of this double-blind, placebo-controlled study found that the oral administration of SAMe proved to be an effective and quick acting antidepressant in patients suffering from major depression.
— B.L. Kagan, et al., ''Oral S-adenosylmethionine in Depression: A Randomized, Double-blind, Placebo-controlled Trial,'' *American Journal Psychiatry,* 147(5), May 1990, p. 591-595.

This double-blind study compared the effects of intravenous SAMe with oral imipramine in the treatment of patients suffering from major depression. Nine patients each received either drug over a period of two weeks. Results showed the SAMe proved more effective, with 66% of those taking it showing significant clinical improvement by the end of the second week compared to just 22% of patients taking imipramine.
— K.M. Bell, et al., ''S-adenosylmethionine Treatment of Depression: A Controlled Clinical Trial,'' *American Journal of Psychiatry,* 145(9), September 1988, p. 1110-1114.

Results of this double-blind, placebo-controlled found SAMe, a natural occurring compound to be an effective treatment against depression comparable to tricylcic antidepressant but with relatively fewer side effects.
— G.M. Bressa, ''S-adenosyl-l-methionine (SAMe) as Antidepressant: Meta-analysis of Clinical Studies,'' *Acta Neurol Scand Suppl,* 154, p. 7-14.

This double-blind, randomized study compared the efficacy of oral SAMe and desipramine administered over a period of 4 weeks in the treatment of major depression. Results showed that 62% of those receiving SAMe experienced significant improvements compared to a 50% improvement rate among patients taking desipramine.
— K.M. Bell, et al., ''S-adenosylmethionine Blood Levels in Major Depression: Changes with Drug Treatment,'' *Acta Neurol Scand Suppl,* 154, 1994, p. 15-18.

This review article notes that both controlled and uncontrolled study results have pointed to antidepressant effects of SAMe.
— S.A. Vahora & P. Malek-Ahmadi, ''S-adenosylmethionine in the Treatment of Depression,'' *Neurosci Biobehav Rev,* 12(2), Summer 1988, p. 139-141.

Results of this study found that the parental administration of 400 mg of SAMe over a period 15 days remitted depressive symptoms in patients suffering from depression.

> —M. Fava, et al., "Rapidity of Onset of the Antidepressant Effect of Parenteral S-adenosyl-L-methionine," *Psychiatry Research,* 56(3), April 28, 1995, p. 295-297.

Results of this single-blind, placebo-controlled study found that the oral administration of 1,600 mg per day of SAMe over a month period significantly improved depressive symptoms in postmenopausal female patients suffering from major depression.

> —P. Salmaggi, et al., "Double-blind, Placebo-controlled Study of S-adenosyl-L-methionine in Depressed Postmenopausal Women," *Psychother Psychosom,* 59(1), 1993, p. 34-40.

General

Results of this study showed that SAMe exerted anti-inflammatory activity in the inhibiting of oedema and pleurisy in rats.

> —M. Gualano, et al., "Anti-inflammatory Activity of S-adenosyl-L-methionine in Animal Models: Possible Interference with the Eicosanoid System," *International Journal of Tissue React,* 7(1), 1985, p. 41-46.

Gonarthrosis

Results of this study found SAMe administered at daily doses of between 800-1200 mg to be equally as effective as naproxen administered at daily doses of between 500 mg-750 mg in the treatment of patients suffering from activated gonarthrosis, with both drugs showing significant improvement across all parameters studied.

> —Z. Domljan, et al., "A Double-blind Trial of Ademetionine vs Naproxen in Activated Gonarthrosis," *International Journal of Clinical Pharmacol Ther Toxicol,* 27(7), July 1989, p. 329-333.

Infantile Porphyria Cutanea Tarda

This article reports on two cases of infantile porphyia cutanea tard, one in a 7-year-old girl and the other in a 12-year-old boy . Combined treatment with low-dose oral chloroquine and oral S-adenosyl-L-methionine led to complete clinical and biochemical recovery within a period of 3 months.

> —A.M. Battle, et al., "Two Cases of Infantile Porphyria Cutanea Tarda: Successful Treatment with Oral S-adenosyl-L-methionine and Low-dose Oral Chloroquine," *British Journal of Dermatology,* 116(3), March 1987, p. 407-415.

Intrahepatic Cholestasis

Results of this study indicated that SAMe administered at doses of 800 mg per day worked as a physiological antidote against estrogen hepatobiliary toxicity in women with prior intrahepatic cholestasis of pregnancy.

> —M. Frezza, et al., "Prevention of S-adenosylmethionine of Estrogen-induced Hepatobiliary Toxicity in Susceptible Women," *American Journal Gastroenterol,* 83(10), October 1988, p. 1098-1102.

Lead Poisoning

Results of this study showed that the administration of SAMe was effective in countering lead poisoning in rats.

> —S.R. Paredes, et al., "S-adenosyl-L-methionine a Counter to Lead Intoxication?" *Comp Biochem Physiol,* 82(4), 1985, p. 751-757.

Results of this study showed that the administration of SAMe was effective in countering lead poisoning in both mice and human subjects.

> —S.R. Paredes, et al., "S-adenosyl-L-methionine and Lead Intoxication: Its Therapeutic Effect Varying the Route of Administration," *Ecotoxicol Environ Safe,* 12(3), December 1986, p. 252-260.

In this study, five patients suffering from lead poisoning received 12 mg/kg body weight, of intravenous SAMe per day over a 22 day period. Results showed a significant recovery of erythrocytic ALA-D was observed in all cases.

> —S.R. Paredes, et al., "Beneficial Effect of S-adenosyl-L-methionine in Lead Intoxication. Another Approach to Clinical Therapy," *International Journal of Biochemistry,* 17(5), 1985, p. 625-629.

Liver Damage

Results of this study showed that the administration of 30 mg of SAMe six times per day coupled with 6000 gamma per day of vitamin B12 produced a significant improvements of biochemical parameters in patients with hepatic cirrhosis or various chronic hepatites.

> —F. Miglio, et al., "Double-blind Studies of the Therapeutic Action of S-Adenosylmethionine (SAMe) in Oral Administration, in Liver Cirrhosis and other Chronic Hepatitides," *Minerva Med,* 66(33), May 2, 1975, p. 1595-1599.

In this study, patients suffering from hepatic cirrhosis were intravenously treated for a period of 30 days with 150 mg per day SAMe and 2000 gamma per day of vitamin B-12 or with vitamin B-12 alone. Results showed significant improvements in the groups of patients receiving the combined treatment only.

> —G. Labo, et al., "Double-blind Polycentric Study of the Action of S-adenosylmethionine in Hepatic Cirrhosis," *Minerva Med,* 66(33), May 2, 1975, p. 1590-1594.

Results of this study showed that the intravenous administration of two daily doses of 15 mg of SAMe over a period of 20 days led to significant improvement in patients hospitalized for chronic hepatitis.

> —L. Cantoni, et al., "Relations Between Protidopoiesis and Biological Transmethylations: Action of S-Adenosylmethionine on Protein Crasis in Chronic Hepatopathies," *Minerva Med,* 66(33), May 2, 1975, p. 1581-1591.

Results of this study found that the intravenous administration of 15 mg 4 times per day of SAMe over a period of one month led to significant improvements in hepatitic cirrhosis patients.

> —G. Ideo, "S-Adenosylmethionine: Plasma Levels in Hepatic Cirrhosis and Preliminary Results of its Clinical Use in Hepatology. Double-blind Study," *Minerva Med,* 66(33), May 2, 1975, p. 1571-1580.

Results of this study found that the slow intravenous administration of 30-45 mg per day of SAMe over a period of 30-60 days led to significant improvements in patients suffering from cirrhosis of the liver and other chronic hepatites.

—G. Labo & G.B. Gasbarrini, "Therapeutic Action of S-adenosylmethionine in Some Chronic Hepatopathies," *Minerva Med,* 66(33), May 2, 1975, p. 1563-1570.

Results of this double-blind, placebo-controlled study found that the short-term administration of 1600 mg per day of SAMe had significant clinical benefits in patients suffering from intrahepatic cholestasis relative to controls.

—M. Frezza, et al., "Oral S-adenosylmethionine in the Symptomatic Treatment of Intrahepatic Cholestasis. A Double-blind, Placebo-controlled Study," *Gastroenterology,* 99(1), July 1990, p. 211-215.

This article reports on the case of patient suffering from danazol-induced cholestasis who experienced immediate resolution after receiving SAMe intravenously for 3 weeks followed up by oral administration of the drug for another 6 weeks.

—G.P. Bray, et al., "Resolution of Danazol-induced Cholestasis with S-adenosylmethionine," *Postgraduate Medical Journal,* 69(809), March 1993, p. 237-239.

Results of this meta-analysis involving 6 controlled studies of the effects of ademethionine in treating intrahepatic cholestasis of liver disease and pregnancy showed that the administration of ademethionine for 15-30 days produced significantly better results than controls.

—M. Frezza, "A Meta-analysis of Therapeutic Trials with Ademetionine in the Treatment of Intrahepatic Cholestasis," *Ann Ital Med Int,* 8 Suppl, October 1993, p. 48S-51S.

This single-blind, placebo-controlled study examined the effects of 800 mg of intravenous SAMe per day on women suffering from intrahepatic cholestasis of pregnancy administered until delivery and over a mean period of 18 days. Results showed that women receiving SAMe exhibited significantly lower levels of total bile acids, serum conjugated bilirubin and aminotransferases than controls. Such patients showed significant decreases in pruritus as well.

—M. Frezza, et al., "S-adenosylmethionine for the Treatment of Intrahepatic Cholestasis of Pregnancy. Results of a Controlled Clinical Trial," *Hepatogastroenterology,* 37, (Suppl 2), December 1990, p. 122-125.

Results of this study showed that the combined therapy of SAMe and Nifedipene significantly inhibited experimentally-induced liver cirrhosis in rats.

—E. Barrio, et al., "Comparative Effect of Nifedipine and S-adenosylmethionine, Singly and in Combination on Experimental Rat Liver Cirrhosis," *Life Science,* 52(20), 1993, p. PL217-20.

This review article notes that clinical studies involving more than 1,000 cholestatic patients have found that the intravenous administration of SAMe at doses of 800 mg/day is an effective and safe means of treating patients suffering from intrahepatic cholestasis.

—M. Coltorti, et al., "A Review of the Studies on the Clinical Use of S-adenosylmethionine (SAMe) for the Symptomatic Treatment of Intrahepatic Cholestasis," *Methods Find Exp Clin Pharmacol,* 12(1), Jan-Feb 1990, p. 69-78.

Male Sterility

Results of this study showed that the administration of 800 mg per day of SAMe over a period of 3 months increased basal motiligy of spermatozoa in 6 out of 10 male infertility cases treated.

—R. Piacentino, et al., "Preliminary Study of the Use of S. adenosyl Methionine in the Management of Male Sterility," *Minerva Ginecol,* 43(4), April 1991, p. 191-193.

Migraine

Results of this study showed that the administration of SAMe alleviated pain in patients suffering from migraines.

—G. Gatto, et al., "Analgesizing Effect of a Methyl Donor (S-adenosylmethionine) in Migraine: An Open Clinical Trial," *International Journal of Clinical Pharmacol Research,* 6(1), 1986, p. 15-17.

Osteoarthritis

This study examined the effects of S-adenosylmethionine (SAMe) administered over a period of 24 months in patients with osteoarthritis of the knee, hip, and spine. Results showed 600 mg of SAMe daily for the first two weeks and 400 mg per day thereafter proved clinically effective and improved feelings of depression often associated with the disease as well.

—B. Konig, "A Long-term (two years) Clinical Trial with S-adenosylmethionine for the Treatment of Osteoarthritis," *American Journal of Medicine,* 83(5A), November 20, 1987, p. 89-94.

Results of this non-controlled study involving 20,641 patients with osteoarthritis of the knee, the hip, and the spine showed ademetionine tablets administered over a period of 8 weeks showed good effectiveness in 71% of patients, moderate effectiveness in 21% and poor in 9%.

—R. Berger & H. Nowak, "A New Medical Approach to the Treatment of Osteoarthritis. Report of an Open Phase IV Study with Ademetionine (Gumbaral), *American Journal of Medicine,* 83(5A), November 20, 1987, p. 84-88.

In this double-blind, placebo-controlled study, patients with osteoarthritis of the knee, the hip, and/or the spine received either 1,200 mg of S-adenosylmethionine (SAMe) per day or 1,200 mg of ibuprofen per day over a period of four weeks. Both treatments proved equally effective in alleviating symptoms of morning stiffness, pain at rest, pain on motion, crepitus, swelling, and limitation of motion of the affected joints.

—H. Muller-Fassbender, "Double-blind Clinical Trial of S-adenosylmethionine Versus Ibuprofen in the Treatment of Osteoarthritis," *American Journal of Medicine,* 83(5A), November 20, 1987, p. 81-83.

In this double-blind, placebo-controlled study, patients with osteoarthritis of the knee, the hip, and/or the spine received either 1,200 mg of S-adenosylmethionine (SAMe) per day or 150 mg of indomethacin per day over a period of four weeks. Both treatments proved effective in alleviating symptoms of morning stiffness, pain at rest, pain on motion, crepitus, swelling, and limitation of motion of the affected joints.

—G. Vetter, "Double-blind Comparative Clinical Trial with S-adenosylmethionine and Indomethacin in the Treatment of Osteoarthritis,'' *American Journal of Medicine,* 83(5A), November 20, 1987, p. 78-80.

In this double-blind, placebo-controlled study, patients with unilateral knee osteoarthritis received either 1,200 mg of S-adenosylmethionine (SAMe) per day or 20 mg per day of oral piroxicam over a period of 84 days. Both treatments produced significant improvements in total pain scores after being administered for 28 days.

>—A. Maccagno, et al., ''Double-blind Controlled Clinical Trial of Oral S-adenosylmethionine Versus Piroxicam in Knee Osteoarthritis,'' *American Journal of Medicine,* 83(5A), November 20, 1987, p. 72-77.

This double-blind, placebo-controlled study involving 734 subjects compared the efficacy of 1,200 mg per day of S-adenosylmethionine (SAMe) with 750 mg per day of naproxen in the treatment of osteoarthritis of the hip, knee, spine, and hand. Both drugs proved more effective than controls and SAMe was significantly more tolerable than naproxen.

>—I. Caruso & V. Pietrogrande, ''Italian Double-blind Multicenter Study Comparing S- adenosylmethionine, Naproxen, and Placebo in the Treatment of Degenerative Joint Disease,'' *American Journal of Medicine,* 83(5A), November 20, 1987, p. 66-71.

This review article discussed findings from clinical trials involving over 22,000 osteoarthritis patients between the years of 1982 and 1987. Results of such studies support the efficacy and tolerability of SAMe in treating those suffering from the disease.

>—C. di Padova, ''S-adenosylmethionine in the Treatment of Osteoarthritis. Review of the Clinical Studies,'' *American Journal of Medicine,* 83(5A), November 20, 1987, p. 60-65.

Results of this study showed that the intramuscular administration of SAMe had chondoprotective effects in rabbits with surgical-induced osteoarthritis.

>—H.A. Barcelo, et al., ''Effect of S-adenosylmethionine on Experimental Osteoarthritis in Rabbits,'' *American Journal of Medicine,* 83(5A), November 20, 1987, p. 55-59.

This study examined the anti-inflammatory effects of SAMe in patients with severe degenerative anthropathies. Results showed that 30 mg of SAMe administered intravenously twice a day over a 2 week period had significant anti-inflammatory effects and no side effects in such patients.

>—E. Polli, et al., ''Pharmacological and Clinical Aspects of S-adenosylmethionine (SAMe) in Primary Degenerative Arthropathy (Osteoarthrosis),'' *Minerva Med,* 66(83), December 5, 1975, p. 4443-4459.

In this double-blind, placebo-controlled study, patients with hip and/or knee osteoarthritis received either 1,200 mg of S-adenosylmethionine (SAMe) per day or 1,200 mg of ibuprofen per day over a period of 30 days. SAMe proved more effective in alleviating symptoms associated with disease than ibuprofen.

>—S. Glorioso, et al., ''Double-blind Multicentre Study of the Activity of S-adenosylmethionine in Hip and Knee Osteoarthritis,'' *International Journal of Clinical Pharmacol Research,* 5(1), 1985, p. 39-49.

Results of this study showed that the intramuscular administration of SAMe had protective effects in rabbits with experimental-induced degenerative arthropathy of the knee.

    —H.A. Barcelo, et al., "Experimental Osteoarthritis and Its Course When Treated with S-Adenosyl-L-methionine," *Rev Clin Esp,* 187(2), June 1990, p. 74-78.

Primary Fibromyalgia

Results of this double-blind, placebo-controlled study found SAMe to be an effective treatment for management of primary fibromyalgia mainly do to its ability to improve the patient's depressive state and reduce the number of trigger points.

    —A. Tavoni, et al., "Evaluation of S-adenosylmethionine in Primary Fibromyalgia. A Double-blind Crossover Study," *American Journal of Medicine,* 83(5A), November 20, 1987, p. 107-110.

This double-blind, placebo-controlled study examined the effects of 800 mg per day of SAMe administered orally on patients suffering from primary fibromyalgia. Results showed improvements with respect to pain, fatigue, morning stiffness, and mood in those receiving the drug.

    —S. Jacobsen, et al., "Oral S-adenosylmethionine in Primary Fibromyalgia. Double-blind Clinical Evaluation," *Scandinavian Journal of Rheumatology,* 20(4), 1991, p. 294-302.

Stroke

Results of this study found that the administration of SAMe protected against energy failure in cerebral ischemia of rats while also increasing recovery time.

    —Y. Katayama, et al., "Effects of S-adenosyl-L-methionine on Experimental Cerebral Ischemia," *No To Shinkei,* 37(3), March 1985, p. 243-247.

Wilson's Disease

Results of this study showed that the oral administration of 30 mg of SAMe 4-5 times per day had significant beneficial effects on liver function in nine brothers suffering from Wilson's Disease.

    —G. Gasbarrini, et al., "On the Therapeutic Combination of S-adenosylmethionine with D-Penicillamine in Wilson's Disease," *Minerva Med,* 66(33), May 2, 1975, p. 1600-1604.

APPENDIX B

HUMAN DOSAGE RANGE

The dosage ranges that follow are calculated upon study results plus what most clinicians have found is the most effective dose. However, every individual is unique and, therefore, there may be a substantial difference in the suggested therapeutic amount given — either more or less than what is suggested here. As these are therapeutic, they should only be offered by licensed clinicians.

(T) = Treatment dose
(P) = Preventive dose

NUTRIENTS

■ ACETYL-L-CARNITINE

AGING
1500 mg to 3 g per day/for up to 90 days (T)

AIDS/HIV
6 g per day for up to 2 weeks (T)

ALZHEIMER'S DISEASE
2 g to 2.5 g per day/for up to 6 months (T)

AMENORRHEA
2 g per day for 6 months (T)

CARDIOVASCULAR/CORONARY HEART DISEASE
3 mg per day intravenous (T)

DEMENTIA
1000 mg per day (T)

DEPRESSION
1500 mg per day (T)

NEUROLOGICAL FUNCTION
3 g per day for 14 days (T)

PARKINSON'S DISEASE
2 g per day for 7 days (T)

STROKE
1.5 g per day intravenous (T)

■ ACIDOPHILUS

GENERAL
250 ml twice a day for 7 days (T)

VAGINITIS
8 ounces of yogurt per day for 6 months (T)

■ ALPHA-LIPOIC ACID

DIABETES
100-1000 mg per day (T)

GLAUCOMA
0.15 g per day for 1 month (T)

■ BETAINE

HOMOCYSTINURIA
6 g to 20 g per day (T)

■ BIFIDUS

CANCER
500 ml per day of Bifodium longum enriched yogurt (P)

GENERAL
lyophilized Bifidobacterium bifidum & Lactobacillus acidophilus capsules 4 times per day for 28 days (T)

NEWBORNS
(10(6)/g of powder) fed for first 2 months (P)

■ BIOTIN

NEUROLOGICAL DISORDERS
10 mg per day (T)

■ BORON

ARTHRITIS
6 mg per day (T)

■ BROMELAIN

DENTAL HEALTH
240 mg per day (T)

IMMUNE ENHANCEMENT
200-300 mg/kg per day (T)

■ CALCIUM

DENTAL FLUOROSIS
250 mg per day (T)

HYPERTENSION
2 g per day for up to 28 weeks (T)

OSTEOPOROSIS
1 g per day for up to 6 months (T/P)

■ CHOLINE

HEMIPLEGIA
250 mg to 1000 mg per day for 8 weeks (T)

HEPATIC STEATOSIS
1 g to 4 g of choline chloride per day for 4 weeks (P/T)

NEUROLOGICAL FUNCTION
6 ml per day (T)

SEIZURES
12-16 g per day (T)

STROKE
1,000 mg intravenous for 14 days (T)

TARDIVE DYSKINESIA
500 mg to 1200 mg per day (T)

■ CHROMIUM

CARDIOVASCULAR/CORONARY HEART DISEASE
200 mcg to 600 mcg per day/for up to 16 months (T)

DIABETES
125 mcg to 200 mcg per day/for up to 3 months (T)

TURNER'S SYNDROME
30 g of brewer's yeast containing 50 mcg of chromium per day for 8 weeks (T)

■ COD LIVER OIL

*CARDIOVASCULAR/CORONARY
  HEART DISEASE*
20-25 ml per day for up to 8 weeks (T)

■ COENZYME Q10

CANCER
1mg/kg to 390 mg per day (P)

*CARDIOVASCULAR/CORONARY
  HEART DISEASE*
3 mg to 150 mg per day/for up to 3 months (T)

KEARNS-SAYRE SYNDROME
120 mg to 150 mg per day (T)

LUNG DISEASE
90 mg per day for 8 weeks (T)

■ FOLIC ACID

ARTHRITIS
1-5 mg to 6400 mcg per day/for up to 2 months (T)

*CARDIOVASCULAR/CORONARY
  HEART DISEASE*
2.5 mg to 10 mg per day for up to 6 weeks (T)

CERVICAL DYSPLASIA
10 mg per day for 3 months (T)

FRAGILE X SYNDROME
0.5 mg/kg to 10 mg per day (T)

GINGIVAL HEALTH
4 mg per day for 30 days (T)

HOMOCYSTINURIA
400 mcg per day for 70 days (T)

KIDNEY DAMAGE
10 mg per day for 3 months (T)

LITHIUM PROPHYLAXIS
200 mcg per day (T)

MULTIPLE SCLEROSIS
200 mcg to 300 mcg per day (T)

PREGNANCY
0.4 mg to 5 mg per day beginning prior to conception and continued up to 10-12 weeks of pregnancy (P) 2 mg to 5 mg per day from day 16 to 3 months (T)

ZINC ABSORPTION
400 mcg every other day for 16 weeks (T)

■ GLUTATHIONE

CANCER
8 g/m2 added to treatment with 100 mg/m2 of cisplatin every 21 days (T) 2.5 g to 5 g in 100-200 ml of normal saline of glutathione over 15 minutes before cisplatin treatment (T) 5 g per day (T)

INFERTILITY
600 mg intravenous every other day for 2 months (T)

■ INOSITOL

CARDIOVASCULAR/CORONARY HEART DISEASE
1.2 g 3 times per day for 4-6 weeks (T)

DEPRESSION
2 g per day though studies show higher (T)

DIABETES
6 g per day for 3 months (T)

OBSESSIVE COMPULSIVE DISORDER
4 g per day though studies show higher (T)

PANIC DISORDER
12 g per day 3 days (T)

RESPIRATORY DISTRESS SYNDROME
120 mg/kg to 160 mg/kg per day inravenous in infants with a birth weight less than 2000 g (P) 70 mg to 240 mg/kg per day in preterm infants (T)

■ IODINE

ANTIBACTERIAL EFFECTS
Povidone-iodine vaginal pessaries twice per day for 2 weeks (T) 1 mg per day though studies show higher (T)

THYROID FUNCTION
200 mg per day of iodized oil (T)

WOUND HEALING
1% povidone-iodine solution (T)

■ IRON

ANEMIA
30 mg to 60 mg per day/for up to 6 months (T)
200 mg intravenous per week for 5 months (T)

COGNITIVE FUNCTION
13 mg per day for 8 weeks (T)

■ MELATONIN

CANCER
10 mg to 50 mg per day (T)
20 mg per day intramuscular followed by 10 oral mg per day in patients experiencing remission (T)

JET LAG
5 mg every three days prior to flight, during flight, and once a day for three days after flight (T)

SLEEP
2 mg to 10 mg per night/for up to 4 weeks (T)

■ NAC

AIDS/HIV
3.7, 11, 33 and 100 mg/kg IV tiw or 6 weeks of oral 600, 1200, 2400 and 4800 mg qd for 6 weeks (T)

CARDIOVASCULAR/CORONARY HEART DISEASE
150 mg/kg-1 (T)
100 mg/kg intravenous (T)
15 g intravenous over a 24 hour period (T)
100 mg/kg followed by a continuos infusion of 20mg/kg (T)

CHRONIC BRONCHITIS
300 mg b.i.d (T)
15 mg/kg to 600 mg/kg per day/for up to 10 days (T)

GLUTATHIONE DEFICIENCY
6mmol/kg to 15 mg/kg per day/for up to 2 weeks (T)

LUNG DAMAGE
40 mg/kg per day intravenous for 72 hours (T)
200 mg t.i.d. for 8 weeks (T)

MUSCLE FATIGUE
150 mg/kg (T)

■ OLIVE OIL

*CARDIOVASCULAR/CORONARY
  HEART DISEASE*
50 g per day (T)

■ OMEGA FATTY ACIDS

ARTHRITIS
2.6 g per day of omega-3 fatty acids per day for
12 months (T)

CANCER
18 g of fish oil per day for 40 days (T)

*CARDIOVASCULAR/CORONARY
  HEART DISEASE*
24 g per day of omega-3 fatty acids for 4 weeks
(P)

DIABETES
3 g per day of omega-3 fatty acids for 8 weeks
(T)

■ PAPAIN

LUNG ABSCESS
Transthoracal injection of a 0.5% solution (T)

■ PANTOTHENIC ACID

HEPATITIS
90 mg to 180 mg per day of pantethein for 3-4
weeks (T)

LIVER DAMAGE
500 mg/kg of pantethine & 100 mg/kg of pantothenic acid for 5 days (T)

■ PHOSPHATIDYLSERINE

ALZHEIMER'S DISEASE
100 mg to 400 mg per day/for up to 12 weeks
(T)

BRAIN FUNCTION
100 mg to 300 mg per day/for up to 12 weeks
(T)

*CARDIOVASCULAR/CORONARY
  HEART DISEASE*
30 to 60 mg intravenous (T)

STRESS
50 to 800 mg per day/for up to 10 days (T)

■ POTASSIUM

*CARDIOVASCULAR/CORONARY
  HEART DISEASE*
2 mg to 100 mmol per day/for up to 2 months
(T)

■ PYCNOGENOL

*CARDIOVASCULAR/CORONARY
  HEART DISEASE*
150 mg per day of procyanidal oligongers preparation (T)

LIGHT VISION
200 mg per day of procyanidal oligongers preparation for 5 weeks (T)

■ SELENIUM

IMMUNE FUNCTION
200 mcg per day to 1500 mcg per week/for up
to 4 months (T)

MOOD
100 mcg per day for 5 weeks (T)

■ SUPEROXIDE DISMUTASE

BURNS
1000 units/kg intravenous within 6 hours of injury (T)

FANCONI ANAEMIA
25 mg/kg per day for 2 weeks (T)

MULTIPLE ORGAN FAILURE
3000 mg per day intravenous for 5 days (T)

■ VITAMIN A/BETA-CAROTENE

ACNE
0.025% vitamin A acid in gel form for 12 weeks (T)
300,000-400,000 IU retinol for 3-4 months (T)

AIDS/HIV
50,000 IU at 1 and 3 months; 100,000 IU at 6 and 9 months; 200,000 IU at 12 and 15 months (T) 60 mg to 180 mg per day of beta-carotene/ for up to 4 months (T)

ANEMIA
2.4 mg retinol (T)

BITOT'S SPOTS
100,000 or 200,000 IU every 6 months in children (T)

BLINDNESS
200,000 IU every 6 months in children (T)

CANCER
2.2 mmol per week of beta-carotene (P)
20 to 30 mg per day of beta-carotene/for up 9 months (P)
30,000 IU to 300,000 IU per day/for up to 12 months (T)

DARIER'S DISEASE
1 X 10(6) IU for 14 days (T)

HAIR LOSS
18,000 IU retinol per day (T)

IMMUNE ENHANCEMENT
30 mg of beta-carotene per day (T)
20 mg of beta-carotene per day for 2 weeks (T)

LIVER DAMAGE/DISEASE
25,000 to 50,000 IU per day for 4 to 12 weeks (T)

LUPUS
100,000 IU per day for 2 weeks (T)

MEASLES
400,000 IU (T)

PNEUMONIA
500,000 IU per day for one week (T)

RETINITIS PIGMENTOSA
15,000 IU per day

WARTS
Vitamin A acid (2% in petrolatum, 1 x day, topically) (T)

XEROPHTHALMIA
60 mg every 6 months (P)
200,000 IU twice a year (P)
50,000 IU-200,000 IU every 4 months (T)

■ VITAMIN B1

ALZHEIMER'S DISEASE
100 mg per day for 12 weeks (T)

CARDIOVASCULAR/CORONARY HEART DISEASE
50 mg/kg to 200 mg per day/for up to 3 months (T)

GENERAL
10 mg per day (T)

LACTIC ACIDOSIS
Two 400 mg doses (T)

LIVER DISEASE
50 mg per capita per day for 30 days (T)
200 mg per day (T)

■ VITAMIN B2

*CONGENITAL
    METHAEMOGLOBINAEMIA*
120 mg per day (T)

DEPRESSION
10 mg per day (T)

MIGRAINE
400 mg single oral dose (T)

SICKLE CELL DISEASE
5 mg twice a day for 8 weeks (T)

■ VITAMIN B6

ANEMIA
180 mg per day for 20 weeks (T)

ASTHMA
200 mg to 250 mg per day/for up to 6 weeks (T)

CARPAL TUNNEL SYNDROME
100 mg to 200 mg per day/for up to 12 weeks
(T)

IMMUNE FUNCTION
50 mg per day for 3 to 5 weeks (T)

INFANTILE SPASMS
0.2-0.4 g.kg-1 (T)
300 mg/kg per day for 4 weeks (T)

MEMORY
20 mg per day for 3 months (T)

PMS
40 to 200 mg per day (T)

PREGNANCY
25 mg every 8 hours for 72 hours (T)

■ VITAMIN B12

AIDS/HIV
250 pg/ml per day (T)

METHYLMALONIC ACIDEMIA
1 mg intravenous on alternate days followed by
15 mg per day oral in infants (T)

MULTIPLE SCLEROSIS
60 mg per day for 6 months (T)

SLEEP
3000 mcg per day (T)
1.5 mg per day t.i.d. (T)

■ VITAMIN C

AGING
2 g per day (T)

AIDS/HIV
50 g to 200 g per 24 hours (T)

ALCOHOL TOXICITY
1 g per day for 3 days (T)

ASTHMA
1 g per day for 6 months (T)

AUTISM
8 g/70 kg per day for 30 weeks (T)

CANCER
1 g to 10 g per day/for up to 9 months (T)

CARDIOVASCULAR/CORONARY HEART DISEASE
60 mg to 2 g per day (T/P)

DIABETES
500 mg to 2 g per day/for up to 3 months (T)

FERTILITY
200 mg per day (T)

GENERAL
2 g per day (T)

GLUTATHIONE DEFICIENCY
0.7 mmol/kg per day for 1-2 weeks (T)

HEPATITIS
300 mg per day (T)

HERPES
500 mg to 1 g per day/for up to 6 weeks (T)

HTLV-I ASSOCIATED MYELOPATHY (HAM)
1.5 g to 3 g per day for 3 to 5 days (T)

IMMUNE ENHANCEMENT
2 g to 3 g per day (T)

IRON ABSORPTION
1500 mg per day for 5 weeks (T)

MENOPAUSE
200 mg following each meal for 2 weeks plus another 100 mg 4 times per day for 4 weeks (T)

NEUTROPHIL DYSFUNCTION
500 mg per day for 30 days (T)

OBESITY
3 g per day for 6 weeks (T)

RESPIRATION
600 mg to 2 g per day (T)

SMOKING CESSATION
300 mg per day

TETANUS
1000 mg per day intravenous

WOUND HEALING
500 to 3000 mg per day

■ VITAMIN D

BONE LOSS
400 IU to 21,000 IU per day/for up to two years (T)

CANCER
3.75 mcg per day (T)

CARDIOVASCULAR/CORONARY HEART DISEASE
1 mcg per day for 6 months (T)

CROHN'S DISEASE
1000 IU per day for 1 year (T)

DIABETES
10,000 IU per day though studies show higher (T)

NEPHROTIC SYNDROME
25 mcg per day (T)

OSTEOPOROSIS
800 IU per day (P)

PREGNANCY
1000 IU per day (P)

■ VITAMIN E

ABETALIPOPROTEINEMIA
800 mg per day though studies show higher (T)

ACNE
10 mg of tocopheryl succinate twice daily for 6-12 weeks (T)

ANEMIA
600 mg per day for 30 days (T)

BREAST IMPLANTS
1000 IU, b.i.d. beginning a week after surgery and lasting for up to 2 years (T)

CANCER
100 IU to 2500 IU per day (T/P)

CARDIOVASCULAR/CORONARY
   HEART DISEASE
300 mg to 900 mg per day/for up to 5 months (T)
200 IU to 1600 IU per day/for up to 2 years (T)

CHOLESTASIS
50-100 mg intravenous every 3 to 7 days for 32 months (T)
15-25 IU/kg per day (P)
25 IU/kg per day for 2.5 years (T)
0.8 to 2.0 IU/kg intramuscular per day (T)

DIABETES
200 mg to 1 g per day/for up to 4 months (T)

EPILEPSY
400 IU per day (T)
600 mg per day (T)

GENERAL
200 mg per day for 4 month (T)
300 IU to 800 IU per day/for up to 6 months (T)

GLUTATHIONE SYNTHESIS
1000 IU per day (T)

HEMOLYSIS
800 IU per day for 2 months (T)
300 mg per day (T)

HEPATITIS
200 mg per day for 10 days (T)

HOMOZYGOUS BETA-THALASSEMIA
300 mg per day 15 days (T)

IMMUNE ENHANCEMENT
25 mg/kg to 800 mg per day/for up to 30 days (T/P)

LEG CRAMPS
400 IU per day (T)

MYOTONIC DYSTROPHY
600 mg per day (T)

NEWBORNS
20 mg/kg to 120 mg/kg per day intramuscular soon after birth (P)

OSTEOARTHRITIS
400 mg to 400 IU per day/for up to 3 weeks (T)

PHYSICAL PERFORMANCE
2 x 200 mg per day for 10 weeks (T)

PMS
150 IU to 600 IU per day (T)

PROLIFERATIVE
   VITREORETINOPATHY
100 microM (T)

RESPIRATION
900 IU per day for 6 weeks (T)

RETROLENTAL FIBROPLASIA
100 mg per day (T)

SEXUAL FUNCTION
300 mg per day for 8 weeks (T)

SHORT BOWEL SYNDROME
400 IU per day (T)

SMOKING
800 mg per day for two weeks (T)

SPONDYLOSIS
100 mg per day for three weeks (T)

STRESS
1200 mg per day for 14 days (P)

TARDIVE DYSKINESIA
1600 IU per day for 6 weeks (T)

ULCERATIVE COLITIS
3 g per day (T)

■ VITAMIN K

*CARDIOVASCULAR/CORONARY
HEART DISEASE*
10 mg intramuscular every 5 days prior to delivery (P)

■ ZINC

ACNE
75-150 mg per day of zinc sulphate though studies show higher (T)

ACRODERMATITIS ENTEROPATHICA
50 mg t.i.d single dose (T)
100 mg per day up to the age of 2.5 years (T)

AIDS/HIV
200 mg per day (T)

ALCOHOL CIRRHOSIS
200 mg per day of zinc sulphate (T)

ANOREXIA
45-90 mg per day (T)
40 mumol per day intravenous for 7 days, reduced to oral intake of 15 mg per day for 60 days (T)

ARTHRITIS
60-150 mg per day of zinc sulphate/for up to 6 months though studies show higher (T)

BIRTH WEIGHT
25 mg per day (P)

CANCER
250 mg oral zinc gluconate per day (T) over 3 week period

*CARDIOVASCULAR/CORONARY
HEART DISEASE*
50-75 mg per day for 12 weeks (T)
60-150 mg per day of zinc sulphate though studies show higher (T)

CHILDHOOD GROWTH
3 mg to 2 mg/kg per day/for up to 6 months (T)

COMMON COLD
Lozenge every two hours containing 13.3 mg (T)

DIAPER RASH
10 mg per day for 4 months (T)

DIARRHEA
20 mg per day (T)

ECZEMA
220 mg oral per day (T)

GONADAL FUNCTION
50 mg per day for 6 months (T)

HERPES
4% topical solution (T)

IMMUNE ENHANCEMENT
440 mg per day (T)

MALE INFERTILITY
60-150 mg per day of zinc sulphate though studies show higher (T)

OBESITY
600 mg per day (T)

ULCERS (LEG)
Gauze compress medicated with 400 mcg of zinc oxide (T)

WILSON'S DISEASE
150 mg to 220 mg per day (T)

HERBAL SUPERSTARS

◼ ALOE

CONTRACEPTION
7.5% and 10% concentrations of lyophilized aloe barbadensis (P)

DIABETES
1/2 teaspoon per day for 4-14 weeks

◼ GARLIC

AIDS/HIV
5 g per day of aged garlic extract for 6 weeks followed by 6 weeks of 10 g per day (T)

*CARDIOVASCULAR/CORONARY
  HEART DISEASE*
10 g of raw garlic per day following breakfast for two months (T) 600 mg to 900 mg of garlic powder per day/for up to 4 months (T) 1.3% allicin at a 2400 mg dose (T)
One fresh clove of garlic per day for 16 weeks (T)

◼ GINKGO BILOBA

ANTI-CLASTOGENIC EFFECTS
120 mg per day for 2 months (T)

BRAIN FUNCTION
150 mg to 600 mg per day (T)

*CARDIOVASCULAR/CORONARY
  HEART DISEASE*
50 mg to 240 mg per day/for up to 12 weeks (T)

CLAUDICATION
120 mg per day for 3 months

NEUROPATHY
87.5 mg intravenous for 4 days

◼ GINSENG

BLOOD ALCOHOL CLEARANCE
3 g/65 kg 40 minutes after last drink (T)

DIABETES
50 to 200 mg per day for 8 weeks

IMMUNE FUNCTION
One capsule every 12 hours for 8 weeks of either 100 mg of aqueous ginseng extract or 100 mg of standardized extract

◼ TURMERIC

*CARDIOVASCULAR/CORONARY
  HEART DISEASE*
500 mg per day for 7 days (T)

◼ YOHIMBINE

*CARDIOVASCULAR/CORONARY
  HEART DISEASE*
5 mg per day (T)

DEPRESSION
4 mg/t.i.d. (T)

NARCOLEPSY
8 mg/kg per day (T)

SEXUAL FUNCTION
15 mg to 42 mg per day/for up to 10 weeks (T)

ADDITIONAL HERBS

■ BLACK WALNUT

*CARDIOVASCULAR/CORONARY
HEART DISEASE*
84 g per day (T)

■ CRANBERRY

URINARY TRACT INFECTION
4 ounces to 16 ounces of cranberry juice per day/
for up to 7 weeks (T) 300 ml per day of cranberry
juice (T)

■ DWARF/SAW PALMETTO

BENIGN PROSTATIC HYPERPLASIA
160 mg twice a day for 3 months (T)

■ EVENING PRIMROSE OIL

ARTHRITIS
20 ml per day for 12 weeks (T)
6 g per day (T)

DIABETES
4 g per day for 4 weeks (T)

■ FLAX

*CARDIOVASCULAR/CORONARY
HEART DISEASE*
40 g of flaxseed oil per day for 23 days

GENERAL
50 g per day of flaxseed for 4 weeks

LUPUS
30 g flaxseed per day (T)

■ HAWTHORN

*CARDIOVASCULAR/CORONARY
HEART DISEASE*
600 mg per day of Hawthorn Extract LI 132 for
8 weeks (T)
100 mg of Crataegus pinnatifida leaves for 4
weeks (T)
600 mg of Crataegus extract for 8 weeks (T)

■ LOVAGE

*CARDIOVASCULAR/CORONARY
HEART DISEASE*
3 g to 9 g daily as an oral decoction, extract, or
tincture (T)

■ PUMPKIN

ACUTE SCHISTOSOMIASIS
80 g of pumpkin seeds 3 times per day for 1
month (T)

■ ST. JOHN'S WORT

DEPRESSION
100 mg to 900 mg per day (T)

■ STINGING NETTLE

BENIGN PROSTATIC HYPERPLASIA
300 mg of Urtica dioica root extract per day for
8 weeks (T)

■ VALERIAN

SLEEP
450 mg and 900 mg per day (T)

THERAPEUTIC AMINO ACIDS

■ ARGININE

CANCER
30 g per day for 3 days (T)

*CARDIOVASCULAR/CORONARY
HEART DISEASE*
5.6 g to 21 g per day/for up to 6 weeks (T)
500 mg/kg to 20 g intravenous (T)

HEPATITIS
3 x 400 tablets mg of arginine tidiacicate over a period of 30 days (T)

MALE INFERTILITY
80 ml of 10% L-arginine HCL daily per os over 6 month period (T)

PAIN
10% solution, 300 ml (30 g)/patient L-arginine intravenous over a 60-70 minute period (T)

■ ASPARTIC ACID

OPIATE ADDICTION
8 g for 7 days following the appearance of opiate withdrawal (T)

■ GLUTAMIC ACID

CANCER
4 g swish and swallow twice per day beginning first day of chemotherapy for up to 28 days (T)

NEUROTOXICITY
1500 mg per day (T)

■ GLYCINE

SCHIZOPHRENIA
0.4-0.8 g/kg/day (T)

■ ORNITHINE

AGING
10 g ornithine oxoglutarate per day for 2 months (T)

CANCER
18 g per day of oral alpha-difluoromethylornithine for 1 month (T)

ENCEPHALOPATHY
34 mmol per day of ornithine salts for 7-10 (T)

■ TYROSINE

DEPRESSION
3,200 mg per day (T)

ESSENTIAL AMINO ACIDS

■ ISOLEUCINE

AMYOTROPHIC LATERAL SCLEROSIS
8 g per day

■ LYSINE

BILIARY COLIC
1.8 g lysine acetylsalicylate via intravenous bolus (T)

HERPES
936 mg to 3,000 per day/for up to 12 months (T)

RHEUMATIC DISORDERS
320 mg per day of ketoprofen lysine (T)

■ METHIONINE

PARACETAMOL POISONING
2 g to 5 g every 4 hours up to 10 total g beginning within ten hours of paracetamol overdose (T)

■ PHENYLALANINE

CANCER
250 mg 3 times per day for 15 days (T/P)

DEPRESSION
75 mg to 250 mg per day/for up to 30 days (T)

VITILIGO
50 mg/kg per day (T)

■ TRYPTOPHAN

DEPRESSION
2 to 8 g per day for 4 weeks (T)

MANIA
3 to 10 g per day for 1 week (T)

MENSTRUATION
6 g per day for luteal phase dysphoric disorder (T)

PAIN
3 g to 6 g per day (T)

PARKINSON'S DISEASE
150-450 mg per day (T)

SLEEP
1-15 g per day (T)

APPENDIX C

The peer review studies that follow are examples of what can happen when otherwise beneficial nutrients are misused. They are provided as a reminder that every individual is unique, as well as a warning to consult a licensed clinician prior to engaging in any therapeutic program of nutritional supplementation.

NUTRIENTS

■ BORON

This review article notes that boron is essential for the growth of many plants and is found in animal and human tissues at trace amounts. Boron poisoning has been reported in humans due to accidental ingestion or use of large doses for burn treatment. Normal levels of boron in soft tissues, urine, and blood range from less than 0.05 ppm to no more than 10 ppm. In cases of poisoning, levels as high as 2000 ppm have been reported.

—R.F. Moseman, "Chemical Disposition of Boron in Animals and Humans," *Environ Health Perspect,* 102 (Suppl 7), November 1994, p. 113-117.

This review article notes that the improper use of boric acid containing antiseptics remains one the primary causes of toxic accidents among infants and newborn children. Such accidents often involve ingestion of insecticides and household products containing borates.

—C. Locatelli, et al., "Human Toxicology of Boron with Special Reference to Boric Acid Poisoning," *G Ital Med Lav,* 9(3-4), May-July 1987, p. 141-146.

This article notes that chronic low-level boron exposure has been shown to cause reduced growth, cutaneous disorders and suppression of male reproductive system function in animals.

—C. Minoia, et al., "Toxicology and Health Impact of Environmental Exposure to Boron. A Review," *G Ital Med Lav,* 9(3-4), May-July 1987, p. 119-124.

Results of this study showed that workers exposed to boron oxide experienced significantly greater levels of eye irritation, dryness of the mouth, nose, or throat, sore throat, and productive cough compared to non-exposed controls.

> —D.H. Garabrant, et al., "Respiratory and Eye Irritation from Boron Oxide and Boric Acid Dusts," *Journal Occup Med,* 26(8), August 1984, p. 584-586.

■ BROMELAIN

This article reports on the case of a 58-year-old pharmaceutical worker who frequently developed asthma and rhinitis when handling bromelain on the job. RAST and prick test showed strong positive reactions to bromelain, and inhalation test with 0.03 mg bromelain as well as peroral challenge by ingestion of 190 g pineapple led to asthmatic reactions.

> —X. Baur & G. Fruhmann, "Allergic Reactions, Including Asthma, to the Pineapple Protease Bromelain Following Occupational Exposure," *Clin Allergy,* 9(5), September 1979, p. 443-450.

This article reports on two cases of bronchial asthma resulting from bromelain inhalation.

> —F. Galleguillos & J.C. Rodriguez, "Asthma Caused by Bromelin Inhalation," *Clin Allergy,* 8(1), January 1978, p. 21-24.

This article reports on four cases of occupational allergy to bromelain by employees of a blood grouping laboratory.

> —G. Gailhofer, et al., "Asthma Caused by Bromelain: An Occupational Allergy," *Clinical Allergy,* 18(5), September 1988, p. 445-450.

This article reports on two cases of occupational allergy to bromelain with respiratory manifestations including allergic bronchial asthma.

> —G. Gailhofer, et al., "Allergic Bronchial Asthma Caused by Bromelin," *Derm Beruf Umwelt,* 35(5), September-October 1987, p. 174-176.

■ CALCIUM

This article reports on the case of severe soft tissue calcification with temporary loss of limb function in a patient with rhabdomyolysis-induced acute renal failure following a high dose of intravenous calcium to treat hypocalcemia

> —E.P. Thyssen, "Temporary Loss of Limb Function Secondary to Soft Tissue Calcification in a Patient with Rhabdomyolysis-induced Acute Renal Failure," *American Journal of Kidney Disease,* 16(5), November 1990, p. 491-494.

This article reports on the case of a 40-year-old woman with previous parathyroidectomy for adenoma who had a serum calcium level of 5.35 mmol l-1 following an inadvertent calcium overdose resulting from her belief that such high doses were beneficial.

> —N.H. McAlister, et al., "Unintentional Self-intoxication with Inorganic Calcium," *Journal of Internal Medicine,* 228(2), August 1990, p. 193-195.

This article reports on the cases of five infants who received 10% calcium gluconate via umbilical artery catheters that led to intestinal bleeding and lesions of the buttock, anus, groin, and thigh.

—L.S. Book, et al., ''Hazards of Calcium Gluconate Therapy in the Newborn Infant: Intra-arterial Injection Producing Intestinal Necrosis in Rabbit Ileum,'' *Journal of Pediatrics,* 92(5), May 1978, p. 793-797.

Results of this study indicated that parenteral calcium treatment in normotensive but moderately ill neonates can increase blood pressure and heart rate to undesirable levels.

—D.J. Salsburey & D.R. Brown, ''Effect of Parenteral Calcium Treatment on Blood Pressure and Heart Rate in Neonatal Hypocalcemia,'' *Pediatrics,* 69(5), May 1982, p. 605-609.

This article reports on the case of a 37-year-old female patient with postoperative hypoparathyroidism who had hypertension and elevated plasma renin activity and subsequent hyperaldosteronism during a two-month hypercalcemic period due to excessive calcium supplements and vitamin D.

—I. Yamamoto, et al., ''Reversible Hypertension Caused by Calcium Overloading in a Patient with Postoperative Hypoparathyroidism,'' *Endocrinol Jpn,* 29(6), December 1982, p. 725-731.

■ CHOLINE

This article notes that the intake of choline and lecithin have been shown to cause acute gastrointestinal distress, sweating, salivation, and anorexia.

—J.L. Wood & R.G. Allison, ''Effects of Consumption of Choline and Lecithin on Neurological and Cardiovascular Systems,'' *Fed Proc,* 41(14), December 1982, p. 3015-3021.

■ CHROMIUM

This article notes that animal studies have shown hexavalent chromium compounds can induce lung cancer while no such effects have been seen with trivalent chromium compounds. In humans, numerous harmful effects of airborne exposure to chromium, primarily in occupational settings, have been shown including irritative lesions of the skin and upper respiratory tract, allergic reactions, and cancers of the respiratory tract.

—World Health Organization, ''Chromium,'' *Environ Health Criteria,* 61, 1988, p. 1-197.

This review article notes that acute and chronic chromium toxicity are primarily attributable to hexavalent as opposed to trivalent compounds. Common detrimental effects include dermatitis, allergic and eczematous skin reactions, skin and mucous membrane ulcerations, perforation of the nasal septum, allergic asthmatic reactions, bronchial carcinomas, gastro-enteritis, hepatocellular deficiency, and renal oligo anuric deficiency.

—F. Baruthio, ''Toxic Effects of Chromium and its Compounds,'' *Biol Trace Elem Res,* 32, January-March 1992, p. 145-153.

This review article notes that hexavalent chromium compounds appear to be 10-100 times more toxic than the trivalent chromium compounds when administered orally.

 —S.A. Katz & H. Salem, "The Toxicology of Chromium with Respect to its Chemical Speciation: A Review," *Journal of Appl Toxicol,* 13(3), May-June 1993, p. 217-224.

■ COD LIVER OIL

This study examined the side effects of cod liver oil in atherogenic dyslipidemia patients. Results showed those patients taking the highest doses experienced the most severe side effects including aggravated chronic gastrointestinal, hepatic and pancreatic disorders.

 —A.L. Vertkin, et al., "Clinical Evaluation of Aiconol Side Effects," *Klin Med,* 72(1), 1994, p. 41-44.

Results of this study showed that unstabilized fish oils consumed as a source of n-3 fatty acids can cause exposure to toxic products of lipid peroxidation in humans.

 —L.A. Piche, et al., "Malondialdehyde Excretion by Subjects Consuming Cod Liver Oil vs a Concentrate of n-3 fatty Acids," *Lipids,* 23(4), April 1988, p. 370-371.

■ DEPRENYL

This article reports on the case of a 70-year-old Parkinson's patient who developed severe hypoglycemia resulting from treatment with selegiline.

 —M.J. Rowland, et al., "Hypoglycemia Caused by Selegiline, an Antiparkinsonian Drug: Can Such Side Effects be Predicted?" *Journal of Clinical Pharmacol,* 34(1), January 1994, p. 80-85.

Results of this study on the administration of selegiline as an adjunct to levodopa-carbidopa in 8 Parkinson's patients showed numerous adverse side effects associated with drug.

 —C.H. Waters, "Side Effects of Selegiline (Eldepryl), *Journal of Geriatric Psychiatry Neurol,* 5(1), January-March 1992, p. 31-34.

■ FOLIC ACID

This review article notes that oral folic acid is generally considered safe; however, studies have shown it to cause neurological injury in patients with undiagnosed pernicious anemia. The authors argue that folic acid should also be administered with care when prescribed to drug-treated epileptics because it has been shown to influence seizure control.

 —C.E. Butterworth, Jr. & T. Tamura, "Folic Acid Safety and Toxicity: A Brief Review," *American Journal of Clinical Nutrition,* 50(2), August 1989, p. 353-358.

This article reports on two cases who experienced an exacerbation of psychotic behavior during folic acid administration.

 —P. Prakash & W.M. Petrie, "Psychiatric Changes Associated with an Excess of Folic Acid," *American Journal of Psychiatry,* 139(9), September 1982, p. 1192-1193.

This article reports on the case of a 36-year-old anephric man who experienced hypersensitivity to folic acid when receiving a dose of 1 mg per day. The patient became febrile and pruritic with symptoms including fever, generalized pain, chills, and urticaria.

—G.P. Sesin & H. Kirschenbaum, "Folic Acid Hypersensitivity and Fever: A Case Report," *American Journal of Hosp Pharm,* 36(11), November 1979, p. 1565-1567.

■ HYDERGINE

This article reports on a case of a patient with Iatrogenic Ergot Vasospastic Angitis induced by the administration of hydergine.

—O.P. Kapoor, "Iatrogenic Ergot Vasospastic Angiitis. A Case Report," *Vasc Surg,* 10(1), January-February 1976, p. 58-60.

■ IODINE

This article reports on the case of a 34-year-old mediastinitis patient who received continuous povidone-iodine irrigation and absorbed toxic amounts of iodine at a level of 9,375 mcg/dl which led to metabolic acidosis, mental deterioration and eventual death.

—P.L. Glick, et al., "Iodine Toxicity in a Patient Treated by Continuous Povidone-iodine Mediastinal Irrigation," *Ann Thorac Surg,* 39(5), May 1985, p. 478-480.

This article reports on the case of a 6-week-old girl with transient congenital hypothyroidism associated with multiple applications of povidone iodine during pregnancy and lactation.

—Y. Danziger, et al., "Transient Congenital Hypothyroidism after Topical Iodine in Pregnancy and Lactation," *Arch Dis Child,* 62(3), March 1987, p. 295-296.

This article reports on the case of a 63-year-old woman with a multinodular goiter. Iodine-induced thyrotoxicosis developed after povidone-iodine was applied to the surface of a granulating hip wound.

—P.E. Reith & D.K. Granner, "Iodine-induced Thyrotoxicosis in a Woman with a Multinodular Goiter Taking Levothyroxine," *Arch Intern Med,* 145(2), February 1985, p. 355-356.

This article reports on the case of iodine poisoning in a patient with chronic obstructive pulmonary disease following 20 years of iodinated glycerol therapy.

—K. Geurian & C. Branam, "Iodine Poisoning Secondary to Long-term Iodinated Glycerol Therapy," *Arch Intern Med,* 154(10), May 23, 1994, p. 1153-1156.

This article reviews the scientific literature on adverse effects of iodine over the past 100 years. The authors note that excessive iodine exposure through foods, dietary supplements, topical medications, and/or iodinated contrast media has resulted in thyroiditis, goiter, hypothyroidism, hyperthyroidism, sensitivity reactions, or acute responses for some individuals.

—J.A. Pennington, "A Review of Iodine Toxicity Reports," *Journal of the American Diet Assoc,* 90(11), November 1990, p. 1571-1581.

■ IRON

This article reports on the case of a 19-year-old male emergency room patient requiring a gastrotomy to remove a large amount of elemental iron. At the time of the procedure, the patient's stomach showed full-thickness inflammation; the entire mucosal surface was hemorrhagic in nature.

  —R. Foxford & L. Goldfrank, ''Gastrotomy—A Surgical Approach to Iron Overdose,'' *Ann Emerg Med,* 14(12), December 1985, p. 1223-1226.

This article reviews the gastrointestinal effects of iron overdose in humans. The authors note that such effects may occur acutely or weeks later and generally occur in the stomach or proximal small bowel. Two adult cases are described, both ingesting enteric-coated iron preparations and suffering from protracted abdominal pain.

  —M. Tenenbein, et al., ''Gastrointestinal Pathology in Adult Iron Overdose,'' *Journal of Toxicol Clin Toxicol,* 28(3), 1990, p. 311-320.

This article notes that iron poisoning is the most common cause of overdose mortality in children under the age of 6. The case of a 22-month-old boy is described who accidentally ingested 50 ferrous sulfate tablets (60 mg elemental iron/tablet). During the child's first four days in the intensive care unit, he developed coma, metabolic acidosis, hypovolemic and cardiogenic shock, liver failure, coagulopathy and adult respiratory distress syndrome.

  —K. Cheney, et al., ''Survival After a Severe Iron Poisoning Treated with Intermittent Infusions of Deferoxamine,'' *Journal of Toxicol Clin Toxicol,* 33(1), 1995, p. 61-66.

This article notes that life-threatening iron overload may occur without severe anemia in patients with sideroblastic disorders.

  —T.E. Peto, et al., ''Iron Overload in Mild Sideroblastic Anaemias,'' *Lancet,* 1(8321), February 19, 1983, p. 375-378.

■ L-DOPA

This article reports on the case of a patient in which malignant melanoma developed in a benign nevus four months following L-Dopa treatment for Parkinson's disease.

  —A.S. Kochar, ''Development of Malignant Melanoma after Levodopa Therapy for Parkinson's Disease. Report of a Case and Review of the Literature,'' *American Journal of Medicine,* 79(1), July 1985, p. 119-121.

This article reports on the cases of 4 idiopathic Parkinson's disease patients who developed subacute confusional state, associated with delusions, hallucinations, and myoclonus following an increase in levodopa dosage.

  —M.Y. Neufeld, ''Periodic Triphasic Waves in Levodopa-induced Encephalopathy,'' *Neurology,* 42(2), February 1992, p. 444-446.

Results of this study found that young-onset Parkinson's patients showed significantly higher frequency for both dyskinesias and fluctuations after both 3 and 5 years of levodopa therapy relative to older-onset patients.

  —V. Kostic, et al., ''Early Development of Levodopa-induced Dyskinesias and Response

Fluctuations in Young-onset Parkinson's Disease,'' *Neurology,* 41(2 (Pt 1)), February 1991, p. 202-205.

■ NAC

This study examined the effects of NAC on nitroglycerin-induced headache and dilation of temporal and radial arteries in healthy subjects. Results showed that NAC potentiated headache response and potentiated temporal artery dilation.

—H.K. Iversen, ''N-acetylcysteine Enhances Nitroglycerin-induced Headache and Cranial Arterial Responses,'' *Clin Pharmacol Ther,* 52(2), August 1992, p. 125-133.

Results of this study showed that intravenous administration of NAC following paracetamol poisoning produced symptoms of skin rash in 14% of the 56 Chinese patients studied.

—T.Y. Chan & J.A. Critchley, ''Adverse Reactions to Intravenous N-acetylcysteine in Chinese Patients with paracetamol (acetaminophen) Poisoning,'' *Hum Exp Toxicol,* 13(8), August 1994, p. 542-544.

This article reports on seven patients with adverse allergic reactions to NAC in the from of Parvolex.

—D.N. Bateman, et al., ''Adverse Reactions to N-acetylcysteine,'' *Hum Toxicol,* 3(5), October 1984, p. 393-398.

This article reports on the case of a 2 1/2-year-old girl who developed status epilepticus and cortical blindness as a result of N-acetylcysteine treatment for paracetamol overdose.

—E. Hershkovitz, et al., ''Status Epilepticus Following Intravenous N-acetylcysteine Therapy,'' *Isr Journal of Medical Science,* 32(11), November 1996, p. 1102-1104.

This article reports on 7 cases of allergic reactions to NAC in patients being treated with the drug intravenously following acetaminophen overdose. All patients were pruritic and reactions consisted of skin rashes and urticaria and/or angioedema.

—M. Tenenbein, ''Hypersensitivity-like Reactions to N-acetylcysteine,'' *Vet Hum Toxicol,* 26 (Suppl 2), 1984, p. 3-5.

■ OLIVE OIL

This article reports on two cases of hypersensitivity to olive oil.

—T. van Joost, et al., ''Sensitization to Olive Oil (olea europeae),'' *Contact Dermatitis,* 7(6), November 1981, p. 309-310.

■ PABA

This article reports on the case of a patient who developed allergic photocontact dermatitis following the use of a commercial sunscreen preparation containing PABA.

—C.G. Mathias, et al., ''Allergic Contact Photodermatitis to Para-aminobenzoic Acid,'' *Arch Dermatol,* 114(11), November 1978, p. 1665-1666.

This article reports on the case of a 6-year-old girl who developed allergic photocontact dermatitis following the use of a commercial sunscreen preparation containing PABA.

—T. Horio & T. Higuchi, "Photocontact Dermatitis from P-aminobenzoic Acid," *Dermatologica,* 156(2), 1978, p. 124-128.

■ PAPAIN

This article reports on the case of a patient who experienced a severe systemic allergic reaction following the consumption of meat tenderizer. Further examination revealed that the reaction was mediated by IgE antibody to papain, an ingredient of the tenderizer.

—L.E. Mansfield & C.H. Bowers, "Systemic Reaction to Papain in a Nonoccupational Setting," *Journal of Allergy Clin Immunol,* 71(4), April 1983, p. 371-374.

This article reports on the case of a non-atopic worker in a factory involved in the packing of papain powder who experienced late-onset asthma following his first exposure to papain dust. Such symptoms stopped when he was not exposed to the papain.

—M.L. Flindt, "Respiratory Hazards from Papain," *Lancet,* 8061, February 27, 1985, p. 430-432.

This article reports on the case of a patient who developed life-threatening anaphylaxix following occupational exposure to papain. The patient's symptoms included urticaria, angioedema, glottic symptoms, intermittent problems mimicking rheumatoid, gastrointestinal, cardiac, and pulmonary disease.

—H.B. Freye, "Papain Anaphylaxis: A Case Report," *Allergy Proc,* 9(5), September-October 1988, p. 571-574.

This article reports on findings from one pharmaceutical plant where 12 of 23 employees experienced respiratory symptoms associated with exposure to papain.

—H.S. Novey, et al., "Pulmonary Disease in Workers Exposed to Papain: Clinico-physiological and Immunological Studies," *Clin Allergy,* 10(6), November 1980, p. 721-731.

This article reports on the study of 7 of 11 workers occupationally exposed to airborne papain who experienced immediate hypersensitive reactions consisting primarily of rhinitis and asthma.

—X. Baur & G. Fruhmann, "Papain-induced Asthma: Diagnosis by Skin Test, RAST and Bronchial Provocation Test," *Clin Allergy,* 9(1), 1979, p. 75-81.

■ POTASSIUM

This article reports on the case of a 77-year-old male who developed extreme hyperkalemia following treatment with a potassium saving diuretic in combination with potassium supplementation.

—B. Hylander, "Survival of Extreme Hyperkalemia," *Acta Med Scand,* 221(1), 1987, p. 121-123.

This article reports on the cases of two patients with underlying heart disease who suffered cardiac arrest following the administration of oral potassium.

—H.N. Hultgren, et al., "Cardiac Arrest Due to Oral Potassium Administration," *American Journal of Medicine,* 58(1), January 1975, p. 139-142.

This article reports on the case of a patient whose electrocardiogram became highly abnormal and developed hypotension while being administered potassium and disopyramide.

—B.D. Maddux & R.B. Whiting, "Toxic Synergism of Disopyramide and Hyperkalemia," *Chest,* 78(4), October 1980, p. 654-656.

This article reports on the cases of two patients who developed severe hyperkalemia and cardiac arrhythmia following excessive intake of potassium-containing salt substitutes.

—V. Yap, et al., "Hyperkalemia with Cardiac Arrhythmia. Induction by Salt Substitutes, Spironolactone, and Azotemia," *JAMA,* 236(24), December 13, 1976, p. 2775-2776.

This article reports on the case of a Bartter's syndrome patient who developed severe hyperkalemia following treatment with a combination of indomethacin and potassium chloride supplementation.

—F. Akbarpour, et al., "Severe Hyperkalemia Caused by Indomethacin and Potassium Supplementation," *Southern Medical Journal,* 78(6), June 1985, p. 756-757.

■ QUERCETIN

Results of this study showed that the IP injection of quercetin led to sperm abnormalities in mice.

—P.B. Rastogi & R.E. Levin, "Induction of Sperm Abnormalities in Mice by Quercetin," *Environ Mutagen,* 9(1), 1987, p. 79-86.

■ S-ADENOSYLMETHIONINE

Results of this study showed that S-Adenosyl-L-methionine caused hypokinesia, tremor, rigidity, and abnormal posture in rats.

—B.G. Crowell, Jr., et al., "S-adenosyl-L-methionine Decreases Motor Activity in the Rat: Similarity to Parkinson's Disease-like Symptoms," *Behav Neural Biol,* 59(3), May 1993, p. 186-193.

Results of this study found that excess brain levels of SAMe induces symptoms in rats similar to those associated with Parkinson's Disease in human subjects.

—C.G. Charlton & B. Crowell, Jr., "Parkinson's Disease-like Effects of S-adenosyl-L-methionine: Effects of L-dopa," *Pharmacol Biochem Behav,* 43(2), October 1992, p. 423-431.

■ SELENIUM

This article reports on two cases of selenium poisoning in children. Both developed severe cystic fibrosis and one died.

—W. Snodgrass, et al., "Selenium: Childhood Poisoning and Cystic Fibrosis," *Clin Toxicol,* 18(2), February 1981, p. 211-220.

This article reports on the case of a 17-year-old male who committed suicide by ingesting excessive amounts of selenium. Autopsy results showed congestion of lungs and kidneys, diffuse swelling of the heart, brain edema, and orange-brown discoloration of the skin and all viscera. Selenium blood and tissue levels exceeded normal range by a factor of 100-1000.
—C. Koppel, et al., "Fatal Poisoning with Selenium Dioxide," *Journal of Toxicol Clin Toxicol,* 24(1), 1986, p. 21-35.

This article reports on the case of a patient who developed hypothyroidism following the intravenous administration of large doses of selenite as a treatment for sepsis secondary to pneumonia.
—L.C. Hofbauer, et al., "Selenium-induced Thyroid Dysfunction," *Postgraduate Medical Journal,* 73(856), February 1997, p. 103-104.

Results of this Italian epidemiological study indicated a positive association between overexposure to selenium via drinking water and the incidence of amyotrophic lateral sclerosis.
—M. Vinceti, et al., "Amyotrophic Lateral Sclerosis after Long-term Exposure to Drinking Water with High Selenium Content," *Epidemiology,* 7(5), September 1996, p. 529-532.

■ VITAMIN A/BETA-CAROTENE

This review article notes that studies have shown that the intake of 25,000-50,000 IU per day of vitamin A for several months or longer can lead to numerous adverse effects. Lower doses of the vitamin have been shown to cause toxicity in children, pregnant women, and in patients with pre-existing liver problems.
—J.N. Hathcock, et al., "Evaluation of Vitamin A Toxicity," *American Journal of Clinical Nutrition,* 52(2), August 1990, p. 183-202.

This article reports on the case of a patient with severe hepatotoxicity due to the intake of 25,000 IU of vitamin A per day in the form of over-the-counter supplements.
—T.E. Kowalski, et al., "Vitamin A Hepatotoxicity: A Cautionary Note Regarding 25,000 IU Supplements," *American Journal of Medicine,* 97(6), December 1994, p. 523-528.

This article reports on the case of a neonate who died following intake of 60 times the daily suggested dose of vitamin A over an 11 day period. Complications resulting from the toxicity included hypercalcemia, hyperphosphatemia, a bleeding disorder, and pulmonary insufficiency.
—M.E. Bush & B.B. Dahms, "Fatal Hypervitaminosis A in a Neonate," *Arch Pathol Lab Med,* 108(10), October 1984, p. 838-842.

Results of this large-scale, double-blind, placebo-controlled study showed an increased 2-week prevalence of diarrhea, rhinitis, cold/flu, cough, and rapid breathing in Haitian children between the ages of 6-83 months following a megadose of supplemental vitamin A.
—S.K. Stansfield, et al., "Vitamin A Supplementation and Increased Prevalence of Childhood Diarrhoea and Acute Respiratory Infections," *Lancet,* 342(8871), September 4, 1993, p. 578-582.

Results of these two trials indicated that beta-carotene supplementation was associated with an increased incidence of lung cancer among smokers in both Finland and the United States.

—L.M. De Luca & S.A. Ross, ''Beta-carotene Increases Lung Cancer Incidence in Cigarette Smokers,'' *Nutr Rev,* 54(6), June 1996, p. 178-179.

■ VITAMIN B1

This article reports on the case of a patient who developed anaphylaxis following the emergency room administration of intravenous thiamine.

—J.M. Stephen, et al., ''Anaphylaxis from Administration of Intravenous Thiamine,'' *American Journal of Emergency Medicine,* 10(1), January 1992, p. 61-63.

Results of this study found that infants dying from sudden infant death syndrome had significantly higher serum levels of thiamine relative to control infants dying from other causes.

—R.E. Davis, et al., ''High Serum Thiamine and the Sudden Infant Death Syndrome,'' *Clin Chim Acta,* 123(3), August 18, 1982, p. 321-328.

This article reports on the case of a patient demonstrating incompatibility following the parenteral administration of a vitamin B1 containing medicament.

—R. Kolz, et al., ''Intolerance Reactions Following Parenteral Administration of Vitamin B,'' *Hautarzt,* 31(12), December 1980, p. 657-659.

■ VITAMIN B6

This article reports on the case of an 81-year-old female patient with mixed motor and sensory neuropathy caused by excessive intake of pyridoxine as a treatment for carpal tunnel syndrome.

—F.J. Foca, ''Motor and Sensory Neuropathy Secondary to Excessive Pyridoxine Ingestion,'' *Arch Phys Med Rehabil,* 66(9), September 1985, p. 634-636.

This article reports on the case of female patient with sensory neuropathy resulting from long-term ingestion of pyridoxine.

—J.A. Waterston & B.S. Gilligan, ''Pyridoxine Neuropathy,'' *Medical Journal of Aust,* 146(12), June 15, 1987, p. 640-642.

This article reports on seven adults cases of ataxia and severe sensory-nervous-system dysfunction resulting from daily intake of high levels of vitamin B6.

—H. Schaumburg, et al., ''Sensory Neuropathy from Pyridoxine Abuse. A New Megavitamin Syndrome,'' *New England Journal of Medicine,* 309(8), August 25, 1983, p. 445-448.

This article reports on two cases of permanent sensory deficit after treatment with excessive doses of parenteral pyridoxine.

—R.L. Albin, et al., ''Acute Sensory Neuropathy-neuronopathy from Pyridoxine Overdose,'' *Neurology,* 37(11), November 1987, p. 1729-1732.

This article reports on 16 cases of neuropathy associated with pyridoxine abuse.

> —G.J. Parry & D.E. Bredesen, ''Sensory Neuropathy with Low-dose Pyridoxine,'' *Neurology,* 35(10), October 1985, p. 1466-1468.

■ VITAMIN B 12

This article reports on the case of an acne patient with an eruption of acne rosacea following ingestion of a high dose vitamin B complex supplement.

> —E.F. Sherertz, ''Acneiform Eruption Due to Megadose Vitamins B6 and B12,'' *Cutis,* 48(2), August 1991, p. 119-120.

This article reports on the case of a patient who experienced an allergic reaction to vitamin B12 which manifested itself in terms of eczematous and exanthematic skin lesions following long-term intake of high doses.

> —I. Pevny, et al., ''Vitamin B 12-(cyanocobalamin)-allergy,'' *Hautarzt,* 28(11), November 1977, p. 600-603.

■ VITAMIN C

This article reports on the case of a patient receiving a single intravenous dose of 45 g of ascorbic acid for treatment of primary amyloidosis and the nephrotic syndrome who experienced acute oliguric renal failure.

> —J.M. Lawton , et al., ''Acute Oxalate Nephropathy after Massive Ascorbic Acid Administration,'' *Arch Intern Med,* 145(5), May 1985, p. 950-951.

This article reports on a patient with severe dental erosion attributable to three years of daily chewing of vitamin C tablets.

> —J.L.Giunta, ''Dental Erosion Resulting from Chewable Vitamin C Tablets,'' *Journal of the American Dental Association,* 107(2), August 1983, p. 253-256.

This article reports on the case of a patient with vitamin C allergy of the delayed type with eczematous skin lesions appearing as a reaction to vitamin C consumed in normal dietary foods. Lesions disappeared following the intake of a vitamin C-free diet.

> —J. Metz, et al., ''Vitamin C Allergy of the Delayed Type,'' *Contact Dermatitis,* 6(3), April 1980, p. 172-174.

Results of this study showed that the overconsumption of vitamin C can result in excessive serum levels causing hyperoxalemia that may contribute to vascular disease in chronic hemodialysis patients.

> —C. Pru, et al., ''Vitamin C Intoxication and Hyperoxalemia in Chronic Hemodialysis Patients,'' *Nephron,* 39(2), 1985, p. 112-116.

This article reports on two cases of Hodgkin's disease and one of bronchial carcinoma where high levels of vitamin C therapy was associated with the onset of dangerous symptoms.

> —A. Campbell & T. Jack, ''Acute Reactions to Mega Ascorbic Acid Therapy in Malignant Disease,'' *Scott Med Journal,* 24(2), April 1979, p. 151-153.

■ VITAMIN D

This article reports on 4 cases of hypervitaminosis D in patients with osteoporosis or osteomalacia who were administered pharmacologic doses of vitamin D and became hypercalcemic with acute renal failure.

> —M.S. Schwartzman & W.A. Franck, "Vitamin D Toxicity Complicating the Treatment of Senile, Postmenopausal, and Glucocorticoid-induced Osteoporosis. Four Case Reports and a Critical Commentary on the Use of Vitamin D in these Disorders," *American Journal of Medicine,* 82(2), February 1987, p. 224-230.

This article reports on the case of a rheumatoid arthritis patient with widespread joint and periarticular calcinosis resulting from supplemental vitamin D.

> —R.C. Butler, et al., "Calcinosis of Joints and Periarticular Tissues Associated with Vitamin D Intoxication," *Ann Rheum Disease,* 44(7), July 1985, p. 494-498.

This article reports on the case of a 43-year-old man with alopecia maligna who received a total of 130 mg vitamin D3 per day for 4 weeks. Two weeks following the end of treatment and after extreme sun exposure, the patient suffered from a hypercalcaemic crisis and died 5 weeks later of acute cardiac failure.

> —F. Laubenthal, et al., "Fatal Vitamin D Intoxication," *Dtsch Med Wochenschr,* 100(9), February 28, 1975, p. 412-415.

This review article notes that the excess consumption of vitamin D can lead to hypercalcemia and that symptoms of this condition include feeding difficulties, polydypsia, polyuria, irritability, lassitude and poor weight gain. A concentration of 100 IU (2.5 g) of vitamin D per 100 kcal ingested is the current (1989) recommended dose provide by the Committee on Nutrition of the American Academy of Pediatrics.

> —R.W. Chesney, "Vitamin D: Can an Upper Limit be Defined?" *Journal of Nutrition,* 119(12 Suppl), December 1989, p. 1825-1828.

■ VITAMIN E

This article reports on the author's own clinical experience involving 50 patients with thrombophlebitis involving the lower extremities brought on, at least in part, by large doses of self-prescribed vitamin E. The author discusses additional side effects associated with large doses of vitamin E including breast tenderness, elevation of blood pressure, a fatigue syndrome, myopathy, intestinal cramps, urticaria, and the possible aggravation of diabetes mellitus.

> —H.J. Roberts, "Thrombophlebitis Associated with Vitamin E Therapy. With a Commentary on other Medical Side Effects," *Angiology,* 30(3), March 1979, p. 169-177.

This article reports on the cases of two patients who developed a generalized erythema multiforme reaction following the topical use of vitamin E on scar tissue.

> —H. Saperstein, et al., "Topical Vitamin E as a Cause of Erythema Multiforme-like Eruption," *Arch Dermatol,* 120(7), July 1984, p. 906-908.

This article reports on two cases of postrhinoplasty epistaxis in patients taking massive doses of vitamin E.

—M.M. Churukian, et al., "Postrhinoplasty Epistaxis. Role of Vitamin E?" *Arch Otolaryngol Head Neck Surg,* 114(7), July 1988, p. 748-750.

This article reports on two cases of gross soft tissue calcification in premature babies following intramuscular administration of vitamin E for prevention of retinopathy of prematurity.

—M. Barak, et al., "Soft Tissue Calcification: A Complication of Vitamin E Injection," *Pediatrics,* 77(3), March 1986, p. 382-385.

This article reports on the cases of 4 adults who developed severe burning sensation and dermatitis following the administration of aloe vera or vitamin E preparations to a skin area that had previously been subjected to a chemical peel or dermabrasion.

—D. Hunter & A. Frumkin, "Adverse Reactions to Vitamin E and Aloe Vera Preparations after Dermabrasion and Chemical Peel," *Cutis,* 47(3), March 1991, p. 193-196.

■ VITAMIN K

This article reports on six cases of chronic liver disease patients who developed cutaneous reactions around the site of vitamin K injection administered as a treatment for the disease.

—A.W. Bullen, et al., "Skin Reactions Caused by Vitamin K in Patients with Liver Disease," *British Journal Dermatol,* 98(5), May 1978, p. 561-565.

This article reports on four patients who developed erytheamtous plaques following intravenous injections of vitamin K.

—M.N. Sanders & R.K. Winkelmann, "Cutaneous Reactions to Vitamin K," *Journal of the American Academy of Dermatology* 19(4), October 1988, p. 699-704.

Results of this study indicated that the administration of vitamin K can induce calcification of soft tissue in hemodialysis patients.

—D. Robert, et al., "Does Vitamin K Excess Induce Ectopic Calcifications in Hemodialysis Patients?" *Clin Nephrol,* 24(6), December 1985, p. 300-304.

This review article cites 52 cases of cutaneous adverse effects to vitamin K injections reported in the scientific literature between the years 1964-1994.

—I. Bruynzeel, et al., "Cutaneous Hypersensitivity Reactions to Vitamin K: 2 Case Reports and a Review of the Literature," *Contact Dermatitis,* 32(2), February 1995, p. 78-82.

This article reports on the case of a 70-year-old woman who developed enlarged annular erythematous plaques at the site of multiple intramuscular vitamin K injections prior to invasive diagnostic procedure.

—M.H. Kay & M. Duvic, "Reactive Annular Erythema after Intramuscular Vitamin K," *Cutis,* 37(6), June 1986, p. 445-448.

■ ZINC

This review article identifies the overt symptoms of zinc toxicity as nausea, vomiting, epigastric pain, lethargy, and fatigue with attendant symptoms of anemia and neutropenia, as well as impaired immune function.

—G.J. Fosmire, ''Zinc Toxicity,'' *American Journal of Clinical Nutrition,* 51(2), February 1990, p. 225-227.

This article reports on the case of a 24-year-old man who accidentally ingested liquid zinc chloride and subsequently suffered from symptoms including erosive pharyngitis, esophagitis, nausea, vomiting, abdominal pain, lethargy, confusion, hypocalcemia and hyperamylasemia.

—S.J. Chobanian, ''Accidental Ingestion of Liquid Zinc Chloride: Local and Systemic Effects,'' *Ann Emerg Med,* 10(2), February 1981, p. 91-93.

This article reports on the case of an adult patient suffering from copper deficiency following ingestion of excessive daily doses of zinc for up to 10 months. Symptoms associated with the condition included hypochromic-microcytic anemia, leukopenia, and neutropenia.

—H.N. Hoffman, et al., ''Zinc-induced Copper Deficiency,'' *Gastroenterology,* 94(2), February 1988, p. 508-512.

In this study, 11 healthy males received 300 mg per day of zinc for a period of six weeks. Results showed a reduction in lymphocyte stimulation response to phytohemagglutinin as well as chemotaxis and phagocytosis of bacteria by polymorphonuclear leukocytes.

—R.K. Chandra, ''Excessive Intake of Zinc Impairs Immune Responses,'' *JAMA,* 252(11), September 21, 1994, p. 1443-1446.

This article reports on the case of an adult sickle cell anemia patient who developed hypocupremia following two years of zinc administration as an antisickling agent.

—A.S Prasad, et al., ''Hypocupremia Induced by Zinc Therapy in Adults,'' *JAMA,* 240(20), November 10, 1978, p. 2166-2168.

HERBS

■ BEE PROPOLIS

This article notes that the number of allergic eczematous contact dermatitis cases has increased in recent years resulting, in part, from nonoccupational exposure to propolis in biocosmetics and other natural products. A case is described of a patient suffering from acute oral mucositis with ulceration caused by a lozenge containing propolis.

—K.D. Hay & D.E. Greig, ''Propolis Allergy: A Cause of Oral Mucositis with Ulceration,'' *Oral Surg Oral Med Oral Pathol,* 70(5), November 1990, p. 584-586.

This article presents 22 cases of patients suffering propolis-induced dermatitis.
> —E. Rudzki & Z.Grzywa, "Dermatitis from Propolis," *Contact Dermatitis,* 9(1), January 1983, p. 40-45.

This article reports on 6 cases of patients with propolis-induced contact dermatitis.
> —T.M. Schuler & P.J. Frosch, "Propolis-induced Contact Allergy," *Hautarzt,* 39(3), March 1988, 139-142.

■ CARROT

This article reports on the case of a 34-year-old female cook who experienced allergic rhinoconjunctivitis and contact urticaria in both hands associated with severe itching following the handling of raw carrots. In addition, she experienced anaphylactic episodes after accidentally eating raw carrots, but had no such reaction to the consumption of cooked carrots.
> —M. Gomez , et al., "Hypersensitivity to Carrot Associated with Specific IgE to Grass and Tree Pollens," *Allergy,* 51(6), June 1996, p. 425-429.

This article reports on the case of carrot addiction in a 49-year-old female under conditions of emotional stress. The authors suggest the source of the addiction is likely to be beta-carotene.
> —R. Kaplan, "Carrot Addiction," *Aust N Z Journal of Psychiatry,* 30(5), October 1996, p. 698-700.

This article reports on three cases of carotenoid dependence with symptoms including irritability and nervousness associated with abstinence. Each of the three patients were smokers and described their dependence as being similar to their addiction to tobacco.
> —L. Cerny & K. Cerny, "Can Carrots be Addictive? An Extraordinary Form of Drug Dependence," *British Journal of Addiction,* 87(8), August 1992, p. 1195-1197.

■ DANDELION

This article reports on 7 cases of dandelion dermatitis all of which measured positive to patch testing of dandelion extracts.
> —C.R. Lovell & M. Rowan, "Dandelion Dermatitis," *Contact Dermatitis,* 25(3), September 1991, p. 185-188.

■ GARLIC

This article reports on the case of an atopic patient who developed severe asthma following exposure to garlic dust as well as the ingestion of garlic.
> —J.A. Lybarger, et al., "Occupational Asthma Induced by Inhalation and Ingestion of Garlic," *Journal of Allergy Clin Immunol,* 69(5), May 1982, p. 448-454.

This article reports on the case of 49-year-old man with superficial pemphigus that appeared following garlic ingestion.

—V. Ruocco, et al., "A Case of Diet-related Pemphigus," *Dermatology,* 192(4), 1996, p. 373-374.

Results of this study found that the administration of garlic bulb aqueous extract over a period of 21 days caused toxic effects in male rats.

—B. Fehri, et al., "Toxic Effects Induced by the Repeat Administration of Allium Sativum L." *Journal of Pharm Belg,* 46(6), November-December 1991, p. 363-374.

This article reports on the case of a spontaneous spinal epidural hematoma causing paraplegia secondary to a qualitative platelet disorder following excessive intake of garlic.

—K.D. Rose, et al., "Spontaneous Spinal Epidural Hematoma with Associated Platelet Dysfunction from Excessive Garlic Ingestion: A Case Report," *Neurosurgery,* 26(5), May 1990, p. 880-882.

■ GINKGO BILOBA

This article reports on 3 cases of contact dermatitis from ginkgo fruit.

—R.R. Tomb, et al., "Mini-epidemic of Contact Dermatitis from Ginkgo Tree Fruit (Ginkgo biloba L.)," *Contact Dermatitis,* 19(4), October 1988, p. 281-283.

■ GINSENG

This article reports on 2 cases of ginseng poisoning. Symptoms included mydriasis and disturbance in accommodation of both eyes, dizziness and semiconsciousness.

—B.Y. Lou, et al., "Eye Symptoms Due to Ginseng Poisoning," *Yen Ko Hsueh Pao,* 5(3-4), December 1989, p. 96-97.

■ GREEN TEA

This article reports on 3 cases of workers in green tea factories who developed asthmatic and nasal symptoms following exposure to green tea dust. Further tests demonstrated that all 3 workers exhibited an immediate skin and bronchial response to EGCg, a component of the green tea leaves.

—T. Shirai, et al., "Epigallocatechin Gallate. The Major Causative Agent of Green Tea-induced Asthma," *Chest,* 106(6), December 1994, p. 1801-1805.

■ LICORICE

This article presents the case of a 36-year-old patient who developed signs of acute rhabdomyolysis following the consumption of five daily licorice sticks over a period of one month.

—A. Berlango Jimenez, et al., "Acute Rhabdomyolysis and Tetraparesis Secondary to Hypokalemia Due to Ingested Licorice," *An Med Interna,* 12(1), January 1995, p. 33-35.

This article reports on the case of a 72-year-old man who developed acute renal failure following severe hypokalemic rhabdomyolysis caused by excessive intake of glycyrrhizin.

> —A. Chubachi, et al., "Acute Renal Failure Following Hypokalemic Rhabdomyolysis Due to Chronic Glycyrrhizic Acid Administration," *Intern Medicine,* 31(5), May 1992, p. 708-711.

This article reports on the case of a 38-year-old woman who was hospitalized due to hypertension and hypokalaemic alkalosis resulting from the consumption of 200 g of licorice per day.

> —M.A. Seelen, et al., "Hypertension Caused by Licorice Consumption," *Ned Tijdschr Geneeskd,* 140(52), December 28, 1996, p. 2632-2635.

This article reports on the case of a 40-year-old female with severe hypertension and hypokalaemic metabolic alkalosis resulting from excessive licorice consumption.

> —J. Heikens, et al., "Liquorice-induced Hypertension—A New Understanding of an Old Disease: Case Report and Brief Review," *Neth Journal of Medicine,* 47(5), November 1995, p. 230-234.

■ MISTLETOE

This article reports on the case of a 49-year-old woman suffering from symptoms of nausea, general malaise, and a dull ache in the right hypochondrium. She presented with the same symptoms again two years later upon which time both illnesses were determined to have resulted from an herbal remedy containing kelp, motherwort, skullcap, and mistletoe. Mistletoe was singled out as the likely cause since it is the only constituent of the remedy that has been shown to contain potential toxins.

> —J. Harvey & D.G. Colin-Jones, "Mistletoe Hepatitis," *British Medical Journal,* 282(6259), January 17, 1981, p. 186-187.

■ SUNFLOWER

This article reports on the case of a man who developed rhinitis and conjunctivitis over a period of 5 years exposure to sunflower pollens, with the onset of asthma during the fifth year. While all such symptoms disappeared upon elimination of exposure, he did experience an allergic attack after consuming honey which contained 30% sunflower pollens.

> —J. Bousquet, et al., "Occupational Allergy to Sunflower Pollen," *Journal Allergy Clin Immunol,* 75(1 Pt 1), January 1985, p. 70-74.

■ TEA TREE OIL

This article reports on 4 adult patients with allergic contact dermatitis caused by 'tea tree' oil.

> —P.G. van der Valk, et al., "Allergic Contact Eczema Due to 'Tea Tree' Oil," *Ned Tijdschr Geneeskd,* 138(16), April 16, 1994, p. 823-825.

■ YOHIMBINE

This article reports on 3 cases of patients experiencing yohimbine-induced manic symptoms.
—L.H. Price, et al., "Three Cases of Manic Symptoms Following Yohimbine Administration," *American Journal of Psychiatry,* 141(10), October 1984, p. 1267-1268.

This article reports on the case of a 62-year-old male who ingested 100, 2.0 mg yohimbine tablets. Short-term symptoms included tachycardia, hypertension, and anxiety, but he appeared to suffer no long-term damage from the overdose.
—K. Friesen, et al., "Benign Course After Massive Ingestion of Yohimbine," *Journal of Emergency Medicine,* 11(3), May-June 1993, p. 287-288.

This article reports on the case of a 42-year-old male who developed a generalized erythrodermic skin eruption, progressive renal failure, and lupus-like syndrome following yohimbine therapy.
—B. Sandler & P. Aronson, "Yohimbine-induced Cutaneous Drug Eruption, Progressive Renal Failure, and Lupus-like Syndrome," *Urology,* 41(4), April 1993, p. 343-345.

AMINO ACIDS

■ ARGININE

This article reports on 2 cases of severe hepatic disease and moderate renal deficiency in which hyperkalemia developed during and after infusion with arginine monohydrochloride. The hyperkalemia was associated with fatal cardiac arrhythmia in one patient. The hyperkalemia in both was believed to be caused by an inability to metabolize the administered arginine and excrete the excess extracellular potassium.
—D.A. Bushinsky & F.J. Gennari, "Life-threatening Hyperkalemia Induced by Arginine," *Annals of Internal Medicine,* 89(5 Pt 1), November 1978, p. 632-634.

Results of this study indicated that subjects with low insulin secretion resulting from diabetes, stress, etc. could be at risk for developing pathological hyperkalaemia if given intravenous infusions of arginine.
—F. Massara, et al., "The Risk of Pronounced Hyperkalaemia after Arginine Infusion in the Diabetic Subject," *Diabete Metab,* 7(3), September 1981, p. 149-153.

■ GLYCINE

This article reports on the case of an immunological adverse reaction to the bladder irrigation fluid, glycine.
—P.E. Moskovits, et al., "A Red Patient: Immunological Reaction to Glycine?" *Anaesthesia,* 42(9), September 1987, p. 962-964.

Results of this study indicated that transurethral prostate resection or endometrial resection with hypotonic glycine can cause symptomatic hyponatremia that is hypo-osmolar and possibly prove fatal.

> —J.C. Ayus & A.I. Arieff, "Glycine-induced Hypo-osmolar Hyponatremia," *Arch Intern Med,* 157(2), January 27, 1997, p. 223-226.

The authors of this article report on a case of transient blindness after bilateral knee arthroscopy and suggest glycine toxicity may be the cause of the blindness following surgery.

> —S.S. Burkhart, et al. "Transient Postoperative Blindness as a Possible Effect of Glycine Toxicity," *Arthroscopy,* 6(2), 1990, p. 112-114.

This article reports on 2 cases of altered consciousness associated with nausea and vomiting following kidney surgery believed to have resulted from the transfer of large amounts of irrigating solution containing glycine 1.5%.

> —P. Tauzin-Fin, et al., "Glycine Poisoning after Percutaneous Kidney Surgery," *Canadian Journal of Anaesth,* 40(9), September 1993, p. 866-869.

■ ISOLEUCINE

Results of this long-term study found L-isoleucine and L-leucine to be promoters of bladder cancer in rats.

> —T. Kakizoe, et al., "L-Isoleucine and L-leucine are Promoters of Bladder Cancer in Rats," *Princess Takamatsu Symp,* 14, 1983, p. 373-380.

■ LEUCINE

Results of this long-term study found L-isoleucine and L-leucine to be promoters of bladder cancer in rats.

> —T. Kakizoe, et al., "L-Isoleucine and L-leucine are Promoters of Bladder Cancer in Rats," *Princess Takamatsu Symp,* 14, 1983, p. 373-380.

■ LYSINE

This article reports on the case of a 44-year-old woman who developed Fanconi's syndrome following L-lysine ingestion.

> —J.C. Lo, et al., "Fanconi's Syndrome and Tubulointerstitial Nephritis in Association with L-lysine Ingestion," *American Journal of Kidney Disease,* 28(4), October 1996, p. 614-617.

■ PHENYLALANINE

Results of this double-blind, placebo-controlled study showed significant increases in involuntary movements following intake of 100 mg/kg of phenylalanine by male schizophrenics.

> —D.M. Mosnik, et al., "Tardive Dyskinesia Exacerbated after Ingestion of Phenylalanine by Schizophrenic Patients," *Neuropsychopharmacology,* 16(2), February 1997, p. 136-146.

■ TRYPTOPHAN

This article reports on 4 cases of patients presenting with pulmonary infiltrates, pleural effusions, hypoxemia, peripheral eosinophilia, dyspnea, fatigue, and weakness following consumption of L-tryptophan-containing products.

> —I.J. Strumpf, et al., ''Acute Eosinophilic Pulmonary Disease Associated with the Ingestion of L-Tryptophan-containing Products,'' *Chest*, 99(1), January 1991, p. 8-13.

This article reports on the case of 51-year-old woman who developed acute febrile illness with respiratory failure following L-tryptophan ingestion.

> —K.E. Mar, et al., ''Bronchiolitis Obliterans Organizing Pneumonia Associated with Massive L-tryptophan Ingestion,'' *Chest,* 104(6), December 1993, p. 1924-1926.

This article reports on the case of a 45-year-old woman with symptomatic gastrointestinal involvement, eosinophils in the cellular infiltrate, and was found to have eosinophilia-myalgia syndrome associated with L-tryptophan consumption.

> —K. De Schryver-Kecskemeti, et al., ''Gastrointestinal Involvement in L-tryptophan (L-Trp) Associated Eosinophilia-myalgia Syndrome (EMS),'' *Dig Dis Sci,* 37(5), May 1992, p. 697-701.

INDEX

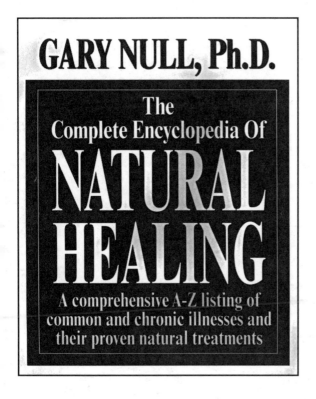

To Order *The Complete Encyclopedia of Natural Healing*

The Complete Encyclopedia of Natural Healing
ISBN # 1-57566-258-2   Price $35.00

(If ordering via mail please complete this order form and mail with remittance to the address provided below):

Quantity of books	Unit Price	Total
	Subtotal	$ _____
	8.25 % Sales Tax (NY only)	$ _____
	8.25 % Sales Tax (TN only)	$ _____
	* Shipping & Handling	$ _____
	Total Order	$ _____

---

*Shipping & Handling depend on the number of books bought—see below:
1 Book-$4.95   2-5 Books-$8.95   6-10 Books $12.95

For orders over 10 books, please call customer service at the phone number below

---

To Order By Telephone (Call Toll-free):
With MC or Visa, call 888-345-BOOK (2665) Mon.-Fri., 9:00-5:00 Eastern Standard Time
http://www.kensingtonbooks.com

To Order By Mail:
Just fill out the information below and send this page with your remittance to:

> **Order Dept.**
> **Kensington Publishing Corp.**
> **850 Third Avenue**
> **New York, NY 10022**

- -

Name _____

Address _____

City _____ State _____ Zip _____

MC/Visa # _____ Exp. Date _____

Signature (cannot process without signature) _____

Check/Money Order enclosed for $ _____ Payable to Kensington Publishing Corp.

Daytime Phone _____

*GNNH98